MRI and CT of the
MUSCULOSKELETAL SYSTEM

MRI and CT of the MUSCULOSKELETAL SYSTEM

HOSSEIN FIROOZNIA, M.D.

Professor of Radiology and
Director, Section of Musculoskeletal Radiology,
New York University Medical Center,
New York, New York

CORNELIA N. GOLIMBU, M.D.

Associate Professor of Radiology,
New York University Medical Center,
New York, New York

MAHVASH RAFII, M.D.

Associate Professor of Radiology,
New York University Medical Center,
New York, New York

WOLFGANG RAUSCHNING, M.D., Ph.D.

Professor of Orthopedics,
University of Uppsala, Uppsala, Sweden

JEFFREY C. WEINREB, M.D.

Professor of Radiology and Director, MRI,
New York University Medical Center
New York, New York

With 2,701 Illustrations and 56 Four-Color Plates

Mosby Year Book

St. Louis   Baltimore   Boston   Chicago   London   Philadelphia   Sydney   Toronto

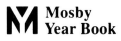

**Mosby
Year Book**

Dedicated to Publishing Excellence

Editor: Anne S. Patterson
Assistant Editor: Maura K. Leib
Manuscript Editor: George B. Stericker, Jr.
Book and Cover Design: Gail Morey Hudson

Printed in the United States of America.

Mosby–Year Book, Inc.
11830 Westline Industrial Drive, St. Louis, Missouri 63146

Library of Congress Cataloging in Publication Data

MRI and CT of the musculoskeletal system / [edited by] Hossein
 Firooznia . . . [et al.].
      p. cm.
    Includes bibliographical references.
    Includes index.
    ISBN 0-8151-3247-6
    1. Musculoskeletal system — Magnetic resonance imaging.
  2. Musculoskeletal system — Tomography. I. Firooznia, Hossein.
    [DNLM: 1. Bone Diseases — diagnosis.   2. Joint Diseases — diagnosis.
  3. Magnetic Resonance Imaging.   4. Musculoskeletal System — anatomy &
  histology.   5. Musculoskeletal System — pathology.   6. Spinal
  Diseases — diagnosis.   7. Tomography, X-Ray Computed.   WE 141 M0387]
  RC925.7.M73   1991
  616.7'0754 — dc20
  DNLM/DLC
  for Library of Congress   91-32730
                                                                        CIP

92 93 94 95 96 CL/MY/ 9 8 7 6 5 4 3 2 1

Artist

NANCY PRENDERGAST, M.D.

Contributors

MICHAEL M. ABROSINO, M.D.

Assistant Professor of Radiology,
New York University Medical Center,
New York, New York

MELVIN H. BECKER, M.D.

Professor of Radiology,
New York University Medical Center,
New York, New York

M. VALLO BENJAMIN, M.D.

Professor of Neurosurgery,
New York University Medical Center,
New York, New York

JOHN J. BONAMO, M.D.

Associate Professor of Orthopedic Surgery,
New York University Medical Center,
New York, New York

HOSSEIN FIROOZNIA, M.D.

Professor of Radiology and
Director, Section of Musculoskeletal Radiology,
New York University Medical Center
New York, New York

NANCY B. GENIESER, M.D.

Professor of Radiology and
Director, Section of Pediatric Radiology,
New York University Medical Center,
New York, New York

GARY GILYARD, M.D.

Fellow in Sports Medicine,
New York University Medical Center,
New York, New York

CORNELIA N. GOLIMBU, M.D.

Associate Professor of Radiology,
New York University Medical Center,
New York, New York

ROY A. HOLLIDAY, M.D.

Assistant Professor of Radiology and
Director, Section of Head and Neck Radiology,
New York University Medical Center
New York, New York

IRVIN I. KRICHEFF, M.D.

Professor of Radiology and
Director, Section of Neuroradiology,
New York University Medical Center,
New York, New York

MYRON M. LEVITT, M.D.

Fellow in Neuroradiology,
New York University Medical Center,
New York, New York

ANDREW W. LITT, M.D.

Assistant Professor of Radiology,
New York University Medical Center,
New York, New York

JEFFREY MINKOFF, M.D.

Associate Professor of Orthopedic Surgery and
Director, Sports Medicine,
New York University Medical Center,
New York, New York

RICHARD S. PINTO, M.D.

Professor of Radiology,
New York University Medical Center,
New York, New York

MAHVASH RAFII, M.D.

Associate Professor of Radiology,
New York University Medical Center,
New York, New York

WOLFGANG RAUSCHNING, M.D., Ph.D.

Professor of Orthopedics,
University of Uppsala, Uppsala, Sweden

NEIL M. ROFSKY, M.D.
Fellow in MRI,
New York University Medical Center,
New York, New York

ORRIN SHERMAN, M.D.
Assistant Professor of Orthopedic Surgery,
New York University Medical Center,
New York, New York

JEFFREY C. WEINREB, M.D.
Professor of Radiology and
Director, MRI,
New York University Medical Center,
New York, New York

Foreword

The discovery of x rays more than 90 years ago was a significant milestone in the history of medicine. In the following 70 years there were numerous refinements and innovations in the field of diagnostic radiology, including introduction of progressively safer contrast media for intravascular injection, myelography, and arthrography. But a quantum leap forward occurred when computed tomography (CT) was introduced into clinical practice in the early seventies. Suddenly, cross-sectional imaging became available. This eliminated the confusing superimposition of shadows in many parts of the body, such as the spine, pelvis, and shoulder, where there are complex curvilinear and overlapping surfaces. CT still has numerous clinical applications, and will probably retain this position for the foreseeable future. It is the modality of choice in the investigation of lesions containing a significant amount of calcification, or osteosclerosis, and when a precise delineation of the extent and location of calcified structures is necessary. An example of the former is a suspected blastic neoplasm; of the latter, presurgical planning for the decompressive surgery of spinal stenosis.

Besides cross-sectional imaging, an additional bonus of CT was its vastly superior sensitivity to soft tissue contrast. Thus, it became the modality of choice for detection of soft tissue tumors. Nevertheless, it still was not possible to evaluate optimally the articular cartilage, ligaments, menisci, and many other soft tissue structures unless a contrast substance was also used.

Magnetic resonance imaging (MRI) became available for clinical use in 1983. Although the first clinical images were far from ideal, it soon became clear that a revolution was in progress. It is now evident that MRI probably represents the most significant advance in diagnostic medicine since the discovery of x rays. Initially, MRI was used almost exclusively for evaluation of CNS lesions. However, shortly afterwards, it became clear that MRI was uniquely suited for evaluation of the musculoskeletal system. This is due to its inherently high sensitivity to soft tissue contrast, its ability to manipulate the signal intensity of various soft tissues by the use of a different pulse sequence, and its ability to generate images directly, rather than by reformatting, in coronal, sagittal, axial, and any other plane desired. It is remarkable that MRI, in less than 10 years, has almost totally supplanted some of our classic diagnostic modalities such as arthrography. It is now seriously challenging both myelography and angiography, and this is just the beginning. For evaluation of the disorders of various structures of the musculoskeletal system, including bone marrow, muscles, tendons, ligaments, fat, articular cartilage, and menisci, and for intervertebral disks in the cervical and thoracic region, spinal cord, nerve roots, it is the diagnostic imaging modality of choice.

CT and MRI are clearly excellent diagnostic tools. However, their judicious utilization requires a working knowledge of the utility and pitfalls of their application in the diagnosis of various disorders in each region of the musculoskeletal system. The contributing authors of this book are all soldiers in the field; no desk generals. All the authors deal, on a daily basis, with the diagnosis and management of various musculoskeletal disorders. They have worked in their chosen special area prior to and since the inception of CT and MRI. The material presented therefore is the result of actual first-hand clinical work; and thus eminently real, doable, and useful in the daily practice of medicine. This book is written in a direct manner, presenting an objective assessment of the true value of CT and MRI and, when appropriate, other modalities, such as myelography, arthroscopy, and CT-arthrography. Therefore, this is not a single-modality thesis pushing what the editors like. The information presented in this volume is very helpful not only to the radiologist but also to the orthopedic surgeon, who, as the physician responsible for the well-being of the patient, must decide to utilize one or more, or none, of these very informative, but costly, modalities.

This volume is the most comprehensive book on CT and MRI of the musculoskeletal system published to date. It brings the reader up to date with a review of the most important and pertinent literature published up to 1991. It treats various disorders of the spine and the extremity joints in great depth, offering new insights, helpful tips, and clear definitions. The data on correlation of the CT and MRI findings with surgical diagnoses of the lesions of the spine are, I believe, the most comprehensive ever published. The data on accuracy and sensitivity of CT and MRI of the two most commonly examined joints, the shoulder and knee, are presented by orthopedic surgeons with extensive experience in their field.

This book is more than 900 pages in length and contains 56 color plates, including original cryomicrosections of cadaver anatomy. There are more than 100 drawings, all very meticulous copies of specimens, photographs of specimens, or diagnostic images, and 2700 state-of-the-art CT and MR images. Accordingly, this book should be of tremendous value not only to radiologists but also to the orthopedists, neurologists, neurosurgeons, and all other physicians who deal with disorders of the musculoskeletal system.

Theodore R. Waugh, M.D., C.M., Ph.D, F.R.C.S.(C)
Walter A.L. Thompson
Professor of Orthopedic Surgery, and
Chairman, Department of Orthopedic Surgery,
New York University School of Medicine

Foreword

The enormous benefits of computerized tomography (CT) to both patient and physician were apparent from the moment of its introduction to clinical medicine in 1971. Its cross-sectional images not only demonstrated the interrelation of organ structures but differentiated tissues from one another on the basis of their x-ray absorption — making CT a unique tool for the envisaging of human anatomy. Early CT machines were devoted to imaging the brain, but within a few years CT technology improved to the point that the technique could be applied to the visualization of support and motor structures of the body. This significantly enhanced the ease and accuracy of the diagnosis of disorders of the spine; and — through the use of systemic and/or local radiographic contrast agents — it improved the evaluation of disorders of the joints, as well as allowing a more accurate evaluation of neoplasms and infections which affect muscle and bone.

The advent of magnetic resonance imaging (MRI) occurred a little over a decade after introduction of CT. Its first use was also the study of the central nervous system. As MRI is both free of the beam hardening artifacts that so frequently cause difficulty in the CT imaging of soft tissues adjacent to bone and able to demonstrate cross-sectional anatomy in almost any plane, the menisci, ligaments, tendons, and muscles could be visualized directly without the use of invasive techniques. This accelerated its application in the diagnosis of pathologic conditions of bones, joints, and muscles. The images produced by MRI rivaled those previously seen in the finest anatomy textbooks. MRI has already replaced many routine and interventional procedures as the diagnostic procedures of choice in many conditions afflicting bones, joints, and muscles

This text — written by Dr. Firooznia and his co-workers — is a remarkable byproduct of the collegial environment which exists among the clinical departments at NYU. It clearly demonstrates the application and usefulness of CT and MRI in the diagnosis of pathologic conditions affecting the musculoskeletal system through an approach which presents these imaging modalities as being complementary — not competitive. An indication in it that one technique is the most effective for making a specific diagnosis is an expression of the combined experience of its clinician/writers, who then proceed to explain what they demand from the two imaging techniques. This superbly illustrated book should be a boon to all physicians interested in disorders of the spine and musculoskeletal system.

Norman E. Chase, M.D.

Professor and Chairman
Department of Radiology
New York University School of Medicine

Preface

MRI and CT are now well established as the most useful modalities for diagnosing disorders of the spine and musculoskeletal system. They have essentially replaced tomography and arthrography, and have significantly reduced the need for myelography. Because the data provided by MRI and CT reveal fundamentally different characteristics of tissues, these modalities are often not competitive but are essentially complementary. For a number of diseases one or the other is the modality of choice, and, understandably, each has its own peculiar pitfalls.

This book is written with the express aim of providing a comprehensive, up-to-date, and practical guide on the utility and pitfalls of MRI and CT in the diagnosis and management of diseases of the musculoskeletal system. It is intended for radiologists, orthopedists, and all other physicians who deal with these disorders. Illustrations and line drawings are used profusely to demonstrate not only the classic and most common imaging characteristics of a particular disorder but also its unusual and difficult-to-appreciate features.

The first part, Chapters 1 through 8, deals with disorders of the spine. We are fortunate to have the incomparable anatomic plates of the spine prepared by the Master himself, Wolfgang Rauschning, M.D., Ph.D., of Uppsala, Sweden. Nancy Prendergast, M.D., a talented artist and radiologist at our institution, meticulously prepared the line drawings. We have tried to present a balanced view of the utility and pitfalls of CT, MRI, and myelography in the work-up of patients with spinal disorders. To this end, a comprehensive comparison of the accuracy of CT, MRI, and myelography is provided.

In the remainder of the book, every attempt has been made to present an objective assessment of the clinical value of CT, MRI, arthroscopy, CT-arthrography, and other modalities, when appropriate, in the work-up of patients with systemic disorders, or diseases of the extremities.

The second part of the book, Chapters 9 through 13, deals with systemic disorders (infection and neoplastic conditions).

The third part, Chapters 14 through 22, deals with disorders of various joints, from the temporomandibular to the ankle and foot.

The fourth part, Chapter 23, is a discussion of operational safety considerations of MRI.

Hossein Firooznia, M.D.
New York, N.Y.
July 1991

Acknowledgments

I speak for all my colleagues in expressing gratitude to everyone who has been a source of inspiration and help in myriad ways to make this book possible. Thanks are due to:

Norman Chase and Theodore Waugh, for creating the optimal milieu in the departments of radiology and orthopedics to foster conditions conducive to this task.

M. Vallo Benjamin, from whom I have learned everything I know about the pathology and behavior of disks.

Lisa Bracy Lomax, whose loyalty, common sense, and word processing skills are second to none.

Martha Helmers and Anthony Jalandoni, of our photoradiology department, for their magnificent photography.

Anne S. Patterson and Maura K. Leib, of Mosby–Year Book, for their encouragement, persistence, understanding, and good humor.

George B. Stericker, senior manuscript editor of Mosby–Year Book, for his meticulous, patient, and thorough editing of this text.

Hossein Firooznia, M.D.

Contents

Color Plates

PART I SPINE

1 Correlative Anatomy of the Spine and Its Contents

HOSSEIN FIROOZNIA
WOLFGANG RAUSCHNING

The important elements that make up a typical vertebra include the vertebral body, facet joints, pedicles, laminae, and spinous process. Other important anatomic landmarks are the neural foramina and the spinal canal.

VERTEBRAL BODY

The bodies of the vertebrae are cylindrical structures composed of trabecular bone encased by a thin shell of cortical bone. Some investigators believe the endplates to be modified trabecular bone. In newborns the vertebral marrow is mostly red marrow.[1] With advancing age, there is a gradual replacement of the red marrow by yellow (fatty) marrow in a diffuse and homogeneous fashion. By the age of 20 the yellow marrow fraction is about 20%, and by 70 or so it is 50% to 60%.[2-4] In many subjects focal areas of fatty deposit are noted in the vertebrae.[5] These

may be more or less spherical, which is the form commonly encountered, or (less commonly) of irregular outline. The incidence of focal fatty deposits increases with advancing age.

There is often some fat present adjacent to and surrounding the main trunk of the basivertebral vein. Our experience with measuring trabecular bone density in the midportion of the vertebral body and comparing it with the trabecular bone of the entire vertebra, utilizing single energy computed tomography in a prospective longitudinal 4-year study, has revealed that in subjects with rapid bone loss (e.g., perimenopausal and early postmenopausal women [1 or 2 years before and up to 7 to 10 years after the menopause]) following oophorectomy, or in patients receiving high doses of corticosteroids, there is a preferential loss of bone in the midportion of the vertebra surrounding the basivertebral vein. In some subjects there is also the suggestion of a concomitant increase in the amount of fat in this region.

Bone loss

Bone loss in the conditions just mentioned probably occurs simultaneously in both cortical and trabecular bone compartments. However, the loss of trabecular bone is significantly more pronounced than that of cortical bone, most likely because of the significantly faster turnover rate of the trabecular bone. The vertebral bodies are the largest reservoir of trabecular bone in the human skeleton. The earliest clinical manifestations of bone loss in the conditions mentioned above are in areas of the skeleton composed predominantly of trabecular bone, particularly the bodies of the vertebrae. The loss of bone in the vertebrae does not occur in a uniform fashion. There is preferential loss in the midportion surrounding the basivertebral vein. Trabecular bone loss begins with resorption of small segments of the most recently formed trabeculae. These appear as spotty lucencies on CT. If a map of trabecular bone density is generated, marked nonhomogeneity will be noted.

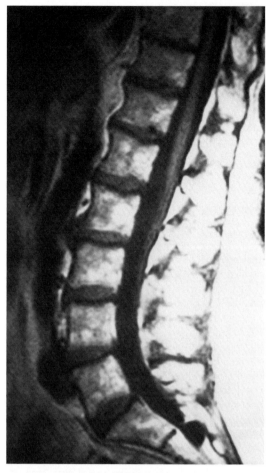

FIGURE 1-1
Midsagittal T1-weighted MRI of the lumbar spine. There are extensive deposits of fat in all the lumbar vertebrae of this 80-year-old woman.

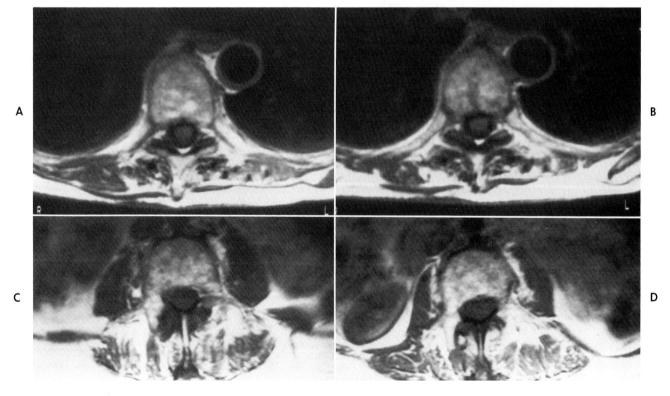

FIGURE 1-2
Focal and diffuse infiltration of the vertebral marrow by fat in an elderly woman, T1-weighted MRI. **A** and **B** are at T7-8 and, **C** and **D**, at L2-3. There is diffuse replacement of the vertebral marrow by fat.

The density of trabecular bone is not uniform throughout the vertebral body; it is highest adjacent to the endplates and the peripheral surfaces[6-9] and decreases gradually toward the central portion. In general, trabecular bone is essentially similar to compact bone. The major difference between the two is that in compact bone the bony lamellae are closely packed together, with very little space between them, whereas in trabecular bone the small bony lamellae are irregularly arranged, with more or less wide marrow spaces between them. In patients with bone loss of an acute and rapid nature, fairly distinct small areas of trabecular bone resorption appear. The tiny spaces thus created are gradually filled with fat, provided no other metabolic disease of bone is present. In advanced cases these may be demonstrated on high-resolution CT images. One may also demonstrate this phenomenon by generating a map of density values on a cross-sectional CT image of the vertebral body. In normal young adults the vertebrae exhibit a fairly homogeneous pattern of density values, except for the normally denser peripheral areas. In subjects with osteopenia a markedly non-homogeneous map of density values may be noted, due mostly to the loss of bone substance and, in varying degrees, to an accumulation of excess fat between the trabeculae. This reduces the measured density value (on CT) of the area under study. In more advanced stages of bone loss, zones of bone resorption merge and a fairly diffuse pattern of bone loss is noted. The density values, however, still show moderate to marked nonhomogeneity (Figs. 1-1 to 1-8).

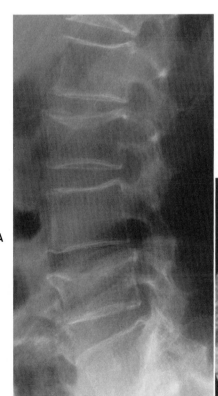

FIGURE 1-3
Osteoporosis. Spotty pattern of bone loss in a patient with the advanced condition.

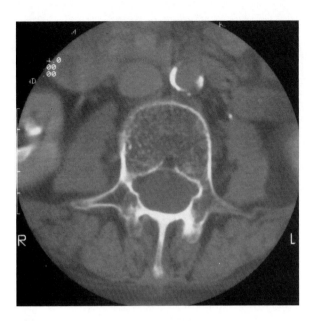

FIGURE 1-4
A, A lateral projection of the lumbar spine reveals osteoporotic compression fractures of L2 and L4. Fairly prominent striations, mimicking a hemangioma, are seen in L3. B, A soft tissue window axial slice through L3 shows marked osteoporosis. The pattern of thickened vertical striations was seen in all lumbar bodies of this patient with advanced osteoporosis.

A

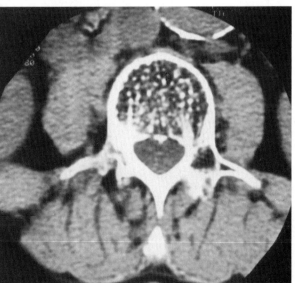

B

FIGURE 1-5
Osteoporosis. A midsagittal T1-weighted MRI cross section of the lumbar spine shows characteristic deformity of the vertebral bodies due to osteoporosis. There is diffuse replacement of the bone marrow by fat.

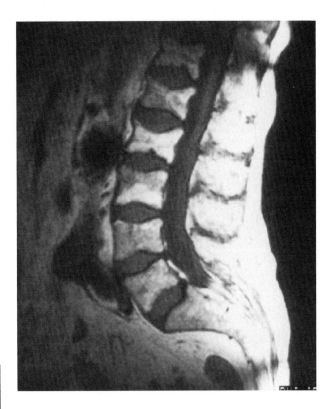

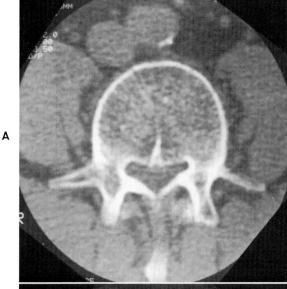

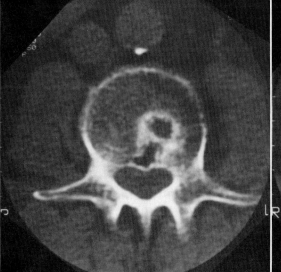

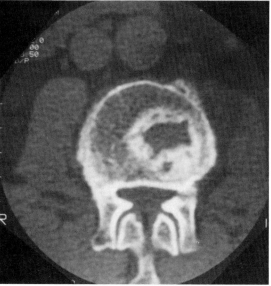

FIGURE 1-6
Osteoporosis. CT slices through L4, **A**, L5, **B**, and L3, **C**. Fine spotty loss of bone in a patient with congenital stenosis and osteoporosis. A Schmorl node is evident in L5 and L3. Schmorl's nodes are more frequent in patients with osteoporosis than in normal subjects.

A   B

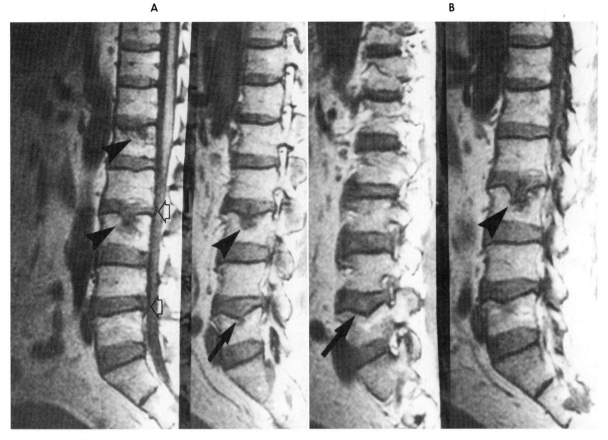

FIGURE 1-7
Schmorl nodes at L1 and L3 in a 65-year-old man with idiopathic osteoporosis, MRI (TR/TE 550/30).
A is a midsagittal and right parasagittal and, **B,** two right parasagittal images. The *arrowheads* denote
the nodes. In **A** and **B** there is a compression fracture of the L5 superior endplate *(arrows)*. Note the
moderate amount of bulging of the disks *(hollow arrows* in **A**).

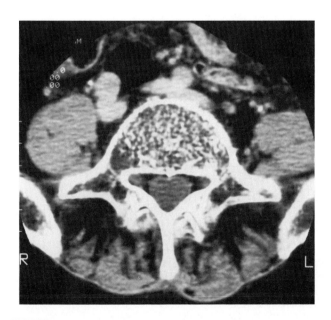

FIGURE 1-8
An axial slice through the body of L5 with severe osteoporosis. There
is thickening of the vertical trabeculae.

MRI signal characteristics of vertebral bodies

The MRI signal characteristics of the vertebral bodies
are dependent on the composition of the vertebral
marrow. In infants and young children, in whom the
vertebral marrow is composed of mostly hematopoietic
tissue (red marrow), the vertebrae have low to medium
signal on T1-weighted spin echo (SE) images. As the
relative fraction of yellow marrow increases with advancing
age, the marrow space becomes brighter (higher
signal intensity). When the marrow is infiltrated by
extraneous cellular elements and substances (e.g., metastasis,
leukemia, hemorrhage, or infection), the signal
characteristics may be altered.[4,10,11,12] In normal adults
the vertebral marrow usually has medium signal intensity
on T1-weighted SE images. As a rule, the normal adult
vertebral marrow has significantly less signal intensity on
T1-weighted images than the nearby epidural and
paraspinal fat does but more than the paraspinal muscles.
On T2-weighted SE images the marrow signal is of
medium to low intensity.

Focal areas of fatty deposit

Focal areas of fat[5] appear in the bodies of the vertebrae
with advancing age. In our experience approximately 45%

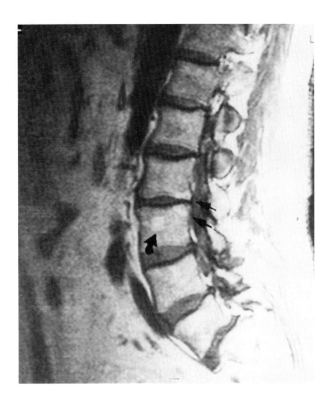

FIGURE 1-9
Focal fatty deposit *(curved arrow)* in the body of L3. The L2-3 disk is narrow due to degenerative disease. Note the accumulation of fat adjacent to the vertebral endplates posteriorly *(arrows)*.

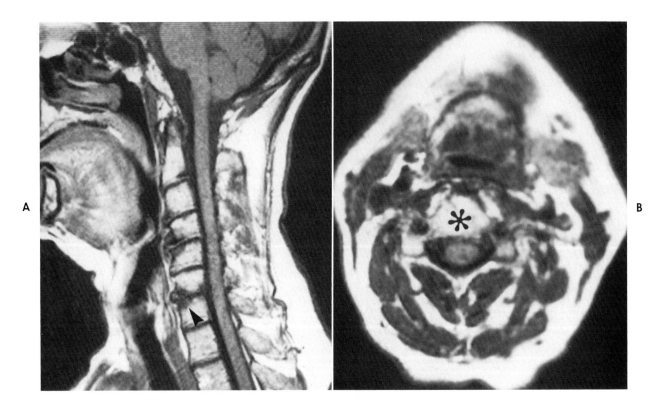

FIGURE 1-10
Fat accumulation in the vertebral marrow of an 85-year-old man. **A** is a midsagittal and, **B,** an axial T1-weighted MR image. There is extensive replacement by fat. The *arrowhead* in **A** denotes osteosclerosis of the vertebral endplate and adjacent marrow at C6-7. This is evidenced by zones of markedly low signal (or signal void). Note also the similar findings at C3-4 and C4-5. In B replacement of the marrow by fat is more noticeable at C3. (The *asterisk* is on the vertebral body.)

of all subjects 50 years or older undergoing entire spine MRI examination for various causes, including work-up of metastases, myeloma, or various neurological disorders, have had at least one (often several) focal area of fatty deposit in their vertebrae. These are more commonly noted in the thoracic and lumbar than in the cervical vertebral bodies. Although they are distributed randomly in the vertebrae, we have noted that they are distinctly less common directly adjacent to the peripheral cortical shell or vertebral endplates (provided the intervertebral disk is healthy). The zones of fat usually appear as areas of high signal intensity on T1-weighted images, and of medium signal on T2-weighted images, showing the same signal characteristics as the epidural fat (Figs. 1-9 and 1-10).

Basivertebral venous trunk

The basivertebral venous trunk is usually well visualized on axial CT and MRI cross sections and on midsagittal MRI cross sections. The confluence of the basivertebral veins is situated behind the posterior surface of the vertebral body, approximately halfway between the superior and inferior endplates. It extends into the vertebral body 1 to 1.5 cm before dividing into branches. The branching may occur at its entrance into the vertebral body, just after its entrance, or deeper within the body. The venous branches often have a V-shaped configuration, the confluence being generally quite clearly identified in the lower three cervical bodies and in almost all the thoracic and lumbar bodies. A distinct calcified venous cap may be noted on the dorsal aspect of the basivertebral vein. On midsagittal T1-weighted MRI cross sections one can usually identify the "orifice" of the vein in the midportion of the posterior vertebral body surface.

The *MRI signal* characteristic of the basivertebral vein–fat complex is dependent upon the pulse sequence utilized, the presence of fat and (slow-moving) venous blood, and the possibility of even-echo rephasing. Often one may note a bandlike horizontal area of medium to high signal, which is due to the fat and venous blood. Occasionally, instead of this pattern, a globular area of medium to high signal intensity will be noted in the center of the vertebral body (Figs. 1-11 to 1-13).

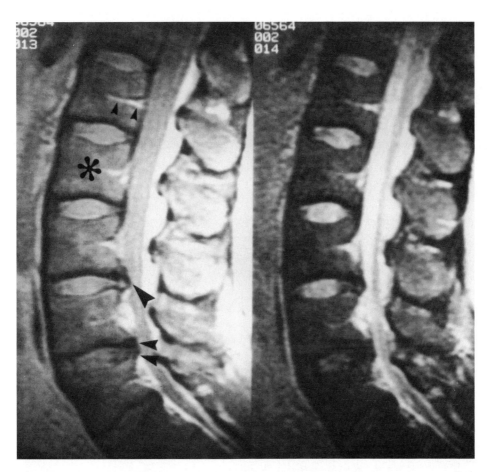

FIGURE 1-11
Normal basivertebral vein of the lumbar spine, midsagittal MR (TR/TE 2000/50 and 100). The *asterisk* is on L2. *Two small arrowheads* denote the vein at L1. There is herniation of both the L3-4 disk *(single arrowhead)* and the L4-5 disk *(bottom two arrowheads).*

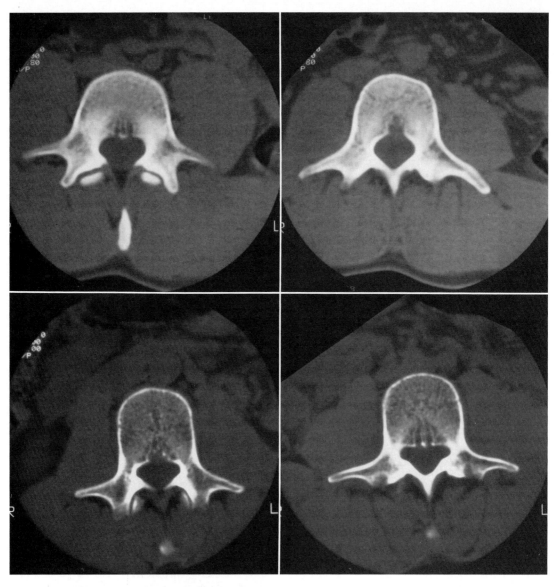

FIGURE 1-12
Normal basivertebral vein of the lumbar spine.

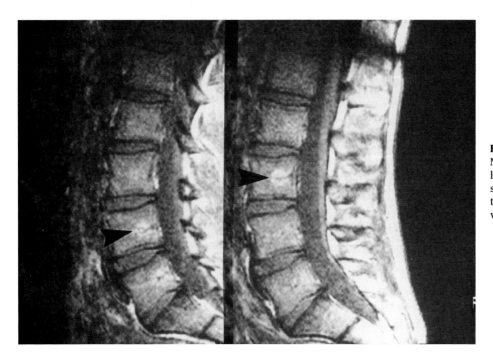

FIGURE 1-13
Normal basivertebral vein of the lumbar spine, sagittal and para-sagittal T1-weighted cross sections. The *arrowheads* point to the vein at L3 and L4.

CERVICAL SPINE
Cervical vertebral bodies

The first and second cervical vertebrae (atlas and axis) are functionally and morphologically distinct. The atlas (C1) is an osseous ring that, unlike the other vertebrae, does not have a body. It has paired articulating facets for matching articular surfaces on the occipital bone above and the axis below. The axis (C2) has an elongated body that continues superiorly as the odontoid process (dens). The odontoid process articulates anteriorly with the anterior arch of C1 in a true synovial joint; posteriorly it is held in place mainly by the transverse ligament and, to a lesser degree, by the cruciform ligament and alar ligaments. There are synovial bursae between the odontoid and these ligaments.[13] Thus the odontoid is encircled by synovial bursae, which explains the fairly frequent involvement of the atlas-odontoid articulation in systemic inflammatory arthritides (e.g., rheumatoid and psoriatic) (Figs. 1-14 and 1-15 and Plate 1-1).

On axial cross sections the cervical vertebrae are circular, or circular with a slight anteroposterior flattening. The lower cervical vertebrae (particularly C4, C5,

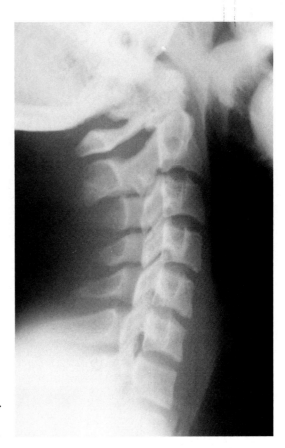

FIGURE 1-14
Normal lateral projection of the cervical spine.

A   B   C

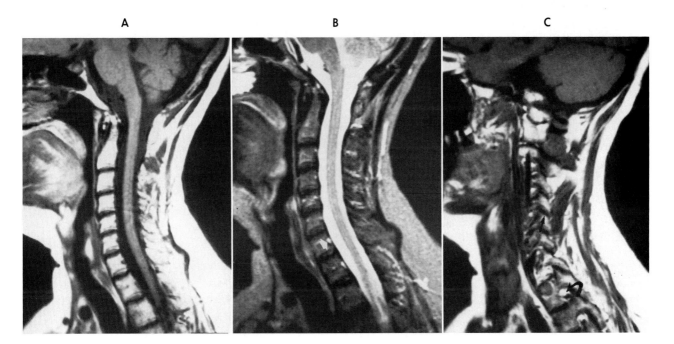

FIGURE 1-15
Normal cervical spine. **A,** Midsagittal T1-weighted image. Note the relationship of the spinal cord to the cervical vertebrae. The cord is of medium signal intensity. It is surrounded by CSF (which is of low signal intensity) and spinal ligaments (also of low intensity). **B,** Midsagittal T2-weighted image. The CSF is now of high signal intensity, providing a myelographic effect. The spinal cord is gray. The width of the subarachnoid space is optimally visible. Note the cervical basivertebral veins, appearing as focal areas of bright signal on the dorsal aspects of the cervical vertebrae. The arrow points to the basivertebral vein at C7. **C,** parasagittal T1-weighted image. The cervical facet joints are visible. The *upper arrow* points to the C3-C4 facet joint on the right side. The *curved arrow* is pointing to fat in the upper portion of the C7-T1 neural foramen. The neural elements are seen as an area of low signal intensity immediately inferior to the tip of the arrow.

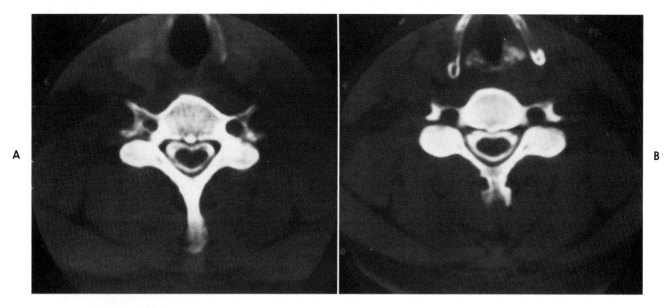

FIGURE 1-16
Normal basivertebral vein. Cervical CT-myelogram. **A,** A calcified venous cap is visible. **B,** Continuation
of the cap as a bony ridge on the posterior aspect of C6.

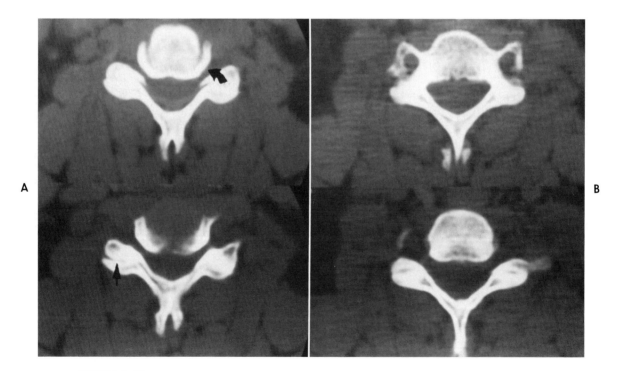

FIGURE 1-17
Normal cervical spine. **A,** C6-C7. The *curved arrow* in the upper figure points to the uncinate process
on the left side, forming the anterolateral wall of the neural foramen. The *straight arrow* in the lower
figure points to the facet joint on the right. **B,** Configuration of the cervical bodies and spinal canal at
C6.

and C6) may be slightly to moderately wedge shaped on midsagittal cross sections. The C5 vertebral body often is the smallest, but this should not cause it to be mistaken for fractured. The superior endplate of most cervical vertebrae is flat. The inferior endplates of the lower three cervical bodies may be moderately concave. The orifice of the basivertebral vein, usually noted in the middle of the posterior surface of the vertebral body, is not especially prominent in the cervical spine, except in the lower two or three vertebrae. In some subjects a small (2 to 4 mm thick) smooth midline ridge is noted on the posterior surfaces of C5, C6, and C7. This is a normal variant and is related to the formation of the basivertebral venous cap. It should not be mistaken for an osteophyte, bony degeneration, or calcification of the posterior longitudinal ligament (Figs. 1-16 and 1-17).

Uncinate processes and Luschka joints

The lateral margins of the superior endplates of C3 to C7 form a short bony wall that extends anteroposteriorly and curves around the posterolateral corner of each endplate (uncinate process). There is an articulating facet on the lateral side of the inferior endplates, usually of C2 to C6, that articulates with the uncinate process of the

next caudad cervical body to form the uncovertebral (Luschka) joint.[14-16] Consequently, the cervical disks are surrounded by a bony wall laterally and posterolaterally. The joints of Luschka may be involved in systemic inflammatory arthritides or degenerative osteoarthrosis. Hypertrophic changes of the uncinate process are usually the most important cause of stenoses of the cervical neural foramina (Figs. 1-17 and 1-18).

The transverse process of each cervical vertebra contains the foramen tranversarium, which is situated anterolaterally and through which the vertebral artery passes. The vertebral artery is anterior to the dorsal root ganglion, which is situated on the superior surface of the posterior bony wall of each foramen.

Cervical facet joints

The cervical facet joints are oriented in their anterior portions at a 10-to-20-degree tilt to the horizontal plane and in their posterior portions at a 10-to-20 degree tilt to the vertical. Thus the anterior portions may not be visualized on axial CT or MRI images to best advantage. Conventional (lateral) tomography may be necessary. The articular pillars and facet joints are usually well seen on parasagittal MRI or reformatted CT images. The facet

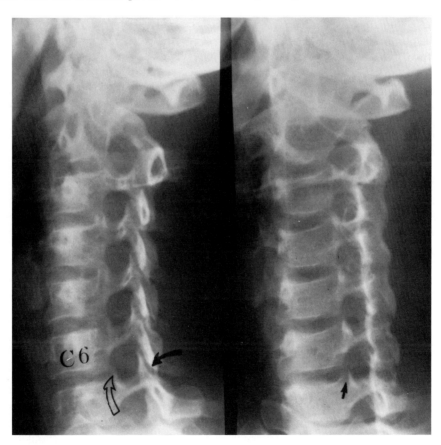

FIGURE 1-18
Anatomy of the normal cervical neural foramina. Oblique projections obtained with slightly different degrees of angulation show the facet joints and their relationship to the neural foramina at C6-C7 (*solid curved arrow*). The *hollow curved arrow* points to the Luschka process of C7. The Luschka processes are better visualized by using a less oblique projection. The *solid straight arrow* points to the Luschka process of C7.

joints, whose capsules are lined by synovial tissue, may be involved in systemic inflammatory arthritides (e.g., rheumatoid arthritis) and spondyloarthropathies. Erosive changes and bony anklyosis with adult rheumatoid arthritis are noted usually in the C2-4 region whereas with juvenile rheumatoid arthritis and spondyloarthropathies they may be seen affecting practically the entire spine.

The cervical spine of an adult who has had juvenile rheumatoid arthritis (JRA) may superficially resemble that of a subject with adult-onset spondyloarthropathy. However, careful inspection will reveal the vertebrae to be significantly smaller in patients with JRA, because the ankylosis has occurred before the affected vertebrae were fully developed whereas in adults the vertebrae have reached their full size by the time the ankylosis occurs (Figs. 1-17 and 1-18).

It is important to note the anatomical relationships of the facet joints to the spinal canal and neural foramina. In the cervical spine the facet joints are situated on the posterior aspect of each neural foramen. Occasionally, marked hypertrophic changes of a facet will cause stenosis of the foramen, but this is uncommon. The usual cause of cervical neural foraminal stenosis is hypertrophic change of an uncinate process and the matching articular facet of the vertebral body cephalad to it (Luschka joint). The cervical facet joints do not participate in formation of the boundaries of the spinal canal; hence they do not ordinarily cause spinal stenosis.[17-25] However, there may be marked synovial thickening, joint effusion, and paraarticular cyst formation affecting the facet joints in patients with long-standing inflammatory arthritis. This has been suspected on CT or MRI and verified at pathological examination (Plate 1-2).

Cervical neural foramina

The cervical neural foramina are at approximately 45 degrees to the sagittal plane. Thus they are not ordinarily appreciated on coronal or sagittal images. However, oblique images obtained at a 45-degree angle to the sagittal usually reveal them.[17-25] They extend from the inferior cortex of the pedicle of one vertebra to the superior cortex of the pedicle of the vertebra immediately caudad to it. Their anteromedial boundaries are formed by the Luschka joint complexes, with the joint itself being approximately at the level of the midportion of the neural foramen. Their posterolateral boundaries are formed by the anterior surfaces of the articular processes, with the superior margin of the facet joint itself being approximately at the level of the upper third of the neural foramen. The neural elements are situated in the lower portion of each foramen. The ventral root is in the lower portion, and the dorsal root directly above it. The upper portion of each foramen is occupied by fat and epidural veins.

The clinically significant part of the neural foramen is

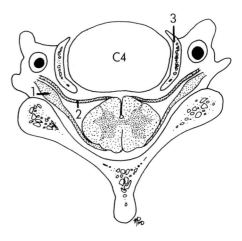

FIGURE 1-19
Schematic through the inferior endplate of a normal C4 vertebra. *1,* Dorsal root ganglion of C5; *2,* ventral root of C5; *3,* uncinate (Luschka) process of C5. This slice, at the level of the lower endplate of C4, shows the relationship of the cervical nerve root to the Luschka process anteriorly and medially.

its lower portion, where the neural elements are situated (Figs. 1-19 and 1-20 and Plate 1-2). For visualization, thin section (1.5 to 3 mm) axial CT images are necessary. Consecutive slices with the gantry tilted appropriately along the plane of the corresponding intervertebral disk are obtained. The true width of the neural foramen can be assessed on these images, but because the clinically important portion is the lowest portion, it is important to pay careful attention to the slices obtained close to the cortex of the foraminal floor (Fig. 1-18).

SIZE OF THE CERVICAL NEURAL FORAMINA

There are no reliable measurements to distinguish a neural foramen that is stenotic from one that is not. In our experience, in patients without any symptoms who have no abnormalities of the spine, the lower portion of the foramen measures 2.5 to 7 mm in width. Compression of the cervical nerves may occur (in the lower half of the foramen) usually when there are hypertrophic changes of the Luschka process, or occasionally with hypertrophic changes of the facet joint. However, neural foraminal stenosis may be asymptomatic. For further discussion, see Chapter 4.

IMAGING

Visualization of the neural elements within the neural foramen usually requires CT-myelography or MRI. On high-resolution CT-myelograms it is usually possible to identify the dorsal and ventral nerve roots entering the foramen. Recently it has become possible to identify the nerve roots on high resolution MRI axial cross sections, although at the present time (1991) this is not consistently achieved. Further improvements in MRI imagers are necessary for this purpose.

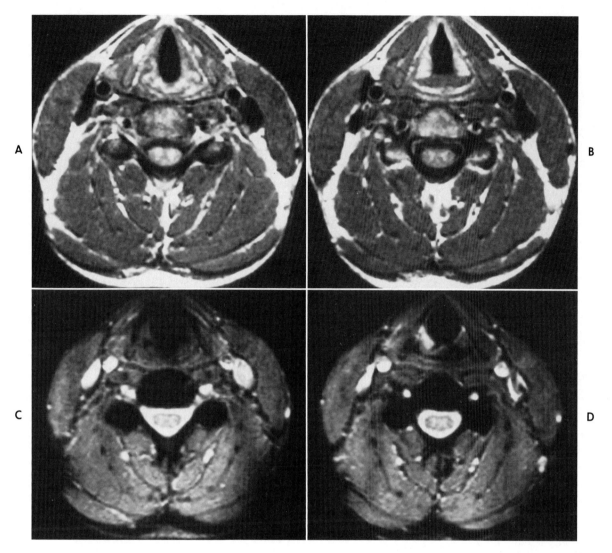

FIGURE 1-20
Normal cervical spine. **A** and **B**, T1-weighted axial cross sections and, **C** and **D**, gradient echo axial cross sections at C5-6. The relationship of the spinal cord to the spinal canal, intervertebral disk, and neural foramina is well shown. The cervical nerve roots and neural foramina are visible in **A**. The epidural venous plexus is better delineated in **B**. The gradient echo images, **C** and **D**, provide a myelographic effect. The vertebral body and neural arch are depicted as areas of markedly low signal (or essentially signal void).

THORACIC SPINE
Thoracic vertebral bodies

The thoracic vertebral bodies are usually somewhat flatter anteroposteriorly than the cervical bodies. On axial cross sections the posterior surface of each vertebra is slightly flat or concave and relatively short compared to the lumbar vertebrae, a feature most prominent in the T3-6 region. The vertebrae gradually increase in width and height from the upper to the lower thoracic region. On midsagittal cross sections they are moderately wedge shaped, conforming to the normal gentle kyphosis of the thoracic spine. The basivertebral vein is fairly prominent and relatively large in the thoracic region. The first three to five thoracic vertebrae may be difficult to visualize on conventional radiography, but they can be clearly seen on sagittal MRI or axial CT and MRI cross sections[26-30] (Fig. 1-21 and Plate 1-3).

An important characteristic of the thoracic vertebrae is their articulations with the rib cage. A costocentral articulation exists between each rib and the body of the vertebra, and a costotransverse articulation between the rib and the transverse process. These joints may be affected by various pathological processes, particularly inflammatory arthritis. However, the region is only poorly visualized on conventional roentgenography. For visualization of the osseous structures thin section axial CT is usually best. We have encountered osteochondroma, posttraumatic deformity, and posttraumatic osteoarthrosis in this region leading to thoracic nerve compression (Figs. 1-22 and 1-23).

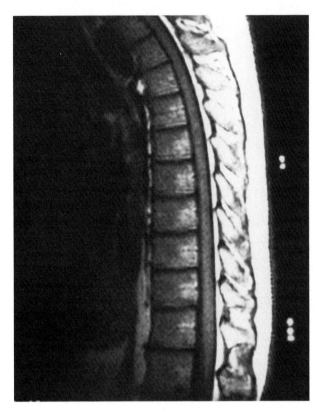

FIGURE 1-21
Normal thoracic spine. Midsagittal T1-weighted cross section in a subject without symptoms.

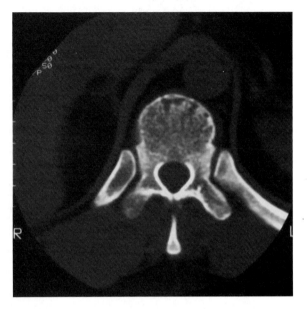

FIGURE 1-22
Normal thoracic vertebral body and costocentral articulation. Note the prominent veins within the vertebral body converging toward the basivertebral vein.

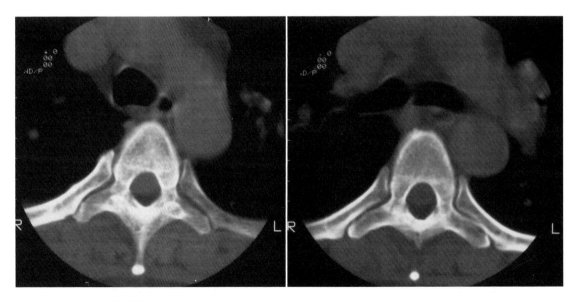

FIGURE 1-23
Normal costocentral and costotransverse articulations of the thoracic spine.

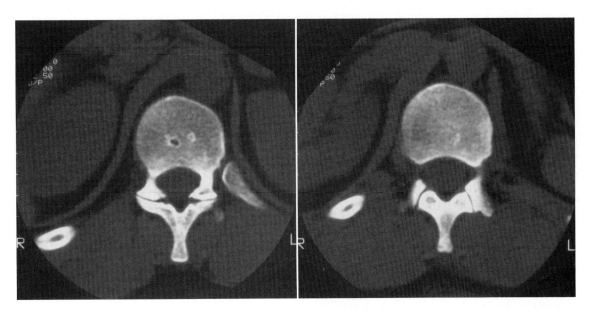

FIGURE 1-24
Normal facet joints of the lower thoracic spine.

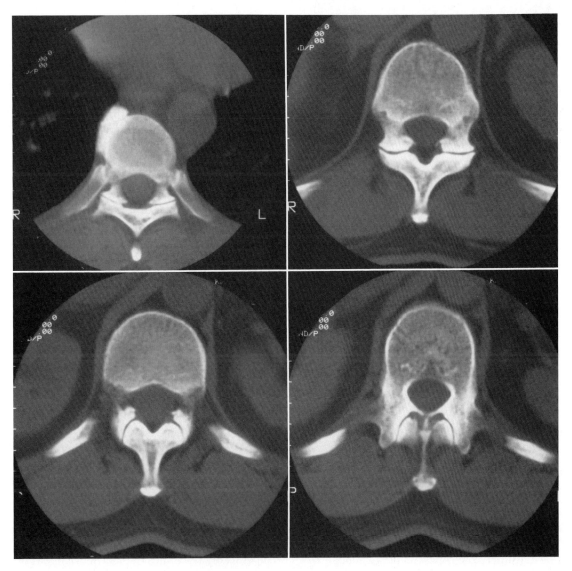

FIGURE 1-25
Normal facet joints of the thoracic spine.

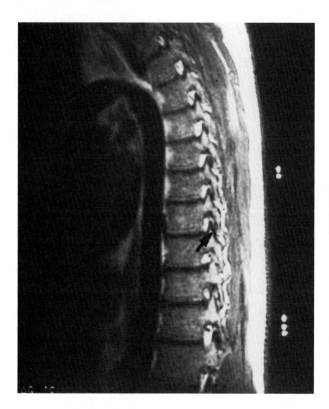

FIGURE 1-26
Normal thoracic facet joints. A parasagittal T1-weighted cross section shows the thoracic facets. The *arrow* is pointing to the superior articular facet of T7.

Thoracic neural foramina

The thoracic neural foramina extend from the spinal canal at an angle of 90 degrees to the sagittal. As in the rest of the spine, they are continuous from pedicle to pedicle. They contain the thoracic nerves and are usually quite well delineated on parasagittal MRI cross sections. On T1-weighted images, it is possible to see that they are filled with fat and the dorsal root ganglion–thoracic nerve complex appears as an area of low signal in their center (Plate 1-3).

Thoracic facet joints

The thoracic facet joints have an oblique axial orientation in the upper thoracic region and gradually become aligned with an oblique coronal orientation in the lower thoracic region. They may not be well seen on axial cross sections (either CT or MRI) of the upper thoracic spine but are better visualized on parasagittal MRI cross sections of the lower thoracic spine, where they start to resemble the lumbar facet joints (Figs. 1-24 to 1-26).

Although the thoracic facet joints can be involved in various inflammatory arthritides, degenerative osteoarthrosis is uncommon.

LUMBAR SPINE
Lumbar vertebral bodies

The lumbar vertebral bodies increase in size progressively from L1 to L4.[27-31] The L5 body may actually be smaller than L4. The posterior surfaces of L1, L2, and L3 usually have a distinct axial concavity in the middle. The posterior surfaces of L4 and L5 may be flat or convex. The superior endplate of each lumbar vertebra is flat, although it may have a gentle symmetrical depression on both coronal and sagittal cross sections. The inferior endplate has a depression generally similar to that of the superior endplate, though slightly more pronounced. The inferior endplates of L3, L4, and L5 in 7% to 16% of patients may have paired parasagittal concavities when viewed in axial cross section. On anteroposterior conventional roentgenographic studies these concavities can be seen to have bilateral symmetry. On lateral projections they lie posteriorly and appear to be superimposed. This has been called *Cupid's bow contour of the spine.*[32,33] On CT, Cupid's bow is visualized in the axial plane as two rounded relatively well-circumscribed areas of hypodensity rimmed by apparent osteosclerosis in the posterior half of the inferior endplates (Figs. 1-27 to 1-29).

The exact mechanism of the formation of Cupid's bow is not known. As Dietz and Christensen[33] state, one is tempted to attribute this finding to a variation in notochordal development since it affects the vertebral endplates posteriorly. However, a careful review of notochordal embryology[34-36] fails to provide a plausible explanation for the peculiar parasagittal position observed (the notochord being a sagittal structure, albeit posteriorly situated).

Deformities of the vertebral endplates occur in a number of disorders, including osteoporosis, anemia, and megalonuclei pulposi (MP). Of these conditions, only MP superficially resembles Cupid's bow contour of the spine,

A   B   C

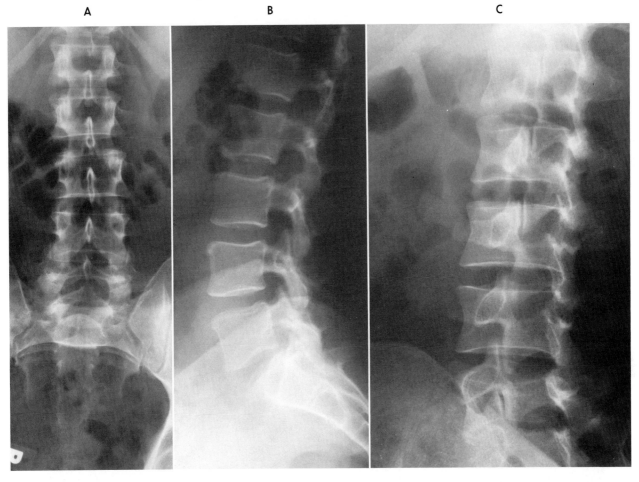

FIGURE 1-27
Normal AP, **A**, lateral, **B**, and oblique, **C**, projections of the lumbar spine.

all others having features that readily differentiate them from this normal anatomic variant. MP is a developmental anomaly, probably related to altered regression of the notochordal tissues,[33,37] consisting of a single broad concavity that affects both the superior and the inferior endplates of multiple thoracic and lumbar vertebrae. The concavity is situated slightly posteriorly, but it affects almost the entire vertebral endplate. The location of the concavity corresponds to that of the notochord and its remnant, the nucleus pulposus, which is situated sagittally, albeit slightly posterior to the central axis of the vertebral column.[33] The radiographic features of MP have been discussed by Dietz and Christensen[33] and are characteristic, which helps differentiate this entity from other conditions causing alterations of the vertebral endplates.

Lumbar neural foramina

The lumbar neural foramina are oriented in the coronal plane. They are usually well seen on axial CT or MRI cross sections and on parasagittal MRI cross sections and normally contain fat. The lumbar dorsal root ganglion, situated directly beneath the pedicle in the upper portion of each foramen, is seen as an area of relatively reduced signal surrounded by fat.

Each lumbar neural foramen has an hourglass configuration and extends from the inferior cortex of the pedicle of one vertebra to the superior cortex of the pedicle of the next caudad vertebra. Its anterior wall consists of the posterior surface of the vertebral bodies and the intervertebral disk. Its posterior wall is formed by the anterior surfaces of the inferior articulating process of the cephalad vertebra and the superior articulating process of the caudad vertebra. The lumbar neural foramina may be reduced in height when there is collapse of an intervertebral disk. Hypertrophic changes of the vertebral endplates and articulating facets produce neural foraminal stenosis. In subjects with degenerative disk disease associated with collapse of the disk, the contents of the lumbar neural foramina are further encroached upon by buckling and redundancy of the ligaments and capsules of the facet joints (Plate 1-4).

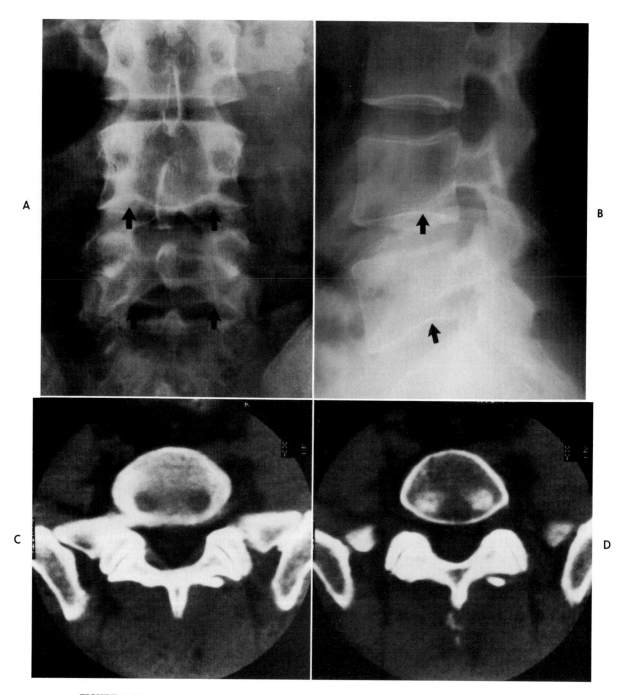

FIGURE 1-28
Cupid's bow contour of the inferior lumbar vertebral endplates, a normal variant. **A,** Anteroposterior and, **B,** lateral projections show the characteristic contour of the inferior endplates of L4 and L5 *(arrows).* **C,** Axial CT slice centered at the inferior endplate of L5. The bilaterally symmetrical areas of hypodensity correspond to concavities in the endplate. **D,** 5 mm above **C.** The vertebral endplate at the base of Cupid's bow is seen as an area of increased density surrounded by the more lucent vertebral trabecular bone and marrow. In patients with scoliosis, when only one side of the vertebral endplate is included in the CT slice, occasionally it will be difficult to make a diagnosis if the examiner is not aware of this normal anatomical variant.

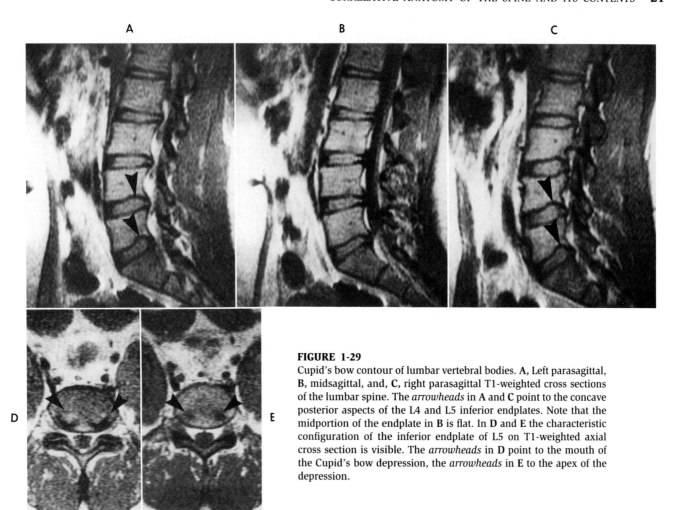

FIGURE 1-29
Cupid's bow contour of lumbar vertebral bodies. **A**, Left parasagittal, **B**, midsagittal, and, **C**, right parasagittal T1-weighted cross sections of the lumbar spine. The *arrowheads* in **A** and **C** point to the concave posterior aspects of the L4 and L5 inferior endplates. Note that the midportion of the endplate in **B** is flat. In **D** and **E** the characteristic configuration of the inferior endplate of L5 on T1-weighted axial cross section is visible. The *arrowheads* in **D** point to the mouth of the Cupid's bow depression, the *arrowheads* in **E** to the apex of the depression.

Lumbar facet joints

The lumbar facet joints are in an oblique plane that changes its orientation from L1 to S1. Part of the facet is oriented at 45 degrees or so to the sagittal. The remainder is in an almost coronal plane. The articular facet of the superior (ascending) articulating process has a concave surface that faces posteriorly and medially. This facet articulates with the inferior (descending) articular process, which has a convex facet on its anterior surface that faces anteriorly and laterally. When a lumbar facet joint is viewed on an axial cross section, the anterior articular facet belongs to the vertebral body sitting below it and the posterior facet belongs to the vertebral body sitting above it (Figs. 1-30 and 1-31).

As in the rest of the spine, the lumbar facet joints are true synovial joints. They are covered by hyaline cartilage that may be 2 to 4 mm in thickness. The fine detail of the subchondral cortex of the facet joints and the hypertrophic changes of the facets due to osteoarthrosis are well appreciated on CT examination of the spine. Articular cartilage is best appreciated on gradient echo MRI axial cross sections. On these images the articular cartilage has a bright signal, standing out in sharp contrast against the gray-black silhouette of the subjacent cortical bone. The capsule of the facet joint is a continuation of the ligamentum flavum. The facet joint cavity has a characteristic configuration as delineated on facet joint contrast injection. Long-standing joint effusion and increased intraarticular pressure may lead to formation of paraarticular synovial cysts, similar to a Baker (or popliteal) cyst in the knee region. Synovial cysts arising from the facet joints may present as a mass in the paraspinal soft tissues or in the epidural space. They may become quite large, occupying half or more of the cross-sectional surface area of the spinal canal, and may extend for about half or more of the height of one vertebral body cephalad and caudad in the spinal canal. There may be calcification in the wall of the cyst.

Lateral recess

The anterolateral portion of the spinal canal is called the lateral recess. It is a more distinct part of the canal in

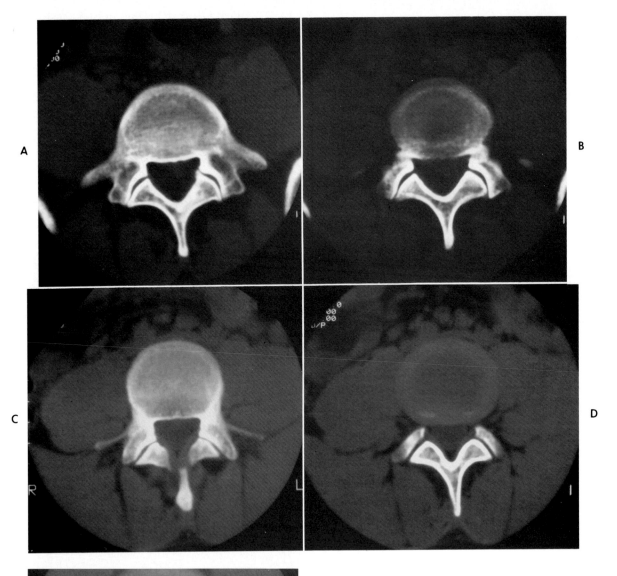

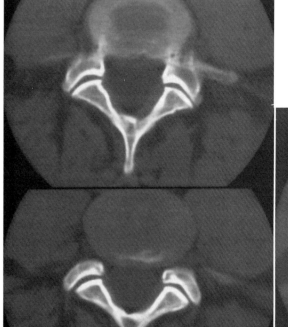

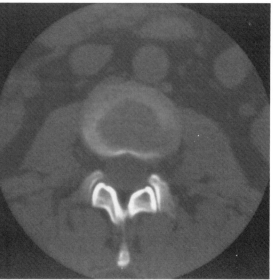

FIGURE 1-30
Normal lumbar facet joints. **A** and **B**, L4-L5. **C**, L3-L4. **D**, L2-L3.

FIGURE 1-31
Normal facet joints of the lumbar spine. **A**, L4-L5. In this patient the joints have a 15-to-20-degree tilt to the coronal plane. **B**, L2-L3. In this patient they are practically in the sagittal plane.

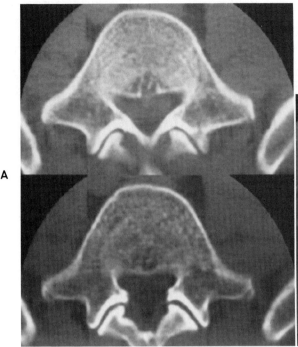

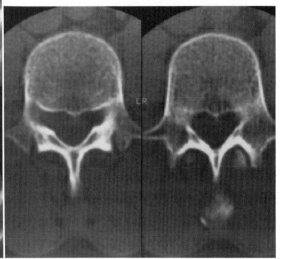

FIGURE 1-32
Normal lateral recess of, A, L4 and, B, L5.

L4, L5, and S1 segments and it contains the descending nerve root. It is bounded anteriorly by the posterior surface of the intervertebral disk and vertebral body, laterally by the pedicle, and posteriorly by the superior articular process.

The most important part of the lateral recess is its superior portion, at its entrance. This is where entrapment of the descending nerve root may occur when hypertrophic changes of the superior articular facet or the vertebral endplates develop. The lateral recess is usually more than 3 mm in anteroposterior diameter. When it is less than 2 to 3 mm, it is considered stenotic.

The lateral recess is best studied with CT. In our experience *a significant number of subjects with stenosis of the lateral recess have no symptoms.* In some of these individuals careful examination will show the descending nerve root to be not entrapped in the stenotic recess but actually pushed medial to its expected position in the recess. We believe that, as gradual stenosis of the lateral recess develops, the hypertrophic changes force the descending nerve root medially and it consequently escapes entrapment in the stenotic recess. Axial CT images with proper window and level settings will usually reveal the precise location of the descending root in these patients (Fig. 1-32).

SACRUM

The sacrum is formed by fusion of the five sacral vertebrae. The spinal canal continues as the central canal of the sacrum, which is triangular-ovoid in cross section. The sacral neural foramina are situated lateral to the sacral canal and have an anteroposterior channel through which the corresponding divisions of the sacral nerves pass.

SPINAL LIGAMENTS
Anterior longitudinal ligament

The anterior longitudinal ligament covers the anterior and part of the lateral surfaces of the vertebrae and extends practically the entire length of the spine. Its fibers are firmly attached to the vertebrae, especially in the vicinity of the vertebral endplates. The fibers of this ligament also merge with the anterior and lateral portions of the annulus fibrosus. Consequently, when degenerative changes of the intervertebral disks occur, leading to bulging or herniation, the fibers of the anterior longitudinal ligament are also forced outward. Centrifugal displacement of the fibers of the annulus, which are attached to the vertebral cortex by Sharpey's fibers, eventually leads to the formation of degenerative osteophytes, which commonly occur anteriorly and laterally (in the lumbar and thoracic spine) but are uncommon posteriorly.[38]

Posterior longitudinal ligament

The posterior longitudinal ligament extends along the posterior surface of the vertebral bodies from the clivus to the sacrum. Superiorly it merges with the tectorial membrane, which is attached to the posterior surface of the clivus. The fibers of this ligament are attached to the vertebral bodies in the vicinity of the vertebral endplates, but not to the midposterior surfaces of the vertebrae, where the veins leading to formation of the confluence of the basivertebral vein are situated. In some subjects a small amount of fat is present between this ligament and the posterior surface of the vertebral bodies. In the cervical and upper thoracic region the ligament is broad and of fairly uniform width. In the lumbar and lower

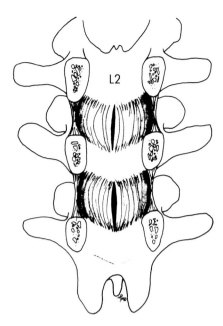

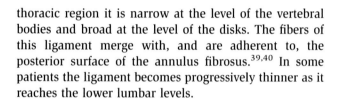

FIGURE 1-33
Schematic of a normal lumbar neural arch. The ligamentum flavum extends from the lamina of one vertebra to the lamina of the next, forming part of the posterior wall of the spinal canal.

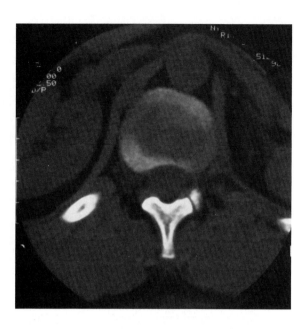

FIGURE 1-34
Normal T11-12 thoracic disk.

thoracic region it is narrow at the level of the vertebral bodies and broad at the level of the disks. The fibers of this ligament merge with, and are adherent to, the posterior surface of the annulus fibrosus.[39,40] In some patients the ligament becomes progressively thinner as it reaches the lower lumbar levels.

Ligamentum flavum

The ligamentum flavum is a fibroelastic structure that covers the bony gaps (between the laminae) in the posterior wall of the spinal canal. There is a right and a left ligament at each level, and each extends from the anteroinferior surface of the lamina above to the posterosuperior surface of the lamina below.[41] Anterolaterally the ligament continues as the capsule of the facet joint. It is rather thin in the cervical spine but becomes progressively thicker in the lower lumbar spine, and may normally be 2 to 4 mm thick in the lower lumbar region on axial CT or MR images. Most investigators believe that the ligamentum flavum does not increase in size after full skeletal maturity. However, it may appear thickened on CT, MRI, or myelography in older subjects, especially patients with degenerative spondylosis. This is probably due, at least in part, to the reduction in length of the spinal column (essentially because of reduced disk thickness), which leads to buckling and redundancy of the ligament (Fig. 1-33).

INTERVERTEBRAL DISKS

There are 23 intervertebral disks in the normal spine. They are thinnest in the thoracic region and thickest in the lumbar region. The thickness of the lumbar interver-

tebral disks increases from L1-2 to L5-S1. However, we have found that the L5-S1 intervertebral disk may be normally thinner than the disk above it, without pathological evidence of degenerative disease. Therefore, diagnosing pathology of this disk solely on the basis of its diminished thickness is unreliable; other evidence of disk disease must be present for the diagnosis to be established (Fig. 1-34 and Plate 1-5).

Each intervertebral disk is composed of three distinct parts:

1. *Cartilaginous plate (endplate).* This is a layer of cartilage that covers the surface of the bony vertebral endplate. The bony endplate has a peripheral part (which corresponds to the apophyseal ring and is covered by fibrocartilage) and a central part (covered by hyaline cartilage). The boundary between the two is not usually distinct.[35]
2. *Annulus fibrosus.* This consists of essentially two sets of fibers, fibrocartilaginous and collagenous, arranged in circular and concentric fashion, that form a limiting membrane for the nucleus pulposus. The annulus fibrosus is the major part of the intervertebral disk. Its fibrocartilaginous fibers (type II collagen) arise from the peripheral portion of the cartilaginous plate and merge imperceptibly with the nucleus pulposus. Its collagenous fibers (type I collagen) are short and form the peripheral part of the annulus. The collagenous fibers insert into the ring apophysis and cross over the edge of the vertebral endplate to insert into the cortex of the vertebral body via Sharpey's fibers. The collagenous fibers also insert into the anterior and posterior

A

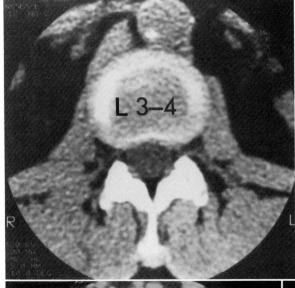

FIGURE 1-35

Normal configuration of the L3-4 disk. **A,** Note the concavity in the posterior disk margin. **B,** A CT-myelogram in another patient shows the posterior margin of the disk to be flat. This individual did not have any complaints related to the lumbar spine; the myelogram was part of the work-up for a fracture of T6. Notice that there is no fat in the midline between the dural sac and the posterior border of the disk and also that the disk is in contact with the dural sac. **C,** Inferior endplate of L3. The configuration of the posterior surface of the L3-4 disk is identical to that of the endplate.

B

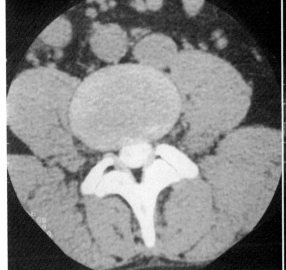

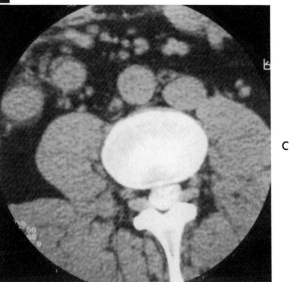

C

longitudinal ligaments. The annulus is significantly stronger anteriorly, where its attachment to the anterior longitudinal ligament (ALL) is substantial, than posteriorly, where its attachment to the posterior longitudinal ligament (PLL) is less extensive. (The PLL itself is significantly narrower than the ALL.[35,41-53])

The *configuration of the intervertebral disks* is, to a great extent, dictated by that of the neighboring vertebral endplates and bodies. The posterior border of the lower thoracic and three upper lumbar disks may be concave, similar to the posterior surfaces of the corresponding vertebrae. The posterior longitudinal ligament probably is, at least partially, responsible for maintaining the concavity of the posterior borders of each disk. The posterior borders of the L4-5 and L5-S1 disks may normally be flat or convex in about 25% to 30% of the adult population (Figs. 1-35 to 1-37).

Although the *vascularity of the annulus fibrosus* is generally considered nonexistent, this is only partially true. Hassler[54] performed microangiography on 28 cadavers, with the specific aim of studying the vascularity of the margins of the intervertebral disks. The vascularity of the peripheral margin of the annulus, where it attaches to the vertebral margins, was found to be abundant, with deep penetration into the disk substance in infants and young children. In adults, however, it was sparse and the vessels were nonpenetrating. The free margin of the annulus — the part between the attachments to the vertebrae above and below — had a rich vascular supply in both children and adults. The existence of vascularity of the outer layer of the annulus has been demonstrated by other investigators also. A microscopic examination of the disks from 88 subjects by Coventry et al.,[35,49-51] in which changes were compared from decade to decade,

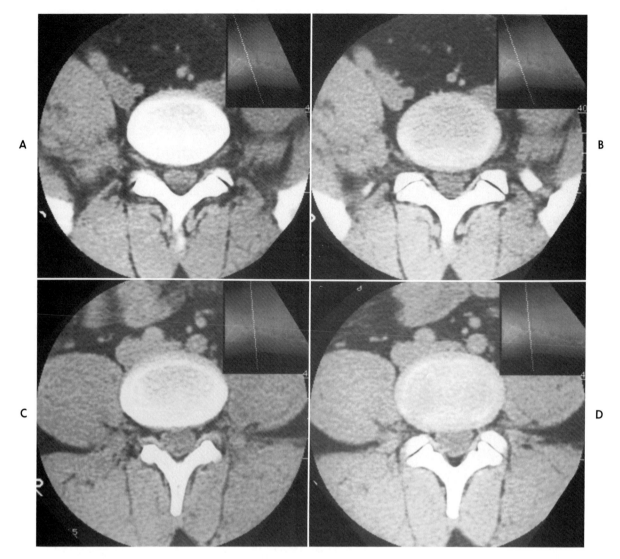

FIGURE 1-36
Configurations of the vertebral endplates and disks. **A** and **B**, L5-S1 and, **C** and **D**, L4-5. Note that the configuration of the disk in **B** and **D** matches that of the posterior aspect of the endplate in **A** and **C**.

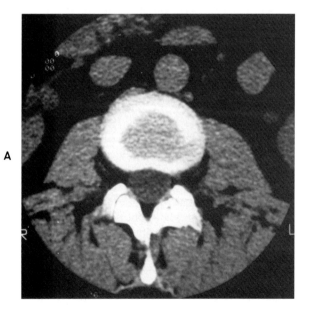

FIGURE 1-37
Normal configurations of the lumbar disks and posterior borders of the lumbar bodies. **A**, Concave (L2-3 disk and endplates).

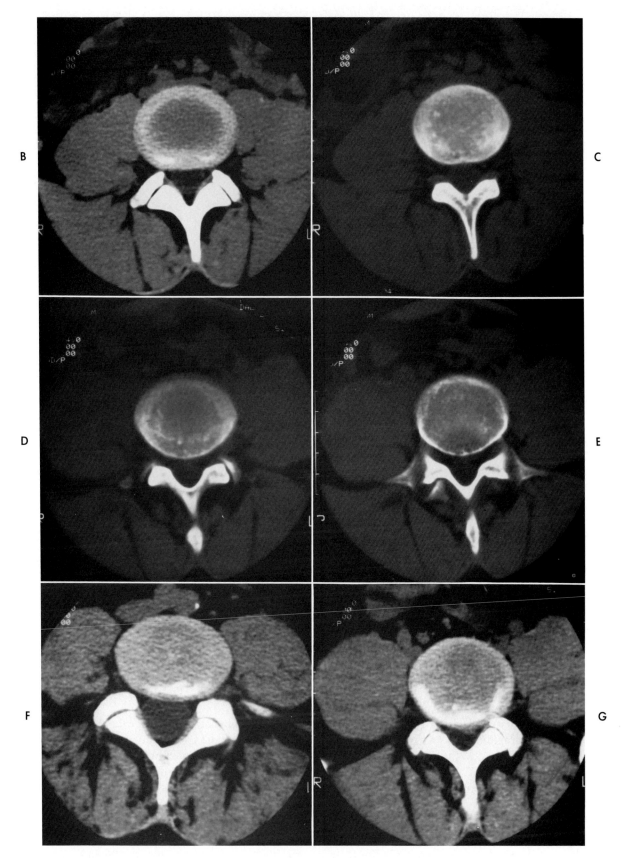

FIGURE 1-37, cont'd
B and C, Flat (L3-4 disk and endplates). D, E, and F, Round (L4-5 disk and L4 endplate). G, Round (L4-5 disk). Note the focal herniation of the disk to the left of midline.

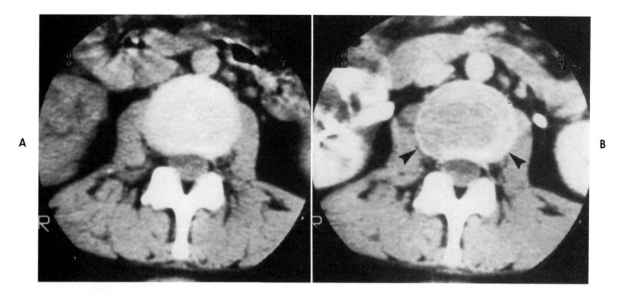

FIGURE 1-38
Normal L3-4 disk. **A,** Precontrast and, **B,** postcontrast CT. Note the enhancement of the disk margins *(arrowheads).*

showed regrowth of vascularity through the cartilaginous plate into the disk concomitant with aging and degenerative changes. The number of vascular channels was noted to increase with each passing decade. Additionally, progressively increasing granulation tissue, edema, and reparative scarring were noted with correspondingly more extensive degenerative changes (Fig. 1-38).

We have had experience with intravenous contrast–enhanced CT of the lumbar spine in 176 patients, 143 of whom have been previously reported.[55] There was distinct enhancement of the margins of normal, bulging and herniated disks in more than 60% of these patients, most prominent in the presence of bulging and herniation. Based on this pattern of enhancement in normal and pathological disks, on the findings at surgery in 77 patients, and on pathological examinations of resected disk substance therefore, we believe that (1) the margin of lumbar disks has at least a moderate degree of vascularity, (2) this vascularity is more pronounced in bulging and herniated disks, and (3) with severe herniation the vascularity (and swelling and granulation tissue) may be quite pronounced and affect several millimeters to a centimeter or so of the herniated portion of the disk.

3. *Nucleus pulposus.* This structure has a semiliquid (gellike) consistency in children and young adults, but with advancing age there is gradual loss of water. Whereas in a full-term newborn the nucleus is 85% to 90% water, in a 70-year-old subject it is 70% to 75%. There is also gradual replacement of the nucleus by fibrocartilaginous material; in the sixth and seventh decades it may be indistinguishable from the annulus fibrosus. It is also noteworthy

that with advancing age there is revascularization through the cartilaginous plate and annulus fibrosus into the nucleus pulposus, which is now essentially fibrocartilaginous.[35,49-53,56-59]

MRI of normal lumbar disks

On MRI imaging, each intervertebral disk shows essentially two more or less distinct regions of different signal intensity. On short TR/short TE images the contrast between the two regions is not pronounced. Peripherally there is a thin gray-black band that corresponds to the outermost fibers of the annulus and the confluence of the annulus with the anterior and posterior longitudinal ligaments. Centrally there is an area of low signal intensity, slightly brighter than the peripheral region, that corresponds to the nucleus pulposus and the inner fibers of the annulus. On long TR/long TE images the central region has a fairly bright signal. This portion corresponds to the nucleus pulposus and the inner (fibrocartilaginous) fibers of the annulus. There is a band of low signal intensity in the peripheral region that corresponds to the outermost fibers of the annulus and longitudinal ligaments (Fig. 1-39).

The signal characteristics of the intervertebral disk on gradient echo images are usually a thin band of low intensity at the periphery of the disk, often thinner than the corresponding area on long TR/long TE images, and a bright central portion.

MRI of cadaver disks

Pech and Haughton[53] correlated MR images with anatomical studies of cadaver vertebral specimens. On short TR/short TE (300/18) images of a 55-year-old specimen there was little contrast in the disk, although the periphery had a slightly more intense signal (shorter

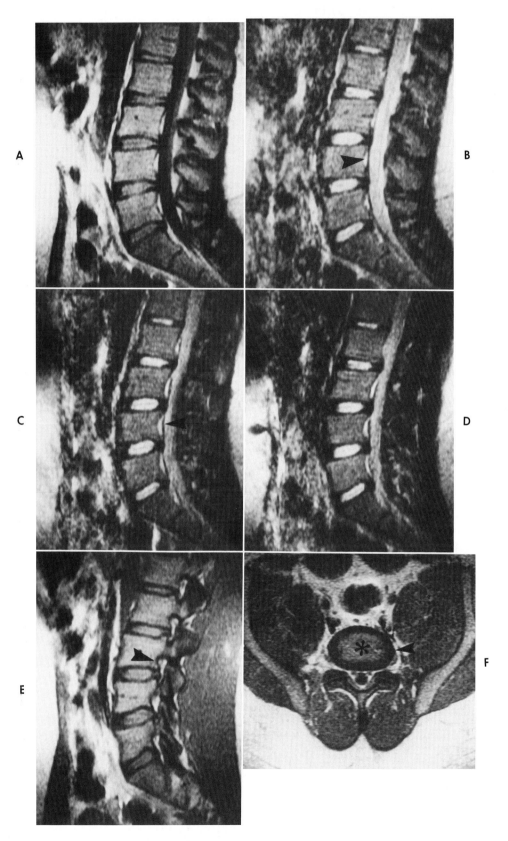

FIGURE 1-39
Normal lumbar spine. **A** is a midsagittal T1-weighted cross section, and **B** is a midsagittal and **C** and **D** are parasagittal T2-weighted cross sections showing the nucleus pulposus and inner fibers of the annulus fibrosus to be of normally bright signal. The *arrowhead* in **B** denotes epidural fat on the posterior surface of L4. The CSF is bright and provides a myelographic effect. The *arrowhead* in **C** designates the posterior longitudinal ligament. Note that the posterolateral surface of the annulus is more prominent and seems to be protruding into the canal in **C** and **D**. This does not represent bulging or herniation, however. **E** is a T1-weighted parasagittal cross section at the level of the pedicles, and **F** is an axial T1-weighted cross section through L5-S1. The *arrowhead* in **E** points to the neural foramen between L3 and L4, and that in **F** points to the outer portion of the annulus. The *asterisk* in **F** denotes the central portion of the disk, corresponding to the nucleus and the inner fibers of the annulus.

T1) than the central portion. The bright signal region was thought to correspond to the collagenous fibers of the annulus, and the central portion to the nucleus pulposus and inner fibers of the annulus. On long TR/long TE images (1500/100) more contrast was noted between the two regions. The peripheral (collagenous) portion appeared as a thin black band. The nucleus and the fibrocartilaginous portion of the annulus appeared as an area of bright signal.

MRI of abnormal lumbar disks

The signal characteristics of intervertebral disks change with advancing age. This is secondary to physical and chemical changes in the disk as well as to loss of water from both the annulus and the nucleus, which in normal young adults are approximately 80% and 90% water respectively. With aging, the nucleus loses proportionately more water than the annulus. In disks with advanced degenerative disease, the signal intensity is diminished and almost uniform; the difference between the central portion (which usually has higher intensity) and the periphery (which usually has lower intensity) is no longer pronounced, or is altogether lost. The loss of signal in degenerative disk disease cannot be explained

solely by the loss of water from the disk. The magnitude of the change is more than can be expected by the amount of water lost. Thus other factors, such as changes in the physical and chemical composition of the disk, are probably also important causes of alteration and loss of signal in degenerative disk disease.[60]

Intranuclear cleft

Diskography in infants and children usually reveals the central portion of the disk to have an ovoid configuration. In adults a septumlike structure may be noted in the middle of the nucleus pulposus. On T2-weighted MRI images of normal lumbar disks there is often a linear area of reduced signal in the central portion of the nucleus. Aguila et al.[61] referred to this as the "intranuclear cleft" and stated that it is caused by an alteration in the nuclear matrix and, more importantly, by invagination of the lamellae of the annulus into the nucleus, the latter process becoming increasingly obvious in the second and third decades of life. These workers further stated that anatomical and histological review of three cadaveric specimens had shown the area with decreased signal intensity on MR to contain a fibrous septum histologically identical to the annulus fibrosus. In their study 93% of all

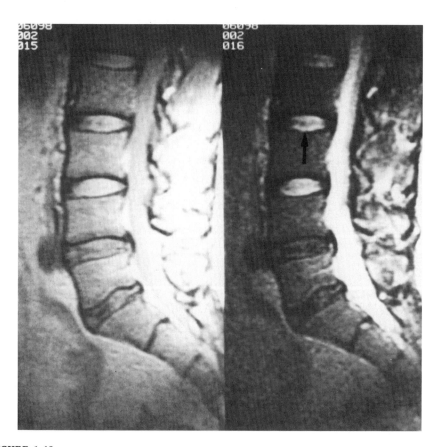

FIGURE 1-40
Intranuclear cleft. Midsagittal proton density–weighted and T2-weighted cross sections of the lumbar spine showing indications of degenerative disk disease at L4-5 and L5-S1. The L2-3 and L3-4 disks are normal. The *arrow* points to the so-called intranuclear cleft, which appears as a horizontal band of decreased signal in the equator of the L2-3 disk.

normal disks demonstrated this decreased signal intensity within the nucleus. If this finding was present in one disk, it was present in 94% of the other disks as well (Figs. 1-40 and 1-41).

However, Pech and Haughton[53] compared MRI findings with autopsy findings in the spines of cadavers and found no definite correlation of this low intensity area in their specimens. Modic et al.,[62] in a study published in 1988, stated that, although it may not be immediately apparent on gross inspection, this area of low signal intensity in the middle of the nucleus pulposus represents a zone of more fibrous tissue than the surrounding nucleus pulposus and is almost universally seen in individuals older than 30 years. Pech and Haughton[53] stated that this probably constitutes a remnant of the collagenous skeleton of the disk.

A linear area of low signal may be noted in the middle of thoracic disks. This has been shown to be a truncation artifact, and it can be made significantly less bothersome by using a larger matrix. Changing the direction of phase encoding gradient also will cause it to appear in a plane along the vertical axis of the spinal canal rather than in an axial plane.[63]

DURAL SAC

In adults the spinal cord extends to the L1-2 region. The dural sac continues to the lower lumbar spine, in some subjects to L4 or L5 and in others to S1 or S2. It may stay constant in size in the lumbar region until the point of its termination, although more commonly it tapers progressively for 2 to 4 cm just proximal to its termination. In the cervical, thoracic, and most of the lumbar spine it is in the center of the spinal canal. At L5 or L5-S1 it moves gradually to the posterior part, especially in subjects in whom there is marked tapering of its distal portion. Consequently the epidural space may be quite capacious, particularly anteriorly, at L5-S1 and to a lesser extent L4-5 (Fig. 1-42).

The signal characteristics of CSF are dependent upon the pulse sequence utilized. On T1-weighted images, CSF has a low signal intensity but the spinal cord has a relatively high intensity and the interface between them is usually crisp and well defined. The signal intensity of CSF progressively increases with lengthening of the TR and TE. On T2-weighted images a myelographic effect is produced. The CSF also has a high signal intensity relative to the spinal cord and extradural structures on gradient echo images.

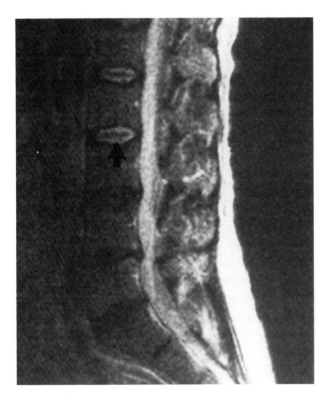

FIGURE 1-41
Intranuclear cleft. Sagittal T2-weighted cross section of the lumbar spine showing a horizontal band of low signal intensity in the equator of the L1-2 and L2-3 *(arrow)* disks. The L3-4, L4-5, and L5-S1 disks are markedly low in signal due to degenerative disease.

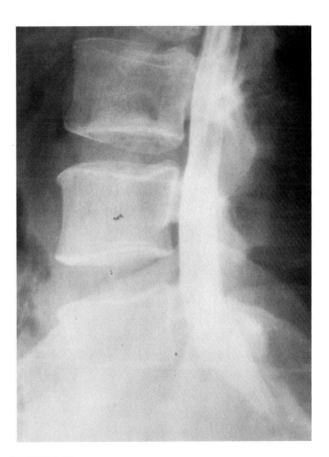

FIGURE 1-42
Lumbar spine, lateral myelogram. The anterior epidural space at L5 and L5-S1, measuring about 10 mm in this patient, is filled with fat. In patients with a relatively wide anterior epidural space, herniation of the L5-S1 disk may not distort the dural sac or root sleeves.

In the cervical spine, artifacts related to the pulsations of CSF are more pronounced than in the thoracic and lumbar spine. In the middle segments of the thoracic region the subarachnoid space is fairly large relative to the spinal cord. Consequently a significant amount of CSF may be present. Several artifacts related to the pulsations of CSF are noted on axial MRI images. Variations in the CSF signal presenting as circular, ovoid, or curvilinear areas of relatively low signal intensity may be seen. In the lumbar region the effects of CSF pulsation are less prominent, although artifacts mimicking a subarachnoid lesion or arachnoiditis may appear as focal areas of increased signal intensity on T1-weighted images.

A particularly troublesome artifact is truncation effect, which may cause the spinal cord to appear significantly smaller than it actually is or may produce linear areas of alternating increased and decreased signal mimicking syringomyelia.[64-66] Truncation artifact is usually more prominent on T2-weighted images and is caused by errors in sampling at the interfaces of tissues with significantly different composition (e.g., CSF and the spinal cord or CSF and a vertebral body). It may be practically eliminated with a larger matrix, and is usually not evident if a matrix of 256×256 is used. It may also be projected at a 90 degree angle to the longitudinal axis of the spinal cord by changing the direction of the phase encoding gradient.

EPIDURAL SPACE

The epidural space contains relatively less fat in the cervical and thoracic region than in the lumbar region. There is practically none in the anterior part of the cervical and thoracic epidural space. In the anterior lumbar epidural space the thickness of the fat increases progressively from L1 to L5. At L4-5 and L5-S1 there may be a significant layer, especially in persons in whom the dural sac has either terminated above the S1 level or tapered significantly. In some persons there is a layer of fat 10 mm or more thick in the anterior epidural space between the posterior border of L4-5 and L5-S1 and the anterior surface of the dural sac. In these persons the L5 and S1 nerve roots are clearly visualized on CT and MRI anterior to the dural sac. Because of abundant epidural fat, a herniated L4-5 or L5-S1 disk is particularly well displayed on CT and MRI; however, on myelography, occasionally even a large (midline) L5-S1 herniation will be missed because the posterior border of the herniated disk may not come into contact with the anterior surface of the dural sac and there may be no abnormality (displacement or distortion) of the dural sac and descending sacral roots (root sleeves).

SPINAL CORD

Magnetic resonance imaging has enabled visualization of the spinal cord to occur directly without the necessity of injecting contrast intrathecally. At present, it is the modality of choice for evaluating spinal cord status in most instances. When proper pulse sequences are used,

fairly accurate estimations of the size and configuration of the cord can be made from sagittal, coronal, and axial images.

Corresponding to the origin of the cervical and brachial plexuses, as well as the lumbosacral plexus, there are two areas of slight expansion: the cervical, from C4 to T2, and the lumbar, from T9-10 to T12. In adults the spinal cord extends from the level of the foramen magnum to about L1. According to Rene Louis[67] it terminates at L1-2 in 36%, at mid-L1 in 26%, at mid-L2 in 20%, and at L2-3 in 6% of normal subjects. However, it may be abnormally low in position and terminate at the lower end of the lumbar canal or, very rarely, even extend to the lower portion of the sacral canal. In some individuals with abnormally low termination, several congenital abnormalities of the vertebral column as well as intrathecal tumors may also be present — diastomatomyelia, lipomas, and dermoid tumors. Most of these are well visualized on MRI.[68]

In the cervical region the spinal cord is elliptical on cross section. In the thoracic region it is more or less circular. It is flattened somewhat anteroposteriorly, with a groove anteriorly, in which the anterior spinal artery is situated. The size of the spinal cord varies from subject to subject. Thus diagnosis of atrophy or enlargement must be made with great caution, particularly when the cord is measured on CT-myelography or MRI. In the case of CT-myelography, empirically derived window and level settings that provide an accurate measure for the specific scanner employed should be used. In the case of MRI, it is also necessary to find the appropriate technical parameters that will yield an accurate measure of spinal cord size. At present, these parameters must be determined separately for the particular MRI imager being used.

The spinal cord is usually well delineated on T1-weighted images, in which the CSF is of relatively low signal intensity and the cord of relatively high intensity. Provided there are no significant artifacts, and with proper window and level settings, the cord can be measured fairly accurately on T1-weighted images. However, further experience with actual measurement of cord specimens on various pulse sequences is necessary before the ideal parameters can be determined. Of several artifacts that may interfere with the accuracy of spinal cord measurement, the truncation artifact is particularly troublesome. In the cervical cord and, to a lesser extent, the thoracic cord it can cause an erroneously small appearance (Figs. 1-15, 1-16, and 1-19 to 1-21) (Plates 1-1 and 1-3).

The transverse diameter of the spinal cord is normally 12 to 13 mm at its widest segment (C3 to T2). At its narrowest segment (midthoracic region) it may be 7 to 8 mm. At the lumbar enlargement (T9-L1) it is about 12 mm. The anteroposterior diameter is 8 to 9 mm at the cervical and lumbar enlargements and 1 to 2 mm less elsewhere.[21,26,41,69,70]

The lower end of the spinal cord is the conus medul-

FIGURE 1-43
Normal conus medullaris. Sagittal T1-weighted cross section showing the configuration of the conus *(arrow)*. Degenerative disk disease at L2-L3 and focal herniation at L4-L5 are also present.

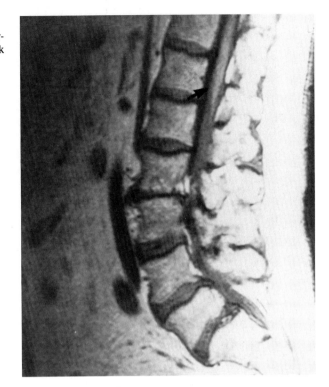

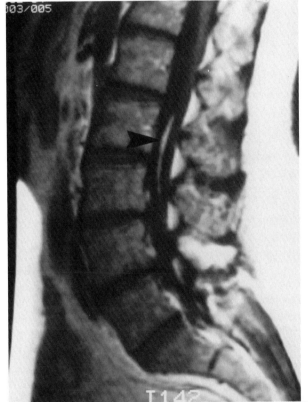

FIGURE 1-44
Thick filum terminale. **A**, Midsagittal and, **B**, axial T1-weighted cross sections showing the filum *(arrowheads)*.

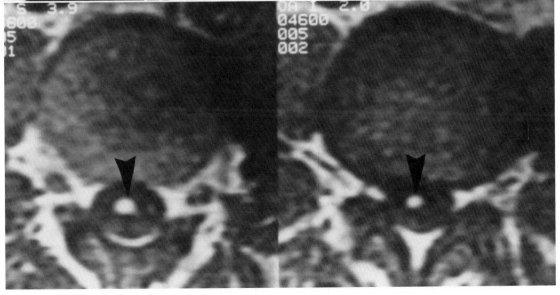

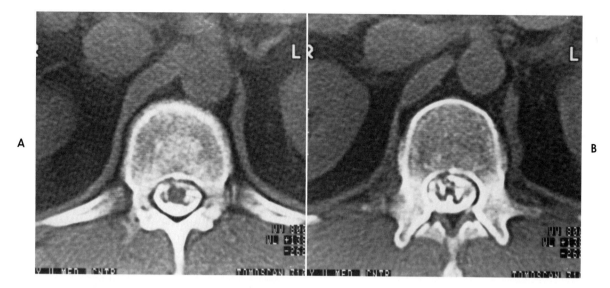

FIGURE 1-45
CT myelograms showing the normal conus medullaris and lumbar nerve roots. **A** is the conus. In **B**, note the W configuration of the nerve roots just distal to the conus.

laris, from which a thin midline prolongation extends, the filum terminale interna. The filum terminale continues inside the dural sac and terminates at the bottom (Figs. 1-43 to 1-45 and Plate 1-6).

The spinal cord is enveloped by the pia mater, arachnoid, and dura. The subarachnoid spaces are filled with CSF. External to the dura is the epidural space, which is filled with fat, areolar tissue, and the epidural venous plexus.

SPINAL NERVES

The spinal nerves emerge from the cord in pairs: 8 in the cervical, 12 in the thoracic, 5 in the lumbar, 5 in the sacral, and 1 in the coccygeal region. Each pair is formed by the union of an anterior (ventral) and a posterior (dorsal) root. The nerve roots, in turn, are formed by the union of multiple rootlets that emerge from the anterolateral and posterolateral surfaces of the spinal cord. The dorsal root has an oval enlargement called the dorsal root (nerve) ganglion. It is usually located in the neural foramen. The union of the dorsal and ventral roots, just after the dorsal root ganglion, forms the spinal nerve, which extends from this point distally.

In fetuses up to about the third month, the spinal cord occupies the entire length of the spinal canal and the spinal nerves exit the canal at right angles. However, the vertebral column grows faster than the spinal cord and, consequently, the lower end of the cord appears to migrate upward. At 5 months it is at about S1, at 6 months at L3, and at birth at L1-2.[71]

In the earlier literature it was stated that the spinal cord ascends throughout childhood, attaining its final position by adulthood.[72,73] According to Wilson and Prince,[71] it was assumed that the lower level of the conus is normally at L3 by birth and ascends to L2-3 by age 5, L2 by age 12, and eventually L1 by adulthood.[72,73] They determined its location on spinal MRI examinations in 184 children ranging from newborn to 20 years of age and found levels from T12 to L2-3 for the 0-to-2-year-old group (with an average of L1-2) and L1 to L2 for the 19-to-20-year-old group (average L1-2).[71] Thus they concluded that the conus medullaris does not ascend throughout childhood but attains its adult level sometime during the first few months of life. However, it is presently agreed that a conus at L2-3 (or one or two levels higher) is normal at any age and one at L3 is indeterminate since it could be normal or tethered.

The apparent upward migration of the conus and the spinal cord as a result of faster growth of the vertebral column most likely is not uniform throughout the length of the cord, as can be surmised from the configuration of the spinal nerves. The least amount of upward migration occurs at the upper cervical cord, and the most at the conus medullaris. Consequently, although the upper cervical nerves exit the spinal canal only slightly below their origin from the spinal cord, the thoracic and lumbar nerve roots must descend a progressively greater distance before they reach their respective neural foramina.

Cervical spinal nerves

There are eight pairs of cervical nerves. The first pair leaves the spinal canal above the arch of C1 laterally, the second pair above C2, the third above C3 (through the C2-3 foramen), and so on to the eighth pair, which leaves above T1 (through the C7-T1 foramen). Another way of remembering this is to think of each cervical nerve as sitting on top of the pedicle of its corresponding vertebral body, except C8, which sits atop T1. For example, C3 is on top of the pedicle of C3 (in the C2-3 neural foramen), and C4 is on top of the pedicle of C4.

The cervical nerve roots emerge from the spinal cord slightly above the level of their corresponding neural foramina — the dorsal roots extending anteriorly and laterally, the ventral roots extending laterally. They then run slightly inferiorly in the subarachnoid space to reach their respective dural sleeves, which are quite short and branch off from the dural sac just above the middle of the neural foramen. The ventral roots are directly posterior to the intervertebral disks and posterolateral to the uncovertebral processes. The dorsal roots are lateral to the ventral roots and run along the anteromedial surfaces of the facet joints. The dorsal root ganglion is situated in a shallow fossa on the superior articulating process.

It is important to note that the cervical neural elements (roots, ganglia, and nerves), unlike their lumbar counterparts, lie in the lower portion of the cervical neural foramen. It is also important that an intimate relationship exists between the uncovertebral process on the anteromedial side (and the facet joint on the posterolateral side) and the inferior portion of the neural foramen. The most common cause of cervical neural foraminal stenosis, osteoarthrosis of the Luschka joints, is partially explained by this strategic juxtapositioning of the cervical roots and Luschka process. Compression of the cervical neural elements is often secondary to degenerative hypertrophic changes in the Luschka joints. Far less commonly, degenerative disease of the facet joints leads to stenosis of the neural foramina. Cervical facet joint osteoarthrosis, when responsible for foraminal stenosis, usually causes stenosis of the upper portion of the foramen, rarely the lower portion (Plates 1-7 and 1-8).

Thoracic spinal nerves

There are twelve pairs of thoracic nerves, each leaving the spinal canal below the pedicle of its respective vertebra. The first pair (T1) leaves below the pedicle of T1, the last (T12) below the pedicle of T12. Because of unequal growth rates between the cord and vertebral column, each cord segment is situated higher than its respective vertebra. The length of this discrepancy is about the height of one vertebral body in the cervical and upper thoracic region, but it increases progressively. Thus the thoracic nerve roots emerge from the spinal cord above the level of their respective neural foramina and travel some distance in the subarachnoid space to reach their corresponding root sleeves. The root sleeves, however, originate from the dural sac only slightly above the level of their respective neural foramina in the thoracic spine. Thus, in the thoracic region, the root sleeves are quite short and the dorsal root ganglion is usually situated in the midportion of the neural foramen.

Lumbar spinal nerves

In the lumbar spine the dural sac contains only lumbar, sacral, and coccygeal nerve roots. In some subjects the roots are grouped together so they resemble the letter H or W on axial cross section when the person is lying supine. This pattern is noted on CT-myelography. On MRI the roots often occupy the posterior half and about one third of the anterior half of the cross-sectional surface area of the dural sac when the person is supine. From this region they move anteriorly, inferiorly, and laterally to reach their respective dural sleeves.

The lumbar root sleeves emerge from the anterolateral dural sac and extend inferiorly, slightly anteriorly, and laterally into the lateral recess. They then continue medially on up to the middle of the pedicle. In some subjects they may extend to the inferior surface of the pedicle. On myelography the nerve roots (within the root sleeves) are usually visualized up to the midportion of the pedicle. However, in subjects in whom the root sleeves continue to the inferior surface of the pedicle, the nerve roots are also visualized up to this point. The roots then curve anteriorly and laterally beneath the pedicle to leave the spinal canal and enter the top of their respective neural foramina. The dorsal root ganglia are formed at this point, shortly distal to the terminations of the root sleeves (Figs. 1-46 to 1-52 and Plates 1-9 and 1-10).

The point of origin of L1, L2, and L3 root sleeves is just below the superior endplate of their respective vertebrae (i.e., below the level of the disk). The L4 root sleeves emerge at the level of the superior endplate of L4 in about 87% of subjects (myelography and CT-myelography); in the remaining 13% they arise slightly higher. The L5 root sleeves originate from the dural sac a few millimeters above the superior endplate of L5 in about 59% of the subjects. The S1 root sleeves usually arise above the inferior endplate of L5 and continue epidurally in the anterolateral portion of the spinal canal directly behind the disk of L5-S1; they then enter the lateral recess of S1. Thus, on axial cross sections, one usually does not see the root sleeves directly behind the L1-2, L2-3, and (in 87%) L3-4 disks because they have not yet separated from the dural sac.

The descending nerve roots at these levels are within the dural sac, having moved now to the anterolateral portion of the sac, and are just below and behind the posterolateral margins of their respective disks prior to entering the corresponding root sleeves. Thus, on axial cross sections obtained at or immediately below the superior vertebral endplate, they can be identified in the lateral recess. Because L5 root sleeves originate from the dural sac a few millimeters above the L5 superior endplate in 59% of subjects, they are distinctly visible in the epidural space posterior to the L4-5 disk just before they enter the lateral recess. At L5-S1 the sacral root sleeves (S1) are clearly identified in the epidural fat anterolateral to the dural sac; they can be seen behind the

Text continued on p. 40.

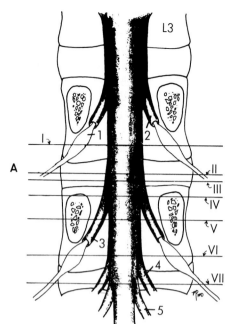

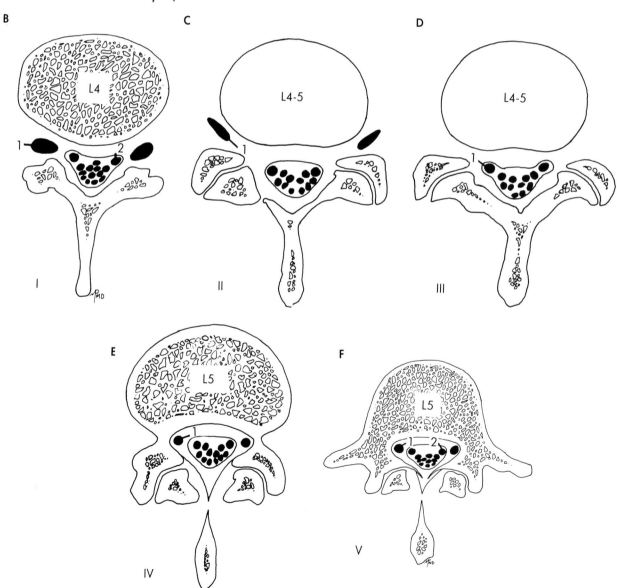

FIGURE 1-46
A, Normal anatomy of the dural sac, descending nerve roots, and spinal nerves in the lumbar region. *1,* Right dorsal nerve root ganglion of L4; *2,* dural sleeve of the left L4 descending nerve root; *3,* dural sleeve of the right L5 descending nerve root; *4* and *5,* dural sleeves of the left S1 and S2 descending nerve roots. (Axial slices *I* through *VII* are shown individually in **B** to **I.**) **B,** Slice *I,* at the upper L4-L5 intervertebral foramen. *1,* Dorsal root ganglion of the right L4 nerve root; *2,* descending left L5 nerve root. **C,** Slice *II,* at the L4-5 disk level. *1,* Right L4 spinal nerve exiting the neural foramen. **D,** Slice *III,* L4-5 disk level. The right L5 descending root is starting to enter its root sleeve. **E,** Slice *IV,* at the superior margin of the L5 pedicles. *1,* Right L5 descending nerve root, surrounded by its sleeve, now in the lateral recess. **F,** Slice *V,* through the midportion of the L5 pedicle. *1,* Right L5 descending nerve root; *2,* left S1 descending nerve root within the dural sac.

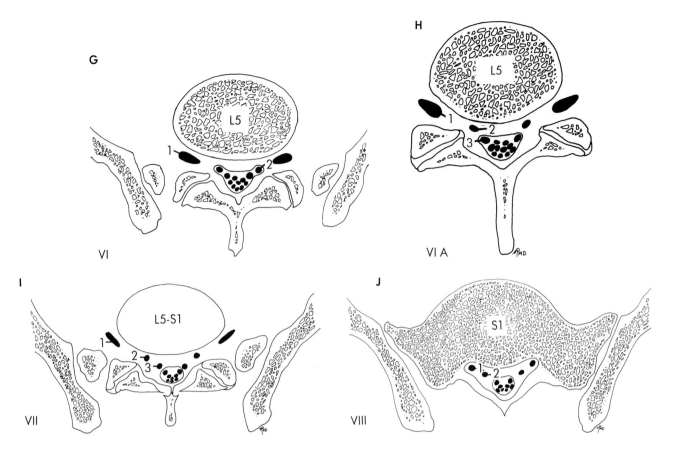

FIGURE 1-46, cont'd

G, Slice *VI*, through the upper portion of the L5-S1 neural foramen. *1*, Right L5 dorsal root ganglion; *2*, left S1 descending nerve root starting to enter its root sleeve. **H,** Slice *VIA* (not shown in **A**, but the same level as *VI*). (In some subjects the S1 root sleeve has already separated from the dura at this level.) *1*, Right dorsal root ganglion of L5; *2*, right descending nerve root in the anterior epidural space; *3*, right descending S2 root in the dural sac. **I,** Slice *VII*, just above the inferior endplate of L5 but encompassing the L5-S1 disk level. *1*, Right exiting L5 spinal nerve; *2*, right descending S1 nerve root; *3*, right descending S2 nerve root. **J,** Axial slice *VIII* (not shown in **A**), through the middle of S1. *1* and *2* are the descending sacral roots (S1 and S2) on the right side.

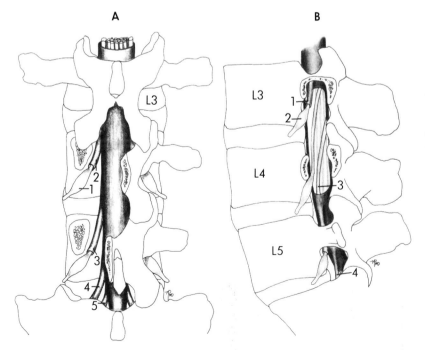

FIGURE 1-47

Normal anatomy of the dural sac and nerve roots in the lumbar region. **A,** Frontal view. A portion of the neural arch at L4 and L5 has been removed. *1*, Dorsal root ganglion of the right L4 descending nerve root; *2*, dural sleeve of the right L4 descending root; *3*, dural sleeve of the right L5 descending root; *4* and *5*, dural sleeves of the right descending S1 and S2 roots. **B,** Lateral view. A portion of the pedicle of L3 and L4 has been removed. *1*, Dural sleeve of the left L3 descending nerve root; *2*, dorsal root ganglion of the left L3 descending nerve root; *3*, left L5 descending nerve root; *4*, dural sleeve of the left S1 descending nerve root.

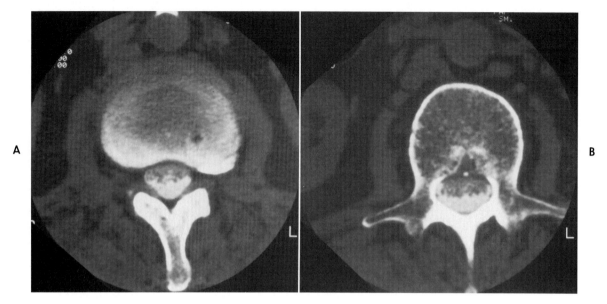

FIGURE 1-48
Normal lumbar nerve roots on a prone CT-myelogram. **A,** L3-4 and, **B,** L4. Note that the lumbar and sacral roots are all in the anterior half of the dural sac when the patient is prone.

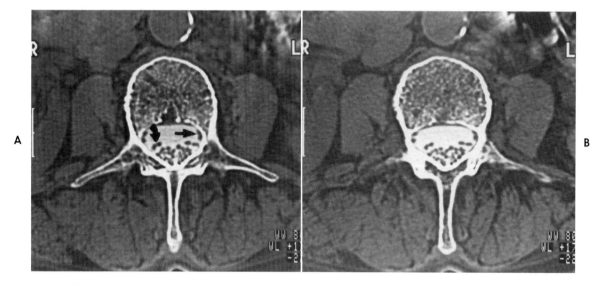

FIGURE 1-49
Descending lumbar nerve roots in a supine patient. **A,** An axial slice through the midportion of the L2 pedicle, normal CT-myelogram. The *horizontal arrow* points to the descending L2 nerve roots on the left. The *curved vertical arrow* points to the descending L3 nerve roots on the right. The remaining lumbar and sacral roots are in the posterior portion of the dural sac. **B,** 3 mm below A.

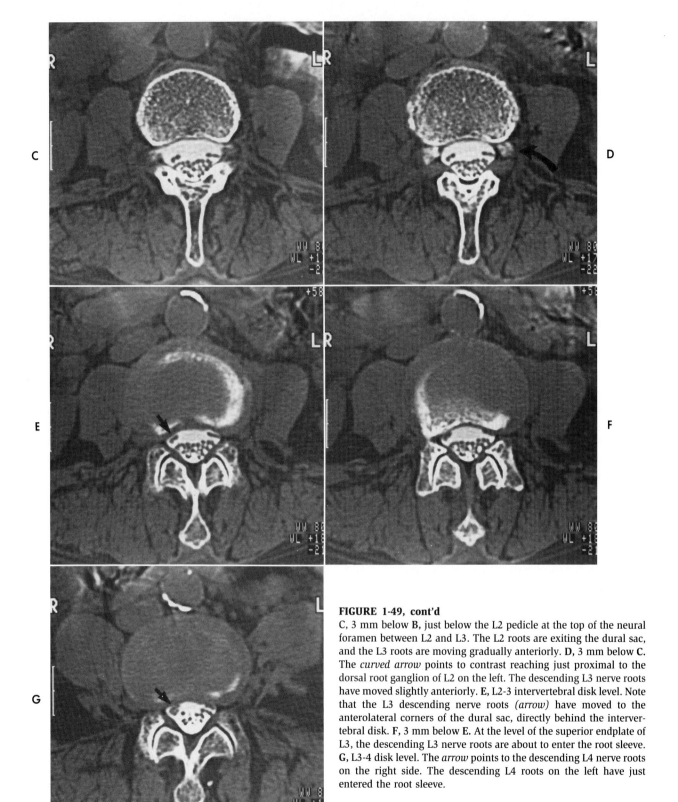

FIGURE 1-49, cont'd

C, 3 mm below B, just below the L2 pedicle at the top of the neural foramen between L2 and L3. The L2 roots are exiting the dural sac, and the L3 roots are moving gradually anteriorly. **D**, 3 mm below **C**. The *curved arrow* points to contrast reaching just proximal to the dorsal root ganglion of L2 on the left. The descending L3 nerve roots have moved slightly anteriorly. **E**, L2-3 intervertebral disk level. Note that the L3 descending nerve roots *(arrow)* have moved to the anterolateral corners of the dural sac, directly behind the intervertebral disk. **F**, 3 mm below **E**. At the level of the superior endplate of L3, the descending L3 nerve roots are about to enter the root sleeve. **G**, L3-4 disk level. The *arrow* points to the descending L4 nerve roots on the right side. The descending L4 roots on the left have just entered the root sleeve.

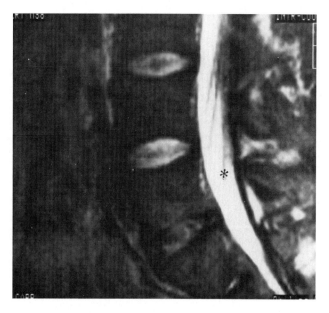

FIGURE 1-50
Normal L4, L5, and S1 descending roots on parasagittal T2-weighted MRI. There is a marked loss of signal at L5-S1, indicating degenerative disease. The *asterisk* is on the S1 descending nerve root on the right side.

posterolateral margin of the L5-S1 intervertebral disk just before they enter the lateral recess of S1.

The spinal nerves are formed immediately after the dorsal root ganglion and extend inferiorly, slightly laterally, and anteriorly in the neural foramen to exit just above the disk. At the disk level they are situated in an oblique horizontal plane anterolaterally in the paraspinal fat.

• • •

There are ordinarily two pairs of lumbar spinal "nerves" that can be affected by the herniation of an intervertebral disk. To avoid confusion, we have designated them the descending nerve root and the exiting spinal nerve.

DESCENDING NERVE ROOT

At each lumbar intervertebral disk level, on each side the descending nerve root is situated anteriorly and laterally in the dural sac. At L1-2 it is L2, which may be compressed by a herniated L1-2 disk; at L2-3 it is L3; at L3-4 it is L4; and at L4-5 and L5-S1 it is L5 and S1, which would be compressed by a herniated disk at these levels.

Each descending nerve root is directly posterior to the posterolateral margin of the disk. It leaves the dural sac through the root sleeve, the root sleeves emerging on the anterolateral aspect of the dural sac just below the superior endplate of the corresponding vertebra. The descending roots travel in the lateral recess and leave the spinal canal through the top of the neural foramina (Figs. 1-50 to 1-52).

EXITING SPINAL NERVE

The dorsal root ganglion lies in the top of the neural foramen, beneath the pedicle of the vertebral body forming the superior boundary of the disk. The exiting nerve extends from the dorsal root ganglion inferiorly, anteriorly, and laterally in the neural foramen. At the disk level it is in the paraspinal fat, far lateral to the posterior aspect of the disk (at about 4 or 8 o'clock in the axial plane). For example, at the L4-5 disk level the exiting nerve would be L4, which is formed just distal to the L4 dorsal root ganglion; at L1-2 it would be L1; and at L5-S1, L5.

EPIDURAL VEINS

Epidural veins form an extensive plexus surrounding the dural sac. In the cervical spine an extensive sinusoidal venous network occupies the space between the dural sac and the bony spinal canal. Anteriorly and laterally on each side, a distinct vertical venous channel is present behind the vertebral bodies just medial to the neural foramen (the anterior longitudinal epidural vein). The right and left vertical venous channels connect via horizontal channels through the neural foramina to a plexus surrounding the vertebral artery. This plexus, in turn, communicates with the perivertebral venous plexus via multiple communicating vessels. The anterior longitudinal epidural veins are connected by horizontally coursing retrocorporeal veins, which themselves communicate with the basivertebral vein in the midposterior surface of each vertebral body. The basivertebral vein may lead into an emissary vein that passes through each vertebra and joins the perivertebral venous plexus. In the

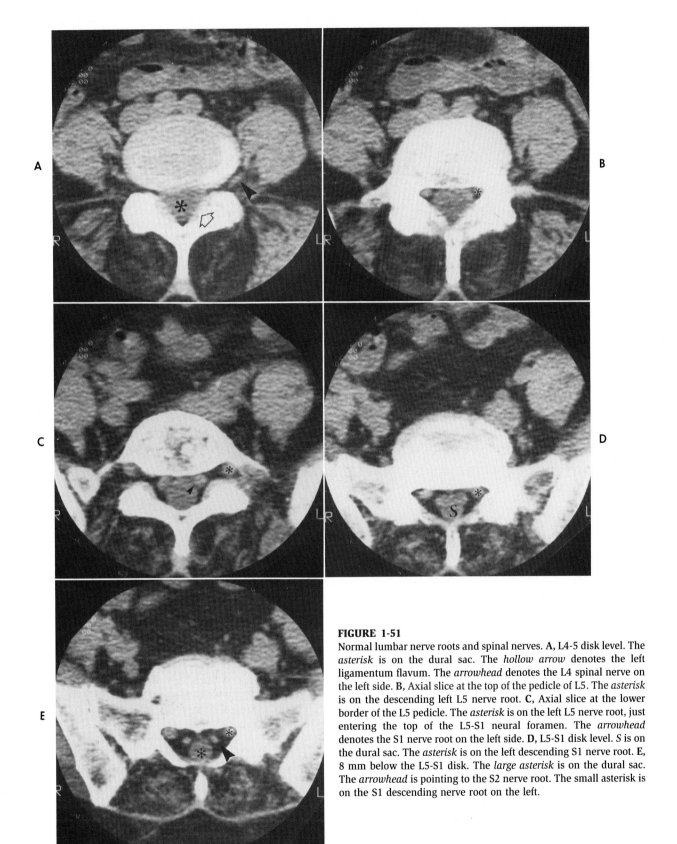

FIGURE 1-51

Normal lumbar nerve roots and spinal nerves. **A,** L4-5 disk level. The *asterisk* is on the dural sac. The *hollow arrow* denotes the left ligamentum flavum. The *arrowhead* denotes the L4 spinal nerve on the left side. **B,** Axial slice at the top of the pedicle of L5. The *asterisk* is on the descending left L5 nerve root. **C,** Axial slice at the lower border of the L5 pedicle. The *asterisk* is on the left L5 nerve root, just entering the top of the L5-S1 neural foramen. The *arrowhead* denotes the S1 nerve root on the left side. **D,** L5-S1 disk level. *S* is on the dural sac. The *asterisk* is on the left descending S1 nerve root. **E,** 8 mm below the L5-S1 disk. The *large asterisk* is on the dural sac. The *arrowhead* is pointing to the S2 nerve root. The small asterisk is on the S1 descending nerve root on the left.

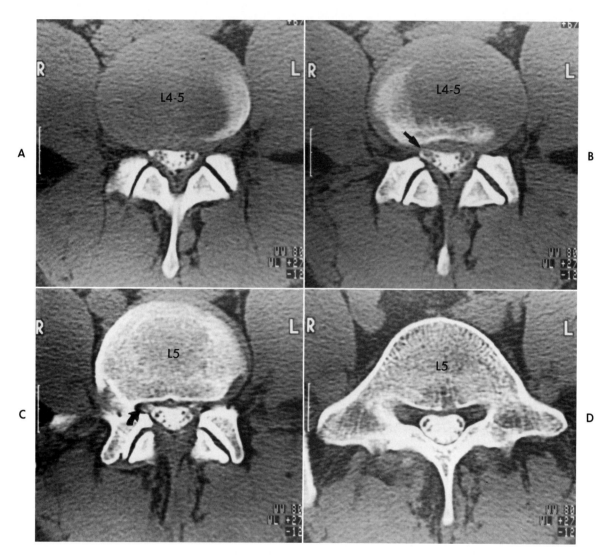

FIGURE 1-52
Normal L5 and S1 nerve roots and exiting spinal nerves. **A,** CT-myelogram, axial slice just below the inferior endplate of L4. There are descending roots in the dural sac anterolaterally. However, the L5 roots have not separated from the sac yet. **B,** Axial slice at the superior endplate of L5. The L5 descending roots are just budding. The *arrow* points to the right L5 root. **C,** 4 mm below **B.** The descending lumbar roots are now completely separated from the dural sac and are within the sleeves. The *arrow* points to the right L5 root. **D,** This slice is distal to the end of the L5 dural sleeve. The descending L5 roots are visible in the lateral recess of L5. The descending sacral roots are close to the anterolateral corners of the dural sac.

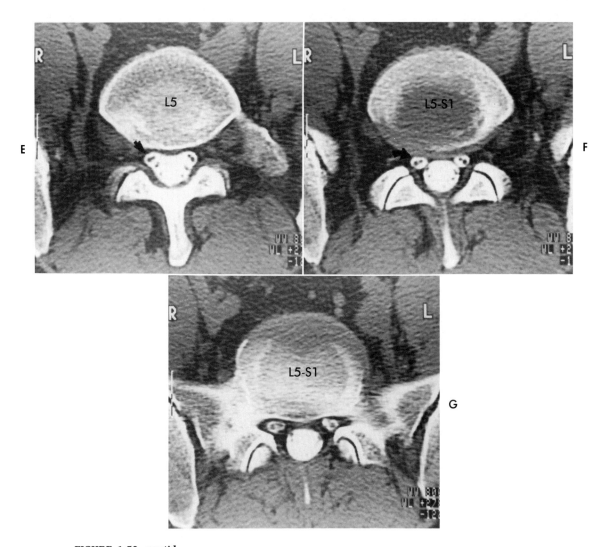

FIGURE 1-52, cont'd
E, 8 mm below **D.** The descending sacral roots have started to bud. The *arrow* points to the right S$_1$ root.
F, 4 mm below **E.** The sacral roots are now in the anterior epidural space posterior to the L5-S1 disk.
G, 8 mm below **F.** The descending sacral roots can be seen in the lateral recess of S1.

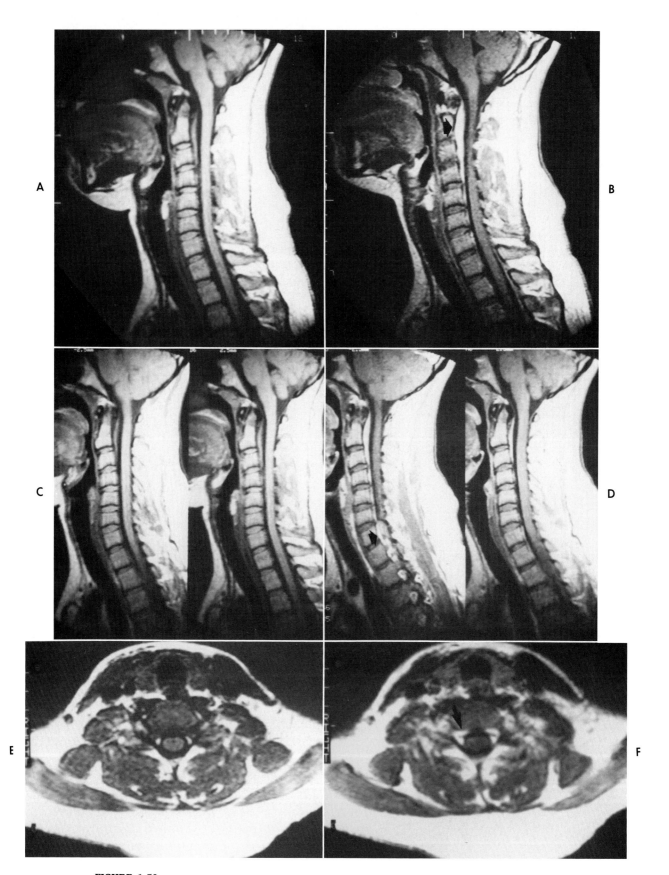

FIGURE 1-53

Normal epidural veins. **A,** Midsagittal T1-weighted MRI of the cervical spine. There is an area of moderately increased signal in the epidural space directly posterior to C2 and C3. **B,** After intravenous gadopentetate note the enhancement of the epidural veins in this region *(arrow).* **C,** Sagittal and parasagittal T1-weighted cross sections prior to the injection of gadopentetate and, **D,** after intravenous gadopentetate. The *arrow* denotes enhancement of the left epidural veins. Similar enhancement to the right was also noted. **E,** Axial slice at C6-7 prior to and, **F,** after the intravenous gadopentetate. The *arrow* in **F** denotes epidural vein enhancement.

posterior aspect of the spinal canal there is also a venous plexus in the epidural space that communicates with an external venous plexus surrounding the neural arch and the spinous processes. In the lower part of the cervical spine most of the anterior epidural venous plexus drains into the vertebral veins on each side[19,22,41,74-82] (Fig. 1-53).

A working knowledge of epidural venous anatomy is important for identifying these structures and differentiating them from other tissues in the epidural space. In the cervical region the epidural venous plexus becomes evident on parasagittal MR images as longitudinal bands of increased signal and on axial images as areas of increased signal anterolaterally corresponding to the position of the anterior longitudinal epidural vein and communicating transforaminal horizontal venous branches.

The anatomy of the epidural venous plexus is less well defined in the thoracic and lumbar spine. Nevertheless,

vertically coursing venous channels similar to the cervical spine are usually present on each side of midline. Extensive communicating channels between these vertically coursing venous channels and the basivertebral veins are also present. There is also communication via horizontally coursing veins that pass through the neural foramina to communicate with the perivertebral venous plexus (Figs. 1-11, 1-16, 1-23, and 1-54 to 1-56).

The epidural venous plexus and the perivertebral venous plexus are valveless systems and part of an important network of venous drainage that communicates with the valveless superficial veins of the extremities, abdominal wall, thoracic wall, and head and neck. The functional anatomy of this system and its importance in the spread of pelvic metastases, embolization, and formation of satellite brain abscesses in patients with a lung abscess were elucidated originally by Oscar Batson.[80-82] The epidural venous plexus is part of a valveless venous system that functions as a shunting channel (only

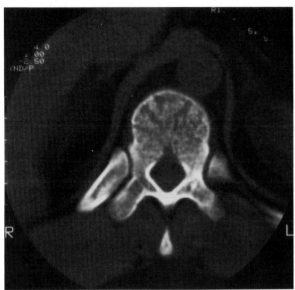

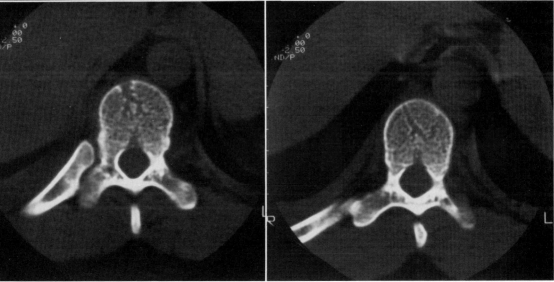

FIGURE 1-54
Normal basivertebral vein of the thoracic spine.

FIGURE 1-55
Normal basivertebral vein of T3.

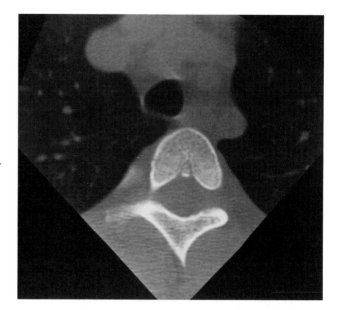

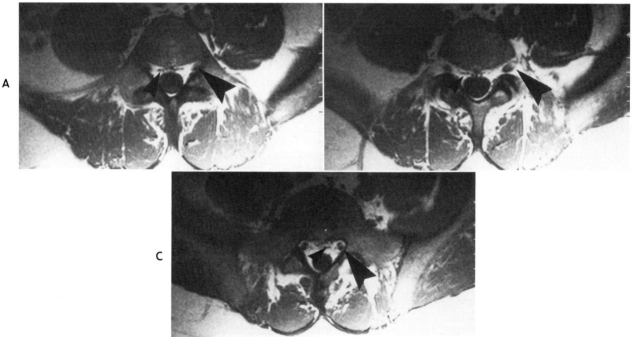

FIGURE 1-56
Normal lumbar spine, axial cross sections at L5-S1, T1-weighted. **A**, Slice through the pedicle of L5. The *arrowhead* on the left is pointing to the left L5 descending nerve root in the lateral recess of L5 just above the neural foramen between L5 and S1. The *arrowhead* on the right is pointing to the epidural venous plexus, which appears as a linear area of low signal in the anterior epidural space between the dural sac and the posterior border of the vertebral body. **B**, Axial slice through the top of the neural foramen between L5 and S1. The *arrowhead* on the left is pointing to the L5 dorsal root ganglion. The *small arrowhead* on the right is pointing to the epidural venous plexus. **C**, S1 level. The *arrowhead* on the left is pointing to the left S1 descending nerve root. The *small arrowhead* on the right is pointing to the epidural venous plexus in the anterior epidural fat between the dural sac and the posterior border of S1.

when needed), a reservoir, and a pressure regulator. Consequently, blood flow in the epidural venous plexus is not unidirectional. Although the general direction of flow is toward the heart, the system can and does have bidirectional flow. In the cervical spine the epidural venous plexus usually flows caudally, showing a close relation to the CSF circulation.

Because the velocity and direction of flow in the epidural venous plexus are variable, sometimes a definitive identification of these venous structures becomes difficult. When gadopentetate (gadolinium [Gd-DTPA]) enhancement is utilized, the epidural venous plexus is clearly identified on sagittal and axial cross sections as areas of increased signal intensity corresponding to the expected anatomical position of the structures. Intravenous injection of iodinated contrast also leads to enhancement of the epidural venous plexus, as demonstrated by Russell et al.[74] on CT examination of the cervical spine. In the thoracic and lumbar spine, occasionally enhancement of the basivertebral vein is obtained by intravenous contrast injection. The veins immediately continuous with the basivertebral vein may appear as a plaque 1 to 2 mm thick and 8 to 10 mm wide on the posterior surfaces of the lumbar vertebrae just above and below the orifices of the basivertebral veins. At the level of the intervertebral disk, however, the epidural veins consist of vertically directed channels situated at least halfway lateral to the midline and usually well identified in the epidural fat at L4-5 and L5-S1.

CONGENITAL ANOMALIES OF ROOT SLEEVES
Conjoined roots (composite nerve root sleeve)

Abnormalities of the spinal nerve roots are said to occur throughout the spine. Usually they do not give rise to clinical complaints or neurological abnormalities, in most instances consisting of a root sleeve with two roots instead of one. So far, the majority of reported cases have been unilateral. The most commonly affected levels, in descending order of frequency, are L4-5, L5-S1, and L3-4.[83-84] In our experience the abnormality has occurred in about 1.6% of all patients undergoing CT examination for low back pain syndrome. Ethelberg and Riishede[83] reported four cases in 1162 patients admitted for lumbar laminectomy (0.3%).

We have noted that the composite sleeve originates from the dural sac at a point halfway between the expected positions of the two sleeves it replaces. It is 1.5 to 2 times bigger than a normal sleeve. The two nerve roots within it *(double root sign)* often leave the spinal canal through individual neural foramina, each traveling in its own sleeve caudally within the canal just lateral to the dural sac and exiting through its own neural foramen. Less commonly the two roots leave the canal through a single neural foramen, usually that of the lower root. On axial images one frequently notes an asymmetrical origin of the root sleeves, a large descending sleeve, and a large ganglion and nerve in the neural foramen (Figs. 1-57 to 1-61).

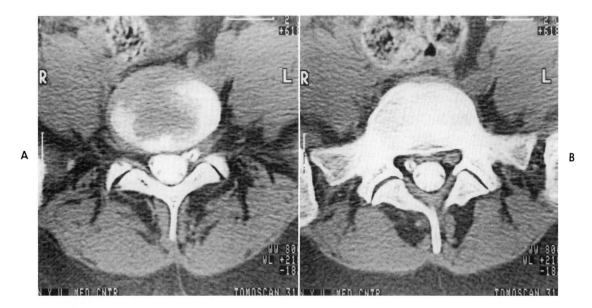

FIGURE 1-57
Asymmetrical lumbar nerve roots and conjoined root sleeves. **A**, CT-myelogram at L5-S1. The right S1 nerve root has not yet separated from the dural sac. The left S1 and S2 sleeves are visible. **B**, 10 mm below **A**. The right S1 root sleeve is now visible. The left S1 and S2 sleeves do not contain contrast, because they have already terminated. *Continued.*

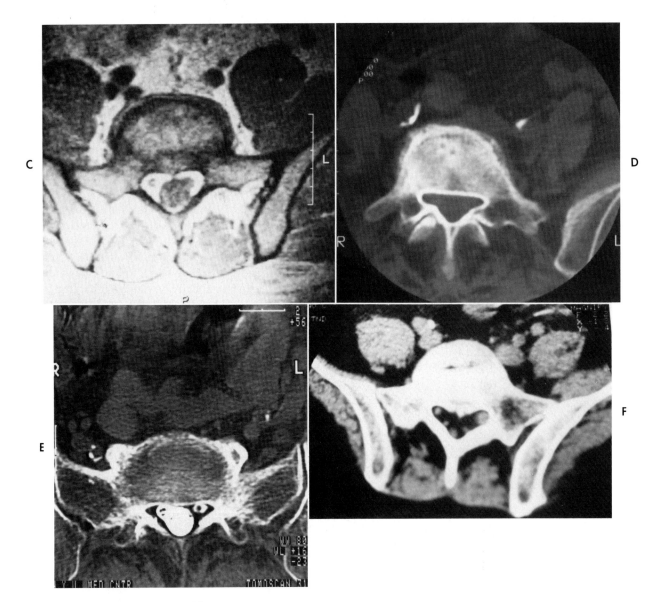

FIGURE 1-57, cont'd
C, Spin density MRI at L5-S1 in another patient showing asymmetry of the S1 root sleeve origins. In a conjoined root sleeve, at least for part of its course, the nerve roots of two levels (e.g., L5 and S1) are approximated. Asymmetry of the origins without actually a conjoined sleeve is a common anatomical variant. In this situation there is some asymmetry of the root sleeve origins, but careful inspection shows only one root inside the sleeve. Root sleeves belonging to the levels above and below are present, although slightly asymmetrical in their origin. Each also contains only its respective nerve root. **D,** Conjoined L5 and S1 root sleeves on the right side in another patient. Note the enlarged lateral recess. **E,** CT-myelogram, S1 level. Conjoined S1 and S2 root sleeves are seen on the right side. **F,** Conjoined S1 and S2 roots on the left in another patient. Note the enlargement of the left lateral S1 recess.

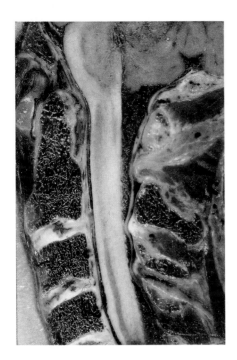

PLATE 1-1
Midsagittal microsection through C1, C2, C3, and C4 showing the relationship of the spinal cord to the odontoid process, bodies of C2 to C4, and posterior wall of the canal. The term microsection has been used throughout this book for anatomy plates prepared by Wolfgang Rauschning (using a technique described elsewhere). Although sectioning of the tissues was performed, usually with a thickness of 1 μm, these plates are photographs of the surface anatomy and are not sections in the true sense of the word.

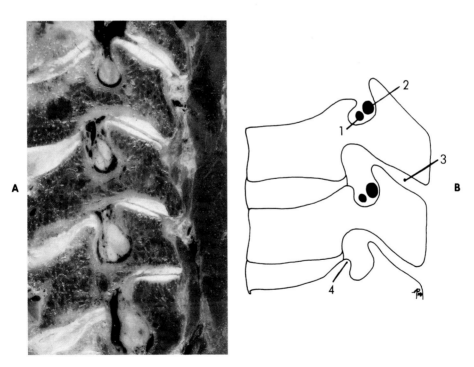

PLATE 1-2
Normal cervical spine. **A,** Oblique cryomicrosection showing the neural foramina and neural elements. **B,** Schematic of a cervical neural foramen. *1,* Ventral root; *2,* dorsal root; *3,* facet joint; *4,* uncinate (Luschka) process.

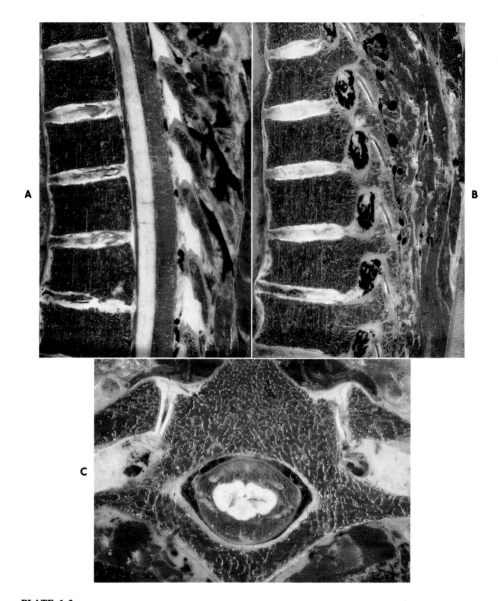

PLATE 1-3
Normal thoracic spine. **A,** Midsagittal microsection showing the overall relationship of the thoracic spinal cord to the thoracic spine and canal. **B,** Parasagittal microsection showing the anatomy of the thoracic neural foramina and facet joints to best advantage. **C,** An axial microsection through a typical thoracic vertebra reveals the overall relationship of the cord to the thoracic vertebral bodies and spinal canal. Note the costocentral articulations.

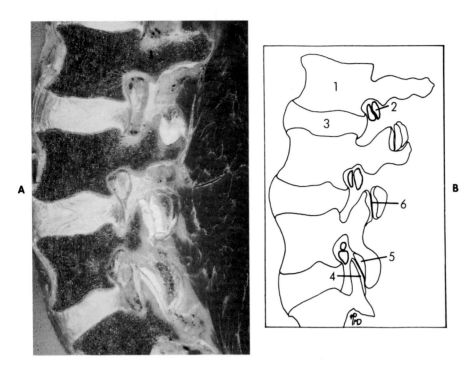

PLATE 1-4
Anatomy of a normal lumbar neural foramen. A is a parasagittal microsection through L2, L3, L4, and L5 and, **B,** a schematic. *1,* L2; *2,* dorsal root ganglion of L2 in the L2-L3 neural foramen; *3,* L2-3 disk; *4,* superior articular facet of L5; *5,* inferior articular facet of L4; *6,* L3-L4 facet joint.

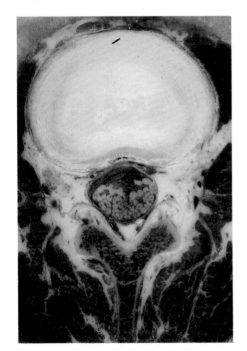

PLATE 1-5
An axial microsection through the L3-4 intervertebral disk shows the normal configuration of the disk, dural sac, neural foramina, descending lumbar and sacral nerve roots, and spinal canal.

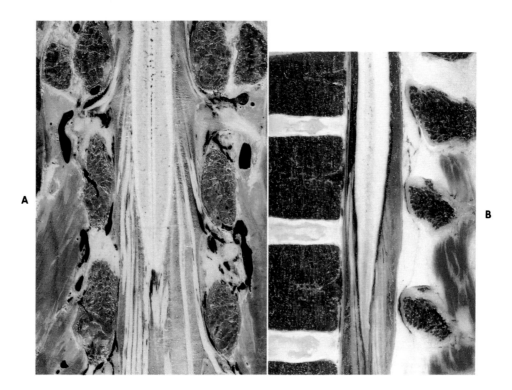

PLATE 1-6
Normal conus medullaris. A, Coronal and, B, sagittal microsections of the spine.

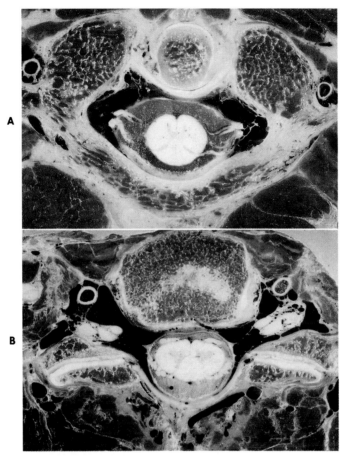

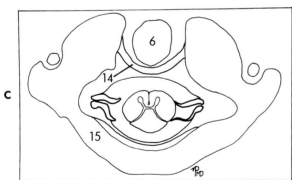

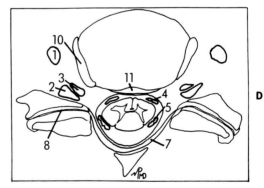

PLATE 1-7

Normal cervical spine, transaxial microsection. **A**, C2 and, **B**, just above the inferior endplate of C4 (at the C4-5 intervertebral disk). **C** and **D** are schematics of **A** and **B**. *1,* Vertebral artery; *2,* dorsal root ganglion; *3* and *4,* ventral roots; *5,* dorsal root; *6,* odontoid process; *7,* ligamentum flavum; *8,* facet joint; *9,* neural foramen; *10,* Luschka process; *11,* posterior longitudinal ligament; *12,* superior articulating process; *13,* inferior articulating process; *14,* transverse ligament; *15,* lamina.

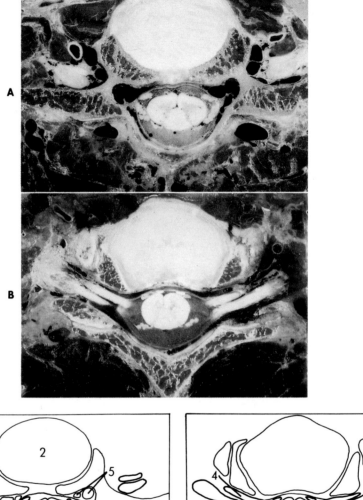

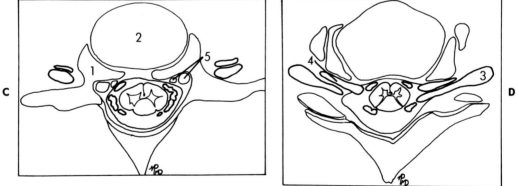

PLATE 1-8
Normal cervical spine. Microsections through the intervertebral disks. **A,** C5-6 and, **B,** C6-7. **C** and **D,** Schematics of **A** and **B.** *1,* Luschka process; *2,* intervertebral disks; *3,* dorsal root; *4,* ventral root; *5,* epidural venous plexus.

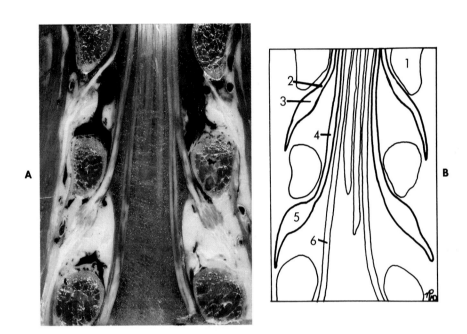

PLATE 1-9

A, Coronal microsection of the lumbar dural sac at L3, L4, and L5; **B,** schematic. The descending right l3 nerve root is directly medial to the L3 pedicle, joining its dorsal root ganglion at the top of the L3-L4 neural foramen. The descending L4 roots and their dorsal ganglia are visible on both sides. The descending L5 roots are also visible. *1,* Left pedicle of L3; *2,* right L3 descending root; *3,* L3 dorsal root ganglion; *4,* right descending L4 root; *5,* L4 dorsal root ganglion; *6,* right descending L5 root.

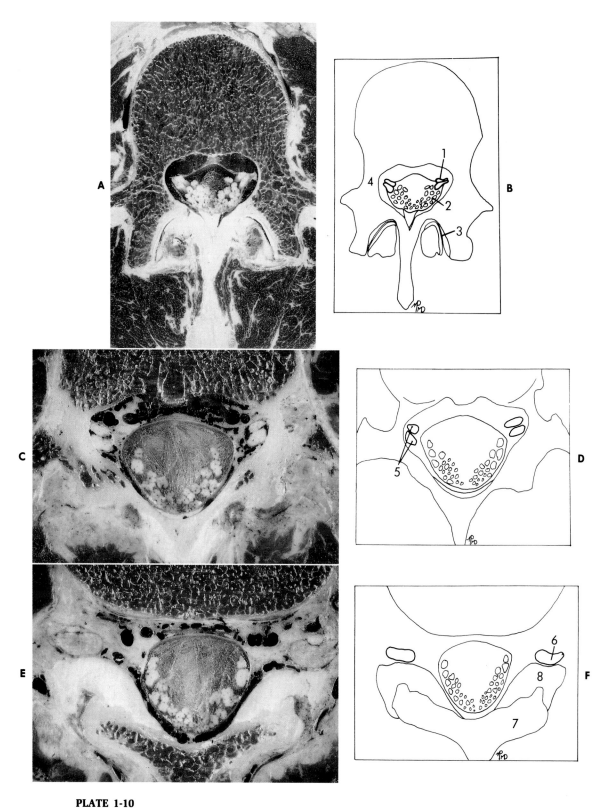

PLATE 1-10

Anatomy of the normal lumbar nerve roots. **A,** Transaxial microsection and, **B,** schematic. *1,* Left descending lumbar root starting to enter its dural sleeve; *2,* descending lumbar and sacral roots in the dural sac; *3,* facet joint; *4,* pedicle. **C** and **E,** microsections and, **D** and **F,** schematics. *5,* Descending lumbar roots now completely separated from the dural sac and running in the lateral recess on the medial side of the pedicle; *6,* dorsal root ganglion; *7,* lamina; *8,* ligamentum flavum joining the capsule of the facet joint.

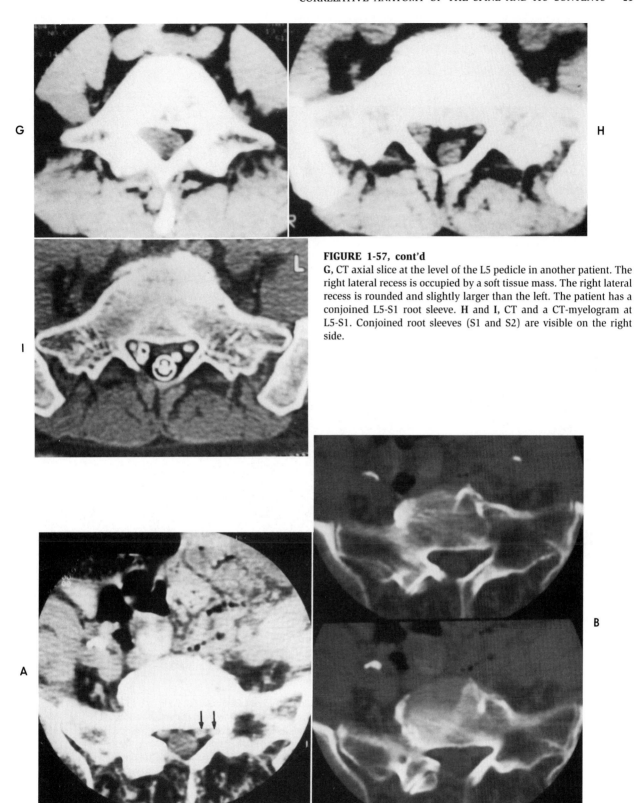

FIGURE 1-57, cont'd
G, CT axial slice at the level of the L5 pedicle in another patient. The right lateral recess is occupied by a soft tissue mass. The right lateral recess is rounded and slightly larger than the left. The patient has a conjoined L5-S1 root sleeve. **H** and **I,** CT and a CT-myelogram at L5-S1. Conjoined root sleeves (S1 and S2) are visible on the right side.

FIGURE 1-58
Conjoined roots. **A,** Soft tissue and, **B,** bone window axial images through L5-S1. Note the two roots *(arrows)* on the left of the dural sac. There is only one on the right. The lumbar and first two sacral root sleeves may arise from the dural sac asymmetrically. This is more common in the lower two lumbar and first sacral roots. One root may start to separate from the dural sac while the one on the other side remains within the sac several millimeters more distally. Asymmetrical roots are sometimes associated with no other abnormality; just the sleeves may be conjoined. In this patient, who had left sided sciatic syndrome, a conjoined sleeve was identified at surgery at about the level of the pedicle of L5.

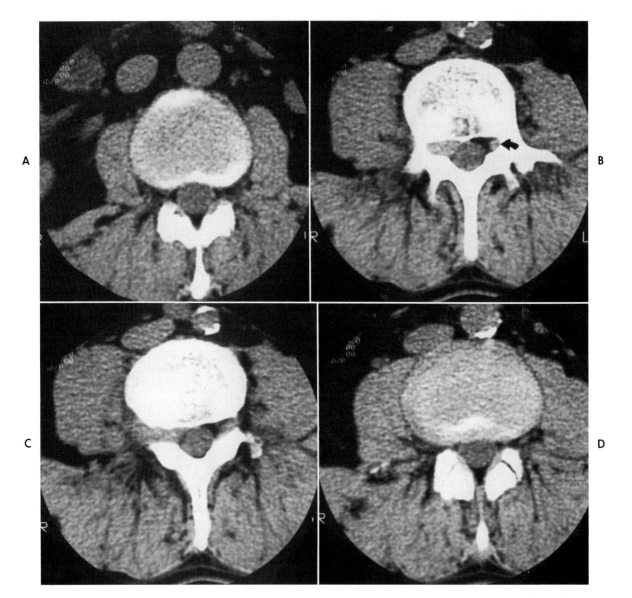

FIGURE 1-59

Conjoined root sleeves (L2 and L3) on the right side. **A,** Normal L2-3 disk. **B,** Axial CT slice through the pedicle of L3. The *arrow* points to the descending left L3 root. The right L3 root is obscured by a soft tissue mass. Note the enlargement of the right lateral recess. **C,** Axial CT slice at the top of the L2-L3 neural foramen. The L3 dorsal root ganglion is visualized on the left side. The right ganglion is obscured by a soft tissue mass in the neural foramen. **D,** Normal L3-4 disk. The differential diagnosis in this patient includes a conjoined root sleeve, an epidural mass (e.g., neurofibroma or metastasis), a migrated fragment of herniated disk, and a root cyst. The enlargement of the lateral recess favors root cyst or conjoined root sleeve, since it is not ordinarily seen in patients with metastases or migrated fragments of herniated disks. In this patient conjoined root sleeves were found at surgery. Myelography and MRI can help to differentiate conjoined sleeves from root cysts by demonstrating fluid within the cyst.

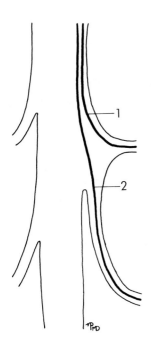

FIGURE 1-60
Schematic of conjoined root sleeves showing, *1*, the L4 and, *2*, the L5 descending nerve roots. In this arrangement, which is the most frequently encountered variation, the root sleeves have a common origin but each root still exits the spinal canal through its own neural foramen.

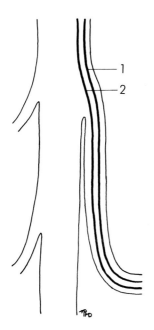

FIGURE 1-61
Another schematic of conjoined root sleeves. *1*, L4 and, *2*, L5 descending nerve roots are shown. This variation is less common. Note that both roots exit the spinal canal through a single neural foramen.

As stated previously, this anomaly is most often asymptomatic. Occasionally there will be clinical findings that suggest sciatica. CT and MRI generally reveal what appears to be a "large" descending root, root sleeve, or dorsal root ganglion. There may be two roots going through a single neural foramen (prior to formation of the ganglion) or lying lateral to the dural sac in the spinal canal; or there may be slight enlargement of the lateral recess in association with the composite sleeve in the spinal canal.[85] An extruded fragment of herniated disk, trapped at the level of the pedicle in the canal, may mimic a conjoined nerve sleeve. However, enlargement of the lateral recess is not usually seen with an entrapped migrated disk fragment.

Occasionally it will be necessary to differentiate a swollen ganglion, root cyst, foraminal disk herniation, neurofibroma, or (rarely) focal nodule of epidural metastasis, either inside the canal or in the neural foramen. The definitive diagnosis depends on other findings and the signal characteristics of these lesions on MRI. For example, a root cyst containing CSF is usually easily identified on MRI. If doubt remains after review of CT and MRI in these patients, myelography may be indicated.[86,87]

Because of the recurrent or intractable nature of the clinical findings, surgical exploration occasionally becomes necessary. The preoperative diagnosis is usually herniated disk. In some patients laminectomy will be followed by almost complete remission of symptoms, possibly due to the decompression of the spinal canal. It is assumed that spinal stenosis effectively exists in these subjects because of (the large size of) the composite sleeve running lateral to the dural sac in the spinal canal or in the neural foramen. (A composite nerve would be less mobile and probably also more likely to become "entrapped and compressed.")

Root sleeve cysts (Tarlov cysts, perineurial cysts)

Root sleeve cysts are anatomical variants that may be seen at all levels. They are generally 15 to 20 mm in width and length but occasionally will grow to quite large size and cause compression of the neural structures. Large perineurial cysts usually involve the first and second sacral roots. Pressure defects (erosions) of the vertebrae may accompany them. Patients who have large lumbar root cysts usually have sacral root cysts as well.

The diagnosis of root sleeve cysts is usually easily established by MRI; myelography also demonstrates them. The cysts are generally well-circumscribed structures situated anterolaterally that arise from the dural sleeve, are filled with CSF, and communicate with the subarachnoid space (Figs. 1-62 to 1-65).

According to Truwit and Harle,[88] perineurial cysts of the spinal nerve roots were first described by Tarlov in 1938.[89] He reported their extradural perineurial location and suggested an inflammatory etiology. Although they

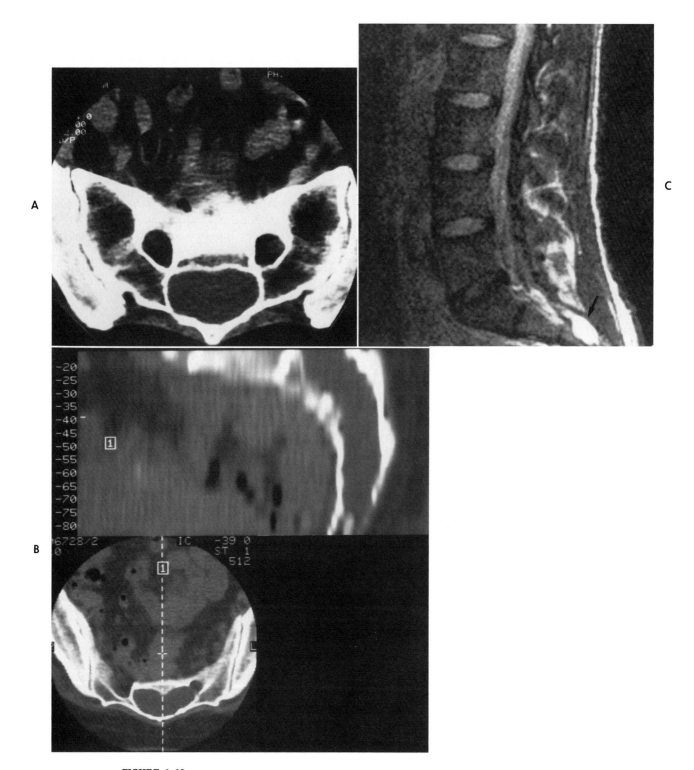

FIGURE 1-62
Sacral root cyst. **A,** Axial CT, soft tissue window setting. There is enlargement of the sacral canal. Note the sclerotic margin of the canal. **B,** Midsagittal reformatted image through the enlarged sacral canal showing the extent of enlargement due to a large sacral root cyst. **C,** Sagittal T2-weighted MRI in another patient. Note the root cyst in the sacral canal *(arrow)*.

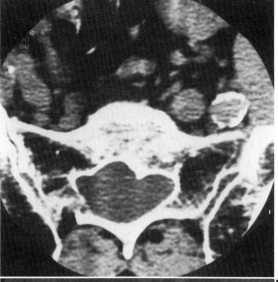

A

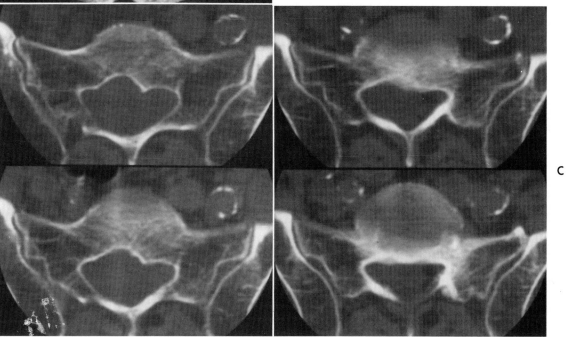

B

C

FIGURE 1-63
Sacral root cysts. **A,** Soft tissue and, **B** and **C,** bone window CT images of the sacrum showing enlargement, deformity, and pressure erosion of the sacral spinal canal due to large root cysts on the right side.

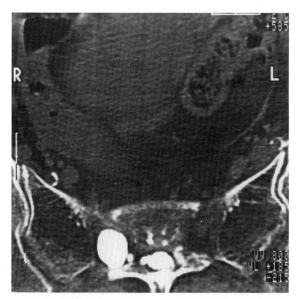

FIGURE 1-64
Sacral root cyst. A CT-myelogram shows the cyst on the right side.

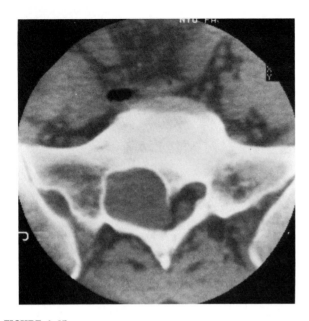

FIGURE 1-65
Neurofibroma, surgically documented. Note the marked erosion of the sacral canal on the right. In some patients erosions produced by neurofibroma can mimic abnormalities produced by large root cysts. Myelography and MRI will help make the diagnosis by demonstrating a fluid-filled sac instead of a solid mass.

are generally asymptomatic, some authors (including Tarlov) have described a variety of clinical findings in patients who have them.[89-91] Schreiber and Haddad[91] reported three patients with symptoms attributable to perineurial cysts and proposed a traumatic etiology. Truwit and Harle[88] had a patient with a large, yet asymptomatic, Tarlov cyst.

The myelographic findings with perineurial cysts have been detailed by numerous investigators — including Schreiber and Haddad,[91] Seaman and Furlow,[92] Smith,[93] and Taheri et al.[94] Initially myelography was thought to offer little since it was felt that the cysts did not communicate intrathecally, in which case myelography would reveal only the extradural defects. However, Siqueira et al.[95] described the CT findings of posterior sacral erosions and enlargement of the sacral canal and reported that water-soluble contrast was seen to layer within the dependent portion of the cysts.

The differential diagnosis of perineurial cysts includes meningocele and arachnoid cysts.[88] A concise but complete discussion of this differential diagnosis has been provided by Truwit and Harle,[88] who state that meningoceles rarely extend anteriorly and those that do are almost always solitary. In addition, at the thoracic level anterior meningoceles are part of the spectrum of neuroenteric cysts, with associated vertebral anomalies the rule, and at the sacral level they usually occur with large sacral defects. Extradural arachnoid cysts can have a radiographic presentation essentially indistinguishable from that of Tarlov cysts. Several points, however, may help to differentiate the two: 85% of arachnoid cysts are typically

posterior or posterolateral to the thecal sac, although some (15%) may lie lateral to the sac; only rarely do extradural arachnoid cysts lie anterior to the canal, and most often these are cervical in location; extradural arachnoid cysts also typically obliterate the epidural fat on CT,[96] may be multiple, and usually communicate with the subarachnoid space (therefore opacifying with intrathecal contrast).

REFERENCES

1. Trubowitz S, Davis S: The bone marrow matrix. In Trubowitz S, Davis S (eds): The human bone marrow: anatomy, physiology, and pathophysiology. Vol 1. Boca Raton Fla, CRC, 1982, pp 43-76.
2. Meunier P, Aaron J, Edouard C, Vignon G: Osteoporosis and the replacement of cell populations of the marrow by adipose tissue. Clin Orthop 1971;80:147-154.
3. Kricun ME: Red-yellow conversion: its effect on the location of some solitary bone lesions. Skeletal Radiol 1985;14:10-19.
4. McKinstry SC, Steiner RE, Young AT, et al: Bone marrow in leukemia and aplastic anemia: MR imaging before, during, and after treatment. Radiology 1987;162:701-707.
5. Hajek PC, Baker LL, Goobar JE, et al: Focal fat deposition in axial bone marrow: MR characteristics. Radiology 1987;162:245-249.
6. Tanaka Y: A radiographic analysis on human vertebrae in the aged. Virchows Arch [Pathol Anat] 1975;366(3):187-201.
7. Atkinson PJ: Variation in trabecular structure of vertebrae with age. Calcif Tiss Res 1967;1:24-32.
8. Dyson ED, Jackson CK, Whitehouse WJ: Scanning electron microscope studies of human trabecular bone. Nature 1970;225:957-959.
9. Whitehouse WJ, Dyson ED, Jackson CK: The scanning electron microscope in studies of trabecular bone from a human vertebral body. J Anat 1971;108:481-496.
10. Smoker WRK, Godersky JC, Knutzon RK, et al: The role of MR imaging in evaluating metastatic spinal disease. AJNR 1987;8:901-908.
11. Moore SG, Gooding CA, Brasch RC, et al: Bone marrow in children with acute lymphocytic leukemia: MR relaxation times. Radiology 1986;160:237-240.
12. Modic MT, Feiglin DH, Piraino DW, et al: Vertebral osteomyelitis: assessment using MR. Radiology 1985;157:157-166.
13. Hadley LA: Anatomico-roentgenographic studies of the spine. Springfield Ill, Thomas, 1964.
14. Frykholm, R: Lower cervical vertebrae and intervertebral discs: surgical anatomy and pathology. Acta Chir Scand 1951;101:345.
15. Compere EL, Tachdjian MO, Kernahan WT: The Luschka joints: their anatomy, physiology, and pathology. Orthopedics 1959;1:159.
16. Hall MC: Luschka's joints. Springfield Ill, Thomas, 1965.
17. Pech P, Daniels DL, Williams AL, Haughton VM: The cervical neural foramina: correlation of microtomy and CT anatomy. Radiology 1985;155(1):143-146.
18. Modic MT, Masaryk TJ, Ross JS, et al: Cervical radiculopathy: value of oblique MR imaging. Radiology 1987;163:227-231.
19. Daniels DL, Hyde JS, Kneelon KN, et al: The cervical nerves and foramina: local coil MR imaging. AJNR 1986;7:129-133.
20. Daniels DL, Grogan JP, Johansen JG, et al: Cervical radiculopathy: computed tomography and myelography compared. Radiology 1984;151:109-113.
21. McMasters DL, deGroot J, Haughton VM, et al: Normal cervical spine. In Newton TH, Potts DG (eds): Computed tomography of the spine and spinal cord. San Anselmo Calif, Clavadel Press, 1983, pp 53-78.
22. Flannigan BD, Lufkin RB, McGlade C, et al: MR imaging of the cervical spine: neural vascular anatomy. AJNR 1987;8:27-32.

23. Yu S, Sether L, Haughton VM: Facet joint menisci of the cervical spine: correlative MR imaging and cryomicrotomy study. Radiology 1987;164:79-82.

24. Czezvionke LF, Daniels DL, Peter SPH, et al: Cervical neural foramina: correlative anatomic and MR imaging study. Radiology 1988;169:753-759.

25. Yenerich DO, Haughton VM: Oblique plane MR imaging of the cervical spine. J Comput Assist Tomogr 1986;10:823-826.

26. McMasters DL, DeGroot J, Haughton VM, et al: Normal thoracic spine. In Newton TH, Potts DG (eds): Computed tomography of the spine and spinal cord. San Anselmo Calif, Clavadel Press, 1983, pp 79-92.

27. Modic MT, Massaryk TJ, Ross JS: Magnetic resonance imaging of the spine, Year Book, Chicago, 1989, pp 56-61.

28. Schmorl G, Junghanns H: The human spine in health and disease. Translated and edited by E.F. Besemann. New York, Grune & Stratton, 2nd Am ed, 1971.

29. Gardner E, Gray DJ, O'Rahilly R: Anatomy. Philadelphia, Saunders, 4th ed, 1975.

30. Latchaw R, Taylor S: CT of the normal and abnormal spine. In Latchaw R (ed): Computed tomography of the head, neck, and spine. Chicago, Year Book, 1985, pp 595-618.

31. Dorwart RH, Sauerland EK, Haughton VM, et al: Normal lumbar spine. In Newton TH, Potts DG (eds): Computed tomography of the spine and spinal cord. San Anselmo Calif, Clavadel Press, 1983, pp 93-114.

32. Firooznia H, Tyler I, Golimbu C, Rafii M: CT of the Cupid's bow contour of the lumbar spine, Comput Radiol 1983;7(6):347-350.

33. Dietz GW, Christensen EE: Normal ''Cupid's bow'' contour of the lower lumbar vertebrae. Radiology 1976;121:577-579.

34. Hamilton WJ, Mossman HW: Human embryology. 4th ed, Baltimore, Williams & Wilkins, 1972, p 530.

35. Coventry MB, Ghormley RK, Kernoman JW: The intervertebral disc: its microscopic anatomy and pathology. I. Anatomy, development, and physiology. J Bone Joint Surg (Am) 1945;27(1):105-113.

36. Firooznia H, Pinto RS: Chordoma. In Ranniger K (ed): Bone tumors. 1st ed, New York, Springer-Verlag, 1977, pp 355-416.

37. de Lorimier AA, Moehring HG, Hannan JR: Clinical roentgenology. Springfield Ill, Thomas, Vol 2, 1954, p 363.

38. Resnick D: Degenerative diseases of the vertebral column. Radiology 1985;156:3-14.

39. Firooznia H, Benjamin MV, Pinto RS, et al: Calcification and ossification of the posterior longitudinal ligament of the spine: its role in secondary narrowing of the spinal canal and cord compression. NY State J Med 1982;82(8):1193-1198.

40. Firooznia H, Rafii M, Golimbu C, et al: Computed tomography of calcification and ossification of the posterior longitudinal ligament of the spine. J Comput Tomogr 1984;8:317-324.

41. Rauschning W: Detailed sectional anatomy of the spine. In Rothman SLG, Glenn WV (eds): Multiplanar CT of the spine. Baltimore, University Park Press, 1985, pp 33-85.

42. Rauschning W: Correlative multiplanar computed tomographic anatomy of the normal spine. In Post MJD (ed): Computed tomography of the spine. Baltimore, Williams & Wilkins, 1983, pp 1-57.

43. Glenn WV Jr, Burnett K, Rauschning W: Magnetic resonance imaging of the lumbar spine: nerve root canals, disc abnormalities, anatomic correlations, and case examples. Milwaukee, General Electric, 1986, pp 1-24.

44. Rauschning W: Surface cryoplaning: a technique for clinical anatomical correlations. Upsala J Med Sci 1986;91:251-255.

45. Monajati A, Wayne RS, Rauschning W, Ekholm SE: The cauda equina: MR imaging considerations. AJNR 1987;8:27-32.

46. Rauschning W: Anatomia del canale spinale e delle strutture nervose lombari. In Postacchini F (ed): Stenosi colonna lombari. New York, Springer Verlag, 1988, pp 21-48.

47. Rauschning W: Detailed anatomy of the lumbar spine. In Cauthen JC (ed): Lumbar spine surgery: indications, techniques,

failures, and alternatives. 2nd ed, Baltimore, Williams & Wilkins, 1988, pp 5-16.

48. Rauschning W: Normal anatomy of the vertebral canal and the lumbar neural structures. In Postacchini F (ed): Lumbar spinal stenosis. New York, Springer Verlag, 1989, pp 21-48.

49. Coventry MB, Ghormley RK, Kernohan JW: The intervertebral disc: its microscopic anatomy and pathology. II. Changes in the intervertebral disk concomitant with age. J Bone Joint Surg(Am) 1945;27:233-247.

50. Coventry MB, Ghormley RK, Kernohan JW: The intervertebral disc: Its microscopic anatomy and pathology. III. Pathological changes in the intervertebral disc. J Bone Joint Surg (Am) 1945;27:406-474.

51. Coventry MB: Anatomy of the intervertebral disk. Clin Orthop Rel Res 1969;67:9-15.

52. Modic MT: Ref 27, pp 49-52.

53. Pech P, Haughton VM: Lumbar intervertebral disk: correlative MR and anatomic study. Radiology 1985;156:699-701.

54. Hassler O: The human intervertebral disc: a micro-angiographical study on its vascular supply at various ages. Acta Orthop Scand 1970;40:765-772.

55. Firooznia H, Kricheff II, Rafii M, Golimbu C: Lumbar spine after surgery: examination with intravenous contrast enhanced CT. Radiology 1987;163:221-226.

56. Ho PSP, Yu S, Sether LA, et al: Progressive and regressive changes in the nucleus pulposus. I. The neonate. Radiology 1988;169:87-91.

57. Yu S, Haughton VM, Ho PSP, et al: Progressive and regressive changes in the nucleus pulposus. II. The adult. Radiology 1988;169:93-97.

58. Kieffer SA, Stadlan EM, Mohandas A, Peterson HO: Discographic-anatomical correlation of developmental changes with age in the intervertebral disc. Acta Radiol [Diagn] 1969;9:733-739.

59. Adams MA, Dolan P, Hutton WC: The stages of disc degeneration as revealed by discograms. J Bone Joint Surg (Br) 1986;68:36-41.

60. Haughton VM: MR imaging of the spine. Radiology 1988;166:297-301.

61. Aguila LA, Piraino DW, Modic MT, et al: The intranuclear cleft of the intervertebral disk: magnetic resonance imaging. Radiology 1985;155:155-158.

62. Modic MT, Masaryk TJ, Ross JS, et al: Imaging of degenerative disk disease. Radiology 1988;168:177-186.

63. Berger RK, Czervionke LF, Kass EG, et al: Truncation artifact in MR images of the intervertebral disk. AJNR 1988;9:825-828.

64. Bronskill MJ, McVeigh ER, Kucharczyk W, Henkelman RM: Syrinx-like artifacts on MR images of the spinal cord. Radiology 1988;166:485-488.

65. Levy LM, Di Chiro G, Brooks RA, et al: Spinal cord artifacts from truncation errors during MR imaging. Radiology 1988;166:479-483.

66. Curtin AJ, Chakeres DW, Bulas R, et al: MR imaging artifacts of the axial internal anatomy of the cervical spinal cord. AJR 1989;152:835-842.

67. Louis R: Topographic relationships of the vertebral column, spinal cord, and nerve roots. Anat Clin 1978;1:3-12.

68. Raghavan N, Barkovich AJ, Edwards M, Norman D: MR imaging in the tethered spinal cord syndrome. AJR 1989;152:843-852.

69. Seibert CE, Barnes JE, Dreisbach JN, et al: Accurate CT measurement of the spinal cord using metrizamide: physical factors. AJR 1981;136:777-780.

70. Resjo IM, Harwood-Nash DC, Fitz CR, Chuang S: Normal cord in infants and children examined with computed tomographic metrizamide myelography. Radiology 1979;130:691-696.

71. Wilson DA, Prince JR: MR imaging determination of the location of the normal conus medullaris throughout childhood. AJNR 1989;10:259-262. AJR 1989;152:1029-1032.

72. Harwood-Nash DC, Fitz CR: Myelography. In Harwood-Nash DC, Fitz CR: Neuroradiology in infants and children. St. Louis, Mosby, 1976, p 1133.

73. Kirks DR: Spine and contents. In Kirks DR: Practical pediatric imaging. Boston, Little Brown, 1984, p 134.

74. Russell EJ, D'Angelo CM, Zimmerman RD, et al: Cervical disk herniation: CT demonstration after contrast enhancement. Radiology 1984;152:703-712.

75. Nordenstrom B: A method of angiography of the azygos vein and the anterior internal plexus of the spine. Acta Radiol 1955;44:201-208.

76. Djindjian R, Pansini A, Dorland P: Phlébographie rachidienne par voie trans-épineuse. Acta Radiol [Diagn] 1963;1:689-701.

77. Braun JP, Tournade A: Le canal de conjugaison cervical (The transverse cervical canal). J Neuroradiol 1979;6:327-334.

78. Théron J, Djindjian R: Cervicovertebral phlebography using catheterization. Radiology 1973;108:325-331.

79. Théron J: Cervicovertebral phlebography: pathological results. Radiology 1976;118:73-81.

80. Batson OV: The vertebral vein system. Am J Roentgenol 1957;78:195-212.

81. Batson OV: Function of vertebral veins and their role in spread of metastases. Ann Surg 1940;112:138-149.

82. Batson OV: Vertebral vein system as mechanism for spread of metastases. Am J Roentgenol 1942;48:715-718.

83. Ethelberg S, Riishede J: Malformation of lumbar spinal roots and sheaths in causation of low backache and sciatica. J Bone Joint Surg 1952;34B:442-446.

84. Keon-Cohen B: Abnormal arrangement of the lower lumbar and first sacral nerves within the spinal canal. J Bone Joint Surg 1968;50B:261-266.

85. Hoddick WK, Helms CA: Bony spinal canal changes that differentiate conjoined nerve roots from herniated nucleus pulposus. Radiology 1985;154:119-120.

86. Helms CA, Dorwart RH, Gray M: The CT appearance of conjoined nerve roots and differentiation from a herniated nucleus pulposus. Radiology 1982;144:803-807.

87. Williams AL, Haughton VM, Daniels DL, Grogan JP: Differential CT diagnosis of extruded nucleus pulposus. Radiology 1983;148:141-148.

88. Truwit CL, Harle TS: Case report 524, Giant Tarlov (perineurial) cysts of lumbosacral spine. Skeletal Radiol 1989;18:75-77.

89. Tarlov IM: Perineurial cysts of the spinal nerve roots. Arch Neurol Psychiatry 1938;40:1067-1074.

90. Abbott KH, Retter RH, Leimbach WH: The role of perineurial sacral cysts in the sciatic and sacrococcygeal syndromes. A review of the literature and report of 9 cases. J Neurosurg 1957;14:5-21.

91. Schreiber F, Haddad B: Lumbar and sacral cysts causing pain. J Neurosurg 1951;8:504-509.

92. Seaman WB, Furlow LT: The myelographic appearance of sacral cysts. J Neurosurg 1956;13:88-94.

93. Smith DT: Multiple meningeal diverticula (perineurial cysts) of the cervical region disclosed by Pantopaque myelography. Report of a case. J Neurosurg 1962;19:599-601.

94. Taheri ZE, Riemenschneider PA, Ecker A: Myelographic diagnosis of sacral perineurial cyst. J Neurosurg 1952;9:93-95.

95. Siqueira EB, Schaffer L, Kranzler LI, Gan J: CT characteristics of sacral perineurial cysts. J Neurosurg 1984;61:596-598.

96. Naidich TP, McLone DG, Harwood-Nash DC: Arachnoid cysts, paravertebral meningoceles, and perineurial cysts. In Newton TH, Potts DG (eds): Modern neuroradiology. Vol 1. Computed tomography of the spine and spinal cord. San Anselmo Calif, Clavadel Press, 1983, pp 383-396.

2 Degenerative Disease of the Lumbar Spine

HOSSEIN FIROOZNIA

Degenerative disease of the spine refers to a constellation of interrelated disorders that may be asymptomatic or associated with myelopathy, neuropathy, and pain. The relationship between degenerative disease of the spine and these clinical manifestations is, at least in a sizable number of patients, only partly understood. Almost all imaging modalities available today provide a set of data that are mainly morphological in nature rather than functional or physiopathological. It is hoped that future improvements in MRI technology, along with other emerging diagnostic modalities, will provide more clinically pertinent information as to the physiopathological changes that occur in degenerative diseases of the spine. We wish to emphasize also that the identification of morphological changes in the vertebral column, intervertebral disks, nerve roots, spinal nerves, and spinal cord (e.g., osteosclerosis, osteophytes, facet joint arthrosis, spinal stenosis, bulging or herniation of the disks, even displacement of the nerve roots or spinal nerves with deformity) do not in themselves constitute proof that the patient's symptoms are due to these disorders. Intuitively, in many instances, particularly when the manifestations fit the nature and location of the abnormalities, we can be fairly certain of a cause-and-effect relationship. However, in many other instances fairly prominent abnormalities of the spine and neural elements will exist in patients who have no symptoms. Conversely, a significant number of patients will suffer back pain, even unilateral radiculopathy of one or more lumbar levels, without seemingly having any detectable abnormalities that are causally related.

Degenerative disorders of the spine are interrelated. Each should ideally be discussed in the context of all other associated abnormalities. However, to facilitate understanding of this complex subject, we will consider the following disorders separately:

Degenerative disk disease with related abnormalities of the
   vertebrae and facet joints
Malalignment and instability of the spine
Spinal stenosis (Chapter 4)

DEGENERATIVE DISK DISEASE WITH RELATED ABNORMALITIES OF THE VERTEBRAE AND FACET JOINTS
Computed tomography
LOW BACK PAIN, SCIATICA, AND STENOSIS

The patient lies supine on the CT table with hips and knees flexed and supported to reduce the lumbar lordosis while providing as much comfort as possible. Elevating the hips by pillows, towels, etc. to decrease the angle of lordosis at L5-S1 is usually counterproductive: it will often be impossible in patients with acute back pain and it may aggravate the pain in others. An uncomfortable patient is less able to stay motionless, and motion degrades the quality of the study. The prone position is not advisable either, for it causes motion of the spine during respiration and is uncomfortable for elderly individuals as well as anyone with respiratory problems.

A lateral localizer image (digital projection radiograph, scout view) of the lumbar spine is obtained. It should include at least the first two sacral segments and the entire lumbar spine. This is necessary for ensuring the accurate identification of all lumbar vertebrae. The CT slices are positioned as follows: At each disk the gantry is angled to obtain axial cross sections parallel to the midplane of that disk. The axial slices should extend from the middle of the pedicle of the cephalad vertebra to the middle of the pedicle of the caudad vertebra. The gantry is then angled appropriately for the next disk, and the axial cross sections are programmed. It is not sufficient to obtain only one or two slices through the intervertebral disks. The spinal canal must be evaluated above and below the disk to detect expansion of the herniation or migration of a sequestered (free) fragment. It is also important to obtain axial slices up to the *level of the pedicle,* because the spinal canal naturally has a moderate degree of constriction at this point and most migrating disk fragments will become entrapped here.

We ordinarily examine the L3-4, L4-5, and L5-S1 levels using the method just described in patients with low back pain and sciatica. However, in patients with spinal stenosis and when the clinical findings suggest pathology at L1-2 and L2-3, pedicle-to-pedicle axial cross sections are obtained at each of these levels as well. The slices are 3 to 5 mm thick and overlapped 1 mm. This arrangement guarantees optimum coverage of the disks and is helpful for obtaining smoother reformatted images if these become necessary. Thinner slices are usually not needed in the lumbar region.

The midplane of the disk in most supine patients at L5-S1, and occasionally also at L4-5, forms an angle with the vertical that is more than 21 degrees. This means that the CT gantry cannot be angled sufficiently to obtain axial cross sections parallel to the midplane of these disks. In such circumstances the axial slices through the disks are obtained with the CT gantry angled to its maximum (usually 20 to 21 degrees). It is generally then possible to interpret the CT images without difficulty, even though the axial cross sections are not parallel to the midplane of the disk but pass through the posterior margin of it at an oblique angle. However, in the exceptional patient in whom the status of the disk is doubtful, reformatted axial images parallel to the midplane and in the sagittal and coronal planes should be obtained for further evaluation.

In our experience it is easier to evaluate the contour of the posterior border of the disks when the slices are parallel to the midplane of the disk. There is also less geometric distortion of the spinal canal if the slices are perpendicular to its long axis. If axial slices cross obliquely through the posterior disk margin, the CT image may lack detail at the posterior margin of the vertebral endplate and a crown of soft tissue density may project into the canal[1] (Figs. 2-1 to 2-3). This artifact (the so-called tilt artifact) is caused by the slanting posterior margin of the disk. Rarely it may be confused with a herniation, although small herniations are generally masked by it (Fig. 2-4). With experience the examiner is usually able to differentiate the two. Nevertheless, any time spent angling the gantry and obtaining reformatted images is well worth the effort in gained confidence.

Extension of an intervertebral disk beyond the margins of the vertebral endplates has traditionally been classified as either a bulging annulus fibrosus or a herniated nucleus pulposus. Strictly speaking, the phrases "bulging annulus" and "herniated nucleus" are not accurate in most instances, but we plan to retain them in this text because they are widely used and have become synonomous, respectively, with bulging and herniation of the disk.

A clearly identifiable annulus, separate from the nucleus, is usually seen only in youngsters, and then only in those with a normal disk. Bulging of the disk is secondary to degeneration, which affects both the annulus and the nucleus. Thus a bulging disk would seem preferable to a bulging annulus. Herniation is also uncommonly limited to the nuclear material. Most herniations occur in disks affected by degenerative disease. In these cases the boundary between the annulus and nucleus is not distinct, and in advanced cases the entire disk consists of a mass of fibrocartilaginous tissue. Consequently most herniations are of fibrocartilaginous tissue derived from both the annulus and the nucleus. In subjects with a relatively normal disk the herniated material may be composed essentially of nucleus pulposus. Herniation of normal disks is rare, but it may occur with trauma.

Bulging annulus fibrosus. The diagnosis of a bulging disk is made when there is generalized and smooth extension of the disk beyond the margins of the vertebral endplates[2-5] (Figs. 2-5 to 2-7). The bulging ordinarily should not extend more than a few millimeters above or below the disk. The posterior borders of normal L1-2, L2-3, and L3-4 disks often have a concavity in their midportion (Fig. 2-7). A bulging disk may follow this contour and have a similar concavity in its midposterior margin. When the posterior margins of these disks are convex, either a herniation or a bulge is present. The posterior margins of the L5-S1 and L4-L5 disks may be normally flat or convex. This should not be mistaken for a bulging or herniated disk.

Although bulging of the disk may be asymmetrical, any extension beyond the vertebral margins should be generalized and smooth.[2] The margin of a bulging disk should not have irregularities. The presence of a focal irregularity indicates herniation.

In patients with scoliosis or other conditions causing slanting of the vertebral endplates, the disk margins often appear to be protruding on one side or the other. This may be caused by a normal, bulging, or herniated disk. The lateral extension becomes clinically significant only when there is herniation into the upper portion of the neural foramen. Cephalad extension of an intraforaminal herniation is usually necessary for clinical manifestations to appear. In scoliotic patients the disk may also appear to protrude into the spinal canal. It is often not possible to determine

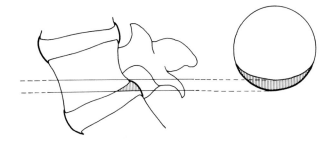

FIGURE 2-1
Tilt artifact. When there is a marked lordosis and axial cross sections cannot be obtained parallel to the midplane of the disk, or when CT slices are obtained with 0 degrees of angulation of the gantry, the slanting posterior border of a normal disk may create a characteristic soft tissue density on the vertebral endplate that resembles a herniated disk. It may also mask a small herniation.

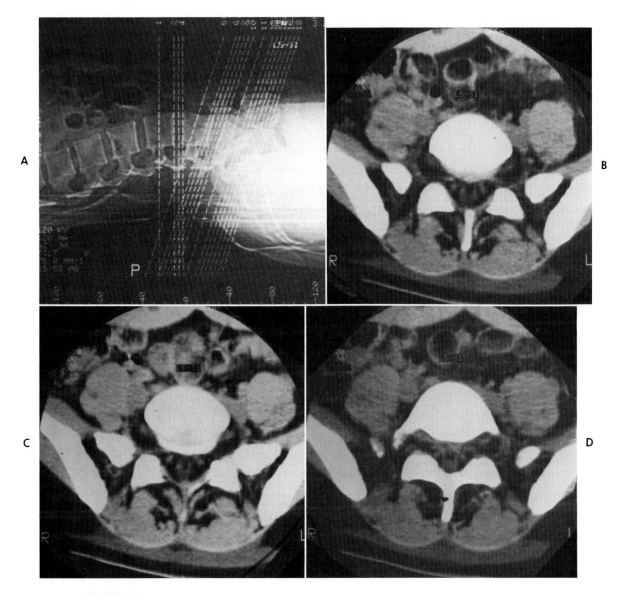

FIGURE 2-2
Marked lordotic angle at L5-S1 causing a soft tissue density at the disk level that mimicks a disk herniation. **A,** Lateral localizer view of the lumbar spine and CT slices with maximum angulation of the gantry at L5-S1. The L5-S1 slices form an angle of approximately 30 degrees with the midplane of the disk. **B,** A crown of soft tissue projects posterior to L5, mimicking a disk herniation. **C,** Partial volume effect, with the superior edge of the posterior S1 margin producing the typical calcification density posterior to the disk. **D,** CT slice just below the inferior cortex of the L5 pedicle. Note the elongation of the anteroposterior diameter of the canal. This is due to the CT slice's not being perpendicular to the longitudinal axis of the spinal canal. Reformatted images through L5-S1 revealed no evidence of a herniated disk.

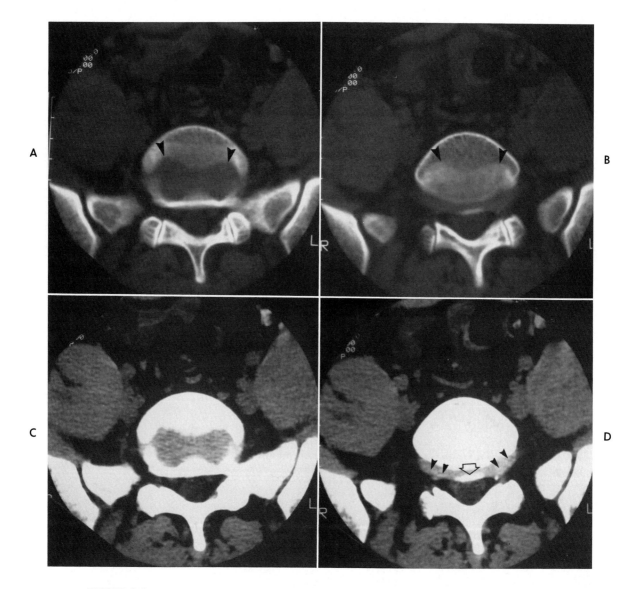

FIGURE 2-3

Tilt artifact resembling a herniated disk in a patient with marked lordosis of L5-S1. **A** and **B,** Bone window and, **C** and **D,** soft tissue window settings, axial CT at the L5-S1 level. Note the crown of soft tissue projecting in a circular fashion posterior to the inferior endplate of L5 in **B** and **D** (*arrowheads* in **D**). The *hollow arrow* in **D** is pointing to bone. This is due to a partial volume effect with the posterior margin of the S1 superior endplate. The *arrowheads* in **A** and **B** point to the typical CT configuration of the Cupid's bow contour (a normal variant) of the L5 endplate.

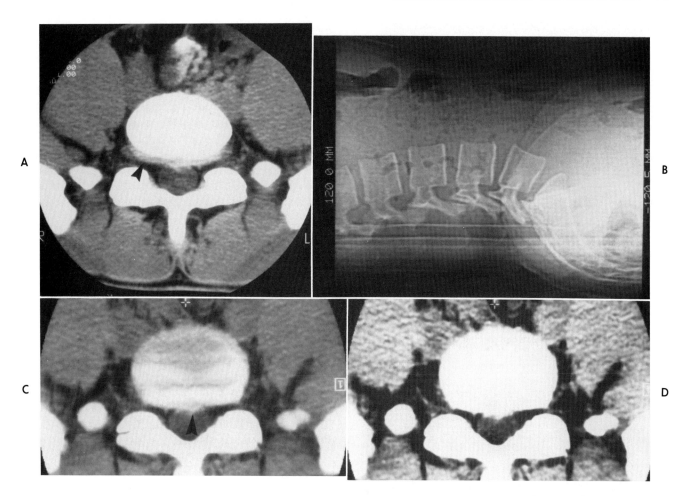

FIGURE 2-4
Midline L5-S1 disk herniation in a patient with marked lordosis at L5-S1. **A,** Axial CT slice showing a crown of soft tissue density *(arrowhead)* projecting posterior to the inferior endplate of L5. This is due to the excessive lordosis at L5-S1, as seen in **B.** A reformatted image parallel to the midplane of L5-S1, **C,** subtracts this soft tissue density. There is an irregular soft tissue density in the midline projecting into the spinal canal *(arrowhead),* the herniation, that was almost completely masked by the tilt artifact. **D,** Narrower window settings show the herniation to better advantage.

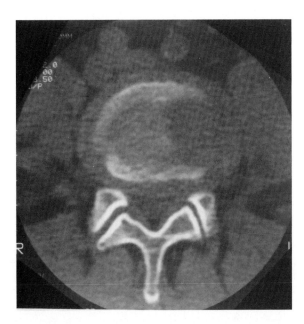

FIGURE 2-5
An axial CT slice through L3-4 shows circumferential bulging of the annulus fibrosus.

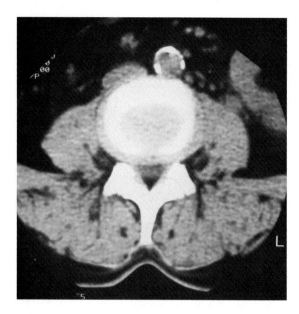

FIGURE 2-6
CT of the spine at L4-5 showing a smooth and symmetrical circumferential bulging of the disk.

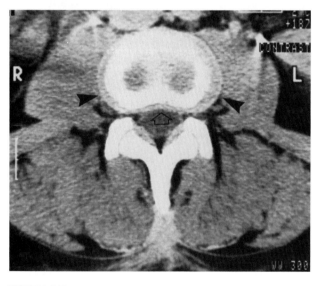

FIGURE 2-7
Postcontrast CT at L3-4 showing circumferential bulging of the disk. Note the enhancement of the disk margins *(arrowheads)*. The normal concavity of the posterior border of the disk is preserved *(hollow arrow)*.

the exact nature of these apparent disk abnormalities on a routine CT examination. Reformatting along the tilted plane of the endplates may be necessary. The patient must be examined with a modified lumbar spine CT technique. We obtain consecutive axial slices, with zero angulation of the gantry, the slices being 3 mm thick and overlapped 1 mm. Reformatting in multiple planes is often necessary for a definitive diagnosis of the presence or absence of disk herniation.

The definitive differentiation between herniation and bulging of a disk is dependent upon visualizing the characteristic deformity of the disk margin, which is best accomplished on axial cross sections. In most patients this differentiation is not possible using sagittal images alone. Bulging of the disk is due to the continuous and relentless process of degeneration that accompanies aging. It occurs gradually over the span of many years. Aging leads to desiccation of the nucleus and annulus. Nuclear desiccation is more severe and causes collapse of the disk space, which leads to bulging of the annulus.[2,6-9] As the degenerative process advances, the annulus loses its elasticity. Multiple cracks, tears, and areas of scarring develop and may calcify. At this stage the disk actually shrinks somewhat.

SPINAL TRAUMA AND BULGING OF THE LUMBAR DISKS

Bulging of a disk is due to desiccation and degeneration. It develops over many years, essentially because of the normal wear and tear of aging. Acute traumatic injuries such as falls or motor vehicle accidents do not cause bulging.

Pathology. The classical studies of Coventry et al.[10,11] are still the best guide to understanding the anatomy, physiology, and pathology of the intervertebral disk. In this section we present first a summary of Coventry's exhaustive study on pathological changes of the disk and then a summary of our own findings in studies of the thoracic and lumbar disks.

The following paragraphs constitute a précis of the articles by Coventry et al.[10,11]:

Beginning even at birth and continuing through the earlier years of growth and development, the body passes through a succession of degenerative stages, reflected in all of its tissues, as part of the aging process. These (retrogressive) stages may seem insignificant compared to the (progressive) developmental stages, but, as growth slows, retrogression accelerates and, in the later years, it eventually dominates. All the body's tissues are affected by these downhill changes, some much more than others.

The intervertebral disks, of course, follow this pattern of progression and retrogression. They are affected early, and they regress more rapidly and severely than do most other tissues of the body. This is usually explained on the basis of excessive wear and tear. At all times the intervertebral disks are actively functioning. They are subject to a great deal of traumatic insult. Their constant use, as well as their susceptibility to trauma and relatively poor blood supply, dooms them to early and advanced degenerative changes.

In the *first decade* of life the cartilaginous plate (hyaline cartilage) is prominent. The cartilage cells are round to oval and microscopically quite clear. In the very early years numerous vascular channels can be seen embedded in and perforating the cartilaginous plate from the vertebral side. By the age of 10 years these channels have largely disappeared (though in some persons they may remain to the age of 20). Fibrosis, followed by the invasion of cartilage cells, obliterates the channels, but their scars remain throughout the life of the disk. These obliterated channels may be areas of weakness, predisposing to herniation of nucleus pulposus into the body of the vertebra.

The various components of the intervertebral disk grow and change according to the stresses and strains of aging, with resulting changes in their function. Thus the annulus has formed by the age of 6 months, for the child is beginning to sit up and needs the spinal column for support, and with continuing development it begins to attach itself to the newly formed anterior and posterior longitudinal ligaments. Stress and strain exert their influences, and by the tenth year the annulus has completely developed as a compact retaining structure. During the first decade the nucleus develops rapidly. Chordal remnants (cells and gelatinous matrix) tend to disappear, and the nucleus consists of a fine interlacing of fibrils in a delicate ground substance of amorphous mucoid material. Fibroblasts in large numbers can be seen, as well as cartilage cells, especially around the periphery.

In the *second decade,* though it has slowed considerably, the growth of bone continues from the base of the cartilaginous plate. Many vascular channels are still present, filled with blood, and can be seen to penetrate deeply into the cartilaginous plate. These channels diminish as age progresses, none being found in subjects older than 19 years. The cartilaginous plate has become somewhat thinner and is fused anteriorly and posteriorly to the apophyseal ring. It has reached maturity and is almost at the end of its phase of progression and development.

The annulus, in response to the vigorous activity of the second decade of life, is further strengthened. Its lamellae are tightly packed together and function more as a whole. In the later years of the second decade, however, there is evidence of annular fiber degeneration — the fibers becoming less distinct, the number of nuclei seeming to decrease, and early hyalinization often appearing.

The nucleus is still undergoing development; nevertheless, the loss of its diffuse character is becoming noticeable. Whereas during the first decade it is a general admixture of cells, fibrils, and homogeneous ground substance, during the second it is more broken up and irregular. There is also evidence of some degeneration in the cartilaginous plate, although these are early changes and microscopic evidence is not abundant. During the second decade wear and tear appear mostly in the annulus. The fibers become coarse and hyalinized, a concentric fissuring of the lamellae occurs, and cellular detail is almost lost. In one specimen out of eight, a moderate amount of edema will be seen between the lamellae, and in approximately one third there will be degenerative changes of the fibrocartilaginous cells. The nucleus is no longer mucoid. Its general composition is cavitary, with vacuoles in a loose fibrillar network. At the periphery are heavier fibers and many more cartilage cells than were seen in the previous decade. The nucleus is beginning to blend more intimately with the annulus.

During the *third and fourth decades* a number of striking and severe retrogressive changes occur. The degenerative defects in the cartilaginous plate range from thinning to complete absence of cartilage. In several places there is bony invasion of the cartilaginous plate from below, with blood channels and marrow elements penetrating into the nucleus. The annulus shows fissuring, hyaline degeneration, cartilage cell proliferation, and nuclear pyknosis. Another interesting finding is vascularization of the annulus, first noticed by Coventry et al. in a specimen from a woman 35 years of age. Several small thin-walled blood vessels were seen to be embedded in the medial layers of the posterior portion of the annulus. They were grouped together and their lumina were filled with blood cells. This invasion of the annular fibrocartilage by blood vessels may be an attempt on the part of the body to strengthen and nourish a structure that

has become weakened and degenerated. The nucleus shows further microscopic evidence of fluid loss: its soft and lacy appearance gives way to a mass of fibrous tissue and cartilage cells, becoming most evident during the fourth decade. Only in occasional sections do remnants of the mucoid ground substance and fibrillar reticulum persist. The distinction between nucleus and annulus becomes less marked. It appears as though the body is attempting to make the disk one solid fibrocartilaginous mass.

In the *fifth decade and beyond* further indications of degenerative changes in the cartilaginous plate appear. The plate becomes generally thin, even perforated in some regions. There are microscopic protrusions of disk substance through the defects and erosions of the plate by bone marrow. Clefts and fissures develop. In older individuals calcified nuclear protrusions may be seen. The annulus, likewise, shows retrogressive changes. Hyalinization is well advanced, and degeneration of the fibrocartilage cells is common. Many of the fibrils are short, thick, and swollen, and sections may show edema fluid in small cavities throughout the annulus. In specimens from patients 60 years of age and older there is both narrowing and compression of the posterior fibers. The junction between annulus and nucleus becomes less distinct. The annulus often appears broken posteriorly, and microscopic slides may show invasion by whorls of new deeply staining fibrous tissue and small blood vessels. This invasion usually occurs in areas where posterior breaking and destruction of the annulus have occurred. In a few cases the disk will protrude posteriorly through the tears.

These invasive elements must be interpreted in the same light as protrusions into the vertebrae — i.e., as mainly an attempt by the body to plug and rebuild the damaged disk tissue. Other changes include calcium plaques, small areas of necrosis, and cross and concentric tears. In older individuals annular tears are usually from an earlier time, as evidenced by the amount of repair that has taken place (invasion by blood vessels and formation of fibrous tissue). Some of these vessels will penetrate well into the nucleus, usually in the posterior segment, where more tears occur, but occasionally in the anterior segment as well. The nucleus in the sixth decade exhibits further evidence of gradual fibrous replacement. It will be of almost the same consistency as the annulus, except for some remnants of the fibrillar reticulum. Edema will be present in a few cases. Although it maintains its mucoid consistency, this is fast disappearing as the nucleus becomes replaced by fibrous tissue, cartilage, and amorphous material.

In later decades the nucleus will be composed almost completely of fibrocartilage, with large longitudinal clefts running through many disks. These occur most often with posterior protrusions. In such cases the nuclear material is lost posteriorly and the fissure is the space formerly occupied by this material. In other cases the clefts will run obliquely down to nuclear protrusions through the cartilaginous plate and into the adjacent vertebral bone. In still other cases, especially in older individuals, one may be impressed by the complete loss of all nuclear structure. Large spaces run horizontally. These are evidence of desiccation.

The borderline between the degenerative changes considered by Coventry et al. to be part of "aging"[10] and those considered "pathological"[11] is not particularly clear. The following synopsis describes the pathological changes of the disk.

THINNING OF THE LUMBAR DISKS

Microscopically, thinned lumbar disks can be classified into two groups:

The first consists of disks whose thinning is of undetermined cause. Despite having an intact annulus and cartilaginous plate, with no evidence of invading fibers or granulation tissue, these disks are desiccated and necrotic. Their fluid content is markedly diminished; and, because fluid normally comprises most of the total disk volume, there is an actual loss of space-occupying material. These disks are collapsed and smaller than normal. Roentgenograms may show thinning with practically no marginal sclerosis of the endplates and very little hypertrophic spurring.

The second group consists of disks whose cause of thinning is more evident. Either the annulus is ruptured (usually posteriorly) or the cartilaginous plate contains many defects, or both. Nuclear material escapes through openings in the annulus or cartilaginous plate, with resulting loss of disk tissue and consequent thinning. This is a purely mechanical phenomenon. In addition, blood vessels and fibroblasts may invade the disk through these openings and serve as avenues for dehydration. In time the invading cells completely replace the normal cells of the disk. Roentgenograms in this group invariably show some marginal sclerosis and quite often osteophytic reaction.

Dehydration is the essential cause, then, of disk thinning. Why this occurs in Group 1 is not entirely clear. In Group 2 it is due obviously to invasion of the disk material by blood vessels and fibrous tissue.

INTRASPONGY NUCLEAR HERNIATIONS (SCHMORL BODIES)

A Schmorl body (or node) may be defined as the herniation of disk substance through a cartilaginous plate defect into the body of an adjacent vertebra. Known also as Schmorl's nodule, cartilage node, or intraspongy nuclear hernia, it was first described by Von Luschka in 1858 and "rediscovered" by Schmorl in 1927.[11] The herniated material extends a varying distance into the cancellous bone of the adjacent vertebra. A reactive change occurs in the bone around the herniation, usually in the form of sclerosis. The prolapsed material tends to change to cartilage, especially at the periphery, and even to ossify. It is thought to be the body's method of attempting to solidify the herniation and plug the hole through which disk material is escaping. Granulation tissue grows from the marrow into the disk and can be seen grossly as a dark reddish infiltration of the nucleus. Such herniations occur in the spinal column of young persons rather rapidly after trauma because of the turgor present in the disk. In older persons, however, with loss of fluid from the nucleus, they occur more gradually and are due mainly to the force of the cephalad vertebra moving against the caudad vertebra.

A Schmorl node is not particularly painful, but herniation of the disk can lead to other complications. If much disk tissue escapes and there is degeneration with thinning, the added strain on the ligaments about the disk maybe exquisitely painful. Furthermore, the axis of motion may be displaced posteriorly, contributing to strain on the articular facets.

POSTERIOR DISK HERNIATIONS

According to Coventry et al.[11] posterior protrusion of the intervertebral disk was recognized as early as 1858 (by Von Luschka). Then, in 1911, Goldthwait described a case of posterior disk protrusion, and in 1929 Schmorl rediscovered posterior protrusions. Bradford and Sperling, in their monograph on the intervertebral disk, gave credit to Mixter and Barr for presenting the first adequate description of herniated disks. When there is a herniation, either the annulus ruptures completely or most of its fibers rupture, leaving only the outermost bands intact. These then protrude into the spinal canal, and through the opening so created are pushed the nucleus pulposus and fragments of the remaining annulus. This material becomes dehydrated and necrotic, and, in addition, hyperplasia of the cartilage cells occurs so that in older protrusions the material is chiefly cartilaginous. Bradford and Sperling stated that invasion of the disk by fibrous tissue and blood vessels is rare. However, Coventry et al.[11] find this to be incorrect. In seven of their patients with definite microscopic evidence of posterior disk herniation, three showed invasion by blood vessels and fibrous tissue through the torn annulus into the disk substance (calcification and ossification of the herniated material also may have occurred and there was evidence of bone formation in one of these specimens.

EROSION OF BONE BY HERNIATED DISK MATERIAL

In the discussion of anterior disk herniation, Coventry et al.[11] describe the case of a 68-year-old woman in whom a herniation occurred at L5-S1 anteriorly. The herniated substance, located between the anterior edge of the first sacral segment and the anterior longitudinal ligament, consisted chiefly of desiccated nuclear material that reacted like proliferating cartilage along the border, attempting to penetrate into the marrow spaces. There was also evidence of invasion by granulation tissue into the herniated material. On roentgenograms erosion of the anterosuperior margin of the vertebral body was seen to correspond to the location of the extruded herniated material.

HYPERTROPHIC BONY SPURS

The cause of osteophytic growth in the spinal column was expounded first by Beneke, in 1897. His theory was that, because of degeneration (with resultant loss of disk substance), there is increased mobility of the vertebral bodies and, as this increases, anterior tension is placed on the attachment of the longitudinal ligament above and below the disk. The anterior longitudinal ligament is deeply implanted in bone as Sharpey's fibers, and this pulling stimulates the periosteum to form new bone, much as tension on the tendinous attachments in children causes characteristic bony ridges and tubercles.

Why osteophyes do not usually occur posteriorly is also explained by Beneke's hypothesis. Since the posterior longitudinal ligament is not attached firmly to bone, tension on it tears the annulus, to which it is adherent, but does not stimulate the periosteum to any great extent.

Donohue modified this hypothesis as to the causation of osteophytic growths by stating that it is the lateral anterior bulging of hypermobile degenerated disks that stretches the ligaments and in turn pulls on the periosteum, causing it to create new bone.

MACROSCOPIC EXAMINATION OF DISK SPECIMENS

Following is our experience with the pathological examination of thoracic and lumbar disks. We examined 21 disks removed from cadavers. One cadaver was of a subject 17 years old, one was 23, and the others were 39

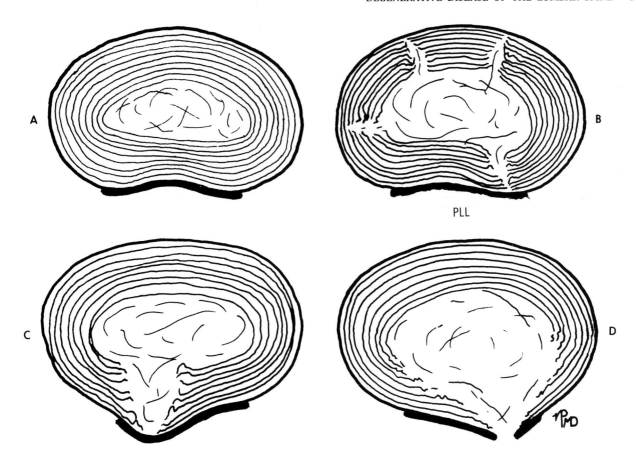

FIGURE 2-8
Schematic of the gross pathology of a degenerated lumbar disk. **A,** The ideal state of a normal disk. This is usually seen only in young subjects. The nucleus and annulus are clearly demarcated, and the contour of the annulus is smooth. **B,** There is disruption of the annulus in multiple areas, with herniation of nuclear material into it (intrasubstance herniation). The disruption has affected most of the fibers but does not reach the outermost ones. The posterior longitudinal ligament *(PLL)* is not torn. The disk contour is normal in this particular case, although with so much disruption of the annulus, irregularity of the disk contour and focal areas of irregularity (denoting herniation) may be present. **C,** Disruption of the annulus and herniation of the disk. Notice that the PLL is not torn. **D,** Disk herniation. Here the annulus-PLL complex is disrupted. The PLL was much thinner in the specimens than what is shown here. It has been purposely accentuated in this schematic to improve its demonstration.

to 67 years of age. Fig. 2-8 is a schematic of the gross pathological changes observed in the 21 disks we examined. The ideal state (a semigelatinous nucleus bounded by a distinct fibrous annulus) was observed in only the two disks from the youngest specimens (Fig. 2-8, *A*). Two other disks had an almost normal internal architecture, and the remaining seventeen had their internal architecture disrupted as follows (the boundary between the annulus and the nucleus was far less distinct in these disks):

In 8 specimens older than 50 years, the disk was essentially a mass of fibrocartilage with no definite boundary between annulus and nucleus.
In 6 specimens the central portion of the disk (nucleus) was transformed into a desiccated featureless zone with calcifications and small cavities (there were a number of cracks and fissures in the substance of these disks extending radially into the peripheral portion).

In about 8 specimens only the central portion of the disk was free of cracks and fissures.
In 9 specimens the peripheral zone of the disk, corresponding to the annulus and constituting about 40% of the disk radius, was partially disrupted and thinned in multiple locations (Fig. 2-8, *B* to *D*) (nuclear and fibrocartilaginous material extended into these cracks and thin zones [intrasubstance herniation]).
In 7 of the 9 specimens the herniated disk material was noted to reach almost to the very edge of the annulus, but the outermost fibers of the APLL complex were not torn (Fig. 2-8, *C*).
In 5 of 7 specimens the disk contour was smooth and circular, despite a considerable amount of intrasubstance herniation (with an intact APLL and normal disk contour); there was a definite focal area of contour deformity (herniation) in the other two disks (also with an intact APLL and a focal disk contour abnormality). In these two the herniated material had reached the periphery of the disk and was accompanied by a focal contour defect (the herniation) with a tear of the APLL complex (Fig. 2-8, *D*) (focal disk contour abnormality).

BULGING IN NORMAL AND DEGENERATED DISKS

Bulging of the disk (i.e., smooth and diffuse extension of the disk margin beyond the endplates) was observed in eight specimens, one in the group of 4 disks that were normal on macroscopic examination and seven in the group of 17 abnormal disks. We believe this to be an important issue that deserves further investigation (i.e., the occurrence of annular bulging in a disk that is unquestionably normal on macroscopic examination). Bulging is generally considered to follow degeneration of the disk. This is most likely correct, because bulging has not been reported in children under 10 years of age (whose disks are normal for all practical purposes)[10,11] but is seen more in older individuals (with a higher incidence of disk degeneration). However, although bulging is almost always accompanied by microscopic evidence of disk degeneration, the disk involved may be normal on macroscopy, CT, and MRI. We have observed bulging in otherwise normal disks on both CT (normal height and configuration) and MRI (normal height, configuration, and signal intensity).

INTRASUBSTANCE HERNIATION

Fissuring of the disk substance, tears and thinning of the inner portion of the annulus, and intrasubstance herniation are important features of a disrupted disk consequent to degenerative disease. The disruption and thinning may become extensive and permit herniation of the nuclear and fibrocartilaginous material peripherally. The outermost fibers of the APLL complex may either not be torn (more commonly encountered) or be torn (less common).

The contour of a disk with intrasubstance herniation may be normal, bulging, or focally abnormal. The most frequently encountered pattern on macroscopy and MRI — herniation extending through a defect in the annulus to the very edge of the annulus and causing extension of the disk margin beyond the endplate borders in an irregular fashion but with an intact APLL complex — should be called just that: hernation. We believe other designations (e.g., protrusion or prolapse) are not helpful unless the person interpreting the study means, and the referring physician understands that these terms mean, herniation. Furthermore, these terms neither imply a less severe form of herniation nor predict the outcome and a suitable treatment (bed rest and antiinflammatory agents vs. surgery). Also, in our experience, long-term follow-up shows that the key factor in predicting the outcome and response to treatment is the presence or absence of spinal stenosis, not the severity of the disk herniation. Thus, in patients without spinal stenosis the response to conservative treatment or surgery is practically the same, regardless of the extent and type of herniation, even when the herniation extends for a significant distance into the spinal canal, or has free (sequestered) fragments.

TERMINOLOGY OF ABNORMAL LUMBAR DISKS

Based on our experiences correlating the abnormalities observed on CT and MRI with surgical findings and our observations of disk specimens, we have adopted the following terminology: normal, bulging, and herniation. Bulging and herniation may coexist, or herniation may occur in a disk with an intact or torn annulus–posterior longitudinal ligament (APLL) complex.

Bulging means smooth and diffuse extension of the disk beyond the endplate margins with minimal or no cephalad or caudad extension. *Herniation* means extension of the disk beyond the endplate margins with a focal or broadbased area of irregularity. The herniated material may spread in various directions (cephalad, caudad, posteriorly into the spinal canal, or laterally into the neural foramen). The phenomenon is called *extension* when the displaced material remains contiguous with the parent disk and a *free fragment* (sequestered) if not.

POSTERIOR LONGITUDINAL LIGAMENT TEAR

The presence or absence of a tear of the posterior longitudinal ligament (PLL) is of no significant clinical, diagnostic, or surgical importance. The PLL is usually very thin and inconspicuous in the lower segments of the lumbar spine. It merges with the outer fibers of the annulus and becomes indistinguishable from it. On MRI a tear of the APLL complex may be identified by visualizing a line of signal void detached from the rest of the disk margin. We have not found other proposed characteristics (e.g., roundness and smoothness of the margin of the herniated material) to be helpful. They do not positively correlate with the findings at surgery.

VACUUM PHENOMENON

In some patients with relatively marked bulging of the disk, there can be severe degenerative changes of the nucleus pulposus but no herniation. The central portion of the disk may be calcified or essentially absent and replaced by a vacuum phenomenon.[13-18] It is interesting that some of the most marked instances of vacuum phenomenon (Figs. 2-9 and 2-10) are noted in patients with fairly obvious bulging of the disk. This is perhaps not surprising since conditions favoring its formation (e.g., long-standing degenerative disease of the disk, a fairly sealed boundary, and a fairly mobile spine) are present in these patients. On the other hand, such conditions do not have to be present in all patients. For example, a vacuum phenomenon may occur in patients with minimal spinal mobility, or no spinal mobility (ankylosis), and in the absence of sustained negative pressure. As is well known, the phenomenon also occurs in more advanced stages of degenerative disk disease with obvious herniation. In these patients the gas may be visible in the herniated portion of the disk, in some cases even seeping into the spinal canal.

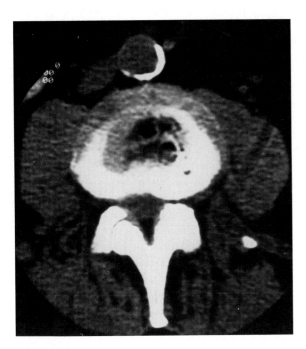

The vacuum phenomenon is due to seepage of gas (92% nitrogen) into the cavities of the degenerated disk. In normal extremity joints traction may induce the phenomenon because gases dissolved in the interstitial fluid percolate into regions that have less than atmospheric pressure.[14] In these joints, even with sustained distraction, fluid replaces the gas within minutes.[15] However, in disks with degenerative disease the gas collected is not ordinarily rapidly replaced by fluid. This may be explained by the absence of fluid sources and of a nearby vascular network to resorb the gas.[16] Restriction of gas absorption, or its inability to escape (or both), suggests at least partial sealing of the disk boundaries. Gas collections may be confined to the central portion of the disk but may also be present in the substance of the herniated segment. These observations agree with the concept that sustained negative pressure, though important, is not absolutely necessary to maintaining intradiskal gas.[14]

FIGURE 2-9
Circumferential bulging of the L3-4 disk associated with the vacuum phenomenon and osteosclerosis of the vertebral endplates.

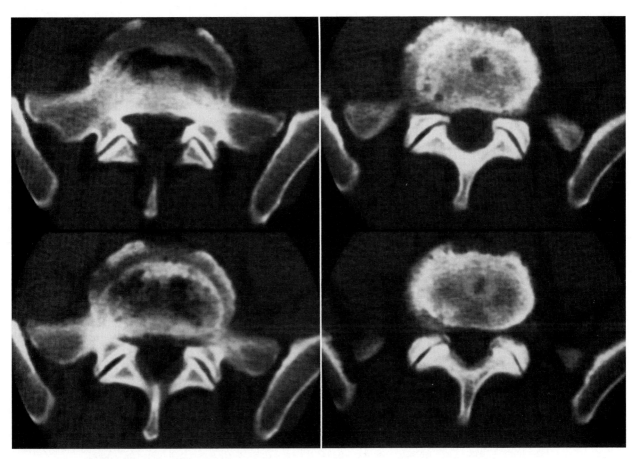

FIGURE 2-10
Axial CT at L5-S1, bone windows, showing circumferential bulging of the disk, which has calcified and ossified. The vacuum phenomenon is also present.

BULGING OF THE DISK IN ADVANCED DEGENERATIVE DISK DISEASE

Bulging of the intervertebral disk is a manifestation of degenerative processes affecting the disk. It is seen in early as well as far-advanced stages of degeneration (Fig. 2-10). In patients with long-standing disk bulges and degenerative disk disease the height of the disk is markedly reduced. The central portion may be calcified or almost totally filled with gas (vacuum phenomenon). The annulus may be bulging along the entire circumference of the vertebral endplate. On gross pathological examination the annulus will usually be rather firm to palpation and not easily compressible, with osteophytes of the endplate margins and calcification of the annulus present.

A bulging disk usually has no clinical significance. However, it may be significant clinically if there is stenosis of the spinal canal or lateral recess.

Stenosis of the spinal canal. In the category of spinal stenoses two groups of patients should be considered: those with a normal disk and those with a bulging disk.

Because of the accentuated concavity of the posterior vertebral borders, patients with a *normal disk* may have the vertebral endplates and annulus appearing to bulge into the spinal canal on axial and sagittal images (Figs. 4-5, 4-6, and 4-7). Similarly, at surgery a normal annulus may be noted to protrude markedly into the spinal canal.

In patients with significant spinal stenosis the dural sac and nerve roots are found to be compressed tightly against the vertebral endplates and intervertebral disk. However, it should be emphasized that this disk configuration in spinal stenosis is not due to any intrinsic pathology and does not require surgical intervention.

In patients with a *bulging disk* (Fig. 2-11), it may be difficult to separate the configuration of the disk (which appears similar to a bulge) from true bulging. This is a judgment call and requires careful assessment of the degree of extension of the disk beyond the vertebral margins. The point is that one should be aware of the normal posterior disk protrusion in patients with spinal stenosis and make any diagnosis of a true bulging or herniation with great caution.

Lateral recess stenosis. The compression of a descending nerve root trapped in a stenotic lateral recess may be further aggravated by a bulging disk.[19,20]

Surgical resection of a bulging disk is rarely indicated, even when the patient has stenosis of the canal or the lateral recess. In these cases a decompressive laminectomy and facetectomy will relieve the symptoms.

HERNIATED NUCLEUS PULPOSUS (HNP)

A diagnosis of HNP is made when the border of the disk extends beyond the margins of the vertebral endplates

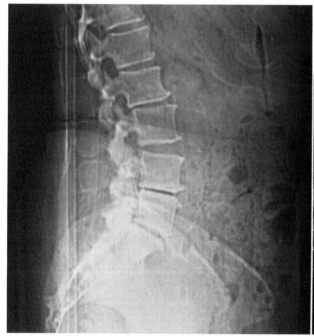
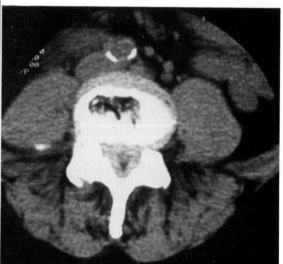

FIGURE 2-11
Bulging of the L4-5 disk and acquired spinal stenosis. **A,** A scout view of the lateral lumbar spine shows significant narrowing of the disk and hypertrophic changes of the vertebral margins. There is also degenerative disease of the other lumbar disks. **B,** An axial CT slice through the disk shows circumferential extension of the disk margin. In addition, the vacuum phenomenon is present and the ligamenta flava are thickened. This combination of a markedly bulging disk and thickened ligaments has produced spinal stenosis in the patient, a 72-year-old woman who presented with gradually worsening neurogenic claudication. She was much improved following surgery.

with a focal or broad-based area of irregularity (Figs. 2-8, C and D, and 2-12, B and C). Herniation of lumbar disks can occur at any point along their circumference. Posteriorly, it may be central (midline), centrolateral, lateral, or far-lateral (foraminal)[3,5,21-23] — with the posterolateral type being most common (probably because of a weakness in the posterolateral annulus).

A central (midline) (Fig. 2-13) or centrolateral (Figs. 2-12, B, and 2-14) HNP may displace or obliterate the epidural fat. The fat is often forced away from the level of the disk, usually to a point above (less commonly, below) the herniation, and there may be indentation or distortion of the dural sac and descending nerve root(s) (Fig. 2-15; see also Figs. 1-54, 1-55, and 1-56). When an HNP is foraminal (far lateral)[22] (Figs. 2-16 to 2-19), the dorsal root ganglion and exiting spinal nerve may be compressed. The diagnosis is missed on myelography (Fig. 2-20) in at least half the patients with this abnormality.

The dural sleeves of the descending nerve roots, as seen on water-soluble contrast myelography, usually terminate somewhere near the midportion of the pedicle (Figs. 2-15 and 2-20, A) or more proximally in about 77% of patients. In the remaining 23% they terminate at the level of the inferior border of the pedicle, or more distally in patients with root cysts (even when the cysts are small). The root sleeve harboring a root cyst is generally wider and longer. Therefore myelography can show the descending nerve root down to the point of termination of its sleeve (i.e., proximal to the dorsal root ganglion). The contrast does not extend beyond this point; and thus the exiting spinal nerve, in the neural foramen and extending anterolaterally into the paraspinal fat, is not visualized. If the HNP

extends upward or there is migration of a free fragment (which is usually trapped at the level of the pedicle), Myelography or CT-myelography (Fig. 2-26, C and D) will show the cutoff and distortion of the root sleeve(s) and dural sac. If the HNP is limited to the neural foramen without extension into the spinal canal, it cannot usually be detected at myelography.[24-27]

An HNP (acute, chronic, soft, or calcified) may exist and be visible on axial and sagittal images without any associated abnormality of the descending nerve roots or dural sac. This usually happens when the spinal canal is quite capacious and a significant amount of epidural fat is present[24-26] (particularly in the L5-S1 region, where the thickness of fat anterior to the dural sac may be 1 cm or more). In these instances a herniated disk may be present without being in contact with the descending nerve roots or dural sac. On the other hand, it should be noted that the posterior border of a normal disk may be in contact with the anterior wall of the dural sac. This is particularly so at the L1-2, L2-3, and L3-4 levels, where the posterior margin of the normal disk is seen not infrequently to be right against the dural sac, without any intervening midline anterior epidural fat. This is normal and does not indicate herniation.

Awareness of the features of normal disks and the characteristics of bulging or herniation on CT and MRI is important from a legal standpoint also. A lumbar HNP means extension of the disk border beyond the margins of the vertebral endplates, with a focal or broad-based area of irregularity. The zone of irregularity corresponds to the apex of a significant intrasubstance herniation, permitting extension of the nuclear and fibrocartilaginous

Text continued on p. 76.

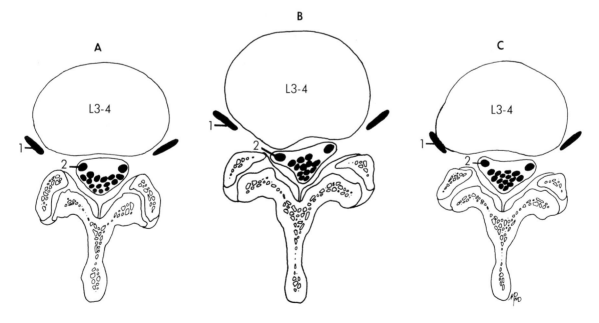

FIGURE 2-12
Schematic of, **A**, a normal disk, **B**, a posterolateral herniation, and, **C**, a far-lateral (intraforaminal) herniation on the right side at L3-4. *1*, The exiting right L3 spinal nerve; *2*, the descending right L4 nerve root.

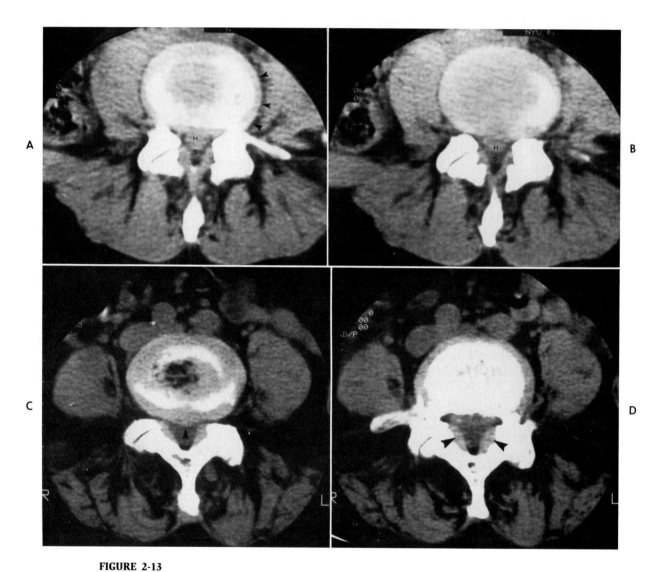

FIGURE 2-13
A and **B**, L4-5. A central herniation *(H)* is visible. *S* denotes the dural sac. There is minimal circumferential bulging of the disk, which is more prominent on the left side *(arrowheads* in **A)** because of a slight scoliosis. **C** and **D**, L4-5 in another patient. There is moderate circumferential bulging in this individual with a small central herniation *(arrowhead* in **C).** The vacuum phenomenon is also present. **D,** Axial slice at the level of the superior endplate of L5. Note here the circumferential bulging of the disk and the thickened ligamenta flava *(arrowheads).*

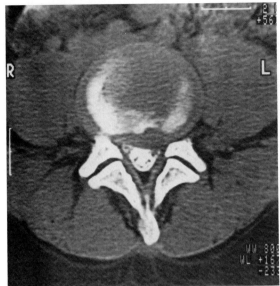

A

FIGURE 2-14

A, A CT myelogram at L4-5 shows circumferential bulging and herniation of the disk to the left of midline. The dural sleeve of the right descending L5 nerve root is normally exiting on the right. It is compressed and has not filled on the left. **B,** Lateral and, **C,** oblique views of the myelogram show the right side to be normal. The obliteration of the sleeve of the left L5 nerve root can be detected at this level. The *asterisk* is on L4.

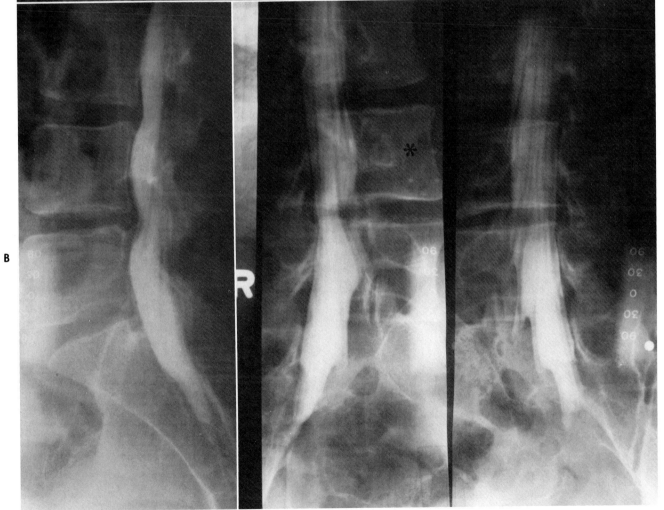

B

C

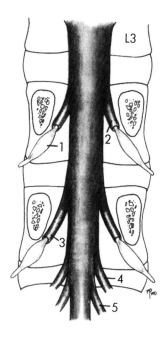

FIGURE 2-15
Schematic of the lumbar thecal sac and nerve roots. *1,* Dorsal root ganglion of the right L4 nerve root; *2,* dural sleeve of the left L4 descending nerve root; *3,* dural sleeve of the right L5 descending nerve root; *4* and *5,* dural sleeves of the left descending S1 and S2 nerve roots.

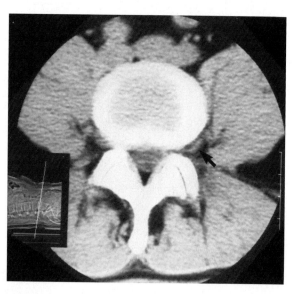

FIGURE 2-16
Herniation of an L4-5 intervertebral disk into the right neural foramen. The *arrow* denotes the normal exiting L4 nerve on the left side. On the right the L4 nerve is obscured by the herniated disk. At surgery the herniation was seen to occupy the right neural foramen.

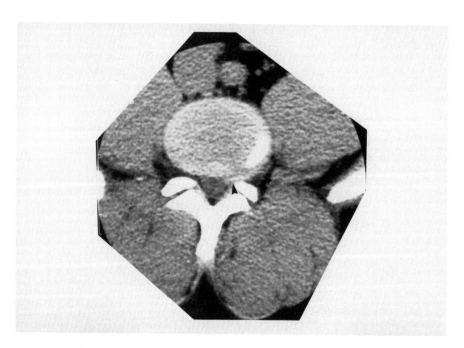

FIGURE 2-17
Left-sided posterolateral and intraforaminal herniation at L4-5 *(arrowhead).*

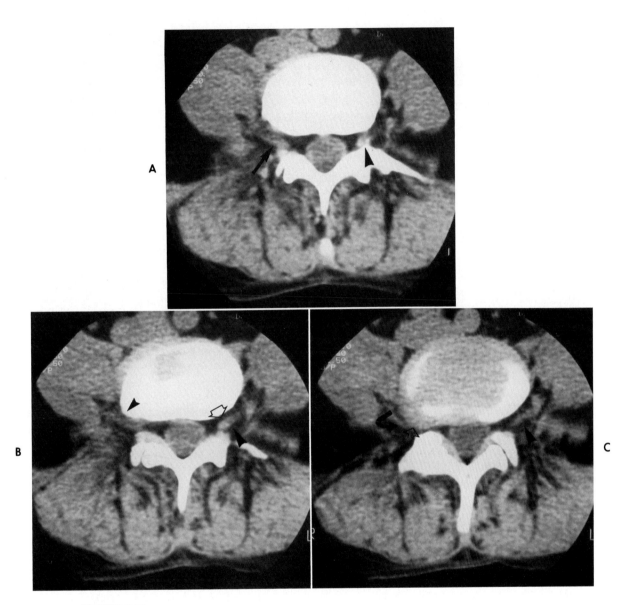

FIGURE 2-18

Right intraforaminal disk herniation. **A,** An axial slice just below the pedicles of L3 shows the normal left dorsal root ganglion *(arrowhead)*. The soft tissue mass has distorted the right neural foramen and dorsal root ganglion *(arrow)*. **B,** An axial slice 4 mm below A shows the origin of the left L3 exiting spinal nerve *(large arrowhead)*, which is normal. Note the small osteophyte arising from the posterolateral margin of the vertebral endplate on the right *(small arrowhead)*. The fat plane between the vertebra and the right exiting L3 spinal nerve is obliterated. Notice also the normal fat plane on the left *(hollow arrow)*. **C,** Another axial slice, 4 mm below **B,** shows the normal left exiting L3 nerve *(arrowhead)*. On the right there is herniation of the disk almost exclusively into the right neural foramen *(hollow arrow)*. The *curved arrow* points to the displaced right exiting L3 spinal nerve. At surgery an intraforaminal herniated disk was found.

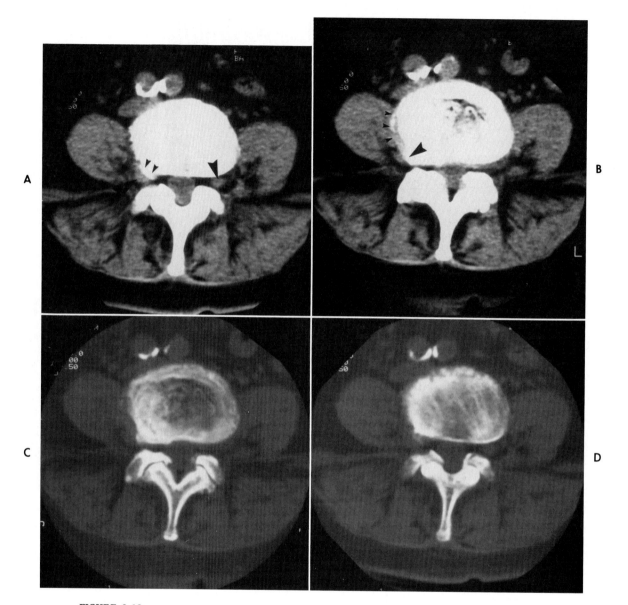

FIGURE 2-19
Neural foraminal stenosis secondary to an old calcified intraforaminal herniated disk. **A** and **B,** Soft
tissue window settings and, **C** and **D,** corresponding bone window settings at L4-5. (In **A,** an axial CT
slice at the top of the L4-5 neural foramen, the *large arrowhead* on the left denotes the dorsal root
ganglion of the left L4 nerve root. The *small arrowheads* on the right point to an osteophyte displacing
the right dorsal root ganglion posterolaterally. The large arrowhead on the right designates the right
dorsal root ganglion. In **B,** an axial slice at L4-5, there is a vacuum phenomenon. Note the calcification
of the herniated disk margin *[small arrowheads].*) The *large arrowhead* on the right points to an
osteophyte arising from the posterolateral border of the inferior L4 endplate, displacing the right
exiting L4 spinal nerve.

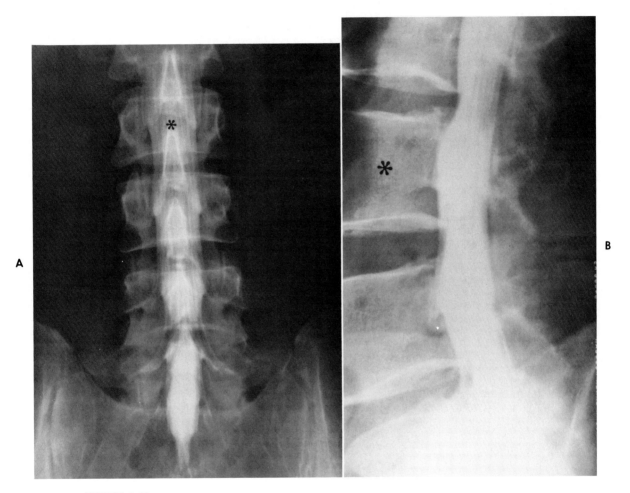

FIGURE 2-20
Intraforaminal disk herniation. **A** and **B**, Frontal and slightly oblique/lateral myelograms reveal no abnormality. The *asterisk* is on L2.   *Continued.*

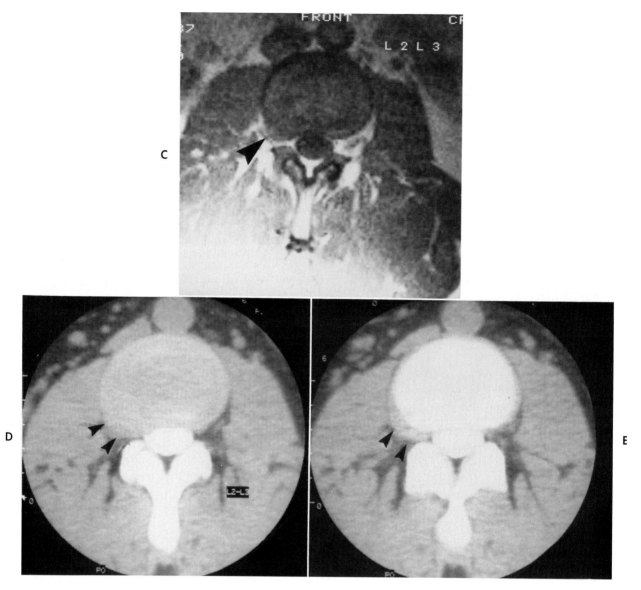

FIGURE 2-20, cont'd
C, A T1-weighted MR, however, and, D and E, CT-myelograms show a pronounced herniation of the L2-3 disk *(arrowheads)*.

material to the very edge of the annulus and causing a focal or broad-based deformity of the disk margin. The APLL complex at the leading edge of the herniation is more commonly not torn than torn and therefore stays attached to the rest of the disk margin. Less commonly the APLL is torn, in which case it may be displaced away from the disk margin with the herniated material.

An HNP may be small and focal (Fig. 2-21) or broad based (Fig. 2-22). However, its margin must be irregular. This is the basic morphological difference between bulging and herniation. The margin of a bulging disk is smooth, that of a herniated disk irregular. Obviously, bulging and herniation both may be present in the same disk (Figs. 2-13, *A* and *C*, and 2-14, *A*), and in these

situations the margin of the bulging segment is smooth and follows the contour of the endplate whereas that of the herniated portion is irregular. A large herniation may cause displacement, distortion, or obliteration of the root sheaths and compression, deformity, or displacement of the dural sac; and yet it may not do any of these things if there is sufficient room in the spinal canal. On the other hand, the mere fact that the posterior border of the disk is in contact with the dural sac (provided there is no displacement or distortion of it) must not be viewed as evidence in favor of herniation. The posterior borders of the L1-2, L2-3, and L3-4 disks are often right against the dural sac without any intervening fat in the midline. In slightly more than 35% of patients there is some fat

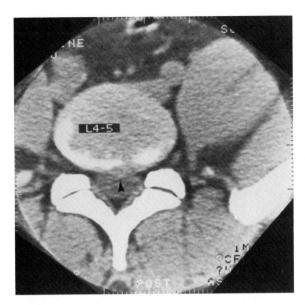

FIGURE 2-21
A small herniation of the L4-5 disk, slightly more prominent to the left of midline *(arrowhead).*

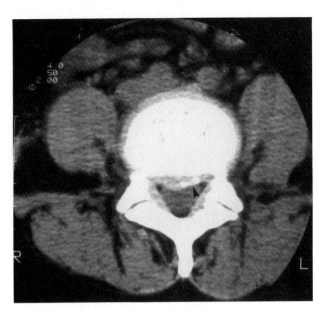

FIGURE 2-22
Calcified disk herniation. An axial slice at the level of the superior endplate of L5 shows slight circumferential bulging of the disk. The contour of the posterior border is irregular, indicating midline herniation. The *arrowhead* denotes calcification of the margin of the disk to the left of midline.

between the dural sac and the posterior border of a normal disk in the midline at L4-5, and in almost all patients at L5-S1. Anterolaterally some epidural fat is seen at every lumbar level.

In patients with advanced degenerative disease of the intervertebral disks there is usually collapse of the disk and the disk height may be reduced to only a few millimeters. Extensive calcification of the disk substance, both the annulus and the nucleus, along with the vacuum phenomenon may also be present. The gas can be seen to reach the very edge of the herniated disk.

Extension and migration beyond the level of the disk. An HNP may extend upward or downward in the spinal canal (Fig. 2-23), usually stopping at the level of the vertebral pedicle because of the natural constriction of the canal in this region.[3,21] Extension means that the herniated segment has extended beyond the level of the disk in the spinal canal but is still attached to the parent disk (Fig. 2-23, *2*). When it becomes separated, it is considered a free fragment (Fig. 2-23, *4*). A free fragment may migrate superiorly or inferiorly, stopping at the level of the adjacent vertebral pedicles. Rarely will it migrate beyond the pedicles. We have found that extension of a herniated disk or migration of a free fragment occurs somewhat more often superiorly than inferiorly, due probably to the fact that there is more room in the canal immediately above the disk than below it.[21] The migrated fragments may contain calcification. The disk from which these fragments have come may be difficult to identify because the margins of the donor disk are deceptively smooth and indistinguishable from normal disk margins. Extension or migration of a herniated disk, in our experience, occurs about 30% of the time.

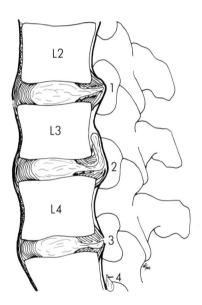

FIGURE 2-23
Schematic of the various kinds of disk herniation. *1*, L2-3. There is rupture of most of the inner fibers of the annulus. The nuclear material has extended through the rupture to the very edge of the APLL complex, which is displaced posteriorly but not ruptured. *2*, L3-4. The pathology of the annulus is similar to that of L2-3, but there is upward extension of the nuclear material beneath the PLL and the ligament is not ruptured. *3*, L4-5. There is a tear of the APLL complex with herniation of nuclear material through the tear. *4*, A free fragment in the spinal canal posterior to the PLL is trapped at the level of the inferior margin of the L5 pedicle.

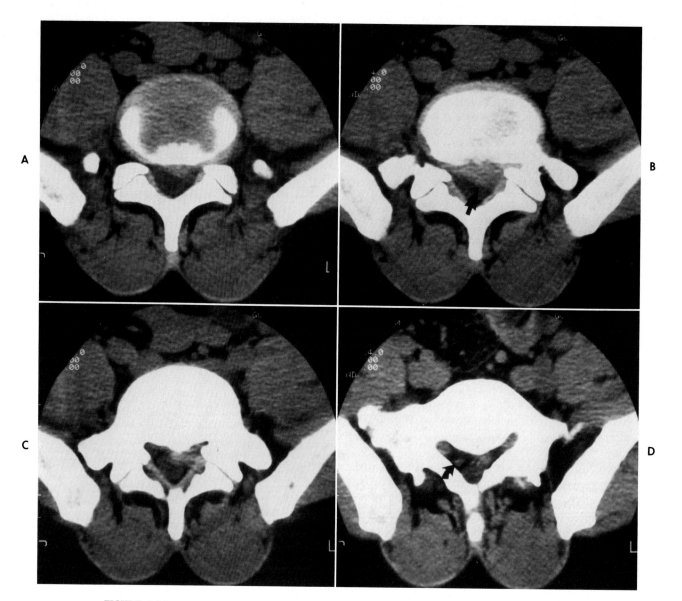

FIGURE 2-24

An L4-5 herniated disk with extension inferiorly and migration of a free fragment affecting the left S1 descending nerve root. **A** and **B,** Axial CT slices show a large herniation with a major component on the left (*arrow* in **B**). **C,** An axial slice through the upper part of the L5 pedicles shows extension inferiorly on the left side. Note the obliteration of epidural fat anteriorly and anterolaterally on the left. **D,** Axial slice 8 mm below **C,** through the lower portion of the L5 pedicles. The *arrow* points to the normal right descending S1 nerve root. A small migrated free fragment is present on the left, engulfing the left S1 descending root. There was no abnormality 4 mm above this level indicating detachment of the fragment (visible in **D**) from the extended herniated disk (visible in **C**).

Extension of an HNP and migration of a free fragment may coexist (Fig. 2-24). The extension is often subligamentous (Fig. 2-23), but this is of no great clinical or surgical significance. A free fragment is more commonly associated with a tear of the APLL complex. It also is more free to move about in the spinal canal and may migrate further from the parent disk. It may move laterally (into the neural foramen) or posteriorly, in which case one may confuse it with other epidural lesions (e.g., neoplasms). Free fragments may also become embedded in bone and cause erosion. A herniated disk extending into the spinal canal often will come to rest just lateral to midline (Fig. 2-55), as reported by Schellinger et al.,[28] although one straddling the midline (Fig. 2-25) is not as rare as those authors report. When a herniated disk extends or free fragment migrates to such an extent

that it is a considerable distance from the parent disk, the clinical manifestations may be confusing. This is because the lumbar roots affected do not correspond to the level of the herniation. A problem in the work-up of patients with a free fragment is the difficulty of identifying small epidural lesions on CT and MRI. In these cases CT-myelography (Fig. 2-26) is the only diagnostic modality to use.

Schellinger et al.[28] described a sagittally aligned fibrous septum dividing the anterior epidural space into right and left halves (Figs. 2-27 and 2-28). The septum extends from the posterior border of the vertebral body to the posterior longitudinal ligament (PLL). At the disk level the PLL is attached to the annulus and the midline septum does not exist. The septum is visualized optimally in the lower lumbar region, because there the PLL is situated further from

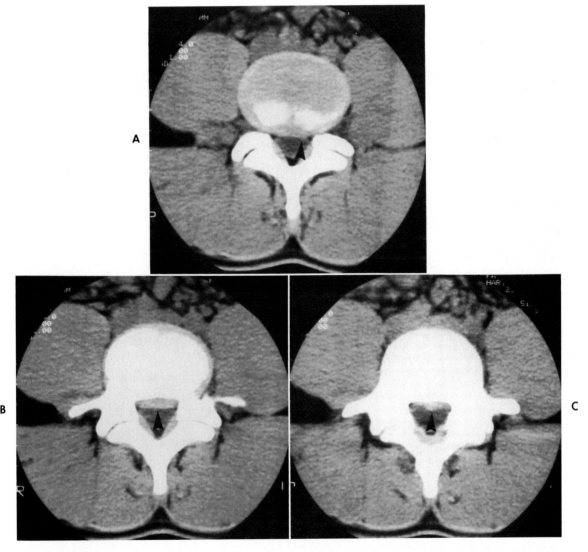

FIGURE 2-25
Small L4-5 disk herniation extending inferiorly. **A,** A CT slice shows moderate extension of the disk margin beyond the vertebral endplate, with a focal area of irregularity to the left of midline *(arrowhead)*. **B,** Another slice 4 mm below **A** and, **C,** a slice 8 mm below **A** show downward extension of the disk material *(arrowhead in **C**)*.

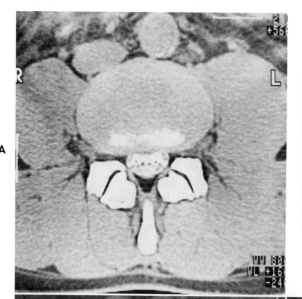

FIGURE 2-26

L3-4 disk herniation. **A,** A CT-myelogram shows moderate asymmetry of the posterior border of the disk, with slight to moderate compression of the anterior dural sac. Another slice, **B,** 6 mm and one, **C,** 9 mm above **A** reveal that there is still minimal asymmetry with probable compression of the anterior dural sac to the right of midline. **D,** A CT-myelogram 12 mm and another, **E,** 15 mm above **A** show obvious compression with deformity of the dural sac on the right side. The L3 descending root sleeve is exiting normally on the left. It is obliterated on the right. A migrated fragment of herniated disk was found at surgery. No abnormalities were detected on CT or MRI in this patient.

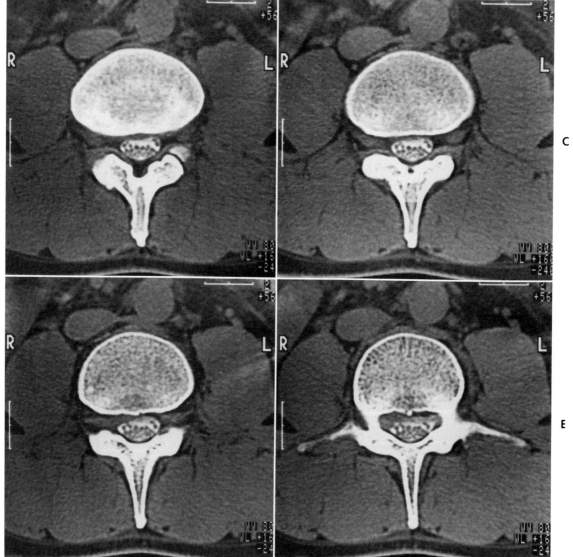

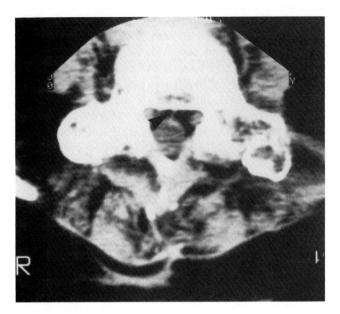

FIGURE 2-27
Right midline septum in the anterior epidural space *(arrowhead)* at the level of the L5 pedicle.

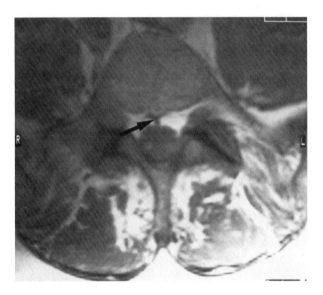

FIGURE 2-28
Normal midline fibrous septum *(arrow)* at L5.

the posterior vertebral border. Schellinger et al. analyzed the path of migration of sequestered (free) disk fragments in 47 patients and found that 42% migrated superiorly and 40% inferiorly. The migrated fragments were trapped most often (94% of the time) in the right or left half of the anterior epidural space, rarely straddling the midline.

Thecal sac and nerve root involvement. The optimal evaluation of an abnormal intervertebral disk by CT or MRI must include axial slices from the middle of the pedicle of the cephalad vertebra to the middle of the pedicle of the caudad vertebra. This region contains the exiting spinal nerves (as they descend in the neural foramina and leave the foramina at about the disk level) and the descending nerve roots (which after emerging

from the dural sac run inferiorly, anteriorly, and laterally in the spinal canal, enter their respective lateral recesses, and curve beneath the pedicles to leave the spinal canal).

The L1, L2, L3, and L4 root sleeves usually emerge from the dural sac just below the superior endplate of their respective vertebrae. The nerve roots themselves, before they enter the root sheaths, are in the anterolateral portion of the dural sac, directly behind the disks. The descending roots leave the dural sac, surrounded by their dural sleeves, just below each disk. The L5 root sleeve may emerge from the dural sac somewhat higher (i.e., above the superior endplate of L5, behind the L4-5 disk) and run directly behind the margin of the L4-5 disk in the anterolateral epidural fat. The S1 root sleeve emerges from the dural sac well above the superior endplate of S1 and runs in the epidural fat directly behind the L5-S1 disk.

A posterolateral HNP without significant superior or lateral extension may cause compression of its descending nerve root. For example, a posterolateral L3-4 herniation may compress the ipsilateral descending L4 nerve root. When there is superior extension of the herniation or migration of a free fragment, the descending root (one level higher) may be compressed as it curves beneath the pedicle. An L3-4 herniated disk fragment migrating superiorly in the spinal canal, then, would compress the L3 descending root(s) and dural sac. When there is herniation of the disk into the neural foramen, it may affect the dorsal root ganglion directly beneath the pedicle and the exiting spinal nerve that leaves the neural foramen in its upper third and descends anterolaterally into the paraspinal fat. Thus, an intraforaminal (far-lateral) L3-4 HNP would compress both the L3 dorsal root ganglion and the L3 exiting spinal nerve. A large central HNP may compress not only its own nerve roots but also the other nerve roots within the dural sac, by marked compression of the dural sac. Large anterior and lateral herniated lumbar disks, displacing the kidney, or other structures are occasionally encountered.

Invasion of the dura. Rarely a herniated lumbar disk, usually one that is calcified, will become adherent to and embedded in the dura, perforating it and partially entering the subarachnoid space.

CT diagnosis. The CT diagnosis of HNP is greatly facilitated by the presence of epidural fat and by differences in the density of the herniated substance and the thecal sac and nerve roots. In most patients the herniated disk is visually denser than the adjacent thecal sac and nerve roots. With a midline or posterolateral herniation, often the symmetry of the soft tissues in the spinal canal will be disturbed. The small amount of epidural fat present in the anterolateral canal and the descending root sleeve within it (which emerges from the dural sac at or just below the disk level) may be obliterated when a posterolateral HNP is present. At the L5-S1 level a significant amount of anterior epidural fat is usually present, and the herniated disk itself will usually be clearly visible, displacing the sacral nerve roots, which have already emerged from the dural sac and are running anterolaterally in the epidural space. At L4-5 in some patients there is enough anterior midline epidural fat to form an interface between the disk and the dural sac. A midline L4-5 HNP may obliterate this fat and displace and deform the dural sac. The descending L5 root sleeves are occasionally identified anterolaterally posterior to the L4-5 disk. This happens in a small number of subjects in whom the L5 descending roots emerge from the dural sac well above the superior endplate of L5.

An HNP may obliterate the anterolateral epidural fat triangles and distort the descending roots. At the L1-2, L2-3, and L3-4 disks the midline anterior epidural fat is usually scant or altogether absent. An interface containing fat or nonfat connective tissue separating the disk from the dural sac may not be present in normal subjects at these levels. Thus the posterior border of the disk may be in contact with the dural sac. This is normal and does not imply herniation of the disk. Herniation is diagnosed when the disk extends beyond the vertebral margins with an irregular border or a focal area of irregularity in its border. A herniated disk may or may not displace or distort the dural sac and the other neural elements.

Anterolaterally within the spinal canal there is some fat at all lumbar vertebral segments (anterolateral fat triangles), usually less at the upper three than the lower two segments. At the first three lumbar disk levels the descending roots are generally not visualized directly posterior to the disks because the L1, L2, and L3 roots have not yet separated from the dural sac (i.e., at the disk level). However, immediately below these disks the root sleeves are visualized as distinct structures in the lateral recess. Obliteration of the anterolateral fat triangles is a helpful sign of disk herniation or infiltration of the epidural space by other elements. A posterolateral HNP may distort the lateral recess and the descending root within it. An intraforaminal HNP may obscure the dorsal root ganglion and/or the exiting spinal nerve. These structures may be displaced, and the fat surrounding them distorted.

It should be emphasized that HNP is an abnormality of the disk itself. Its diagnosis should be made when the disk margin extends beyond the vertebral endplates with a focal or broad-based area of irregularity. This diagnosis, however, depends neither on the coexistence of abnormalities in the neural elements nor on the presence of clinical findings. Compression, displacement, and distortion of the neural elements are complications of HNP and their presence or absence is dependent on a number of other factors besides disk herniation (e.g., the size of the herniation, the strategic juxtaposition of the herniation and neural elements, and the size of the spinal canal). For example, when the spinal canal is large there may be no compression or displacement of the neural elements; however, there may be marked compression of the dural sac and nerve roots (even with a small herniated disk) in patients with spinal stenosis.

Most HNPs have a higher Houndsfield number than the thecal sac or the nerve roots. We usually do not rely on densitometry for differentiation between these elements. However, in doubtful cases one may take advantage of this. Utilization of *blink mode* enhances the usefulness of this feature. Occasionally an isodense HNP will be encountered. This is more likely to occur in patients with moderate to marked spinal stenosis and is probably due to paucity of CSF.[21] In these patients CT differentiation of the HNP from the thecal sac may not be possible. At times a massive HNP will occupy a large portion of the spinal canal and compress the thecal sac against the posterior wall of the canal (Figs. 2-29 and 2-30). Then the CT diagnosis of disk herniation may not be possible because there is no detectable, displaced, or distorted epidural fat and no visible interface between the HNP and the contents of the spinal canal.

The CT diagnosis of HNP may be particularly difficult in the following conditions:

1. Spinal stenosis: The herniated disk may be missed in spinal stenosis because of overcrowding of the soft tissues within the spinal canal, leading to difficulty in identification of the herniated material (Figs. 2-29 to 2-31).

2. Previous spinal surgery: In these patients there may be distortion of the epidural fat or significant scarring. It may not be possible to differentiate a recurrent herniation from scarring following surgery.

3. Pantopaque in the canal: In patients who have undergone myelography with iophendylate (Pantopaque) and a significant amount of contrast remains within the spinal canal, there may be marked degradation of the CT image. For these patients MRI is the modality of choice. We have used MRI in several patients with Pantopaque in the spinal canal, and the examination was quite satisfactory.

4. Marked congenital deformity and scoliosis: In these patients because of the slanting plane of the vertebral endplates, kyphoscoliosis, or other deformities, a definitive diagnosis of HNP often is difficult on CT, MRI, or myelography. The technique of CT examination must be modified and tailored to the shape of the spine. We have found the following modifications helpful: Consecutive 3 mm thick slices, overlapped 1 mm, without any angulation of the gantry should be obtained. If the area of pathology is limited to a small segment of the spine, thinner slices (on the order of 1 mm) may be obtained. It may be necessary to use reformatted sagittal, coronal, and axial cross sections. If a definitive diagnosis is not established after obtaining high-resolution reformatted images, CT-myelography or MRI may be needed. Reformatting of CT-myelography images in the sagittal, coronal, and axial planes often will help elucidate the abnormalities present.

5. Obese patients: There usually is no significant problem in examining obese patients if the CT examination is performed on the most recent state-

of-the-art imagers. However, artifacts may be produced because of the excessive volume of fat in the path of the CT beam. One possible solution is to obtain an MRI, but care must be exercised not to exceed the weight limitations of the MRI imager. We have examined patients weighing 350 pounds without any apparent harmful effect to the MR imager (Philips, 1.5 tesla). Nevertheless, although the problem of artifacts due to photon deficiency is not present with MRI, in markedly obese patients the MRI image is not ideal either.

6. Patients with conjoined root sleeves and root cysts (Tarlov cysts)[29-34] (Figs. 2-31 to 2-33): See pp. 49 to 54.

7. Neurofibroma, epidural neoplasm, and abscess: CT-myelography or MRI may become necessary for a definitive diagnosis in these patients (Fig. 2-34).

8. Tethered cord, lipomas, and other intraspinal neoplasms: Confusion can arise in these patients.

9. Spondylolisthesis and disk herniation: Patients with spondylolisthesis may have significant distortion of the epidural fat. At the posterior margin of the disk a density can be present on axial CT images that

Text continued on p. 89.

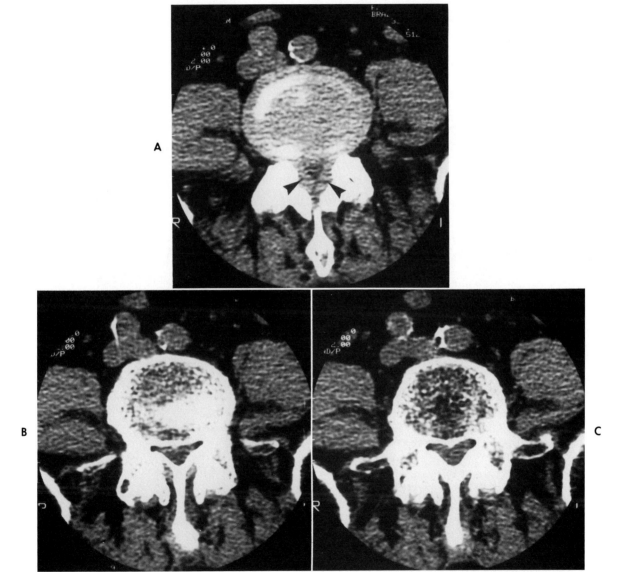

FIGURE 2-29
Congenital spinal stenosis and a herniated disk at L4-5. **A,** Axial CT, 3 mm thick, parallel to the midplane of the disk. There is circumferential bulging, and the definition of soft tissues within the spinal canal is poor. A diagnosis of disk herniation, or lack thereof, could not be made. At surgery a herniated disk was found. Note the thickening of the ligamentum flavum *(arrowheads)*. The patient also has degenerative disease of the facet joints, with a slight to moderate protrusion of the hypertrophic facets into the spinal canal. **B** and **C,** Axial CT cross sections through the pedicles of L5 show marked congenital spinal stenosis and degenerative disease of the facet joints.

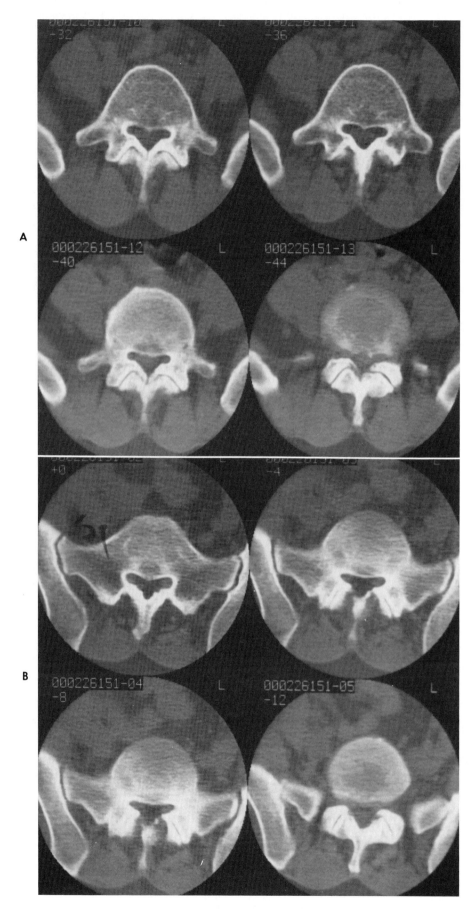

FIGURE 2-30
For legend see opposite page.

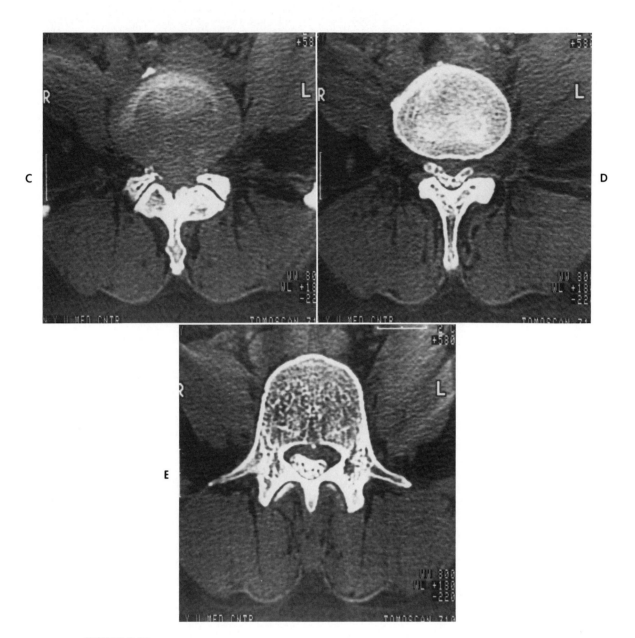

FIGURE 2-30

Congenital spinal stenosis localized to L5 and S1 and an L4-5 disk herniation. **A** and **B,** Computed tomography at L4-5, L5, L5-S1, and S1 shows the diminished surface area of the canal, with thickened pedicles and laminae. At L4-5 (**A**) the soft tissue definition within the canal is poor. No interface can be detected between the disk and the dural sac. The tissues within the canal appear to be of uniform density. It was suspected that this patient had a herniated disk, but this could not be shown conclusively. **C** to **E,** CT myelography. (At L4-5 [**C**] the dural sac is not recognizable. There is only minimal contrast in a root sleeve at the entrance to the right neural foramen, and none can be seen in the dural sac. A large herniated disk, occupying practically the entire spinal canal, was suspected. The laminae are thickened, consistent with a congenital stenosis. Just above the inferior endplate of L4 [**D**] and through the L4 pedicles [**E**] the anterior surface of the dural sac is compressed, more prominent on the left side, secondary to extension of herniated disk material to the level of the pedicles.)

Continued.

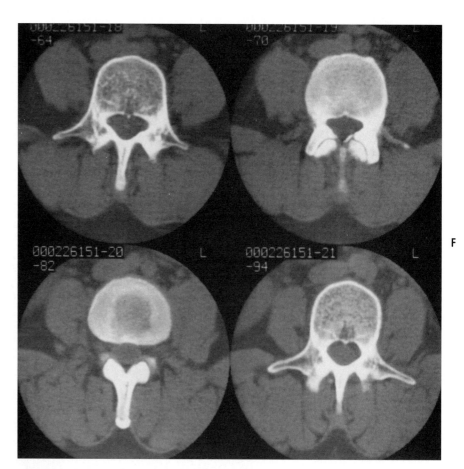

FIGURE 2-30, cont'd

F, L3 and the L4 disk. Computed tomography shows the spinal canal to be of normal size and configuration at this level. The congenital stenosis was limited to L5 and S1. (Stenosis affecting L5-S1 is distinctly unusual. In most patients the L5-S1 region is normal.)

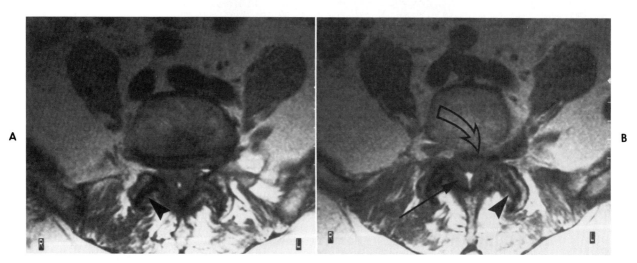

FIGURE 2-31

Severe degenerative disease of the facet joints, spinal stenosis, and disk herniation at L4-5. A and B are T1-weighted axial MRIs showing severe degenerative disease of the facet joints *(arrowhead)* and stenosis of the spinal canal. There is marked hypertrophy of the ligamentum flavum *(straight arrow in B)*. The definition of soft tissues within the canal is poor. No definite disk herniation is identified. A Grade I spondylolisthesis was present, which would account for the configuration of the posterior border of the disk in **A**. The focal areas of signal void in **B** *(curved hollow arrow)* are due to a partial volume effect with osteophytes. A herniated disk was found at surgery.

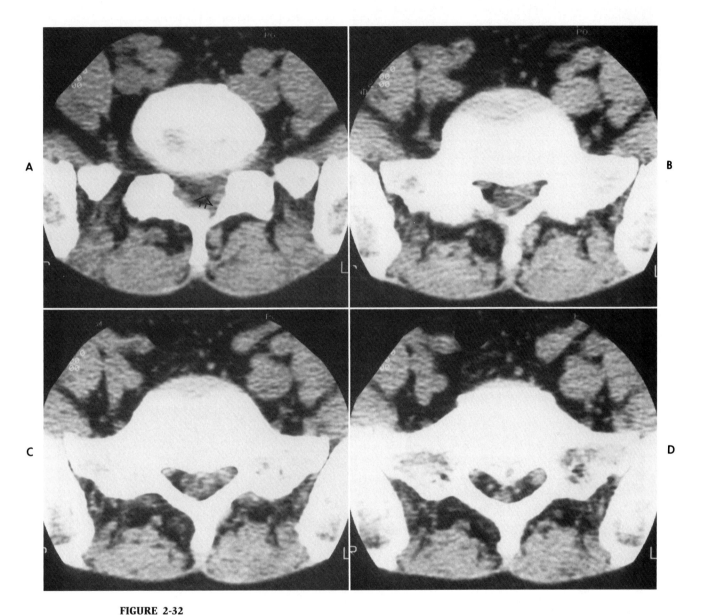

FIGURE 2-32
Herniation of L5-S1 to the left of midline and conjoined S1 nerve roots on the left. CT axial slices, soft tissue windows, show posterior extension on the medial side of the ligamentum flavum (*hollow arrow* in **A**). Note the obliteration of anterolateral epidural fat by the herniation on the left. **B**, A CT slice 8 mm below **A**, **C**, a slice 4 mm below **B**, and **D**, another slice 4 mm below **C**, at the S1 level. At surgery a conjoined left S1 root sleeve and a herniated disk were found. The left S1 root sleeve was larger than the right, and there was asymmetry of its origin along with a slight enlargement of its left lateral recess.

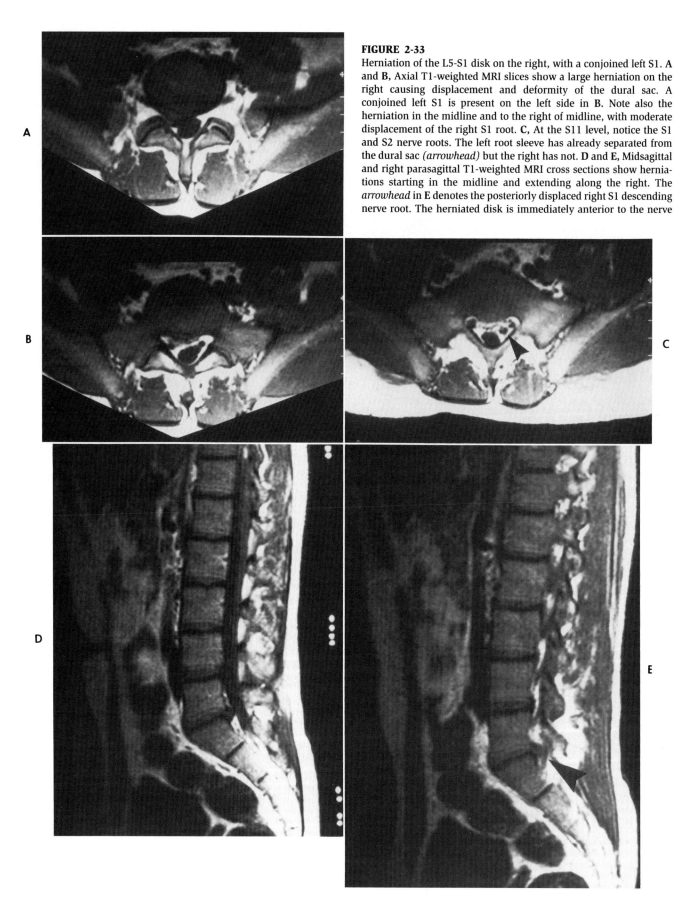

FIGURE 2-33
Herniation of the L5-S1 disk on the right, with a conjoined left S1. **A**
and **B,** Axial T1-weighted MRI slices show a large herniation on the
right causing displacement and deformity of the dural sac. A
conjoined left S1 is present on the left side in **B.** Note also the
herniation in the midline and to the right of midline, with moderate
displacement of the right S1 root. **C,** At the S11 level, notice the S1
and S2 nerve roots. The left root sleeve has already separated from
the dural sac *(arrowhead)* but the right has not. **D** and **E,** Midsagittal
and right parasagittal T1-weighted MRI cross sections show herniations starting in the midline and extending along the right. The
arrowhead in **E** denotes the posteriorly displaced right S1 descending
nerve root. The herniated disk is immediately anterior to the nerve

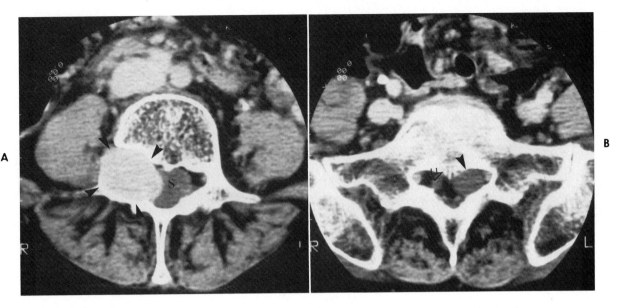

FIGURE 2-34

Neurofibroma and root cyst in the same patient. **A,** An axial CT slice through the pedicle of L5, soft tissue window setting, shows a soft tissue mass on the right *(arrowheads)*. (**S** is on the dural sac.) The right pedicle has been eroded. Note the sclerotic margin of the eroded bone anteriorly and posteriorly, indicating a long-standing pressure defect due to the slow-growing neoplasm. The lesion did not fill with contrast on myelography. At surgery a neurofibroma was found. **B,** At the S1 level the *arrowhead* denotes an enlarged S2 root sleeve on the left (root cyst). The *hollow arrow* is pointing to the normal S2 root sleeve on the right.

occasionally resembles an HNP but may not be one[35] (Fig. 2-35). There are least three reasons for this:

a. In patients whose disk height is preserved, the posterior margin of the disk must necessarily extend from the vertebral endplate below to the endplate of the anteriorly displaced vertebra above. Therefore at least some of the disk will be situated behind the endplate of the vertebra above and axial cross sections that encompass it will show it to be protruding into the spinal canal behind the vertebral endplate, simulating a herniated disk (Fig. 2-35). This is a normal configuration and not due to HNP.

b. In patients whose disk is significantly narrowed, a partial volume effect with the vertebral endplate(s) occurs. Depending upon the thickness of the disk and the presence or absence of scoliosis or tilting of the vertebral endplates, one or two partially calcified (bilateral or unilateral) densities may be noted at the posterior disk border[35] (Fig. 2-36). A herniated disk will be obscured by these superimposed densities.

c. In patients whose spondylolisthesis is long standing, disruption of the annulus may lead to herniation of the disk (Figs. 2-37 and 2-38). A herniated disk in these cases has the same imaging characteristics as in the other cases, but careful analysis will usually reveal a focal irregularity on the posterior disk surface indicating superimposition of the herniation on the

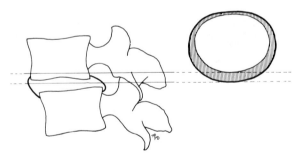

FIGURE 2-35

Schematic representation of spondylolisthesis. An axial slice encompassing the inferior endplate of the verterbral body that has slipped forward will show a soft tissue density posterior to the endplate. This is the intervertebral disk, which (of necessity) is posterior to the endplate (which has slipped forward). Note the oblique posterior disk margin. The image of the disk may be confused with the image of the herniation, and a small herniation may thus be missed. An axial slice encompassing the superior endplate of a vertebra that has not slipped anteriorly will show no significant extension of the disk margin posterior to it as long as the disk is normal. If the disk is narrow, a 4 to 5 mm slice may encompass both endplates and will show two rings of density (containing bone).

Text continued on p. 95.

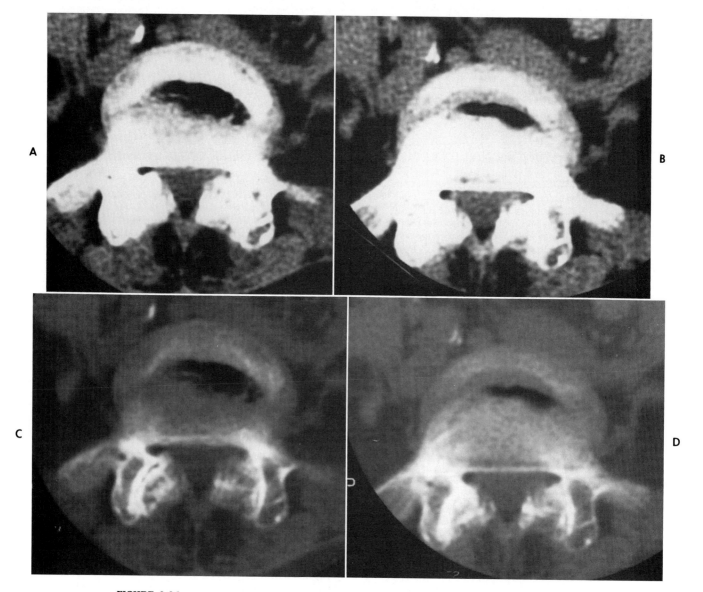

FIGURE 2-36
Stenosis of the spinal canal and lateral recess due to degenerative spondylolisthesis. A to D, Soft tissue and bone windows at L5-S1 show a vacuum phenomenon, degenerative disease of the facet joints, and spinal stenosis. There is also a slight anterior slipping of the L5 facets, which has caused stenosis of the lateral recess.

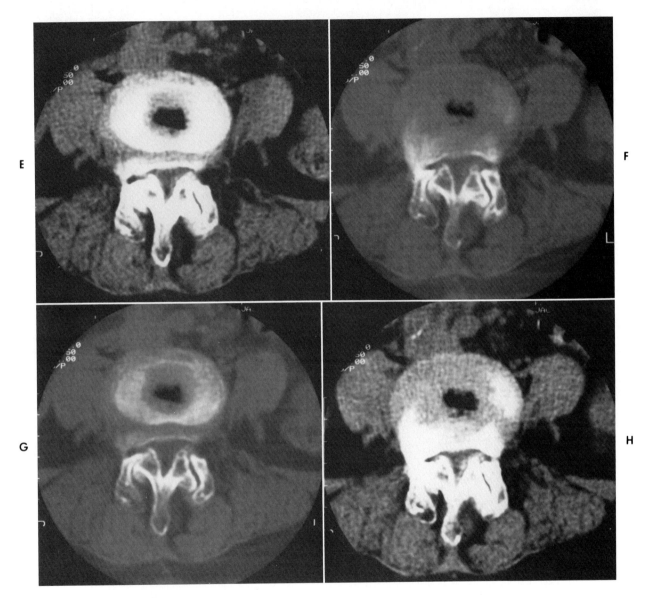

FIGURE 2-36, cont'd
E to H, Soft tissue and bone windows at L4-5 reveal the vacuum phenomenon, along with degenerative disease of the facet joints. There is also a spinal stenosis resulting from the anterior slippage of L4 and the lateral recess stenosis secondary to anterior slippage of the L4 facets.

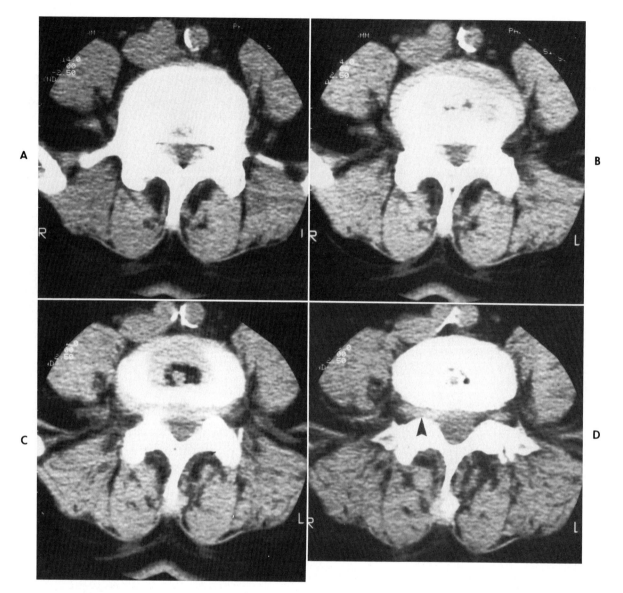

FIGURE 2-37

Degenerative spondylolisthesis and disk herniation at two levels. **A** to **D,** Soft tissue windows at L4-5 and, **E** to **H,** corresponding bone windows, CT examination. There is chronic degenerative disk disease, evidenced by the vacuum phenomenon (best seen in **C** and **G**). Note the spondylolisthesis at L4-5, accounting for the soft tissue density on the posterior disk margin that projects posterior to the posterior margin of the inferior L4 endplate (see Fig. 2-35). (**A, B, E,** and **F** show the L5 superior endplate with stenosis of the canal at that level. Notice also the degenerative disease of the facet joints [**E, F, G,** and **H**].) The soft tissue mass in **D** *(arrowhead)* occupies the right L4-5 neural foramen and distorts the ganglion of the right L4 spinal nerve root. Compare this with the normal left side. It proved to be an intraforaminal disk herniation. **I** and **J,** Axial CT slices at L5-S1 show herniation of the disk to the left of midline *(arrow in J),* causing posterior displacement and distortion of the left S1 nerve root. The *arrow* in **I** denotes the normal right S1 nerve root. This case illustrates some of the difficulties encountered in pinpointing the exact cause of clinical findings in spondylolisthesis.

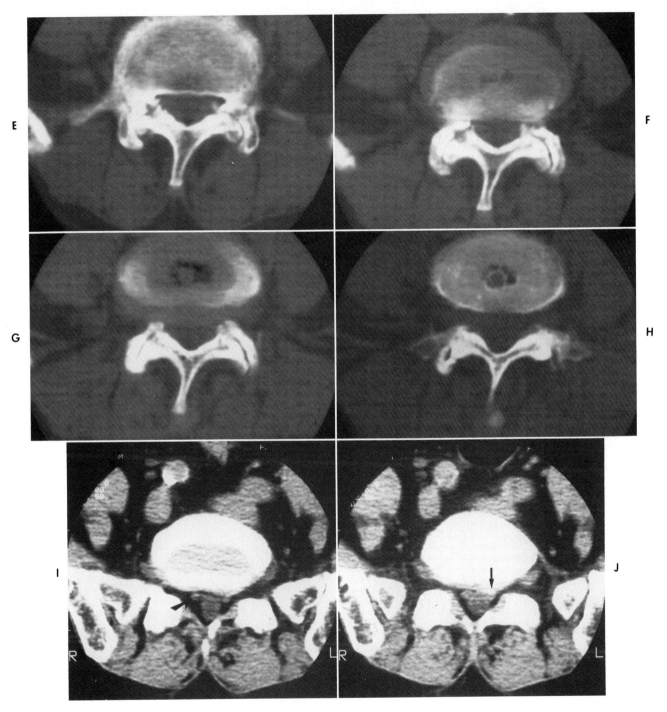

FIGURE 2-37, cont'd
For legend see opposite page.

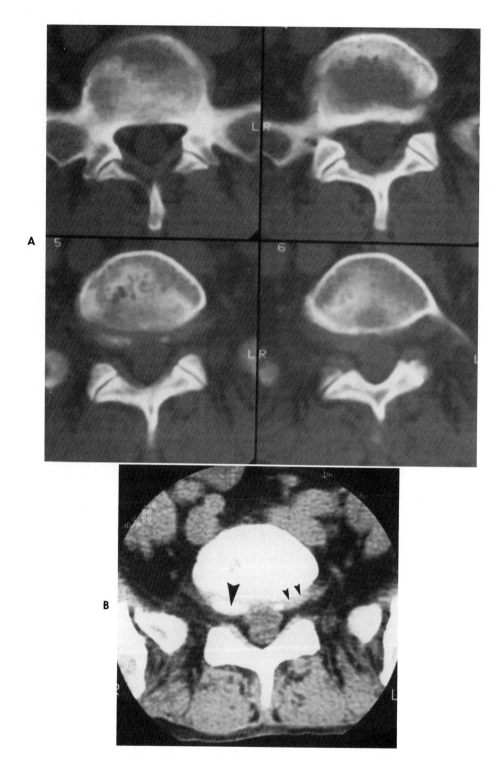

FIGURE 2-38
Herniated disk in spondylolisthesis. **A,** Bone windows at L5-S1 and, **B,** a soft tissue window at this level show the crown of soft tissue density (*small arrowheads* in **B**) that projects posterior to the inferior L5 endplate. It contains calcification and is secondary to marked lordosis at this level as well as a slight spondylolisthesis. The calcific density in **B** *(large arrowhead)* is due to a partial vacuum effect with the posterior edge of the superior S1 endplate. **C,** A soft tissue window through L5 just below the pedicles and another, **D,** through the pedicles show a fragment of the herniated L5-S1 disk *(arrow)* trapped in the right lateral recess of L5. It extends inferiorly into the top of the neural foramen *(arrow* in **C)** and obscures the right L5 dorsal root ganglion.

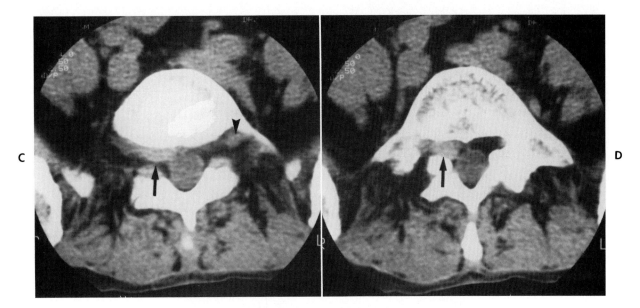

FIGURE 2-38, cont'd
For legend see opposite page.

spondylolisthesis. CT detection of an HNP in these patients may be difficult.

• • •

We have examined two groups of patients with spondylolisthesis and compared our preoperative diagnoses with the findings at surgery.

CT and CT-myelography. Among 179 patients with spondylolisthesis studied by CT, we found 112 with the condition secondary to degenerative arthrosis of the facet joints and 67 with the condition due to a defect in the neural arch (spondylolysis). Forty-six patients underwent surgery for back pain, sciatica, or spinal stenosis. Their preoperative CT reports were retrieved and compared to the findings at surgery:

> 8 herniated disks, 37 spinal stenoses, and 6 neural foraminal stenoses were recorded on CT prior to surgery whereas 14 disk herniations, 42 spinal stenoses, and 3 neural foraminal stenoses were noted at surgery.
>
> 8 herniated disks observed at surgery were in patients in whom this diagnosis had been made preoperatively; six were missed preoperatively.
>
> In 38 cases CT-myelography was performed and furnished additional information indicative of disk herniation or spinal stenosis in 6.
>
> The correlation between CT-myelography and surgery was better than 95%.

Although disk herniation at the level of a spondylolisthesis was once thought to be rare,[36] in our experience it has not been. Rothman and Glenn[35] noted herniation in 26% of patients with spondylolisthesis and a pars defect. We discovered it in 37% of our patients (both degenerative spondylolisthesis and spondylolysis) (Fig. 2-39). Preoperative CT diagnosis of disk herniation in spondylolisthesis is difficult because of distortion of the

spinal canal, spinal stenosis, the partial volume effect of the vertebral endplates, and the inevitable oblique slant of the posterior disk margin. The overall accuracy of preoperative CT diagnoses in these patients is about 70%. Myelography is even less helpful. However, CT-myelography increases the accuracy of the diagnosis to better than 95%.

MRI. Among 132 patients with spondylolisthesis evaluated by MRI, we found 97 with the condition due to degenerative arthrosis of the facet joints and 45 with it secondary to a defect in the neural arch. Computed tomography of the spine was performed in 113 of these patients, and 21 underwent surgery. Comparison of CT and MRI revealed the two modalities to be almost equal in their ability to elucidate the diagnosis in these patients.

> 11 patients had documented disk herniation at surgery; 7 were diagnosed by CT and 8 by MRI prior to surgery.
>
> In 2 patients CT diagnosis of a herniated disk was made prior to surgery; MRI failed to reveal the herniation.
>
> In 3 patients MRI detected a surgically verified herniated disk that was missed at preoperative CT.

Correlation. All told, an accurate diagnosis of disk herniation preoperatively was made in 10 of 11 patients with spondylolisthesis and disk herniation when CT and MRI results were considered together. Comparison of the two groups reveals a noticeable improvement in diagnostic accuracy when both modalities are used.

Myelography. Myelography was performed in 12 patients (57%) who underwent surgery and had received preoperative CT and MRI. In these patients no significant additional information was noted. The accuracy of CT and MRI combined was almost equal to that of CT-myelography. The optimal work-up therefore seems to be CT or MRI as the initial examination and if the diagnosis is not established with either of these then the other is per-

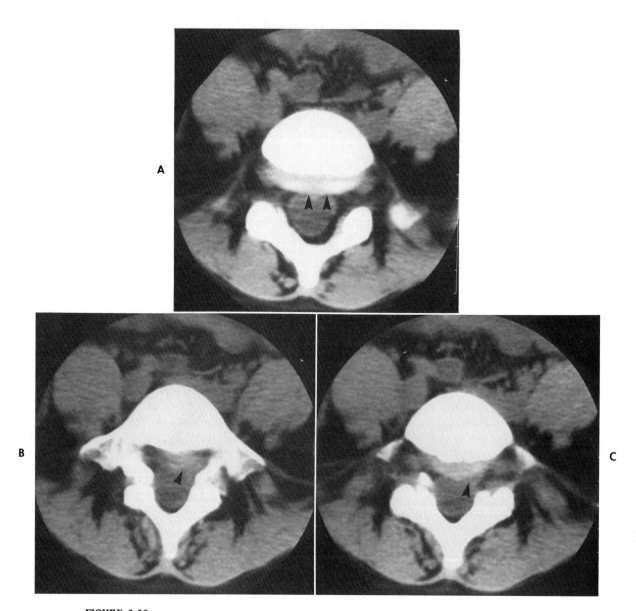

FIGURE 2-39
Spondylolysis and spondylolisthesis complicated by disk herniation at L5-S1, CT examination. **A,** The
arrowheads indicate the characteristic deformity produced by spondylolisthesis and also the marked
lordosis of the L5-S1 angle in this patient. Note the anteroposterior elongation of the spinal canal. **B** and
C, Just above L5-S1. The *arrowhead* points to a disk herniation in the midline and slightly to the left
of midline.

formed. Myelography should be done only when the diagnosis is not established following both CT and MRI examination.

Magnetic resonance imaging
LOW BACK PAIN, SCIATICA, AND STENOSIS

To reduce patients' anxiety and apprehension, we try to explain the MRI procedure to them. For those who are markedly apprehensive or claustrophobic, explanation and reassurance by the physician may be helpful. Some do remarkably well if they are taught relaxation exercises a few days prior to the examination. When necessary, a mild short-acting sedative may be given before the procedure. If a patient is bothered by the noises of the MRI imager, we offer earplugs (to block the noise) or headphones (for listening to music). To ensure cooperation, we make the patients as comfortable as possible with pillows and cushions.

Then we obtain the following:
1. Coronal T1 (scout)
2. Sagittal T1
3. Sagittal T2
4. Axial T1

Additional sequences and alternatives are
1. A sagittal gradient echo, along with (or instead of), T2
2. An axial gradient echo, along with T1, to differentiate an osteophyte from a herniated disk
3. A sagittal and axial proton density
4. A midsagittal serial multiecho

The patient is placed on the spine surface coil and moved into the magnet. A set of coronal T1-weighted images (T1-WI) is obtained for localization purposes (scout). With a fairly short TR/TE, a reduced matrix, and a 25 to 30 cm field of view, these images are obtained in 1 to 2 minutes. Utilizing the coordinates from the coronals, we program sagittal T1- and T2-weighted images (T2-WI) to extend from neural foramen to neural foramen. To ensure an accurate counting of the lumbar vertebrae, sagittal cross sections must include the conus medullaris region and the lower thoracic cord as well as the sacrum.

The choice of technical parameters is dependent upon the MRI imager used and the preference of the physicians. The protocol must take into consideration the required number of slices, the slice thickness, interslice gap, and signal to noise ratio (S/N), and the number of excitations (NEX) (also called signal averages [NSA]). For the T1-WI sequence, a TR of about 500 to 700 msec, a TE of 20 to 25 msec, a slice thickness of 4-5 mm, and a matrix of 256×256 are used. On a high field (1.5 tesla) T1-WI sagittal cross sections of acceptable quality would take 4 to 6 minutes, given the technical capabilities of the high field MRI imagers in 1991. T1-WI sagittal cross sections are useful for an overall evaluation of the morphology of the vertebrae, bone marrow, intervertebral disks, spinal cord, spinal canal, and conus medullaris. T2-WI sagittal cross sections are useful for a myelographic effect,

visualization of the subarachnoid space, and detection of signal abnormalities of the disks and spinal cord. Intermediate, or "balanced," TR/TE images (proton density [PD] or spin density[SD]) may also be obtained as part of the sequence of T2-WI cross sections (Fig. 2-40); however, when T1-WI cross-sections are also obtained PD images are not usually necessary. Furthermore, on some MRI imagers the T2-WI images will be of higher quality without the first sequence (PD) images. T2-weighted sagittal cross sections with a TR of about 1800 to 2400 msec and a TE of 80 to 100 msec may then be utilized. Axial cross sections are necessary for a reliable evaluation of lumbar disk contour. In most instances T1-WI axial cross sections are sufficient. Gradient echo axial images may be needed for differentiating an osteophyte from a herniated disk. On these images osteophytes are black whereas noncalcified herniated disks are bright. T2-WI axial cross sections may become necessary when T1-WI axial views are not diagnostic.

Each disk is examined by means of axial slices angled parallel to its midplane. Furthermore, obtaining one or two slices through an abnormal disk is not sufficient for a meaningful evaluation of that disk level. The axial slices must extend from pedicle to pedicle to ensure that cephalad or caudad extension of a herniation or other pathological process within the spinal canal and neural foramina is identified. In short, the technique for MRI axial examination of the lumbar spine is similar to that for CT lumbar examination. At present, a full package of axial T1-WI slices can be obtained for three or four abnormal disks without markedly prolonging the MRI examination time.

Gradient echo imaging is an alternative method that can be used to obtain a myelographic effect in a shorter period as compared to the routine spin echo T2-WI sequence. Gradient echo images are also more helpful in visualizing the facet joints.

There are presently a number of devices and technical innovations[37-42] that can help improve overall image quality and eliminate artifacts in the lumbar spine. They include specially designed surface coils, fold-over suppression, gradient refocusing, cardiac gating, flow compensation, and presaturation techniques. The pace of technical improvements in MRI has been astonishing during the first few years of its widespread clinical application. It is to be hoped that in the near future, examination times can be significantly reduced. At that time we would be able to perform MR imaging in multiple planes, utilizing several angles and pulse sequences in every patient. This (hopefully) will help uncover disorders that currently escape detection. They escape not so much because of the limitations of MRI as because there is an inability to obtain these pulse sequences in a reasonably short time interval.

Normal lumbar disk: MRI characteristics. The normal lumbar disk has essentially two more or less distinct regions of signal intensity.

On short TR/short TE images (T1-weighted) the differ-

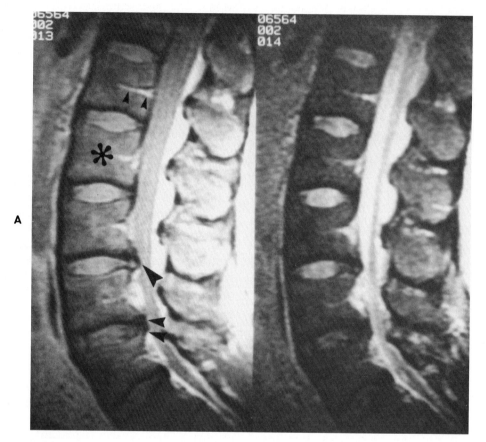

FIGURE 2-40

Normal and herniated lumbar disks. **A,** Midsagittal MRI, TR 2000/TE 50 and 100. The *asterisk* is on L2. *Two small arrowheads* denote the normal basivertebral vein of L1. There is herniation of the L3-4 disk *(arrowhead).* Note that the signal void of the APLL complex is not disrupted. There is also midline herniation of L4-5 *(two medium-sized arrowheads).* **B** to **G,** Axial slices, TR 1000/TE 20. (**B,** Normal L1-2 disk, **C,** normal L2-3 disk, and, **D** to **F,** normal L3-4 disk. There is herniation of the L3-4 disk, with the *arrowhead* in **E** pointing to a signal void at the margin of the herniated material [which corresponds to the intact outermost fibers of the APLL complex]. **D** is 5 mm below **E** through the pedicles of L4. The *arrowhead* denotes the herniated material, which has extended inferiorly and is indenting the anterior wall of the dural sac. **F,** 5 mm above **E,** at the level of the L3 dorsal root ganglion *[two small arrowheads on the left].* The *larger arrowhead* designates the midline herniation. This slice crosses through the superior portion of the herniated material, consisting mainly of annulus fibrosus and the posterior longitudinal ligament, which accounts for the markedly low signal of this region. **G,** Normal L4-5 disk. The *large arrowhead on the left* denotes the disk herniation. The *small arrow on the right* is pointing to the normal right exiting spinal nerve.)

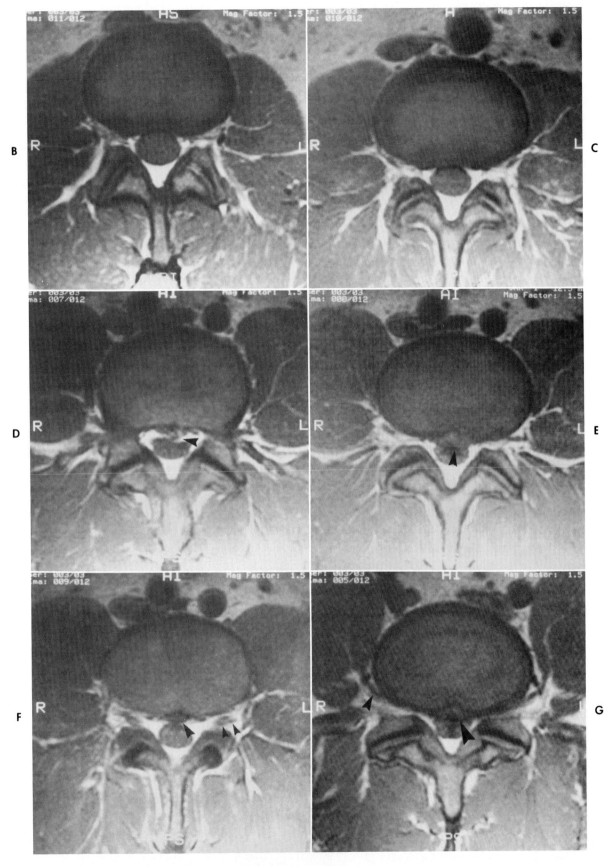

FIGURE 2-40, cont'd
For legend see opposite page.

ence between the two regions of signal is not pronounced; in fact, it may be nonexistent. The outermost fibers of the annulus and the confluence of the annular fibers with the anterior and posterior longitudinal ligament fibers appear as a gray-black band outlining the peripheral margin of the disk (Fig. 1-44). The remainder of the disk (i.e., the inner fibers of the annulus and the nucleus) are of low signal intensity but may be slightly brighter than the peripheral region. In many patients the entire disk is of a homogeneously low signal intensity and the peripheral margin cannot be differentiated from the rest of the disk. The signal pattern of the vertebral bodies (vertebral marrow) is dependent on the age of the patient and the extent of fat replacement within the marrow. In children and young adults, in whom nonfatty cellular elements predominate, the marrow may be quite low in signal. With advancing age and an increase in the yellow marrow fraction, the signal intensity increases. In middle-aged subjects the vertebral body signal is of intermediate strength, somewhere between the signals of paraspinal fat and muscle. The vertebral cortex and endplates appear as a thin band of low signal, or signal void. In older individuals there may be extensive fatty infiltration of the marrow (Figs. 1-1 to 1-3). The signal characteristics of the basivertebral venous plexus are dependent on the amount of fat surrounding the venous channels, the size of the channels, and in certain instances the status of venous flow (Figs. 1-13 and 2-40). The intervertebral disk is of lower signal intensity than the vertebral bone marrow. Cerebrospinal fluid (CSF) is usually indistinguishable from ligaments and the cortex of the vertebral bodies, all appearing as black areas of signal void. The ligamentum flavum may have moderately higher signal intensity than the other spinal ligaments. The conus medullaris is usually well seen, with its moderately bright signal

surrounded by dark CSF, dura, and the cortex of the bony spinal canal.

On T2-weighted images the central portion of the intervertebral disk is bright. A black line may be noted in the equator of the disk, the so-called intranuclear cleft. The central high signal intensity region corresponds to the nucleus pulposus and the cartilaginous fibers of the inner portion of the annulus fibrosus. The outer fibers of the annulus remain as a band of gray-black. The vertebral marrow loses some of its brightness because of the moderate T2 of fat. The CSF becomes intensely bright, with a myelographic effect. The spinal cord and conus medullaris have relatively lower signal but still stand out clearly against the bright CSF. The width of the subarachnoid space is well delineated on this pulse sequence.

The MRI features of normal and abnormal vertebrae and intervertebral disks on gradient echo sequence (T2*) are dependent upon (among other factors) the TR/TE and the flip angle chosen (Fig. 2-41). However, as a rule, the following pertain:

There is a thin band of low signal intensity at the periphery of the disk, often thinner than the corresponding area on long TR/long TE images.

The central portion of the disk has a bright signal and the intranuclear cleft is usually not visible.

The vertebral marrow is quite low in signal,[43] but the facet joints are fairly well delineated.

The articular cartilage is of moderately high signal and stands out clearly against the black articular cortex.

Some MR imagers permit a single slice to be imaged in sequentially lengthening echo times (TE). This is useful for a survey type of study, when several TR/TE combinations may be employed. We select a midsagittal slice (usually 10 mm thick), a TR of about 900 msec, and eight echos (at a TR/TE of 900/30, 900/60. . .900/240). As

A   **B**

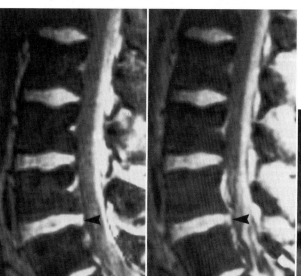

C

FIGURE 2-41
Disk herniation at L4-5. **A,** Midsagittal and, **B,** immediately parasagittal MRI cross sections of the lumbar spine (gradient echo). The *arrowheads* point to the herniation. **C,** Axial cross section at L4-5. In this image the herniation is better appreciated *(arrowhead).*

the TE is increased significantly, T2-weighting becomes evident even though the TR is not long. At a TE of approximately 120 msec a prominent T2 effect is obtained. The signal falls rapidly, of course, with long TEs and the image is degraded. This sequence may be useful when a puzzling signal pattern of the spinal cord, disk, bone marrow, or surrounding soft tissues is encountered. Examples include vertebral hemangioma, particularly when associated with acute trauma, cysts and abscesses of the vertebral body, vascular abormalities of the cord, and questionable zones of abnormal signal in the cord.

On long TR/short TE images (spin density or proton density) the CSF is gray and the spinal cord and bone marrow are of intermediate signal strength (Fig. 2-40). This sequence takes less time but is a poor substitute for T2-weighted images. In some patients the differences between disk, CSF, and neural elements may not be great enough to permit a definitive diagnosis.

MRI of the abnormal lumbar disk. Degeneration of the lumbar intervertebral disks leads to a reduction of signal from the central portion of the disk on T2-WI. However, gradient echo images are not particularly sensitive to disk pathology in most instances because a degenerated disk may appear as bright as a normal disk. In advanced stages the contrast between the central and peripheral portions of the disk is lost on T2-WI and the entire disk is of low signal intensity. Although there is a loss of water from the disk, this fact alone cannot explain the full extent of the signal loss.

In addition to the loss of water, other physical and chemical changes occur in degenerative disk disease[7,44-47] and most likely play a role in the reduction of signal from the disk. The reduced signal is often associated with a decrease in the height of the disk (though this is not a constant finding). A disk with clearly low signal on MRI may appear normal for all practical purposes on conventional radiography. It may also be normal on CT. Despite the lack of unequivocal proof (i.e., pathological evidence of degeneration in a large number of disks with low signal), the general assumption is that the loss of signal on T2-WI indicates degenerative disease.

A lumbar disk with low signal intensity on T2-WI may not exhibit any other abnormality. There may be no associated bulging or herniation. In our experience, reduced signal from the L4-5 and L5-S1 intervertebral disks without associated bulging or herniation is seen in many adults referred for back pain and sciatica. The clinical significance of this, however, remains to be determined. At present, the exact prevalence of disk degeneration (low signal on T2) in a large number of adults without any symptoms is not known. Boden et al.[48] reported their MRI findings in 67 asymptomatic individuals. Some 34% of 20-to-39-year-olds, 59% of 40-to-59-year-olds, and all 60-to-80-year-olds but one had degeneration of the lumbar disks. We have observed diminished signal from L4-5, L5-S1, and other disks on MRI examination in 19 of 60 adult patients (30%) 37 to 69 years of age (mean 57 years) referred for other than back pain and sciatica. As documented by Coventry et al.,[10,11] degenerative changes of the disk occur as early as the second and third decades and become quite common with advancing age. MRI demonstration of low signal intensity (on T2-WI) from intervertebral disks probably represents in vivo evidence of degenerative changes.

It should be noted that on gradient echo images a degenerated disk may be indistinguishable from a normal disk. Although identification of a herniated disk (which has a bright signal on gradient echo images) and differentiation of it from an osteophyte (which is usually low in signal) are facilitated by gradient echo imaging, one should be aware of the disadvantages of this technique. There is an inherently lower signal to noise ratio, an increased susceptibility to motion artifacts and field non-homogeneity, and a masking of vertebral (marrow) pathologies. Gradient echo images, however, are usually more sensitive than spin echo sequences in detecting calcification and gas (vacuum phenomenon) within the disk.

• • •

The criteria for diagnosing a herniated disk on MRI are similar to those for making such a diagnosis on CT and have been discussed earlier in this chapter. We will now consider the findings that are especially pertinent to MRI. A clear advantage of MRI is that it provides direct sagittal as well as axial cross sections and these facilitate and improve the evaluation of disk diseases.

Bulging of the disk. The peripheral margin of the annulus fibrosus of a normal lumbar disk is usually convex in both the cephalocaudal and the horizontal plane. This means that the disk margin extends beyond the edge of its vertebral endplates by as much as (depending upon how it is measured) 2 to 3 mm. In patients with spinal stenosis, because the posterior vertebral surface often has an exaggerated concavity, the endplate margins and disks appear to protrude prominently into the canal. This is an exaggeration of the normal configuration and is normal for these subjects (Figs. 4-5, 4-6, and 4-7). However, even though the vertebral endplates and disk are protruding into the spinal canal, the disk itself does not extend beyond the endplates more than it normally should. Thus, in spinal stenosis, it appears to be bulging although in reality it is normal.

Bulging of a lumbar disk is recognized on MRI when the disk extends in a diffuse and symmetrical fashion beyond the margins of the adjacent vertebral endplates (Fig. 2-42). The margin of a bulging disk is smooth, without a focal irregularity. However, it is not usually possible to evaluate the characteristics of the posterior disk margin or to differentiate bulging from herniation on sagittal images alone. Axial cross sections are essential for this.

Most bulging disks have low signal intensity on T2-weighted images, indicating degeneration. However, approximately a third will be of normal height and have a normal signal pattern. In disks with intrasubstance

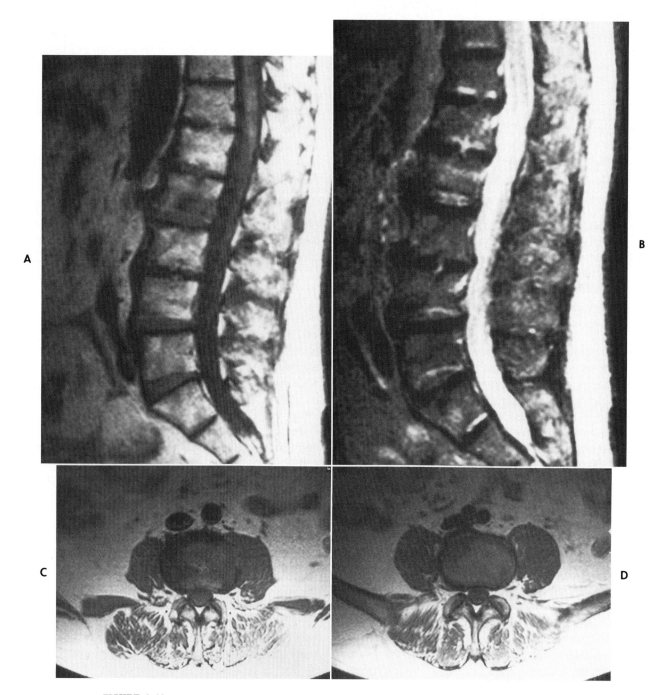

FIGURE 2-42
Bulging of the L3-4 and L4-5 intervertebral disks. **A,** A midsagittal T1-weighted cross section and, **B,** a midsagittal T2-weighted cross section show degenerative disease in practically all lumbar disks, along with moderate bulging. Note the prominent chemical shift artifact at the endplates, accounting for the bright band of signal at the upper margins of the disks and the band of low signal at the lower margins. The band of high signal intensity mimics an intradiscal effusion. An axial T1-weighted cross section at L3-4, **C,** and another at L4-5, **D,** show circumferential bulging. The concavity of the posterior disk margin is preserved. Note the hypertrophic bony ridges and the osteophytes anteriorly, especially to the right of midline, at L4-5.

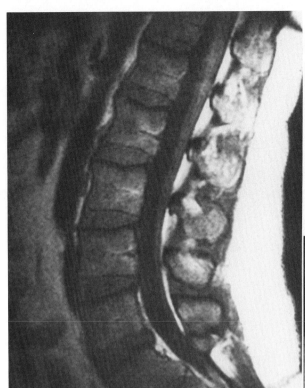

A

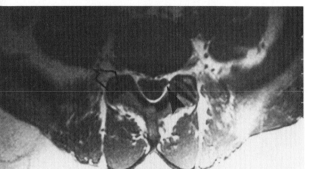

B

FIGURE 2-43
Midline bulge or a small herniation at L5-S1. **A,** Midsagittal and, **B,** axial T1-weighted cross sections show the posterior border of the disk to project more than would be expected normally beyond the margins of the vertebral endplates (better seen on the sagittal view). The dural sac is normal. The axial projection confirms these findings. The descending S1 nerve roots *(arrowhead)* have just started to emerge from the dural sac and are normal. The *hollow arrow on the right* denotes the dorsal root ganglion and origin of the right L5 spinal nerve, which are both normal.

disruption the outer portion of the annulus, which is normally gray-black on T2-weighted images, may be significantly thinner posteriorly. The central portion of the disk, which is usually of higher signal intensity, may be seen to extend into the thinned out zones of the annulus (intrasubstance herniation) without causing a focal deformity of the disk margin. Occasionally cracks and fissures, appearing as linear areas of increased signal, will be seen crossing through the annulus. In general, the contour of a normal disk is similar to that of its vertebral endplates: if the edges of the endplate are round, so are those of the disk; if the endplate has a midline posterior concavity, so should the disk. When a disk has lost its posterior midline concavity, even though it is normal otherwise, bulging is present. If the sole abnormality is a loss of the posterior midline concavity with a questionable focal extension of the midposterior border, it may not be possible to differentiate a small midline herniation from a bulge at L4-5 and L5-S1 (Fig. 2-43).

Although in most bulging disks the height is diminished, in the initial phase of bulging a disk may be of normal height. The various types of marrow changes attributed to disk degeneration may be present with a bulging disk, and the margins of such a disk may be seen extending into the neural foramina on both sides. This is a fairly common phenomenon and in most instances has no clinical significance. Likewise, the posterior margin of a bulging disk may create a smooth rounded impression on the dural sac, usually well seen on T2-weighted sagittal and axial cross sections, but in subjects without spinal stenosis this is usually of no clinical significance. Only when there is severe spinal stenosis may a bulging

disk contribute to the compression of neural elements and thereby become clinically significant.

In patients with advanced degenerative disk disease the height of the disk is markedly diminished and the volume is reduced. The signal intensity on T2-WI is also reduced. In fact, the whole disk may be essentially a zone of signal void when there is resorption or calcification of the central portion of the disk. Many patients with long-standing degenerative disk disease have bulging disk margins that may be calcified or accompanied by vertebral osteophytes. However, to qualify for the designation of bulging, the disk margin must be *smooth* and *rounded*.

There are a number of explanations for this loss of disk volume. Several episodes of herniation followed by displacement and resorption of the disk material probably occur. The herniation process may incite a vascular granulation tissue to form that digests the herniated material and induces scar formation. The locus of the annular rupture fills in, and the disk margin may be only minimally irregular (with no configuration that indicates disk herniation). Gradual desiccation of the disk, from a total average of 85% to 90% water to about 70% or 75%, is responsible for some loss of volume. The nucleus pulposus loses proportionately more water and may become nonexistent.

Disk herniation. The diagnosis of a herniated disk is made on MRI[28,49-51] when the disk margin extending beyond the edge of the vertebral endplate has an irregular contour, often with a focal deformity (Figs. 2-44 to 2-50). The deformity is usually better recognized on axial (Figs. 2-44, *B* and *C,* and 2-45) than on sagittal cross sections. Sagittal cross sections, however, may show an interrup-

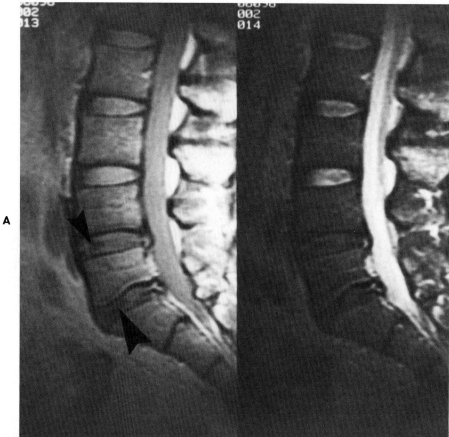

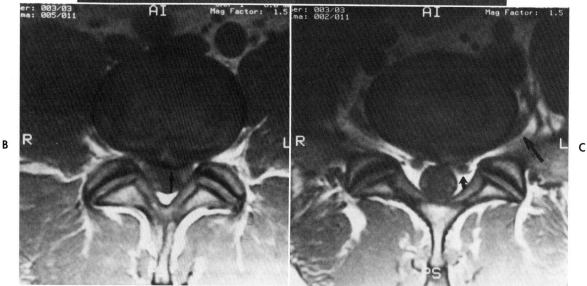

FIGURE 2-44
Herniation of the L4-5 and L5-S1 disks. Midsagittal MR of the lumbar spine, **A** (TR 1800/TE 30 and 80), **B,** L4-5 (TR 1000/TE 20), and, **C,** L5-S1 (TR 1000/TE 20). Sagittal cross sections show the loss of signal from L4-5 and L5-S1 best. The posterior borders of L4-5 and L5-S1 extend beyond the vertebral endplates and are indenting the anterior surface of the dural sac. There is an area of signal void in the anterior portion of the L4-5 *(small arrowhead* in **A**) and L5-S1 *(large arrowhead)* disks. On CT examination some calcification as well as gas (a vacuum phenomenon) could be seen. In **B,** note the L4-5 disk herniation *(arrow),* with an irregular contour. Note also the area of medium-increased signal in its center and the adjacent black line (signal void). This corresponds to the APLL complex, which is intact at this level. In **C,** notice the herniation of disk material in the midline and to the left, with displacement of the left S1 nerve root posteriorly *(small curved arrow).* The *large arrow* denotes the origin of the left L5 exiting spinal nerve, which is normal.

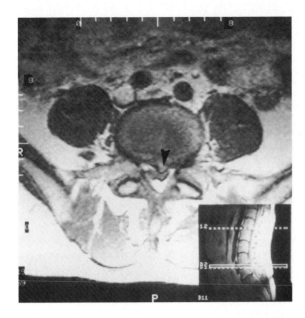

FIGURE 2-45
L4-5 herniated disk. A T1-weighted cross section MRI through the disk shows herniation to the left of midline *(arrowhead)*. The herniated material is hyperintense relative to the disk and confined by a line of signal void (representing the annulus fibrosus and posterior longitudinal ligament).

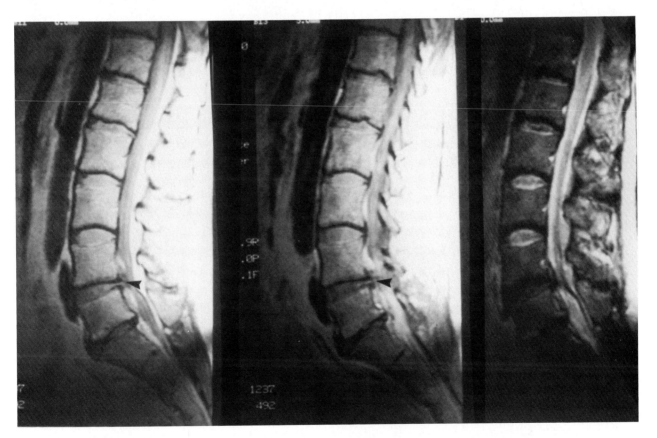

FIGURE 2-46
Tear of the annulus–posterior longitudinal ligament (APLL) complex associated with a herniated disk. Midsagittal and left parasagittal MRI cross sections of the lumbar spine (TR 2000/TE 20) and a midsagittal cross section (TR 2000/TE 80) show marked reduction of signal from the L4-5 disk and reduction of both signal and height from L5-S1, indicating degenerative disk disease. The *arrowhead* is pointing to the APLL tear at L4-5.

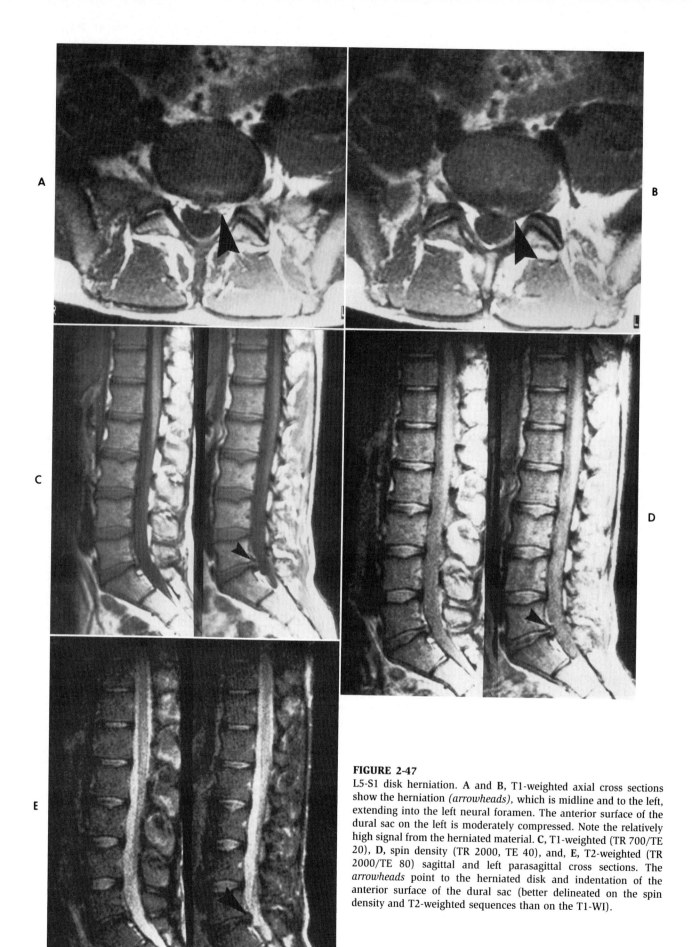

FIGURE 2-47

L5-S1 disk herniation. **A** and **B**, T1-weighted axial cross sections show the herniation *(arrowheads)*, which is midline and to the left, extending into the left neural foramen. The anterior surface of the dural sac on the left is moderately compressed. Note the relatively high signal from the herniated material. **C**, T1-weighted (TR 700/TE 20), **D**, spin density (TR 2000, TE 40), and, **E**, T2-weighted (TR 2000/TE 80) sagittal and left parasagittal cross sections. The *arrowheads* point to the herniated disk and indentation of the anterior surface of the dural sac (better delineated on the spin density and T2-weighted sequences than on the T1-WI).

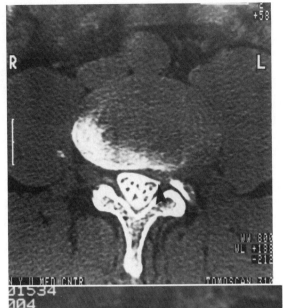

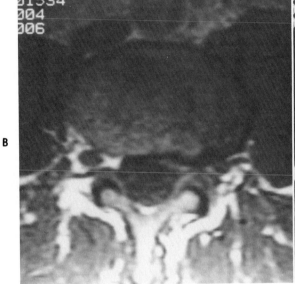

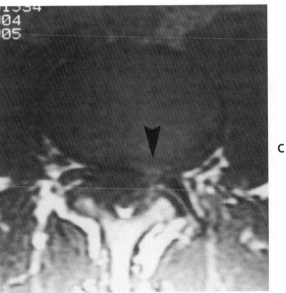

FIGURE 2-48
Small disk herniation. **A,** A CT-myelogram at L3-4 shows the left anterolateral dural sac *(arrowhead)* compressed, with a small epidural defect. At surgery the herniation was found to extend into the left neural foramen. **B** and **C,** Corresponding T1-weighted MRI examinations at L3-4 show the herniated disk material as an area of medium-low signal in the anterolateral epidural space on the left *(arrowhead* in **C**).

tion or tear of the annulus–posterior longitudinal ligament (APLL) complex to better advantage (Fig. 2-46). Disruption of the APLL complex can be identified on any of the routine pulse sequences utilized (T1-weighted, proton density, T2-weighted) or gradient echo sequences, though it usually is more prominent on one set of parameters than on another. It is seldom possible to predict which parameters will show the disruption to best advantage, nevertheless, we have found the overall extent of compression and deformity of the dural sac to be better displayed on sagittal cross sections. The effacement of nerve roots and spinal nerves, on the other hand, is better seen on axial cross sections (Fig. 2-50).

Most herniations occur in disks that are already degenerated, but this is not invariably the case. A herniation may develop in a disk that is of normal configuration and signal intensity (usually in a young patient after significant trauma to the spine), though it is

much less likely in the lumbar region. On T2-WI, and on other pulse sequences as well, the herniated material in degenerative disk disease may be isointense, hypointense, or hyperintense relative to the disk of origin (Figs. 2-44, 2-45, and 2-47). The APLL complex may be identified as a line of signal void, often not torn, at the leading edge of the herniated material (Figs. 2-44, *B* and 2-45). A less frequently encountered pattern is a herniation in which there is disruption of the APLL-complex with extension of the hyperintense disk material through the defect beyond the confines of the disk (Fig. 2-46). The herniated material, which on histological examination is usually found to consist of both annulus and nucleus, may extend into the spinal canal in a cephalad or caudad direction and become detached from the parent disk (free fragment or sequestered fragment). Free fragments often are hyperintense on T2-WI. The parent disk itself is frequently of low intensity and may have a markedly nonhomogenous

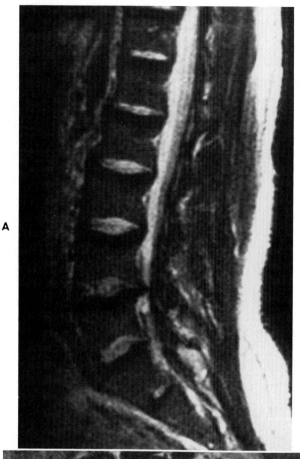

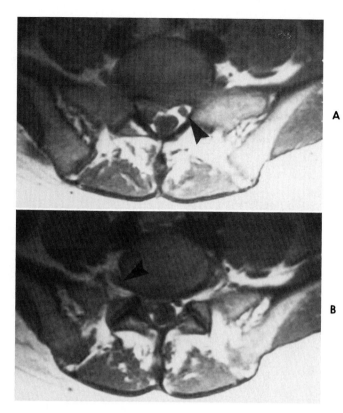

FIGURE 2-50
L5-S1 herniation on the right side. A and B, T1-weighted axial MR slices show distortion of the anterior epidural fat and displacement of the right S1 nerve root posteriorly. The *arrowhead* in A denotes the normal S1 descending root on the left, surrounded by epidural fat. In B the *arrowhead* points to the normal exiting L5 spinal nerve on the right.

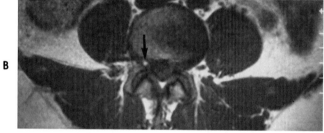

FIGURE 2-49
Focal disk herniation on the posterior left side. A, Parasagittal T2-weighted MRI of the lumbar spine. Note the herniation at L4-5. B, An axial T1-weighted image shows normal epidural fat in the anterolateral spinal canal *(arrow)*. There is a posterolateral herniation on the left, which has obliterated the fat.

signal because of calcification and zones of fibrosis or scarring and the vacuum phenomenon. These abnormalities may not be clearly delineated on spin echo imaging; gradient echo is more sensitive in delineating calcification and the vacuum phenomenon.

On sagittal cross sections there will often be displacement of epidural fat away from the level of the herniated disk (Fig. 2-46). The disk material pushes the fat to a point above or below the disk. Occasionally a herniated disk will distend and displace the epidural veins, and in this situation one may see a 2 to 3 mm thick layer of

moderately bright signal on the posterior surface of the vertebral body; this is soft tissue with signal characteristics of a vein on various pulse sequences, including enhancement following intravenous gadopentetate administration. These venous channels are usually more conspicuous on parasagittal cross sections. Unlike epidural fat, which can be interrupted and displaced cephalad and caudad, the epidural veins are displaced only posteriorly or to the sides. The pattern of disk disruption and intradiskal herniation, often clearly visible on macroscopic inspection of degenerated disks, is occasionally identified on T2-weighted axial cross sections. Future improvements in spatial resolution of MRI, particularly in the axial plane, may make it possible to study internal disruption of the disk in more detail.

An intraforaminal herniation (Fig. 2-51) is diagnosed on MRI when the herniated material is seen encroaching into the neural foramen. The dorsal root ganglion is usually engulfed by the material, and the fat within the foramen may be completely obliterated. These features are equally well displayed on axial and sagittal cross sections (Figs. 2-20 and 2-51).

FIGURE 2-51
Intraforaminal disk herniation. **A,** T1-weighted axial at L5-S1 showing herniation of the disk into the right neural foramen, obliterating the fat and the dorsal root ganglion of L5. The *arrowhead* denotes the normal L5 ganglion on the left. **B,** Parasagittal T1-weighted cross section. Note the herniation and partial obliteration of the dorsal root ganglion *(large arrowhead)*. Compare this with the normal L5-S1 neural foramen, containing fat and surrounding the L5 dorsal root ganglion on the left side (*large arrowhead* in **C**). The *smaller arrowhead* in **B** denotes the dorsal root ganglion of L3 on the right side. **D,** T1-weighted axial cross section at S1. The descending S1 nerve roots were not affected. The *arrowhead* is pointing to the normal descending nerve root.

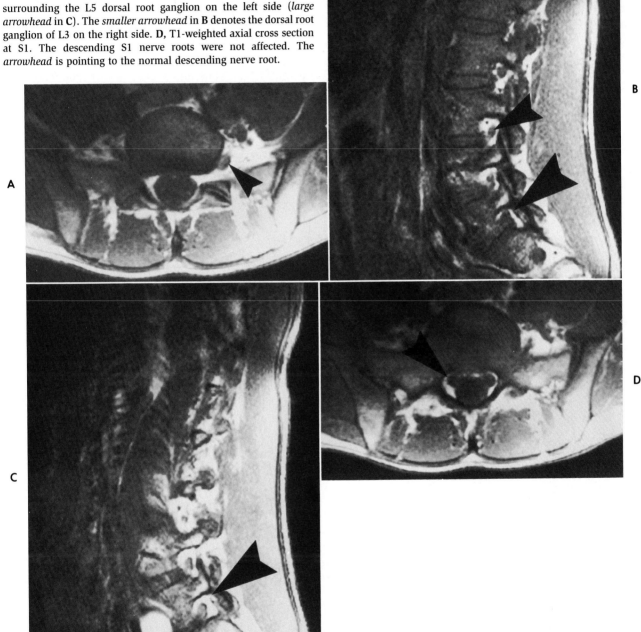

In some patients the herniated disk material has markedly low signal intensity on both T1- and T2-weighted images, possibly because of calcification and/or osteophytes. To differentiate these lesions from a herniated disk, we often use gradient echo images. On this pulse sequence the disk material usually has medium to high signal intensity while calcification and osteosclerotic osteophytes stay as zones of signal void. We use gradient echo imaging in addition to spin echo in most instances because a small herniated disk (which may be isointense with CSF) often will be missed when gradient echo imaging is the sole pulse sequence utilized.

Intravenous gadopentetate[42] is not ordinarily used in patients without a history of previous disk surgery. However, in difficult cases it may be helpful. For example, it may be beneficial in patients with degenerative disk disease to enhance the disk margins, and occasionally it

highlights the substance of the disk itself, similar to what occurs with intravenous contrast CT. The enhancement is due to the normally existing vascularity of the annular margin[12] and to vascular granulation tissue that forms in response to the disruption and tearing of the annulus with herniation. We have noted granulation tissue throughout the substance of the disk (annulus and nucleus) at autopsy.

VERTEBRAL ENDPLATE AND MARROW ABNORMALITIES IN DEGENERATIVE DISK DISEASE

DISRUPTION AND FISSURING OF THE ENDPLATES (TYPE I CHANGES)

In some patients with severe degenerative disk disease pathological examination reveals the endplate to be markedly irregular, with zones of disruption and fissur-

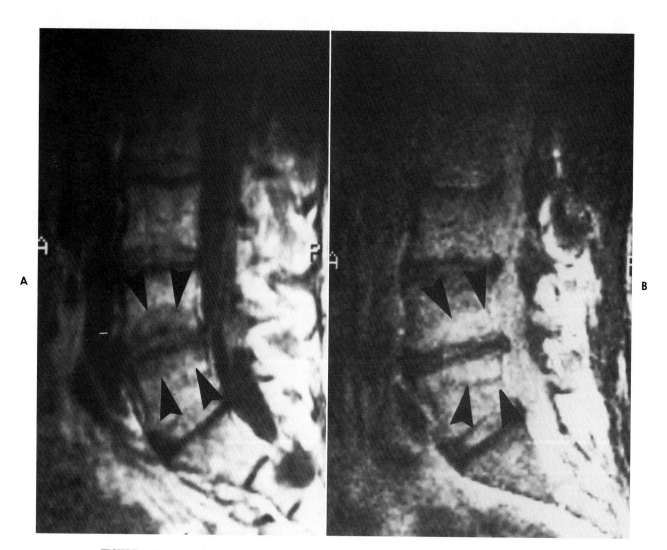

FIGURE 2-52
Marrow abnormalities associated with degenerative disk disease. **A,** A T1-weighted parasagittal MRI of the lumbar spine shows an area of low signal intensity in the marrow of L4 and L5 adjacent to the L4-5 disk *(arrowheads)*. **B,** A T2-weighted MRI of the spine shows moderately to markedly increased signal of the L4 and L5 marrow adjacent to the degenerated disk *(arrowheads)*.

ing.[52] There is granulation tissue with moderately prominent vascularity as well as edema in the endplate and immediately adjacent to the endplate. The histological presentation suggests an inflammatory process affecting the endplate and the bone marrow adjacent to it. On MRI, reduction of T1-weighted signal and increase in T2-weighted signal are evident (Figs. 2-52 and 2-53). We have seen this characteristic signal abnormality in patients with instability and abnormal motion of the vertebrae. The pattern persists for as long as the abnormal spinal motion persists. When the motion is restricted or completely lost, fatty deposits often appear adjacent to the endplates and remain more or less permanently.

The pattern of low signal on T1-WI and high signal on T2-WI must be differentiated from the osteomyelitis pattern. In some patients with advanced degenerative disk disease a thin linear area of increased signal will be noted on T2-WI, probably due to granulation tissue or fluid in the cracks and fissures of the disk or endplate. The boundaries of the disk will be fairly well preserved in most cases. In patients with disk infection and osteomyelitis, however, the signal void of the vertebral endplates may be lost. The zone of increased signal on T2-WI (from pus and inflammation) often obliterates the endplate and extends through the disk and into the adjacent vertebral body as well. The pus may be seen dissecting beneath the anterior longitudinal ligament, from one vertebral body to the next.

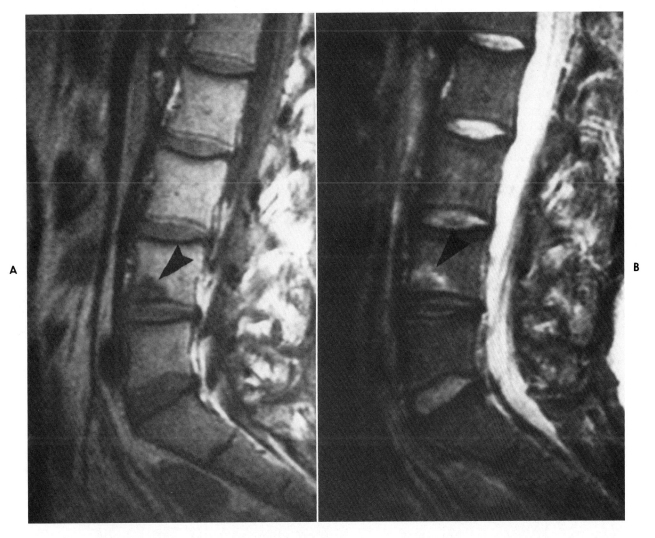

FIGURE 2-53
A, On a T1-weighted parasagittal MRI of the lumbar spine (TR 505/TE 20) there is an area of low signal affecting the L4 marrow adjacent to the anterior portion of the inferior endplate *(arrowhead).* **B,** Corresponding parasagittal T2-weighted MRI (TR 2100/TE 75). Note the increased signal of the L4 marrow adjacent to the inferior endplate. Notice also the minimal area of reduced signal immediately above the endplate surrounded by increased signal, indicative of minimal osteosclerosis with a large area of granulation tissue (and probably edema) of the L4 marrow *(arrowhead).*

FATTY DEPOSITS ADJACENT TO THE ENDPLATES (TYPE II CHANGES)

In some patients with long-standing degenerative disease of the lumbar spine there are accumulations of fat in the marrow immediately adjacent to the endplates[52,55] (Fig. 2-54) that may be several millimeters or more thick. They are identified on CT when a density map of the vertebral body is generated. On MRI they show increased T1 signal and isointense or moderately hyperintense T2-weighted signal.

VERTEBRAL ENDPLATE OSTEOSCLEROSIS

Osteosclerosis of the vertebral endplate is often seen with degenerative disk disease. In most patients it is limited to a few millimeters of the substance of the endplate and adjacent vertebral body, but in some it is significantly more extensive and may occupy more than half the vertebra. It is often noted on both sides of a degenerated disk. The osteosclerotic region of the vertebral body may have a distinctly convex and smooth border. Its extent often seems far out of proportion to the degree of degeneration of the disk, which, though reduced in height, may be normal in all other respects on conventional radiography. In some patients with endplate osteosclerosis diskography reveals extravasation of contrast into the substance of the vertebral body.

The exact mechanism by which osteosclerosis is produced in association with degenerative disk disease is not understood. Likewise, the significance of the vertebral endplate defects leading to extravasation of contrast into

the substance of the vertebral body (on diskography) is not clear. Vertebral endplate osteosclerosis has been thought by some investigators to be a complication of degenerative disk disease. Although this hypothesis is probably correct in most instances of slight to moderate osteosclerosis, it is difficult to accept as the sole explanation in patients with the advanced condition. Possibly a primary degenerative disease of the vertebrae themselves (perhaps aseptic necrosis or a chronic inflammatory process of bone) is leading to this osteosclerosis and this, in turn, interferes with the physiological function of the endplate-disk interface (i.e., transfer of oxygen and nutrients)[56] to cause, at least in some patients, degenerative disease of the disk itself.

Vertebral endplate osteosclerosis is easily identified at conventional radiography and CT by the demonstration of markedly increased bone density. There is also reduced MRI signal on T1- and T2-weighted cross sections.

One must be aware of chemical shift artifacts, which can produce bands of increased and decreased signal at tissue interfaces (e.g., the vertebral endplates). This phenomenon occurs when the frequency encoding axis is aligned parallel to the vertical axis of the spinal column. The band of low signal may cause the endplate to appear unusually thick. Conversely, the band of high signal projected onto the midportion of an intervertebral disk may give a false impression of a torn annulus and in some cases appear as fluid in the substance of the disk on T2-weighted images. It should not be mistaken for a Type I change (disruption and fissuring of the endplates),

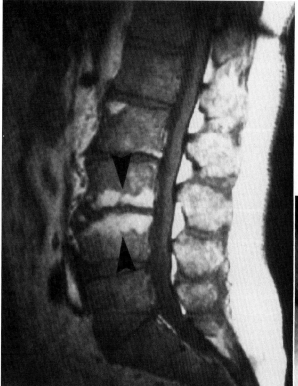
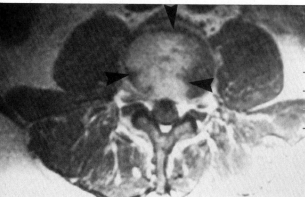

FIGURE 2-54
Fat replacement of marrow in degenerative disk disease. **A,** A sagittal T1-weighted cross section of the lumbar spine shows moderately to markedly reduced height of the L1-2, L2-3, and L3-4 disks. There is fat replacement of the marrow adjacent to the L3 and L4 endplates *(arrowheads).* **B,** An axial T1-weighted cross section just above the L3-4 disk shows fat replacement of the marrow adjacent to the inferior L3 endplate *(arrowheads).*

which is sometimes associated with a small amount of fluid in the substance of the disk.

OSTEOSCLEROSIS ADJACENT TO THE ENDPLATE (TYPE III CHANGES)

In some patients with degenerative disk disease the vertebral marrow immediately adjacent to the endplates will show reduced signal on T1- and T2-weighted images because the marrow elements (i.e., hematopoietic tissue and fat that reside in the spaces between the bony lamellae) are crowded out by the increased calcium containing fraction of the tissues within the vertebral body. In advanced sclerosis there may be little or no marrow elements left in the affected zone. Correlation of MRI findings with conventional roentgenographic findings in osteosclerosis reveals an apparent discrepancy, due to the different sensitivity of the x rays versus magnetic resonance to the composition of tissues making up the vertebral body (i.e., the quantity of bone containing trabeculae and the content of the marrow[hematopoietic cells, other soft tissues, and fat]). When there is replacement of the marrow elements by fat, even though there may be some degree of osteosclerosis, the increased signal from the fat on T1-weighted images makes the affected regions hyperintense. The radiographic examination of these patients may disclose a moderate degree of osteosclerosis because of the increased sensitivity of the x rays to calcium containing tissues. However, when osteosclerosis is severe and the marrow elements (particularly fat) have been crowded out, the MR image will show a zone of reduced signal on T1- and T2-weighted images.

In our experience the majority of patients with degenerative disk disease have not had any of the marrow changes just described. If all patients examined for back pain and sciatica are included, only about 35% have had the marrow abnormalities described. A Type I abnormality (fissuring, disruption, and granulation tissue formation of the endplate and marrow adjacent to the endplate) has been the least commonly encountered (making up less than 2% of our cases). Types II and III, in roughly equal proportions, have made up the remainder. The Type I abnormality appears to be a transitory phenomenon; we have seen it change to a Type II. Type I marrow alterations have been more common in patients with spondylolisthesis and degenerative disk disease. There is an instability of the spine in these patients that can be demonstrated with fluoroscopy. We have seen Type I signal convert to Type II in several patients when, on follow-up examination, hypertrophic changes causing restriction of motion developed. Type I signal abnormality has also been seen in postoperative patients in whom extensive laminectomy and facetectomy led to instability and a progressive spondylolisthesis. Following successful interbody or posterolateral fusion, Type I signals disappeared and fat signals took their place. In patients with interbody fusion, fat has been noted to cross the site of fusion, indicating that a solid state was achieved. Conversely, when the bony fusion was not solid, Type I signal changes have been noted adjacent to the vertebral endplates.

VERTEBRAL EROSION AND HERNIATED LUMBAR DISKS

Erosion of the midposterior margin of the vertebral endplate is occasionally seen with herniation of an intervertebral disk (Figs. 2-55 and 2-56), particularly in children and teenagers. In some of these young patients

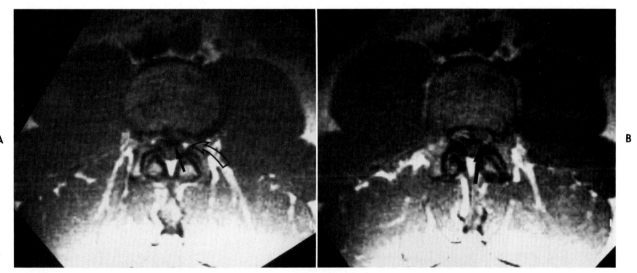

FIGURE 2-55
Herniated L1-2 disk with inferior extension. **A** and **B**, T1-weighted axial MRI. (In **A** [L2-3] the *solid arrow* designates the herniation to the left of midline. In **B** [an axial slice through the L3 pedicle] the *arrow* denotes extension of the herniation to the left of midline. Note the line of markedly low signal [a midline fibrous septum] limiting the herniation to the left.)   *Continued.*

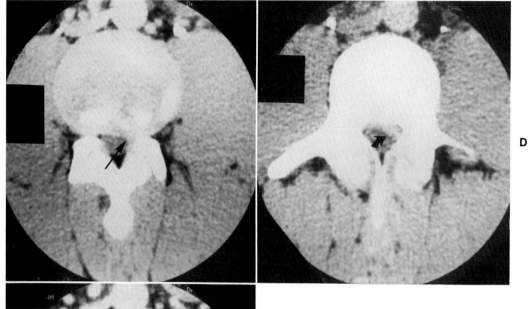

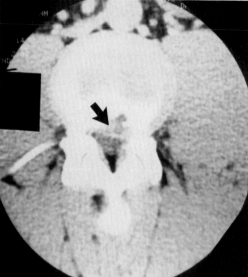

FIGURE 2-55, cont'd
C and D, Corresponding CT axial slices obtained 6 months later. (In C the anterolateral epidural fat is obliterated by the disk on the left *[arrow]*. It was not obliterated at the time the MRI was obtained, however *[curved hollow arrow in A]*. In D the *curved arrow* denotes extension of herniated disk material to the left of midline.) E, Axial slice through the superior L3 endplate. A bony defect on the posterior border of the endplate *(arrow)* can be seen. It is occasionally found in children, teenagers, and young adults following an acute herniation. In some of these patients it will be due to an avulsion fracture of the posterior border of the vertebral endplate associated with the herniation.

FIGURE 2-56
Degenerative disk disease and a defect in the vertebral endplate. **A** and **B**, Soft tissue and bone windows at L4-5, including the superior L5 endplate. (In **A** there is herniation of the disk, more prominent on the right *[arrowhead]*. In **B** the defect and the endplate are better delineated on the bone window *[arrowheads]*.) This 18-year-old youth had a history of acute back pain and right-sided sciatica 7 months prior to the CT examination.

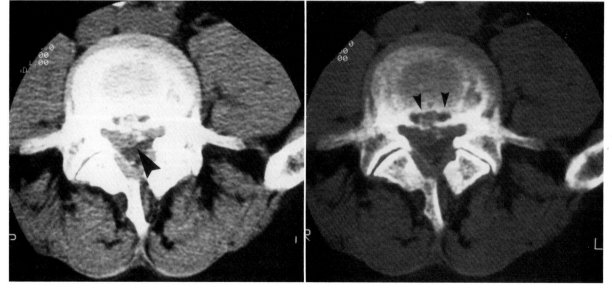

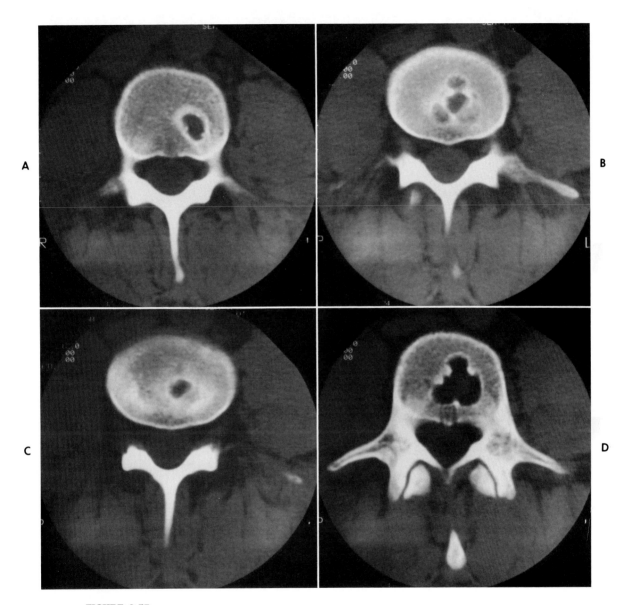

FIGURE 2-57
Schmorl-Scheuermann disease. A to D show the characteristic configuration of the Schmorl node on axial CT examination.   *Continued.*

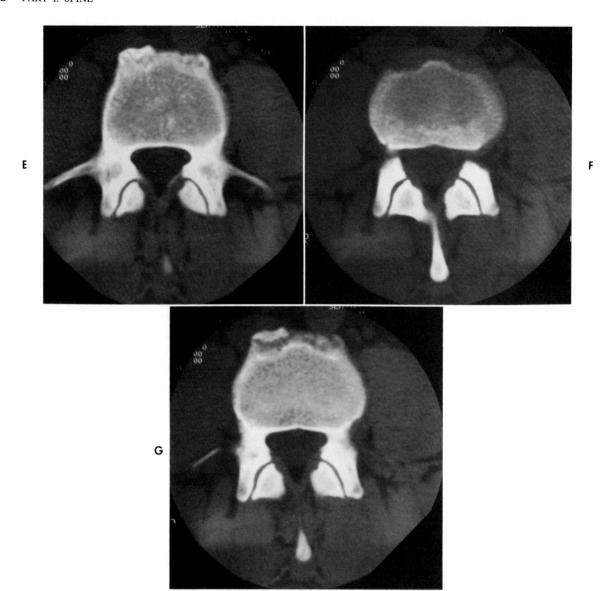

FIGURE 2-57, cont'd
E to G show the configuration of the deformity (ring apophysis) in Scheuermann's disease. Schmorl's nodes are due to herniation of the disk material through the endplate into the vertebral body. When it occurs in youngsters, before the ring is fused, disk material may herniate between the ring and the vertebral body, preventing fusion of the apophysis to the endplate and body. This leads to the characteristic deformity of the anterior vertebral endplate margin in Scheuermann's disease.

the herniation may be due to acute trauma and the defect may be a fracture of the vertebral endplate, which is displaced posteriorly into the spinal canal.

In adults, erosion of the vertebral margins or the vertebral endplate is uncommon. Nevertheless, erosion of the vertebral cortex (anterior wall of the spinal canal) or the neural arch may be seen with an acute nontraumatic disk herniation (Fig. 2-56) or when a free fragment has become embedded in bony cortex. This probably occurs because the fragment is enveloped by granulation tissue, which can extend into the adjacent tissues by eroding and digesting them; and on surgical exploration with pathological examination, the herniated disk fragment will

usually be found embedded in the cortex and surrounded by granulation tissue and/or fibrosis.[11] This is a rare phenomenon that, when present, may cause confusion in the differential diagnosis. If there is herniation of disk material into the substance of a vertebral body, as occurs in Schmorl-Scheuermann disease (Fig. 2-57), a vertebral endplate defect may be identified.

TRAUMATIC LUMBAR DISK HERNIATION

Surgically documented acute herniation of a previously normal lumbar disk is extremely rare. There were none in our 256 surgically explored disks. In fact, during the past 15 years we have seen just two cases of acute lumbar disk herniation that were likely due to trauma. One patient was 18, and the other 23, years old. They had had no symptoms prior to the trauma, and an acute sciatic syndrome developed within hours after the incident. Herniation of a lumbar disk was shown unequivocally on CT in both patients and on MRI in one patient. The lumbar spine was otherwise normal. There were no vertebral osteophytes, bony ridges, vacuum phenomenon, or other abnormalities to indicate long standing degenerative disease of the spine. On MRI the involved disk, as well as all other disks, were of normal size and signal intensity. The herniated material was isointense with the parent disk (nucleus pulposus) on all pulse sequences.

Trauma may aggravate a previously existing degenerative disease of the spine. However, an objective documentation and quantification of the extent of aggravation requires pre- and posttrauma radiographic, CT, and MRI studies. These are rarely available.

Radiographic work-up of patients with back pain and sciatica

In our experience CT is a proven modality for evaluating lumbar disk herniation, particularly in patients without prior spinal surgery.[3] In patients with back pain or clinically suspected stenosis we advocate not myelography as the initial diagnostic procedure but CT or MRI. There is a gradual but sure trend at our institution for surgeons to feel confident enough to operate solely on the basis of abnormalities identified at CT and/or MRI without preoperative myelography. This has been particularly true in patients in whom a definite herniated disk was identified and there was an obvious positive correlation with the clinical findings. The main argument in favor of myelography has been the (understandable) insistence by almost all surgeons that the region of the conus medullaris be visualized and the possibility of a neoplasm in it, or of any neoplasms, be excluded. It is generally accepted that neoplasms of the conus medullaris and lumbar region may be responsible for ill-defined back pain and may mimic the sciatic syndrome. Fortunately, at present, there is no need for myelography to visualize the contents of the spinal canal and conus region. This objective is easily achieved by high resolution MRI. We therefore recommend MRI in all cases being worked up for lumbar spinal disk surgery. CT and MRI are complementary, and both may be necessary for a definitive diagnosis; but, regardless of the ultimate findings, the initial diagnostic modality in patients with back pain, sciatica, or suspected stenosis should always be CT or MRI. If a definite diagnosis is not established, we do MRI in those for whom CT was the initial diagnostic procedure and vice versa. In the preoperative work-up of sciatica or stenosis, an MRI examination is indicated for most patients who have had only a CT examination, to exclude the possibility of disease in the conus region and lower lumbar canal.

Accuracy of computed tomography in the diagnosis of lumbar disk herniation

Computed tomography has an accuracy rate of 90% to 92% when it comes to predicting HNP in patients who have not had prior disk surgery. In 1984 we reported our experience[3] with 100 patients who had undergone CT of the lumbar spine followed by surgery for sciatica. The 61 men and 39 women were 19 to 76 years of age (mean 49 years) and had been referred for back pain or radiculopathy, usually recurrent or of several years' duration. Preoperative CT reports were retrieved and compared with the findings at surgery. All patients were operated on by the same neurosurgeon at New York University Medical Center. A drawing of the surgical findings was prepared after each of 116 disk explorations. Presurgical accuracy of CT in predicting HNP was as follows: 97 true-positives, 7 true-negatives, 4 false-positives, and 8 false-negatives. The CT diagnosis and surgical findings of HNP agreed in 89 patients. Among these 100 patients, 9 had had prior spinal surgery. If we exclude them from the study, then CT was accurate 93% of the time in predicting the presence or absence of HNP prior to surgery (100 of 107 disk explorations).

Thus there was a discrepancy between the preoperative CT diagnosis and the findings at surgery in

1. Patients who had had prior spinal surgery
2. Patients with combined disk herniation and spinal stenosis
3. Patients with combined disk herniation and spondylolisthesis
4. Patients whose CT had been incorrectly interpreted

Difficulty interpreting a CT study of the spine may be due to several factors—marked obesity of the patient, motion during the examination, presence of Pantopaque in the spinal canal from previous myelography, and marked deformity or scoliosis.

Correlation of surgical findings with CT, MRI, myelographic, and CT-myelographic findings

The surgical and preoperative radiographic findings were compared in 217 patients. In 91 of these who were previously reported on,[3] and in an additional 126 who did not have a history of prior spinal surgery, a total of 256 disk explorations were performed. These patients were all referred for back pain, sciatica, and/or clinically suspected spinal stenosis, usually of a long-standing or recurrent nature. The original 91 patients were operated on by the same surgeon at NYU Medical Center and the additional 126 were done by a group of 16 neurosurgeons and orthopedic surgeons. All patients had a CT examination performed at NYU Medical Center. Some of these subjects had had other studies prior to their referral to the Medical Center—including CT, MRI, myelography, and CT-myelography. CT-myelography in 73 patients and MRI in 54 patients were obtained at the Medical Center in addition to the studies performed at outside institutions. Comparison of the preoperative diagnoses and the findings at surgery will be discussed.

CORRELATION OF CT AND SURGICAL FINDINGS

A correct diagnosis, either the presence or the absence of herniation (true positive or true negative), was made by CT prior to surgery in 234 of 256 disk explorations, for an accuracy rate of 91%. There were 221 true-positives, 13 true-negatives, 12 false-positives, and 10 false-negatives.

CORRELATION OF MRI AND SURGICAL FINDINGS

In 63 patients MRI was also performed and a correct diagnosis was established in 54, for an accuracy rate of 85%.

CORRELATION OF MYELOGRAPHIC AND SURGICAL FINDINGS

Myelography was performed in 143 patients, with a correct diagnosis of disk herniation (or lack thereof) being reached in 112 (accuracy rate 78%). Comparison of myelographic and CT findings in these cases revealed a slightly superior accuracy for myelography at L1-2 and L2-3. At L3-4, L4-5, and L5-S1 the accuracy rates for myelography and CT were 83% vs. 89%, 76% vs. 91%, and 72% vs. 93%. The superiority of CT over myelography at L5-S1 most likely stems from the fact that there is a significant amount of epidural fat present anteriorly in this region, facilitating the diagnosis of herniation on CT but interfering with it on myelography.[14,15,16] There were 21 patients in whom a foraminal (far-lateral) disk herniation was diagnosed on CT and verified at surgery. The herniation was missed on myelography in 13 of these patients (62%). The superiority of CT in detecting intraforaminal disk herniation is well known. The difficulty with myelography appears to arise from the fact that a purely intraforaminal disk herniation does not indent the dural sac or disturb the descending nerve root. An intraforaminal herniation may compress the dorsal root ganglion and exiting spinal nerve, but these structures are distal to the terminal end of the root sleeve and thus myelography is deceptively normal. If the herniation extends superiorly in the neural foramen as well as into the spinal canal, however, the descending root (one level higher) may become compressed between it and the pedicle. The dural sac is usually also indented, and thus the cutoff of the descending root sleeve, along with indentation of the dural sac, is detected on myelography.[14,17,19]

CORRELATION OF CT-MYELOGRAPHIC AND SURGICAL FINDINGS

CT-myelography was performed in 129 patients. (The smaller number is due to the fact that some patients underwent myelography but not CT and a small number had CT-myelography but no routine myelography films were available.) CT-myelography correctly predicted the presence or absence of disk herniation in 123 patients (of a total 129), for an accuracy rate of 95%. In addition, both myelography and CT-myelography were helpful in identifying patients with root sleeve cysts and conjoined root sleeves.[16,19,22-26,35,36]

CORRELATION OF CT/MRI AND SURGICAL FINDINGS

CT and MRI examinations of the spine were performed in 63 patients. When CT alone was evaluated, a preoperative diagnosis of HNP was made correctly in 92%. The accuracy of MRI alone was 85%. When CT and MRI were both considered, a definitive diagnosis was established in 60 patients, for an accuracy rate of 96%.

In 39 patients myelography was also performed, but a retrospective evaluation of these showed nothing additionally helpful. Although one case with a conjoined root was clearly diagnosed at myelography, and this was not obvious on either CT or MRI, the overall accuracy of myelography (excluding the findings at CT-myelography) was 83% as compared to 96% for CT and MRI combined. The accuracy of CT-myelography in this group was 96%.

Multiple lumbar herniated disks

Among 217 patients with 256 disk explorations, there were 19 multiple lumbar disk herniations: 17 patients with two and 2 with three (Fig. 2-58).

Multiple lumbar herniations are fairly commonly noted on CT and MRI in patients with symptoms. Among 211 patients with sciatica referred for CT of the lumbar spine, 37 had one lumbar HNP, 4 had two, 4 had three, and 2 had four (though without surgical proof).

Utility and pitfalls of CT, MRI, and myelography

Computed tomography is particularly useful in the evaluation of patients in whom there are significant bony hypertrophic changes, osteophytes, and ligamentous calcifications. A calcified herniated disk is clearly visualized, as is a vacuum phenomenon. MRI, however, may pose occasional difficulties in the identification of calcified ligaments and herniated disks and also in discerning a vacuum phenomenon. On the other hand, MRI is particularly helpful in studying the spinal canal and conus region, and we routinely recommend it for preoperative work-ups when it has not been previously performed. Myelography can establish the diagnosis of conjoined root sleeves and Tarlov cysts on a definitive basis,* despite the fact that these may be suspected on CT and MRI. On MRI a definitive diagnosis is established when CSF can be demonstrated in the cyst and a solid mass lesion is excluded.

Myelography, however, is significantly less accurate in detecting disk herniations at L4-5 and L5-S1.[19] In addition, more than 50% of all foraminal herniations are

---

*References 22-26, 29-34, 57, 58.

missed (Fig. 2-20). If the surgeon is not forewarned of this, a foraminal HNP may be overlooked at laminectomy.[27] We currently find CT-myelography to be the most accurate modality, although when CT and MRI are each performed in the same patient their accuracy of diagnosis approaches that of CT-myelography. In fact, on retrospective analysis, when CT and MRI were both available, usually no additional information was obtained from the added performance of myelography. Therefore we recommend CT and MRI, if indicated clinically, as complementary procedures for clarification of the diagnosis, in preference to myelography. We believe myelography should be performed only when both CT and MRI have been done but a definitive diagnosis has not been established.

Disk herniation in sacralization and spondyloarthropathy

When the last lumbar vertebra resembles the sacral vertebrae and its transverse process becomes fused to the sacrum, the condition is known as sacralization. If the bony ankylosis is progressing, in a patient between 16 and 22 years of age, for example, a chronic and localized form of low back pain associated with a moderate degree of lumbosacral stiffness can be expected. Usually there is no radicular pain radiation, but the clinical presentation may nevertheless be confusing. When the process is completed, the back pain disappears. In addition, there is usually no herniation of the L5-S1 disk. Disks do not herniate when there is ankylosis between the vertebrae. Herniation occurs only when movement is possible between the neighboring vertebrae.

We have seen disk herniations in many patients with unfused vertebrae just below or just above vertebrae that were fused (congenitally or surgically) though not in the anklyosed segment itself.

Herniation of a lumbar intervertebral disk in patients with ankylosing spondylitis is extremely uncommon. According to Burkus,[58] who reported such a case in 1988, nerve root impingement secondary to intervertebral disk herniation had not been previously reported in a patient with ankylosing spondylitis. With classic ankylosing spondylitis, or other forms of spondyloarthropathy, there is bony ankylosis of the spine and facet joints as well as the sacroiliac joints. Restriction of spinal motion is a well-known clinical characteristic of these conditions.

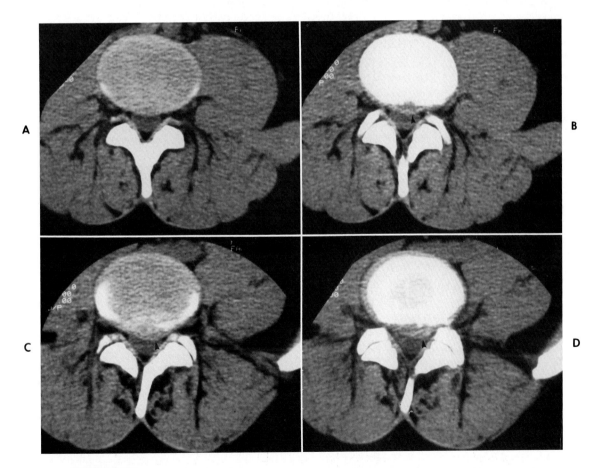

FIGURE 2-58
Three herniated disks in the same patient. **A,** An axial CT slice through the L3-4 disk and, **B,** another taken 4 mm below it reveal a central herniation that is slightly more prominent to the left of midline. (The irregularity of contour is better appreciated in **B** [*arrowhead*].) **C** and **D,** Axial slices at L4-5. Note the central herniation, more prominent to the left (*arrowhead*). *Continued.*

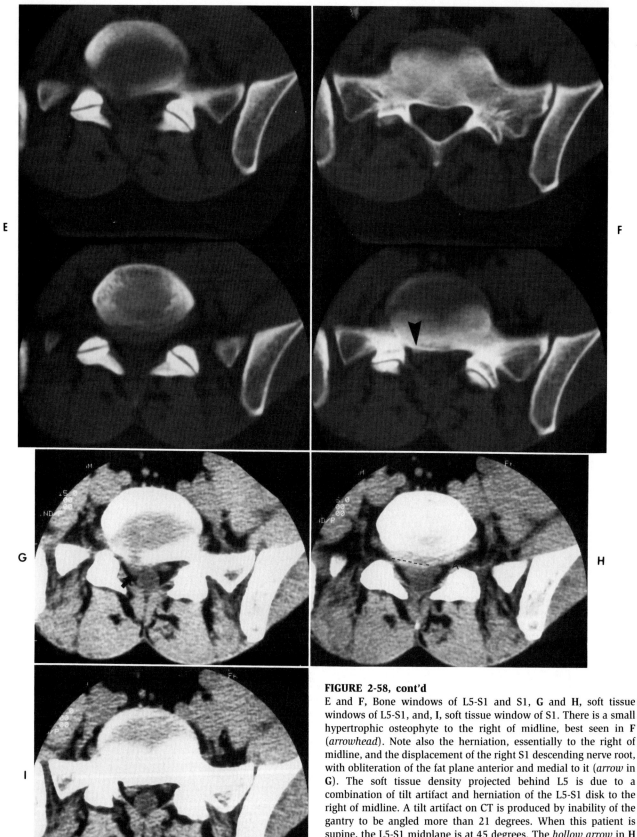

FIGURE 2-58, cont'd

E and F, Bone windows of L5-S1 and S1, G and H, soft tissue
windows of L5-S1, and, I, soft tissue window of S1. There is a small
hypertrophic osteophyte to the right of midline, best seen in F
(*arrowhead*). Note also the herniation, essentially to the right of
midline, and the displacement of the right S1 descending nerve root,
with obliteration of the fat plane anterior and medial to it (*arrow* in
G). The soft tissue density projected behind L5 is due to a
combination of tilt artifact and herniation of the L5-S1 disk to the
right of midline. A tilt artifact on CT is produced by inability of the
gantry to be angled more than 21 degrees. When this patient is
supine, the L5-S1 midplane is at 45 degrees. The *hollow arrow* in H
denotes the crown of soft tissue density projecting into the neural
foramen and spinal canal as a result of the excessive L5-S1 lordosis.
This patient also has some scoliosis, which accounts for the slight
asymmetry of visualized structures. A crown of soft tissue density is
to be expected in patients with marked lordosis and does not
represent disk herniation; it will disappear on reformatted images
parallel to the midplane of the disk. The posterior border of the
crown is obscured by the herniation extending from midline to the
right. The *broken line* points to the boundary between the herniated
disk and the soft tissue density resulting from the tilt artifact. Behind
it are the herniated tissues.

Herniation of a disk usually does not occur when there is ankylosis of the spine and practically no motion is occurring at the disks. However, if the ankylosis is segmental (i.e., if there are intervening vertebrae not fused), then the fulcrum of motion may be shifted to them and these disks, which are under increased stress, may show evidence of herniation.

To illustrate this point, two brief case histories will be given:

A young woman with ankylosis of the spine (C2 to C5) and a herniated disk was seen by us. She had had juvenile rheumatoid arthritis. At surgery a C5-6 herniation was identified. On MRI there was degeneration of this disk, although the other disks were typically smaller, fused, and free of degenerative changes.

The patient reported by Burkus,[59] a 45-year-old black man with a clinically established diagnosis of ankylosing spondylitis, had had an acute onset of pain radiating from his right buttock into the right leg. Physical examination indicated nerve root impingement (right first sacral root), and roentgenograms showed syndesmophytes extending across the margins of the lumbar disk spaces from L1 to L5 with fusion of the facet joints. Although the L5-S1 disk was free of syndesmophytes and the L5-S1 facet joints were not fused, there was bilateral fusion of the sacroiliac. Myelography and CT were performed and revealed a herniated L5-S1 disk, with displacement of the right S1 nerve root posteriorly. This was confirmed at surgery. The postsurgical follow-up examination revealed that the radicular symptoms had subsided, but the patient's chronic low back pain continued without change.

Involvement of the spine in spondyloarthropathy generally consists of an inflammatory process affecting the sacroiliac joints, the facet joints, the spinal ligaments, and the annulus fibrosus. In classic ankylosing spondylitis the sacroiliac joints are generally the first structures involved. Low back pain and stiffness are prominent clinical manifestations, although the pain usually does not radiate into the lower extremities. Involvement of the facet joints and other spinal structures is also associated with pain and stiffness of the spine, but the pain characteristically is not radicular.[60] Erosion of the vertebral margins, which typically occurs anteriorly (Romanus lesion), produces squaring of the vertebrae.[61] During the healing phase of the inflammatory process osteosclerosis affects the anterior discovertebral junctions, associated at each level with ossification of the adjacent annulus. When bony ankylosis of the facet joints is complete, practically all motion is eliminated within the affected spinal segment. There is seldom radiographic evidence of the degenerative process, the disk heights are maintained, and no osteophytes appear. These findings are seen in fused spinal segments regardless of etiology, but only when ankylosis occurs *before* there have been degenerative changes of the disks. Otherwise, a mixed pattern is present.

Occasionally, in patients with long-standing ankylosing spondylitis, there will be extensive osteosclerosis that seems to affect just a single disk space (often in the vicinity of the thoracolumbar junction). The margins of the vertebrae are markedly irregular, with associated osteolysis and fractures in the fused spinal segment. The fractures likely occur through or just adjacent to the involved disk.[62-65] This phenomenon (Andersson lesion) may also follow excessive motion in an unfused segment of the spine between two completely ankylosed segments. The intervertebral disk in this situation is at the fulcrum of motion, similar to the disk located either above or below a fused segment. This disk is thus under increased mechanical stress, and thus susceptible to degenerative disease, and in such circumstances herniation becomes a definite possibility.

Long-term follow-up of the herniated lumbar disk

Included in this report are 136 patients, 89 men and 47 women, 31 to 64 years of age (mean 47 years), with a history of sciatica. The interval between the first episode of back pain and the time of interview averaged 11 years, 4 months, with a range of 3 to 26 years. These patients were selected from a larger group with back pain, sciatica, or clinically suspected spinal stenosis who had been referred for CT examination of the spine. The requirements for inclusion in the study were as follows:

1. The patient had to be able to give a reliable history.
2. The first episode of back pain had to have occurred 3 or more years prior to the interview.
3. A myelogram or CT documenting disk herniation had to be available.
4. Surgery had to have been recommended as the procedure of choice for treatment of the herniation but had *not* to have been performed for a medical reason or refusal of the patient.

In 97 patients, myelography was the only diagnostic procedure performed during the initial work-up (Group I); in 19, CT was the only modality (Group II); and in 20, CT and myelography both were performed (Group III). Follow-up myelography was available in 73 patients from Group I. The epidural defect corresponding to the herniated disk was moderately smaller in 53 of these: in 33 it was markedly reduced; in 11 it was no longer detectable at the site of the previous herniation; in 9 it remained virtually unchanged (osteophytes, bony ridges, or calcified old herniations were identified in 7 of these).

A CT examination of all patients was obtained at the time of interview. Comparing this with the old CT examination(s) in patients from Groups II and III revealed a number of interesting findings:

In 11 patients a herniated disk with significant calcification was present on the initial CT examination (no significant change was noted on follow-up CT in the calcified portion of the herniation).
A vacuum phenomenon, reduced disk height, or the development of osteophytes was observed in 7 patients (average follow-up 9 years).
The remaining 28 patients had herniation without calcification on the initial examination.

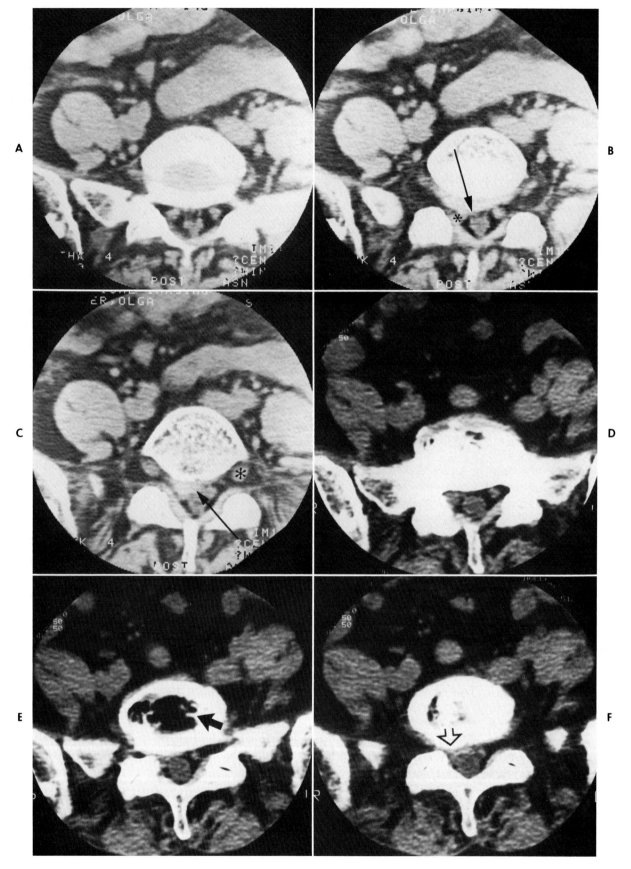

FIGURE 2-59
For legend see opposite page.

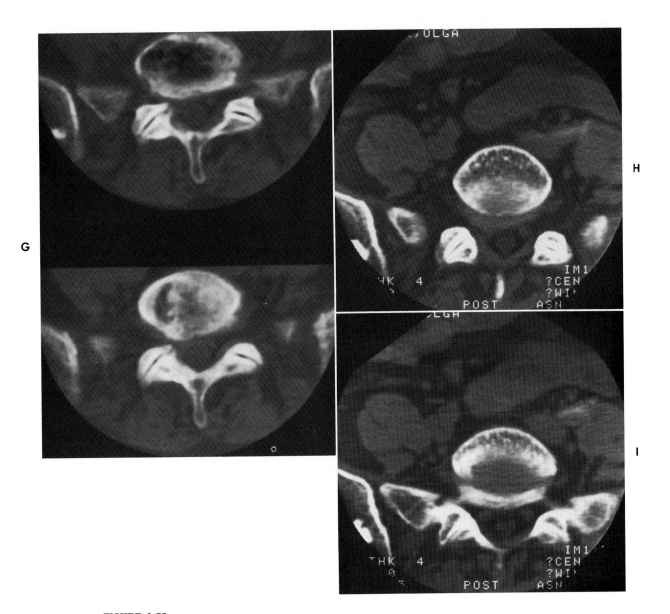

FIGURE 2-59
Follow-up of a herniated L5-S1 disk without surgery. **A** to **C**, Soft tissue window axial slices. The *arrow* in **B** denotes the herniation to the right of midline, displacing the right S1 nerve root posteriorly *(asterisk)*. The *arrow* in **C** points to an upward extension of the disk herniation to the right of midline. (The *asterisk* is on the left L5 dorsal root ganglion, which is normal, just below the L5 pedicle.) **D** to **F**, Corresponding axial CT slices obtained 3 years, 2 months, later in this 67-year-old man. The axial slices (**A** to **C**) were obtained with 0 degrees of angulation of the gantry, resulting in elongation of the spinal canal and the apparent difference between the two sets of images. The slices obtained parallel to the midplane of the disk (**D** to **F**) show the true size of the spinal canal. The *arrow* in **E** points to a vacuum phenomenon that developed. There are also hypertrophic changes in the posterior border of the vertebral endplates, to the right of midline, at the site of the previous disk herniation. The right S1 nerve root is displaced posteriorly, and a small soft tissue component of the herniated disk is associated with the hypertrophic osteophytes. The *hollow arrow* in **F** denotes hypertrophic changes. **G**, Bone windows at L5-S1 show the hypertrophic changes of the vertebral margins to better advantage. Compare with **H** and **I**, which are corresponding bone windows obtained 38 months prior to the current examination. Notice also the development of degenerative disease of the right facet joint, with hypertrophic osteophytes and the vacuum phenomenon.

Follow-up CT in 13 patients (out of 28) revealed a moderate to severe reduction in size of the herniated portion, and, in addition, the descending nerve roots (which had been swollen, obscured, or displaced by the herniated disk on the original CT examination) were now in almost normal position, without displacement, and free of swelling.

A marked reduction in disk height and a vacuum phenomenon were seen in 3 patients, and a small amount of calcification was present in the herniated portion of 3 disks.

In the remaining 15 patients (of the 28) there was slight to moderate reduction of the herniated portion (in 8) or no significant change (in 7). Osteophytes or calcification of the herniated portion of the disk were noted in 7 of the 15, and a vacuum phenomenon had developed in 6 (Figs. 2-59 to 2-61).

Follow-up CT examination of patients in Group I (in whom myelography was the initial radiographic examination) also showed a spectrum of findings similar to the findings in Groups II and III; the reduction in size of the herniated disk corresponded well to the decrease in size of its epidural defect. However, CT was often more helpful in making a precise identification of the lesion(s) responsible for the defect (e.g., soft herniated disks, osteophytes, bony ridges, or calcified ligaments). These abnormalities were not as clearly identifiable on conventional myelography.

We believe that acute herniation of a lumbar disk may

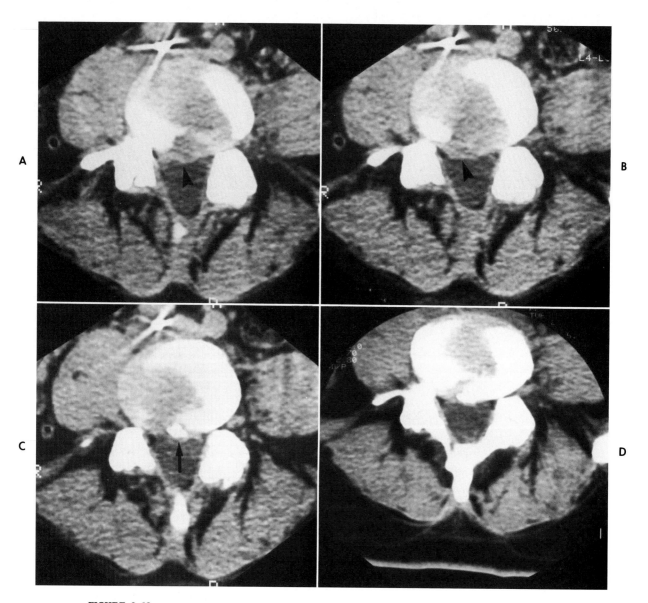

FIGURE 2-60
Follow-up of a herniated L4-5 disk without surgery. **A** and **B**, Axial CT scans reveal the herniation centrally and to the right of midline *(arrowheads)*. **C** and **D**, taken approximately 44 months later, show calcification in the midline on the posterior disk border *(arrow in* **C***)*. The herniation has shrunk significantly and is practically invisible.

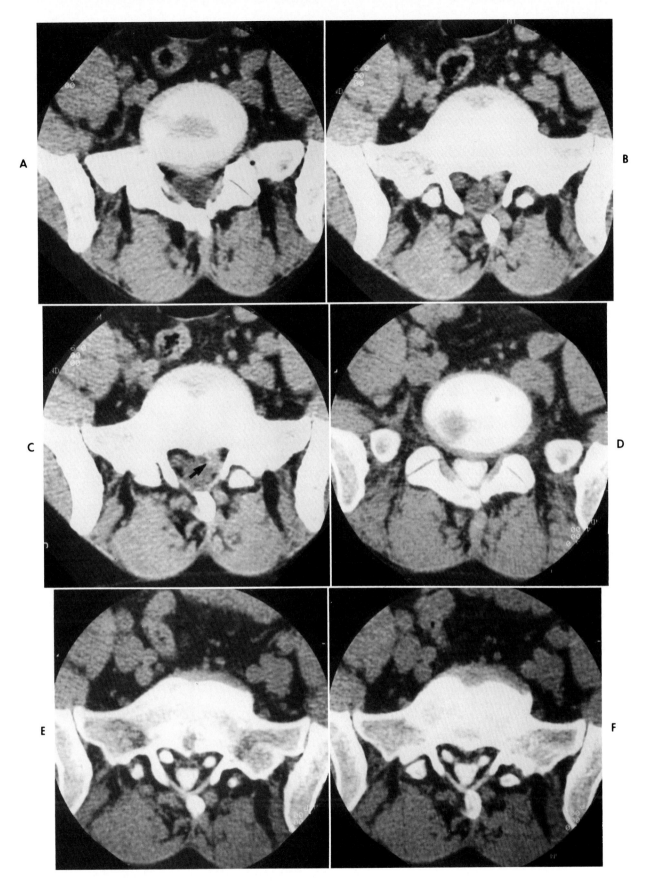

FIGURE 2-61
Follow-up of an L5-S1 herniated disk without surgery. **A** to **C** show the herniation with a fragment displacing and distorting the descending S1 nerve root on the left (*arrow* in **C**). **D** to **F**, A CT myelogram 3 years later shows moderate bulging of the disk, with minimal irregularity of its posterior border due to the previous herniation. (In **E** and **F** the previous disk fragment is no longer present, and the S1 descending nerve roots are normal.)

be associated with some inflammation and edema, at times quite pronounced, as evidenced by the granulation tissue observed at pathological examination of resected segments. The observation also of inflamed, red, and angry nerve roots at surgical exploration[66] supports this opinion. We have seen (on intravenous contrast–enhanced CT) marked enhancement of the disk margins and a considerable portion of the entire substance of the disk in several patients with surgically documented herniations. In all these cases granulation tissue of varying thickness was present in the resected fragments and in 6 of 30 disks there was inflammation with edema.

We also have observed enhancement of herniated disk margins and free fragments on gadopentetate-enhanced MRI. We believe the reduced size of a protruding herniation at follow-up CT examination is at least partly due to the resolution of this inflammation and edema. The regression of a protruded disk segment at short-term follow-up after bedrest and the administration of antiinflammatory agents, likewise, is probably due to resolution of the inflammatory process. In long-standing herniations it is likely that fragmentation of at least a portion of the protruded disk, along with mechanical displacement of any resulting fragments, occurs; and there probably is resorption of the herniated material as well by granulation tissue.[67] In addition, particularly when there have been repeated episodes of herniation, the resected segment may show mature granulation tissue formation and scarring with or without calcification. Granulation tissue and its accompanying vascularity are most likely instrumental in the digestion and shrinkage of the herniated portion of the disk.

Short-term radiographic follow-up of disk herniation

Among the 67 patients included in this group, with a follow-up ranging from 4 to 16 weeks (mean 8 weeks), two CT examinations were available: one at the time of the most recent acute episode of back pain, and one at the conclusion of short-term follow-up.

> There were 26 patients in whom a significantly smaller herniation was noted.
> A vacuum phenomenon, not present on the initial CT examination, was clearly visible in 7 patients (average follow-up 8 weeks).
> Calcification of the herniated portion, also not present on the initial examination, occurred in 5 patients (average follow-up 15 weeks).
> There was a marked reduction of disk height in 5 patients (average follow-up 8 weeks).

CT of the lumbar spine in subjects with no symptoms

Among the 200 patients included in this report, there were 121 women and 79 men, ranging in age from 36 to 87 (mean 58 years), who had been free of back pain for at least 1 year prior to the examination, which was performed for a known intraabdominal malignancy or metastasis. Two slices, 5 mm thick and appropriately angled, were obtained through the L3-4, L4-5, and L5-S1 disks in each patient.

> Bulging of the disk without calcification was noted in 34, and bulging with calcification in 45, patients.
> Soft disk herniations (without calcification) were seen in 9 patients; 4 had, and 5 did not have, compression or displacement of the nerve roots or dural sac.
> A herniated disk containing calcification or ossification and extending into the spinal canal or neural foramina was present in 38 patients.
> Osteophytes or bony ridges projecting into the spinal canal or neural foramina were noted in 43.
> Various degrees of diminished disk height, with or without osteosclerosis of the vertebral endplates and with or without a vacuum phenomenon, were noted in 41.
> Osteophytes and bony ridges of the anterior and lateral borders of the vertebral endplates were present in 85.
> There was moderate to marked degenerative disease of the facet joints in 58, and 9 had severe degeneration of the facet joints (4 with the vacuum phenomenon).
> Spinal stenosis of at least a moderate degree was present in 21.
> A Grade I degenerative spondylolisthesis was noted in 15 subjects.
> There were 87 patients 60 to 87 years old among the 200 studied.

No soft herniations were detected in this group, despite the moderate to marked degrees of degenerative disease (evidenced by diminished disk heights, bulging, a vacuum phenomenon, calcified margins, osteophytes, and bony ridges) in 73 patients.

Myelography in subjects with no symptoms

Hitselberger and Witten[68] studied 300 patients who had undergone myelography for evaluation of an acoustic neurilemmona. They were 18 to 76 years of age, with a mean of 52 years. Each examination included an AP view of the cervical and lumbar spine. When an abnormality was noted during fluoroscopy, additional pertinent views were obtained. In addition, the patients were questioned regarding back pain. Anyone with a history suggesting a radicular syndrome was excluded from the study. There were abnormalities consistent with various degrees of degenerative disk disease in 110 examinations (or 37%). The defect was single in 56 and multiple in 54. A lumbar abnormality was present in 71, and a cervical abnormality in 63.

MRI of the lumbar spine in subjects with no symptoms

Boden et al.[48] performed MRI on 67 individuals who had never had low back pain, sciatica, or neurogenic claudication. The subjects were 20 to 80 years of age (mean 42). At least one bulging disk was seen in 54% of the 35 who were less than 60 years of age and in 79% of the 14 who were 60 years or older. Disk herniation was present in 24%, and stenosis of the spinal canal in 4%. The prevalence of abnormal scans was 20% among the 20-to-59-year-olds and 57% among the 60-to-80-year-olds.

In a retrospective evaluation of MRI examinations in 60 patients 37 to 69 years of age (mean 57) referred for reasons other than sciatica and stenosis, we found the following:

> Diminution or almost complete loss of signal from at least one lumbar disk in 19 patients
> Bulging of at least one disk in 12 patients
> One or more herniated disks (presence or absence of calcification not ascertainable) in 18 patients

Clinical significance of abnormal CT and MRI findings in subjects with and without symptoms

The relatively high prevalence of abnormal CT and MRI findings in pain-free individuals emphasizes the fact that, before any significant therapeutic decision can be made, these abnormalities must be correlated with the clinical manifestations in each case. It must be emphasized also that specific abnormal CT or MRI findings are not, in and of themselves, false-positive events. For example, bulging or bony ridges do represent objective pathological processes but are not necessarily the cause of a patient's symptoms. Examiners are handicapped in trying to link abnormal findings to clinical manifestations; imaging tools can provide a representation of the gross pathological anatomy but very little, if any, information as to the pathophysiology of the tissues examined. Nevertheless, the following observations may be helpful in assessing the significance of abnormal CT and MRI findings:

> Reductions in height and signal intensity of lumbar disks are signs of disk degeneration.
> The incidence of these abnormalities increases with age; in 60-year-olds and older they are present in practically all individuals.
> Osteophytes, bony ridges, and calcified bulging or herniated disks are seen with increasing frequency in older age groups; in 50-year-olds and older at least two thirds have one or more calcified bulging or herniated disk.
> All the abnormalities mentioned so far may be totally asymptomatic and frequently they are. Actually, the incidence of back pain peaks at about 50 years but the incidence and extent of degenerative disk changes continue an unbroken upward course.[66]
> In the case of calcified abnormal disks or bony ridges, the determining factor in their clinical significance is the presence or absence of spinal stenosis. Without spinal stenosis, even a large calcified herniated disk or bony ridge, even one that displaces the nerve root or dural sac, may be (and usually is) asymptomatic.

These observations indicate that the mere mechanical displacement of neural elements, particularly when it occurs gradually over many years, does not lead to clinical manifestations. The lumbosacral nerve roots can be moved 10 to 12 mm in a cephalocaudad or other direction without deleterious effect. The trouble starts when there is *tethering* of the roots, as for example by a distal stenosis or herniation or when the roots are stretched beyond their tolerance. Then motor and sensory neurological deficits appear in the territory served by the affected nerve roots.

Bulging is a frequently encountered abnormality of lumbar disks. We have found its incidence to increase with advancing age, up to 55 or so years. After that there is no more increase, and may actually be a decrease, in the relative number of noncalcified bulging disks. In our experience a true bulging (diffuse and symmetrical extension of the disk margin beyond the vertebral endplates) is not usually associated with significant clinical findings. A bulging disk becomes problematical when spinal stenosis is also present. Then the bulging disk contributes to the compression of neural elements and this worsens the stenosis.

Disk herniation and acute clinical manifestations

In our experience soft disk herniations (noncalcified) are distinctly uncommon in asymptomatic individuals. Among 200 subjects who had been asymptomatic for at least a year, 9 (or 4.5%) had soft disk herniations (all but two small and focal) and 7 had a spinal canal that was normal (or large, with plenty of epidural fat). Thus, we feel that the discovery of a noncalcified herniated disk is an important finding and one that is more likely than others, in the absence of stenosis, to be accompanied by clinical manifestations.

The cause of acute clinical manifestations in patients with disk herniation is not known, but we are almost certain that mechanical compression or displacement of the neural elements is not in itself the key offending mechanism. An acute back episode may be precipitated by any of the following: displacement of diseased facets, the sudden entrapment of neural elements associated with abnormal motion of the spine, the stretching of or injury to the spinal ligaments, an acute herniation of a disk. (Although a full discussion of this subject is beyond the scope of the present chapter, we will review briefly the association of a soft herniation and clinical findings.)

Herniation of the disk is secondary to disruption of its internal structure, leading to intrasubstance (intradiskal) herniation. Tearing and fissuring of the disk occur as part of the degenerative process. Eventually the peripheral zone (annulus) tears and nuclear material with fibrocartilaginous disk tissue from the more central portion pushes through the tear to the very edge of, but not through, the APLL-complex, creating a focal contour deformity; however, the APLL complex is not torn. Less commonly tearing of the disk substance extends through the APLL complex and permits disk material to escape into the space beyond. The tearing of disk substance leads to the formation of granulation tissue, with focal areas of scarring, bleeding, necrosis, and eventual calcification in some cases. These abnormalities are usually seen in the outer portion of the annulus, which corresponds to the peripheral 5 or 10 mm of the disk radius.[69] Although distinctly uncommon, we have seen granulation tissue, scarring, necrosis, and calcification involve practically the entire substance of severely degenerated disks.

But why should disk herniation be accompanied by (intense) pain? Many investigators have attempted to answer this question. At present, the best that can be offered are speculations and educated guesses. Bobechko and Hirsch[70] proposed an autoimmunological origin. Hirsch[71] and Hirsch et al.[72] suggested leakage of acid metabolites from the interior of the degenerated disk. Nachemson[73] found lower pH values, and Hakelius[74] did likewise, following negative surgical exploration. Macnab[66] found the affected nerve roots at surgical exploration to be "inflamed, red, and angry." We have seen granulation tissue in surgically resected disk fragments of practically all acute disk herniations. In addition, we have seen evidence of inflammation and edema in 6 of 30 specimens (though we feel it is probably much more common than this). Inflammation is not usually seen in disk fragments removed at surgery because the surgical intervention has been done, in most cases, following a few weeks of bed rest and the administration of antiinflammatory agents. Thus, in all likelihood, a pathological process (or processes), still not understood but probably of an inflammatory nature, along with the by products of inflammation and autoimmune reactions, plays a major role in irritating the APLL complex and nearby neural elements. This then leads to generation of pain signals in the APLL complex and sensitizes the nerve roots to mechanical pressure, leading to back pain and sciatica.

Yoshizawa et al.[69] confirmed the presence of an extensive axonal network of free nerve terminals in the anterior and posterior longitudinal ligaments and outer portion of the annulus fibrosus. The free-lying terminals described conform with the generally accepted morphology of pain receptors.[75] Thus a histologically documented anatomical basis exists for pain generation in the diseased annulus–posterior longitudinal ligament complex. The pain may be local or referred. As stated by Macnab,[66] pressure on a peripheral nerve does not produce pain, it produces paresthesia; but compression of an "inflamed, red, and angry" nerve root secondary to a herniated disk does reproduce sciatic pain. Macnab[66] demonstrated this by placing one catheter beneath an inflamed nerve root and another beneath a normal nerve root at the conclusion of lumbar laminectomy; when the catheters were distended, the pressure beneath the inflamed root reproduced the sciatic pain but that beneath the normal root caused only paresthesia.

Radiographic findings in subjects with back pain and sciatica

Among the 473 patients included in this report, there were 327 men and 146 women 22 to 84 years of age (mean 51 years) who had all been referred for CT examination of the spine as part of the work-up for back pain, clinically suspected stenosis, or sciatica.

138 patients had a history of back pain, but the pain did not radiate into their thighs or legs. In these individuals, 84 (or 61%) were without detectable abnormality on CT that could have explained their symptoms and 33 (24%) had facet joint arthrosis (mild or moderate in 27, marked in 6).
We are uncertain as to the relationship between facet joint degenerative arthrosis and back pain. In our experience

approximately 29% of patients who have no symptoms will have facet joint arthrosis. Osteophytes arising from the vertebral margins anteriorly and laterally may also be seen. Old calcified herniated disks, osteophytes, and bony ridges projecting into the spinal canal but not causing significant stenosis are also seen with equal frequency in asymptomatic patients.
Thus, in 61% of subjects with back pain, CT examination did not disclose a relevant disorder that could have accounted for their symptoms. In the remaining 39% a soft herniated disk, stenosis, or evidence of spinal instability or other abnormality was discovered that could have been responsible for the patients' back pain.

Among the remaining 335 patients with findings clearly indicative of radiculopathy, 57% (192 subjects) had either a herniated disk or spinal stenosis, or both, that correlated with their clinical findings and 43% (143 subjects) had no significant pathology, or the detected abnormality did not correlate positively with the clinical findings.

FACET JOINT DISEASE AND DEGENERATIVE DISEASE OF THE LUMBAR SPINE

Degenerative disease of the facet joints is described in Chapter 4.

MALALIGNMENT AND INSTABILITY OF THE SPINE AND DEGENERATIVE DISEASE

Degenerative disk disease can lead to malalignment of the spine. Some of the most common abnormalities are loss of lordosis, straightening, reversal of normal curvature, scoliosis, deviations to the right or left, and spondylolisthesis-like displacement of the vertebrae. Malalignment of the spine may be lateral, anterior, or posterior (retrolisthesis). There may also be instability associated with degeneration of the disks and facets. In the lumbar spine, degenerative disk disease and facet disease may be accompanied by abnormal motion of the spine. In patients with advanced degenerative disease of the facet joints, spondylolisthesis may also be present. There may be abnormal spinal motion in an anteroposterior direction because of articular facet deformity and laxity of the spinal ligaments. In a normal person the lumbar facet joints have an oblique orientation, with a component in the coronal plane. This prevents anteroposterior movement of one vertebral body relative to its neighbors. In a patient with advanced degenerative disease there is deformity of the articular facets, which leads to erosion and destruction of the coronal component of the facets and is more prominent in an individual with congenitally deformed facets or one who is congenitally prone to deformity and fragmentation of the facets with aging. When the facets are deformed, there is no longer a barrier to movement of the vertebrae in an anteroposterior or side-to-side direction.

Evaluation of abnormal motion of the lumbar spine is easily achieved with fluoroscopy. (It is advisable to record the findings on videotape.) The procedure is done with the patient standing, first flexing and then extending the spine. Bending to the sides should also be performed. Fluoroscopy is helpful in identifying the specific motion of the spine that causes the most pain.

CT and MRI are usually not necessary for evaluating instability of the spine. However, in trauma cases CT helps identify fractures through the pedicles and laminae that may be responsible for the instability. Motion studies of the lumbar spine are not routinely possible on CT and MRI at present. Furthermore, the lumbar flexion and extension views, though helpful, are generally inferior to those obtained by fluoroscopic motion studies.

Rigidity versus instability of the spine in degenerative disease

In many patients with moderately advanced degenerative disease of the intervertebral disks and facet joints, there will be varying degrees of reduced range of motion of the spine. When one can see osteophytes bridging the disks and calcification of the ligaments, the spine is probably completely rigid. On conventional radiography and CT one often notes such calcifications, bridging, and hypertrophic ridges. Another sign of lost spinal motion is the presence of fat at, and immediately adjacent to, the ankylosis. On MRI the fat can be seen to have accumulated next to the vertebral endplates in the anklyosed area. On the other hand, there will be areas of low signal on T1- and high signal on T2-weighted cross sections directly adjacent to the area of spinal instability. Histological examination reveals disruption of the vertebral endplates, with fissuring, edema, and granulation tissue formation in these regions, accounting for the interesting signal patterns produced on MRI.

REFERENCES

1. Hirschy JC, Leue WM, Berninger WH, et al: CT of the lumbosacral spine: importance of tomographic planes parallel to vertebral endplate. AJNR 1980;1:551-556. AJR 1981;136:47-52.
2. Williams LA, Haughton VM, Meyer GA, Ho KC: Computed tomographic appearance of the bulging annulus. Radiology 1982;142:403-408.
3. Firooznia H, Benjamin V, Kricheff II, et al: CT of lumbar spine disk herniation: correlation with surgical findings. AJNR 1984;5:91-96. AJR 1984;142:587-592.
4. Yu SW, Sether LA, Ho PS, et al: Tears of the anulus fibrosus: correlation between MR and pathologic findings in cadavers. AJNR 1988;9:367-370.
5. Kieffer SA, Sherry RG, Wellenstein DE, King RB: Bulging lumbar intervertebral disk: myelographic differentiation from herniated disk with nerve root compression. AJNR 1982;3:51-58. AJR 1982;138:709-716.
6. Coventry MB, Ghormley RK, Kernohan JW: The intervertebral disc: its microscopic anatomy and pathology. Anatomy, development, and physiology. J Bone Joint Surg 1945;27:105-112.
7. Brown MD: The pathophysiology of disc disease. Orthop Clin North Am 1971;2:359-370.
8. McRae DL: Asymptomatic intervertebral disc protrusions. Acta Radiol 1956;46:9-27.
9. Harris RI, Macnab I: Structural changes in the lumbar intervertebral discs. J Bone Joint Surg (Br) 1954;36:304-322.
10. Coventry MB, Ghormley RK, Kernohan JW: The intervertebral disc: its microscopic anatomy and pathology. II. Changes in the intervertebral disc concomitant with age. J Bone Joint Surg (Am) 1945;27:233-247.
11. Coventry MB, Ghormley RK, Kernohan JW: The intervertebral disc: its microscopic anatomy and pathology. III. Pathological changes in the intervertebral disc. J Bone Joint Surg (Am) 1945;27:460-474.
12. Hassler O: The human intervertebral disc: a microangiographical study on its vascular supply at various ages. Acta Orthop Scand 1970;40:765-772.
13. Larde D, Mathieu D, Frija J, et al: Spinal vacuum phenomenon. CT diagnosis and significance. J Comput Assist Tomogr 1982;6:671-676.
14. Orrison WW, Lilleas FG: CT demonstration of gas in a herniated nucleus pulposus. J Comput Assist Tomogr 1982;6:807-808.
15. Fuiks DM, Grayson CE: Vacuum pneumarthrography and the spontaneous occurrence of gas in joint spaces. J Bone Joint Surg (Am) 1950;32:933-938.
16. Ford LT, Gilula LA, Murphy WA, Mokhtar G: Analysis of gas in vacuum lumbar disc. AJR 1977;128:1056-1057.
17. Resnick D, Niwayama G, Guerra J Jr, et al: Spinal vacuum phenomena: anatomical study and review. Radiology 1981;139:341-348.
18. Gulati AN, Weinstein ZR: Gas in the spinal canal in association with the lumbosacral vacuum phenomenon: CT findings. Neuroradiology 1980;20:191-192.
19. Mikhael MA, Ciric I, Tarkington JA, Vick NA: Neuroradiological evaluation of lateral recess syndrome. Radiology 1981;140:97-107.
20. Ciric I, Mikhael MA, Tarkington JA, Vick NA: The lateral recess syndrome. A variant of spinal stenosis. J Neurosurg 1980;53:433-443.
21. Fries JW, Abodeely DA, Vijungco JG, et al: Computed tomography of herniated and extruded nucleus pulposus. J Comput Assist Tomogr 1982;6:874-887.
22. Williams AL, Haughton VM, Daniels DL, Thornton RS: CT recognition of lateral lumbar disk herniation. AJNR 1982;3:211-213. AJR 1982;139:345-347.
23. Williams AL, Haughton VM, Daniels DL, et al: Differential CT diagnosis of extruded nucleus pulposus. Radiology 1983;148:141-148.
24. Epstein BS: The spine, 4th ed. Philadelphia, Lea & Febiger, 1976, pp 634-647.
25. Finneson BE: Low back pain. Philadelphia, Lippincott, 1973, pp 59-60.
26. Shapiro R: Myelography, 3rd ed. Chicago, Year Book, 1975, p 377.
27. Macnab I: Negative disc exploration — an analysis of the cause of nerve-root involvement in 68 patients. J Bone Joint Surg (Am) 1971;53:891-903.
28. Schellinger D, Manz HF, Vidic B, et al: Disk fragment migration. Radiology 1990;175:831-836.
29. Truwit CL, Harle TS: Case report 524, Giant Tarlov (perineurial) cysts of lumbosacral spine. Skeletal Radiol 1989;18:75-77.
30. Schreiber F, Haddad B: Lumbar and sacral cysts causing pain. J Neurosurg 1951;8:504-509.
31. Seaman WB, Furlow LT: The myelographic appearance of sacral cysts. J Neurosurg 1956;13:88-94.
32. Siqueria EB, Schaffer L, Kranzler LI: CT characteristics of sacral perineurial cysts. J Neurosurg 1984;61:596-598.
33. Helms CA, Dorwart RH, Gray M: The CT appearance of conjoined nerve roots and differentiation from a herniated nucleus pulposus. Radiology 1982;144:803-807.
34. Ethelberg S, Riishede J: Malformations of lumbar spine roots and sheaths in the causation of low backache and sciatica. J Bone Joint Surg 1952;34:442-446.
35. Rothman SLG, Glenn WV: Spondylolysis and spondylolisthesis. In Newton TH, Potts DG (eds): Modern neuroradiology, Vol 1, San Anselmo Calif, Clavadel Press, 1983, pp 267-280.

36. Epstein BS, Epstein JA, Jones MD: Lumbar spondylolisthesis (with lysis or due to degenerative disease). Radiol Clin North Am 1977;15:261-287.

37. Edelman RR, Atkinson DJ, Silver MS, et al: FRODO pulse sequences: a new means of eliminating motion, flow, and wraparound artifacts. Radiology 1988;166:231-236.

38. Haacke EM, Lenz G: Improving MR image quality in the presence of motion by using rephasing gradients. AJR 1987;148:1251-1258.

39. Tyrrell RL, Diemling M: Fast three-dimensional MR imaging: clinical application. JNMR Med 1987;6:240-252.

40. Axel LL: Surface coil magnetic resonance imaging. J Comput Assist Tomogr 1984;8:381-384.

41. Enzmann DR, Rubin JB, Wright A: Use of cerebral spinal fluid gating to improve T2-weighted images. I. The spinal cord. Radiology 1987;162:763-767.

42. Hueftle M, Modic MT, Ross JS, et al: Lumbar spine: postoperative MR imaging with Gd-DTPA. Radiology 1988;167:817-824.

43. Winkler ML, Ortendahl DA, Mills TC, et al: Characteristics of partial flip angle and gradient reversal MR imaging. Radiology 1988;166:17-26.

44. Eyring JE: The biochemistry and physiology of the intervertebral disk. Clin Orthop Rel Res 1969;67:16-28.

45. Hendry NGC: The hydration of the nucleus pulposus and its relation to intervertebral disc derangement. J Bone Joint Surg 1958;40B:132-144.

46. Lindahl U, Roden L: The chondroitin 4-sulfate−protein linkage. J Biol Chem 1966;241:2113.

47. Lipson SJ, Muir H: Proteoglycans in experimental intervertebral disc degeneration (1980 Volvo award in basic science). Spine 1981;6:194-210.

48. Boden SD, David OD, Dina ST, et al: Abnormal magnetic resonance scans of the lumbar spine in a semtamatic subjects; a prospective investigation. J Bone Joint Surg 1990;72A:403-408.

49. Yu SW, Haughton VM, Sether LA, Wagner M: Comparison of MR and diskography in detecting radial tears of the anulus: a postmortem study. AJNR 1989;10:1077-1081.

50. Masaryk TJ, Ross JS, Modic MT, et al: High-resolution MR imaging of sequestered lumbar intervertebral disks. AJNR 1988;9:351-358. AJR 1988;150:1155-1162.

51. Modic MT, Masaryk T, Boumphrey F, et al: Lumbar herniated disk disease and canal stenosis: prospective evaluation by surface coil MR, CT, and myelography. AJR 1986;147:757-765.

52. Modic MT, Masaryk TJ, Ross JS, et al: Imaging of degenerative disk disease. Radiology 1988;168:177-186.

53. Modic MT, Steinberg PM, Ross JS, et al: Degenerative disk disease: assessment of changes in vertebral body marrow with MR imaging. Radiology 1988;166:193-199.

54. de Roos A, Kressel H, Spritzer C, Dalinka M: MR imaging of marrow changes adjacent to endplates in degenerative lumbar disk disease. AJR 1987;149:531-534.

55. Hajek PC, Baker LL, Goobar JR, et al: Focal fat deposition in axial bone marrow: MR characteristics. Radiology 1987;162:245-249.

56. Brodin H: Paths of nutrition in articular cartilage and intervertebral disc. Acta Orthop Scand 1954-1955;Q24:177-183.

57. Haughton VM, Eldevik OP, Magnaes B, Amundsen P: A prospective comparison of computed tomography and myelography in the diagnosis of herniated lumbar disks. Radiology 1982;142:103-110.

58. Raskin SP, Keating JW: Recognition of lumbar disc disease. Comparison of myelography and computed tomography. AJR 1982;139:349-355.

59. Burkus JK: Herniated nucleus pulposus in a patient with ankylosing spondylitis. Spine 1988;13:103-106.

60. Wilkinson M, Bywater EGL: Clinical features and course of ankylosing spondylitis as seen in a follow-up of 222 hospital referred cases. Ann Rheum Dis 1958;17:209-228.

61. Romanus R, Yden S: Destructive and ossifying spondylitic changes in rheumatoid ankylosing spondylitis (pelvospondylitis ossificans). Acta Orthop Scand 1952;22:88-99.

62. Dihlmann W, Delling G: Disco-vertebral destructive lesions (so-called Andersson lesion) associated with ankylosing spondylitis. Skeletal Radiol 1978;3:10-16.

63. Rivelis M, Freiberger RH: Vertebral destruction at unfused segments in late ankylosing spondylitis. Radiology 1969;93:251-256.

64. Wholey MH, Pugh DG, Bickel WH: Localized destructive lesions in rheumatoid spondylitis. Radiology 1960;74:54-56.

65. Veerapen K, Dieppe PA, Verrapen R, Griffith HB: The "last joint" syndrome in ankylosing spondylitis. Br Med J 1986;293:368.

66. Macnab I: Backache. Baltimore, Williams & Wilkins, 1981, p 94.

67. Lindblom K, Hultqvist G: Absorption of protruded disk tissue. J Bone Joint Surg 1950;22:557-560.

68. Hitselberger EW, Witten RM: Abnormal myelograms in asymptomaic patients. J Neurosung 1968;28:204-206.

69. Yoshizawa H, O'Brien JP, Smith WT, et al: The neuropathology of intervertebral discs removed for low back pain. J Pathol 198;132:95-104.

70. Bobechko WP, Hirsch C: Auto-immune response to nucleus pulposus in the rabbit. J Bone Joint Surg 1965;47B:574-582.

71. Hirsch C: Studies on the pathology of low back pain. J Bone Joint Surg 1959;41B:237-243.

72. Hirsch C, Ingelmark BE, Miller M: The anatomical basis for low back pain. Acta Orthop Scand 1963;33:1-17.

73. Nachemson A: Intradiskal measurements of pH in patients with lumbar rhizopathies. Acta Orthop Scand 1969;40:23-42.

74. Hakelius A: Prognosis in sciatica. A clinical follow-up of surgical and non-surgical treatment. Acta Orthop Scand, suppl 129, 1970;1-76.

75. Ham AW: Histology. 7th ed, Philadelphia, Lippincott, 1974, p 939.

3 Myelography and CT-Myelography in Degenerative Disease of the Lumbar Spine

RICHARD S. PINTO
HOSSEIN FIROOZNIA

The gold standard for diagnostic imaging of lumbar disk herniation is the CT-myelogram. Although noninvasive diagnostic imaging modalities (CT and MRI) are highly accurate in diagnosing disk herniation when there is no history of previous disk surgery, spinal stenosis, or spondylolisthesis,[1-7] they can be complicated by these conditions and the visualization of intraspinal anatomy and an accurate assessment of the patient's symptoms lost. CT-myelography may be the only modality able to clarify the confusing pathological anatomy in these situations.[1,3,5] We also utilize it when there is a discrepancy between clinical findings and the apparent diagnosis on CT and MRI.

CT-MYELOGRAPHY TECHNIQUES AND STRATEGIES
Myelographic contrast agents
PANTOPAQUE

During the past 10 years a number of new myelographic contrast agents have been introduced. Prior to the widespread use of metrizamide, iophendylate (Pantopaque) was the standard contrast for myelography. It is an oily substance that invariably produces adhesive arachnoiditis (although fewer than 1% of the patients receiving it develop symptoms); and when adhesive arachnoiditis is severe, it is clinically devastating because no medical or surgical procedure is available to alleviate its symptoms. Thus iophendylate has tended to fall out of favor. In addition, there are other drawbacks to its use. Rarely a hypersensitivity reaction of the meninges (aseptic meningitis) is noted following its intrathecal instilla-tion. Respiratory distress syndromes may occur when an epidural vein is injected, resulting in embolization to the segmental pulmonary arteries. Remnants of iophendylate in the spinal canal can interfere with visualization of the anatomy on CT (though not on MRI).

METRIZAMIDE

Metrizamide, a water-soluble contrast agent, has allowed myelography to be performed without fear of the chronic adverse reactions of Pantopaque. It is totally excreted via the kidneys within 24 hours. However, it is not without its own adverse reactions.[2] These include nausea, vomiting, acute neuropsychiatric changes (e.g., confusion, visual loss, dementia, and[rarely] seizures). Phenothiazime restriction is also necessary since available data suggest potentiation of post-myelographic seizures with metrizamide. Adverse reactions occur in 40% of patients undergoing metrizamide myelography. The mechanism of these reactions is thought to be an interruption of glucose metabolism in the brain.

SECOND-GENERATION NONIONIC CONTRAST AGENTS

Recently a second generation of myelographic contrast agents has been introduced (iohexol and iopamidol). Several studies demonstrate a lower incidence of adverse reactions with these substances, particularly less nausea and vomiting. Only about 10% of patients undergoing myelography with iohexol or iopamidol report adverse effects. The neuropsychiatric reactions encountered following metrizamide administration have been virtually eliminated, and seizure potential has been markedly reduced. Because of the (remote) continuing possibility of post-myelographic seizure, however, the lowest amount and concentration of contrast are recommended.

DOSAGE OF CONTRAST

For lumbar myelography a volume of 8 to 10 ml of 180 to 200 mg/100 ml iodine is sufficient to opacify the lumbar subarachnoid space. The contrast is injected slowly through a small-bore (22-gauge) spinal needle, since the incidence of post–spinal tap headache is quite likely related directly to the size of the needle.

Imaging technique

Conventional myelographic imaging is used primarily to locate the disk space for lumbar CT scanning. The classic views include AP, lateral, and two oblique. Conventional myelography is performed in 45- and 60-degree upright, as well as 0-degree (prone horizontal), positions so the contrast will layer behind each lumbar disk space. Upon completion of the prone portion of the imaging sequence, the patient is placed supine; this allows the contrast to flow into the dorsal thecal sac region to outline the thoracic cord and conus medullaris. Generally the patient should be in a head-up position, approximately 15 degrees, for adequate visualization of the conus region.

As part of a conventional myelographic series, we obtain an AP and a lateral view up to the level of T6 or T7. If the conus medullaris is not optimally visualized, CT slices are obtained from T9 to L1. Post-myelography CT scanning is performed at regions of documented disease on the myelogram. Subtle abnormalities of the root sleeves (e.g., amputation or splaying) should be further clarified by CT scanning at those levels. Patients with dermatomal signatures of a specific lumbar root should have a scan covering the course of that root even if the conventional myelography study fails to demonstrate a lesion. After a review of the images, CT scanning is prescribed for regions of interest that have been demonstrated on the myelogram or related to the patient's clinical presentation. We obtain 3 mm thick slices for any observed epidural lesion demonstrated. If there is a bulge or apparent disk herniation at one level, we encompass the entire region from pedicle to pedicle.

The CT scanning is done with the patient supine. In a pilot study at our institution we discovered that the prone position accentuates the appearance of annular bulging. Another disadvantage of the prone position is that the study is degraded by respiratory motion. To allow the contrast to diffuse passively throughout the spinal subarachnoid space, CT-myelography is usually performed 30 minutes to 1 hour after myelography. This causes the contrast density of the CSF to be reduced, thereby avoiding overshoot CT artifacts. Prior to transferring the patient into the CT gantry, we roll him (or her) 360 degrees to prevent layering of the contrast.

CT-MYELOGRAPHIC FINDINGS IN LUMBAR DISK DISEASE

The radiological signs of a herniated disk on CT-myelography include the following:
1. An extradural soft tissue density (Fig. 3-1), which displaces the thecal sac and ipsilateral nerve root away from the disk [1,4]

    There may be nonopacification of the ipsilateral root sleeve. The epidural defect is localized to the disk space but may extend above or below it in the spinal canal.
2. Extension into the ipsilateral neural foramen (Fig. 3-2)

    In patients with intraforaminal disk herniation occasionally the epidural defect will have a nonhomogeneous density with tiny bubbles of gas in it. This usually is associated with diminution of the height of the disk, rarely with focal erosion of bone.
3. Location of a migrated fragment at the level of the pedicle of the superjacent or subjacent vertebral body (Fig. 3-3)

    The parent disk may appear normal on CT examination, but slices above or below the disk will show the epidural defect. The adjacent osseous structures must be carefully evaluated to rule out a metastatic focus.
4. Focal configuration

    The epidural defect is usually focal and frequently found to reside in the anterolateral aspect of the spinal canal.

Advantages of CT-myelography

CT-myelography is particularly useful in the following conditions:

Conjoined root sleeve and root cysts: These congenital anomalies not infrequently present as "mass" lesions on non–contrast CT.[8] Enlargement of the lateral recess is sometimes seen with conjoined root sleeves. Root cysts may be associated with erosion of the vertebral bodies. Although in most cases the diagnosis is easily established on CT or MRI, occasionally a patient will present with confusing soft tissue densities in the spinal canal, particularly when a herniated disk and conjoined root sleeve coexist. CT-myelography clearly delineates the involved anatomy and helps delineate the herniation, if present.[1,5]

Spinal stenosis: In these patients there is a paucity of epidural fat and the density of the dural sac (Houndsfield units) may be higher than usual because of the lower CSF fraction in the sac.[6,7] These factors reduce the contrast between soft tissue components of the spinal canal and make the diagnosis of a herniated disk more difficult on CT examination. MRI may not be helpful either. CT-myelography, however, delineates the presence of a herniated disk as well as osteophytes, calcified ligaments, or other factors responsible for compression of the neural elements in these patients (Fig. 3-4).

Migrated disk fragments: CT-myelography is often helpful in establishing the diagnosis in these patients. It also clearly delineates abnormalities of the root sleeve or thecal sac secondary to disk herniation (Fig. 3-3, 2).

Osseous or calcified lesions: Occasionally confusion will

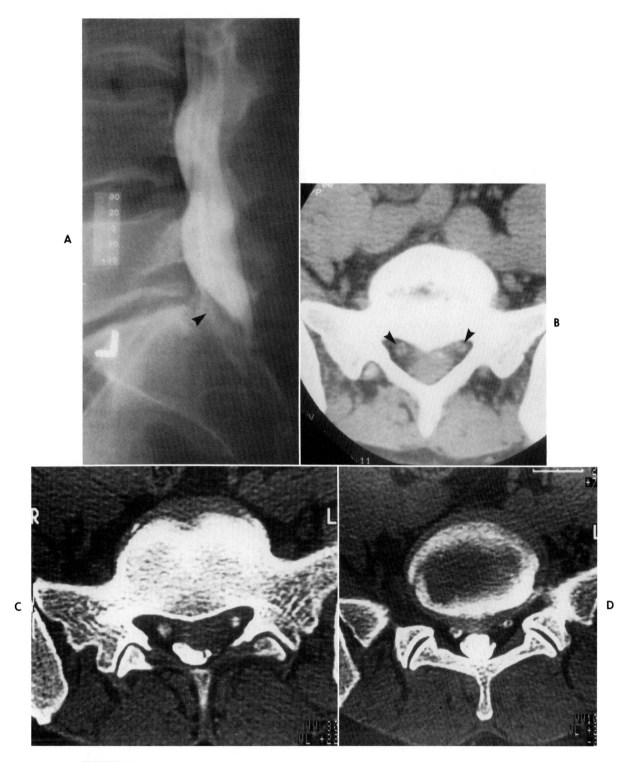

FIGURE 3-1
A, A water-soluble contrast myelogram demonstrates decreased height of the L5-S1 disk space. A short thecal sac can be seen, and an insensitive ventral epidural space is also present *(arrow)*. **B,** A CT slice without intrathecal contrast obtained at the vertebral end plate level of S1 shows the descending roots in the lateral S1 recesses *(arrows)*. The thecal sac is present centrally and appears unremarkable. A small fleck of calcification is visible to the left of midline anteriorly within the thecal sac. **C,** A postmyelographic CT scan at the same level reveals a large epidural defect, indicative of an extruded herniated disk, situated anterolaterally to the left of midline and displacing the left S1 root laterally. It compresses the thecal sac focally (especially to the left of midline). **D,** Another postmyelographic CT slice, this time through the disk space of L5-S1, demonstrates a mild focal epidural defect centrally without distortion of the thecal sac or the right S1 root sleeve. The left S1 root sleeve is displaced laterally.

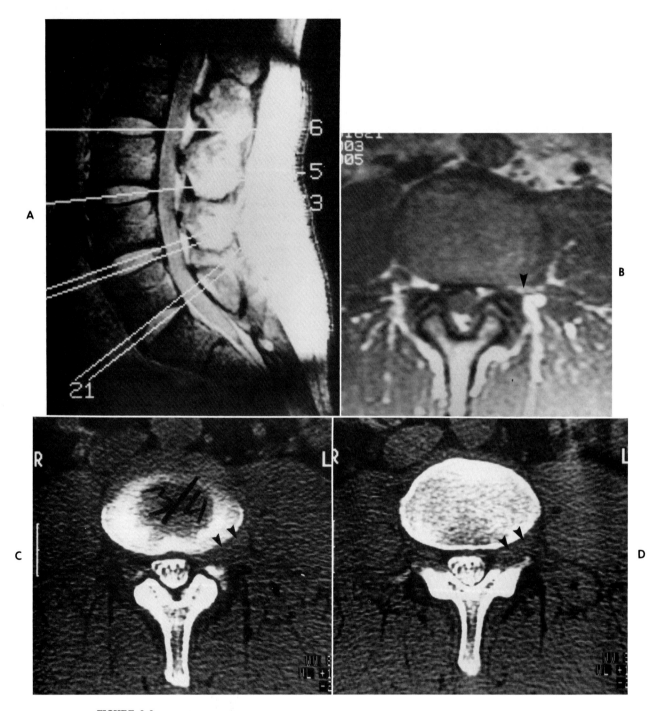

FIGURE 3-2
A 36-year-old patient presenting with left thigh pain. **A,** Sagittal midline MR with image annotation of slices performed in the axial plane. **B,** A single axial slice through L3-4 demonstrates asymmetry of signal from the intraforaminal epidural fat (not initially recognized because it was partially obliterated on the left by a small focal epidural defect [*arrow*]). **C,** An axial postmyelographic CT slice shows the defect, indicative of an intraforaminal herniated disk on the left, obliterating the fat *(arrows).* **D,** Another CT slice through the superjacent intervertebral foramen of L3-4 clearly demonstrates a disk fragment, within the left intervertebral foramen, obliterating the left foraminal fat completely *(arrows).* Note that there is no distortion of the contrast-filled thecal sac with a purely intraforaminal herniated disk.

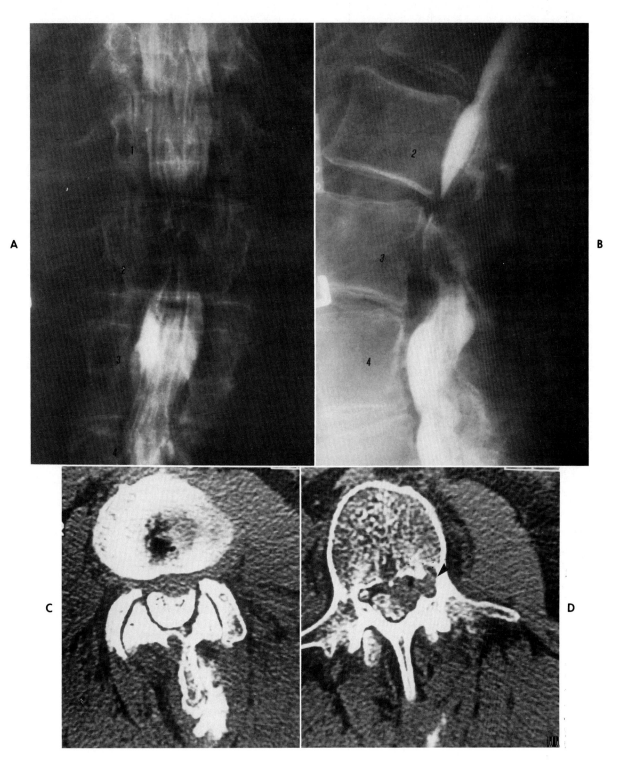

FIGURE 3-3
A and B, AP and lateral projections of a myelogram demonstrate a high-grade epidural block present at L1-2 extending inferiorly to L2-3 on the right. Other epidural changes are evident including a defect posterolaterally on the left of L3-4. C, A postmyelographic CT scan through the L2-3 disk space demonstrates the defect, centrally and to the left of midline, mildly distorting the ventral aspect of the thecal sac. D, At the level of the L2 pedicle there is a large soft tissue mass in the epidural compartment compressing the thecal sac focally and eroding the pedicle and posterior margin of the vertebral body on the left *(arrow)*. This represents a sequestered fragment of disk material that has produced osseous erosive changes, an uncommon occurrence.

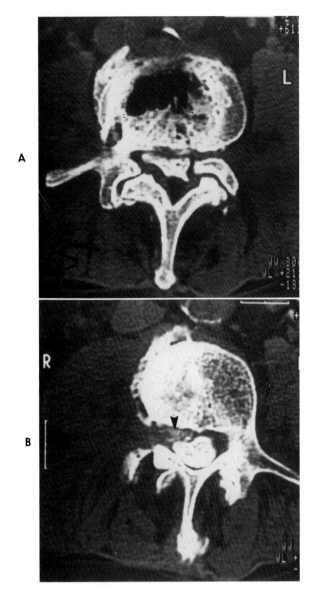

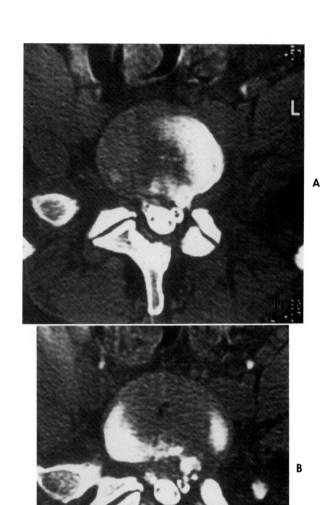

FIGURE 3-4

An elderly man with many years of low back pain who presents with a 6-week history of right leg pain and in whom lumbar stenosis is discovered. **A,** The CT slice after intrathecal administration of contrast demonstrates a degenerative disk, with a vacuum phenomenon intradiscally and a small calcific ridge ventrally. The anterior aspect of the thecal sac is flattened. Posterolaterally on the right a prominent hypertrophied ligamentum flavum compresses the posterolateral aspect of the thecal sac. **B,** A CT slice superjacent to **A** reveals an epidural hyperdensity situated anterolaterally on the right *(arrow)*, producing focal compression of the thecal sac. This indicates extension of the herniated disk.

FIGURE 3-5

A 47-year-old woman who underwent left hemilaminotomy and facetectomy for radicular pain, without improvement. **A,** CT scan after the intrathecal administration of contrast material. A calcific mass is present anterolaterally on the left and displaces the left S1 root sleeve posteriorly without distortion of the thecal sac. **B,** A slice at the superjacent inferior vertebral plate of L5 shows the calcific ridge originating from the inferior vertebral endplate and encroaching on the left anterolateral epidural space. The left S1 root sleeve is mildly displaced at this level. Note the absence of a left ligamentum flavum and the bony defect indicative of the hemilaminotomy. Note also the changes of a medial facetectomy.

arise at MRI examination in patients who have calcified lesions within the spinal canal. Examples include a calcified ligamentum flavum, osteophytes, calcified epidural and intradural neoplasms, a calcified herniated disk, and metastases. CT-myelography is often helpful for these (Fig. 3-4).

Intradural versus extradural lesions: CT-myelography enhances the traditional areas of strength of myelography in differentiating these lesions. For example, a neurofibroma is easily distinguished from a herniated disk.

Osteomyelitis and epidural abscess

Postoperative lumbar spine: In these patients CT-myelography has all the advantages already enumerated for diagnosing disk herniations and differentiating them from conjoined root sleeves, root cysts, and epidural or intradural neoplasms. In addition, in some patients, the differentiation of recurrent disk herniation from an epidural scar[9] may not be possible on CT with intravenous contrast or MRI with gadopentetate. Because these two procedures are less invasive than myelography, and because they both can

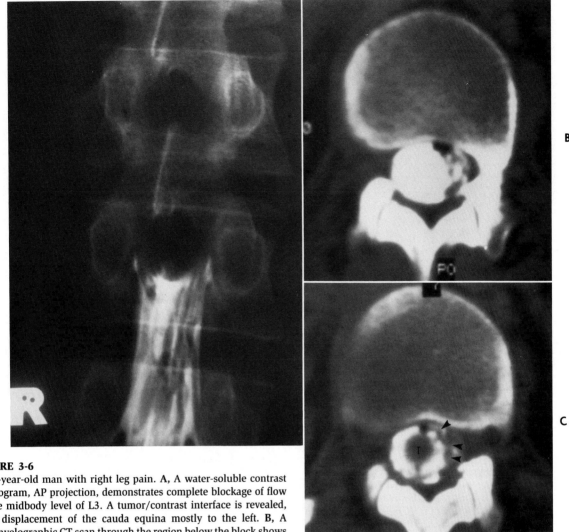

FIGURE 3-6

A 37-year-old man with right leg pain. **A,** A water-soluble contrast myelogram, AP projection, demonstrates complete blockage of flow at the midbody level of L3. A tumor/contrast interface is revealed, with displacement of the cauda equina mostly to the left. **B,** A postmyelographic CT scan through the region below the block shows displacement of the cauda to the left, with a widened subarachnoid space centrally and to the right. **C,** Another CT scan, through the inferior aspect of the tumor *(T)* at L1, demonstrates the widened subarachnoid space with displacement of the cauda to the left *(arrows).* The tumor is present within the contrast-filled subarachnoid space. These findings are diagnostic for a neurofibroma.

delineate the pathology in most failed back syndrome cases, we prefer them to myelography as the initial diagnostic radiology procedure in the work-up of failed back syndrome.

However, if CT with intravenous contrast and MRI with gadopentetate have both been performed and a definitive diagnosis is still not established, we resort to myelography. CT-myelography is especially helpful in differentiating a recurrent disk herniation from scarring in these patients. When an epidural soft tissue density is present but it is not clear whether it represents disk herniation or scarring, CT-myelography may solve the puzzle. In patients with epidural scar the nerve roots are identified as distinct structures within a soft tissue density (Fig. 3-5). In other words, the soft tissue density of scar surrounds the root sleeve, often without displacing or obliterating it. On the other hand, if the epidural mass is a herniated disk, the root sleeve is displaced away from it and may be obliterated. The dural sac is also displaced away from a herniated disk whereas a mature scar pulls the dural sac toward itself.

Lesions of the conus medullaris: It is important to exclude pathology of the conus medullaris region (Figs. 3-6 to 3-9) in patients with sciatic syndrome. At present, MRI of the lumbar spine delineates the conus optimally; thus myelography solely for this purpose is not indicated. However, in questionable instances, CT-myelography can further improve the imaging of pathological anatomy in this region and clarify the diagnosis.

Disadvantages of CT-myelography

Invasiveness of the procedure: The major disadvantage is its invasive nature, which necessitates a spinal tap and instillation of myelographic contrast in the subarachnoid space.

Post–spinal tap headache: This complication is seen in approximately 10% of patients undergoing myelography, even with a small (22-gauge) needle. Spinal tap headaches are disabling to the patient and frequently interfere with normal function because they are worse when the patient is

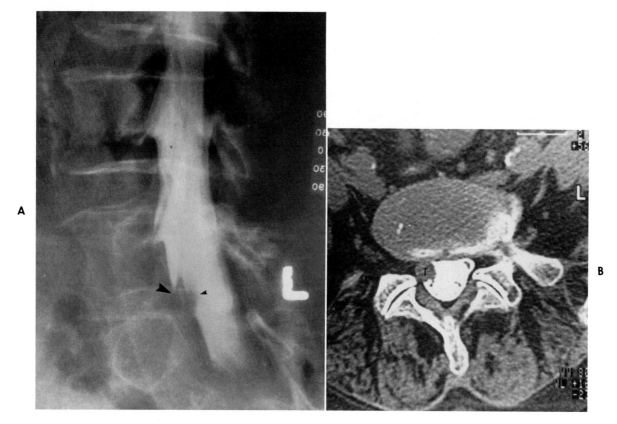

FIGURE 3-7
A 73-year-old man complaining of right leg pain. **A,** An oblique projection of a myelogram demonstrates amputation of the right S1 root sleeve *(arrow)* and a small focal defect *(small arrow).* **B,** A postmyelographic CT scan at the disk space level clearly shows an intradural mass *(T),* with clear separation from the disk space at the origin of the right S1 root sleeve. The differential diagnosis includes neurofibroma and drop metastasis. Past clinical history documented surgical removal of a glioblastoma, which has remained asymptomatic for 3 years. Because of continued pain, even after a course of radiation therapy, this intradural lesion was removed and found to represent a drop metastasis from the prior glioblastoma multiforme.

upright and are relieved only when supine. They can persist for 3 to 7 days (the longest in our series was 30 days); treatment is complete bed rest.

Postmyelographic adverse reactions: The introduction of second-generation nonionic intrathecal contrast agents has lessened the incidence of immediate postmyelographic adverse reactions[2] (headache and nausea). Nevertheless, generally 10% of patients will have mild headache or feeling of nausea. These occur usually 2 to 8 hours after myelography.

Seizure: Uncommonly a patient may have a seizure after myelography. This is reported to occur in 0.7% of the patients undergoing a nonionic water-soluble myelographic procedure (the incidence is probably lower with second-generation agents).

Missed intraforaminal disk herniation: Purely intraforaminal herniated disks[6,7,10] can be missed on myelography because the dural sac or root sleeve may not be distorted. However, this is not usually a problem on CT-myelography (Fig. 3-2) since intraforaminal lesions are readily identified.

Insensitive epidural space: In some patients there is a layer of fat, sometimes more than 10 mm thick, between the posterior surface of L5 and the L5-S1 disk and the anterior aspect of the dural sac. A herniated disk in this region, even when large, may not contact the descending sacral roots or dural sac (Fig. 3-1) and may therefore be missed on myelography. However, this is usually not a problem on CT-myelography because the thick epidural fat provides an excellent contrast, with clear delineation of the sacral roots and dural sac, making identification an easy matter.

COMPARISON OF CT, MRI, AND CT-MYELOGRAPHY

In our experience computed tomography has been able to establish the diagnosis of disk herniation in about 89% of consecutively seen nonselected patients referred for back pain and/or sciatica.[6] This includes patients with previous spinal surgery (Fig. 3-5), stenosis, or other abnormalities. If patients with previous spinal surgery are excluded, the diagnostic accuracy approaches 93%.[6] When a state-of-the-art high-resolution MRI examination in 1991 is compared to a CT examination, the accuracy of MRI approaches that of CT. However, we believe that CT and MRI are complementary procedures; each has special advantages and disadvantages. The choice of the initial

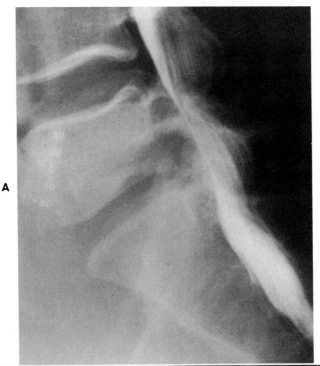

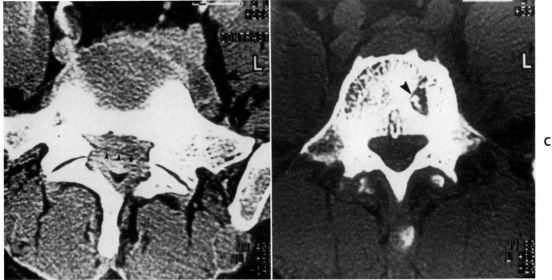

FIGURE 3-8

A, A water-soluble contrast myelogram, lateral projection, demonstrates a large ventral epidural defect extending from the L4-5 to the L5-S1 disk space and inferiorly to the midbody of S1. The patient had complained of low back pain with 2 months of radicular pain in both legs, worse on the left. **B,** A CT scan at the inferior vertebral endplate of L5 performed after intravenous and intrathecal administration of contrast shows an epidural mass *(small arrows)*, greater to the left of midline, compressing the ventral aspect of the thecal sac to a moderate degree. A low-density paraspinal mass *(arrow)* is also seen on the left. **C,** Bone window imaging clearly reveals a sequestrum of bone within the body of L5 *(arrow)*. L5 is also extremely osteoblastic. A paraspinal mass can be detected anterior to the vertebral body, and an epidural lesion is markedly compressing the thecal sac. The finding of an osseous sequestrum with epidural and paraspinal masses strongly supports the diagnosis of a chronic osteomyelitis with paraspinal and epidural spread. Percutaneous fluoroscopically directed needle biopsy demonstrated tuberculosis.

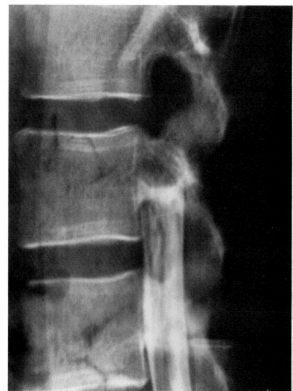

A

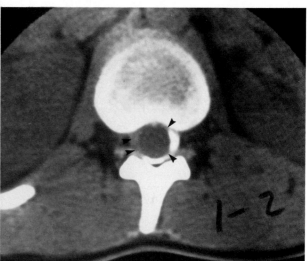

B

FIGURE 3-9

A 21-year-old patient complaining of back pain radiating to both legs, more so to the right. **A,** The lateral projection of a water-soluble contrast myelogram demonstrates complete blockage at L2 with sharp tumor/contrast interface. **B,** A CT scan after intrathecal contrast administration reveals the mass centrally within the spinal canal and the cauda splayed along its circumference *(arrows).*

diagnostic procedure to be utilized is dependent on the preferences of the referring physician and patient, the availability of equipment, and financial considerations. When a definitive diagnosis is not established after one procedure, we use the other as the next diagnostic test. If a definitive diagnosis is still not established, we recommend CT-myelography. Thus CT-myelography may be viewed as the final radiological modality either confirming or excluding lumbar pathology. Since myelography is an invasive procedure, with well-known complications, every effort must be made to obtain the best possible examination the first time. Thin sections, on the order of 3 mm or so, should be obtained both through clinically symptomatic levels (or where dermatomal or root signatures dictate) and through apparently insignificant myelographic epidural defects. The lower thoracic cord to T7, including the conus medullaris, must be visualized.

The diagnostic accuracy of CT-myelography should, in theory, be 100%, limited only by technical factors. In reality, this goal is not achieved in patients with a markedly stenotic canal or spinal deformity or when there have been multiple surgeries.

REFERENCES

1. Anand AL: Plain and metrizamide CT of lumbar disk disease: comparison with myelography. AJNR 1982;3:567-571.
2. Hauge O, Falkenberg H: Neuropsychologic reactions and other side effects after metrizamide myelography. AJR 1982;139:357-360.
3. Haughton VM, Eldevik OP, Magnaes B, Amundsen P: A prospective comparison of computed tomography and myelography in the diagnosis of herniated lumbar disks. Radiology 1982;142:103-110.
4. Kieffer SA, Sherry RG, Wallerstein ED, King RB: Bulging lumbar intervertebral disk: myelographic differentiation from herniated disk with nerve root compression. AJR 1982;138:709-716.
5. Dublin AB, McGahan JP, Reid MH: The value of computed tomographic metrizamide myelography in the neuroradiological evaluation of the spine. Radiology 1983;146:79-86.
6. Firoozonia H, Benjamin V, Kricheff II, et al: CT of lumbar spine disc herniation: correlation with surgical findings. AJR 1984;142:587-592.
7. Fries JW, Abodeely DA, Vjungo JG, et al: Computed tomography of herniated and extruded nucleus pulposus. J Comput Assist Tomogr 1982;6:874-887.
8. Bouchard JM, Copty M, Langelier R: Preoperative diagnosis of conjoined root anomaly with herniated lumbar disks. Surg Neurol 1978;10:229-231.
9. Schubiger O, Valavanis A: CT differentiation between recurrent disc herniation and postoperative scar formation: the value of contrast enhancement. Neuroradiology 1982;22:251-254.
10. Williams AL, Haughton VM, Daniels DL, Thornton RS: CT recognition of lateral lumbar disk herniation. AJNR 1982;3:211-213. AJR 1982;139:345-347.

4 Spinal Stenosis

HOSSEIN FIROOZNIA

Spinal stenosis is a condition in which the spinal cord, cauda equina, nerve roots, or spinal nerves are compressed due to either constriction of the bony canal or enlargement of the soft tissue contents of the canal (or both).[1-6] It is essentially of two kinds: (1) congenital-developmental and (2) acquired. The majority of patients with symptoms suffer from a combination of congenital stenosis and superimposed degenerative changes.

CONGENITAL-DEVELOPMENTAL SPINAL STENOSIS

Congenital-developmental spinal stenosis may be either (a) idiopathic, an isolated anomaly of the spine (with no other significant skeletal dysplasia), or (b), less commonly, associated with congenital skeletal abnormalities.

Idiopathic congenital stenosis

Congenital spinal stenosis may involve many or only one or two vertebrae. It is encountered with almost equal frequency in the cervical spine, usually affecting three or four vertebrae (mostly C3 to C6), and the lumbar spine (usually L2 to L4 but rarely L5-S1). It is uncommon in the thoracic spine.

Congenital stenosis with congenital skeletal abnormalities

Achondroplasia, Morquio's disease, Down's syndrome, and congenital craniovertebral junction anomalies (e.g.,

fusion of C1 to the base of the skull and stenosis of the foramen magnum) may be associated with congenital spinal stenosis.

ACQUIRED SPINAL STENOSIS
CERVICAL SPINE

1. C1-2 instability (erosion of the odontoid process, destruction of the ligaments, erosion of the facet joints) due to
   a. Inflammatory arthritides (noninfectious): rheumatoid arthritis, psoriatic arthritis, anklylosing spondylitis, related conditions
   b. Pyogenic or tuberculous infection of the atlantoaxial complex
2. C3 to C7 malalignment secondary to
   Inflammatory arthritides (rheumatoid, psoriatic, ankylosing spondylitis)
   Degenerative arthritis
   Trauma
3. Calcification and ossification of the posterior longitudinal ligament
4. Degenerative spondylosis
   a. Bony ridges and osteophytes due to degenerative disease of the disks, Luschka joints, and facet joints
   b. Hypertrophy and redundancy of the intraspinal ligaments
5. Paget's disease

6. Postsurgical: overgrowth of bone or slippage of bone graft following anterior decompression and interbody fusion

THORACIC SPINE

1. Trauma
2. Calcification and ossification of the posterior longitudinal ligament
3. Paget's disease
4. Calcified thoracic disk herniation
5. Facet joint degenerative disease, calcified ligamentum flavum, calcified facet joint capsule
6. Vertebral hemangioma

LUMBAR SPINE

1. Degenerative spondylosis
   a. Degenerative disease of the facet joints
   b. Degenerative disk disease with the formation of posterior vertebral endplate osteophytes and bony ridges
   c. Buckling, redundancy, and calcification of the ligamentum flavum and capsule of the facet joints
   d. Degenerative spondylolisthesis
2. Spondylolysis with or without spondylolisthesis
3. Postsurgical
   a. Bony overgrowth following posterolateral fusion
   b. Gradual worsening of spondylolisthesis in a patient with preoperatively normal spinal alignment
   c. Worsening of preexisting degenerative spondylolisthesis, after (wide) laminectomy and facetectomy
4. Posttraumatic

OTHER CONDITIONS

1. Forestier's disease (DISH)
2. Acromegaly
3. Pseudogout
4. Composite nerve root sleeve
5. Epidural lipomatosis

PATHOLOGY AND PATHOLOGICAL ANATOMY OF SPINAL STENOSIS
Achondroplasia

Achondroplasia is the classic form of congenital spinal stenosis (Fig. 4-1). A disturbance of enchondral bone growth leads to premature fusion of the cartilaginous growth plates, with resulting short bones. The vertebral bodies may be diminished in height. The pedicles are short, and consequently the anteroposterior diameter of the spinal canal is decreased. The posterior surfaces of the vertebral bodies have an accentuated concavity. The laminae are thick and broad. The epidural fat may be markedly diminished. Another finding is reduction of the interpedicle distance, which decreases from L1 to L5. This is opposite to what is found in normal subjects. The curvature of the spine is also abnormal: the lumbar spine generally has an exaggerated lordosis, the thoracic spine an exaggerated kyphosis. Spinal stenosis in achondroplasia is usually limited to the lumbar and lower thoracic spine. Less commonly it may be encountered in the cervical spine, or even the entire spine.[5-7]

The clinical manifestations in these patients generally develop earlier than in patients with other forms of spinal stenosis; some individuals need decompressive laminectomy and facetectomy in the second or third decade of life. Axial cross sections of the lumbar spine may show markedly narrowed lumina in the lower thoracic and lumbar region. The surface area of the canal may become progressively smaller, instead of larger, from L1 to L5. The pedicles are practically nonexistent, and the canal may have an anteroposteriorly narrow channel instead of its normal rounded configuration.

Idiopathic congenital spinal stenosis

In patients with idiopathic congenital spinal stenosis the pathology of the condition is similar to that of achondroplasia: the pedicles are thick and short, the laminae are thick and broad, and overlap one another (producing a shingling effect), and the cross-sectional area of the canal is diminished. The cervical canal (Figs. 4-2 to 4-4) may appear flattened anteroposteriorly, but the lumbar canal, though stenotic, usually has a normal configuration.[1,2,4,5,8]

The pedicles are short, and the sagittal diameter of the canal is reduced (Figs. 4-5 to 4-11). The posterior surfaces of the vertebrae, particularly in the lumbar region, have an accentuated concavity (Figs. 4-6, 4-7, and 4-11). Thus the vertebral endplates and disks appear to protrude into the spinal canal on axial cross sections (Fig. 4-8). Often several disks appear to bulge into the canal. Although these apparently bulging disks do not require surgical intervention, they may be an important factor in aggravating stenosis, which will require decompressive laminectomy and facetectomy.

Inflammatory spondylitis
RHEUMATOID ARTHRITIS, PSORIATIC ARTHRITIS, AND RELATED CONDITIONS

In these conditions, recurrent synovitis leads to erosion of the odontoid process and destruction of its stabilizing ligaments, producing C1-2 dislocation and cord compression. We have encountered cord compression with malalignment of the midcervical spine secondary to inflammatory spondylitis (rheumatoid and psoriatic arthritides), causing destructive changes of the Luschka joints and adjacent portions of the disks, facet joints, and neural arches. Neurological symptoms may also be caused by compression of the cord secondary to atlantoaxial subluxation, pannus formation about the odontoid process, and craniovertebral settling[9-12] (Figs. 4-12 and 4-13).

Text continued on p. 152.

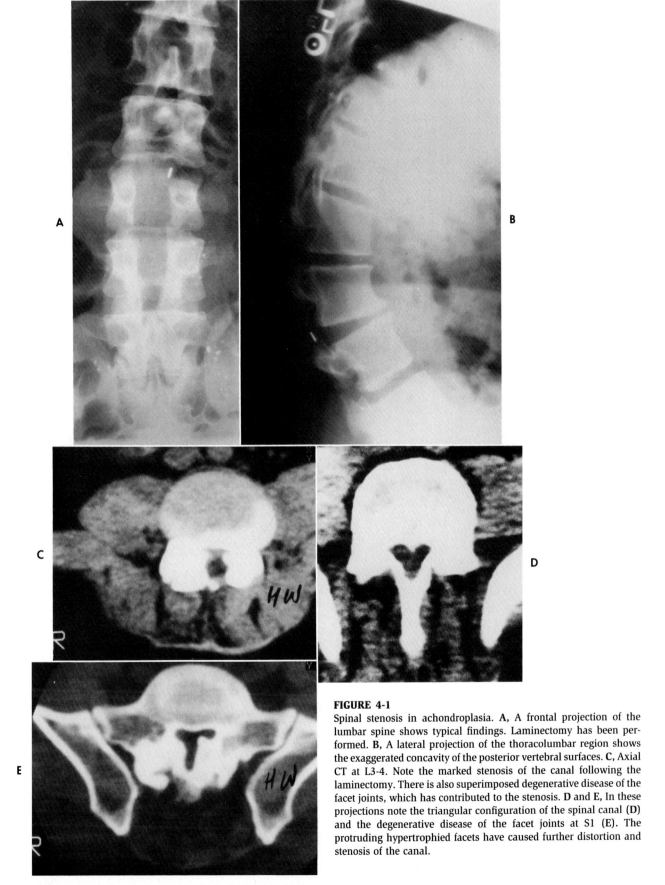

FIGURE 4-1

Spinal stenosis in achondroplasia. **A,** A frontal projection of the lumbar spine shows typical findings. Laminectomy has been performed. **B,** A lateral projection of the thoracolumbar region shows the exaggerated concavity of the posterior vertebral surfaces. **C,** Axial CT at L3-4. Note the marked stenosis of the canal following the laminectomy. There is also superimposed degenerative disease of the facet joints, which has contributed to the stenosis. **D** and **E,** In these projections note the triangular configuration of the spinal canal (**D**) and the degenerative disease of the facet joints at S1 (**E**). The protruding hypertrophied facets have caused further distortion and stenosis of the canal.

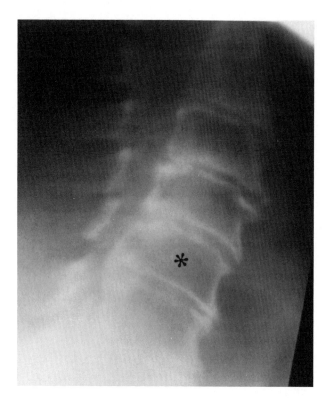

FIGURE 4-2
Congenital stenosis of the cervical spine complicated by acquired stenosis. A lateral tomogram of the cervical spine shows the stenosis at C4-5 and C6. (The *asterisk* is on C5.) A bony bar extends from C5 to C6. Note the marked stenosis of the canal. Congenital stenosis is usually encountered at C4 to C6; it is uncommon at C1 to C3. It may be seen best at the foramen magnum region associated with fusion of a rudimentary C1 to the occipital bone. This combination occurs more often with congenital abnormalities of the odontoid process.

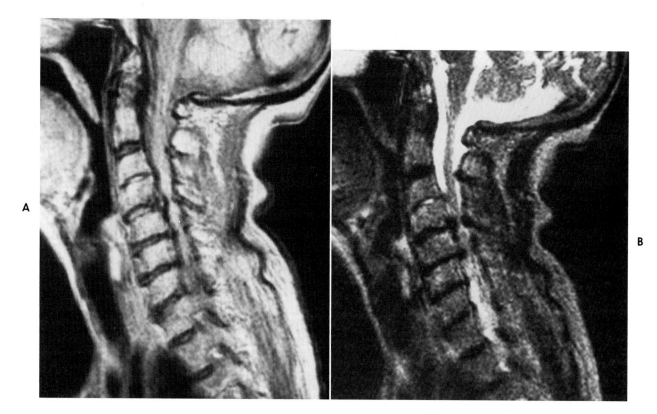

FIGURE 4-3
Congenital spinal stenosis with superimposed degenerative disease. A sagittal MRI, **A** (TR 1200/TE 30), and another, **B** (TR 1200/TE 180), show the stenosis extending from C4 to C7. Note the thoracolumbar scoliosis starting at C7, with the midline of the cervical spine no longer visible below that level. Hypertrophic changes are superimposed on the disk disease, aggravating the C4-7 stenosis. Notice also the hypertrophic ridges with the herniated disk. This patient has a relatively pronounced compression of the cord with long-standing progressive myelopathy.

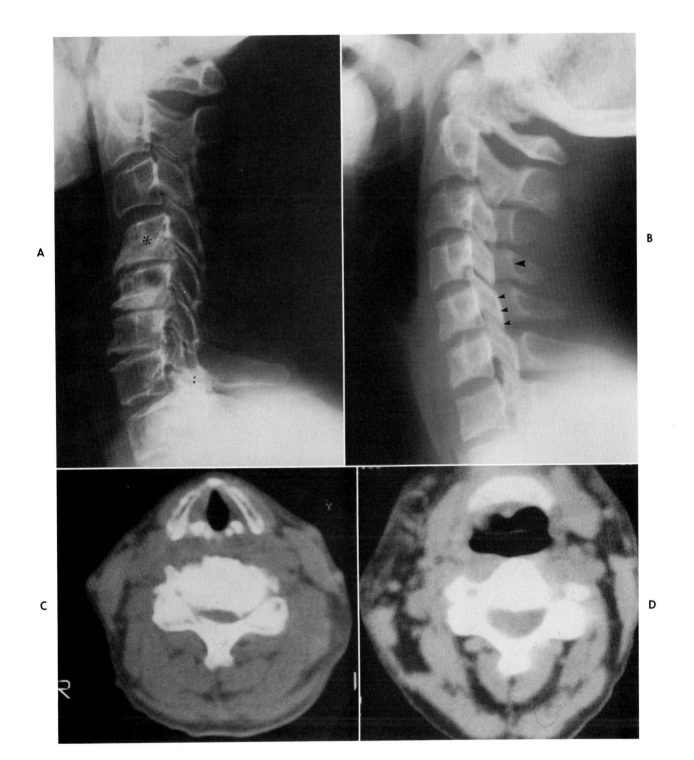

FIGURE 4-4
Congenital stenosis of the cervical spine, C4 to C7, complicated by an acquired stenosis. **A,** There is marked degenerative disease at C4-5, C5-6, and C6-7 involving both the disks and the Luschka joints. Note the spinal malalignment due to it. The cortex of the posterior wall of the canal is only minimally posterior to the cortex of the articulating pyramids. **B,** In this lateral view of the normal cervical spine of another subject, the posterior wall *(single arrowhead)* projects well posteriorly of the articular pyramids *(three arrowheads)*. When the laminae are short and oriented more or less coronally rather than 45 degrees off-coronal, the canal is flattened anteroposteriorly and stenotic. **C,** A CT examination through C5 (same patient as in A) shows the spinal stenosis. Note the thickness of the laminae and their orientation. **D,** Another CT of this patient shows the normal size of the canal at C3.

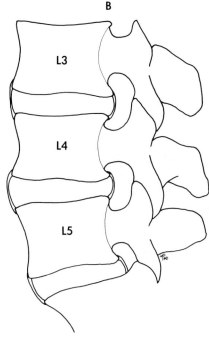

FIGURE 4-5
Normal spine versus congenital stenosis of the lumbar spine. **A**, The normal configuration of the vertebral body and annulus fibrosus. **B**, The configuration in a patient with congenital stenosis. Note the exaggerated concavity of the posterior surfaces of the vertebral bodies. This causes the endplates and annulus to protrude into the canal markedly. Thus axial images will show an apparently bulging disk when, in fact, the configuration is normal for a patient with spinal stenosis.

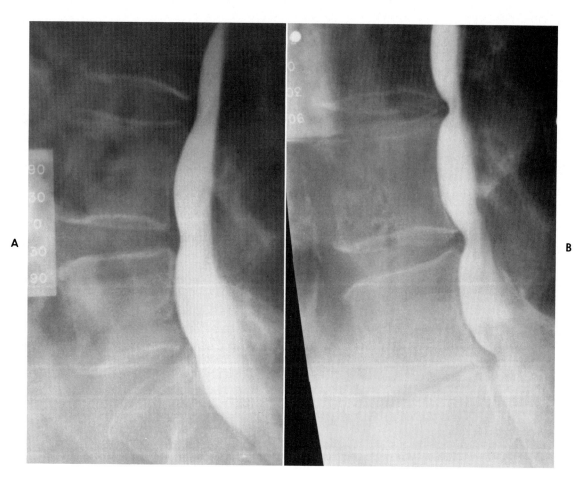

FIGURE 4-6
Normal spine versus spinal stenosis, lateral myelograms. **A**, Normal subject in the prone position. Note the gentle impression of the annulus fibrosus on the anterior surface of the contrast-filled dural tube. **B**, Patient with stenosis in the prone position. Here the posterior surfaces of the vertebral bodies are more concave and the endplates and annulus protrude more noticeably into the canal.

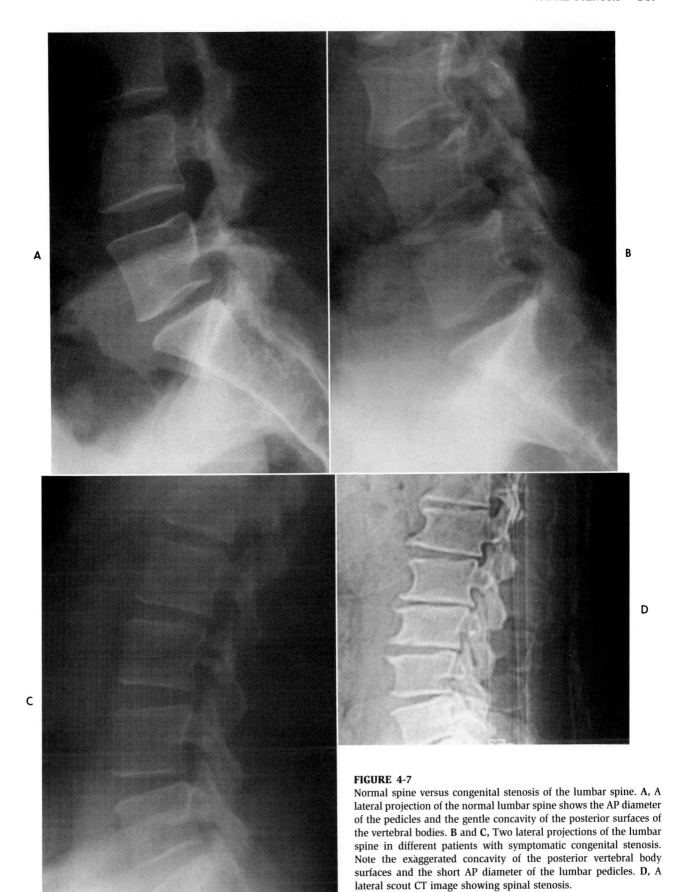

FIGURE 4-7
Normal spine versus congenital stenosis of the lumbar spine. **A,** A lateral projection of the normal lumbar spine shows the AP diameter of the pedicles and the gentle concavity of the posterior surfaces of the vertebral bodies. **B** and **C,** Two lateral projections of the lumbar spine in different patients with symptomatic congenital stenosis. Note the exaggerated concavity of the posterior vertebral body surfaces and the short AP diameter of the lumbar pedicles. **D,** A lateral scout CT image showing spinal stenosis.

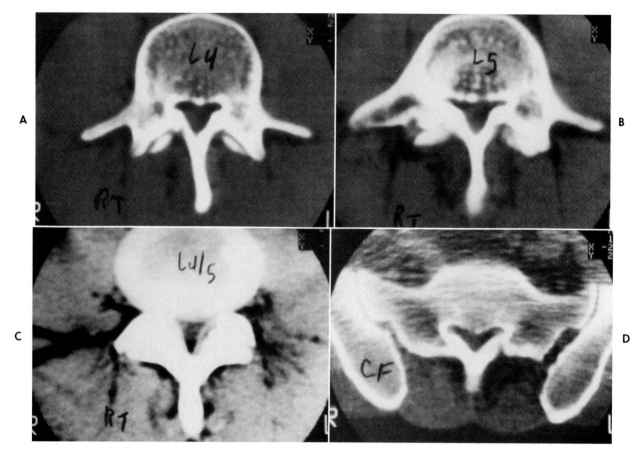

FIGURE 4-8
Congenital lumbar stenosis. **A**, L4, **B**, L5, and **C**, L4-5. **D** is S1 in another patient. Congenital L5-S1 stenosis is uncommon. In the patient shown in **A** to **C**, L5-S1 was normal.

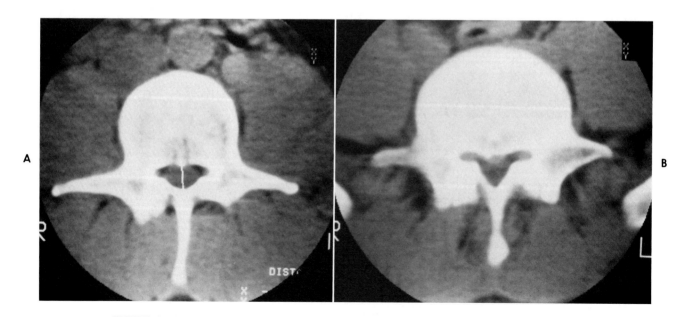

FIGURE 4-9
Congenital lumbar stenosis. **A** is at L4, **B** at L5. There is also minimal to moderate degenerative disease of the facet joints, with protrusion into the spinal canal.

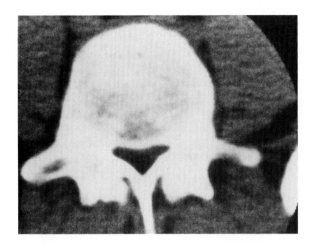

FIGURE 4-10
Congenital lumbar stenosis at L5. Note the exaggerated triangular configuration of the canal and the broad thick elements of the posterior arch.

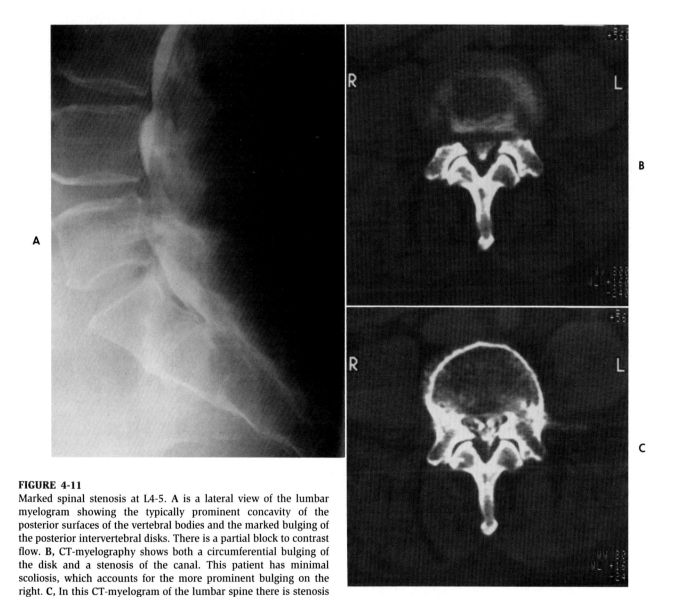

FIGURE 4-11
Marked spinal stenosis at L4-5. A is a lateral view of the lumbar myelogram showing the typically prominent concavity of the posterior surfaces of the vertebral bodies and the marked bulging of the posterior intervertebral disks. There is a partial block to contrast flow. **B,** CT-myelography shows both a circumferential bulging of the disk and a stenosis of the canal. This patient has minimal scoliosis, which accounts for the more prominent bulging on the right. **C,** In this CT-myelogram of the lumbar spine there is stenosis and a small amount of contrast has been retained between the nerve roots in the dural sac. In addition, there is considerable crowding of the descending nerve roots.

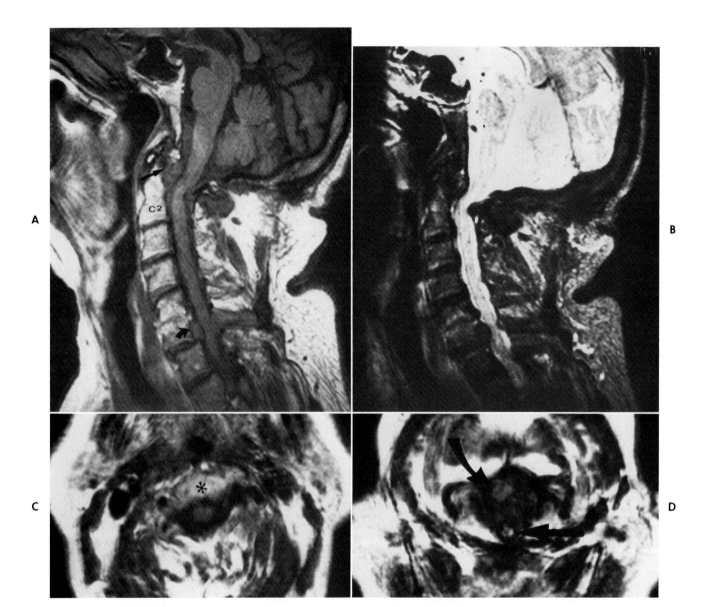

FIGURE 4-12

Pannus in the atlantoaxial region of a patient with long-standing rheumatoid arthritis. **A,** A sagittal T1-weighted cross section shows erosion of the odontoid process, with a soft tissue mass *(arrow)* posterior to the odontoid causing displacement and compression of the cord. **B,** A T2-weighted sagittal cross section shows the mass to be of very low signal intensity, excluding the possibility of effusion. Joint effusion presents with increased signal, similar to CSF, on T2-weighted images. **C,** An axial T1-weighted cross section through the body of C2 *(asterisk)* shows the cord directly behind C2 in the canal. **D,** Another axial T1-weighted slice, this time at the tip of the odontoid process *(straight arrow)*, shows the cord displaced posteriorly and to the left *(curved arrow)* by a large low-signal mass (the pannus) between the odontoid and the cord. Note the extensive fat replacement of marrow at C2 through C6. There is also malalignment at C6-7, and the C5-6 disk is practically fused. Fat has crossed the disk space, which indicates solid bony fusion. The *arrow* denotes a large herniation at the posterior surface of C6. In addition, the anterior surface of the cord is compressed.

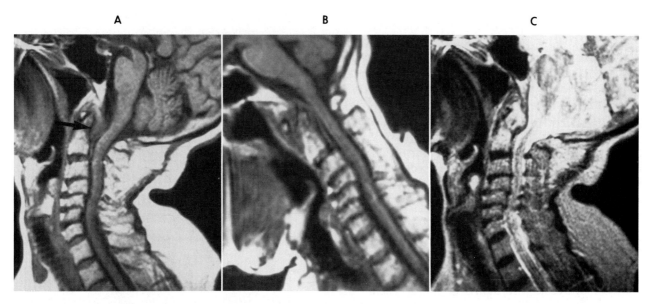

FIGURE 4-13
Atlantoaxial joint effusion in a patient with long-standing rheumatoid arthritis and secondary degenerative disease. **A,** A midsagittal T1-weighted cross section obtained in extension shows a low-intensity mass posterior to the odontoid process *(arrow).* The cord is bent and displaced posteriorly. There is moderate malalignment at C3 to C6, with slight compression of the cord at C4-5. **B,** A midsagittal T1-weighted cross section in flexion shows the soft tissue mass posterior to the odontoid to have disappeared. However, there is still some atlantoaxial dislocation. **C,** Midsagittal MRI (TR 1400/TE 150), with the neck in extension. The mass posterior to the odontoid is of the same signal intensity as CSF, which shows that it is joint effusion.

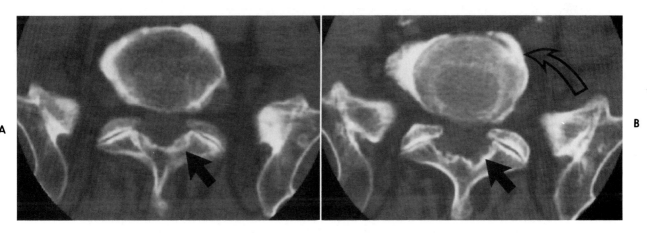

FIGURE 4-14
Spondyloarthropathy. Bone window axial CT slices through L5-S1 in a patient with long-standing inflammatory spondyloarthropathy. The cortex of the neural arch is almost completely eroded *(solid arrow),* and the sacroiliac joint almost completely fused. The facet joints, however, are not fused at this level. The *hollow curved arrow* in **B** denotes calcification of the anterior longitudinal ligament.

ANKYLOSING SPONDYLITIS

Compression of the neural elements in ankylosing spondylitis may occur by a mechanism similar to that described for rheumatoid arthritis, and by two other mechanisms: angular kyphosis, with destructive and sclerotic changes of the intervertebral disks and vertebral bodies (Andersson lesions),[13-15] and arachnoid diverticulae, which usually form in the lower lumbar and sacral region.[16-18] Both these lesions are accompanied by fibrosis and erosive changes of the surrounding bones and may induce the cauda equina syndrome (usually 10, 20, up to 40 years after the spondylitis has been quiescent). On CT or MRI examination the dural sac is seen to have a markedly irregular outline in the lumbar region, and there may be small diverticulumlike outpocketings in it. The bony cortex of the inner wall of the canal is quite irregular due to erosive changes (Fig. 4-14).

Spinal stenosis secondary to degenerative disease

CERVICAL SPINE

Stenosis of the cervical spine occurs secondary to degenerative disease of the intervertebral disks, Luschka joints, and facet joints.

Degenerative disease of the disks is often associated with relatively prominent osteophytes arising from the anterior edges of the vertebral endplates. The lateral and posterolateral borders of the cervical disks are covered by the Luschka processes. Osteophytes do not arise from these. Posteriorly, degenerative disk disease can lead to the formation of vertebral osteophytes and bony ridges (Figs. 4-15 to 4-18). In some patients hypertrophic changes extend along practically the entire posterior surface of the vertebral bodies (Fig. 4-16), rather than being limited to the endplate regions.

Degenerative disease of the uncovertebral (Luschka) joints (Fig. 4-18) is often associated with degenerative disease of the disks. The Luschka processes form the anteromedial walls of the neural foramina. Osteophytes of the Luschka processes extend into the lower part of the cervical neural foramina and are the major cause of cervical neural foraminal stenosis. Hypertrophic changes of the Luschka processes also often extend posterolaterally into the spinal canal and may appear on both sides of midline (Fig. 4-18). In patients with marked Luschka joint degenerative disease, stenosis of the canal may also be present in addition to the neural foraminal changes.

Degenerative disease of the facet joints does not usually cause stenosis of the cervical spinal canal. It is also only rarely the cause of cervical neural foraminal stenosis. However, degenerative disease of the disks, uncovertebral joints, and facet joints may exist simultaneously; and in advanced stages there may be severe stenosis (Figs. 4-19 and 4-20) with malalignment, restriction of motion, or spondylolisthesis (Figs. 4-21 and 4-22).

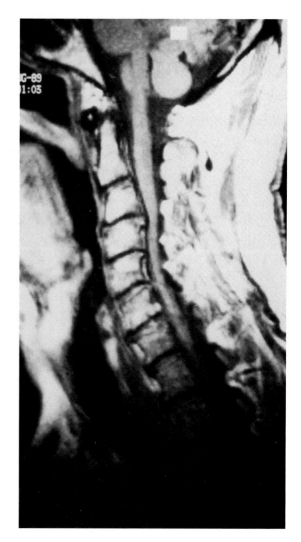

FIGURE 4-15
Cervical canal stenosis due to degenerative disk disease. Note the fairly prominent hypertrophic change in the posterior surface of C3-4 associated with the degenerative disease. There is also a marked stenosis of the canal, with compression of the cord, from C3-4 to C5-6.

THORACIC SPINE

Degenerative disease of the thoracic disks is often associated with hypertrophic osteophytes and bony ridges. A significant number of patients with herniated thoracic disks will have calcification of the disk, which may produce moderate to marked stenosis of the canal. A patient with thoracic disk herniations, calcified or uncalcified, often presents with progressive myelopathy due to long-standing compression of the cord.

Stenosis of the spinal canal may be noted with severe degenerative disease of the thoracic facet joints. This is an extremely rare pathological entity, there being only a few reported cases (Fig. 4-23). Degenerative facet joint disease is associated with hypertrophic changes of the articular facets, which protrude into the spinal canal and

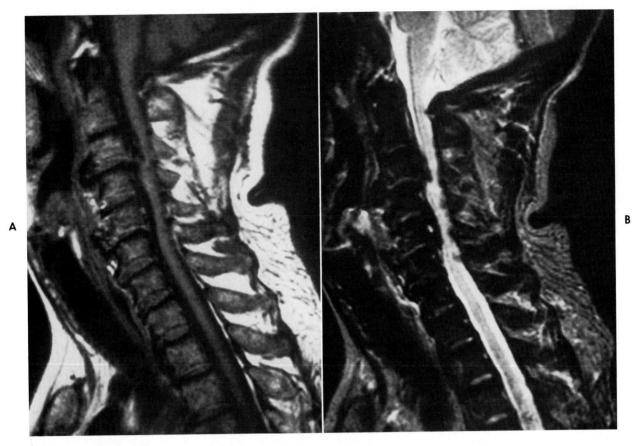

FIGURE 4-16
Marked spinal stenosis due to extensive bony ridges secondary to degenerative disease of the cervical spine. **A,** Midsagittal T1-weighted (TR 600/TE 20) and, **B,** midsagittal T2-weighted (TR 2100/TE 80) MRI examination. This elderly man has severe degenerative disease of all the cervical disks. Broad bony ridges on the posterior surfaces of C3 and C4-5 have produced stenosis of the canal and compression of the cord. The patient also has a gradually evolving myelopathy.

cause stenosis. In addition, hypertrophy and calcification of the ligamentum flavum and calcification of the capsule of the facet joints may be seen.[19-22]

LUMBAR SPINE

The most important causes of lumbar spinal stenosis are degenerative disease of the facets and disks (Fig. 4-24) and hypertrophy of the spinal ligaments[1,3,23] (Fig. 4-25). Degenerative disease of the facet joints leads to protrusion of the articular facets into the canal, causing distortion and stenosis. Hypertrophy of the superior articulating facets is responsible for stenosis of the lateral recess.[23] In these patients the spinal canal has an exaggerated cloverleaf configuration and the descending nerve roots may be compressed in the lateral recess between the vertebral body and the disk anteriorly, the pedicle laterally, and the hypertrophied superior articulating facet posteriorly. In some patients the degenerative changes produce stenosis of the canal only, without causing simultaneous stenosis of the lateral recess. Degenerative hypertrophic spurs arising from the posterior and posterolateral edges of the vertebral endplates secondary to degenerative disk disease may significantly narrow the canal, lateral recess, or neural foramina. In some patients a marked redundancy of the ligamentum flavum leads to its enlargement, occasionally with calcification. A moderately bulging disk, ordinarily of no significance in patients with a normal-sized canal, may contribute to the generation of clinical findings in patients with spinal stenosis. However, this is not an indication for diskectomy; the treatment of choice is surgical decompression (laminectomy and [hemi]facetectomy).

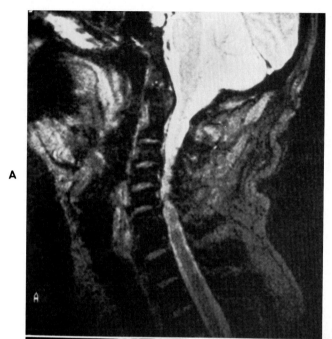

FIGURE 4-17

Spinal stenosis and cord compression with degenerative hypertrophic changes of the vertebral endplates and bony ridges. **A,** A midsagittal gradient echo MRI of the cervical spine (TR 450/TE 20, flip angle 20) shows prominent bony ridges on the posterior surfaces of C3-4, C4-5, and C5-6. The C6 and C7 bodies are fused. There is moderate to marked compression of the cord, along with a gradually worsening myelopathy. **B** and **C,** Gradient echo MRI axial cross sections at C4-5 and C5-6. The *arrows* point to a large calcific bridge on the posterior surfaces of the vertebrae.

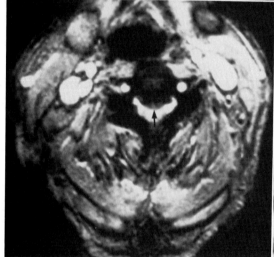

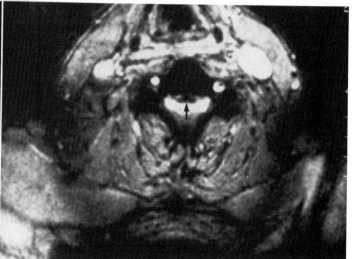

FIGURE 4-18

Stenosis of the cervical canal in a patient with severe degenerative hypertrophic change of the uncinate processes and ossification of the posterior longitudinal ligament (OPLL), causing cord compression and myelopathy. A to D are a CT-myelography study. (Note in **A,** at C4-5, the hypertrophic uncinate changes and the bony ridges, which have caused a marked stenosis of the canal. The cord is compressed and atrophic. In **B,** C5, **C,** C5-6, and, **D,** C7, OPLL has caused compression and deformity of the spine.) **E** is a midsagittal MRI of the cervical spine (TR 900/TE 30). There is atrophy of the cord posterior to C4-7, confirmed by parasagittal and axial cross sections. Note the area of signal void between the cord and the posterior surfaces of C4-7, the area occupied by OPLL. **F,** A midsagittal T1-weighted MRI shows the results of anterior decompression and interbody fusion of C4-7, with resection of OPLL.

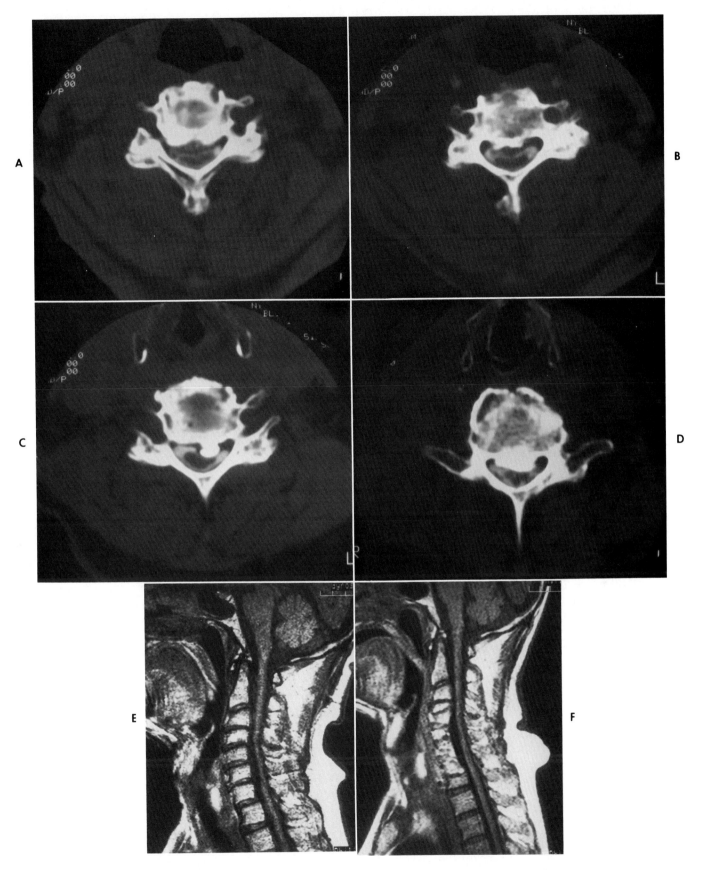

FIGURE 4-18
For legend see opposite page.

A   B   C

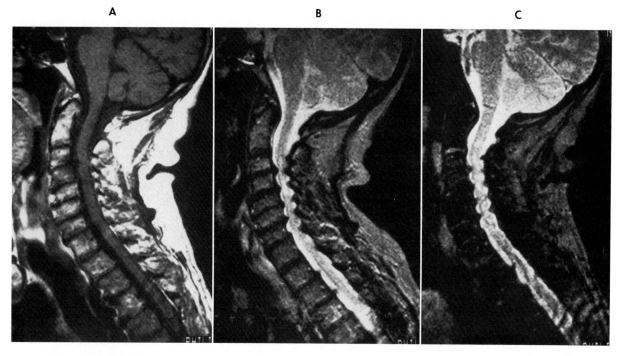

FIGURE 4-19
Spondylosis of the cervical spine. **A**, T1-weighted (TR 600/TE 20), **B**, T2-weighted (TR 2116/TE 80), and, **C**, gradient echo (TR 450/TE 20, flip angle 20) midsagittal cross sections of the cervical spine in an elderly woman with extensive degenerative disease of all cervical disks and moderate to marked hypertrophic changes of the posterior aspects of the disks starting at C3-4 and extending to C6-7. In addition, there is extensive degeneration of the Luschka joints and facet joints. Note the characteristic impression of the hypertrophic changes on the subarachnoid space.

Degenerative spondylolisthesis

In some patients with marked degenerative disease of the facet joints there may be an associated spondylolisthesis[24,25] (Figs. 4-26 to 4-30). This often occurs at L4-5 and is more common in women. The height of the disk may be significantly diminished because of the associated degenerative disease. The thecal sac may be compressed between the posterior arch of an anteriorly displaced vertebra and the posterior surface of the superior endplate of the vertebra caudad to it (Figs. 4-27 and 4-28). Contrary to some reports, herniation of an intervertebral disk at the level of the spondylolisthesis does occur; in fact, it is fairly common in chronic cases and may be responsible for at least some of the clinical findings in these patients.

However, a definitive diagnosis of disk herniation in these patients may be difficult on CT, myelography, or MRI because there is distortion of the canal and epidural fat due to listhesis. Furthermore, because of listhesis, a cross-sectional CT or MR image obtained through the disk may show a soft tissue density projecting behind the posterior edge of the inferior endplate of an *anteriorly* displaced vertebral body (Fig. 4-28). This is produced by the obliquely slanting posterior border of the disk and is

normal. However, it may obscure a herniation in this region.

The patient with spondylolisthesis may have no symptoms for years; and when clinical manifestations do develop, it may be a challenge (sometimes impossible) to pinpoint the cause. If there is forward displacement of the vertebral body, the descending nerve roots will be stretched because the root sleeve and dorsal root ganglion almost always travel forward with the vertebral body. Thus stretching and tethering of the nerve roots are important causes of symptoms in these patients. There is also stenosis of the canal with compression of the dural sac, which may be severe. Stenosis occurs at the disk level. On myelograms (Fig. 4-28) and MRI studies the dural sac is noted to be compressed between the anteriorly displaced neural arch of the slipped vertebra and the posterior surface of the nondisplaced (caudad) vertebra. There is also severe degenerative disease of the facet joints, and the facets are fragmented (Figs. 4-27 and 4-30). Finally, there may be thickening and calcification of the facet joint capsule and ligamentum flavum (Fig. 4-30).

All these factors contribute to further narrowing of the canal and compression of the dural sac. In patients with

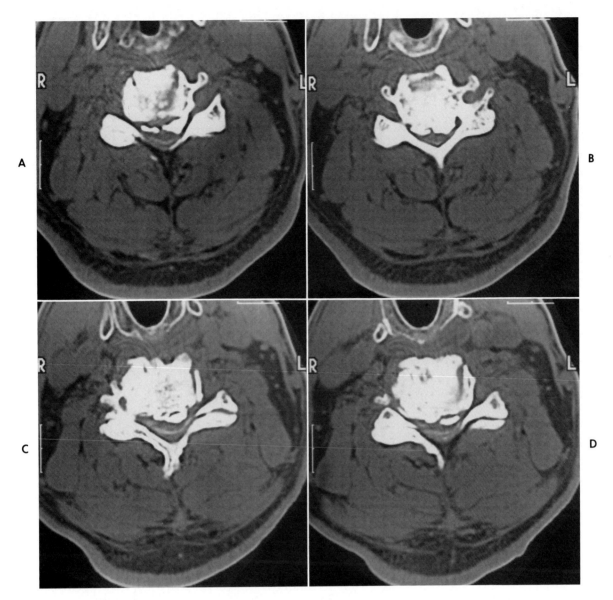

FIGURE 4-20
Severe spinal stenosis due to an old calcified herniated disk with hypertrophic bony ridges. A and B, C4-5 and, C and D, C5-6 CT-myelographic studies show spinal stenosis and atrophy of the cord in a patient with a long-standing history of progressive myelopathy.

severe degenerative disease and marked fragmentation of the facets there may also be osteosclerosis and fractures through the pars interarticularis. A mass of fibrocartilaginous callus may form posterolaterally adjacent to the defect of the posterior arch and protrude into the neural foramen, contributing to the entrapment of exiting spinal nerves.

Degenerative disease of the intervertebral disk, at the level of a spondylolisthesis (or above or below it) and leading to herniation, calcification, or formation of a vacuum phenomenon, occurs in a significant number of patients. The herniation may be an important cause of symptoms, particularly when an acute episode is encountered. Another cause of acute back pain in these patients

is a sudden increase in the extent of spondylolisthesis and stenosis. Minor fractures of the edges of articular processes may facilitate further anterior slippage and precipitate acute symptoms.

Spondylolysis with and without spondylolisthesis

Spondylolysis is most common at L5, and spondylolisthesis with lysis occurs most commonly at L5-S1 (Figs. 4-31 and 4-32). The conditions are usually seen in men. There may be a fibrocartilaginous mass at the site of a pars interarticularis defect that protrudes into the

Text continued on p. 170.

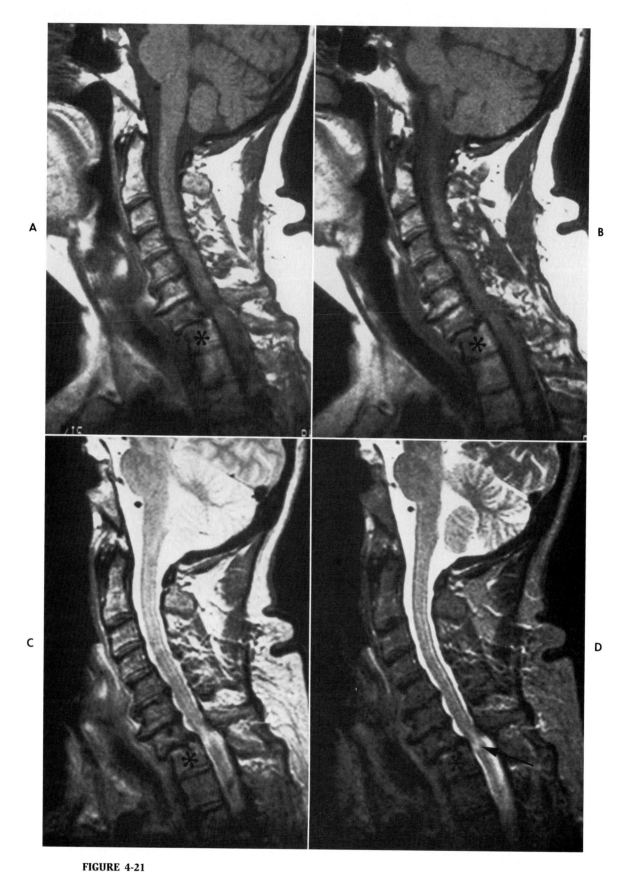

FIGURE 4-21
Degenerative spondylolisthesis of the cervical spine. **A** and **B** are T1-weighted midsagittal and parasagittal MRI studies of the cervical spine. The *asterisks* are on T1. There is a moderate spondylolisthesis at C7-T1 associated with severe degenerative disk disease. **C** and **D** are midsagittal spin density and T2-weighted MRI studies of the cervical spine showing a focal area of increased signal in the substance of the cord (better appreciated in **D** *[arrow]*). These areas, in association with long-standing stenosis and cord compression, are believed to represent zones of edema or myelomalacia, the precursor of cord cavitation, although long-term follow-up is not yet available.

A

B

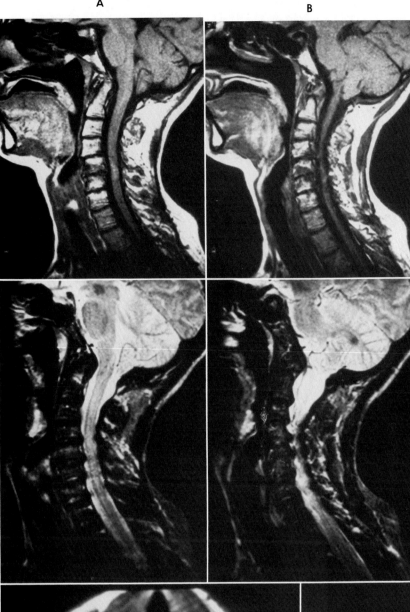

C

D

E

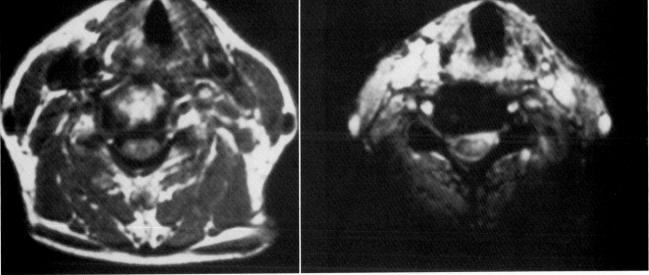

F

FIGURE 4-22

Acquired stenosis with a large spinal canal. Moderate degenerative disk disease and malalignment have caused stenosis on the right with C5-6 radiculopathy. A and B are T1-weighted midsagittal and right parasagittal MRI studies of the cervical spine (TR 600/TE 20). C and D are corresponding T2-weighted cross sections (TR 2000/TE 75) showing the degenerative disease from C4 to C7. There is malalignment of C5 and C6, which are slightly posteriorly displaced, with compression of the anterior surface of the cord. Laterally, note the more significant compression of the cord (parasagittal images, B and D). Fat has replaced marrow adjacent to C6-7 in A. Notice also the moderate osteosclerosis at C5-6 (best seen in A). E is an axial T1-weighted cross section at C5-6 (TR 785/TE 20) and, F, a corresponding gradient echo image (TR 750/TE 20, flip angle 25) showing hypertrophic changes of the posterior surfaces of the endplates on the right, with stenosis of the neural foramina.

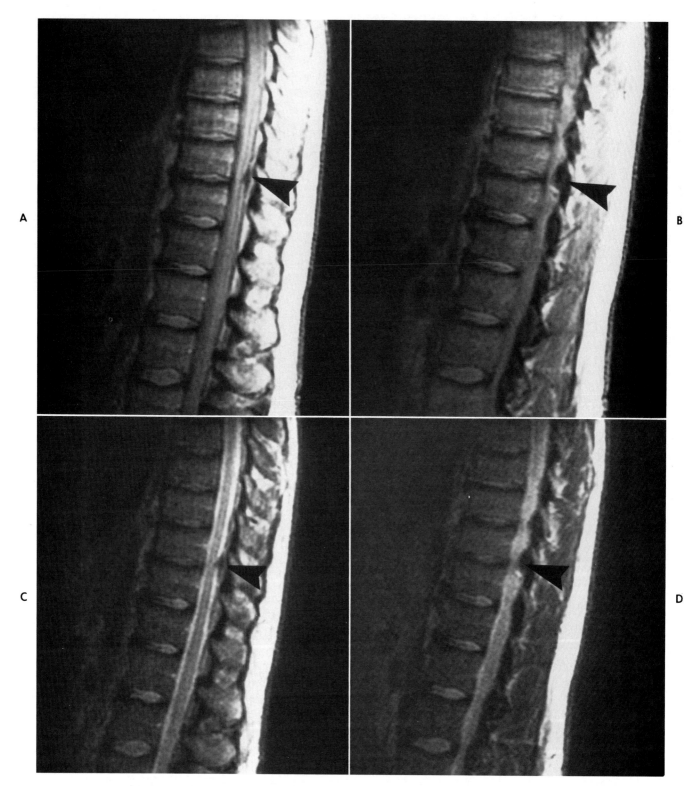

FIGURE 4-23
Thoracic spinal stenosis. A to D are sagittal and parasagittal MRI studies of the thoracic spine (TR 1900/TE 30 and 80). The *arrowhead* in each points to an area of decreased signal corresponding to calcification of the ligamentum flavum at T8-9.

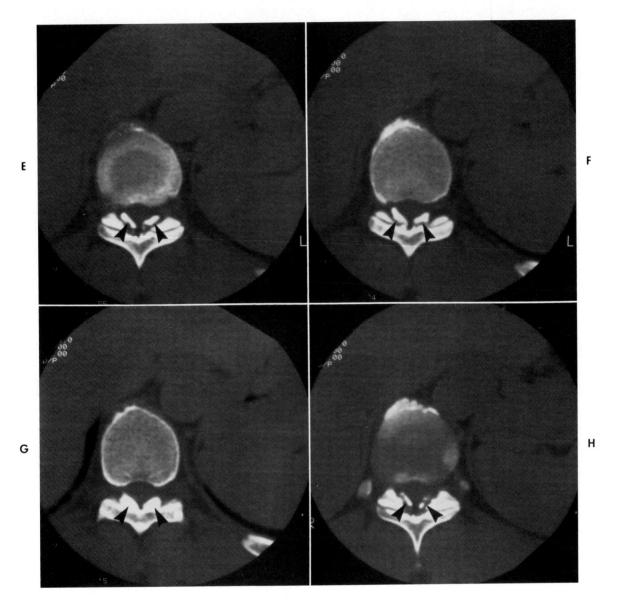

FIGURE 4-23, cont'd
E to H, CT slices at T8-9 showing the calcified ligamentum flavum on the right and left sides
(arrowheads).

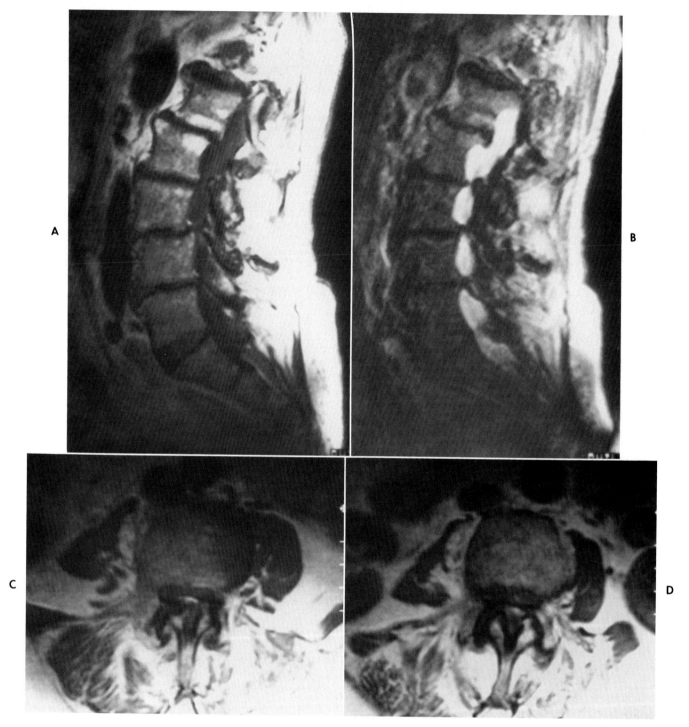

FIGURE 4-24
Severe lumbar spinal stenosis. A and **B**, Midsagittal T1-weighted and T2-weighted (TR 505/TE 20 and
TR 2000/TE 80) and, **C** and **D**, T1-weighted (TR 600/TE 20) MRI studies of L3 and L4. There is
degenerative disease of all the lumbar disks, and all have diminished signal intensities. Note the
marked replacement of marrow by fat adjacent to the L1-2 disk. There are also hypertrophic changes
of the vertebral endplates and facet joints due to the long-standing degenerative processes. These have
induced stenosis of the canal at multiple levels. The distortion and stenosis, in turn, with the
hypertrophic changes in the facet joints, are confirmed on the axial cross sections (**C** and **D**).

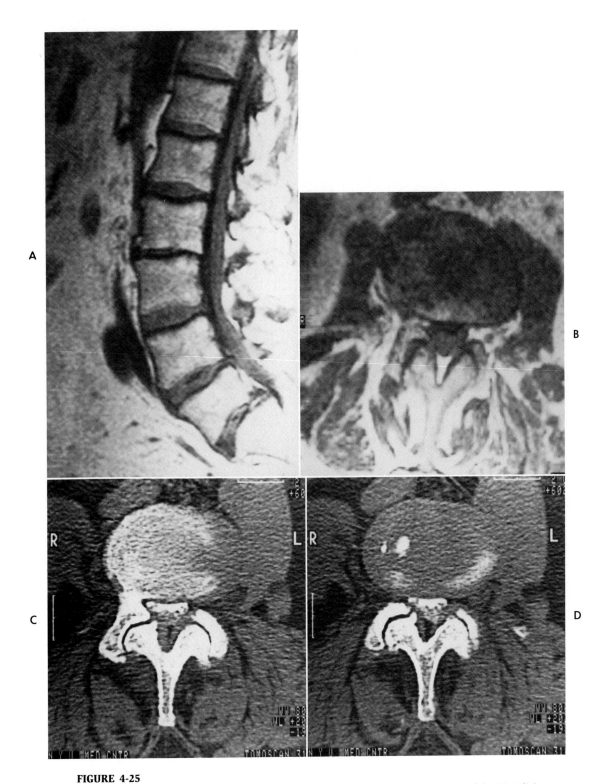

FIGURE 4-25
Spinal stenosis. **A,** A sagittal T1-weighted MRI of the lumbar spine reveals narrowing of the L2-3 disk due to degenerative disease. There is also narrowing of L4-5, with a focal midline herniation, and degenerative disease is present in the L5-S1 disk. Notice the marked stenosis of the canal at L3-4. **B,** An axial T1-weighted through L3-4 shows degenerative disease of the facet joints and compression of the dural sac, which is flattened anteriorly behind the intervertebral disk. Compare with **C** and **D,** CT-myelograms through L3-4. **C** is at the same level as **B.** Note the hypertrophic change of the ligamenta flava and the marked dural sac compression.

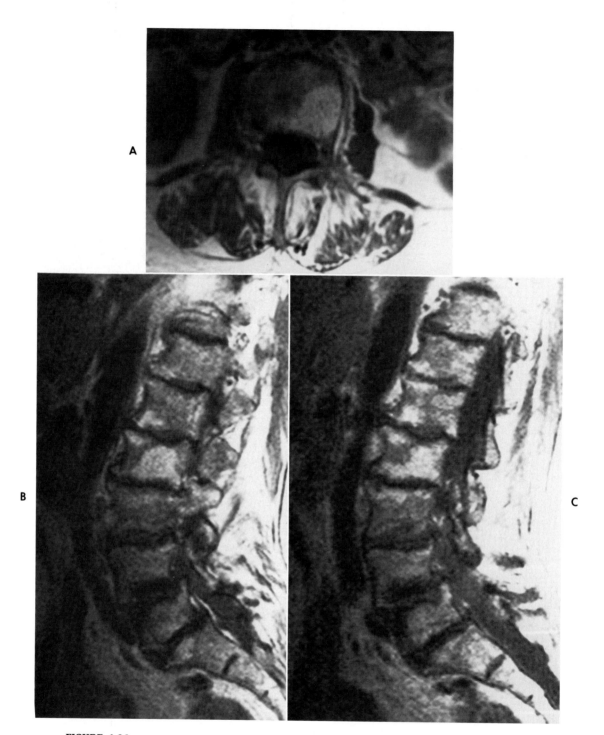

FIGURE 4-26
A, An axial T1-weighted cross section through L2 shows prominent fat replacement of the marrow on the left side. Note also the paraspinal muscle atrophy and the fat infiltration, more prominent on the left. B and C, Sagittal T1-weighted show relatively marked fatty infiltration of T12, L1, and L2. In addition there is a Grade I spondylolisthesis at L4-5. Note the zone of markedly low signal adjacent to the deformed endplates of these vertebrae. On T2-weighted cross sections (not shown) the signal intensity in this region was of medium strength. Anteroposterior instability of the spine at the L4-5 disk was documented at fluoroscopy.

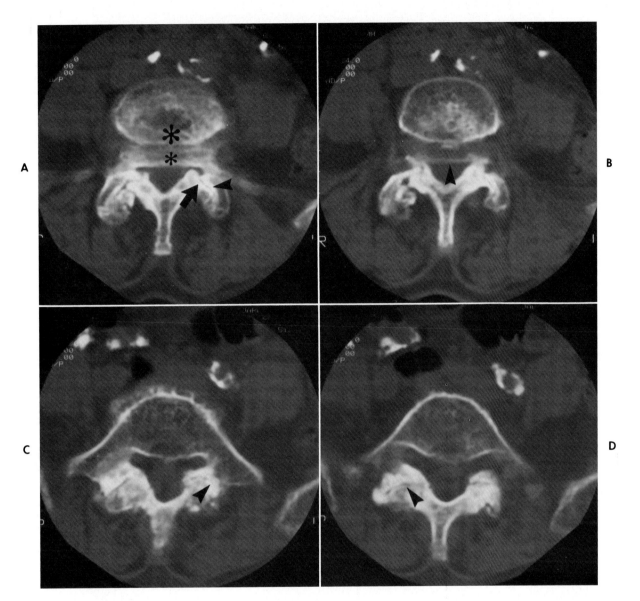

FIGURE 4-27

Spinal stenosis at L4-5 secondary to spondylolisthesis as a consequence of severe facet joint degenerative disease. **A** and **B,** Axial CT slices at L4-5, bone windows. There is a Grade I spondylolisthesis of L4 on L5. The *large asterisk* is on the inferior endplate of L4, which has moved anteriorly. The *small asterisk* is on the superior endplate of L5, which has stayed in place. The disk is markedly narrow, permitting inclusion of both endplates in one 5 mm slice. The posterior arch of L4 has moved anteriorly. The *arrow* denotes the articular facet of the L4 inferior articular process. Note that this facet has slipped anteriorly relative to its matching facet on the superior articular process of L5 *(arrowhead).* There is stenosis of the spinal canal at this level. The dural sac is trapped between the anteriorly displaced posterior arch of L4 and the posterior surface of L5, which has not moved. The maximum degree of stenosis is at the level of the L5 superior endplate **(A).** **B** (4 mm above the L4-5 disk) shows severe facet joint degenerative disease. There is some partial volume effect with the posterior edge of the L5 inferior endplate *(arrowhead).* **C,** A slice 4 mm below the L4-5 disk, through the pedicle of L5, shows severe facet joint degenerative disease *(arrowhead).* The facets are in a coronal plane, and this has prevented slippage of the neural arch anteriorly. **D,** Just below the pedicle of L5. There is severe degenerative disease of the facet joints *(arrowhead),* with marked osteosclerosis.

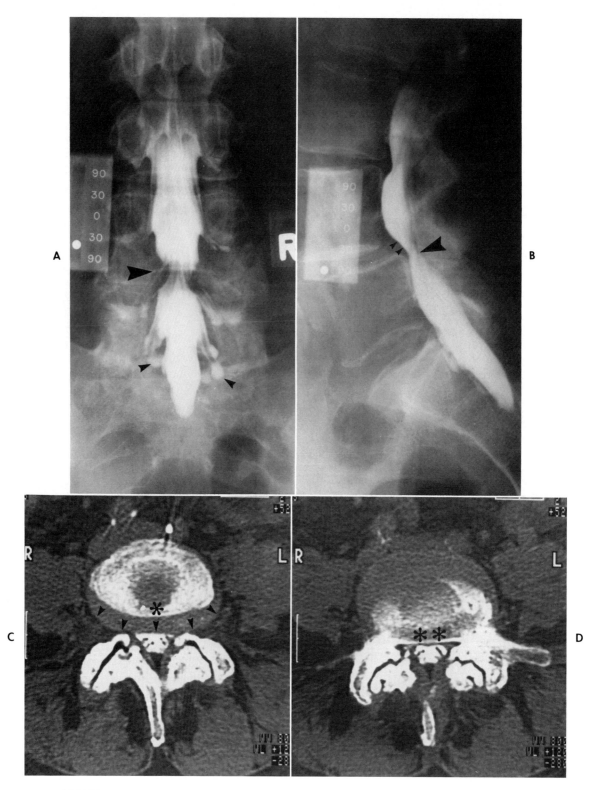

FIGURE 4-28

Degenerative spondylolisthesis at L4-5 causing spinal stenosis. **A,** An AP view of a lumbar myelogram reveals constriction of the contrast-filled dural sac *(large arrowhead)*. The *small arrowheads* denote small root sleeve cysts, an incidental finding. **B,** A lateral projection of the myelogram reveals stenosis of the canal and constriction of the dural sac at the level of the L5 superior endplate. This patient has L4-5 degenerative spondylolisthesis *(large arrowhead)*. Note the characteristic contour of the posterior disk surface *(small arrowheads)* at the level of the spondylolisthesis. This configuration of the disk, and its corresponding axial image, C, are normal for a disk that is not disrupted (at the level of the spondylolisthesis). Compare to Fig. 2-35. In this patient there was also bulging of the L3-4 disk, but the L5-S1 was normal. **C,** A CT-myelogram, axial slice through the L4-5 disk, shows the configuration of a normal disk at this level *(arrowheads)*. This slice includes a portion of the inferior L4 endplate *(asterisk)*. **D,** An axial slice of the CT-myelogram at L4-5 obtained just above the L5 superior endplate and incorporating the posterior surface of the L5 endplate *(two asterisks)* shows degenerative disease of the facet joints (notable also in **C**).

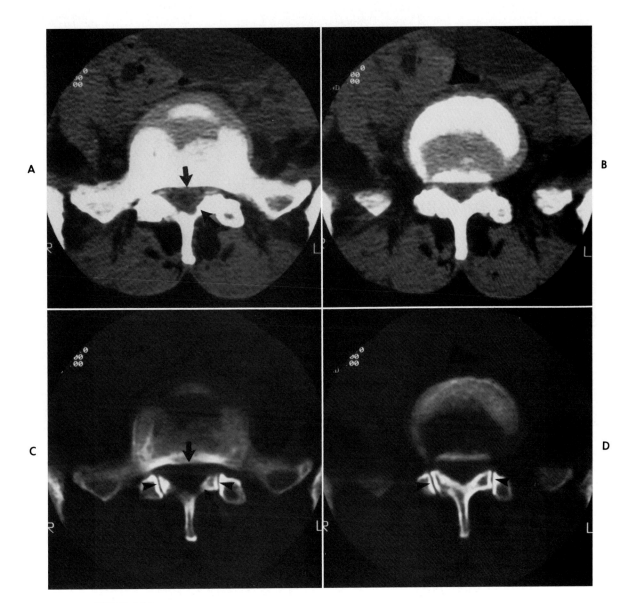

FIGURE 4-29

Spondylolisthesis and stenosis at L5-S1, CT examination. **A** and **B** are soft tissue windows and, **C** and **D,** bone windows showing an almost sagittal orientation of the facet joints *(arrowheads)*. This is a congenital anomaly in this patient, who also has nonunion of accessory centers and subcenters of the articulating pyramids. Note the stenosis of the spinal canal at the level of the S1 superior endplate *(straight arrow* in **A**), caused by the anteriorly displaced L5 neural arch *(oblique arrow* in **A**). The lumbar facets usually have an oblique orientation, often with a coronal component, which prevents the anterior (forward) movement of the proximal (upper) vertebra relative to the distal (lower) one. Occasionally there is a congenital anomaly of the facets, including an abnormal almost sagittal orientation without a coronal component, along with nonunion and fragmentation of the pyramids, that, in combination, permits anterior slippage of the vertebra and causes spondylolisthesis.

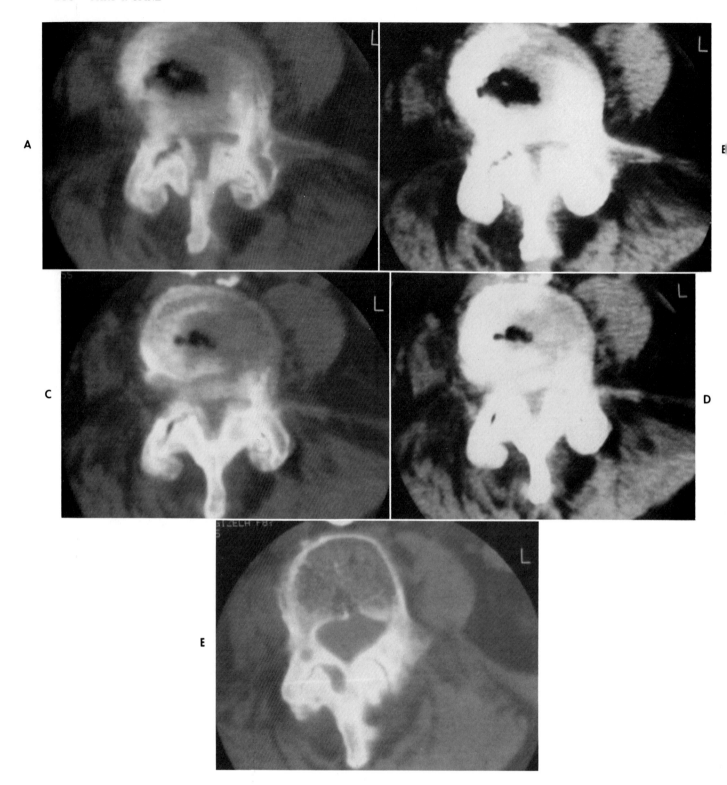

FIGURE 4-30
Spinal stenosis secondary to degenerative spondylolisthesis. **A** to **D,** Marked facet joint degeneration, spondylolisthesis at L4-5, degeneration of the disk, and severe stenosis of the canal due to spondylolisthesis. (**A** and **C** are bone windows; **B** and **D,** soft tissue windows.) **E,** Note the normal-sized spinal canal at the level of the L4 pedicle.

A   B   C

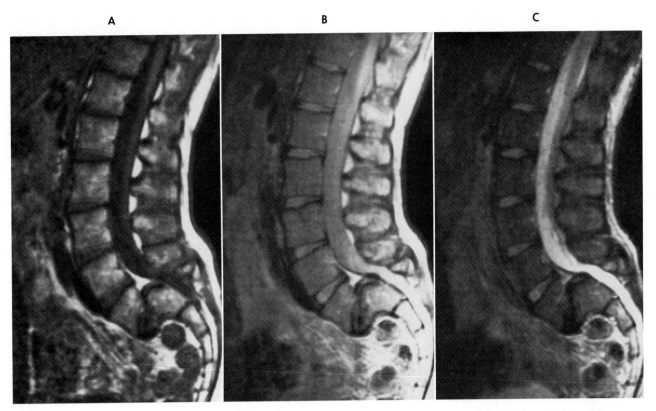

FIGURE 4-31
L5-S1 spondylolisthesis. Sagittal MRI studies (**A,** T1-weighted [TR 466/TE 19], **B,** proton density [TR 2216/TE 29], and, **C,** T2-weighted [TR 2216/TE 80]) reveal spondylolisthesis at L5-S1. Note the loss of signal and the marked distortion of the L5-S1 disk. Hypertrophic changes can be seen on the anterior aspect of S1, forming a shelf for L5. Bilateral spondylolysis was also present in this patient.

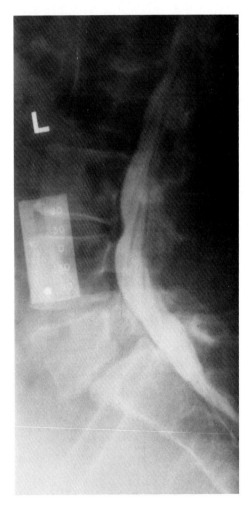

FIGURE 4-32
Spondylolysis and spondylolisthesis. A lateral view of a lumbar myelogram shows spondylolisthesis at L5-S1. This patient had bilateral defects of the neural arch of L5 (spondylolysis). Note the increased AP diameter of the spinal canal; the dural sac is not compressed.

lateral canal and neural foramen and causes compression of the neural elements (Fig. 4-53) regardless of whether or not the patient also has an associated spondylolisthesis.[3,25-28]

Marked compression of the dural sac is uncommon in these patients, because the neural arch is not pulled anteriorly. However, when the listhesis becomes quite pronounced, the sac is angulated and compressed. Also stretching of the descending nerve roots may occur, and there may be herniation of the disk at the level of the listhesis.

Stenosis secondary to thickening and calcification of the intraspinal ligaments

In some patients the most important cause of spinal stenosis is an apparent thickening of the soft tissues within the canal. This is usually due to redundancy and buckling of the ligaments, particularly the ligamentum flavum (Fig. 4-33). Synovial cysts arising from the diseased facet joints may also extend into the canal and compress the neural elements.

Thickening and redundancy of the intraspinal ligaments are noted with degenerative disease of the intervertebral disks and facet joints. The reduced height of the disks causes shortening of the canal and redundancy of the ligaments. Collapse of the disks also exerts pressure on the facets, inducing an upward migration of the superior articulating facet and downward migration of the inferior articulating facet. This then exacerbates the degenerative disease of the facets and reduces the height of the neural foramen. In addition, the available space in the neural foramen is further reduced by thickening, redundancy, and calcification of the ligamentum flavum and capsule of the facet joint. In most patients with thickened intraspinal ligaments, osteophytes and bony ridges due to degenerative disease also develop. However, this is not a constant finding; in some patients with significant ligamentous thickening the size and configuration of the bony canal may be normal, with no osteophytes or protruding facets.

When the diagnosis of spinal stenosis is being contemplated, it is important to remember that the dimensions of the bony canal are only one contributing factor. The thickness of the soft tissues within the canal is at least equally significant.

CALCIFICATION OF THE LIGAMENTUM FLAVUM AND CAPSULE OF THE FACET JOINTS

Calcification of the ligamentum flavum and facet joint capsules (which are continuations of the ligamentum flavum) (Fig. 4-34) can occur in patients with longstanding spondylosis. These thickened and calcified ligaments then contribute to the stenosis. Calcification of the ligamentum flavum, commonly seen with degenerative spondylosis, has also been recorded in patients with pseudogout.

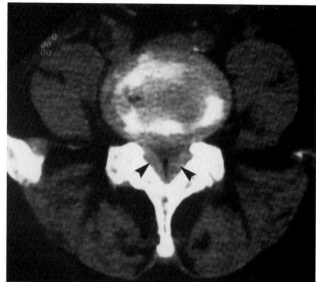

A

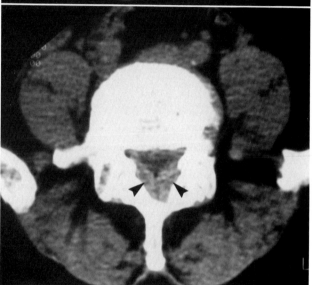

B

FIGURE 4-33
Spinal stenosis. A and B, CT axial slices at L4-5 show marked hypertrophy of the ligamenta flava *(arrowheads)* and circumferential bulging of the disk. The space remaining for the dural sac is severely restricted.

Calcification and ossification of the posterior longitudinal ligament

Calcification and OPLL (ossification of the posterior longitudinal ligament) are seen most commonly among the Japanese, although they may be encountered as well in non-Japanese orientals and in caucasians. The cervical spine is usually affected (Figs. 4-35 to 4-38), but the thoracic (Fig. 4-39, *B*) and lumbar (Fig. 4-39, *C*) spine also may be involved. Symptomatic spinal stenosis generally occurs in the cervical and thoracic, rarely the lumbar, spine.[29-33] The calcification is usually of a few millimeters' thickness, although it may become massive. It may adhere to the dura, penetrate it, and become

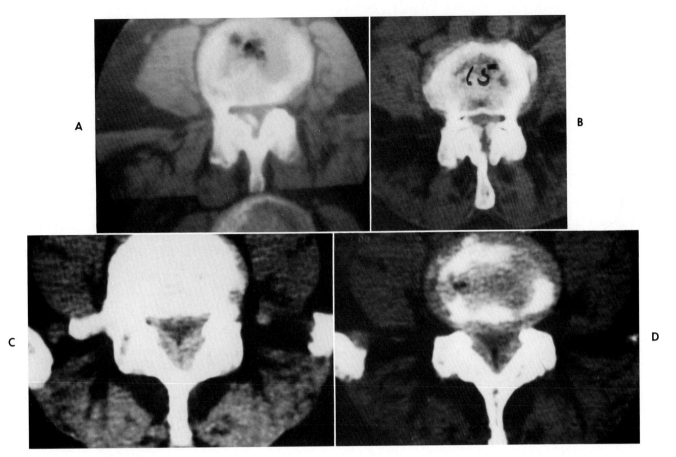

FIGURE 4-34
Spinal stenosis secondary to facet joint degenerative disease with thickening and calcification of the ligamentum flavum. **A,** Marked degeneration of the facet joints and calcification of the ligamentum on the right. Note also the spinal stenosis. **B,** Facet joint degeneration with hypertrophic change of the ligamentum flavum and capsules of the facet joints, causing severe stenosis. **C and D,** Soft tissue and bone windows at slightly different levels show severe stenosis with circumferential bulging of the L4-5 intervertebral disk and hypertrophic change of the ligamentum flavum.

attached to the spinal cord (Fig. 4-38) and may occupy as much as 80% to 90% of the surface of the canal (Fig. 4-40, E to G). The condition may be asymptomatic, or it may lead to compression (Figs. 4-35 and 4-38), causing pain with sensory and motor deficits that are intermittent at first but become progressively worse, resulting in spasticity and paralysis.

Another group of patients will have no symptoms until some minor injury leads to a neurological catastrophe, such as paraplegia or quadriplegia, and a stenosis of the canal is discovered.[34] The spinal cord seems able to tolerate slowly progressive mechanical pressure, as occurs in OPLL, adjusting to the distorted shape of the canal and filling most of the available space, but when there is absolutely no more room any additional encroachment (e.g., by swelling and edema from minor trauma, even without an associated fracture or dislocation, or a minor disk herniation) is enough to precipitate compression and its neurological sequelae. We have seen many patients in whom stenosis (either congenital or acquired) was discovered after such a mishap.

Forestier's disease (diffuse idiopathic skeletal hyperostosis)

Forestier's disease is fairly common, having an incidence of 3%[35] in the general population over 50 years of age, and may occur in as many as 12% of older persons.[36] Anklyosing spinal hyperostosis of Forestier and Rotes-Querol,[37-39] or DISH, is characterized by abnormal bony bridging on the anterolateral surface of the spine that may involve virtually the entire vertebral column but seems most prominent in the lower cervical area (Figs. 4-39 and 4-40). Not uncommonly these excrescences will exhibit a peculiarly continuous (flowing) pattern and occasionally become quite massive (Fig. 4-37). Although spondylosis may coexist, in the classic form osteophytes and marked narrowing of the disk spaces are not usually seen. The extraspinal manifestations include prominent and enlarged bony excrescences, generally at the sites of attachment of major tendons and ligaments and sometimes with calcification.

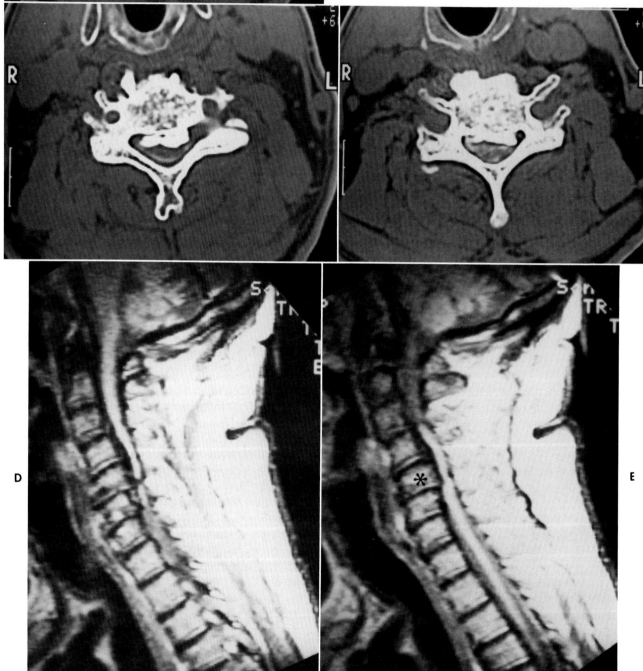

FIGURE 4-35

Spinal stenosis and compression of the cord secondary to degenerative disease, ridges, and calcification of the posterior longitudinal ligament. CT-myelograms at C4-5, **A** and **B**, and C5-6, **C**, reveal a large calcific density posterior to the vertebrae. It has occupied 50% or more of the canal; the cord is compressed and displaced posteriorly. **D** and **E**, Midsagittal MRI studies (TR 1500/TE 45) show malalignment of the cervical spine due to degenerative disease at C4-5 and C5-6. The cord is compressed, flattened, and displaced posteriorly, and there is an area of signal void (calcification) between it and the posterior surfaces of C4 and C5 (best seen in **D**). Compression of the cord by the posterior surface of C5 is best seen in **E**. (The *asterisk* is on the C5 vertebra.)

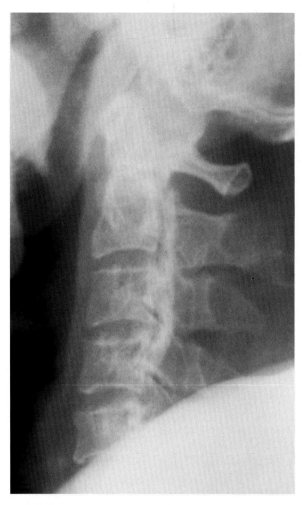

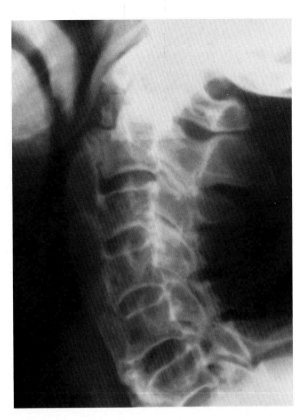

FIGURE 4-37
A lateral projection of the cervical spine shows massive calcification of the anterior longitudinal ligament extending from C2 to C6 in a patient with Forestier's disease (DISH). The disks are normal in this patient, but the canal is borderline stenotic.

FIGURE 4-36
Calcification of the posterior longitudinal ligament extends from C2 to C4.

The first reports of DISH did not emphasize calcification of the posterior longitudinal ligament,[37,40] although it was subsequently found that several patients had moderate to severe calcification (Figs. 4-39 and 4-40). In one series[41] there were 37 patients, out of 74 (50%), who had calcification. Mitsui et al.[38] reported on 71 patients with DISH, of whom 30% had calcification of the posterior longitudinal ligament (PLL), mostly in the cervical spine. Arlet et al.[42] analyzed 40 patients, 43% of whom had both DISH and stenosis of the cervical canal secondary to osteophytosis and calcification of the PLL. Finally, Onji et al.[43] investigated 166 patients, of whom 44% demonstrated concomitant calcification of the PLL and hyperostosis of the anterior vertebral column.

We reviewed 126 patients with DISH affecting the cervical spine or the cervical and thoracic spine[31,32,44] and found definite calcification of the PLL, extending across at least two disk spaces, in 16. Looking at the problem in a different way, we have seen the following relationship between such calcification and DISH: in 29

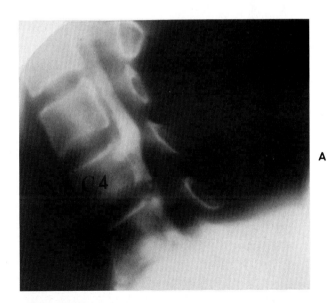

FIGURE 4-38
Calcification of the posterior longitudinal ligament. **A,** A lateral tomogram of the cervical spine reveals a thick calcified PLL, extending to C5-6. *Continued.*

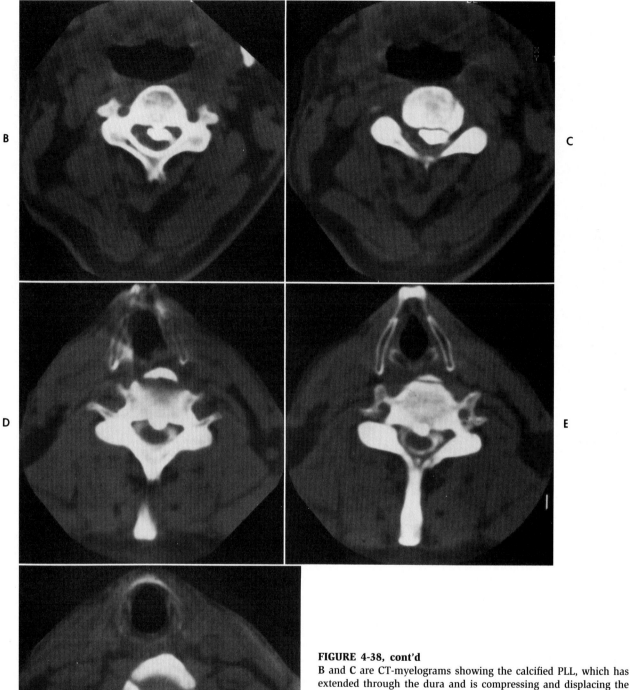

FIGURE 4-38, cont'd
B and C are CT-myelograms showing the calcified PLL, which has extended through the dura and is compressing and displacing the cord. In some patients the calcification gradually becomes embedded in the dura, works through the dura, and attaches itself to the cord. D to F, CT-myelograms of the lower cervical spine show calcification of the PLL, which is gradually decreasing in size. At C7-T1 there is no significant compression of the cord.

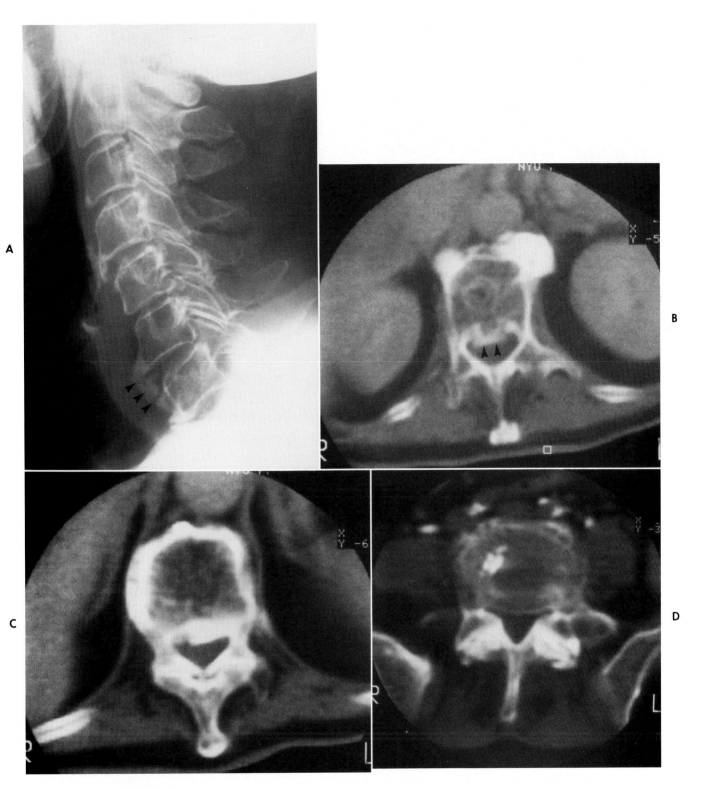

FIGURE 4-39
Forestier's disease. **A,** Cervical spine. Note the characteristic calcifications anterior to C6 and C7 *(arrowheads)*. **B,** Thoracic spine. There is calcification of the posterior longitudinal ligament *(arrowheads)*. **C** and **D,** Lumbar spine. Note the moderate (congenital) stenosis at L5. There is also a superimposed acquired stenosis secondary to degenerative disease of the facet joints **(D)** and calcification of the PLL **(C)**.

A   B   C

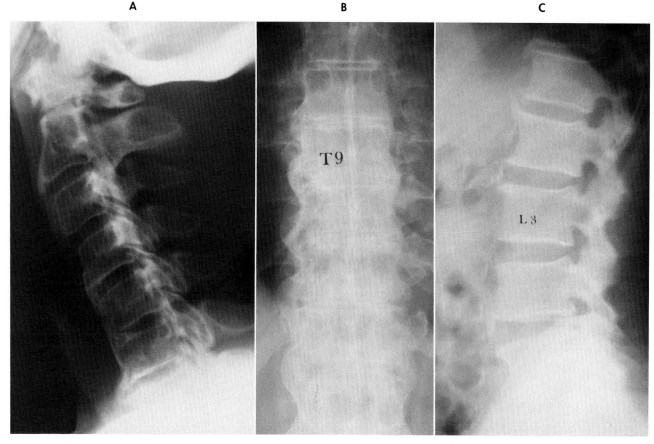

FIGURE 4-40
Forestier's disease and calcification of the posterior longitudinal ligament. **A,** A lateral projection of the cervical spine shows calcification of the PLL from C1 to C6-7. Note the bony bar at the anterior margins of C4-5 and C5-6. **B,** A frontal projection of the thoracic spine reveals typical ossification of the ALL and adjacent tissues. **C,** A lateral projection of the lumbar spine shows moderate congenital stenosis. Note the short pedicles.
                                                                        Continued.

patients with calcification of the PLL there were 16 with DISH.

Spinal stenosis was present in 19 of these 126 patients with DISH, and 14 had calcification of the PLL. The stenosis was due to (1) a developmentally smaller spinal canal, (2) calcification of the PLL, (3) hypertrophy and calcification of the ligamentum flavum, or (4), less commonly, hypertrophic osteophytes and bony ridges (Figs. 4-39 and 4-40).

Paget's disease

Spinal stenosis, particularly in the cervical and thoracic regions (Figs. 4-41 and 4-42), may be seen with Paget's disease.[45] Usually there are two reasons for this:

1. Enlargement of the vertebrae, pedicles, and laminae, as well as softening of bone, may lead to distortion of the canal and stenosis.
2. Deposition of pagetoid and poorly ossified tissue in the epidural space immediately adjacent to the vertebral body and neural arch may occur. This can cause constriction of the dural sac and lead to compression of the neural elements.

Hemangioma

Vertebral hemangiomas (Figs. 4-43 to 4-45) are fairly common, having been noted in 11% of spine specimens obtained at autopsy. They can be cavernous or capillary and are generally encountered in the thoracic spine though they also may be seen in the cervical or lumbar spine and the sacrum. In most cases they are asymptomatic and are discovered incidentally on diagnostic imaging studies of the spine. However, local symptoms (pain and tenderness) may occur. Uncommonly compression of the cord, usually the thoracic (Fig. 4-45) but also the cervical cord, is noted.[46-52] According to McAllister et al.[46] compression of the cord may be due to (1) expansion of an involved vertebra, leading to narrowing and deformity of the canal, (2) extension of a tumor into the extradural space, (3) a compression fracture of an involved vertebra (rare)[47,53] or (4) an extradural hematoma secondary to hemangioma.

McAllister et al.[46] reported eight symptomatic vertebral hemangiomas. Compression of the cord was due to a soft tissue mass in the epidural space, definitely identified in 3, and most likely the cause in 2, cases. In two patients

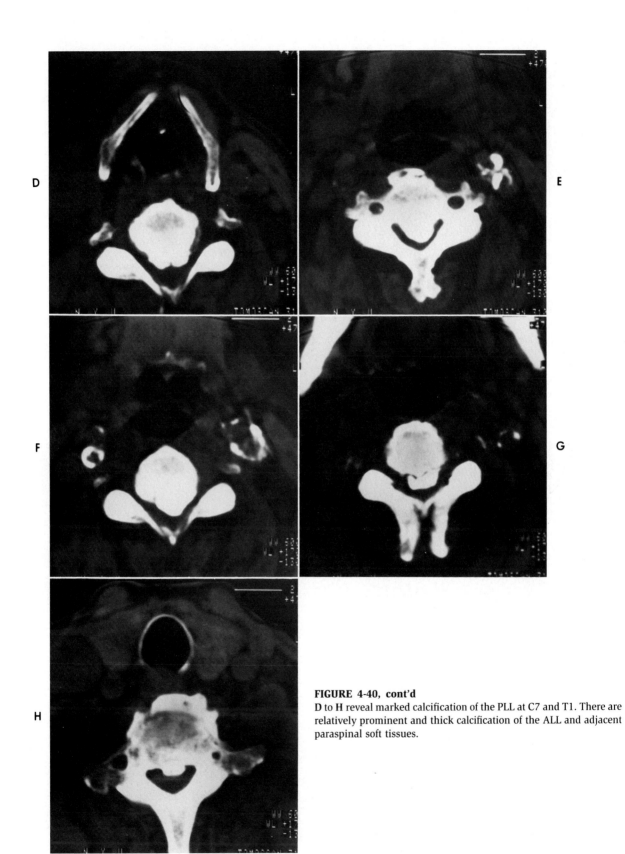

FIGURE 4-40, cont'd
D to H reveal marked calcification of the PLL at C7 and T1. There are
relatively prominent and thick calcification of the ALL and adjacent
paraspinal soft tissues.

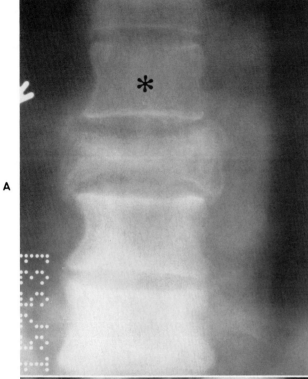

A

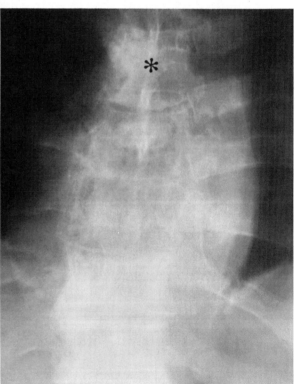

FIGURE 4-41
Paget's disease and stenosis. **A,** A tomogram of the thoracic spine in 1974 shows T8 with a compression fracture (*asterisk* is on T7). The vertebral body is notably expanded and the trabeculae are thick, rough, and prominent. T9 and T10 are sclerotic. **B,** A lateral projection and, **C,** an AP projection in 1981 reveal compression fractures of T8, T9, and T10 (*asterisk* on T7). There is thickening and roughening of the visible trabeculae, but the vertebral bodies are markedly lucent. Note the expansion anteriorly and laterally, with perispinal ossification of the soft tissues, and the suggestion of a paraspinal soft tissue mass.

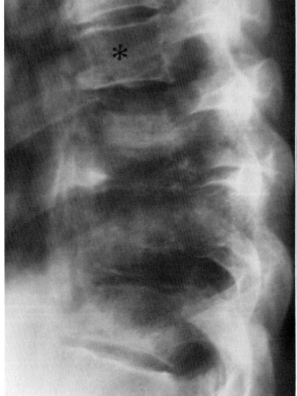

B

C

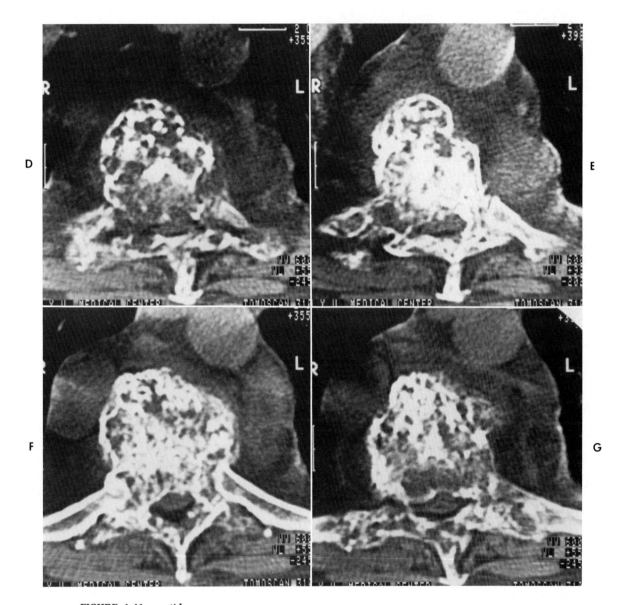

FIGURE 4-41, cont'd
D to **G,** Computed tomograms at T8, T9, and T10 show the markedly deformed vertebral architecture, with severe flattening anteroposteriorly of the canal. A spinal stenosis is present in this patient, and a large paravertebral soft tissue (partially ossified) mass represents the deposition of Paget's tissue. The nonossified paravertebral tissues were prominently enhanced on intravenous injection of contrast.

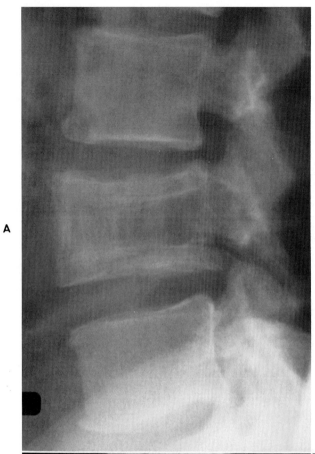

A

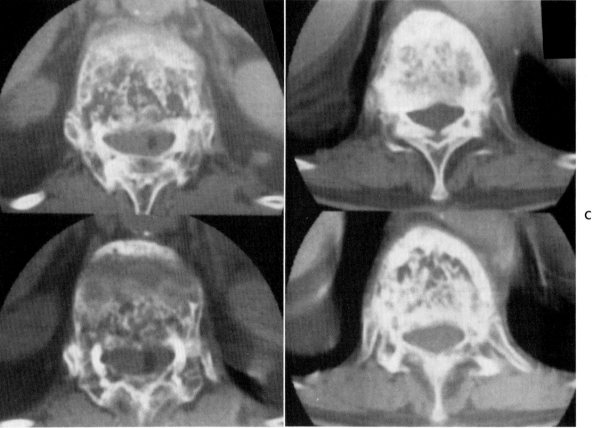

B

C

FIGURE 4-42
Paget's disease of the spine and spinal stenosis. **A,** Note the characteristic picture-frame configuration of L4, with enlargement of the vertebral body causing stenosis of the lumbar spine. This is uncommon. **B** to **E,** T6 and T7. Note here the marked deformity of the canal and the spinal stenosis.

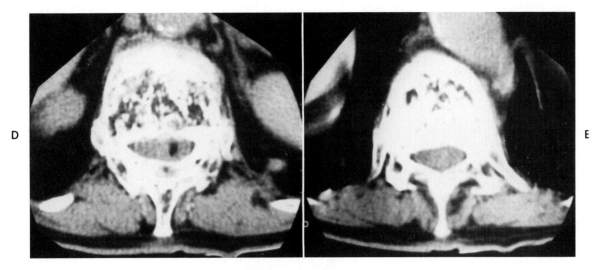

FIGURE 4-42, cont'd
For legend see opposite page.

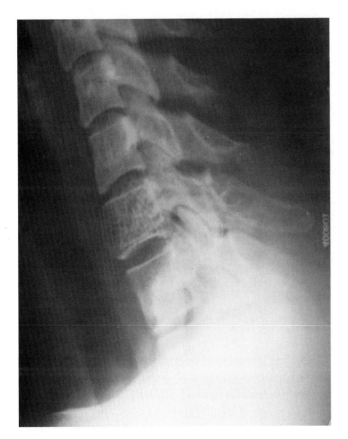

FIGURE 4-43
Hemangioma of C7. There was involvement of the vertebral body, pedicles, laminae, and spinous process. Note the expansion of the vertebral body.

there was expansion of the vertebral body and other bony elements, causing stenosis of the canal; in one case this was due to a combination of the extradural mass and bony expansion. Surgical exploration and histological examination showed the extradural mass to be hemangioma, identical in histology to a vertebral hemangioma.

The epidural component of a hemangioma (Fig. 4-45) may extend into the spinal canal for several centimeters. Large draining veins and occasionally an arteriovenous malformation may also be present. Vertebral hemangiomas have been reported in the multisystem Klippel-Trenaunay-Weber[48,54] and Kasabach-Merritt[48,55] syndromes.

Not uncommonly, multiple vertebral hemangiomas will occur in one subject. They have a fairly characteristic pattern on roentgenograms of the spine — usually vertical striations interspersed with areas of radiolucency (Figs. 4-43 and 4-44), the thickened vertical trabeculae standing out sharply against the lucent background of surrounding bone because of associated fat in the hemangioma. The pattern is fairly characteristic on CT (Fig. 4-44, *C*), with a localized area of lucency (due to excess fat) and dense sclerotic cross sections of the thickened vertical trabeculae (which appear as "dots"). A hemangioma may extend into the pedicles, laminae, and spinous process, and there may be enlargement of the vertebral body and vertebral elements leading to stenosis of the canal. The extraosseous component of a hemangioma is also fairly well visualized on CT, along with the paraspinal soft tissue mass and its epidural extension. We have seen 13 patients with a paraspinal soft tissue component, 7 of whom also had epidural extension. Although there was a significant amount of fat in the vertebral hemangioma, none was noted in the extravertebral component.

The findings on MRI (Fig. 4-44, *A* and *B*) usually

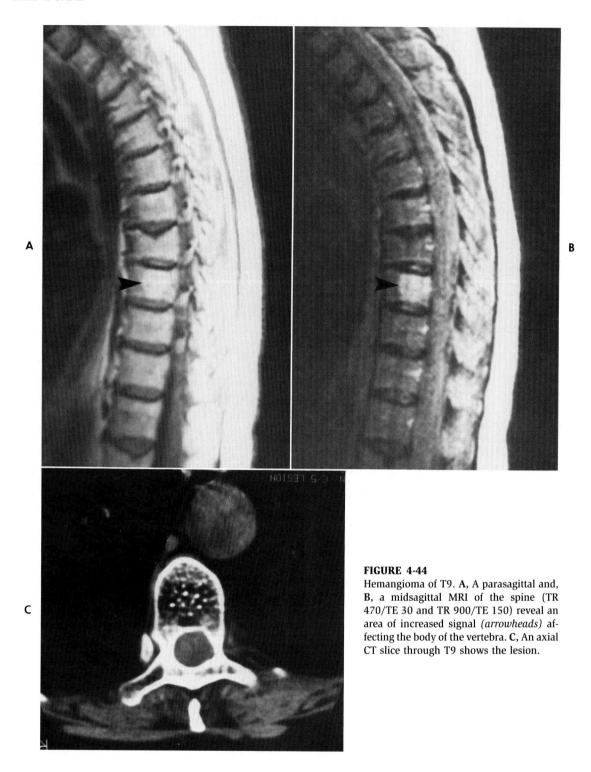

FIGURE 4-44
Hemangioma of T9. **A,** A parasagittal and, **B,** a midsagittal MRI of the spine (TR 470/TE 30 and TR 900/TE 150) reveal an area of increased signal *(arrowheads)* affecting the body of the vertebra. **C,** An axial CT slice through T9 shows the lesion.

consist of a fairly localized area of increased signal on T1-weighted cross sections with a moderate degree of mottling or nonhomogeneity due to the presence of thickened trabeculae. There is also increased signal in the lesion on T2-weighted cross sections. The extravertebral component may have medium signal intensity on both pulse sequences. Ross et al.[56] reported intermediate signal on T1-WI and increased signal on T2-W1 in three patients with extravertebral extension of the soft tissue component of a hemangioma.

The pattern of signal described for hemangioma is seen only in cases without superimposed complications. It is important to keep in mind the possibility of acute fracture, old fracture, acute bleeding, and old bleeding in patients with hemangioma, because the MR features of hemangioma will be altered by any of these superimposed complications.

• • •

We have included vertebral hemangiomas in the discussion of spinal stenosis because they are often

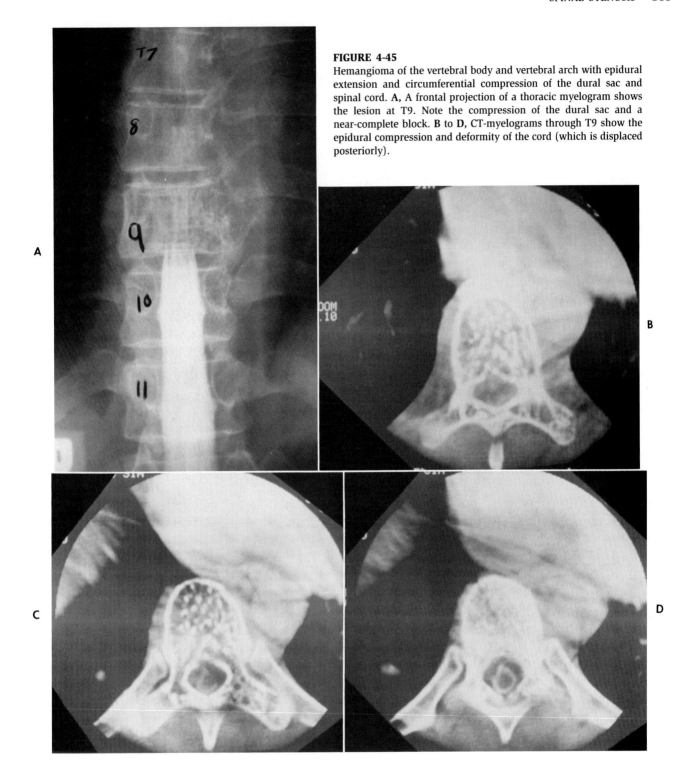

FIGURE 4-45
Hemangioma of the vertebral body and vertebral arch with epidural extension and circumferential compression of the dural sac and spinal cord. **A,** A frontal projection of a thoracic myelogram shows the lesion at T9. Note the compression of the dural sac and a near-complete block. **B** to **D,** CT-myelograms through T9 show the epidural compression and deformity of the cord (which is displaced posteriorly).

overlooked as a cause of cord compression in patients with symptomatic thoracic hemangioma. Stenosis of the thoracic spine usually leads to progressive myelopathy, less commonly to radiculopathy. Symptomatic thoracic hemangiomas also produce spinal stenosis and progressive myelopathy. Acute cord compression, due to bleeding or a compression fracture, is less common.[53] We have seen two young women with thoracic vertebral hemangiomas who reported acute episodes of transient paraparesis during pregnancy (one lasting for 6 days, the other 9

days), with complete recovery. Thoracic hemangiomas, without an apparent extravertebral component, were found in these patients. No other etiological factor was discovered for their transient neurological abnormalities.

Liu and Yang[57] reported on a 25-year-old woman 22 weeks pregnant who presented with progressive paraparesis. Myelography and CT showed a complete block at T4 due to an enlarged vertebra containing a lytic lesion, which was found histologically to be a cavernous hemangioma. We also have seen three patients, all middle-aged women with thoracic hemangiomas, with recurrent symptoms of meningeal irritation lasting several days and subsiding gradually, who had no associated residual neurological deficit. We are uncertain as to the cause-and-effect relationship between the thoracic hemangiomas and clinical manifestations in these patients. The possibility of minimal subarachnoid bleeding, perhaps from associated vascular lesions, was considered, but we had no histological evidence for it.

Epidural lipomatosis

Epidural lipomatosis is seen in patients receiving long-term oral corticosteroid therapy. There seems to be no threshold; the condition can occur even with low doses. It apparently does not occur, however, with endogenous Cushing's disease. Epidural lipomatosis is manifested by increased fat in the epidural space leading to compression of the dural sac and nerve roots. The increased fat is better appreciated when serial studies are compared.

CLASSIFICATION OF SPINAL STENOSES

Spinal stenoses can be regarded as affecting the canal (central stenosis) or the lateral recess and neural foramen (lateral stenosis). The significance and pathogenesis of the symptomatology of neural foraminal and lateral recess stenosis are discussed in the section ''Radiographic diagnosis'' (p. 185).

CLINICAL FINDINGS

Most patients with spinal stenosis are usually asymptomatic until the fifth and sixth decades of life. However, it is not unusual to encounter a 75-year-old individual (or even older) whose symptoms began only a few months previously. The clinical manifestations appear when degenerative disease of the disks and facets, with enlargement of the intraspinal ligaments, causes further limitation of the available space in the spinal canal and compression of the neural elements.

In the cervical and thoracic region spinal stenosis may cause myelopathy, less commonly radiculopathy.[2,58,59] The clinical manifestations in the lumbar region[18] usually consist of back pain with pain and dysesthesias spreading from the lower lumbar region into one or both lower extremities. These findings may last for several years before any objective neurological deficit appears.

Two factors play an important role in the development of clinical findings with spinal stenosis:

1. The actual space available for the neural elements, which itself is dependent on (a) the size of the bony canal and (b) the space occupied by osteophytes and thickened intraspinal ligaments
2. The speed with which the stenosis develops

When spinal stenosis develops fairly rapidly (e.g., in a case of progressive spondylolisthesis following laminectomy in a patient with preexisting degenerative disease of the facets and minimal to moderate degenerative

spondylolisthesis), the clinical manifestations also develop rapidly; but when stenosis develops slowly (over many years, as in a patient with degenerative spondylosis), there may be moderate to marked narrowing of the canal without significant neurological deficits or subjective complaints. It seems that the slow pace of the stenosis allows the cord and nerve roots to adjust gradually to the limited space within the canal. Thus, despite a severe stenosis, these elderly patients may be asymptomatic. However, with advancing age the available space progressively diminishes and, depending on the degree, the patients become more prone to suffering pain and neurological deficit with any additional factor that further compromises the canal (e.g., a minor disk herniation or trauma). The clinical manifestations, nevertheless, are usually not as severe and almost always respond to conservative measures.

The reduction of available space in the spinal canal with advancing age is due to a number of factors. The most important is diminished height of the disks and vertebrae, which leads to shortening of the canal and buckling and redundancy of the intraspinal ligaments. There is also true enlargement of the intraspinal ligaments, occasionally with calcification, in degenerative disease of the spine. Furthermore, bulging and herniation with bony ridges may be present at multiple levels.

A subgroup of patients with spinal stenosis should be mentioned here. These are individuals who have a marked congenital stenosis with superimposed, very slowly evolving, degenerative disease (Figs. 4-2 and 4-4) or calcification and ossification of the posterior longitudinal ligament (Fig. 4-38) who, despite the severity of their stenosis, are asymptomatic. However, even though there may be no clinically detectable findings in these patients, their spinal cord and neural elements are in a precarious state. The slightest additional encroachment into the canal by a herniated disk, even if very small, or some minor swelling can lead to a neurological catastrophe (paraplegia or quadriplegia).

INTERMITTENT NEUROGENIC CLAUDICATION

This is the classic clinical presentation of lumbar stenosis.[60] The patient suffers pain and dysesthesia followed by motor weakness during standing and walking. However, the manifestations of neurogenic claudication, unlike those of ischemic claudication, actually worsen when the patient is standing still. Their intensity is reduced by walking. Also they tend to disappear when the patient sits, squats, or lies down. Dysesthesias, particularly numbness, almost always precede weakness.

In most patients with spinal stenosis there is usually no significant persistent motor or sensory deficit. However, in patients with a long history or in elderly patients with significant degenerative changes, some degree of neurological deficit may be present. We have encountered pure classic neurogenic claudication in only about *20%* of patients as the dominant presenting manifestation of lumbar spinal stenosis. It is relatively more common in patients who also have lateral recess or neural foraminal stenosis than in those with stenosis limited to the spinal canal.

Intermittent neurogenic claudication may also occur secondary to compression of the neural elements in a normal-sized canal. This, however, is unusual. Most cases are seen in patients with a *midline disk herniation* or, less commonly, a foraminal disk herniation. Presumably, weight bearing causes increased protrusion of the disk, leading to further compression of the neural elements and an acquired stenosis in which the canal is narrowed by a herniation large enough to reduce the space available for all the neural elements.

Neurogenic claudication is probably due to ischemia of the neural elements produced by increased mechanical pressure during standing and, less frequently, walking. The specific pattern of presentation of manifestations (i.e., sensory deficits prior to motor weakness) is also characteristic of ischemic neuritis.

RADIOGRAPHIC DIAGNOSIS

Craniovertebral junction. The radiographic diagnosis of disorders of the craniovertebral junction may require tomography, CT, CT-myelography, or MRI. Tomography is often helpful in evaluating erosive changes of the odontoid process and facet joints at the occipitocervical junction (inflammatory arthritis), although the same information can also be obtained from reformatted coronal and sagittal images of a high-resolution 1 or 2 mm thick CT study of this region. However, the fine detail of bony erosion and fracture healing is best revealed by complex-motion conventional tomography. MRI and CT-myelography, often as complementary procedures, are indispensable for an axial display of the shape, size, and nature of various abnormalities of the foramen magnum and spinal canal. Nevertheless, horizontal fractures of the odontoid process and vertebral bodies may be missed on axial CT images and, for this reason, when CT is being used in the evaluation of a fracture-dislocation of the spine, coronal and sagittal reformatting should be routinely obtained.

MRI is most helpful in evaluating the extent of compression of the spinal cord as well as detecting other neurological disorders of this region (e.g., the Arnold-Chiari malformation). MRI should also be used as the initial *screening* procedure despite the fact that CT and CT-myelography may become necessary when calcified or bony lesions are encountered.

Cervical spine

In the remainder of the cervical spine the transverse and sagittal diameters of the canal have been used as indicators of stenosis.[61] The sagittal diameter in normal subjects is usually reported to be more than 13 mm, with diameters of 10 to 13 mm considered borderline and below 10 mm diagnostic of stenosis.

We have found the sagittal diameter of the cervical canal, measured on CT, in asymptomatic individuals who did not have calcification of the intraspinal ligaments, osteophytes, or bony ridges to be as low as 6 mm. Computed tomography is useful for a definitive visualization and measurement of the bony canal, calcified ligaments, and osteophytes. Sagittal T2-weighted and gradient echo MRI cross sections reveal the extent of stenosis as well as atrophy of the cord, if present. One can also evaluate the extent of compression of the subarachnoid space as well as the presence of compression and displacement of, or abnormal signal within, the cord. Focal zones of increased signal on T2-weighted cross sections (Fig. 4-21) are thought to be due to edema or myelomalacia. In a follow-up of patients with increased signal in the cord secondary to chronic compression,[62] it was noted that the signal disappeared in some cases following decompression and the patient's condition improved (implying edema as the cause of the increased signal) but that when the signal did not disappear the patient's clinical condition also did not improve (implying myelomalacia).

Thoracic and lumbar spine

Assessing the sagittal diameter of the thoracic and lumbar spine may be difficult on conventional lateral views or lateral tomograms because the posterior wall of the canal often is not in the coronal plane and therefore cannot be visualized on-end in the lateral projection. Indeed, on CT of the spine the posterior boundary of the canal in the lumbar and lower thoracic region is often a narrow triangle, formed by the inner surfaces of the laminae, and extends as a narrow slit into the bases of the spinous processes. When it can be measured, however, the sagittal diameter is a rough indicator of lumbar stenosis (being reduced in most patients with clinical manifestations). In these cases the pedicles are short and thick and the posterior surfaces of the vertebrae have an accentuated concavity.

In the cervical, thoracic, and upper lumbar segments the spinal canal is usually rounded or ovoid. In the L4, L5, and S1 region, it may be triangular normally, or even trefoil (cloverleaf).

In patients with *congenital stenosis* there is a generalized diminution in size of the canal, but there may be no significant deformity of configuration. The canal may be flattened in the cervical region and more triangular in the lumbar region.

In patients with *acquired stenosis* due to degenerative disease the most important factors causing stenosis are osteophytes, bony ridges, enlargement, and occasionally calcification of the intraspinal ligaments. In the lumbar spine these same factors as well as hypertrophic changes of the facet joints are responsible. Lumbar hypertrophic facet joints protrude into the canal and cause an exaggerated trefoil configuration with significant reduction in size of the canal and lateral recess. Osteophytes and bony ridges arising from the vertebral margin can also cause stenosis of the canal, lateral recess, or neural foramen.

These findings are usually not well seen on conventional roentgenography and tomography, but are displayed clearly on CT and MRI. Furthermore, bulging or herniation of a disk and "thickening" of the ligamentum flavum are usually well evaluated on CT and MRI.

In patients with *severe spinal stenosis*, whether congenital or acquired, there is usually a paucity of epidural fat. This is one of the factors that render detection of a herniated disk difficult in these patients.

Spinal canal stenosis: measurements

When evaluating spinal stenosis, it is important not to rely solely on bony dimensions. Generally a sagittal diameter measuring less than 10 mm is considered significant and may indicate stenosis. However, according to Ullrich et al.,[63] the lumbar canal area can vary from 2 to 4.5 cm². In that case a canal measuring less than 1.5 cm² would have to be considered stenotic. Obviously, soft tissue dimensions are just as important as bony dimensions in giving a true picture of canal area.

Generally speaking, a great deal of emphasis should not be put on measurements. Frequently patients with a relatively marked stenosis will have no clinical manifestations. We have found that the *soft tissue/bony canal ratio* (size of the thecal sac and other nonfatty intraspinal contents relative to the size of the bony canal) is a more helpful finding. Thus, when the canal appears to be totally full of soft tissue structures (Figs. 4-34, *A* and *B*, and 4-24, *C* and *D*), with minimal or no anterior epidural fat (Figs. 4-62, *D*, and 4-63, *F* and *G*), it is likely that the patient has stenosis; on the other hand, if there is sufficient anterior epidural fat, even though the bony canal appears stenotic, clinically significant spinal stenosis probably does not exist. However, it must be emphasized that evaluation of this finding should be performed on high-resolution CT or MR images.

Absence of epidural fat is a particularly useful sign in confirming stenosis of the lumbar region, because anterior epidural fat is normally present in the lumbar region but scant or nonexistent in the thoracocervical region. There is usually a small amount of fat present directly posterior to the dural sac between the ligamenta flava, but it seems to have no diagnostic value.

Diminished width of the subarachnoid space can be equally well demonstrated on MRI and CT-myelography (Figs. 4-19, 4-20, and 4-25). However, in patients with severe stenosis and atrophy of the cord, when water-soluble contrast agents are used for myelography, the contrast often passes around the cord (even in the most severely stenotic region). On MRI, T2-weighted cross sections show the extent of encroachment of osteophytes and other elements into the canal as well as diminution or distortion of the subarachnoid space and compression or displacement of the cord. Sagittal cross sections reveal an overall picture of stenosis. Axial cross sections may show distortion or rotation and displacement of the cord.

When the decision is made to go to surgery for the relief of spinal stenosis, the surgeon must know the precise location and size of various structures causing the stenosis, calcified or uncalcified, and for this assessment computed tomography is by far the procedure of choice. Up to now (1991), CT-myelography was also needed to show the precise extent and nature of compression and/or distortion of the neural elements. However, the availability of high-resolution MRI in recent years has significantly decreased the need for CT-myelography.

In most cases CT supplemented by MRI provides all the information needed for optimal surgical planning. MRI has the added advantage of showing intrinsic pathology of the cord (e.g., edema, myelomalacia, and cavitation [Fig. 4-21], which in their early stages are not detected by myelography). At present, because of favorable experience with MRI in the short time it has been widely available and the confidence gained by radiologists and surgeons in the validity of its findings, an increasing number of surgeons are willing to operate on patients with stenosis based solely on the information supplied by CT and MRI, without insisting on a preoperative myelogram. We believe that CT and MRI in most instances provide all the information necessary prior to surgery in patients with stenosis, and we therefore recommend them, as needed, and add myelography only when CT and MRI both have been performed but the diagnosis is still not established (less than 20% of the time).

A retrospective review of 76 patients who had received MRI and CT-myelography prior to surgery for spinal stenosis revealed the following:

> In 9 patients CT-myelography provided additional information that was not clearly evident on CT or MRI. The additional findings were helpful in clarifying or narrowing the diagnoses — which included arachnoiditis of the lumbar spine, a synovial cyst with partially calcified walls compressing the dural sac at L3, several L3 root cysts, one neurofibroma, and two calcified herniated thoracic disks adherent to the dural sac (one with complete penetration of the dura).

Neural foraminal stenosis

In the *cervical region* the most common cause of neural foraminal stenosis is hypertrophic changes of the Luschka processes (Figs. 4-46 to 4-48). The cervical neural elements are situated in the lower half of the neural foramen (Fig. 4-47, *F* and *G*), and one must be careful to identify stenosis of this portion of the neural foramen.

Stenosis of the neural foramina identified on conventional roentgenographic studies often does not correlate positively with clinical findings. A significant number of patients with neural foraminal stenosis are asymptomatic. In our experience, however, when the width of the neural foramen (measured on CT) is reduced to 2 mm or less, the chance of recurrent cervical symptomatology is distinctly increased. A second, though significantly less common, cause of cervical neural foraminal stenosis is hypertrophic degenerative changes of the facet joints (Figs. 4-49 and 4-50). These should be evaluated by thin sec-

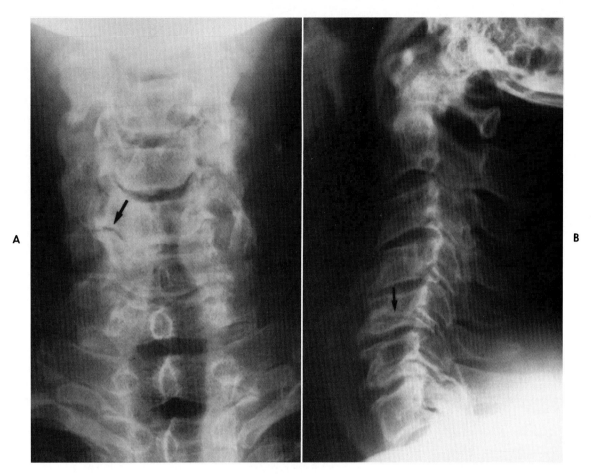

FIGURE 4-46

A and B, Frontal and lateral projections of the cervical spine showing extensive degenerative disease of the Luschka joints (*arrows*) and intervertebral disks.

tion (1 to 2 mm) high-resolution CT or CT-myelography. Consecutive slices, preferably angled along the plane of the disk, should be obtained through the neural foramen. The lower portion of the foramen is identified when the slices touch the cortex of the superior surface of the pedicle, which is the floor of the foramen. The cervical roots are visualized on high-resolution CT-myelography axial cross sections. They are not consistently identified on MRI axial cross sections in routine studies. Oblique MRI cross sections, though appealing in theory, have not been useful in our experience. It is hoped that future improvements in MRI, facilitating acquisition of a three-dimensional Fourier transform with 1 mm thick slices, will make evaluation of the foramina and visualization of the nerve roots a routine procedure.

In the *thoracic region*, neural foraminal stenosis is uncommon. However, it may be seen when patients have multiple hereditary exostoses, a traumatic deformity, or severe posttraumatic facet joint arthrosis.

In the *lumbar spine*, marked hypertrophic changes of the facet joints and osteophytes arising from the vertebral endplates may cause stenosis of the neural foramina

(Figs. 4-51 to 4-53). This is particularly true when collapse of an intervertebral disk has led to reduced height of the foramina. The superior articulating facet is forced upward, leading to reduction in the anteroposterior diameter of the foramen as well. The dorsal root ganglion just beneath the pedicle and the spinal nerve extending from this point inferiorly, anteriorly, and laterally are compressed, usually in the upper portion of the foramen. In our experience surgically documented cases of nerve compression in the *lumbar* neural foramen secondary to bony ridges and osteophytes have been rare, even in patients with severe degenerative disease. (This should not be confused with spinal nerve involvement secondary to a foraminal disk herniation, which is a well-known cause of lumbar radiculopathy.)

On CT, neural foraminal stenosis (Figs. 4-51 and 4-52) is identified by means of axial cross sections. Reformatted parasagittal cross sections are only occasionally helpful. On MRI, both axial and parasagittal cross sections may be beneficial, the parasagittals in particular revealing not only distortion of the normally teardrop-shaped neural foramen but also obliteration of the epidural fat and compression of the dorsal root ganglion or spinal nerve.

Text continued on p. 193.

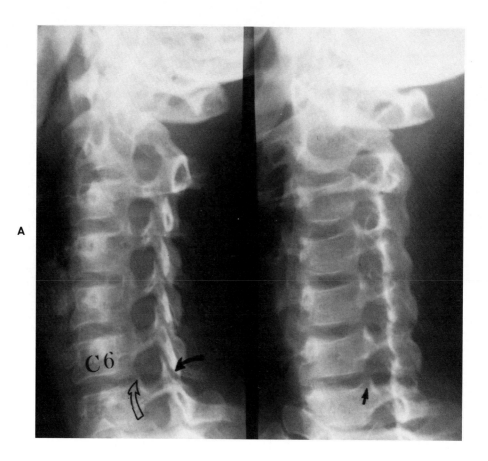

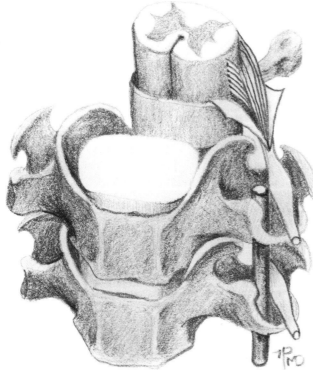

FIGURE 4-47

Cervical neural foraminal stenosis. **A,** Oblique projections of the cervical spine obtained with slightly different degrees of angulation show the foramina. The *solid curved arrow* denotes the facet joint and its relation to the C6-7 foramen. The *hollow curved arrow* points to the Luschka process of C7. **B** is a schematic of the relationships of the cervical nerve roots, dorsal root ganglion, neural foramen, and Luschka process. **C,** Vertebral specimen. Hypertrophic changes of the Luschka process have caused stenosis of the neural foramen. **D** shows stenosis of the C5-6 neural foramen secondary to hypertrophic changes of the C5-6 Luschka process on the left side. Note that the lower portion of the foramen, where the neural elements are, is stenotic. **E,** Hypertrophic change in the Luschka process, causing stenosis of the foramen on the left. **F,** Oblique section showing the relationship of the neural elements to the foramen in the cervical spine. *1,* Ventral root; *2,* dorsal root; *3,* facet joint; *4,* uncinate (Luschka) process. **G,** Axial section of the cervical spine. *1,* Dorsal root ganglion of the right C5; *2,* ventral root of C5; *3,* uncinate (Luschka) process of C5. This slice is at the level of the lower endplate of C4. Note the relation of the cervical nerve root to the Luschka process anteromedially and to the superior articular process of C5 (directly posterior to the dorsal root ganglion) posterolaterally.

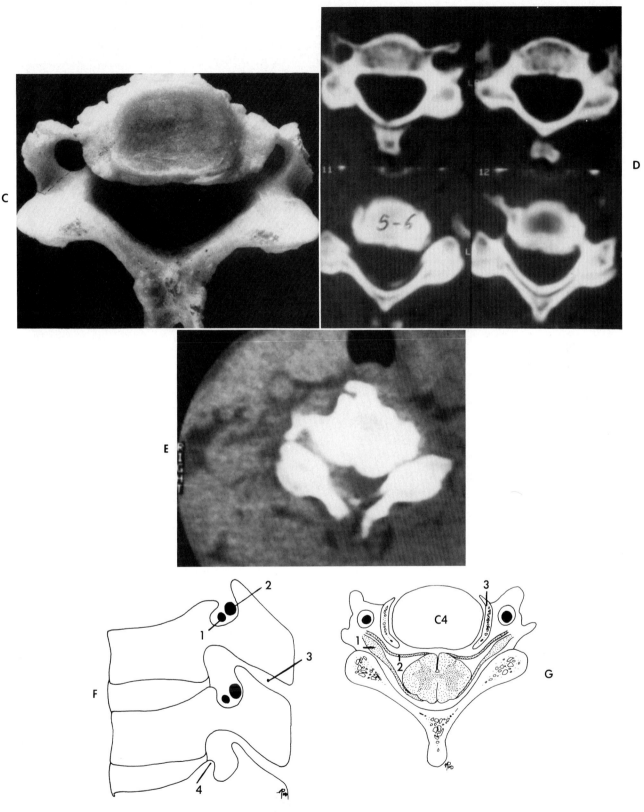

FIGURE 4-47, cont'd
For legend see opposite page.

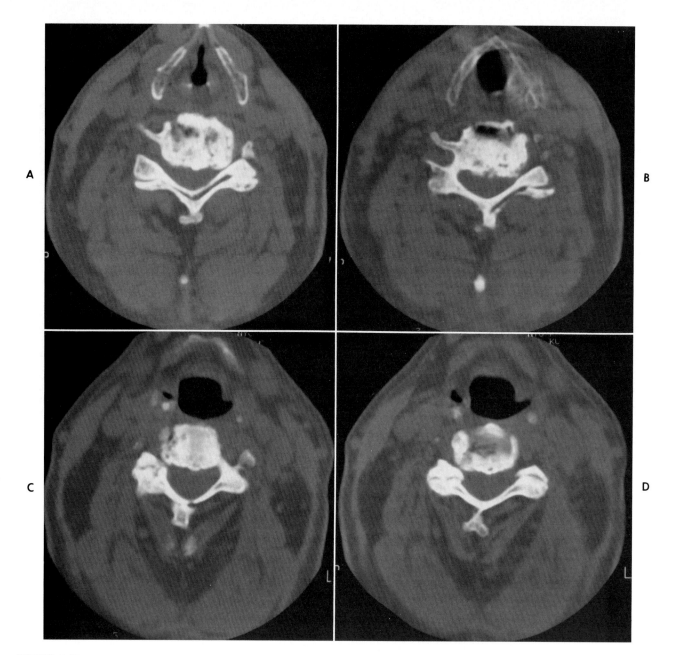

FIGURE 4-48
Neural foraminal stenosis. **A** and **B** show the left neural foramen at C5-6 affected by degenerative hypertrophic changes of the Luschka process. This patient also has chronic degenerative disk disease and bony ridges. The right neural foramen, however, is normal, as are the facet joints. **C** and **D** show the foramen at C4-5 affected by degenerative hypertrophic changes of the Luschka process and facet joint. Such involvement of the facet joints is uncommon as a cause of cervical neural foraminal stenosis. The right facet joint is normal.

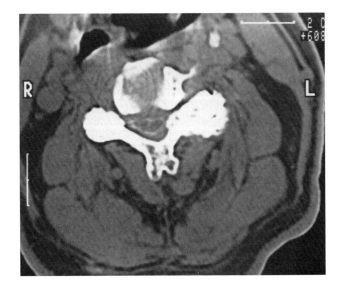

FIGURE 4-49
Neural foraminal stenosis in the cervical spine is usually caused by hypertrophic changes of the Luschka processes. In rare instances it may be due to hypertrophic changes in the facet joints. CT-myelography shows markedly hypertrophic alterations bilaterally in the facet joints. The stenosis was also present bilaterally, though considerably more on the left. A moderate-sized herniation was present in this patient, which accounted for the displacement and deformity of the spinal cord.

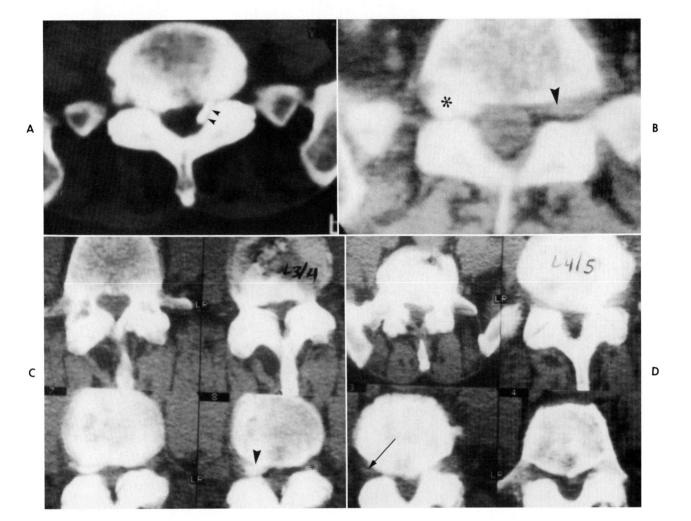

FIGURE 4-50
Lumbar neural foraminal stenosis in four patients. **A,** Affecting the right L5-S1 foramen, just below the pedicle of L5, and the dorsal root ganglion. This was documented at surgery. Note the calcification of the capsule of the left facet joint *(arrowheads)*. **B,** A large calcified osteophyte *(asterisk)* arising from the posterolateral surface of L5 on the right, just below the pedicle. The dorsal root ganglion on the left is normal *(arrowhead)*. At surgery there was marked compression of the ganglion and the exiting L5 nerve on the right. **C,** Four axial slices covering the superior-to-inferior span of the L3-4 neural foramen. Notice the calcified hypertrophic changes on the posterolateral border of L3 on the right *(arrowhead)*. There is also stenosis of the canal secondary to degenerative disease of the facet joints. The left L3 dorsal root ganglion *(asterisk)* is normal. However, the right L3 ganglion is markedly compressed, proven at surgery. **D,** Hypertrophic changes of the posterolateral aspect of L4 on the left, just below the L4 pedicle, causing stenosis of the left foramen. There is hypertrophic facet joint change, which also has contributed to the foraminal stenosis. Notice the normal exiting L4 spinal nerve *(arrow)* on the right. The left exiting nerve was found to be compressed at surgery.

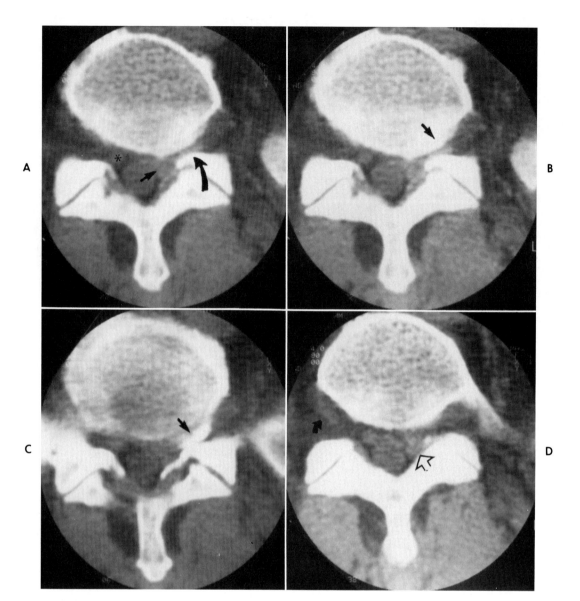

FIGURE 4-51

Neural foraminal stenosis. **A** and **B,** Two window settings of a CT examination obtained just above the inferior endplate of L5. There are hypertrophic changes of the posterolateral border of L5 on the left, which have caused stenosis of the lower portion of the L5-S1 foramen. The *curved arrow* in **A** denotes the stenotic foramen. The *asterisk* is on the normal descending right S1 nerve root, which has already separated from the dural sac. The *straight arrow* designates a soft tissue density in the epidural space occupying the anterolateral portion of the spinal canal on the left. It is a migrated fragment of herniated disk. The left descending S1 nerve root is obscured by the herniated disk. The *arrow* in **B** points to hypertrophic changes on the posterolateral border of L5. **C,** An axial slice obtained 4 mm below **A** and **B,** shows the hypertrophic changes and a calcified ridge *(arrow)*. A soft tissue density, representing herniated disk material, obscures the left anterior epidural fat and extends laterally. In so doing it also obscures the left descending S1 nerve root and lateral recess. **D,** An axial slice just below the L5 pedicle, shows the neural foramen to be normal at this level. The dorsal root ganglion also is normal *(curved arrow)*. The *hollow arrow* denotes the fragment of herniated disk obscuring the descending the left S1 nerve root. In this patient, with marked stenosis of the lower portion of the neural foramen, there is no evidence of compression of the L5 dorsal root ganglion, situated in the upper part of the foramen. The exiting L5 spinal nerve is more anterior and lateral to the site of the stenosis and is not involved.

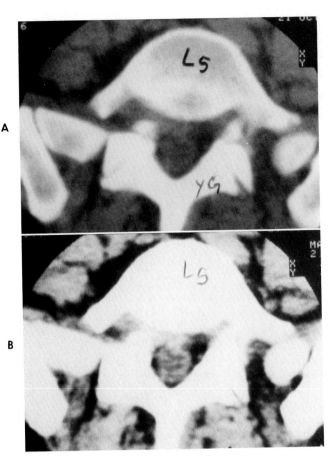

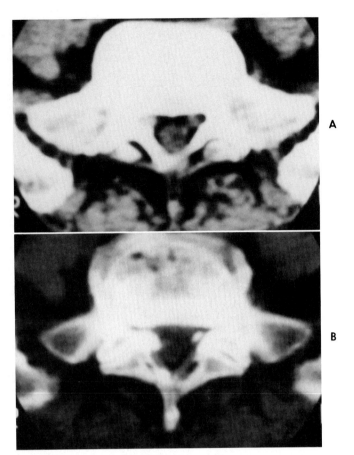

FIGURE 4-52
Neural foraminal stenosis in a patient with spondylolysis and spondylolisthesis. A and B, Bone and soft tissue windows, CT examination at L5-S1. Note the soft tissue density in the anterior and anterolateral spinal canal on the right. At surgery a fibrocartilaginous mass was found at the site of the defect in the arch. The exiting L5 nerve was encased by it. The spinal canal is elongated anteroposteriorly.

FIGURE 4-53
Lateral recess stenosis. A shows moderate stenosis of the right lateral recess, which contains the right descending S1 nerve root. B reveals markedly hypertrophic facet joints, which have created a severe stenosis of the right lateral recess. There is also calcification of the capsule of the facet joints on the left. In many patients with lateral recess stenosis there is no entrapment of the descending nerve root, because the root may not be within the recess (having gradually become medially displaced as the stenosis evolved).

Lateral recess stenosis

The lateral recess (i.e., the anterolateral compartment of the spinal canal that contains the descending nerve root) is bordered anteriorly by the posterolateral surfaces of the disk and the vertebral body below the disk, laterally by the medial surface of the pedicle, and posteriorly by the anterior surface of the superior (ascending) articulating facet. The nerve root descends in the lateral recess, crosses beneath the pedicle, and leaves the spinal canal to reach the ganglion at the top of the neural foramen.

The lateral recess may be narrowed by hypertrophic changes of the superior articulating facet (Figs. 4-54 and 4-59, *B*), by extension of the superior articulating facet into the spinal canal (creating a narrow groove between itself and the vertebral body in front of it), or by vertebral margin hypertrophic changes or a bulging disk (causing further compression of the descending root in the recess). Although vertebral margin osteophytes or old calcified herniated disks can cause stenosis of the lateral recess (Figs. 4-55 to 4-57), *the most significant narrowing occurs from hypertrophic changes at the cephalic end (i.e., at the superior border of the pedicle),* where the sagittal diameter of 3 mm or more may be reduced to 2 mm or less. In most patients with lateral recess syndrome, the sagittal diameter of the recess is less than 2 mm. (For further discussion see Chapter 1.)

Facet joint disease

Facet joints are true synovial joints and may be affected by systemic inflammatory arthritis, infectious arthritis, or degenerative disease. Manifestations appear in the cervical, thoracic, and lumbar spine.

CERVICAL SPINE

The cervical facet joints may be affected by rheumatoid arthritis, psoriatic arthritis, and similar conditions. Erosive changes of the facet joints from C1 to C3-4 are noted in adult-onset rheumatoid arthritis as well as other inflammatory spondyloarthropathies. Marked erosion and destructive changes leading to malalignment and

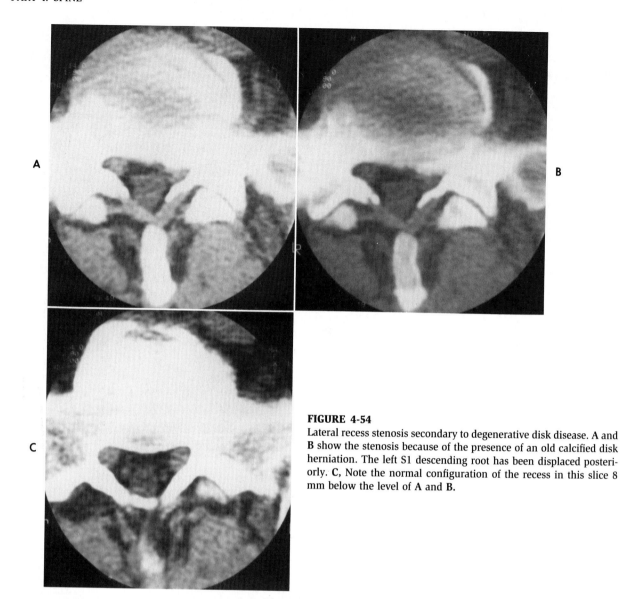

FIGURE 4-54
Lateral recess stenosis secondary to degenerative disk disease. A and B show the stenosis because of the presence of an old calcified disk herniation. The left S1 descending root has been displaced posteriorly. **C,** Note the normal configuration of the recess in this slice 8 mm below the level of **A** and **B.**

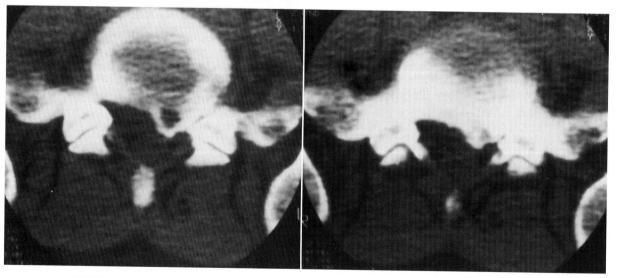

FIGURE 4-55
Lateral recess stenosis secondary to old degenerative disk disease and osteophyte formation. Soft tissue windows at L5-S1 showing almost complete obliteration of the left lateral recess due to hypertrophic changes of the vertebral margin.

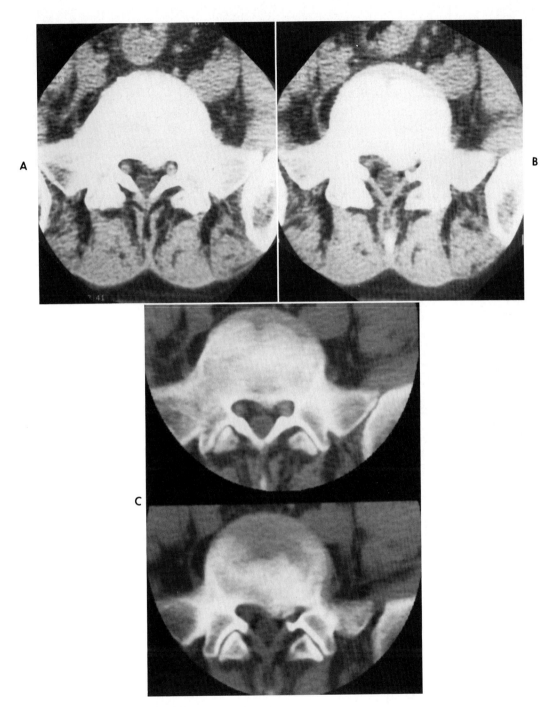

FIGURE 4-56
Degenerative disk disease at L5-S1. **A** and **B** are soft tissue and, **C**, bone windows of a CT examination showing hypertrophic changes of the vertebral endplate. The left S1 descending nerve root is compressed in the left lateral recess.

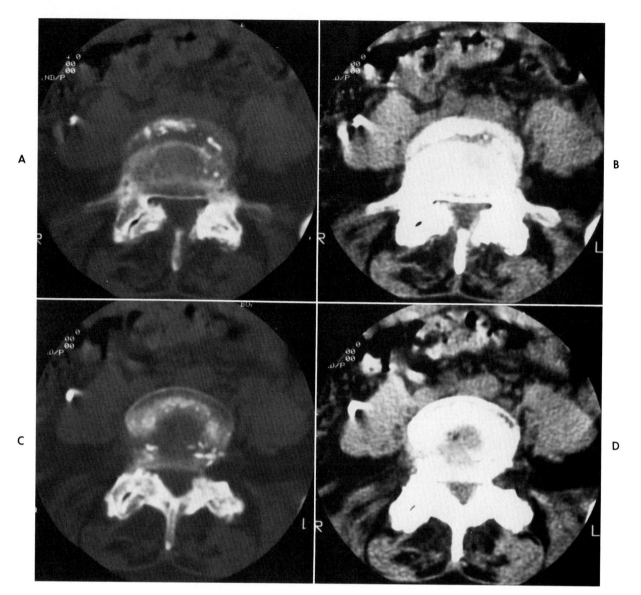

FIGURE 4-57
Severe lumbar spinal facet joint degenerative disease (L4-5). **A** and **B** are bone windows and, **C** and **D**,
soft tissue windows showing hypertrophic changes, osteosclerosis, and the vacuum phenomenon.
There is also a moderate degree of spinal stenosis and spondylolisthesis.

subluxation of the cervical spine may result. Significant inflammatory arthritis of the facet joints below C3-4 is not common in adult-onset rheumatoid arthritis. However, in psoriatic arthritis and other inflammatory spondyloarthropathies extensive inflammatory disease of the facet joints can lead to ankylosis, malalignment, and subluxation in practically the entire cervical spine.

Degenerative disease of the facet joints, though common, is not a significant cause of stenosis in the cervical spinal canal or neural foramina. The facet joints form the posterolateral border of the cervical neural foramen and only occasionally produce stenosis of a foramen.

THORACIC SPINE

Erosive change or ankylosis of the facet joints secondary to inflammatory spondyloarthropathy may be noted in the thoracic spine and lead to ankylosis of the thoracic cage. Inflammatory arthritis of the facet joints is not usually associated with spinal canal or neural foraminal stenosis in the thoracic region. However, one should be aware of the existence of a rare entity consisting of facet joint degenerative disease and thickening with calcification of the ligamentum flavum and facet joint capsules leading to stenosis of the canal in the thoracic region. These patients may suffer from a slowly progressive myelopathy.

LUMBAR SPINE

In the lumbar region the most important abnormality of the facet joints is degenerative disease, which can cause stenosis of the spinal canal, neural foramina, or lateral recesses.

Spinal canal stenosis secondary to facet joint degenerative disease. Degenerative disease of the lumbar facet joints is a major cause of stenosis of the spine (Figs. 4-58 to 4-62). It may present with osteosclerosis (Fig. 4-58), hypertrophic changes (Fig. 4-60), and irregularity of the articular cortex, sometimes with fragmentation of the facets. The vacuum phenomenon (Fig. 4-59) may be present. Some patients with the most extensive facet joint degenerative disease will have marked deformity and abnormality of the facets, osteosclerosis of the pars interarticularis, and fragmentation and fractures of the surfaces of the facets and pars interarticularis.

Part of the facet surface deformity and abnormality of its orientation is secondary to long-standing degenerative disease, causing erosion and fragmentation of the facets. There are also patients in whom the facets are congenitally abnormal in orientation (i.e., almost sagittal) (Fig. 4-29). These individuals are prone to spondylolisthesis. A particularly severe form of deformity and degenerative disease seems to occur in patients with preexisting congenital deformity of the facets or congenital predisposition to fragmentation and defects of the facets and adjacent portions of the neural arch. Facet joint degenerative disease causes hypertrophic change of the facets, which protrude into the spinal canal and cause deformity with stenosis of the canal (Fig. 4-60). The canal may be reduced to a narrow channel between the enlarged facets, or it may have an exaggerated cloverleaf configuration. Hypertrophic changes of the ligamentum flavum and facet joint capsules with or without calcification (Fig. 4-59) may also be present. The combination of these factors often leads to a severe stenosis of the canal.

Facet joint disease may also cause degenerative spondylolisthesis (Figs. 4-26 to 4-28, 4-61, and 4-62). The degenerative process erodes the facet surface, particularly its coronal component, which leads to instability of these joints and permits forward slippage of the posterior facets with spondylolisthesis and spinal stenosis.

Synovial cysts may be seen in association with long-standing degenerative disease or inflammatory arthritis of the lumbar facet joints. A synovial cyst may extend into the spinal canal and compress the dural sac, often posterolaterally. It may contain calcification in its wall and extend 3 or 4 cm in the epidural space. It may extend into the neural foramen and compress the dorsal root ganglion or the exiting spinal nerve.

Hypertrophic changes of the facet joints may cause stenosis of the lateral recess and neural foramina. Neural foraminal stenosis in the lumbar spine is secondary to a combination of factors: degenerative disk disease and loss of disk height exert pressure on the facet joints, forcing the inferior articulating facet of the upper vertebral body downward and the superior articulating facet of its partner upward; this reduces the height of the neural foramen and creates redundancy with buckling of the ligaments; hypertrophic changes and osteophytes arising from the facets or vertebral margins contribute to the stenosis. In extreme cases the dorsal root ganglion and exiting lumbar nerve may be compressed. In our experience surgically documented instances of lumbar neural foraminal stenosis, even in the most severe forms of degenerative disease of the facets, have not been a common finding.

Low back pain and facet joint degenerative disease. Degenerative disease of the facet joints plays an important role in stenosis of the spinal canal, lateral recesses, and neural foramina. Thus it is an indirect, but important, contributor to low back pain and other clinical findings secondary to stenosis.

However, if facet joint disease is present without spinal stenosis, a definitive cause-and-effect relationship between it and the patient's clinical manifestations is difficult to establish. Intuitively, it is reasonable to assume that a diseased facet joint can cause pain, either local or referred, as can any other joint; but because fairly severe degenerative disease of the facet joints may be seen (in our experience) in as many as 27% of asymptomatic subjects, incrimination of the facet joint disease as the cause of a patient's clinical findings becomes complicated. The situation is no more unusual than, for example, tying knee pain to long-standing degenerative disease of the knee. In both situations exclusion of other causes of pain and clinical evaluation are necessary. The facet joints, posterior longitudinal ligament, and for all practical purposes at least the posterior margin of the annulus are innervated by pain fibers. The facets receive their innervation from the dorsal primary ramus. The existence of pain (nociceptive) fibers in facet joints provides an anatomical basis for accepting the concept that pain can be generated and transmitted from the facets and adjacent tissues. The problem is how to identify this subgroup of patients.

According to Helbig and Casey,[64] Ghormley[65] introduced the term "facet syndrome" in 1933 and the role of lumbar facet joint as a source of low back pain and sciatica was emphasized by Badgely[66] in 1941. Ever since, opinions regarding the importance of facet joint disease and its relationship to low back pain have run a cyclical course. CT and MRI in recent years have facilitated the identification of patients in whom facet joint disease is responsible for spinal stenosis and the compression of neural elements. However, a significant number of patients are encountered who have various degrees of facet joint disease, sometimes severe, but no definite stenosis. Some of these individuals undoubtedly have back pain secondary to degenerative disease of the facets. There are also many with various degrees of facet joint degenerative disease, sometimes severe, who are asymptomatic. It is therefore not possible to identify, by radiographic means alone, the subgroup of patients in whom facet joint degenerative disease, without associated stenosis or instability, will be responsible for low back pain and sciatica. The clinical identification of this subgroup and their segregation from the large pool of

Text continued on p. 204.

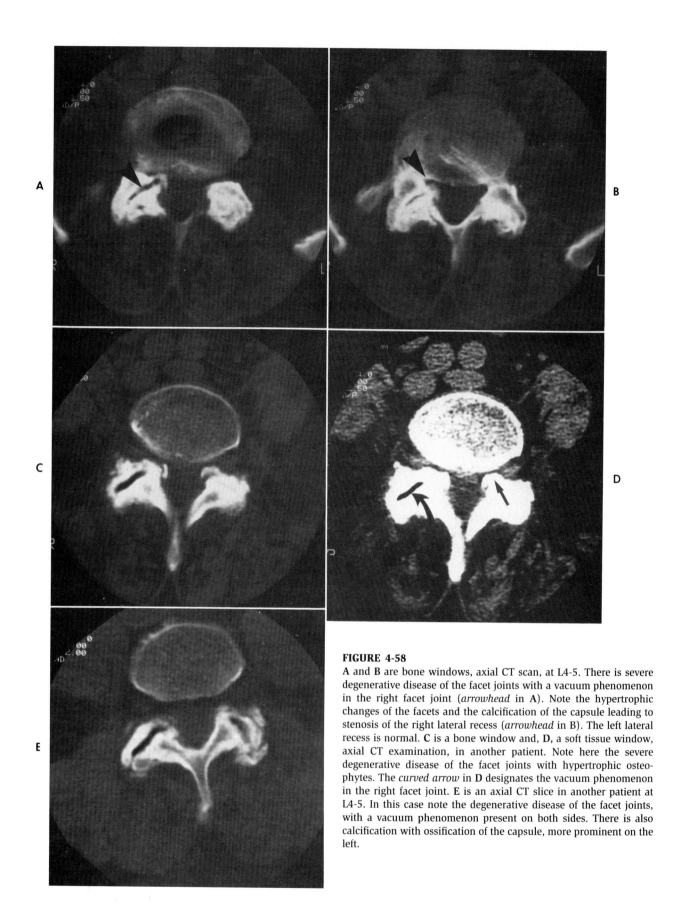

FIGURE 4-58

A and B are bone windows, axial CT scan, at L4-5. There is severe degenerative disease of the facet joints with a vacuum phenomenon in the right facet joint (*arrowhead* in **A**). Note the hypertrophic changes of the facets and the calcification of the capsule leading to stenosis of the right lateral recess (*arrowhead* in **B**). The left lateral recess is normal. **C** is a bone window and, **D**, a soft tissue window, axial CT examination, in another patient. Note here the severe degenerative disease of the facet joints with hypertrophic osteophytes. The *curved arrow* in **D** designates the vacuum phenomenon in the right facet joint. **E** is an axial CT slice in another patient at L4-5. In this case note the degenerative disease of the facet joints, with a vacuum phenomenon present on both sides. There is also calcification with ossification of the capsule, more prominent on the left.

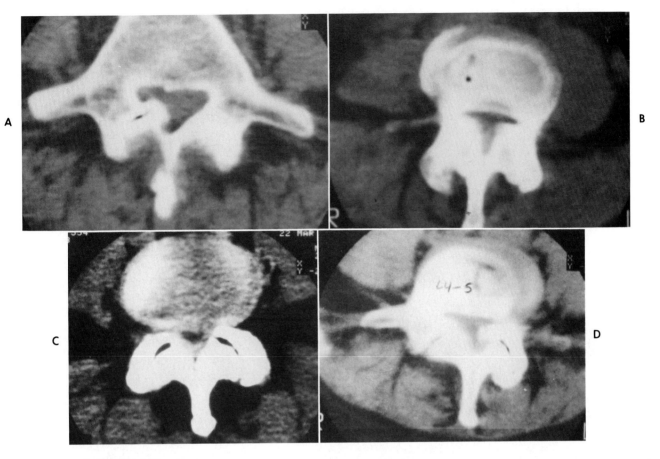

FIGURE 4-59
Acquired spinal stenosis secondary to facet joint degenerative disease in four patients. **A** to **D** show severe facet joint disease, consisting of hypertrophic changes, osteosclerosis, and the vacuum phenomenon. There is also a marked stenosis of the canal in all four individuals.

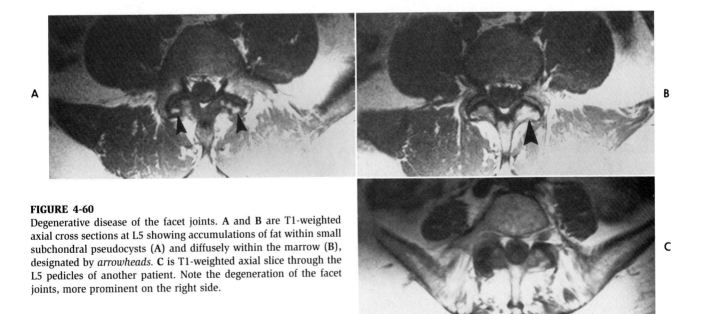

FIGURE 4-60
Degenerative disease of the facet joints. **A** and **B** are T1-weighted axial cross sections at L5 showing accumulations of fat within small subchondral pseudocysts (**A**) and diffusely within the marrow (**B**), designated by *arrowheads.* **C** is T1-weighted axial slice through the L5 pedicles of another patient. Note the degeneration of the facet joints, more prominent on the right side.

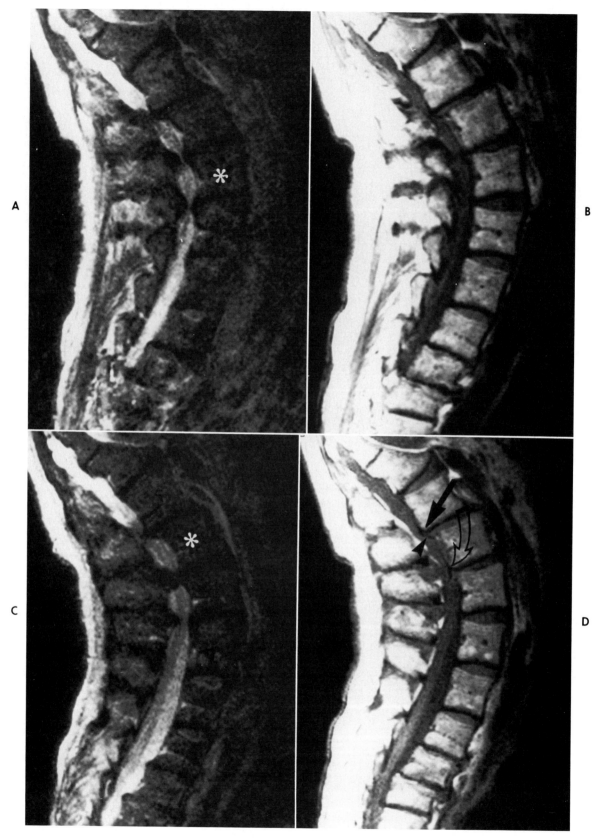

FIGURE 4-61
For legend see opposite page.

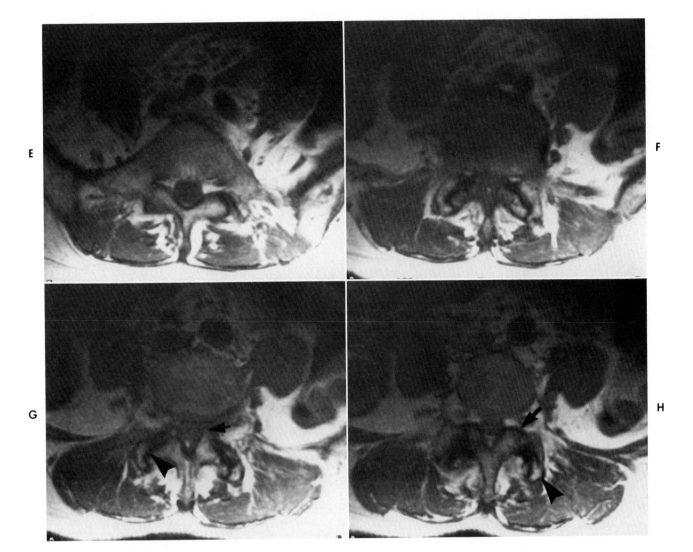

FIGURE 4-61

Spinal stenosis secondary to degenerative spondylolisthesis at L3-4 and L4-5. **A** is a T1-weighted midsagittal and, **B**, a corresponding T2-weighted midsagittal MR of the lumbar spine. There is spondylolisthesis with compression of the dural sac at L4 (*arrow* in **A**). The *arrowhead* in **A** points to dural sac compression at L4-5, at the level of the L5 superior endplate. Note the slanting posterior L4-5 disk surface, consequent to the anterior slippage of L4 on L5. (The *asterisk* in **B** is on L4.) Notice also the severe spinal stenosis at L3-4 and L4-5, due to the spondylolisthesis. **C** and **D** are T1- and T2-weighted parasagittal cross sections showing the extent of stenosis to the right of midline. (The *asterisk* in **D** is on L3.) Notice that the L2-3 stenosis is more prominent to the right of midline. Moderate to severe stenosis is also evident in the midsagittal plane at L2-3 (**B**). In **E** to **H**, T1-weighted (axial) cross sections from the L5 pedicle to just below the L4 pedicle, it is possible to see a number of interesting features. **E** shows the size and configuration of the canal to be within normal limits. **F**, just below the L4-5 disk, shows bilateral facet joint disease, with severe stenosis. In **G**, at the L4-5 disk level, facet joint disease is present. The *short arrow* denotes the tip of the anterior articular facet of the L4 inferior articular process, which has slipped anteriorly relative to the superior articular process of L5 *(arrowhead)*. There is a marked stenosis of the canal. In **H**, just below the L4 pedicle, note the facet joint degenerative disease. The *short arrow* points to the anteriorly displaced L4 inferior articular process relative to the superior articular process of L5 *(arrowhead)*.

A   B   C

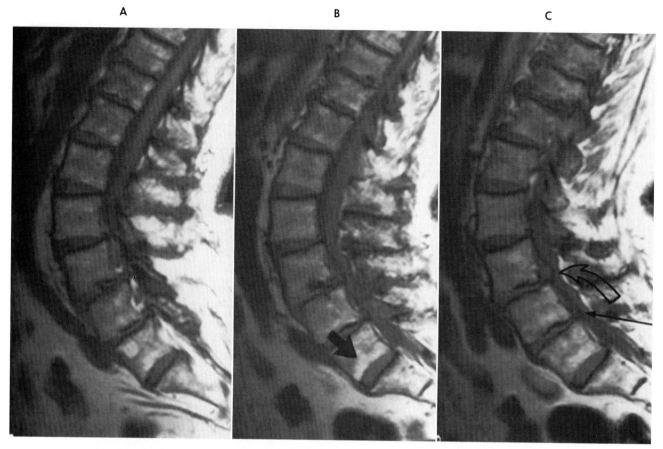

FIGURE 4-62

Spinal stenosis, degenerative disease of the facet joints, and disk herniation. **A** to **C**, T1-weighted sagittal and left parasagittal MR of the lumbar spine (TR 600/TE 20). **D** to **I**, Axial images at L2-3 and L3-4 (TR 900/TE 30). There is moderate spondylolisthesis of L2 relative to L3, and of L3 relative to L4, also of L4 relative to L5 (best seen in the midsagittal cross sections [**A**]). The patient has moderate scoliosis, which would explain why L3-5 are in a parasagittal position. Note the narrowing and degenerative disease of L3-4 and L4-5. The *arrow* in **B** points to fat adjacent to the L5 inferior endplate, a manifestation of the degenerative disease. Note also the herniation of the L3-4 disk extending superiorly behind the body of L3 (*curved hollow arrow* in **C**). At surgery the herniated material was seen to be anterior to the PLL. **D**, at the L3-4 disk, shows moderate to severe stenosis of the canal. It is difficult to identify the herniated disk, however, and to differentiate it from the dural sac. The *large arrowhead* points to degenerative disease of the facet joints. The *small arrowhead* designates a line of signal void defining the posterior extent of the herniated material compressing the dural sac between the ligamenta flava. The posterior border of the dural sac is not ordinarily so distinct (i.e., it does not have such a clearly demarcated signal void boundary). This proved to be the posterior border of the APLL complex (**C**). A slice 7 mm above the L3-4 disk, **E**, at the level of the L3 dorsal root ganglion shows the herniated material extending superiorly (*arrow*) behind the body of L3. The *arrowhead* denotes severe hypertrophic change in the facet joints due to degenerative disease. **F** and **G**, Slices through the L3 pedicle, show facet joint degenerative disease *(arrowheads)* and, **H**, just below the L2-3 disk, shows a signal void (representing the APLL complex, posteriorly displaced by the herniated L2-3 disk *[curved hollow arrow]*). The herniation extends inferiorly. **I**, at the L2-3 disk level, does not show well the soft tissues within the canal (which is stenotic); the herniation is poorly identified, but at surgery it was found to be associated with a minor disk herniation at L4-5 (*small arrow* in **C**). This patient also has severe stenosis at L2-3 and L3-4 secondary to the degenerative facet joint disease, ligament hypertrophy, and spondylolisthesis. The malalignment, consisting of scoliosis and spondylolisthesis, is due to degenerative disease of the disks and facet joints.   *Continued.*

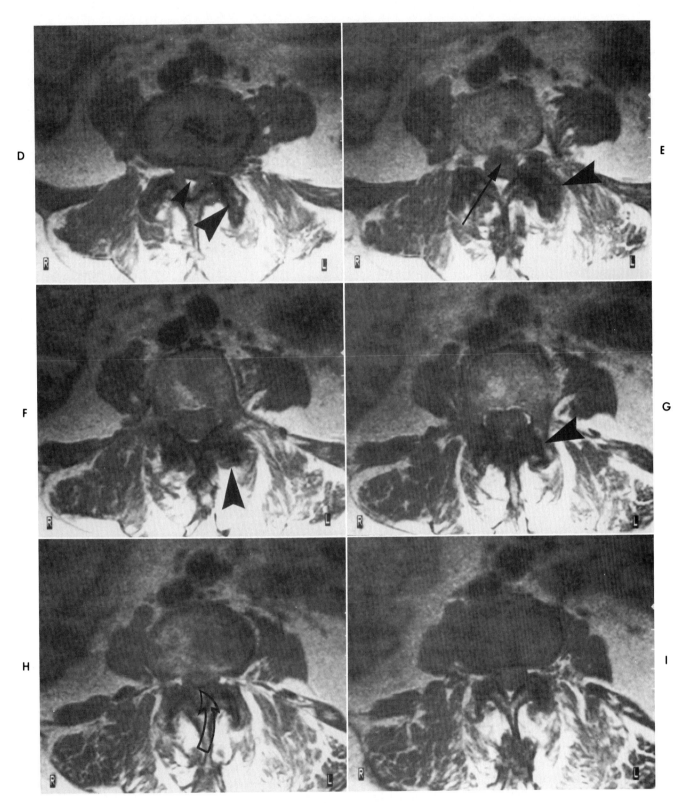

FIGURE 4-62, cont'd
For legend see opposite page.

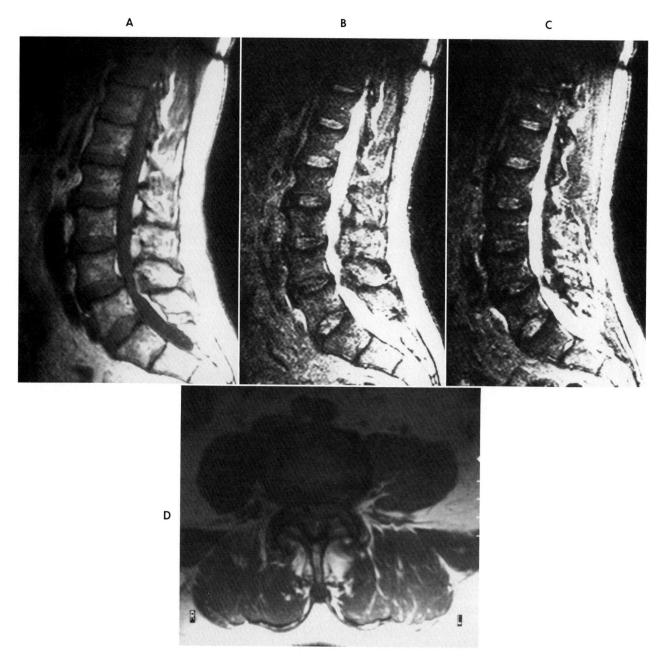

FIGURE 4-63
Severe spinal stenosis due to degenerative disease of the facet joints at L4-5. **A** is a T1-weighted midsagittal (TR 500/TE 20); **B** and **C** are mid-sagittal and parasagittal T2-weighted (TR 2100/TE 80); and **D** is an axial T1-weighted (TR 700/TE 20). There is severe stenosis of the canal, which can be best seen on T2-weighted images. (**D**, the axial cross section, shows the canal totally filled with low-density soft tissue without definite interface or practically any epidural fat.) These findings are typical of marked spinal stenosis. The hypertrophic changes in the facet joints are evident on the axial as well as the T2-weighted sagittal and parasagittal cross sections.

patients with back pain and sciatica are also difficult, because the clinical criteria for making the diagnosis of lumbar facet syndrome are still not well defined.[66-72] (For discussion of spinal instability and facet joint disease see Chapter 2.)

REFERENCES

1. Arnoldi CC, Brodsky AE, Cauchoix J, et al: Lumbar spinal stenosis and nerve root entrapment syndromes. Definition and classification. Clin Orthop Rel Res 1976;115:4-5.

2. Epstein BS, Epstein JA, Jones MD: Cervical spinal stenosis. Radiol Clin North Am 1977;15:215-226.

3. Epstein BS, Epstein JA, Jones MD: Lumbar spinal stenosis. Radiol Clin North Am 1977;15:227-240.

4. Verbiest H: A radicular syndrome from developmental narrowing of the lumbar vertebral column. J Bone Joint Surg 1954;36B:230-237.

5. Roberson GH, Llewellyn HJ, Taveras JM: The narrow lumbar spinal canal syndrome. Radiology 1978;107:89-97.

6. Kirkaldy-Willis WH, Paine KWE, Cauchoix J, McIvor G: Lumbar spinal stenosis. Clin Orthop 1974;99:30-50.

7. Pyeritz RE, Sack GH Jr, Udvarhelyi GB: Cervical and lumbar laminectomy for spinal stenosis in achondroplasia. Johns Hopkins Med J 1980;146:203-206.

8. Epstein JA, Carras R, Hyman RA, Costa S: Cervical myelopathy caused by developmental stenosis of the spinal canal. J Neurosurg 1979;51:362-367.

9. Aisen AM, Martel W, Ellis JH, McCune WJ: Cervical spine involvement in rheumatoid arthritis: MR imaging. Radiology 1987;165:159-163.

10. Beltran J, Caudill JL, Herman LA, et al: Rheumatoid arthritis MR imaging manifestations. Radiology 1987;165:153-157.

11. Martel W: The occipito-atlanto-axial joints in rheumatoid arthritis and ankylosing spondylitis. Am J Roentgenol 1961;86:223-240.

12. Martel W: Cervical spondylitis in rheumatoid disease: a comment on neurologic significance and pathogenesis. Am J Med 1968;44:441-446.

13. Cawley MID, Chalmers TM, Kellgren JH, Ball J: Destructive lesions of vertebral bodies in ankylosing spondylitis. Ann Rheum Dis 1972;31:345-358.

14. Dihlmann W, Delling G: Disco-vertebral destructive lesions (so-called Anderson lesions) associated with ankylosing spondylitis. Skeletal Radiol 1978;3:10-16.

15. Rivelis M, Freiberger RH: Vertebral destruction at unfused segments in late ankylosing spondylitis. Radiology 1969;93:251-256.

16. Bartleson JD, Cohen MD, Harrington TM, et al: Cauda equina syndrome secondary to long-standing ankylosing spondylitis. Ann Neurol 1983;14:662-669.

17. Bowie EA, Glasgow GL: Cauda equina lesions associated with ankylosing spondylitis. Br Med J 1961;2:24-27.

18. Thomas DJ, Kendall MJ, Whitfield AGW: Nervous system involvement in ankylosing spondylitis. Br Med J 1974;1:148-150.

19. Barnett GH, Russell W, Little JR, et al.: Thoracic spinal canal stenosis. J Neurosurg 1987;66:338-344.

20. Kodama T, Okubo K, Matsukado Y: Myelopathy due to ossified ligamenta flava in lower thoracic region. No Shinkei Geka 1979;7:867-873.

21. Marzluff JM, Hungerford DG, Kempe LG, et al.: Thoracic myelopathy caused by osteophytes of the articular process. Thoracic spondylosis. J Neurosurg 1979;50:779-783.

22. Yamamoto I, Matsumae M, Ikeda A, et al.: Thoracic spinal stenosis: experience with 7 cases. J Neurosurg 1988;68:37-40.

23. Ciric I, Mikhael MA, Tarkington JA, et al: The lateral recess syndrome. A variant of spinal stenosis. J Neurosurg 1980;53:433-443.

24. Epstein BS, Epstein JA, Jones MD: Degenerative spondylolisthesis with intact neural arch. Radiol Clin North Am 1977;15(2):275-287.

25. Macnab I: Spondylolisthesis with an intact neural arch — the so-called pseudo-spondylolisthesis. J Bone Joint Surg [Br] 1950;32B:325-333.

26. Wiltse LL: The etiology of spondylolisthesis. J Bone Joint Surg 1963;44A:539-569.

27. Wiltse LL, Widell EH Jr, Jackson DW: Fatigue fracture: the basic lesion in isthmic spondylolisthesis. J Bone Joint Surg [Am] 1975;57A:17-22.

28. Epstein BS, Epstein JA, Jones MD: Lumbar spondylolisthesis with isthmic defects. Radiol Clin North Am 1977;15:261-274.

29. Yoshihiro H, Tokuro N: Calcification of the posterior longitudinal ligaments of the spine among Japanese. Radiology 1971;100:307-312.

30. Minagi H, Gronner AT: Calcification of the posterior longitudinal ligament: a cause of cervical myelopathy. Am J Roentgenol 1969;105:365-369.

31. Firooznia H, Benjamin MV, Pinto RS, et al: Calcification and ossification of the posterior spinal ligament: its role in secondary narrowing of the spinal canal and cord compression. NY State J Med 1982;82(2):1193-1198.

32. Firooznia H, Rafii M, Golimbu C, et al: Computed tomography of the calcification and ossification of the posterior longitudinal ligament of the spine. J Comput Tomogr 1984;8:3117-3124.

33. Firooznia H, Golimbu C, Rafii M: Progressive paralysis in a woman with pseudo-hypoparathyroidism. Skeletal Radiol 1985;13:310-313.

34. Firooznia H, Ahn JH, Rafii M, Ragnarssn KT: Sudden quadriplegia after a minor trauma: the role of pre-existing spinal stenosis. Surg Neurol 1985;23:165-168.

35. Julkunen H, Heinonen OP, Knekt P, et al: The epidemiology of hyperostosis of the spine together with its symptoms and related mortality in a general population. Scand J Rheumatol 1975;4:23-27.

36. Resnick D, Shapiro RF, Wiesner KB, et al: Diffuse idiopathic skeletal hyperostosis (DISH) (ankylosing hyperostosis of Forestier and Rotes-Querol). Semin Arthr Rheum 1978;7:153-187.

37. Forestier J, Rotes-Querol J: Senile ankylosing hyperostosis of the spine. Ann Rheum Dis 1950;9:321-330.

38. Mitsui H, Sonozaki H, Juji T, et al: Ankylosing spinal hyperostosis (ASH) and ossification of the posterior longitudinal ligament (OPLL). Arch Orthop Trauma Surg 1979;94:21-23.

39. Seze Syde, Claisse R: Hyperostose vertébrale lombaire juvénile. Rev Rhum 1960;27:219-225.

40. Forestier J, Lagier R. Ankylosing hyperostosis of the spine. Clin Orthop 1971;74:65-83.

41. Resnick D, Guerra J Jr, Robinson CA, et al: Association of diffuse idiopathic skeletal hyperostosis (DISH) and calcification and ossification of the posterior longitudinal ligament. AJR 1978;131:1049-1053.

42. Arlet J, Pujol M, Buc et al: Rôle de l'hyperostose vertébrale dans les myelopathies cervicales. Rev Rhum Mal Osteoartic 1976;43:167-175.

43. Onji Y, Akiyama H, Shimomura Y, et al: Posterior paravertebral ossification causing cervical myelopathy. A report of 18 cases. J Bone Surg 1967;49:1314-1328.

44. Alenghat JP, Hallett M, Kido DK: Spinal cord compression in diffuse idiopathic skeletal hyperostosis. Radiology 1982;142:119-120.

45. Feldman F, Seaman WB: The neurologic complications of Paget's disease of the cervical spine. AJR 1969;105:375-378.

46. McAllister VL, Kendall BE, Bull JWD: Symptomatic vertebral hemangiomas. Brain 1975;98:71-80.

47. Bell RL. Hemangioma of dorsal vertebrae with collapse and compression myelopathy. J Neurosurg 1955;12:570-576.

48. Feuerman T, Dwan PS, Young RF: Vertebrectomy for treatment of vertebral hemangioma without preoperative embolization. J Neurosurg 1986;65:404-406.

49. Melot CJ, Brihaye J, Jeanmart L, Compel C: Les hemangiomes du rachis cervical. Acta Radiol [Diagn] 1966;5:1067-1078.

50. Mohan V, Gupta SK, Tuli SM, et al: Symptomatic vertebral hemangiomas. Clin Radiol 1980;31:575-579.

51. Greenspan A, Klein MJ, Bennett AJ, et al: Hemangioma of the T6 vertebra with a compression fracture, extradural block and spinal cord compression. Skeletal Radiol 1983;10:183-188.

52. Hekster REM, Luyendijk W, Tan TI: Spinal-cord compression caused by vertebral hemangioma relieved by percutaneous catheter embolization. Neuroradiology 1972;3:160-164.

53. Holta O: Hemangioma of the cervical vertebra with fracture and compression myelomalacia. Acta Radiol [Stockh] 1942;23:423-430.

54. Gourie-Devi M, Prakash B: Vertebral and epidural hemangioma with paraplegia in Klippel-Trenaunay-Weber syndrome. Case report. J Neurosurg 1978;48:814-817.

55. Lozman J, Holmblad J: Cavernous hemangiomas associated with scoliosis and a localized consumptive coagulopathy. A case report. J Bone Joint Surg (Am) 1976;58:1021-1024.

56. Ross JS, Masaryk TJ, Modic MT, Carter JR, et al: Vertebral hemangiomas: MR imaging. Radiology 1987;165:165-169.

57. Liu CL, Yang DJ. Paraplegia due to vertebral hemangioma during pregnancy. Spine 1988;13(1):107-108.

58. Hinck VC, Sachdev NS. Developmental stenosis of the cervical spinal canal. Brain 1966;89:27-36.

59. Paine KWE: Clinical features of lumbar spine stenosis. Clin Orthop Rel Res 1976;115:77-82.

60. Blau JN, Logue V: Intermittent claudication of the cauda equina. An unusual syndrome resulting from central protrusion of a lumbar intervertebral disc. Lancet 1961;1:1081-1086.

61. Wolf BS, Khilnani M, Malis LI: Sagittal diameter of the bony cervical spinal canal and its significance in cervical spondylosis. J Mt Sinai Hosp 1956;23:283.

62. Takahasi M, Yamashita Y, Sakamoto Y, et al: Chronic cervical cord compression. Clinical significance of increased signal intensity on MR images. Radiology 1989;173-219-224.

63. Ullrich CG, Binet EF, Sanecki MG, et al: Quantitative assessment of the lumbar spinal canal by computed tomography. Radiology 1980;134:137-143.

64. Helbig T, Casey KL: The lumbar facet syndrome. Spine 1988;13(1):61-64.

65. Ghormley RK: Low back pain with special reference to the articular facets with presentation of an operative procedure. JAMA 1933;101:1773-1777.

66. Badgely CE: The articular facets in relation to low back pain and sciatic radiation. J Bone Joint Surg 1941;23:481-496.

67. Mixter WJ, Barr JS: Rupture of intervertebral disc with involvement of the spinal cord. N Engl J Med 1934;211:210-215.

68. Carrera GF: Lumbar facet injection in low back pain and sciatica. Preliminary results. Radiology 1980;137:665-667.

69. Destouet JM, Murphy WA: Lumbar facet block: indications and technique. Orthop Rev 1985;14:57-65.

70. Fairbank JCT, Park WM, Mccall IW, O'Brian JP: Apophyseal injection of local anesthetic as a diagnostic aid in primary low back syndrome. Spine 1981;6:593-605.

71. Hirsch D, Inglemark B, Miller M: The anatomical basis for low back pain. Act Orthop Scand 1963;33:1.

72. Lippett AB: The facet joint and its role in spine pain: Management with facet joint injection. Spine 1984;9:746-750.

5 Postoperative Lumbar Spine: General Considerations and Evaluation by CT

HOSSEIN FIROOZNIA
IRVIN I. KRICHEFF

RADIOLOGICAL EXAMINATION OF PATIENTS WITH PRIOR SPINAL SURGERY

Diagnosis and treatment of recurrent or persistent pain and/or neurological deficit following surgery for lumbar disk herniation and/or spinal stenosis are difficult for the clinician as well as the radiologist. The incidence of surgical failure varies from 5% to 25%. The failed back syndrome has been associated with a number of abnormalities, including

1. Inaccurate preoperative diagnosis
2. Inappropriate surgery
3. Persistence or recurrence of disk herniation at the operated level
4. Disk herniation at a new level
5. Postoperative scar
6. Failure to treat a spinal stenosis that existed prior to surgery but was not detected
7. Spinal stenosis following surgery
8. Mechanical instability: occurring or worsening after surgery in patients with preexisting facet joint arthrosis and degenerative spondylolisthesis (Fig. 5-1)
9. Infection (Fig. 5-2)
10. Pseudomeningocele (Fig. 5-3)
11. Arachnoiditis
12. Nerve injury
13. Neural arch and facet fracture
14. Failure of interbody or posterolateral fusion

Evaluation of fusion and stability

Conventional roentgenography is useful for a rapid overall evaluation of spinal alignment. In some patients, although uncommon, it also helps make the diagnosis of failed posterolateral fusion. Comparison of pre- and postoperative lateral films may reveal the extent of postoperative spondylolisthesis. If there is a suspicion of spinal instability, fluoroscopy of the spine in motion (recorded on videotape) is usually indicated. Fluoroscopy should be performed in the lateral and AP projections while the standing patient performs flexion and extension of the spine and bends to the left and to the right. The videotape recording facilitates repeat viewing and comparison with future studies.

If failure of bony fusion is suspected, CT with reformatting of images in the sagittal and coronal planes may help. As a rule, axial cross sections 3 to 4 mm thick (overlapped 1 mm) from the level of the fusion are necessary. It may be possible to obtain direct coronal CT images of the lumbar spine. This can be done only in patients with a small or medium body frame, however, and with a CT unit that has a fairly large gantry opening.

Recent experience has shown the usefulness of MRI in evaluating patients with failure of a bony fusion. When there is solid interbody bony fusion, sagittal T1-weighted cross sections show moderate to significant amounts of fat crossing the region. If there is a lack of fusion, however, with motion of the spine at the site, fat does not accu-

207

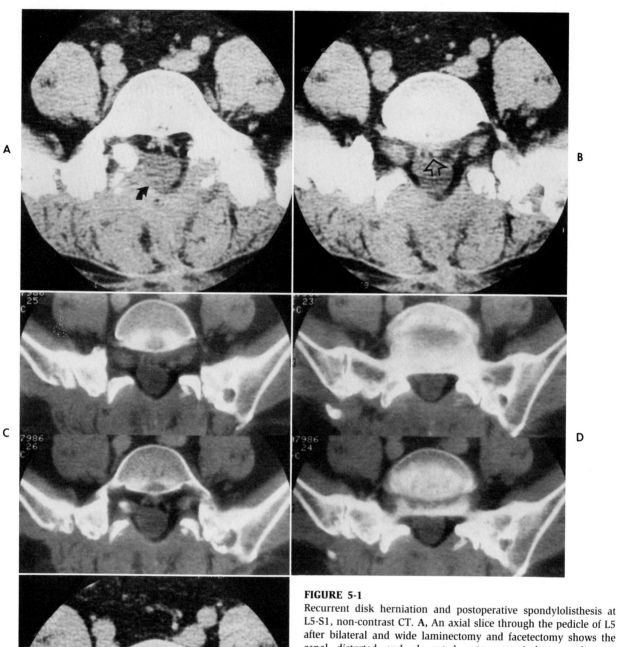

FIGURE 5-1

Recurrent disk herniation and postoperative spondylolisthesis at L5-S1, non-contrast CT. **A,** An axial slice through the pedicle of L5 after bilateral and wide laminectomy and facetectomy shows the canal distorted and elongated anteroposteriorly secondary to spondylolisthesis. The dural sac is retracted to the right. The arrow denotes the site of obliterated epidural fat on the right. **B,** Another slice, 8 mm below A, shows a migrated fragment of herniated disk *(hollow arrow).* **C,** Bone windows reveal the extent of the laminectomy and facetectomy. Note the marked distortion and fragmentation of the facets. **D,** There is a partial volume effect with the vertebral endplates showing the extent of the spondylolisthesis. The dural sac is retracted slightly to the right. The preoperative studies had shown extensive degenerative disease of the facet joints with fragmentation of the articular facets at L4-5 and L5-S1. There was minimal spondylolisthesis at this level prior to surgery. Patients with severe facet joint arthrosis and deformity with fragmentation of the facets are more prone to spondylolisthesis if they are subjected to extensive laminectomy and facetectomy. **E,** Axial slice at L5-S1 showing the combination of disk herniation and posterior projection of the disk secondary to the spondylolisthesis. The posterior border of the soft tissue density is projecting into the canal and is irregular due to the herniation. (Notice again the migrated free fragment in **B.**)

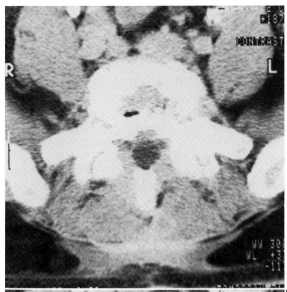

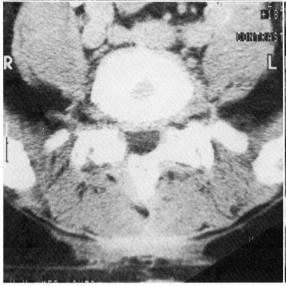

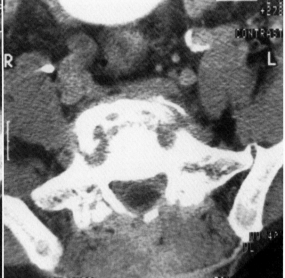

FIGURE 5-2
Postoperative osteomyelitis. Axial slices at L5-S1 after intravenous contrast show destructive change of the vertebral endplates and soft tissue swelling 4 weeks after an L5 laminectomy for L5-S1 disk herniation. The inflammatory process extends into the retrospinal soft tissues and continues into the site of surgery through to the skin.

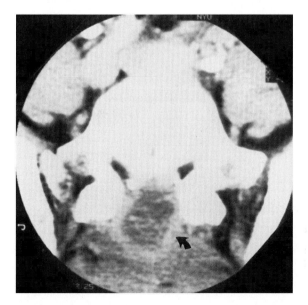

FIGURE 5-3
Pseudomeningocele. A CT examination after intravenous contrast at L5-S1 shows extensive bilateral laminectomy. A large sac (the pseudomeningocele) extends beyond the posterior limit of the canal. The *arrow* points to the enhanced wall of the lesion.

mulate. Instead, there is an area of low signal intensity immediately adjacent to the region on T1-weighted sagittal cross sections and a region of high signal intensity on T2-weighted cross sections. This is probably due to fissuring, edema, and granulation tissue formation secondary to motion of the spine at the site of the failed fusion.

CT of the postoperative lumbar spine

Recurrence of disk herniation and proliferative surgical scar formation are two of the important causes of postoperative pain and neurological deficit.[1-3] Differentiation of the two is usually impossible clinically but, nevertheless, often is useful in making a decision regarding the advisability of further surgical intervention. This is because most patients with extensive surgical scar formation do not benefit from surgery; most scars recur after surgery.[4-9] In our experience, lysis of the scar may offer some relief, though not dramatic. On the other hand, when a herniated disk is definitively identified, the chances of significant postoperative improvement are distinctly increased. Intravenous contrast-enhanced CT of the lumbar spine has been used in differentiating recurrent disk herniation from scar formation,[4,10] with accuracies ranging from 67% to 100%.[10-15]

We studied 168 patients who had previously undergone lumbar disk surgery and had had recurrent or persistent symptoms. The 62 women and 106 men ranged in age from 21 to 79 years (mean, 51 years). The complaints were present immediately after surgery in 19 patients and developed 2 months to 9 years after surgery in 149. Of the total, 143 were reported on in 1987[15] and 25 have since been added.

Lumbar CT was performed with five or six consecutive parallel axial cross sections, 5 mm thick and 4 mm apart, at each intervertebral disk parallel to the plane of the disk from pedicle to pedicle, encompassing L2 to S1. The examination was then repeated with intravenous contrast enhancement. All patients received a rapid-drip infusion (for 8 to 10 minutes) of diatrizoate meglumine USP 30% (Reno-M-DIP), 4.44 ml/kg of body weight (maximum, 300 ml). The CT examination was started when half the infusion had been injected. An additional 50 ml bolus of contrast was given to 31 subjects (delivered in 2 minutes or less) at the midpoint of the drip infusion.

Seventy-seven patients underwent reexploration of the previously operated disk and at least one disk above or below it.

NORMAL AND BULGING DISKS

Enhancement of the margins of a normal disk, anteriorly, laterally, and posteriorly (Fig. 5-4), occurred in 24 of the 77 patients (31%).

18 had bulging of the disk. This diagnosis was made when a smooth, symmetrical, and generalized extension of the margin was noted beyond the vertebral endplate margins.[16] Enhancement occurred in 12 (66%) (Fig. 5-5).

HERNIATED DISKS

At surgical exploration there were 34 instances of recurrent herniation and 16 of herniation at a site other than the previously explored levels.

Enhancement occurred in 36 instances (or 72%) (Figs. 5-6 to 5-9). In most patients it was linear and 2 to 3 mm thick. Often it was present along the entire circumference of the disk (i.e., anteriorly and laterally as well as posteriorly).

In 9 patients there was patchy enhancement of the entire substance of the disk, with near-uniform enhancement of the entire (10 to 13 mm) portion of herniated disk that protruded into the canal.

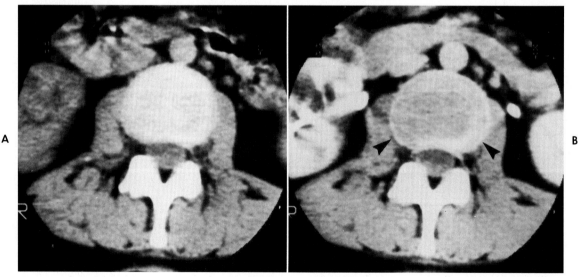

FIGURE 5-4
A normal L3-L4 intervertebral disk. **A** is precontrast and, **B**, postcontrast. Note the enhancement of the margin of the disk *(arrowheads)*. (From Firooznia H, Kricheff II, Rafii M, Golimbu C: Radiology 1987;163:221-226.)

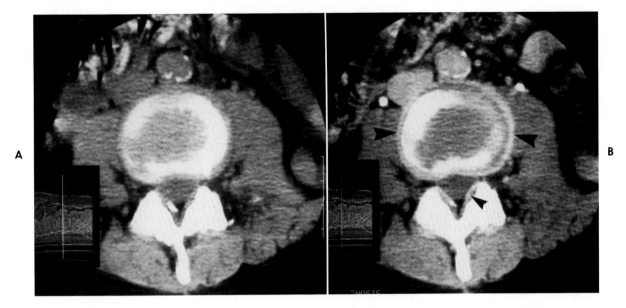

FIGURE 5-5
Generalized bulging of the annulus fibrosus at L3-4. A is a precontrast and, B, a postcontrast study.
Note the markedly enhanced margin of the bulging disk and the ligamenta flava *(arrowheads)*. (From
Firooznia H, Kricheff II, Rafii M, Golimbu C: Radiology 1987;163:221-226.)

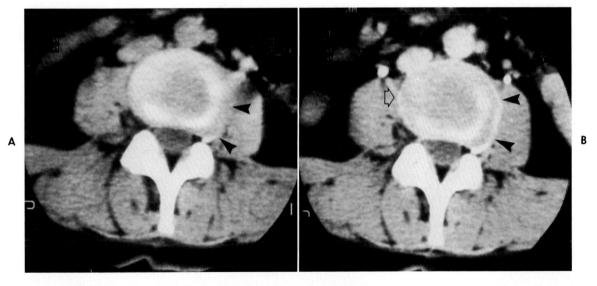

FIGURE 5-6
Herniated disk on the left side. A is a precontrast study. Note the herniation *(arrowheads)* extending
into the neural foramen. B, a postcontrast study, shows the enhanced margins *(arrowheads)* with
enhancement also of the right side *(hollow arrow)*. (From Firooznia H, Kricheff II, Rafii M, Golimbu C:
Radiology 1987;163:221-226.)

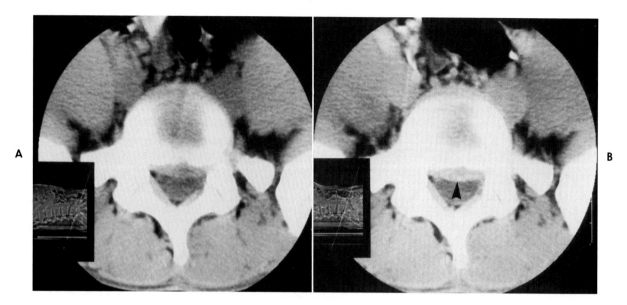

FIGURE 5-7
Herniated disk at L5-S1 **A,** A precontrast and, **B,** a postcontrast study show enhancement of the herniated portion of the disk *(arrowhead).* (From Firooznia H, Kricheff II, Rafii M, Golimbu C: Radiology 1987;163:221-226.)

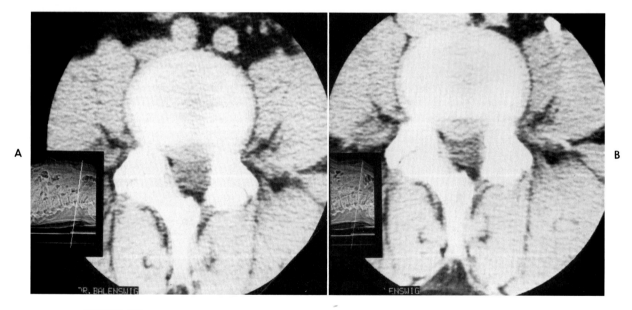

FIGURE 5-8
Recurrent disk herniation at L4-5. Laminectomy was performed on the left side. **A,** Precontrast and, **B,** after intravenous contrast. Note the near homogeneous enhancement of the entire width of the protruding portion. (From Firooznia H, Kricheff II, Rafii M, Golimbu C: Radiology 1987;163:221-226.)

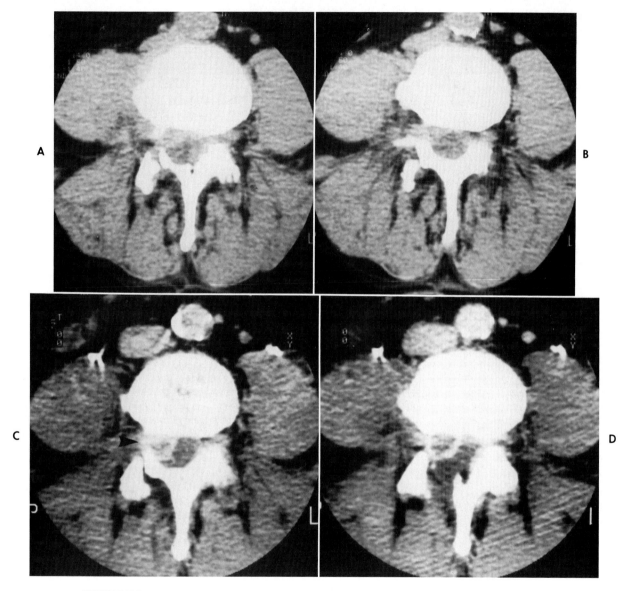

FIGURE 5-9
Recurrent herniation of a disk on the right at L4-5. Laminectomy was performed on the right side. **A** and **B,** Precontrast studies showing the soft tissues within the canal to be not particularly well defined. The dural sac is obscured. **C** and **D,** Postcontrast studies. (In **C,** note the enhancement of soft tissues anterolaterally in the canal *[arrowhead].* In **D** the ring of enhancement surrounds a zone of nonenhancement.) At surgical reexploration a fragment of a recurrent herniated disk was found enveloped by granulation tissue, along with a minimal amount of mature scar. (From Firooznia H, Kricheff II, Rafii M, Golimbu C: Radiology 1987;163:221-226.)

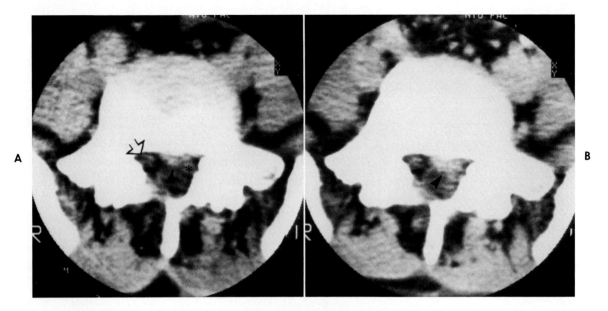

FIGURE 5-10
An enhanced migrated disk fragment. **A,** Precontrast study at L5-S1 in a patient who had had surgery once before. Note the soft tissue density in the midline, extending to the left *(arrowhead),* with posterior displacement of the S1 descending nerve root *(asterisk).* The normal right S1 descending root is indicated by the *hollow arrow.* **B,** Postcontrast study. There is marked enhancement of the epidural soft tissue mass *(arrowhead).* The enhancement obscures the left S1 descending root. At surgical reexploration a fibrocartilaginous fragment of disk intermixed with granulation tissue was found.

In 8 patients there were sequestered fragments (migrated or free [i.e., not attached to the donor disk]) that appeared as indistinct areas of increased density in the canal.

After intravenous contrast administration, in 4 there was marked enhancement of a 2 to 3 mm thick layer of tissue surrounding a less enhancing central nidus; in the other 4 there was nonhomogeneous enhancement affecting 50% to 70% of the free fragments (Fig. 5-10).

We used the same criteria for diagnosing a herniated disk in patients who had had diskectomy as in patients who had not. The diagnosis was made when the disk margins extended with a generally irregular contour or a focal area of irregularity beyond the endplate margins.[16] Unlike postsurgical scars, which may pull the dural tube and neural elements toward them, herniated disks generally push these structures away. A herniated disk does not usually appear as a soft tissue density with a straight linear margin, and it does not extend in linear fashion along the lateral wall of the canal; these are features of postoperative scars.

SURGICAL SCARS

Postoperative scarring was noted at the diskectomy site and/or along the lateral wall of the canal in 48 subjects (Figs. 5-11 and 5-12). A laminectomy scar (Fig. 5-13) was noted in all subjects.

Prominent scar formation without a coexisting herniated disk was seen in 21 patients at reexploration.

A combination of recurrent disk herniation and scarring at the diskectomy site (Figs. 5-13 to 5-16) was found at surgery in 27 patients.

Enhancement occurred in 31 (64%) of these 48 scars.

The laminectomy scar (Fig. 5-13, *E* and *F*), present in all patients, was enhanced in 52 (67%).

A laminectomy scar was identified in all subjects whereas a definite diskectomy scar was identified in only 76%.

The laminectomy scars were less prominent, and enhanced progressively less intensely, as the postoperative follow-up was lengthened.

Laminectomy scars seem to have no positive correlation with a patient's symptoms. On the other hand, the intensity of enhancement and the percentage of scars enhancing did not seem to vary with postoperative time for diskectomy scars. In particular, we have not seen a discernible change in the magnitude of enhancement of diskectomy scars as the number of postoperative follow-up years increased. Gross pathological and microscopic examination of nonenhancing diskectomy scars showed essentially a dense fibrotic tissue with scant vascularity and, in some patients, scattered foci of calcification. The enhancing diskectomy scars consisted of a mixture of mature scar (dense fibrous tissue) and granulation tissue, and had a more generous blood supply.

We have no histological proof of the composition and maturation rate of laminectomy scars. However, extrapolation from observations on diskectomy scars would seem to support the following speculations:

Laminectomy scars mature faster and appear to be

Text continued on p. 220.

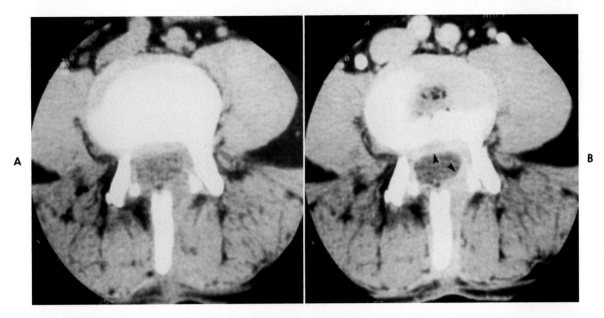

FIGURE 5-11
Surgical scar at a diskectomy site, along the wall of the spinal canal, and at a laminectomy site. **A,** Precontrast study. There is moderately increased density of the soft tissues behind the disk and on the left wall of the canal. **B,** Postcontrast study. Note the enhancement of the soft tissue density representing the diskectomy and laminectomy sites *(arrowheads).* (From Firooznia H, Kricheff II, Rafii M, Golimbu C: Radiology 1987;163:221-226.)

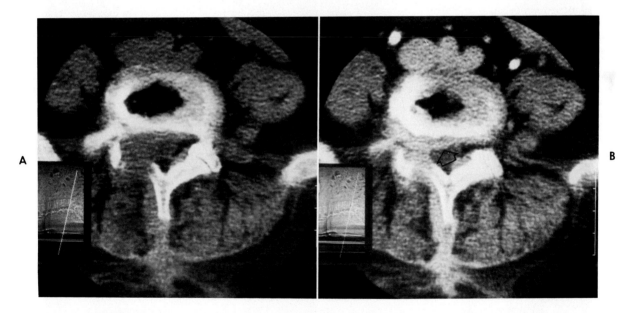

FIGURE 5-12
Postoperative scar. **A,** A CT slice without intravenous contrast shows a laminectomy site on the right, at L4-5. The epidural fat between the dural sac and the wall of the canal on the right is obliterated by the scar. **B,** After intravenous contrast, there is enhancement of the scar *(hollow arrow),* which can be seen to extend into the right neural foramen and along the wall of the canal. A small herniation, surrounded by granulation tissue and mature scar, cannot be ruled out. At reexploration and subsequent pathological examination, granulation tissue and mature scar were found. There was no herniated disk fragment.

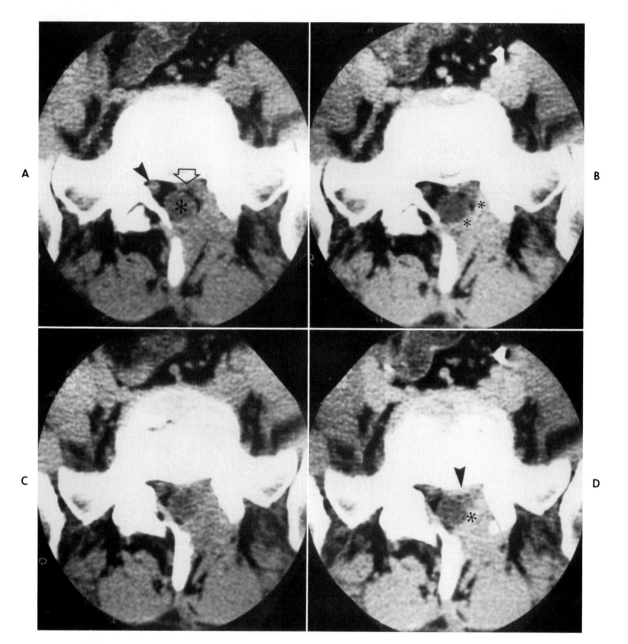

FIGURE 5-13
Recurrent disk herniation and an enhanced surgical scar. **A,** Precontrast study (CT) at L5-S1. Laminectomy on the left side. The *arrowhead* designates the normal right descending S1 nerve root, and the *asterisk* the dural tube. The *hollow arrow* is pointing to a soft tissue density in the epidural space, in the midline and to the left of midline, obscuring the outline of the left descending S1 nerve root. **B,** Postcontrast study. The scar tissue along the left wall of the canal is enhanced *(asterisks)*. Note that the tissue in the epidural space anteriorly on the left is not enhanced. At surgical reexploration a small fragment of herniated disk enveloped by granulation tissue was found. **C,** Precontrast and, **D,** postcontrast CT examinations 4 mm below **A.** Notice the soft tissue enhancement in the epidural space *(arrowhead* in **D**). This most likely is the granulation tissue that was found at pathological examination surrounding the disk fragment. Notice also the enhancement of scar tissue along the left lateral canal wall *(asterisk* in **D**). The dural sac is pulled to the left, and the epidural fat on the left is obliterated.

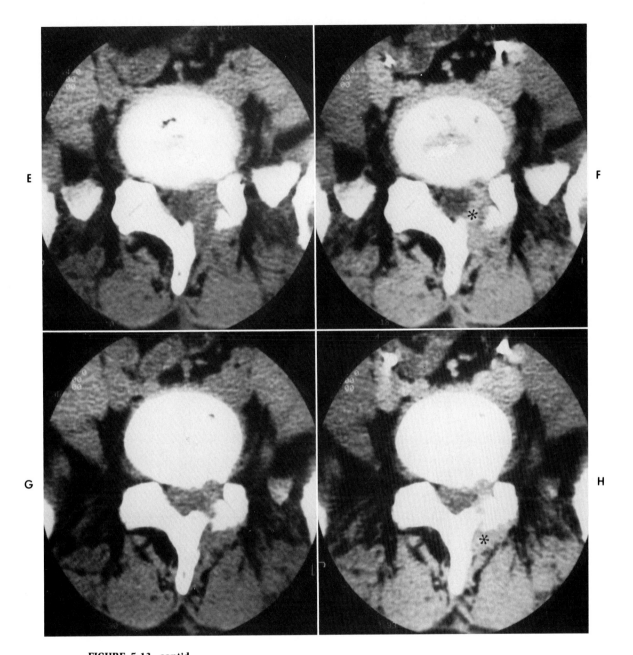

FIGURE 5-13, cont'd
E, Precontrast and, F, postcontrast CT examinations 4 mm below C. Further enhancement of the scar along the left lateral canal wall (*asterisk* in F) can be seen. Notice also the enhanced scar at the laminectomy site, *just posterior to the asterisk.* G is a precontrast and, H, a postcontrast CT examination 4 mm below E. The soft tissues posterior to the laminectomy site are well enhanced *(asterisk)* in H.

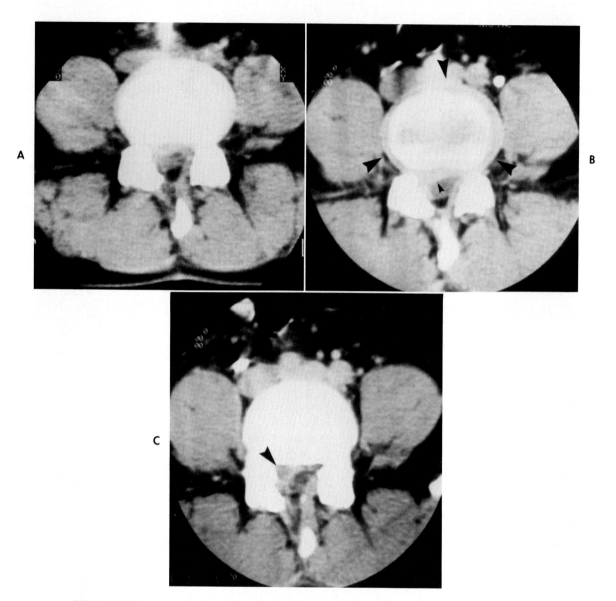

FIGURE 5-14

Enhanced margins of a bulging disk and recurrent herniation with scarring. **A,** Precontrast study at L4-5 in a patient with previous disk surgery showing a poorly defined soft tissue density in the anterior aspect of the canal. The definition of soft tissues within the canal is extremely poor. **B,** Postcontrast study showing the enhanced margins of the disk *(large arrowheads).* The definition of soft tissues has improved. Note the enhanced soft tissue mass in the anterior epidural space. It has a linear margin extending from the left to the right side in oblique fashion *(small arrowhead).* **C,** Another postcontrast study (4 mm below **B,** at the level of the superior L5 endplate) shows an area of nonenhancement anterolaterally on the right *(arrowhead).* At surgery a recurrent herniated disk fragment to the right of midline was surrounded by a layer of granulation tissue. There was also a moderate amount of mature scar tissue.

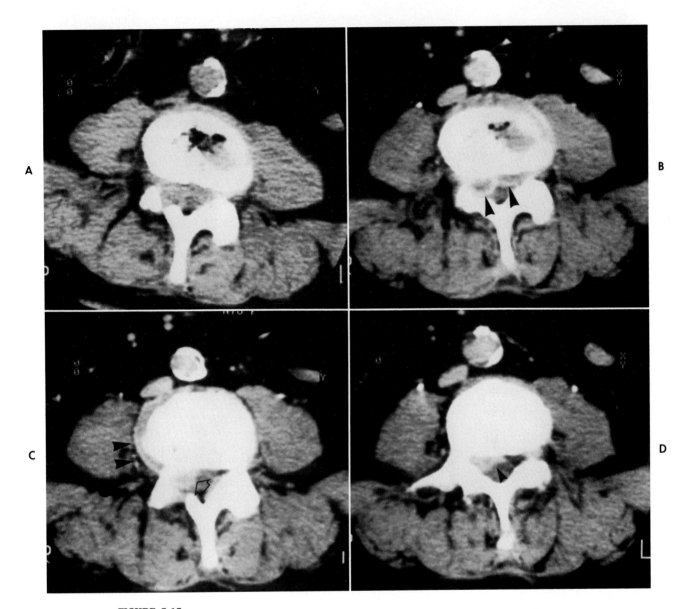

FIGURE 5-15
A recurrent disk herniation with scarring at L4-5. Laminectomy on the right side. **A,** Precontrast study. The soft tissues in the canal are poorly defined. A vacuum phenomenon has developed in the disk. **B,** Postcontrast study. There are two areas of nonenhancement, separated by enhanced margins *(arrowheads).* At surgery two recurrent disk herniation fragments, completely enveloped by granulation tissue and some mature scar, were found. **C,** A slice 5 mm above and, **D,** another 5 mm below the L4-5 disk. There is enhancement of the disk margin, which is bulging on the right *(arrowheads* in **C).** The *hollow arrow* in **C** points to a similarly enhanced soft tissue density on the right of the canal. The enhanced soft tissues in **C** and **D** represent the top and bottom of a sphere of granulation tissue and scar surrounding the disk, which is not enhanced, corresponding to the nonenhanced region in **B.** (From Firooznia H, Kricheff II, Rafii M, Golimbu C: Radiology 1987;163:221-226.)

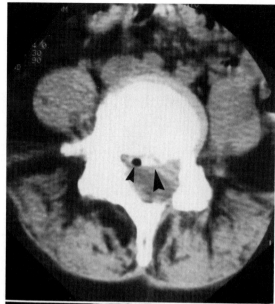

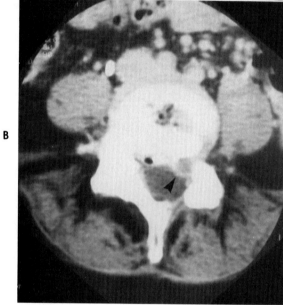

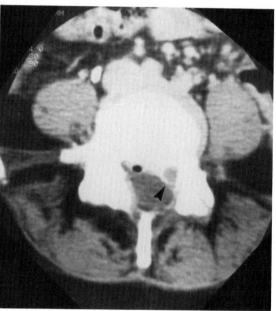

FIGURE 5-16
Recurrent disk herniation and scarring. **A,** Noncontrast CT at L4-5. Laminectomy on the left side. There is calcification of the disk *(large arrowhead)*, which contains a bubble of nitrogen *(smaller arrowhead)*. The remaining soft tissues in the canal are poorly defined, and the epidural fat is obliterated. **B** and **C,** Postcontrast CT examinations show the calcified herniation and nitrogen bubble unchanged. Note, however, the area of nonenhancement in the anterior portion of the canal on the left, surrounded by a ring of enhancement *(arrowhead)*. At surgery a fibrocartilaginous fragment of disk enveloped in granulation tissue, with minimal scar (fibrous tissue), was found corresponding to the lesion in the left anterolateral corner of the canal.

unaffected by events occurring at the posterior border of the disk (repeated herniations or quiescence). These features have been commented upon by other investigators also.

Diskectomy scars are, in some respects, significantly different from laminectomy scars. In patients in whom there is complete healing of the posterior border of an operated disk, with no recurrence of herniation, the diskectomy scar matures naturally and becomes composed essentially of mature fibrous tissue; but unlike the laminectomy scar (which is residing in a quiescent and distant location), it is on the battlefront, so to speak, and thus exposed to repeated episodes of herniation, rupture of disk substance, inflammation, and granulation tissue formation in patients with repeated episodes of disk herniation. In these patients it does not mature. Histological examination confirms the presence of granulation tissue and, occasionally, edema and hemorrhage in the diskectomy scar of these patients.

If a major episode of disk herniation is followed by almost complete healing and years of quiescence, with either surgery or conservative treatment, the scar adjacent to the posterior disk border will have a chance to mature and may even contain foci of calcification. A new episode of disk herniation under these circumstances may incite formation of a new scar on top of the old one. Then there may be mature fibrous tissue, foci of calcification, and foci of young granulation tissue. These factors are most likely responsible for the complex behavior of diskectomy scars, and of the disk itself, when intravenous enhancement is attempted.

There was no definite enhancement of the diskectomy scar and/or the scar along the wall of the spinal canal in 21 subjects (27%).

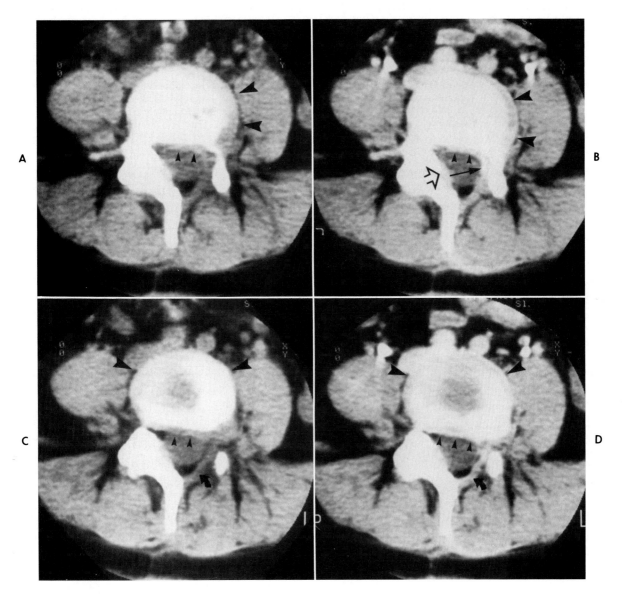

FIGURE 5-17
Enhancement of the margins of a bulging disk with scar. **A,** Precontrast study at L4-5. Laminectomy on the left side. There is moderate scoliosis, which accounts for the asymmetrical bulging on the left *(arrowheads)*. The soft tissues in the canal are not particularly well defined. The *small arrowheads* denote the site of previous diskectomy. **B,** Postcontrast study. Note the pronounced enhancement of the bulging margins on the left *(arrowheads),* along with the soft tissues at the diskectomy site *(small arrowheads)*. A thin layer of scar tissue along the left wall of the canal is also enhanced *(arrow)*. The *hollow arrow* points to marked enhancement of the ligamentum flavum on the right. (The left ligamentum has been resected.) **C,** Another precontrast study, in which the *large arrowheads* denote the margins of the disk. The soft tissues immediately posterior to the disk in the canal are better seen on this slice *(small arrowheads)*. The *curved arrow* denotes the diskectomy scar. **D,** Another postcontrast study. Notice the enhanced margins of the disk *(large arrowheads)*. The soft tissues at the diskectomy site are also enhanced *(three small arrowheads)*. The *curved arrow* points to the laminectomy scar, which is sharply enhanced.

In most instances, enhancement of the diskectomy scar was nearly homogeneous and affected the whole width of the scar, although the margins in some patients appeared to be more prominently enhanced.

The scar usually appeared as a band of soft tissue density posterior to the intervertebral disk, often extending as a straight linear density along the lateral wall of the canal on the laminectomy side (Fig. 5-17).

The lateral recess and its corresponding nerve root were often obscured, although no instance of displacement of the nerve root away from the scar was noted.

The thecal sac in 23 patients was retracted toward the scar along the lateral wall of the canal (Fig. 5-18); in no instance was it displaced away from the scar.

In 9 patients the surgical scar appeared as a focal or nodular area of soft tissue density; in 4 of these patients there was near-uniform enhancement of the scars, and in the remaining 5 the scar did not show definite enhancement. It was not possible to differentiate these scars from a fragment of a herniated disk.

In 2 patients there was scarring shaped like an irregular band of enhancing soft tissue extending anteroposteriorly from the intervertebral disk to the laminectomy defect (Fig. 5-19).

In 9 patients no definitive differentiation between disk herniation and scarring could be made on the CT scans both with and without contrast enhancement; 7 of these 9 also had at least one of the following disorders: spinal

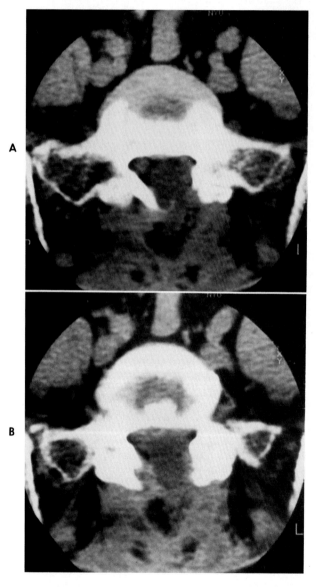

FIGURE 5-18
Noncontrast CT at L5-S1. Status postlaminectomy on the left side. There is retraction of the dural sac to the left, and the epidural fat on the left of the canal is obscured by scarring. The left S1 descending nerve root is partially obscured as well.

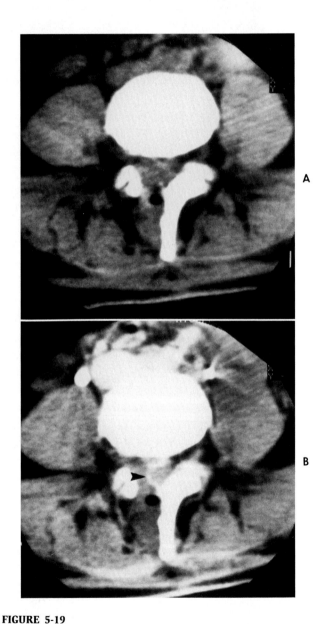

FIGURE 5-19
Postoperative scar. A precontrast study, **A**, at the L4-5 level, status postlaminectomy on the right, reveals gas at the laminectomy site and in the spinal canal. The definition of soft tissues within the canal is poor. A postcontrast study, **B**, shows the scar appearing as an enhanced curvilinear density extending from the site of the diskectomy to that of the laminectomy *(arrowhead)*. (From Firooznia H, Kricheff II, Rafii M, Golimbu C: Radiology 1987;163:221-226.)

stenosis, spondylolisthesis, or remnants of myelographic contrast (Pantopaque) in the dural sac and epidural region.

DURAL SAC AND LIGAMENTUM FLAVUM

Enhancement of the thecal membrane, presumably dura, and ligamentum flavum occurred in 24 subjects (32%). No significant difference was noted in the incidence or intensity of enhancement between those who received only drip infusion and those who received drip infusion and bolus injection. However, the degree of enhancement appeared to be somewhat more prominent in the latter group.

A retrospective analysis of the CT findings in all 168 subjects disclosed no significant differences in the relative frequency of enhancement of various structures between the 77 subjects who underwent reexploration and those who did not.

Evaluation of CT findings in the postoperative lumbar spine

CT of the lumbar spine is a proven modality for detecting lumbar disk herniation and has an accuracy of 90% to 93% in patients without previous disk surgery.[16] It is less useful in patients with histories of surgery for lumbar disk herniation or stenosis.

In our study CT without intravenous contrast was sufficient for establishing the diagnosis of normal postoperative status (Fig. 5-20), a herniated disk at either the level operated on or another level, scar formation, or other abnormalities in 60% of the patients. Intravenous contrast-enhanced CT did not provide additional information that was useful and did not cause us to change our

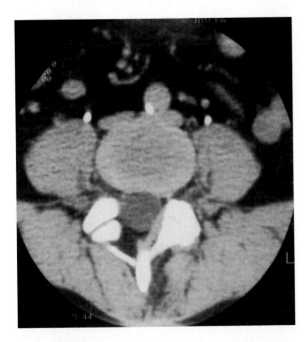

FIGURE 5-20
Normal postoperative status. CT examination after intravenous contrast at L4-5. There has been laminectomy on the right. Notice the absence of lamina and ligamentum flavum on that side. The disk is normal, with no evidence of herniation or scarring.

diagnoses. In the remaining patients, intravenous contrast-enhanced CT helped establish or exclude the diagnosis of disk herniation or scar formation in an additional 23%. Thus the overall accuracy of CT was 83%.

In patients with complicating features such as severe spinal stenosis (Fig. 5-21), spondylolisthesis, diffuse scarring, retained Pantopaque, or other abnormalities, a definitive diagnosis of the presence or absence of disk herniation was usually not possible with noncontrast CT. After intravenous administration of contrast a definitive diagnosis was made in one third of the patients in this group.

Intravenous contrast-enhanced CT was particularly helpful in patients in whom a focal or nodular soft tissue density was present at the diskectomy site or a combination of disk herniation and scarring was suspected (Figs. 5-14 to 5-16). In these patients differentiation of scarring from disk herniation often was not possible with noncontrast CT. Intravenous administration of contrast led to near-uniform enhancement of 65% of the scars, helping to differentiate them from herniated disks, in which enhancement was usually limited to a thin (2 to 3 mm thick) band at the periphery.

Although the differences in enhancement patterns will usually help differentiate scarring from disk herniation, there are limitations to their reliability. In 24 patients (31%) of this series no definite enhancement of surgically verified scars or the margins of recurrent disk herniation was observed. On the other hand, enhancement of the entire margin of normal bulging, and herniated disks occurred in a significant number of patients. Furthermore, there was near-uniform enhancement (10 to 13 mm thick) of the protruding margins and patchy enhancement of the entire body of the disk in 9 surgically verified herniated disks.

The enhancement of normal (Fig. 5-4), bulging (Fig. 5-5), or herniated (Figs. 5-6 and 5-22) lumbar disk margins at a previously unexplored site, along with enhancement of the anterior and lateral margins of a recurrent herniated disk, to our knowledge, had not been reported prior to the publication of an investigation by Firooznia, Kricheff, et al.[15] Although enhancement of the anterior and lateral margins of lumbar disks is evident in the images published by Schubiger and Valavanis,[4] it was not recorded in their text. This observation raises a number of questions regarding the nature of the enhancing rims of disks. According to Schubiger and Valavanis,[4] enhancement noted along the margin of a recurrent lumbar disk herniation is due to the presence of a thin layer of surgical scar tissue. This explanation is consistent with pathological findings in some patients who have undergone exploration, but it does not explain the nature of the enhancement seen along the anterior and lateral margins of a disk or that seen at the margins of a normal, bulging, or herniated disk at a previously unexplored level. In our patients, rimlike enhancement of the protruding margin of a recurrent herniation occurred in 65%.

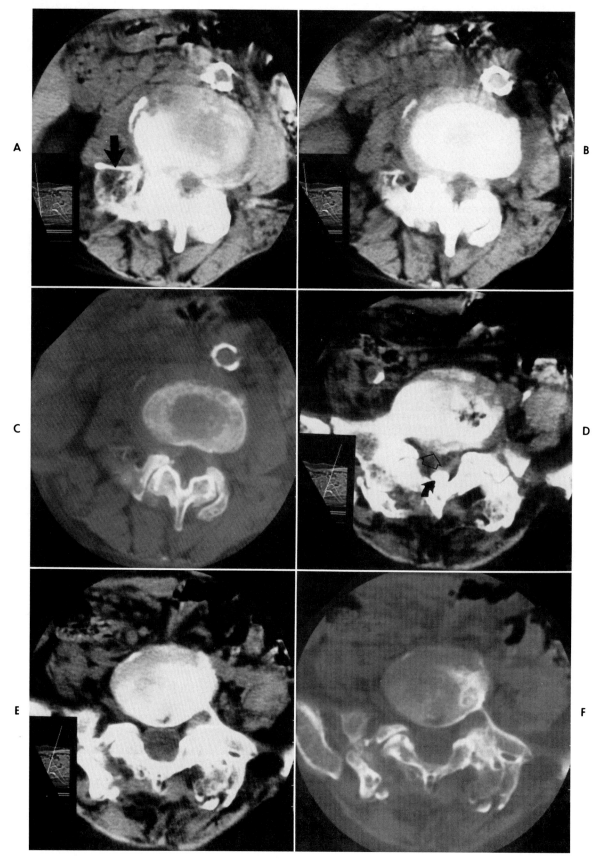

FIGURE 5-21
For legend see opposite page.

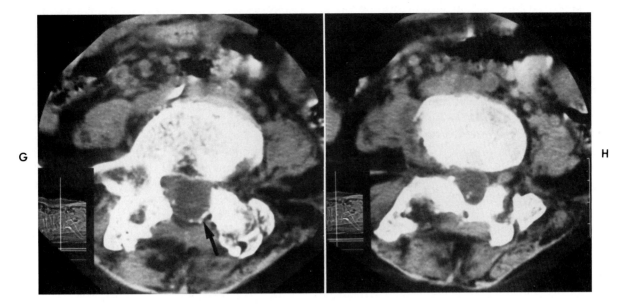

FIGURE 5-21

Spinal stenosis and disk herniation in a patient with previous disk surgery. **A,** L4-5 disk. Note the slight scoliosis with bulging of the disk, more prominent on the left. The margins of the disk are calcified, and the concavity of the posterior disk surface is maintained. The stenosis is secondary to markedly hypertrophic changes in the facet joints. The *arrow* denotes a posterolateral bone graft. **B** and **C,** Inferior endplate of L3. The bulging of the disk is now more noticeable to the right because of the scoliosis. Stenosis of the canal is also evident. **D,** L5-S1. There is a vacuum phenomenon with a calcified herniated disk *(hollow arrow).* The *curved arrow* denotes myelographic contrast in the dural sac secondary to a previous myelographic examination. Notice the hypertrophic changes and degenerative disease in the facet joints. Posterolateral bone fusion can also be seen. **E** and **F,** Soft tissue and bone windows 8 mm above **D.** Note the solid bony fusion on the left. **G,** Another slice, 14 mm above **F,** through the L5 pedicle. There is solid posterolateral bony fusion. Laminectomy has left a scar, and there is calcification of the dural sac *(arrow).* **H,** An axial slice through the L4-5 disk shows the site of previous surgery, with marked narrowing of the disk. There is no evidence of recurrent herniation, however.

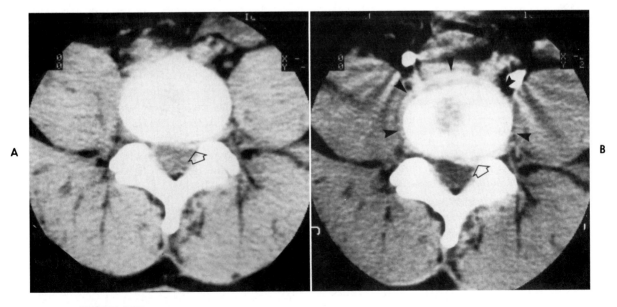

FIGURE 5-22

Enhancement of a bulging herniated disk at L4-5. **A,** Precontrast study at a previously unexplored level. There is a questionable soft tissue density to the left of midline in the anterior epidural space of the spinal canal *(hollow arrow).* **B,** Postcontrast study. Note the markedly enhanced margins of the disk, which is bulging circumferentially *(arrowheads).* The *hollow arrow* denotes the herniation to the left of midline, extending into the neural foramen. At surgery a herniated disk was found.

However, enhancement of similar intensity and configuration also occurred along the posterior margins of herniated disks at previously unexplored levels. Similar enhancement was noted, though less frequently, along the lateral and anterior margins of normal, bulging, and herniated disks.

Thus, although we believe that surgical scar is often a contributing factor in the rimlike enhancement of the posterior margin of a recurrent herniation, we do not believe that in our patients it is the only cause of such enhancement. It certainly is not the cause of enhancement of previously unexplored disks, nor is it the reason why the anterior and lateral margins of any disk enhance. We do not have histological verification of the exact cause of enhancement in unexplored disks, and for anterior and lateral margins of explored disks, but we strongly feel that the following factors are responsible for this phenomenon:

1. Vascularity of the margins of normal and herniated disks
2. Granulation tissue and scar formation at the margins of nonoperated herniated disks, and in the substance (body) of the disk itself
3. Granulation tissue and scar formation at the margins of recurrent disk herniations, and in the substance of the disk itself
4. Enhancement of the epidural venous plexus

Intervertebral disks are generally considered to be avascular. This is only partially correct. Hassler[17] performed microangiography on 28 cadavers, with the specific aim of studying the vascularity of intervertebral disk margins. The vascularity of the peripheral margin of the annulus fibrosus, where it attaches to the vertebral margins, was found to be abundant and to penetrate deeply into the substance of the disk in infants and young children, but in adults it was sparse and the vessels were nonpenetrating. However, the free margin of the annulus fibrosus — the part between the attachments to the vertebral margins above and below — was found to have an equally rich vascular supply in both children and adults. The existence of vascularity of the outer layer of the annulus has also been demonstrated by other investigators.[18-21] A microscopic examination of intervertebral disks from 88 subjects by Coventry[21] and Coventry et al.,[18-20] in which pathological and age-related changes were compared from decade to decade, showed regrowth of vascularity through the cartilaginous endplate into the disk concomitant with aging and with degenerative changes. The number of vascular channels was noted to increase with each passing decade. Additionally, progressively increasing granulation tissue and reparative scarring were seen with correspondingly more extensive degenerative changes.

Based on the pattern of enhancement noted in our patients, the anatomical and pathological evidence cited above, and our own evaluation of surgically resected disk fragments from patients with or without a history of previous disk surgery, and on lumbar disks obtained from cadavers, we believe that the enhancement of normal disk margins results mostly from the vascularity of the outer layer of the annulus fibrosus. This enhancement is more common and more intense in bulging and herniated disks than in normal disks, because the vascularity of degenerated disks is significantly more prominent than that of normal disks. In addition, in degenerative disks there are multiple areas of rupture of the annulus and replacement with granulation tissue and mature fibrous tissue (scar). A careful examination of resected segments of herniated disks confirms this. In addition, there is more prominent regrowth of vascularity through the cartilaginous endplate into the substance of degenerated disks (often with development of Schmorl nodes in cadaver specimens) as well as formation of granulation tissue and scarring with repeated episodes of herniation (which accounts for the occasionally marked enhancement of disk substance seen in these specimens).

Nor is the enhancement limited to disk margins. In some of our patients a patchy, irregular, and nonhomogeneous enhancement was seen to involve the entire body of a herniated disk. Histological examination disclosed the presence of granulation tissue along the margins of these herniations and surrounding the free fragments. The granulation tissue and scar formation were seen more frequently in subjects with a history of longstanding and repeated episodes of disk herniation, although they were also noted in four instances of acutely symptomatic herniation. In some patients with a longstanding herniation, without previous disk surgery, we found extensive scar formation, sometimes with calcification, at the margin of the herniation. In patients who have undergone disk surgery, during the early postoperative period there may be significant soft tissue swelling, edema, granulation tissue formation, and bleeding in the epidural space, causing a mass effect with displacement of the dural sac away from the site of scarring. Gradually, however, there is resolution of the epidural inflammatory mass and the granulation tissue matures to form an epidural scar. At this stage the dural sac is usually pulled toward the epidural scar.

Enhancement of the margins of a nonoperated herniated disk is due to the existence of granulation tissue, occasionally with edema and inflammation, and the more prominent vascularity of the margins of degenerated disks in these patients. These same factors are also responsible for the sporadic enhancement of disk substance occasionally seen. A ring of enhancement surrounding the sequestered fragments (free fragments) of a herniated disk in several patients in our series was shown histologically to be due to the presence of granulation tissue. A mixture of granulation and fibrocartilaginous tissue was found in the free fragments with nonhomogeneous enhancement. Enhancement of the margins and substance of a recurrent herniated disk is also due to these factors.

When recurrent herniation and scarring coexist, postoperative epidural fibrosis may extend in a continuous fashion from the site of diskectomy along the lateral wall of the canal to the laminectomy site. Enhancement, therefore, may be seen as a continuous band extending from the posterior border of the disk, along the lateral wall of the spinal canal, to the diskectomy site. Small recurrent disk herniations are sometimes masked by fibrosis in these patients. In most cases, however, when disk herniation and postsurgical scarring coexist, the herniated disk appears as a soft tissue density extending focally into the spinal canal or neural foramen.

The radiographic characteristics of herniated disks are the same regardless of whether the patient has had previous disk surgery. When there is only a postoperative epidural scar, the soft tissue mass usually has a straight border that blends with a similar epidural density along the lateral wall of the canal (i.e., along the path of surgery on the laminectomy side). In our experience disk herniations have not produced this pattern. In some patients postoperative scarring has been nodular or irregular, and then differentiation from herniation has been more difficult or even impossible. Often, after contrast administration, we have seen linear enhancement surrounding nodular fragments of nonenhancing material. This is a pattern characteristic of recurrent disk herniations surrounded by granulation tissue and scar.

ENHANCEMENT OF THE EPIDURAL AND PERIVERTEBRAL VENOUS PLEXUS

Enhancement of the epidural venous plexus must be taken into account when there is enhancement of a herniated lumbar disk margin that protrudes into the spinal canal. Enhancement of the perivertebral venous plexus[22] must be considered when enhancement is noted along the anterior and lateral margins of a disk. Russell et al.[23] showed that a scarlike pattern with linear or marginal enhancement could occur without previous surgery in cervical disk herniations and stated that this was due to visualization of the displaced cervical epidural veins. A similar process may be responsible for some instances of enhancement in the lumbar region.

ENHANCEMENT OF THE DURA

We have noted that dural enhancement may be focal or ringlike, as has also been noted by Teplick and Haskin.[5] Schubiger and Valavanis[4] suggested that a constricting ringlike scar surrounding the dural sac was responsible for this finding. In our patients enhancement of the dura has occurred with equal frequency at disk levels previously explored and not explored. In none of the patients in this series was a ringlike constricting epidural scar found at surgical reexploration. However, we have seen dural thickening and calcification in postoperative patients.

MYELOGRAPHIC EXAMINATION IN PATIENTS WITH PRIOR LUMBAR SPINAL SURGERY
Conventional myelography

Conventional myelography is particularly helpful in making a diagnosis of conjoined root sleeve, root cyst, or arachnoiditis. Although these diagnoses may be strongly suggested on CT, with even stronger evidence on MRI, they are definitively established on conventional myelography. The epidural defect at the site of surgery with scar formation and a recurrent disk herniation is usually larger on myelography than what is seen in patients with disk herniation without prior spinal surgery. However, distortion of the dural sac secondary to arachnoiditis may be a complicating factor in the detection of a recurrent disk herniation on myelography; and, in addition, a definitive differentiation between recurrent disk herniation and scar formation often is not possible.

CT-myelography

CT-myelography is still the best modality overall for establishing the definitive diagnosis in postoperative patients. Nevertheless, because of its invasive nature, we recommend it only when CT with intravenous contrast enhancement and MRI with gadopentetate have been performed but the diagnosis is still in doubt. CT-myelography establishes the diagnosis in an additional 1% or 2% of these patients and is helpful in differentiating a disk herniation from a scar (Figs. 5-23 and 5-24) and elucidating the cause of radiculopathy when herniation, osteophytes (Fig. 5-25), and scar (Fig. 5-26) are present, singly or in combination, in one patient.

CT-myelography is particularly helpful in patients in whom a significant amount of surgical scar is present. There may be a uniform density occupying the spinal canal, with poor differentiation between the thecal sac and margins of the disk and the descending nerve root sheaths obscured. On CT-myelography the root sheaths will be obliterated (Figs. 5-23 and 5-24) or displaced away from the mass if it is a herniated disk; but if it is scar tissue, they will usually be right in the center of it (Fig. 5-26). CT-myelography also clearly shows the herniated disk, with displacement and distortion of the dural sac. On the other hand, when the mass is essentially surgical scar, the dural sac will often be drawn toward it along the side of the spinal canal.

RADIOLOGICAL WORK-UP OF POSTOPERATIVE PATIENTS

The radiological work-up of patients with previous disk surgery who have no symptoms is still a challenge. Noncontrast computed tomography has, in our experience, been sufficient to establish the diagnosis in 60% of patients. When intravenous contrast has been used, the

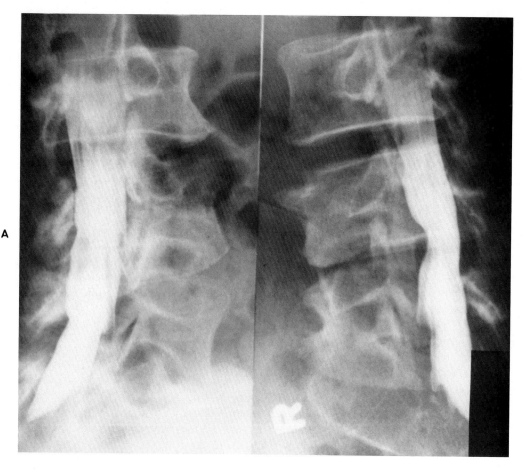

FIGURE 5-23
For legend see opposite page.

A

accuracy of diagnosis approaches 83%. MRI examination with gadopentetate has had an accuracy of about 90%.

As in patients with no previous spinal surgery, CT and MRI should be looked upon as complementary procedures. Both may be necessary if the diagnosis is not established after only one has been performed. The work-up may be started with either modality, depending on availability, cost considerations, and preference of the patient and physicians. A patient with severe low back pain may not be able to tolerate the MRI procedure because it can still take more than 20 minutes, even with the latest state-of-the-art imagers available (1991). The patient may have to change position or get up and walk around for a few minutes before being able to tolerate another 5 to 10 minutes of supine immobilization. In these cases CT is more suitable, for patient motion can degrade only the specific slices obtained during the motion and not the entire sequence, as with MRI. Furthermore, it is easier to position the patient with sufficient flexion of the hips and knees in the larger opening of the CT gantry than in the more confining environment of the MRI magnet.

If a definitive diagnosis is not established after MRI with gadopentetate, we recommend CT with contrast, and vice versa. When both CT with contrast and MRI with gadopentetate have been utilized in unselected patients, the diagnostic accuracy has approached 90%. We believe CT-myelography should be performed only after both

contrast-enhanced CT and gadopentetate-enhanced MRI have been obtained but the diagnosis is not still established. CT-myelography in this particular group is helpful in an additional 1% to 2% of patients.

There is no uniform agreement on what constitutes the ideal sequence of diagnostic modalities in the work-up of postoperative patients. At present (1991) no published comparisons of MRI and CT in failed back syndrome have appeared (i.e., no prospective study with a statistically significant number of patients). Recent studies on MRI of the spine[11,24-30] report accuracies ranging from 79% to 94%.

Experience with the work-ups of postoperative lumbar spine patients has been markedly different from institution to institution. A major reason for this seems to be the competence of the operating surgeons and the specific surgical techniques utilized. For example, where posterolateral fusion is performed, failure of fusion may be an important cause of failed back syndrome. In some institutions extensive laminectomy and facetectomy are done, with a consequential increase in the incidence of postsurgical spinal instability and progressive spondylolisthesis. In others laminotomy and fragment removal are done. Although there is less chance of instability and scarring in these latter patients, the incidence of recurrent herniation is increased. Also the mix of patients seen by each institution plays an important role. It is generally known that the selection criteria used for inclusion of

FIGURE 5-23

Recurrent L4-5 disk herniation. Previous laminotomy on the right at L4-5. **A,** Conventional myelography, oblique views. Note the epidural defect on the right, causing compression of the dural sac and displacement with compression of the right descending L5 root sleeve. **B,** CT-myelography, an axial slice just below the pedicle of L4. There is distortion of the dural sac on the right *(arrow)* secondary to a recurrent herniation. **C** and **D,** Axial slices at L4-5. Note the circumferential bulging of the annulus fibrosus, with irregularity of the posterior vertebral endplate due to previous surgery. The dural sac is posteriorly displaced, with deformity of its anterior and right lateral surface. Note the origin of the left L5 descending root sleeve *(arrow in* **C**). The right L5 descending root sleeve is obliterated by the herniation. The *hollow arrow* in **C** denotes the normal ligamentum flavum on the unoperated side. **E,** An axial slice just below the L5 superior endplate shows the left L5 descending root sleeve *(arrow)* to be normal. The right L5 descending root sleeve is distorted and contains significantly less contrast than the left. **F,** An axial slice through the top of the L5 pedicle shows the L5 descending root sleeves to be normal.

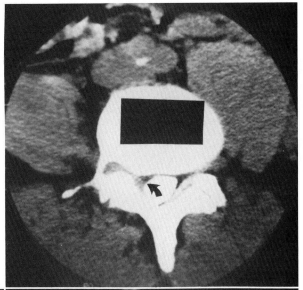

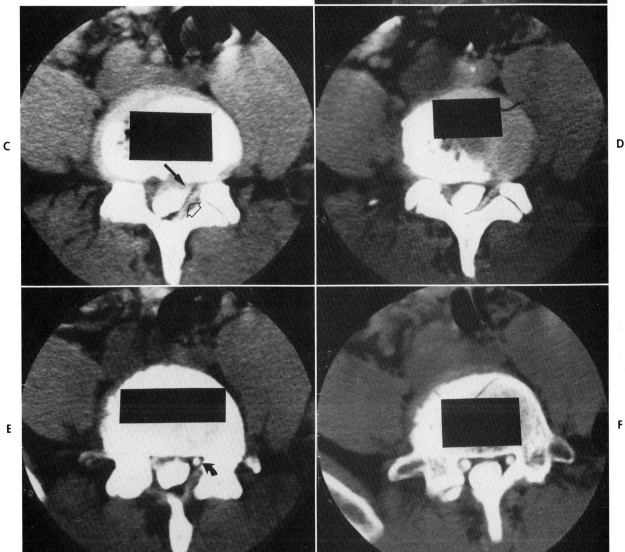

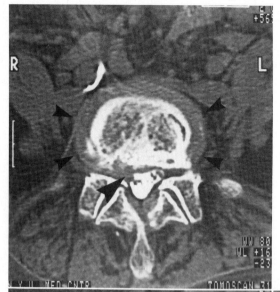

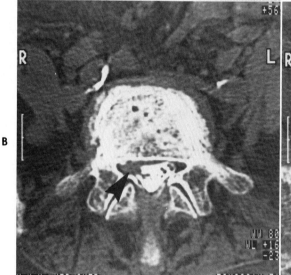

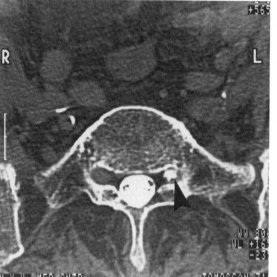

FIGURE 5-24

Recurrent disk herniation. **A**, A CT-myelogram at L4-5 shows a vacuum phenomenon, with marked bulging of the disk *(small arrowheads)*. There is lack of filling of a portion of the dural sac at the origin of the right L5 descending root sleeve *(large arrowhead)* secondary to a herniation. The patient had had a diskectomy for an L4-5 herniation 2 years previously. **B**, Another slice, 5 mm below **A**, shows lack of filling of a portion of the dural sac adjacent to the root sleeve origin *(arrowhead)* secondary to the herniation. **C**, A third slice, 5 mm below **B**, through the midportion of the L5 pedicle, shows the contrast-filled root sleeve in the lateral L5 recess. The right root sleeve contains no contrast.

FIGURE 5-25

A, A lateral projection of the lumbar spine in a patient who underwent resection of a herniated L4-5 disk 2 years prior to this study shows narrowing of the L4-5 disk, with bridging osteophytes *(arrowhead)*. **B** to **D**, Myelograms of the lumbar spine. The *arrowheads* in **B** point to an epidural L4-5 defect extending inferiorly below the L5 superior endplate. Note the anterior epidural defect produced by the bridging osteophytes *(arrowhead* in **C** and **D**). In **E**, a CT-myelogram at L4-5, and **F**, just below the superior L5 endplate, a calcified herniated disk can be seen *(arrow* in **E**). Note the lack of filling on the right of the dural sac *(arrow* in **F**), corresponding to the epidural defect noted at myelography. At surgery a recurrent herniated disk was found; it was partially calcified. **G**, A CT-myelogram at L5-S1. There is a new disk herniation at this site that is calcified.

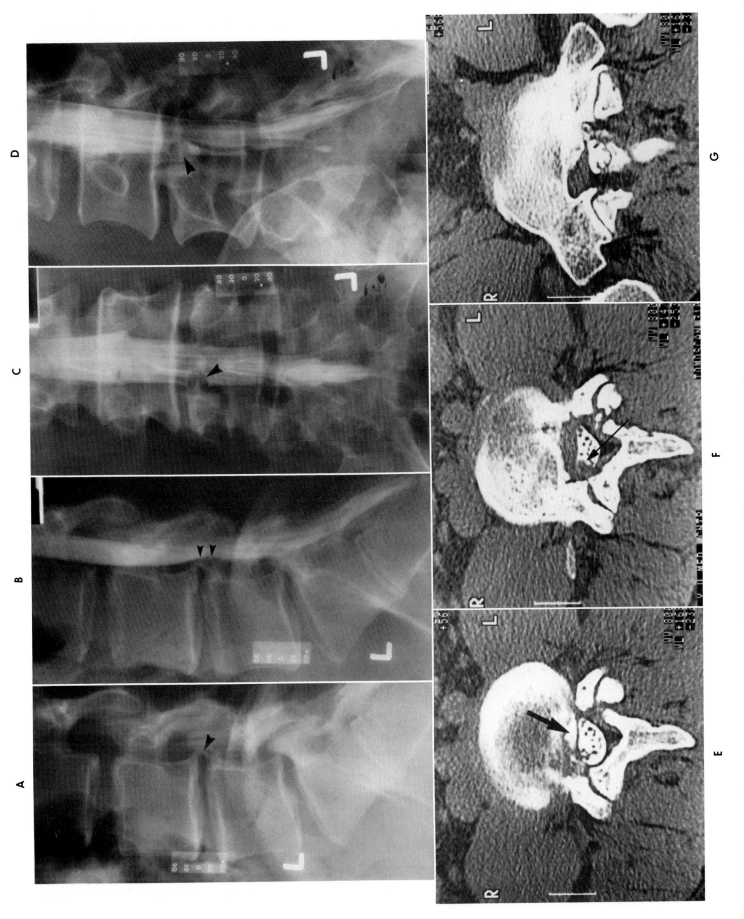

FIGURE 5-25
For legend see opposite page.

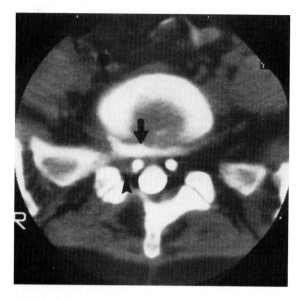

FIGURE 5-26

Postoperative scar at L5-S1. Laminectomy on the right side. A CT-myelogram shows findings indicative of a moderate spondylolisthesis *(arrow)*. There is also moderate scoliosis, which accounts for the asymmetry. An epidural soft tissue density extends from the midline to the right, occupying the right lateral recess and extending along the spinal canal on the right *(arrowhead)*. Notice that the descending sacral nerve roots are in normal position, with the right S1 descending root situated in the substance of the soft tissue density (which at surgery proved to be epidural scar).

patients in the group for surgical treatment of disk herniation and/or stenosis significantly influence the outcome. Generally women, persons who are gainfully and happily employed, and persons whose herniated disk is prominent at one level but no significant pathology exists at other levels are more likely to obtain significant relief from surgery. Conversely, individuals with multilevel pathology or borderline or indefinite disk herniation, and those with secondary gain in mind are less likely to become completely or significantly asymptomatic after surgery. The success rate for each reoperation is usually much less than for the preceding operation. Similarly, the extent of spinal canal deformity, epidural scar formation, or other abnormality increases with each successive operation.

REFERENCES

1. Jacobs RR, McClain O, Neff J: Control of postlaminectomy scar formation. Spine 1980;5:223-229.
2. Burton CV, Kirkaldy-Willis W II, Yong-Hing K, Heithoff KB: Causes of failure of surgery on the lumbar spine. Clin Orthop 1981;157:191-199.
3. Naylor A: Late results of laminectomy for lumbar disc disease. J Bone Joint Surg [Br] 1974;56:17-29.
4. Schubiger O, Valavanis A: CT differentiation between recurrent disc herniation and postoperative scar formation: the value of contrast enhancement. Neuroradiology 1982;22:251-254.
5. Teplick JG, Haskin ME: CT of the postoperative lumbar spine. Radiol Clin North Am 1983;21:395-420.
6. Law JD, Lehman RA, Kirsch WM: Reoperation after lumbar intervertebral disc surgery. J Neurosurg 1978;48:259-263.
7. Finnegan WJ, Fenlin JM, Marvel JP, et al: Results of surgical intervention in the symptomatic multiply operated back patient. J Bone Joint Surg [Am] 1979;61:1077-1082.
8. Benoist M, Ficat C, Baraf P, Cauchoix J: Postoperative lumbar epiduro-arachnoiditis: diagnostic and therapeutic aspects. Spine 1980;5:432-436.
9. Hardy RW Jr: Repeat operation for lumbar disc. In Hardy RW Jr (ed): Seminars in neurological surgery: lumbar disc disease. New York, Raven, 1982, pp 193-202.
10. Braun IF, Hoffman JC Jr, Davis PC, et al: Contrast enhancement in CT differentiation between recurrent disk herniation and postoperative scar: prospective study. AJNR 1985;6:607-612. AJR 1985;145:785-790.
11. Sotiropoulos S, Chafetz NI, Lang P, et al: Differentiation between postoperative scar and recurrent disc herniation. Prospective comparison of MR, CT, and contrast-enhanced CT. AJNR 1989;10:639-643.
12. Weiss T, Treisch J, Kazner E: CT of the postoperative lumbar spine: the value of intravenous contrast. Neuroradiology 1986;28:241-245.
13. Yang PJ, Seeger JF, Dzioba RB, et al: High-dose IV contrast in CT scanning of the postoperative lumbar spine. AJNR 1986;7:703-707.
14. Teplick JG, Haskin ME: Intravenous contrast–enhanced CT of the postoperative lumbar spine: improved identification of recurrent disk herniation, scar, arachnoiditis, and diskitis. AJNR 1984;5:373-383. AJR 1984;143:845-855.
15. Firooznia H, Kricheff II, Rafii M, Golimbu C: Lumbar spine after surgery: examination with intravenous contrast–enhanced CT. Radiology 1987;163:221-226.
16. Firooznia H, Benjamin V, Kricheff II, et al: CT of lumbar spine disk herniation: correlation with surgical findings. AJNR 1984; 5:91-96. AJR 1984;142:587-592.
17. Hassler O: The human intervertebral disc: a micro-angiographical study on its vascular supply at various ages. Acta Orthop Scand 1969;40:765-772.
18. Coventry MB, Ghormley RK, Kernohan JW: Intervertebral disc: its microscopic anatomy and pathology. I. Anatomy, development, and physiology. J Bone Joint Surg [Am] 1945;27:105-112.
19. Coventry MB, Ghormley RK, Kernohan JW: Intervertebral disc: its microscopic anatomy and pathology. II. Changes in the intervertebral disc concomitant with age. J Bone Joint Surg [Am] 1945;27:233-247.
20. Coventry MB, Ghormley RK, Kernohan JW: Intervertebral disc: its microscopic anatomy and pathology. III. Pathologic changes in the intervertebral disc. J Bone Joint Surg [Am] 1945;27:460-474.
21. Coventry MB: Anatomy of the intervertebral disk. Clin Orthop Rel Res 1969;67:9-15.
22. Batson OV: The vertebral vein system. AJR 1957;78:195-212.
23. Russell EJ, D'Angelo CM, Zimmerman RD, et al: Cervical disk herniation: CT demonstration after contrast enhancement. Radiology 1984;152:703-712.
24. Nguyen CM, Ho KC, Yu SW, et al: An experimental model to study contrast enhancement in MR imaging of the intervertebral disk. AJNR 1989;10:811-814.
25. Hueftle MG, Modic MT, Ross JS, et al: Lumbar spine: postoperative MR imaging with Gd-DTPA. Radiology 1988;167:817-824.
26. Bundschuh CV, Modic MT, Ross JS, et al: Epidural fibrosis and recurrent disk herniation in the lumbar spine: MR imaging assessment. AJNR 1988;9:169-178. AJR 1988;150:923-932.
27. Bundschuh CV, Stein L, Slusser JH, et al: Distinguishing between scar and recurrent herniated disk in postoperative patients: value of contrast-enhanced CT and MR imaging. AJNR 1990;11:949-958.
28. Frocrain L, Duvauferrier R, Husson J-L, et al: Recurrent postoperative sciatica: evaluation with MR imaging and enhanced CT. Radiology 1989;170:531-533.
29. Hochhauser L, Kieffer SA, Cacayorin ED, et al: Recurrent post diskectomy low back pain: MR-surgical correlation. AJR 1988;151:755-760.
30. Ross JS, Masaryk TJ, Schrader M, et al: MR imaging of the postoperative lumbar spine: assessment with gadopentetate dimeglumine. AJR 1990;155:867-872.

6 MRI of the Postoperative Lumbar Spine

MYRON M. LEVITT
RICHARD S. PINTO
HOSSEIN FIROOZNIA

The goal of imaging in failed back syndrome is to identify the cause of a patient's clinical manifestations — which can be due to recurrence (or persistence) of disk herniation, spinal stenosis, excessive epidural scar, instability, infection, and arachnoiditis. MRI may be utilized for assessing these, particularly disk herniation, epidural fibrosis, stenosis, and spinal instability.[1-8] The relative suitability of CT, myelography, and CT-myelography has been discussed in the preceding chapters.[9-18] The following paragraphs will deal with the role of MRI in differentiating disk herniation from epidural scar.

Whereas CT scanning offers advantages in the demonstration of calcified herniated disks, calcified ligaments, bony ridges, and gas (the vacuum phenomenon), and also provides better spatial resolution, MRI avoids the need for ionizing radiation and the necessity of administering iodinated contrast intravenously. In addition, a larger region of the spine can be examined with MRI and images in multiple planes can be directly generated, facilitating a more complete evaluation of the canal and its contents.[19-20] The accuracy of noncontrast MRI in the assessment of postoperative herniations and scar has ranged from approximately 75% to nearly 100%,[12,19-22] which compares favorably with the accuracy reported for contrast-enhanced CT. The introduction of gadopentetate* as a paramagnetic contrast agent for MR imaging represented the next stage in the evolution of imaging of the post-operative lumbar spine. A study on the use of contrast-enhanced MRI to differentiate postoperative herniation from epidural scar (published in 1988[20]) reported an accuracy of 100%.

TECHNIQUE

The technical goal of imaging the postoperative lumbar spine is to maximize the contrast between epidural fibrosis and disk material. Since scar tissue enhances immediately after the intravenous injection of gadopentetate, in contradistinction to disk material (which enhances inconsistently and more slowly), optimal scar/disk contrast is achieved on images obtained immediately following injection of gadopentetate.[20]

Our protocol for examination is designed to maintain a constant patient position, so the enhancement patterns on pre- and postcontrast sequences can be documented on identical images, and to facilitate immediate imaging after contrast injection.

A short catheter is placed in a peripheral vein and connected via a long infusion line to a bag of normal saline. The patient is then positioned on a spine surface coil and moved into the magnet. The long infusion line serves as a portal for injection outside the confines of the magnet so contrast can be introduced at the appropriate time without altering the position of the patient.

Our examinations are performed on a 1.5 tesla system. An initial short TR/short TE coronal series (scout) is obtained rapidly (one measure with a reduced number of phase encoding steps). This enables us to prescribe the sagittal sequence along the main axis of the lumbar spine, correcting as much as possible for faulty patient positioning and/or scoliosis. An axial sequence is subsequently prescribed at the appropriate level, based on the sagittal examination establishing angulation and offset. Gadopentetate is then injected (0.2 ml/kg or 0.1 mmol/kg) and an axial sequence identical to the series performed prior to injection is obtained. The original sagittal sequence is

---

*Magnevist (gadolinium dimeglumine).

then rapidly repeated, thereby completing the examination. It should be noted that the immediate postcontrast sequence (which is the most critical diagnostically) may be performed in either the axial or the sagittal plane according to the radiologist's preference. Our sagittal T1-weighted sequence takes approximately 3½ minutes and utilizes a TR/TE of 500/20, two signal averages, a 204 × 256 matrix, 5 mm thick slices at 6.5 mm intervals, and a 325 mm field of view. Phase encoding is selected in the anteroposterior direction to avoid aliasing or wrap-around artifact. The axial T1-weighted sequence utilizes similar parameters with the exception of the field of view (which is reduced to 220 mm), and the number of signal averages (which is increased to four, to improve the signal/noise ratio of the image). Phase encoding is performed in the left to right direction. A fold-over suppression option, available on our unit, is utilized to avoid wrap-around artifact; and a flow artifact reduction capability is employed to presaturate tissue volumes above and below the imaged sections, to prevent ghosting artifact from inflowing blood or CSF. The axial sequence takes approximately 7 minutes to complete. Total examination time, including interscan processing and programming, is about 45 minutes. Filming is performed with constant window and level settings on the pre- and postcontrast sequences.

MRI CHARACTERISTICS OF THE POSTOPERATIVE SPINE

The radiological appearance of the postsurgical spine reflects the surgical procedure performed, which in a typical case of disk surgery involves hemilaminectomy with diskectomy and possible facetectomy with foraminal exploration. Asymmetry of the extravertebral soft tissue of the back is typical, with distortion of muscle and fat planes (Figs. 6-1 to 6-3). The laminectomy defect becomes apparent as the intermediate-signal marrow and the dark-signal cortex of the lamina are unilaterally replaced by enhancing scar tissue (Figs. 6-1 to 6-4). The ligamentum flavum is characteristically absent unilaterally (Figs. 6-1, 6-4, and 6-5). Fat packing or pedicle fat graft, occasionally placed over the laminectomy site to reduce scar formation,[23] is recognized on nonenhanced T1-weighted sequences as a focal area of bright signal in the posterior epidural space (Figs. 6-1 and 6-5).

The evolution of postsurgical changes in the epidural space has been studied by Ross et al.[24,25] In the immediate postoperative period (under 10 days) bright epidural fat is replaced by edematous soft tissue (intermediate and bright signal intensity, respectively, on T1- and T2-weighted sequences) both ventral and lateral to the dural tube as well as in the neural foramen (when surgical exploration of the foramen has been conducted). This abnormal epidural soft tissue characteristically exerts a mass effect on the thecal sac that regresses over several months as cicatrization occurs and varying amounts of epidural fibrosis remain (characterized by more homoge-

neous signal on T1-weighted sequences [Figs. 6-1, 6-4, and 6-6] and persistently bright signal on T2-weighted sequences [Fig. 6-1]). It is not uncommon for the thecal sac to be distorted as it is drawn toward a region of epidural scar (Figs. 6-1 and 6-5).

Enhancement of the parent disk on postgadopentetate MRI has been reported to occur in linear, diffuse, or mottled patterns.[20] The disk is generally thought to be avascular. However, this is only partially correct. Firooznia and Kricheff[13] et al. reported enhancement of the margins of normal, bulging, and herniated disks at operated as well as nonoperated levels on CT following intravenous contrast injection. Enhancement of both operated and nonoperated herniations, extending up to 13 mm toward the center of the disk, was also noted in some patients. As discussed in the preceding chapters, further work with herniated disks from patients with and without previous surgery has revealed the presence of granulation tissue, focal areas of edema, hemorrhage, necrosis, calcification, and scarring on gross and microscopic examination of surgically resected fragments.

We believe therefore that enhancement of the disk margin on contrast-enhanced CT is due to vascularity of the annulus fibrosus. The more frequent and intense enhancement noted in bulging and herniated disks is due to the disk margin's more prominent vascularity as well as to other pathological changes noted in the disk (described above). The enhancement of disk substance, including free fragments, is due mainly to the presence of vascular granulation tissue, although other pathological changes also contribute.

In the case of the parent disk the enhancement observed postoperatively on MR examination often involves the substance of the disk. It has been speculated[20] that such enhancement may occur secondary to vascular ingrowth from bone adjacent to the degenerated disk through the cartilaginous endplate, ingrowth of vascular scar (precipitated by surgical curettage), or diffusion from adjacent vascular structures into the disk. We believe that, in addition to these factors (which are most likely operative as described), the same pathological changes observed in the herniated portion of a disk are quite likely present in the substance of the disk adjacent to the area of herniation and contributing to the enhancement of the body of the disk on MRI. We believe also that the herniated disk fragments recovered at surgery are probably very similar histologically to the parent disk. In other words, granulation tissue, fibrosis, calcification, and hemorrhage are all present in the parent disk also.

When scar tissue is compared to fragments of a resected disk herniation or to a cadaver disk with signs of degeneration, the following differences will be noted: Surgical scars are composed mainly of a fairly homogeneous fibrosis (mature granulation tissue) whereas degenerated disks are composed mainly of a markedly nonhomogeneous tissue with areas of fibrocartilage, calcification, scarring, fibrosis, and focal bleeding. Surgi-

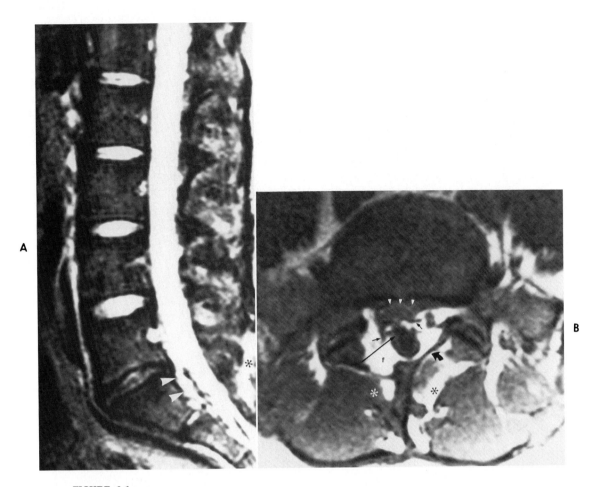

FIGURE 6-1

Postoperative scar. The patient is status post-right L5-S1 hemilaminectomy and diskectomy. **A,** A sagittal T2-weighted image shows signal loss consistent with degenerative change in the L5-S1 disk. The bright signal in the ventral epidural space *(arrowheads)* not contiguous with the disk represents a combination of epidural fibrosis and ventral epidural venous plexus. The *asterisk* denotes high-signal granulation tissue within the posterior extravertebral soft tissues. **B,** An axial T1-weighted image demonstrates asymmetrical distortion of the posterior extravertebral soft tissue *(asterisk)* and a right hemilaminectomy defect. The ligamentum flavum is identified in the left posterolateral canal *(curved arrow)* but is absent on the right side, where the bright epidural signal *(f)* of a surgical fat packing is visible. Ventrally there is displacement of the fat to the center and right by homogeneous intermediate-intensity soft tissue *(arrowheads)*, representing the epidural scar. Areas of linearity *(small arrows)* associated with the scar are characteristic. Note the distorted dural tube *(long arrow)*, which appears retracted by the scar.

cal scar is fairly vascular and rarely calcifies whereas degenerated disks generally have scant vascularity. However, chronically active herniated disks have islands of vascular granulation tissue and foci of congestion, edema, and hemorrhage.

DIFFERENTIATION OF A HERNIATED DISK FROM EPIDURAL SCAR
Histopathology and enhancement dynamics

The differing enhancement characteristics of scar and disk material — the single most important MRI criterion — have been related to the biodistribution of gadopentetate and the differing histopathology of scar and disk.[20,26,27] Gadopentetate is a relatively small molecule, similar in size to iothalamate, a radiographic ionic contrast medium. Its pharmacokinetics adhere to a two-compartment model, with rapid diffusion into the extravascular space followed by rapid equilibration between the intra- and extravascular spaces and elimination by glomerular filtration. Scar enhancement curves have been shown to be similar to those describing the extravascular compartment dynamics for iothalamate.[26]

Tissue enhancement requires three conditions:

1. A vascular supply
2. Endothelial discontinuities through which contrast molecules can extravasate
3. An extravascular compartment where molecules of contrast can accumulate

The brisk enhancement of scar tissue has been attributed to the histopathological fulfillment of these criteria. India-ink injections into dogs, as well as light and electron microscopic examinations in dog and human

Text continued on p. 243.

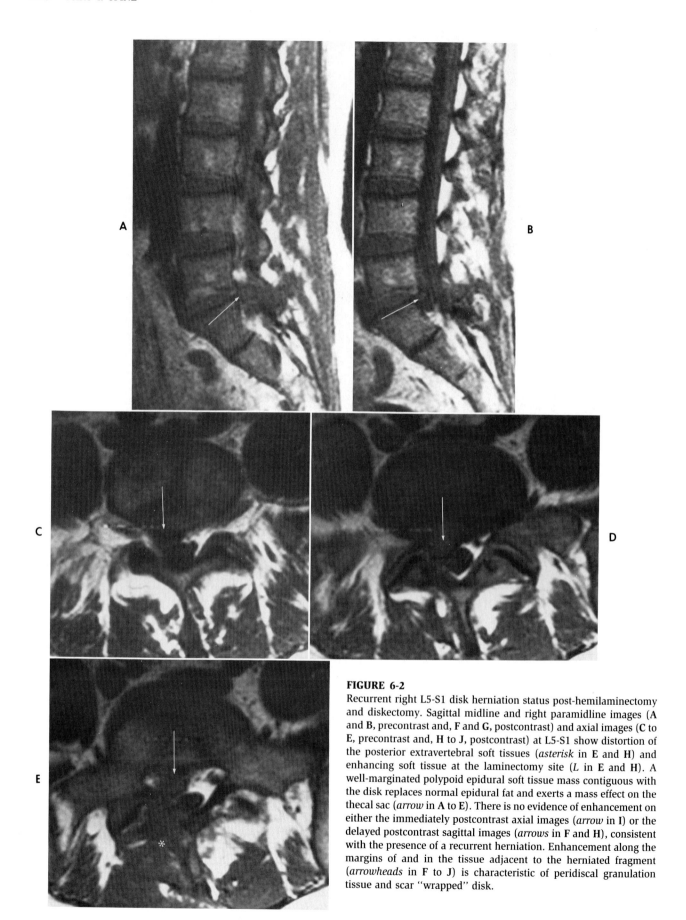

FIGURE 6-2
Recurrent right L5-S1 disk herniation status post-hemilaminectomy and diskectomy. Sagittal midline and right paramidline images (**A** and **B**, precontrast and, **F** and **G**, postcontrast) and axial images (**C** to **E**, precontrast and, **H** to **J**, postcontrast) at L5-S1 show distortion of the posterior extravertebral soft tissues (*asterisk* in **E** and **H**) and enhancing soft tissue at the laminectomy site (*L* in **E** and **H**). A well-marginated polypoid epidural soft tissue mass contiguous with the disk replaces normal epidural fat and exerts a mass effect on the thecal sac (*arrow* in **A** to **E**). There is no evidence of enhancement on either the immediately postcontrast axial images (*arrow* in **I**) or the delayed postcontrast sagittal images (*arrows* in **F** and **H**), consistent with the presence of a recurrent herniation. Enhancement along the margins of and in the tissue adjacent to the herniated fragment (*arrowheads* in **F** to **J**) is characteristic of peridiscal granulation tissue and scar "wrapped" disk.

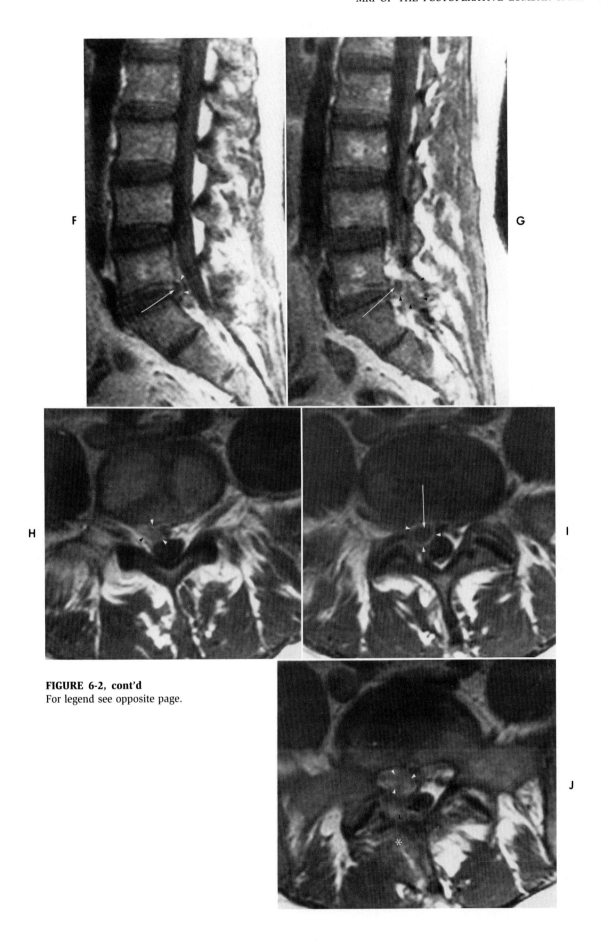

FIGURE 6-2, cont'd
For legend see opposite page.

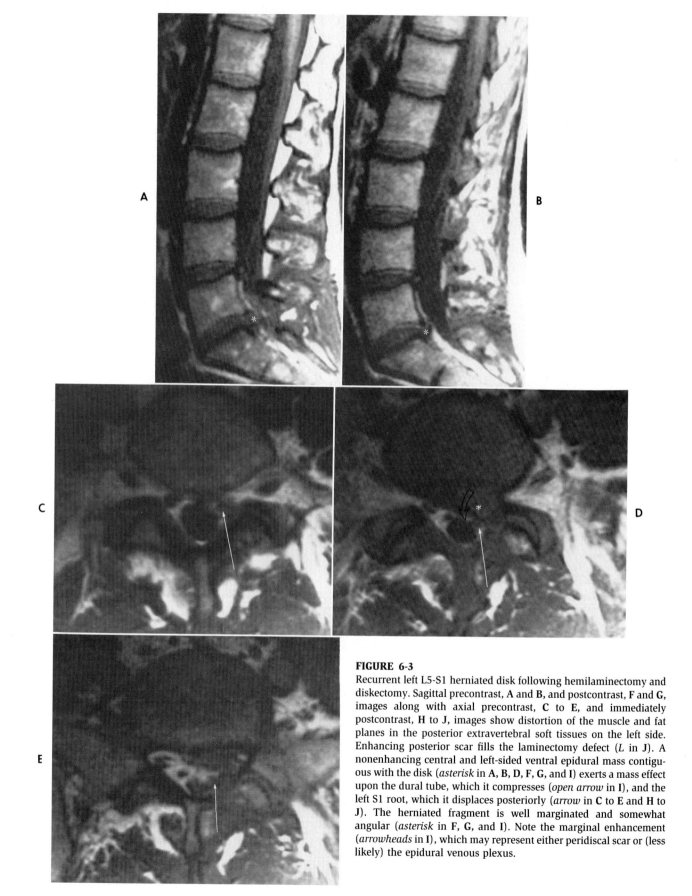

FIGURE 6-3
Recurrent left L5-S1 herniated disk following hemilaminectomy and
diskectomy. Sagittal precontrast, **A** and **B**, and postcontrast, **F** and **G**,
images along with axial precontrast, **C** to **E**, and immediately
postcontrast, **H** to **J**, images show distortion of the muscle and fat
planes in the posterior extravertebral soft tissues on the left side.
Enhancing posterior scar fills the laminectomy defect (*L* in **J**). A
nonenhancing central and left-sided ventral epidural mass contiguous with the disk (*asterisk* in **A, B, D, F, G,** and **I**) exerts a mass effect
upon the dural tube, which it compresses (*open arrow* in **I**), and the
left S1 root, which it displaces posteriorly (*arrow* in **C** to **E** and **H** to
J). The herniated fragment is well marginated and somewhat
angular (*asterisk* in **F, G,** and **I**). Note the marginal enhancement
(*arrowheads* in **I**), which may represent either peridiscal scar or (less
likely) the epidural venous plexus.

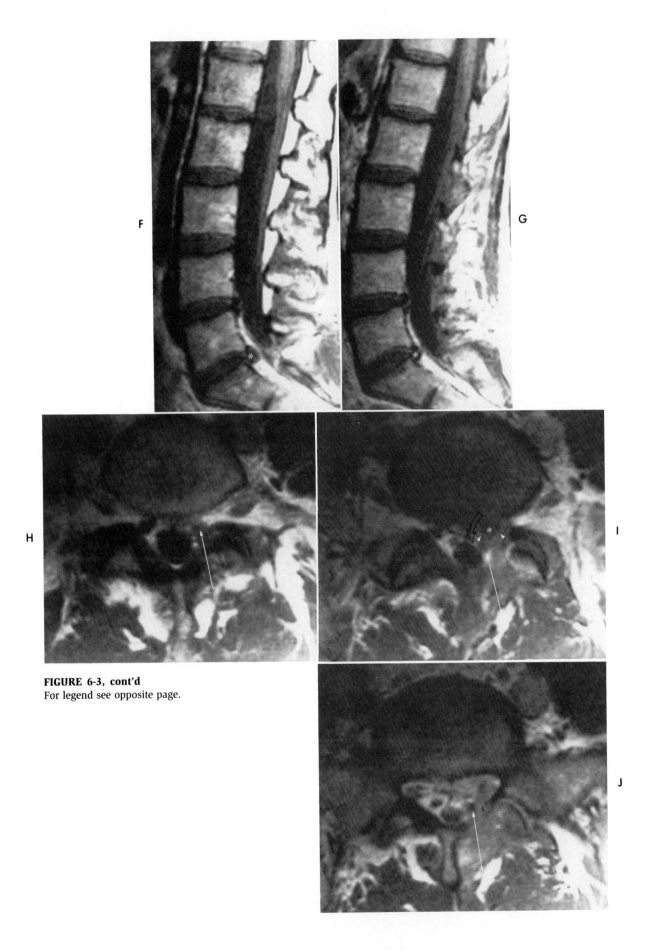

FIGURE 6-3, cont'd
For legend see opposite page.

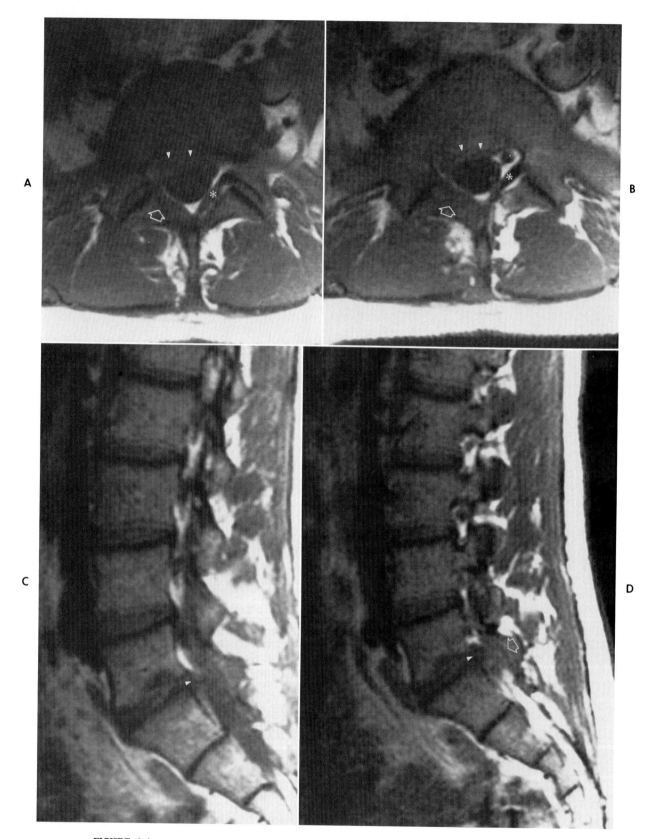

FIGURE 6-4
Epidural scar status post-right L5-S1 hemilaminectomy and diskectomy. Axial T1-weighted images prior to, **A** and **B**, and immediately following, **E** and **F**, gadolinium injection and right-sided sagittal precontrast, **C** and **D**, and 15-minute postcontrast, **G** and **H**, images show the right lamina replaced by enhancing posterolateral scar (*open arrow* in **A** to **F** and **H**). The ligamentum flavum is identified on the left (*asterisk* in **A**, **B**, **E**, and **F**) but absent on the right. Homogeneous intermediate-signal scar replaces epidural fat in the ventral canal centrally and to the right (*arrowheads* in **A** to **D**).

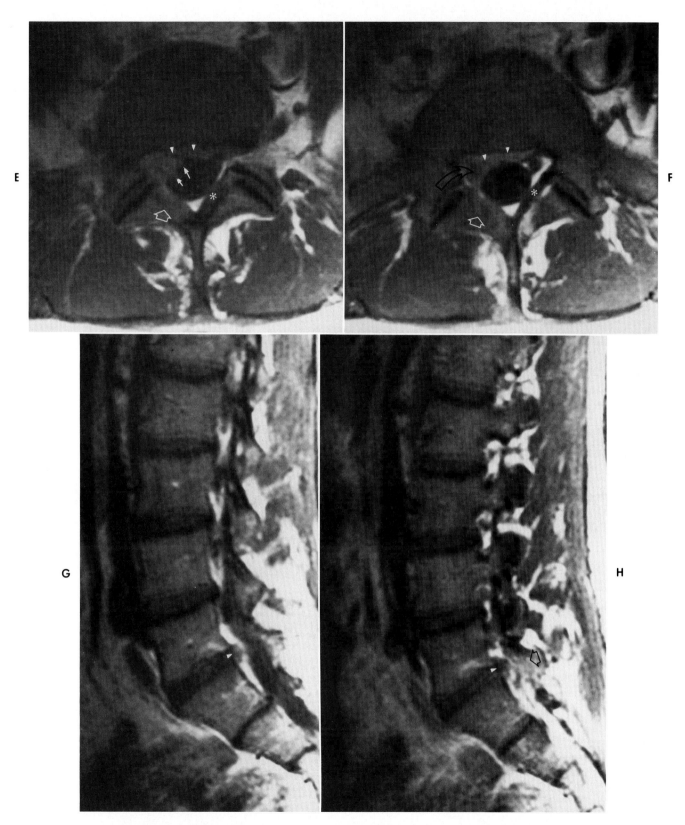

FIGURE 6-4, cont'd
Following gadolinium injection there is brisk uniform enhancement of the scar (*arrowheads* in **E** to **H**). Note both the characteristically irregular margins of the ventral scar (*arrows* in **E**) and the manner in which it conforms to the available space of the lateral recess and vertebral canal. The nonenhancing round structure in the right lateral recess (*curved arrow* in **F**) is easily recognized as the right S1 root by comparison with the left side.

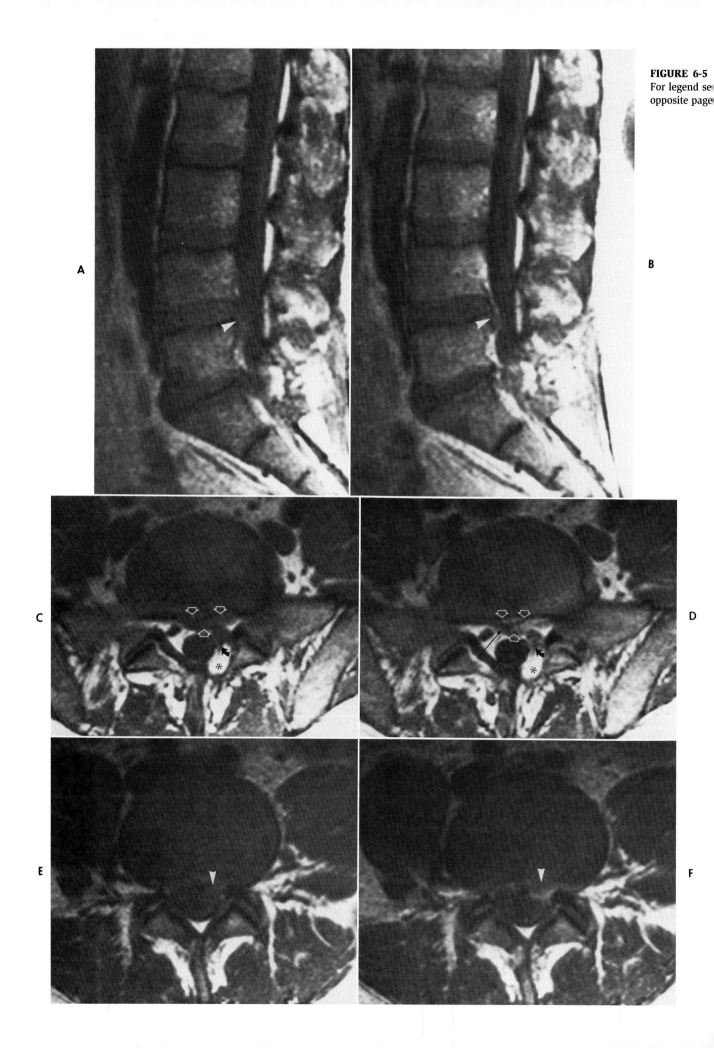

FIGURE 6-5
For legend se
opposite page

FIGURE 6-5

Epidural fibrosis at L5-S1 with an L4-5 herniated disk. The patient is status post-left hemilaminectomy and diskectomy at L5-S1. Sagittal precontrast, **A,** and postcontrast, **B,** along with axial pre- and postcontrast images at L5-S1 (**C** and **D**) and L4-5 (**E** and **F**). Bright-signal fat packing replaces the ligamentum flavum in the left posterolateral epidural space at L5-S1 (*asterisk* in **C** and **D**). Abnormal ventral epidural soft tissue, **C,** undergoes heterogeneous enhancement, **D.** A small nonenhancing focus may represent a tiny disk fragment (*long arrow* in **D**). Enhancing soft tissue anterior to the fat packing (*curved arrow* in **C** and **D**) most likely represents a focus of epidural scar since it slightly retracts both the adjacent left S1 root posteriorly and the dural tube laterally toward itself. At the L4-5 level a nonenhancing left ventral epidural structure, exerting a mass effect upon the thecal sac (*arrowhead* in **A, B, E,** and **F**), represents the herniation (at a previously unexplored level). Its surrounding rim is probably granulation tissue that has developed in response to herniation.

---

epidural scar,[26] have demonstrated numerous small capillaries within a fibrous stroma, endothelial tight junctions with varying degrees of fusion between adjacent cell membranes, and a large interstitial space. Peak epidural scar enhancement was shown at 5 minutes in humans, predicating the necessity of immediate postinjection scanning. The observation of early heterogeneous enhancement evolving into a pattern of more homogeneous enhancement by 30 minutes was tentatively explained by variable rates of diffusion into the extravascular space secondary to regional variations in endothelial integrity (i.e., varying degrees of "loosening" of the tight junctions).

Geographical differences in scar location can lead to histopathological variations in epidural scar and hence spatially variant enhancement dynamics. It has been implied[21] that scar becomes less vascular with age and its enhancement may diminish over time. Anterior epidural scar, however, has been noted[27] to enhance as late as 30 years after surgery, in contradistinction to posterior (laminectomy) epidural scar (which has been shown in dog models[27] to undergo maximum enhancement at 1 month following surgery and to decline rapidly by 4 months, at which time the degree of enhancement is comparable to that of the adjacent paraspinal muscles).

Light and electron microscopy[27] has demonstrated granulation tissue with "leaky" endothelial junctions at 1 month following laminectomy, which was replaced by mature collagenous scar with tight endothelial junctions by the fourth postsurgical month. It was speculated that anterior epidural scar, located in a biomechanically stressful region (at the disk space and endplate), is subject to cycles of trauma and inflammation, which produce scar in various stages of maturation, but that posterior scar, geographically removed from the disk and endplate, would be able to mature without mechanical interruption. Hueftle et al.[20] and Ross et al.[26] called attention to a histopathological difference between scar (which is vascular) and herniated disk (which has scant vascularity) while at the same time noting that both have a capacious extracellular compartment.

The delayed enhancement occasionally seen with recurrent disk herniation is speculated[20,26] to result from diffusion into its extracellular compartment from the adjacent vascular stroma (e.g., peridiscal scar or granulation tissue) related to degenerative changes in the disk. We have observed the characteristic pattern of scar and herniated disk enhancement (early enhancement of scar, but not of disk) following intravenous gadopentetate in 75% to 80% of patients. In some without an apparent reason, in others with calcified herniation and scar, multiple previous operations, and postoperative infection, this characteristic pattern may not be seen.

Radiological criteria

The lack of enhancement in the immediate postcontrast MRI examination is the single most important criterion for diagnosing residual/recurrent disk in the postoperative lumbar spine. An abnormal epidural soft tissue that undergoes immediate enhancement is consistent with epidural scar (Figs. 6-4 and 6-6) whereas a nonenhancing focus of epidural soft tissue implies the presence of a recurrent herniated disk (Figs. 6-2, 6-3, and 6-8). It is not uncommon for peripheral enhancement to be identified along the margins of a herniated disk (Figs. 6-2, 6-3, and 6-7), a finding that has been amply described in the CT literature.[13,15,28] The occasional tendency for disk material to undergo enhancement on delayed examination emphasizes the need for *immediate* postinjection scanning, to avoid misinterpreting a late-enhancing herniation for an epidural scar (Fig. 6-7).

The presence of a mass effect is important in differentiating disk herniation from an epidural scar. Disk herniation characteristically produces a positive mass effect on the adjacent thecal sac and nerve roots, displacing the sac and nerves away from the abnormal mass (Fig. 6-7). Scar tissue, on the other hand, may conform to the surrounding space (Fig. 6-4) and exert a negative mass effect as cicatrization induces retraction of the adjacent structures toward it (Figs. 6-1 and 6-5). Thus, although this sign is often helpful, in our experience and in the reported experience of others using MR[20] and CT,[9,16] scar tissue can also rarely produce a misleading positive mass effect.

Contiguity of abnormal epidural soft tissue with the parent disk has been reported[20] as suggesting disk herniation (Figs. 6-2, 6-3, and 6-8), in contradistinction to noncontiguity, which has been considered more a sign of

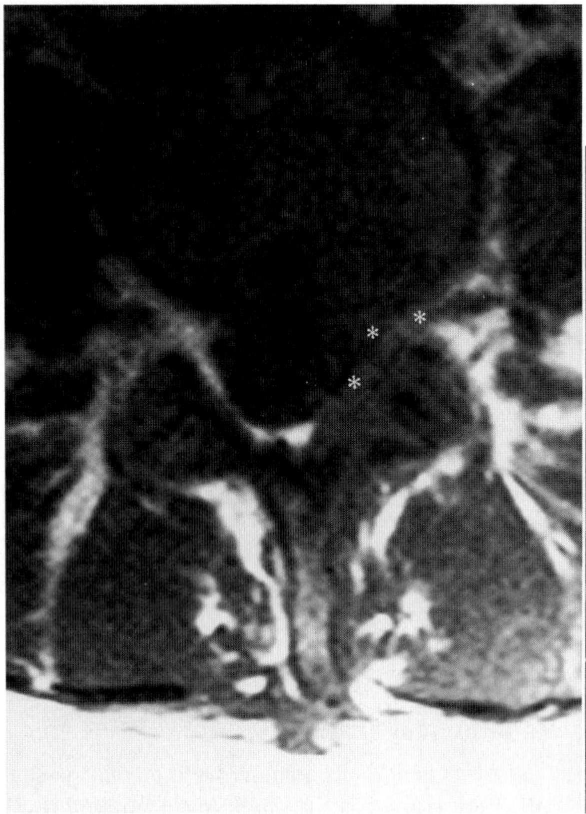

FIGURE 6-6
For legend see opposite page.

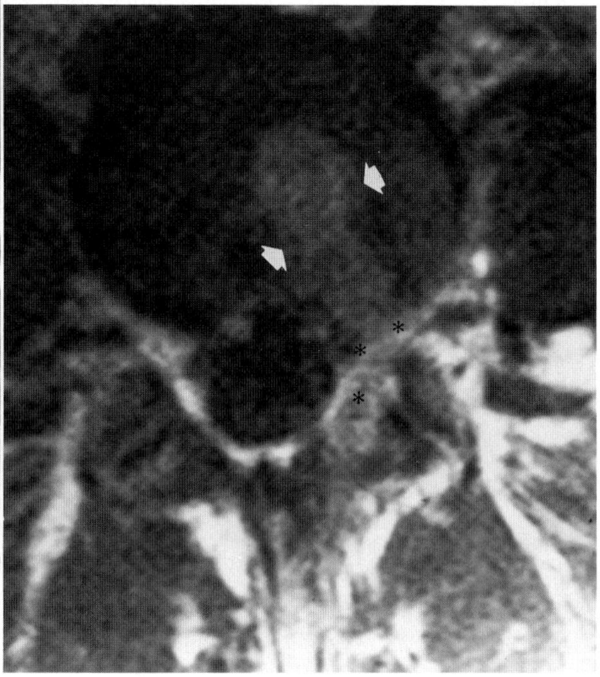

scar formation (Fig. 6-1). Obviously, however, scar tissue can be present at the disk space level and appear contiguous with the disk (Fig. 6-6) while a sequestered or free disk fragment is ostensibly noncontiguous with the disk.

Signal characteristics are generally felt not to be reliable in distinguishing herniation from scar. Several series[12,19,21,22] have compared the signal from abnormal epidural soft tissue with that from the parent annulus, parent disk, and thecal sac and concluded that anterior epidural scar is consistently hypointense or isointense on T1-weighted images (T1-WI) and hyperintense on T2-weighted images (T2-WI). The signal intensity of scar became more variable, however, in the posterolateral epidural space. Herniated disk material, in contradistinction, was consistently hypointense or isointense on T1-WI and T2-WI. The free fragments compared to the parent disk were consistently isointense to hyperintense on T1-WI and hyperintense on T2-WI. It was speculated that they could represent extrusion of relatively more nuclear than annular material.

We have histological documentation in four patients with free fragments on intravenous contrast — enhanced CT that were found to be composed of fibrocartilaginous masses of disk with zones of granulation tissue. These findings would nicely explain the enhancement noted on intravenous contrast CT, and they might also be responsible in some patients for the hyperintense T2-WI and iso- to hyperintense T1-WI MR images observed.

Another series[22] has reported less consistent signal characteristics. Epidural scar (located not far from the disk) was found to be highly variable in signal characteristics on both T1-WI and T2-WI while the disk was slightly less variable, appearing mainly to be isointense on T1-WI, though somewhat less so on T2-WI, with a rim of low signal outlining it on both T1-WI and T2-WI. Compared to the thecal sac on T2-WI,[12] scar usually was hypointense but occasionally was isointense to hyperintense.

In the largest series reported[21] it was stated that fibrous tissue generally has decreased signal on T2-WI and T2-WI. However, the authors did not identify a control tissue to which this signal could be compared, did not chart individual cases, and did not provide photographs of the scar cases. In our series[29] of 19 extruded disk fragments, all were isointense to neural tissue (i.e., conus medullaris) on T2-WI. Among the 11 cases in which a T2-WI was obtained, 5 fragments were hyperintense to CSF, 4 were hypointense, 1 was isointense, and 1 demonstrated mixed signal intensity.

Considering this wide variability of signal characteristics from disk and epidural scar, we believe that their differentiation cannot be reliably made by the use of signal criteria.

FALSE-POSITIVES

A false-positive impression of recurrent disk herniation, with the potential for negative surgical exploration,

B　　　　　　　　　　　C　　　　　　　　　　　D

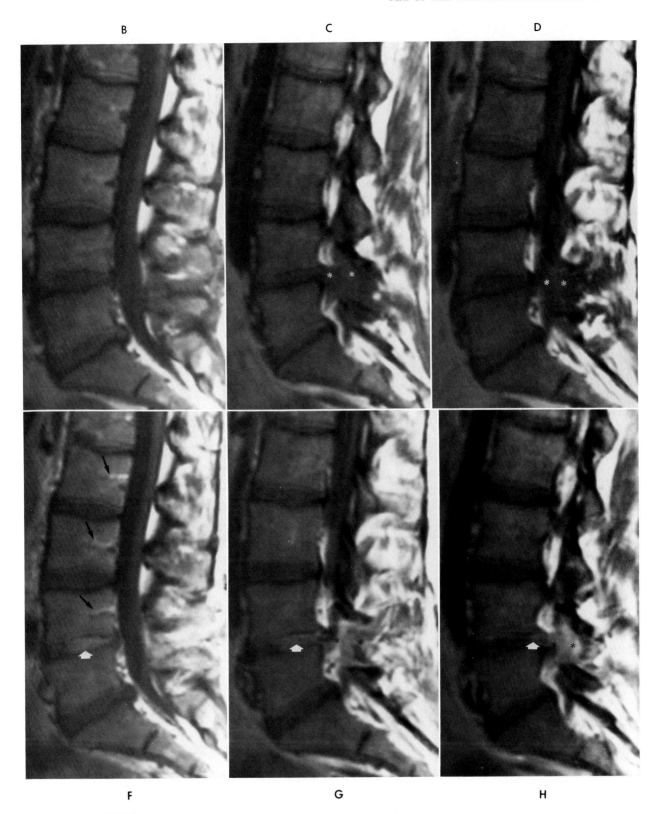

F　　　　　　　　　　　G　　　　　　　　　　　H

FIGURE 6-6
Epidural scar status post-left L4-5 laminectomy and diskectomy. Axial precontrast, **A**, and immediately postcontrast, **E**, images as well as sagittal precontrast, **B** to **D**, and postcontrast, **F** to **H**, images in the midline and left paramidline planes show abnormal soft tissue replacing epidural fat in the lateral recess, intervertebral foramen, and posterolateral epidural space (*asterisks* in **A**, **C**, and **D**). Following contrast administration there is uniform enhancement of both the scar (*asterisks* in **E**, **G**, and **H**) and a focal portion of the contiguous native disk (*white arrow* in **E** to **H**), presumably representing granulation tissue incited by diskectomy. Note the normal enhancement of the basivertebral vein on the midline sagittal image (*black arrows* in **F**). A small central L5-S1 disk herniation was found incidentally at surgical reexploration.

can occur because of several circumstances that may produce a real or apparent epidural focus of nonenhancement — the presence of ventral ridges as well as diskal or ligamentalous calcification, the misidentification of a nerve root as disk material, the heterogeneity of an anterior epidural scar, a technical error in filming or contrast administration, and magnetic susceptibility artifacts.

A ventral ridge may appear darker or brighter on T1-WI (depending on, respectively, its content of cortical bone and marrow) and may not undergo appreciable contrast enhancement. Similarly, calcification of the posterior longitudinal ligament or disk margin may produce abnormal and nonenhancing epidural foci. If these cannot be excluded by morphological considerations, then CT examination, with its superior sensitivity for the identification of calcification, can be definitive.

The descending nerve root in the lateral recess, the

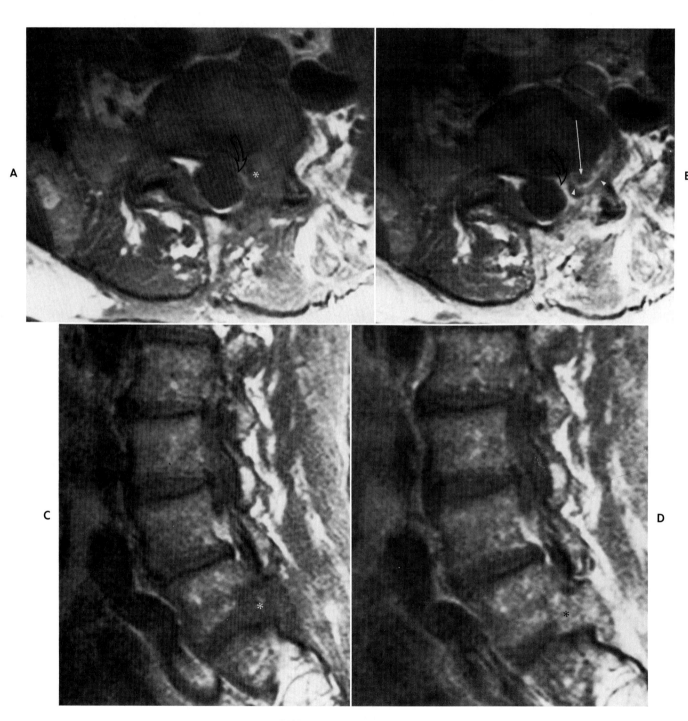

FIGURE 6-7
For legend see opposite page.

dorsal root ganglion, and the exiting spinal nerve in the neural foramen will not enhance appreciably relative to surrounding scar and may be confused with disk material. The distinction can usually be made anatomically by identification of the nonenhancing epidural structure in the appropriate anatomical position of the nerve root compared to both the contiguous images and the contralateral side (Fig. 6-4). In cases of persistent confusion, delayed images may be helpful[20,25] because the disk material undergoes delayed enhancement, thereby establishing the diagnosis (Fig. 6-7). Lack of enhancement on delayed images does not resolve this problem in differential diagnosis, however.

Anterior epidural scar is histologically heterogeneous, containing both mature and immature elements.[20,27] Since enhancement is known to be heterogeneous on early postcontrast imaging,[20] the implicit diagnostic hazard of early heterogeneous enhancement is that an

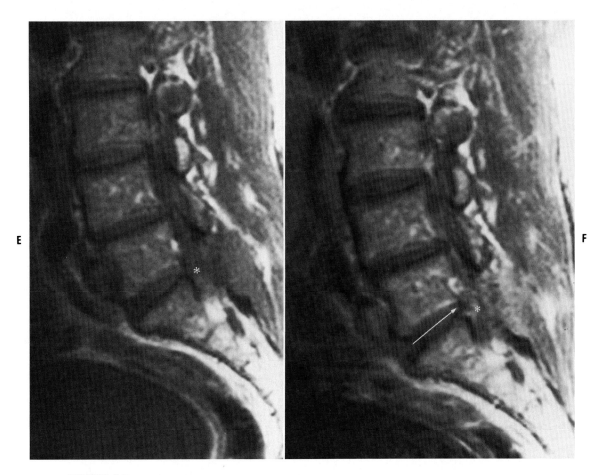

FIGURE 6-7
Recurrent left lateral recess herniation at L5-S1. Axial precontrast, **A**, and immediately postcontrast, **B**, along with sagittal pre- and delayed postcontrast, **C** and **D**, and sagittal pre- and immediately postcontrast, **E** and **F**, examinations the following day show abnormal soft tissue replacement of epidural fat in the left lateral recess (*asterisk* in **A**) and flattening of the anterolateral thecal sac (*curved arrow* in **A** and **B**). Immediately after contrast administration there is a nonenhancing focus (*long arrow* in **B**) partially surrounded by a margin of enhancing tissue (*arrowheads* in **B**) that suggests a herniated disk fragment within a bed of peridiscal scar (although a nonenhanced left S-1 root cannot be entirely excluded, because the root anatomy is not clearly depicted). On the delayed postcontrast sagittal image there is uniform enhancement of the lateral recess (*asterisk* in **D**, compare with **C**), suggesting delayed enhancement of the disk fragment, which now appears isointense with the adjacent scar. (The delayed enhancement eliminates the possibility of mistaking this mass for the nerve root.) The patient was brought back subsequently for precontrast and immediately postcontrast sagittal images, **E** and **F**, which revealed heterogeneous enhancement in the lateral recess (*asterisk* in **F**, compare with **E**), and evidence of a nonenhancing focus (*arrow* in **F**). This corroborated the diagnosis, which was confirmed at surgical reexploration. Note that the disk fragment is entirely invisible on delayed images, **D**, emphasizing the need for immediate postinjection scanning (**B** and **F**) to identify the disk, which could undergo delayed enhancement and be mistaken for a scar.

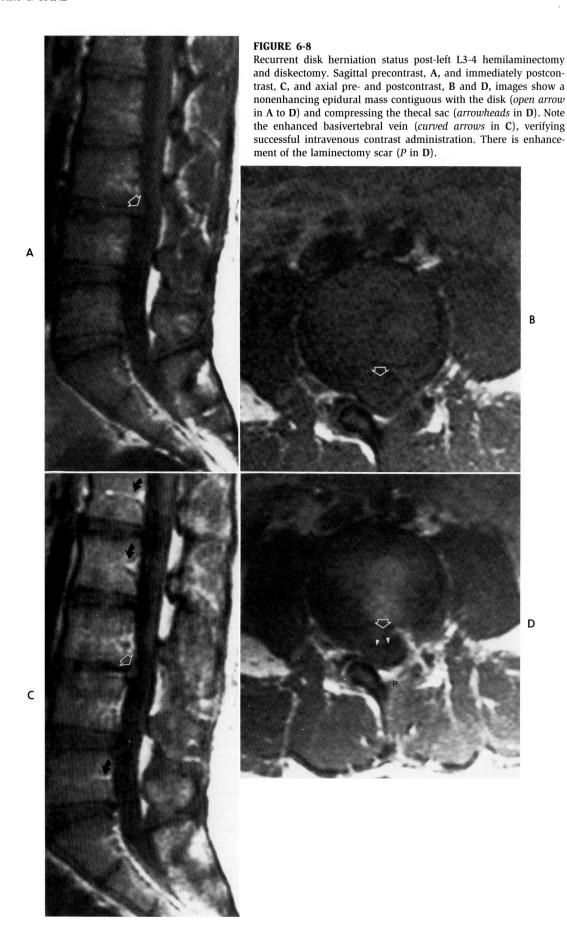

FIGURE 6-8
Recurrent disk herniation status post-left L3-4 hemilaminectomy and diskectomy. Sagittal precontrast, **A**, and immediately postcontrast, **C**, and axial pre- and postcontrast, **B** and **D**, images show a nonenhancing epidural mass contiguous with the disk (*open arrow* in **A** to **D**) and compressing the thecal sac (*arrowheads* in **D**). Note the enhanced basivertebral vein (*curved arrows* in **C**), verifying successful intravenous contrast administration. There is enhancement of the laminectomy scar (*P* in **D**).

epidural focus of relatively low-grade enhancement will be mistakenly identified as a fragment of nonenhancing disk material. A detailed comparison of pre- and postcontrast images will help determine whether this focus undergoes either no enhancement (suggesting disk material) or minimal enhancement (suggesting a relatively more mature epidural scar). Additional criteria such as mass effect (displacement vs. retraction of the dural tube and nerve roots) and morphology (sharply marginated, polypoid, and angular vs. irregular and linear) may be useful.

Filming of the pre- and postcontrast images with inconsistent window and level settings can make a focus of epidural enhancement appear spuriously nonenhanced and create a misimpression of recurrent herniation. This is easily avoided by strict maintenance of constant settings when filming precontrast and postcontrast injection sequences.

Technical failure of intravenous contrast administration will, of course, leave scar tissues nonenhanced and liable to being mistaken for a recurrent herniation. Successful injection of contrast is easily verified by recognizing enhancement of the basivertebral vein (Figs. 6-6 and 6-8) and posterior epidural scar (Fig. 6-8).

A focus of nonenhancement in the postoperative spine may be caused by magnetic susceptibility artifact produced by metallic particles. It is known that tiny metallic particles (not identifiable on plain film or CT) generated by contact of a surgical drill with untempered surgical instruments are deposited at the time of surgery and create metallic artifacts manifested as signal voids.[25,30,31,32] The artifact should be easily recognized by the high peripheral signal halo associated with the signal void as well as by the focal field distortion. In the rare case of persistent confusion it may be exaggerated and hence confirmed on a T2-weighted spin echo sequence or a T2*-weighted gradient refocused echo sequence (the latter producing the most dramatic exaggeration of susceptibility artifact).

FALSE-NEGATIVES

The sources of potential false-negative diagnosis of recurrent disk herniation are related to potentially small disk fragment size, timing of the scan relative to contrast injection, and technical factors of image filming.

Small nonenhancing disk fragments may be missed because of interscan gaps as well as partial volume averaging[20] within a slice containing a large volume of enhancing scar. The potential for missing such small fragments can be minimized by using relatively thin slices and gap thicknesses to the extent that the signal/ noise tradeoff is endurable and by imaging in both the sagittal and the axial plane.

The tendency for some herniated disks to undergo delayed enhancement creates the potential for overlooking a disk fragment on images obtained relatively late following contrast administration, at which time an enhancing herniation may be misinterpreted as a scar. This is avoided by imaging *immediately after* contrast administration. When more than one postcontrast sequence is obtained, diagnostic weighting should be placed on the set of images obtained earliest following injection (Fig. 6-7).

It is important to reemphasize the necessity of obtaining constant window and level settings on pre- and postcontrast images. Varying the settings may create a false visual appearance of enhancement, leading to misinterpretation of nonenhancing disk material as enhancing scar tissue.

REFERENCES

1. Burton CV, Kirkaldy-Willis WH, Yong-Hing K, Heithoff KB: Causes of failure of surgery on the lumbar spine. Clin Orthop 1981;157:191-199.
2. Jacobs RR, McClain O, Neff J: Control of postlaminectomy scar formation: an experimental and clinical study. Spine 1980;5:223-229.
3. Naylor A: Late results of laminectomy for lumbar disk prolapse. J Bone Joint Surg 1974;56B:17-29.
4. Teplick JG, Haskin ME: Review: Computed tomography of the postoperative lumbar spine. AJR 1983;141:865-884.
5. Law JD, Lehman RA, Kirsch WM: Reoperation after lumbar intervertebral disc surgery. J Neurosurg 1978;48:259-263.
6. Finnegan WJ, Fenlin JM, Marvel JP, et al: Results of surgical intervention in the symptomatic multiply-operated back patient. J Bone Joint Surg (Am) 1979;61:1077-1082.
7. Benoist M, Ficat C, Baraf P, Cauchoix J: Postoperative lumbar epiduro-arachnoiditis: Diagnostic and therapeutic aspects. Spine 1980;5:432-436.
8. Hardy RW Jr: Repeat operation for lumbar disc. In Hardy RW Jr (ed): Seminars in neurological surgery. Lumbar disc disease. New York, Raven, 1982, pp 193-202.
9. Teplick JG, Haskin ME: CT of the postoperative lumbar spine. Radiol Clin North Am 1983;21:395-420.
10. Shapiro R: Myelography. Chicago, Year Book, 1975, p 203.
11. Quencer RM, Tenner M, Rothman L: The postoperative myelogram. Radiographic evaluation of arachnoiditis and dural/ arachnoidal tears. Radiology 1977;123:667-679.
12. Sotiropoulos S, Chafetz NI, Lang P, et al: Differentiation between postoperative scar and recurrent disk herniation. Prospective comparison of MR, CT, and contrast-enhanced CT. AJNR 1989;10:639-643.
13. Firooznia H, Kricheff II, Rafii M, Golimbu C: Lumbar spine after surgery: examination with intravenous contrast-enhanced CT. Radiology 1987;163:221-226.
14. Weiss T, Treisch J, Kazner E: CT of the postoperative lumbar spine: the value of intravenous contrast. Neuroradiology 1986;28:241-245.
15. Yang PJ, Seeger JF, Dzioba RB, et al: High-dose IV contrast in CT scanning of the postoperative lumbar spine, AJNR 1986;7:703-707.
16. Braun IF, Hoffman JC Jr, Davis PC, et al: Contrast enhancement in CT differentiation between recurrent disk herniation and postoperative scar: prospective study. AJR 1985;145:785-790.
17. Teplick JG, Haskin ME: Intravenous contrast–enhanced CT of the postoperative lumbar spine: improved identification of recurrent disk herniation, scar, arachnoiditis, and diskitis. AJR 1984;143:845-855.
18. Schubiger O, Valavanis A: CT differentiation between recurrent disk herniation and postoperative scar formation: the value of contrast enhancement. Neuroradiology 1982;22:251-254.
19. Bundschuh CV, Modic MT, Ross JS, et al: Epidural fibrosis and

recurrent disk herniation in the lumbar spine: MR imaging assessment. AJR 1988;150:923-932.

20. Hueftle MG, Modic MT, Ross JS, et al: Lumbar spine: postoperative MR imaging with Gd-DTPA. Radiology 1988;167:817-824.

21. Frocrain L, Duvauferrier R, Husson J, et al: Recurrent postoperative sciatica: evaluation with MR imaging and enhanced CT. Radiology 1989;170:531-533.

22. Hochhauser L, Kieffer SA, Cacayorin ED, et al: Recurrent postdiskectomy low back pain: MR-surgical correlation. AJR 1988;151:755-760.

23. Gill G, Scheck M, Kelley ET, Rodrigo JJ: Pedicle fat grafts for the prevention of scar in low-back surgery. Spine 1985;10:662-667.

24. Ross JS, Masaryk TJ, Modic M, et al: Lumbar spine: postoperative assessment with surface-coil imaging. Radiology 1987; 164:851-860.

25. Ross JS, Hueftle MG: Postoperative spine. In Modic M, et al (eds): Magnetic resonance imaging of the spine. Chicago, Year Book, 1989, pp 120-148.

26. Ross JS, Delamarter R, Hueftle MG, et al: Gadolinium-DTPA-enhanced MR imaging of the postoperative lumbar spine: time course and mechanism of enhancement. AJR 1989;152:825-834.

27. Ross JS, Blaser S, Masaryk TJ, et al: Gd-DTPA enhancement of posterior epidural scar: an experimental model. AJNR 1989; 10:1083-1088.

28. Raininko R, Törmä T: Contrast enhancement around a prolapsed disk. Neuroradiology 1982;24:49-51.

29. Schlesinger SD, Elkin C, Pinto R, Firooznia H: Lumbar and cervical osseous erosions secondary to herniated disks: comparison of CT and MR imaging. Presented at the 75th Scientific Assembly and Annual Meeting of the RSNA, Chicago, 1989. Radiology 1989;173(P):44.

30. Heindel W, Friedmann G, Bunke J, et al: Artifacts in MR imaging after surgical intervention. J Comput Assist Tomogr 1986; 10:596-599.

31. Norman D: The spine. In Brant-Zawadzki M, Norman D (eds): MRI of the central nervous system. New York, Raven, 1987, pp 289-328.

32. Levitt MM, Benjamin V, Kricheff II: Potential misinterpretation of cervical spondylosis with cord compression caused by metallic artifacts in magnetic resonance imaging of the postoperative spine. Neurosurgery 1990;27:126-130.

7 Degenerative Disease of the Thoracic Spine

HOSSEIN FIROOZNIA
M. VALLO BENJAMIN
RICHARD S. PINTO

INCIDENCE

Clinically symptomatic thoracic disk herniation is a rare occurrence. Its true incidence is not known, although it certainly is more common than one would expect from a review of the literature. To help convey an idea of its incidence, various authors have given the ratio of thoracic disk herniations operated on at their institutions to the total number of operations performed for disk herniations in all segments of the spine. This, of course, is dependent upon the mix of patients referred for surgery, the index of suspicion by the consulting surgeons, and the excellence of the radiology department in pursuing the diagnosis. Nevertheless, it is useful to review the incidence reported to gain an overall view of this disease.

The percentages of surgery performed for thoracic disk herniations relative to the total number of disk surgeries performed have been published as follows: Fineschi[1] (0.1% of 1048 cases), Love and Kiefer[2] (0.2% of 5500 cases), Arseni and Nash[3] (0.77% of 2979 cases), and Kite et al.[4] (0.87% of 1145 cases). If the patients reported by Schönbauer[5] (91), O'Connell[6] (115), Logue[7] (250), Kroll and Reiss[8] (350), and Abbott and Retter[9] (600) are also added, a total of 12,078 surgeries for herniated disks have been performed, and of these some 81 have been for thoracic disk herniations, bringing the mean percentage of surgery for that condition to 0.67%. In other words,

there was approximately 1 surgery for thoracic disk herniation in every 150 performed for disk herniations in general.

Another study has estimated that the average surgeon treating patients with disk herniations may see two to four cases of thoracic herniation during his professional lifetime. Carson et al.[10] think it an advantage therefore to consider the frequency of thoracic disk herniations in relation to the entire population rather than in relation to the numbers of patients treated for herniated lumbar and cervical disks. They maintain that only in this way can the search for previously undetected cases receive the necessary impetus. These authors state that in a population of 1 million about one patient per year can be expected to have a recognizable cord compression syndrome from a herniated thoracic disk. Indeed, they suggest that unless the diagnosis has been made as often as the foregoing numbers suggest some of these lesions are being misdiagnosed.

A review of the more recent literature on thoracic disk herniations discloses a higher percentage than has been reported, due most likely to the availability of CT (and more recently MRI). Also the significantly improved surgical results when a transthoracic approach is used rather than a laminectomy have served to heighten the interest in diagnosing, treating, and reporting thoracic disk herniations. Thus, compiling data from the larger series reported shows that there have been 1.6 surgeries performed for thoracic disk herniation in every 100 done for all other disk herniations.

Anatomical dissections

According to Arseni and Nash[3] the investigator Andrae found 15.2% thoracic disk herniations in a random postmortem examination of 368 cadavers. In another study, by Haley and Perry,[11] an examination of 99 cadavers revealed two cases of thoracic disk herniation more than 4 mm in extent. The significance of these reports is not clear. What is clear, however, is that the population at large does not generally suffer from clinically symptomatic thoracic disk herniation of this magnitude.

Radiographic studies

Reliable indications of a herniated thoracic disk on radiographic studies are (1) direct visualization of the herniation by MR, (2) visualization of a calcified herniation by CT, or (3) identification of an epidural defect at the disk space by myelography or CT-myelography. In most patients a definitive diagnosis cannot be made on conventional radiographic studies. However, because many thoracic herniations are associated with calcification of the disk, it might be useful to study the prevalence of the abnormality.

We did a retrospective review of 287 thoracic spinal radiographic studies in patients who had had examination of the thoracic spine for various disorders, including metastasis, trauma, infection, and spondyloarthropathy. Twelve instances of thoracic disk calcification were found (for a prevalence of 4%) in these patients, who were asymptomatic. (See p. 266 for a further discussion of the radiographic findings in thoracic disk herniation.)

A retrospective review of sagittal T1-weighted cross sections of the thoracic spine in 129 patients who had undergone an MRI examination for various diseases (not including suspicion of thoracic disk disease but including metastasis, infections, and trauma) revealed herniation of the thoracic disk (of more than 4 mm) in two patients. The affected disks were T7 and T11. None of the 129 patients had clinical findings indicating a thoracic herniation.

Site of involvement

Thoracic disk herniations can occur at any level but are more common at T8-9, T9-10, T10-11, and T11-12. A T12-L1 herniation also is rather common. As in the cervical and lumbar regions, thoracic herniations occur predominantly in spinal segments that are mobile and subject to excessive stress. The upper thoracic segments, which are relatively immobile, seem less prone to herniations. Arseni and Nash[3] compiled the incidence of thoracic herniations from the literature up to 1963. Including their own 23 patients, they collected 148 for a total of 171 patients. We have added 129 patients from the following series in which the site of involvement was specified: Fisher,[12] Love and Schorn,[13] Arumugasamy,[14] Feiring,[15] Carson et al.,[10] Alberico,[16] Benson and Byrnes,[17] Gelch,[18] and Kretschmer and Gustorf.[19] An additional 85 patients of our own are included, bringing the total to 385. The distribution of thoracic disk herniations in these patients was as follows: 279 at T7 to T12, 101 at T3 to T7, and the remaining 3 at T1 to T3.

Age and sex

The great majority of the patients are in their fourth and fifth decades, but patients as young as 12 and as old as 76 years have been reported. The disease seems to be slightly more common among men, with the male/female ratio at about 59 to 41.

Thoracic disk herniation and Scheuermann's disease

The prevalence of degenerative disk disease, both thoracic and lumbar, is higher in subjects who have Scheuermann's disease. Taveras and Wood,[20] in their classic textbook (1964) on neuroradiology, made the statement that thoracic disk herniations are often seen in relatively young individuals who have Scheuermann's disease with exaggerated thoracic kyphosis. The herniation usually occurs at the apex of the kyphosis, which, along with the higher incidence of disk degeneration, seems to contribute to the increased chances of disk herniation in these subjects.

Paajanen et al.,[21] reporting on 21 cases of Scheuermann's disease, noted that in 55% of their patients the disks were abnormal on MRI compared to 10% in controls. These patients were 13 to 36 years of age (mean 20 ± 3.5 years), and the authors felt that their study confirmed the observation that in patients with Scheuermann's disease, even at an early age, the thoracolumbar disks tend to be abnormal. They synopsized current thinking on the natural history of Scheuermann's with the following observations: one study[22] has hypothesized that the disease is simply a stress spondylodystrophy induced by static loading in a flexed position, with the prolonged load causing growth arrest and endplate fractures; another[23] has suggested that prolapses of disk tissue through the endplates are secondary to reduced mechanical strength in the defective areas; and several others[24-27] support the theory that axial compressive forces can cause Schmorl nodes in the thoracolumbar spine, with the disks becoming more vulnerable to desiccation after vertebral collapse.

In fact, an epidemiological study of patients with Scheuermann's disease[28] has shown twice the prevalence of lumbar spondylosis as in symptom-free controls, leading the investigators to conclude that Scheuermann's is an important etiological factor in spondylosis. Two additional studies, using microradiography[29] and diskography,[30] have pointed to the coexistence of Schmorl nodes and disk degeneration in Scheuermann patients.

Our own studies have produced 12 patients with

Scheuermann's disease and herniated disks in the thoracic region (out of 55 with surgically documented thoracic disk herniations).

CLINICAL FINDINGS

The clinical findings in patients with a thoracic herniation are dependent upon the following:
1. The specific disk or disk levels involved
2. The location of the herniation—median (central), paramedian, or lateral
3. The size of the herniation
4. The duration of illness
5. The size of the canal, and the presence or absence of thoracic spondylosis causing spinal stenosis

In the thoracic spine, because of moderate normal kyphosis, the cord resides in the anterior portion of the canal, but is not stretched against the anterior wall of the canal (Fig. 7-1). In patients with increased kyphosis (e.g., due to Scheuermann's disease [Fig. 7-2], but also to other causes [Fig. 7-3]) the cord is stretched against the anterior

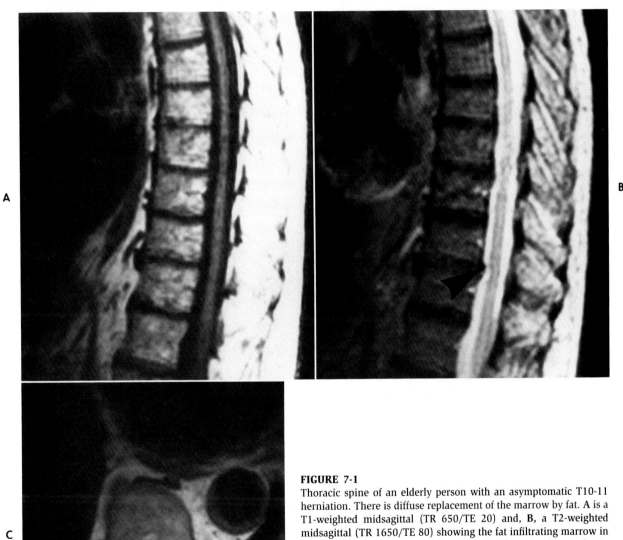

FIGURE 7-1
Thoracic spine of an elderly person with an asymptomatic T10-11 herniation. There is diffuse replacement of the marrow by fat. A is a T1-weighted midsagittal (TR 650/TE 20) and, **B**, a T2-weighted midsagittal (TR 1650/TE 80) showing the fat infiltrating marrow in **A** and the herniation *(arrowhead)* in **B**. There is also moderate degenerative hypertrophy at T8-9, and a slight thoracic scoliosis is present. **C** is an axial MRI at T9. Note the fat infiltrating marrow. The cord is slightly displaced to the left of midline.

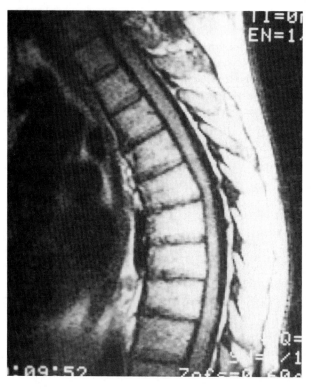

FIGURE 7-2
Scheuermann's disease of the thoracic spine. The cord is pressing against the posterior surface of the vertebral column at the apex of the kyphosis.

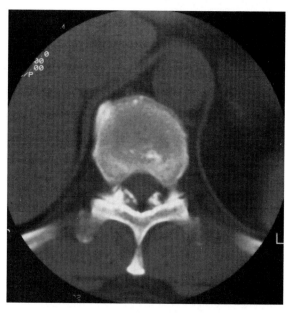

FIGURE 7-4
Thoracic spinal stenosis. Calcification of the ligamenta flava and degeneration of the facet joints are evident. Note also Fig. 4-23.

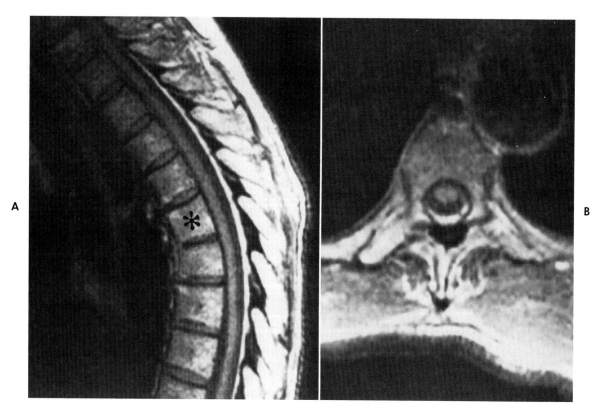

FIGURE 7-3
Kyphotic thoracic spine. **A,** A midsagittal and, **B,** an axial T1-weighted cross section through T5 showing the apex of the kyphosis at T6. The *asterisk* in **A** is on T5. The cord, in the anterior portion of the canal, appears draped against the posterior surfaces of the vertebrae.

wall of the canal. Thus, even a small herniation can cause compression and focal atrophy of the spinal canal.

Young subjects who have a relatively marked kyphosis or one with a sharp angulation (as, for example, after traumatic vertebral fracture) are more likely to develop herniations at the apex of the kyphosis. The cord in these patients is stretched against the posteriorly protruding surfaces of the vertebrae and is more prone to compression, even with small disk protrusions. Thus, although the size of the canal is an important factor, one should not overlook the degree of thoracic kyphosis. The thoracic canal may be normal, or even capacious, relative to the size of the cord; but because the cord is relatively fixed in the anterior canal, it can become compressed by even a small herniated disk.

Generally, when the canal is fairly large and has no exaggerated kyphosis, small thoracic herniations can exist without manifestations; a marked kyphosis or stenosis predisposes the cord to earlier and more severe injury. Congenital stenosis in the thoracic region is rare. Acquired stenosis also is rare, but it does occur secondary to degenerative disease of the facet joints and calcification of the ligamentum flavum (Fig. 7-4) (see also Fig. 4-23).

In patients with C7-T1, T1-2, and T2-3 herniations a syndrome consisting of radiculopathy and myelopathy affecting the shoulder, arm, and chest wall is noted; Horner's syndrome may also be present. Gelch[18] has described a typical case:

A 40-year-old patient admitted to hospital with severe pain in the right side of his neck and chest wall and medial aspect of his right arm, as well as weakness of his right hand and Horner's syndrome, had weakness of the first dorsal and other interosseous muscles of the right hand with hypesthesia along the ulnar aspect of the forearm to the ring and small fingers. On oblique and AP myelograms a smooth epidural defect was seen on the right side, obliterating the nerve root at T1-2. The cord was not displaced, and the neural foramen was not enlarged. The lateral view was normal. At surgery three sequestered disk fragments were removed anterior to the origin of the T1 root. The patient made an uneventful recovery.

A herniation of the T1-2 disk is uncommon. Love and Schorn[13] described only one in 61 cases of thoracic herniation. Murphey et al.[31] reported 4 cases among their 648 patients with "lateral ruptured cervical disk." The clinical findings in these patients often resembled, but did differ from, a cervical root compression syndrome.

Pathogenesis of Horner's syndrome in thoracic disk herniation

According to Gelch[18] the manifestations in Horner's syndrome most likely result from compression of the anterior root of T1, which contains the myelinated axons of sympathetic nerve cells that originate in the mediolateral columns of the C8 and T1 cord segments. The white ramus communicans, which these axons form, has preganglionic fibers that are interrupted before they course upward through the sympathetic chain to the superior cervical ganglion. The anastomotic body has a nonmedulated axon that runs with the carotid plexus to the cavernous sinus, where it enters the right orbit through the superior orbital fissure to the levator palpebrae superioris, dilator pupillae, and musculus orbitalis (Müller) (which maintains the normal position of the eye). Thus compression of the anterior root of T1 by a herniated disk can result in a complete Horner's syndrome.

Vertebral level and location of the herniation

According to Gelch[18] the T1 root compression syndrome consists of pain in the neck, medial border of the scapula, anterior chest, and medial aspect of the upper arm and forearm. There may be hypesthesia along the ulnar aspect of the forearm, weakness in the intrinsic hand muscles, and Horner's syndrome.

The disks from T2 to T9 may be associated with pain surrounding the scapula and tip of the shoulder as well as the chest wall that is at times mistaken for gallbladder disease, disorders of other intraabdominal organs, or diseases of the scapula or shoulder joint. Most patients have a slowly evolving myelopathy. Those with T11-12 and T12-L1 herniation may also have a conus syndrome (i.e., lumbar neuropathy with bladder and rectal sphincter disturbances).

The location of disk herniation is to some extent responsible for the pattern of clinical manifestations. Most patients with central or centrolateral disk herniation present with an essentially progressive myelopathy. Those with strictly lateral herniation may have localized thoracic neuropathy, but this is uncommon and occurs in only 13% to 15% of cases.

Duration of the herniation

The duration of the disease is usually reflected in a long-standing cord compression syndrome secondary to untreated thoracic herniation with paraparesis or paralysis. In patients with long-standing cord compression, after surgery an initial remission may develop, sometimes with almost complete recovery of the neurological deficit, lasting for several months to a few years; however, this may be followed by delayed degenerative changes of the cord (i.e., syringomyelia with paralysis). This is sometimes seen even in patients who present with moderate neurological deficit prior to surgery.

The size of the spinal canal and the presence of stenosis are important factors. Patients who have a large canal may tolerate a herniated disk for a fairly long time. On the other hand, patients whose canal is stenotic to begin with are usually less able to tolerate such compression. This is true whether the stenosis is congenital or acquired. An acquired stenosis (Figs. 4-23 and 7-4) occurs in patients who have extensive degenerative disease of the facet joints with infolding of the ligamentum flavum (which may be calcified) and calcification of the facet joint capsules.

Pain

Except for patients who have T1-2 and T2-3 herniations or those with a lateral herniation, the pain felt generally is dull, ill defined, and migratory. A review of cases in the literature reveals that some 55% to 60% of patients complain of vague and diffuse, but not severe, pain affecting the thoracic, thoracolumbar, or lumbar area with occasional radiation to the lower extremities. The pain usually does not have a definite radicular nature, except in patients with strictly lateral herniations, and in these cases it may be felt along the chest wall with a fairly specific distribution. The pain may be sharp, even at times excruciating. It may also be felt deep within the chest or abdomen, particularly in the retrogastric area, and then the clinical picture is so confusing that patients have been surgically explored for investigation of an intraabdominal disease.

Approximately 20% of patients describe a dull backache with radiation into the posterior and lateral aspect of the thigh. Radiation into the calf and foot is relatively uncommon, and into the toes extremely uncommon. Nevertheless, back pain with radiation into the lower extremities can mimic the lumbar disk syndrome. The problem is further complicated by the fact that a significant number of these patients will indeed have extensive degenerative disease of the lumbar spine as well as herniation of one or more disks. However, myelopathy is not ordinarily a manifestation of lumbar disk disease, and its presence should suggest involvement of a higher segment of the spine.

Also it is important to be careful in patients with T12-L1, and occasionally L1-2 disk herniation, because a conus syndrome may be present. Furthermore, the manifestations of spinal cord involvement may appear in patients with an abnormally low cord termination. Sciatica was noted in two of 23 patients from Arseni and Nash's study,[3] in five of our 85 patients, and in 16% of 242 patients collected from the literature.

Myelopathy

The cardinal manifestation of thoracic disk herniation is a slowly evolving myelopathy. The clinical manifestations of this resemble the manifestations of cord compression secondary to tumors within the thoracic spinal canal. There may be no significant pain, and differentiation from a neoplasm causing compression of the cord may be impossible. Indeed, according to Arseni and Nash,[3] there have been about 10 cases of intrathoracic neoplasm causing compression of the cord for every 1 thoracic disk herniation causing cord compression.

Abbott and Retter[9] distinguished three large groups of thoracic disk herniations—midline and paramedian (causing classic progressive myelopathy), T11-12 and T12-L1 (causing a cauda equina syndrome), and lateral (with a clear-cut syndrome of root compression and minor or no cord compression). The lateral herniations were most frequently mistaken for various visceral disorders, as also reported by Epstein,[32] Kroll and Reiss,[8] and Arseni and Nash.[3] A review of the literature indicates that some 8% to 10% of patients present with symptoms mimicking those of visceral disorders.

The various signs of thoracic cord compression consist of the following:

1. Contraction of the paravertebral muscles (30% to 42%)
2. Sensory disturbances (practically 100%)
3. Motor weakness (usually about 85%)

The sensory disturbances may be noted in higher thoracic dermatomes than the level at which the herniation is discovered. They are not due to ischemia from compression of the anterior spinal artery, as was thought in the past, because the anterior spinal artery is not an end-artery. Rather they probably arise from myelomalacia with syrinx formation at the site of compression as well as proximal and distal to the apex of compression. The artery has multiple radicular branches at various levels of the spinal column, and thus a focal block of the artery is not likely to cause ischemia of the more proximal cord segments. However, the precise mechansim of myelomalacia of the proximal cord segments is not known.

Motor weakness

The patient may complain of heaviness in the feet, dragging of the feet, stumbling, poor control of leg and foot motion, and frequent falling. Physical examination reveals various degrees of motor loss. In more advanced stages paraparesis and paralysis may be noted. Bladder and sphincter control is impaired in slightly more than half the patients.

Trauma

The role of trauma in the pathogenesis of thoracic disk herniation is controversial. We have seen two patients (out of 85) who had a history of significant trauma. A motor vehicle accident preceded the diagnosis of thoracic herniation in one by 8 years and in the other by 2.

Arseni and Nash[3] believe that trauma plays a significant role in this disease. In 5 of their 23 patients it was considered the initiating cause. Other investigators—including Logue,[7] Love and Schorn,[13] and Tovi and Strang[33]—have also reported thoracic herniations following major trauma to the spine. This is usually encountered in young people, who immediately or shortly after a more or less violent traumatic incident involving the spine (with or without vertebral fracture) develop pain and neurological deficit. Progression to a clear-cut cord compression syndrome seldom takes longer than 6 or 7 months, although (less commonly) it may take several years and follow multiple episodes. Arseni and Nash[3] considered 11 of their 23 patients to fit into this category (i.e., due to repeated trauma).

A fairly distinct category of patients prone to traumatic disk herniation consists of those with relatively acute angle thoracic kyphosis. Thus it is advisable to keep this possibility in mind when examining patients with thoracic kyphosis (e.g., Scheuermann's disease, old healed tuberculous spondylitis, or other causes).

RADIOGRAPHIC FINDINGS
Conventional roentgenography and tomography

The abnormalities on conventional roentgenography and tomography are subtle and require technically superb studies. Calcification of one or more disks was noted in 19 patients in our series (Figs. 7-5 and 7-6), and Baker et al.,[34] who reviewed 43 surgically documented cases, found 12 instances. (Interestingly, the calcification was noted in more than two disks in 10 of their patients.) In our series, 14 patients had more than two calcified disks and all but six were herniated, whereas in the series of Baker et al. all but three calcified disks were herniated. Thus, although calcification of thoracic disks is common, it is not diagnostic of disk herniation.

We reviewed 287 thoracic spine studies in patients seen for various spinal disorders and noted thoracic calcification in 12 patients. Thoracic intradiskal calcification generally indicates the presence of disk degeneration and is likely to be seen in older individuals, often involving more than one disk. Most herniations are found in calcified disks, although even in patients who have intradiskal calcification herniation may occur in a disk that is not calcified.

When a calcified disk protrudes into the spinal canal or a calcified herniation extends cephalad or caudad beyond

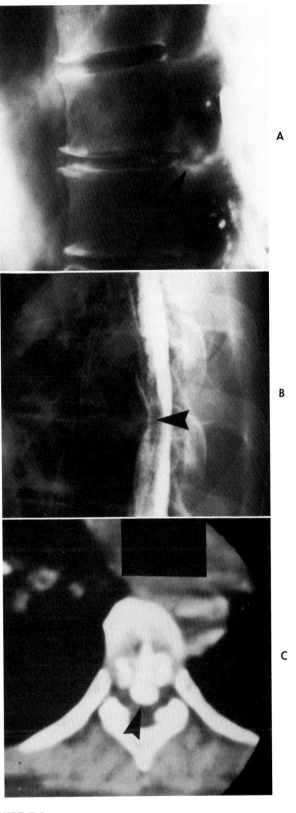

A

B

C

FIGURE 7-6
Calcified herniated T8-9 disk. **A,** Lateral tomogram of the thoracic spine. The *arrowhead* points to a large density within the canal on the posterior aspect of the disk. There is calcification within the disk substance also. **B,** Lateral view of a myelogram. The calcification is compressing the anterior surface of the dural sac and displacing the cord posteriorly *(arrowhead).* **C,** A computed tomogram shows the calcification *(arrowhead).*

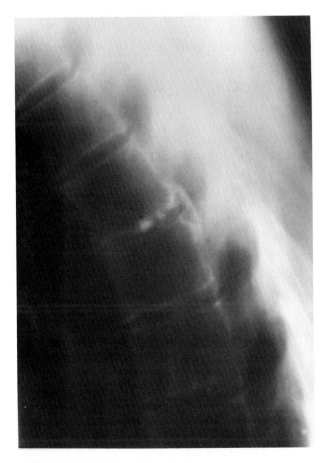

FIGURE 7-5
A calcified herniated thoracic disk on lateral tomography is clearly outlined.

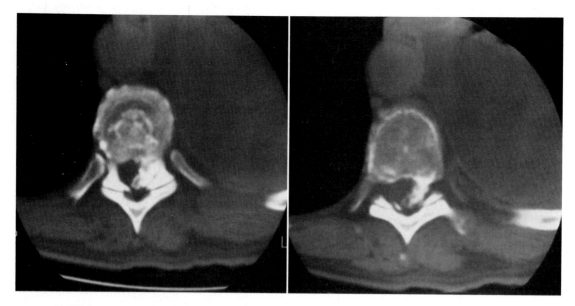

FIGURE 7-7
Calcified herniated thoracic disk. The calcified herniated material occupies nearly 50% of the canal at T9-10.

the disk level, the diagnosis of thoracic disk herniation becomes increasingly likely (Fig. 7-6) on conventional radiography. Other possibilities, however, are calcification and ossification of the posterior longitudinal ligament and calcified intraspinal tumors (e.g., a meningioma and, occasionally, a neurofibroma). Differentiation of calcified neoplasms from calcified herniated disks in the spinal canal may not be possible on conventional radiography. One needs to determine whether the calcification is continuous with the disk (if so, a calcified herniation becomes likely), and for this computed tomography is better (Figs. 7-7 to 7-10). Among our patients 4 had calcified thoracic disks with an extruded fragment in the spinal canal detected by CT. Among the 43 patients reviewed by Baker et al.,[34] 5 had an extruded calcified disk detected on retrospective analysis (three detected on a prospective preoperative review).

Tomography of the thoracic spine often is helpful in more precisely delineating a calcified thoracic disk, and particularly a calcified extruded fragment of a disk (Figs. 7-5 and 7-6). The fragment is usually situated in the anterior portion of the canal, occupying 20% to 30% of the canal, although in long-standing cases it may occupy 80% to 90% of the canal (Figs. 7-9 and 7-11). Then the cord is markedly compressed. Nevertheless, the clinical findings in some of these patients may not be impressive. The situation is similar to cord compression in a patient with calcification and ossification of the posterior longitudinal ligament (OPLL), who may have a massive calcified ligament causing compression of the cord but no clinical findings. We believe that whether or not a person with spinal stenosis is symptomatic depends upon the size of the canal and the speed with which the stenosis develops.[57] If the canal is large, relatively large calcified

herniations, osteophytes, or OPLL may be asymptomatic, particularly if stenosis develops very slowly. If the canal is narrow, even small lesions, particularly those that develop rapidly, may produce evidence of myelopathy. It seems that the cord has a high degree of tolerance to slowly developing mechanical pressure, as in OPLL and some thoracic disk herniations.[57] In these patients the cord conforms to the distorted canal, filling most of the available space, and despite marked deformity of the cord there may be no neurological findings. However, when there is absolutely no more room, any additional pressure (e.g., swelling and edema secondary to a minor trauma) may be sufficient to alter the precarious balance and cause just enough compression to precipitate a neurological catastrophe.

In some patients a fairly specific pattern of vertebral hypertrophic change is seen. There may be hypertrophic changes of the endplates and half of the vertebral bodies adjacent to a herniated disk. This should alert the observer to the possibility of a thoracic disk herniation.

Myelography

Until relatively recently, myelography was the only modality able to disclose the presence of a thoracic herniated disk. At present MRI is gradually replacing it for this purpose. As stated by Baker et al.,[34] if the diagnosis of a thoracic disk herniation is to be made at all one must keep the possibility in mind to ensure that appropriate roentgenographic studies are obtained. Myelography of the thoracic region is more demanding than of the cervical and lumbar regions: the contrast is difficult to position, and at least 10 cc (often more) must be used; after administration it must be watched carefully during

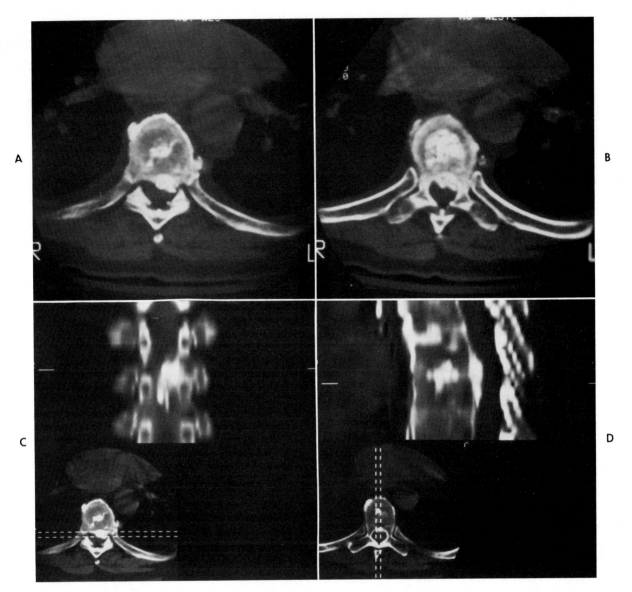

FIGURE 7-8
A herniated T7-8 disk. **A** and **B**, Computed tomograms show calcification of the disk substance as well as the herniated portion, which is in the midline and to the left of midline. **C** and **D**, Sagittal and coronal reformatting reveals that the disk extends superiorly and inferiorly in the canal, mostly to the left of midline.

fluoroscopy, and multiple projections (supine, prone, oblique, and lateral) may be needed; in most cases similar views with the overhead x-ray tube must be used at the conclusion of the study (transtable horizontal, supine, prone, oblique, and lateral); lateral and frontal projections may also be needed for a more precise delineation of the abnormality. In our series myelography was available in 50 patients and showed an epidural defect against the disk in 47.

When the herniated disk is of moderate size, there is usually no problem in its identification. However, when it is large or even medium sized, with congenital or acquired stenosis, there may be a complete block. At first, only the caudal aspect of the defect will be visualized. It

may also be necessary to inject contrast via a C1-2 lateral puncture. The myelographic configuration may suggest an intradural extramedullary tumor (Fig. 7-12, *A*) such as meningioma or neurofibroma. When the cord is compressed against the wall of the spinal canal, it may appear wider, superficially resembling an intramedullary tumor. However, myelographic views at a 90-degree angle to this plane (Figs. 7-11, *A*, 7-12, *B*, and 7-13, *M*) will show the extramedullary nature of the defect.

In some patients the extruded thoracic disk is attached to the dura and gradually becomes embedded in and may even perforate it. This is rare but has been reported by Fisher[12] and others.[14] Even more uncommon is for the calcified disk to perforate the cord. As the thoracic

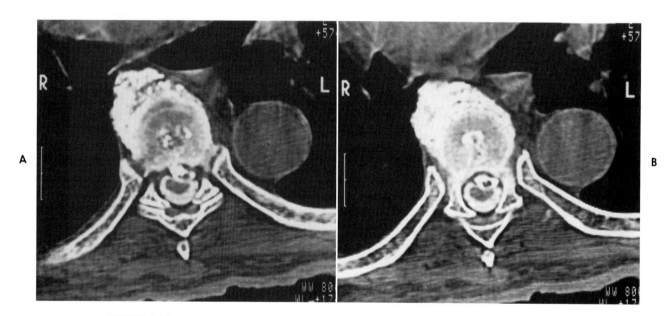

FIGURE 7-9
A calcified herniated T7-8 disk. **A** is an axial CT, bone window setting, showing the intradiskal calcification *(arrowheads)*. **B,** A midsagittal reformatted image shows the calcified herniated disk in the canal.

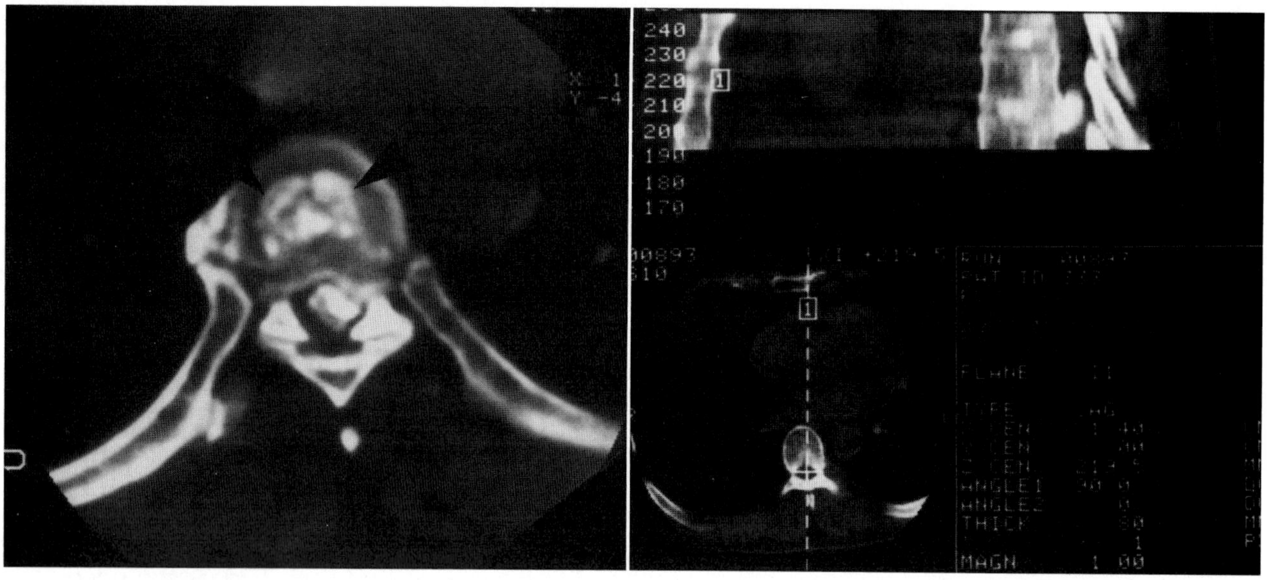

FIGURE 7-10
A patient with Forestier's disease. **A** and **B** are CT-myelograms at T6-7. In **A** there is intradiskal calcification with herniation to the left of midline. The cord is slightly rotated to the left. In **B** the calcification can be seen extending through the dura and in contact with the cord. A large calcification is present on the anterolateral surface of the vertebral body on the right side.

herniation enlarges, it displaces the dura posteriorly, but dural attachments remain on its lateral aspects and may become infolded. On myelography a pattern indistinguishable from that of an intradural extramedullary mass, at least in one view, is seen. This was noted by Baker et al.[34] and was present in four patients of our series (Fig. 7-12, *A*).

In some patients the calcified herniated disk attaches to

the dura and causes fixation of the dura at that point. It may extend superiorly and inferiorly into the spinal canal, moving to a different position (e.g., right to left and sometimes posteriorly) as it extends above and below the level of the herniated disk. Thus the dural sac and spinal cord may remain in one position and then move to the other side, anteriorly, or posteriorly.

In some patients the calcified material will not produce

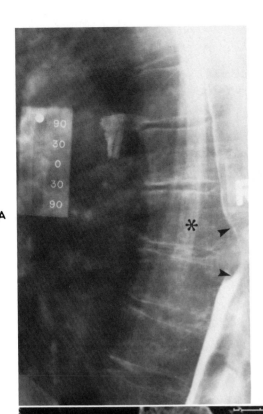

FIGURE 7-11

A calcified herniated T6-7 disk. **A,** Lateral view of a thoracic myelogram with the patient prone. The *asterisk* is on T6. Note that the cord has been posteriorly displaced against the posterior wall of the canal by an epidural defect *(arrowheads)*. **B** and **C,** CT-myelograms show the calcified disk, with a herniation occupying some 70% of the canal. The cord is posteriorly displaced and forced against the left lateral wall of the canal. **D** and **E,** Immediately adjacent to the disk. (The *arrowheads* point to displacement of the cord.) The *curved arrow* in **E** points to the herniated disk, and the *arrow* to contrast in the posterior subarachnoid space on the right.

Continued.

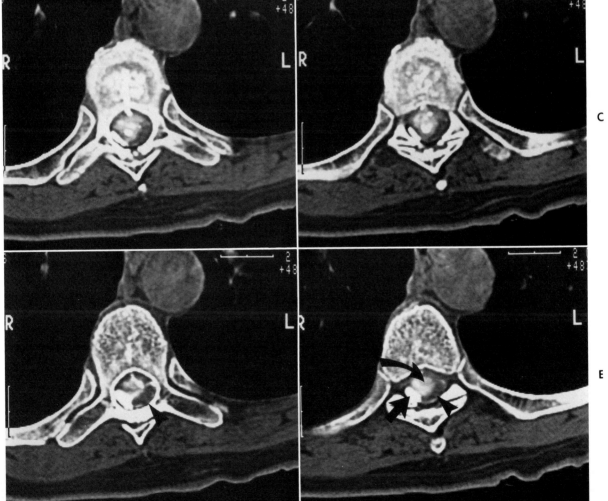

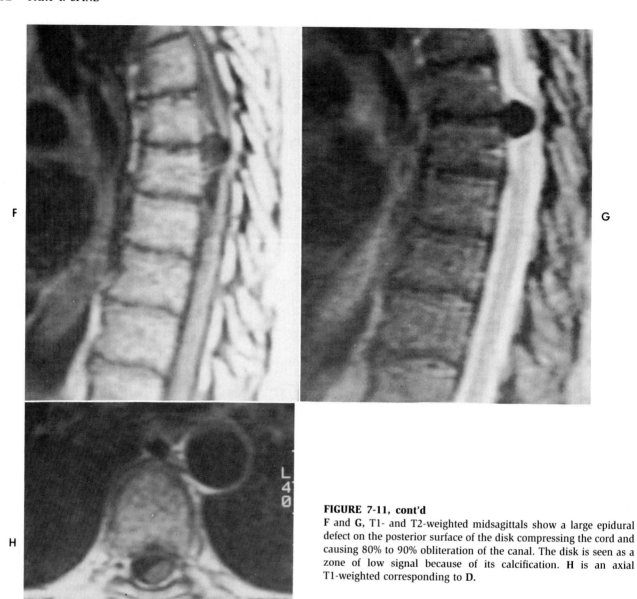

FIGURE 7-11, cont'd
F and G, T1- and T2-weighted midsagittals show a large epidural defect on the posterior surface of the disk compressing the cord and causing 80% to 90% obliteration of the canal. The disk is seen as a zone of low signal because of its calcification. H is an axial T1-weighted corresponding to D.

an anterior epidural mass but, instead, may extend to one side of the canal and posteriorly. The dural sac may become fixed against the posterior surfaces of the disk and vertebral body, without displacement posteriorly, but the cord may be compressed and flattened or deviated (Figs. 7-7 and 7-13). Careful examination with CT and CT-myelography is necessary to understand the nature of this abnormality and the puzzling tortuous course that the dural sac and cord can assume, particularly when there is no epidural defect and the bulk of the mass is on

one side of the canal or even posteriorly. In these cases the sac and cord may be fixed anteriorly, usually with some deviation to either side.

To visualize the extent of the calcification in the spinal canal, and to avoid any confusion between contrast and a poorly calcified herniated disk or neoplasm, it is important to do a CT examination before obtaining a myelogram or CT-myelogram. The myelogram may be normal even in the presence of a herniated disk verified at surgery. On three of a total 50 myelograms in our series,

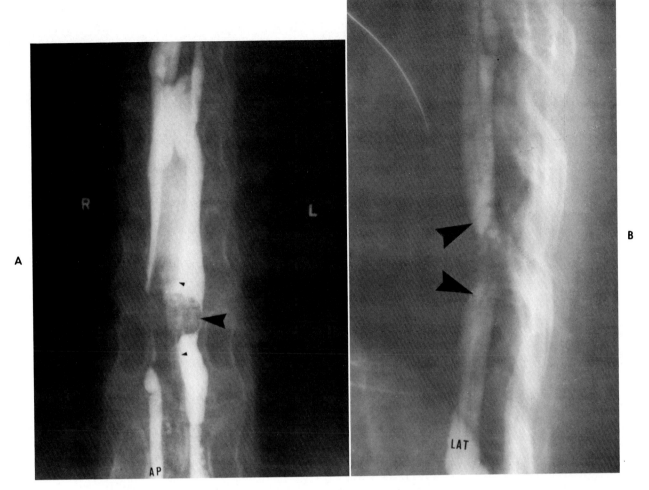

FIGURE 7-12
A T8-9 herniated disk. A is an anteroposterior view of a thoracic myelogram showing a defect in the contrast column that resembles an intradural defect *(large arrowhead)*. The *small arrowheads* denote displacement of the cord to the right. The subarachnoid space is widened on the left side and obliterated on the right, findings that suggest an intradural mass. B, A lateral view of the myelogram clarifies the position of the lesion. A definite epidural defect *(large arrowheads)* is visible against the posterior surface of the disk.

this happened when the disk was small and the curvature of the spine such that it would not permit the herniation to be delineated. To lessen this possibility, the myelographer should be alert to the probable location of an extradural lesion. Baker et al.[34] recommend fluoroscopy in the oblique and lateral positions or obtaining prone lateral overhead films. We also believe fluoroscopy in multiple positions is helpful, with simultaneous recording of findings on videotape.

Myelography in 36 surgically verified thoracic herniated disks has been reported on by Baker et al.[34] Nothing abnormal was found in three of the studies, despite the subsequent finding at surgery of well-defined though small herniations. This is not uncommon. Others — including Abbott and Retter,[9] Arseni and Nash,[3,36] and Terracciano and Ambrosio[37] — have reported similar findings. Myelography showed a central defect in 27, a centrolateral defect in 11, and a lateral defect in 6 patients in our series. In the larger reported series from the

literature, the approximate distribution of these lesions has been central 55%, centrolateral 33%, lateral 12%.

The introduction of water-soluble contrast medium for myelography has facilitated thoracic myelography. The number of patients manifesting a complete block is significantly less with water-soluble contrast and, on delayed films, almost all patients show passage of contrast beyond the point of block.

Computed tomography

Computed tomography was available in 45 patients in our series and showed the presence of a calcified herniated disk (Figs. 7-7 to 7-10, 7-11, 7-13, and 7-14) in 36, all verified at surgery. It must be noted, however, that CT may not show uncalcified soft thoracic herniations and reformatted coronal or sagittal images (Figs. 7-8 and 7-9) will be needed for a precise three-dimensional localization of calcified herniations. In some patients axial CT cross sections show what seems to be a channel

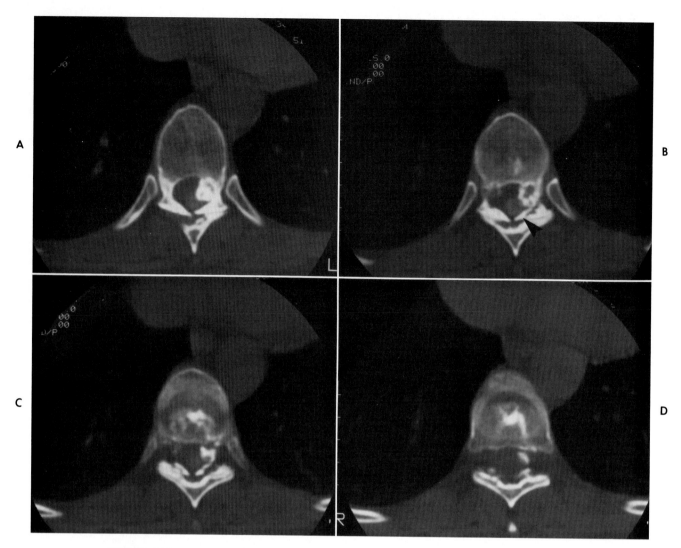

FIGURE 7-13
A calcified herniated T9-10 disk causing displacement and fixation of the cord in the anterolateral canal. **A** and **B,** Axial CT slices through T10 show a calcified lesion on the left side. The ligamentum flavum also is calcified *(arrowhead).* **C** and **D** are CT slices showing the intradiskal calcification along with calcification of the lesion in the canal and the ligamentum flavum.

in the disk substance, through which herniation has occurred.

CT-myelography

CT-myelography is still the gold standard in diagnosing thoracic disk herniations (Figs. 7-10, 7-11, 7-13, and 7-14). It can be performed with a small amount of water-soluble contrast instilled into the subarachnoid space. Computed tomographic slices can then be obtained any time from a few minutes to several hours after the instillation. Depending on the nature of abnormalities detected by the initial set of CT images, one may want to repeat the CT in several hours. Reformatted coronal and sagittal cross sections of CT-myelography (Fig. 7-14) are helpful for delineating these abnormalities three-dimensionally.

Magnetic resonance

The introduction of high-resolution MRI examination has changed the work-up of patients suspected of having thoracic disk herniation, thoracic neoplasms, or myelopathy.[38] It is the modality of choice for initially screening these patients and demonstrate herniated thoracic disks, either calcified or not in practically all cases (Figs. 7-11 and 7-13).

We have had experience with 18 MRI examinations of the thoracic spine in which the diagnosis of a herniated thoracic disk was made and subsequently verified at surgery. The examination is performed with a high-resolution imager and slices 4 to 5 mm thick in the sagittal plane. We have found T1-weighted and gradient echo images to be helpful for screening purposes. When the abnormal disk levels are identified, sagittal and axial

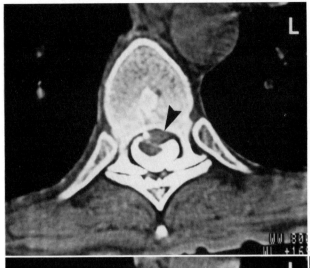

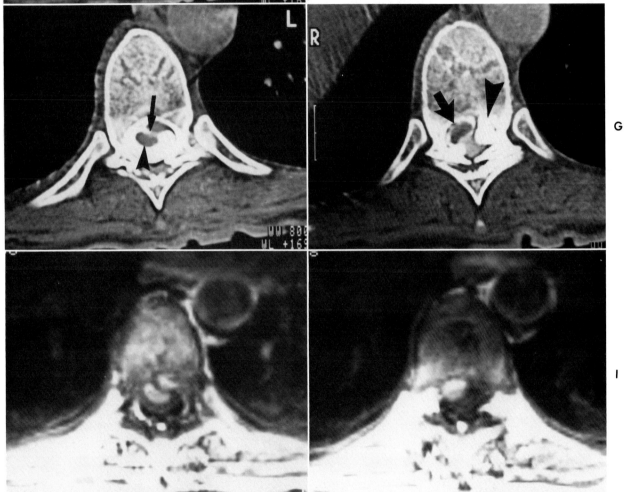

FIGURE 7-13, cont'd

E to G are CT myelograms. The *arrowhead* in E points to herniation extending superiorly behind T9. The cord is deformed, rotated, and displaced to the right. There is also calcification adjacent to the dura. The *arrow* in F points to opacified CSF in the subarachnoid space (which is being compressed by the herniation). The *arrowhead* denotes the cord. G, just above the disk, shows the cord displaced to the right *(arrow)*, with a calcified fragment *(arrowhead)* on the left. H, A T1-weighted axial cross section shows the rotated and displaced cord identical to that seen in E and F. The herniated material is hyperintense relative to the disk and is separated from the cord by the signal void of CSF and dura (note the *arrow* in F). I shows the cord displaced to the right in the anterior part of the canal. In this position the disk was adherent to the dura and cord.

Continued.

cross sections 3 to 4 mm thick and utilizing multiple pulse sequences, including T1 and T2 weighted, are obtained. On T1-weighted sagittal cross sections the posterior border of the involved thoracic disk can be seen to protrude into the spinal canal for at least 3 or 4 mm often significantly more.

The herniated material is usually of extremely low signal intensity, often a zone of signal void (Figs. 7-13, *H* to *K,* and 7-11, *F* to *H*), that appears as a spherical or ovoid mass of similar signal intensity to the annulus–posterior longitudinal ligament complex (Figs. 7-13, *K,* and 7-11, *G*). It may mimic a calcified neoplasm within the canal, compressing, deforming, rotating, or displacing the cord. Axial sections will show the precise relationship of the

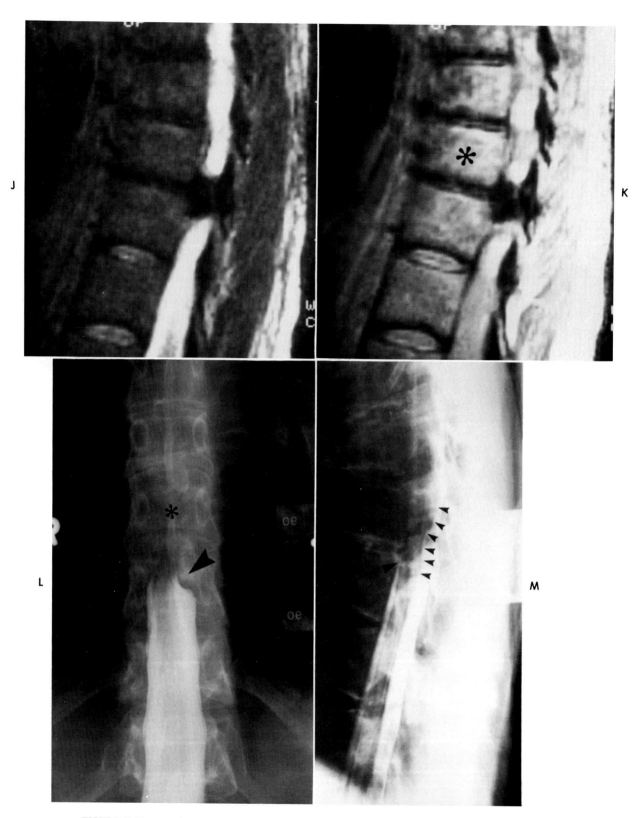

FIGURE 7-13, cont'd
J is a T2-weighted left parasagittal and, **K,** a proton density parasagittal cross section. The *asterisk* in
K is on T9. Note the reduced signal from the disk because of degenerative disease. The large area of
signal void corresponds to the region of calcification. **L,** An AP view of a myelogram. The *asterisk* is on
T9, and the *arrowhead* points to widening of the subarachnoid space on the left, which mimicks an
intradural lesion. The cord is displaced to the right. **M,** A lateral view shows moderate widening of the
cord due to the left-to-right compression. (The smaller *arrowheads* indicate the cord.) There is a curved
configuration to the cord, which returns to the midportion of the canal in the AP dimension. (The *lower
three arrowheads* denote the widening, and the *upper three arrowheads* the cord's return to the central
part of the canal.) Note the expansion of the cord with obliteration of the subarachnoid space *(large
arrowhead).*

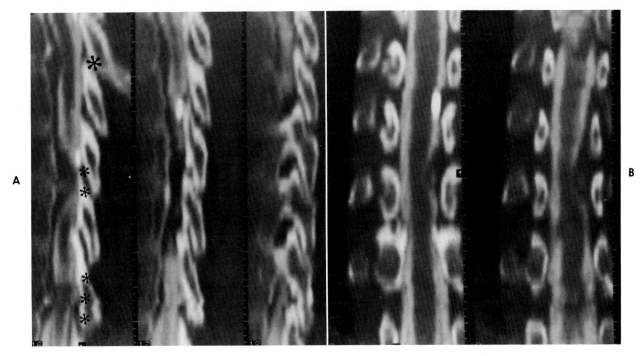

FIGURE 7-14
Three herniated thoracic disks in the same patient. **A,** Reformatted sagittal and parasagittal image of a CT-myelogram. There is an anterior epidural defect, which has caused compression of the subarachnoid space and displacement of the cord posteriorly at T6-7 *(large asterisk)*. A larger epidural defect contains calcification with compression of the cord at T7-8 *(two asterisks)*. Another small epidural defect as T8-9 *(three asterisks)* is visible. **B,** Coronal reformatted image showing the large epidural defect on the right side, patient prone, with the right side corresponding to the observer's right.

disk to the cord. The T2-weighted cross sections provide a myelographic effect with delineation of the extent of subarachnoid compression and separation of CSF from the calcified mass. The disk itself exhibits low signal, indicating degeneration and calcification. Gradient echo images provide information somewhat similar to that from T2-weighted cross sections and seem to offer no diagnostic advantage, although they require less imaging time.

MRI of the thoracic spine is a challenging procedure due mainly to the peculiar anatomy of the thoracic region, the CSF pulsations, and cardiac and respiratory motion. Thus it is essential to utilize gating, spatial presaturation, and other features to obtain the best possible images. Obviously, a surface coil is a must. It is also important to include the cervical spine or the lumbar spine, depending on the suspected level of the thoracic lesion, to assure accurate counting of the thoracic vertebrae. This can easily be done on the initial scout (plan scan), which ordinarily takes a minute or so.

In all 18 patients with thoracic disk herniation in whom we have performed MRI, the herniated material was either of very low signal intensity or no signal on T1-weighted cross sections. Although MRI examination is helpful in most patients, in some the features noted on axial cross sections may be confusing. This is partly due to the low signal intensity of the herniated material and

the difficulty of differentiating it from other intraspinal soft tissues (Figs. 7-11, *H,* and 7-13, *H*). However, CT-myelography usually clarifies the confusion (Figs. 7-11, *C* and *D,* and 7-13, *F* and *G*).

MRI is strongly recommended for all patients with thoracic disk herniation prior to surgical intervention. It is necessary for evaluating the status of the cord. When there is long-standing cord compression, increased signal may appear on T2-weighted cross sections within the cord because of edema or myelomalacia. Although extensive long-term follow-up is still not available, it is felt that when abnormally increased signal is due to edema it disappears along with improvement in the patient's neurological condition, but when the abnormal signal is secondary to myelomalacia it usually shows no change and there is no improvement in the patient's condition.

Some patients with long-standing cord compression will have advanced myelomalacia and intramedullary cysts (syringomyelia). It is important to be aware of this possibility prior to any surgical intervention. The prognosis in patients who already have syringomyelia is poor, and chances of neurological improvement after surgery slim. Thus an accurate assessment of the prognosis is dependent mainly upon the presence or absence of syringomyelia.

Direct mechanical injury to the cord at the time of surgery can cause significant neurological deficit, and in these patients syringomyelia may be noted. Injury to the cord usually occurs when the technique of canal decompression is not optimal. Mechanical injury results when laminectomy is performed and an attempt is made to remove a midline calcified herniation from in front of the cord. The chances of injury are extremely high in this situation.

Some patients with long-standing cord compression, even after decompression and without surgical mechanical injury, are prone to late-onset neurological deterioration (usually with syringomyelia). It is possible that the long-standing compression prior to surgery has produced injury to the cord sufficient to allow the development of myelomalacia, even after the decompression.

Thus not all instances of intramedullary cavitation are secondary to direct mechanical injury during surgical decompression. Another factor that should not be overlooked is the possibility that the patient may have had a nondetectable cord abnormality prior to surgical decompression.

INDICATIONS FOR SURGERY

Progressive signs and symptoms of spinal cord dysfunction due to thoracic disk herniation are absolute indications for surgical intervention, because pressure on the cord must be relieved without delay if progressive myelopathy is to be halted and the chances of late-onset neurological deterioration reduced.[39-41] Patients with strictly lateral herniations may have only radicular pain, without evidence of cord compression. We do not recommend surgery for them unless they are unable or unwilling to live with the disease.

A number of surgical techniques exist for decompressing the thoracic spinal canal:

1. Transthoracic transpleural approach[39-44]
2. Anterolateral extrapleural approach, or a modified costotransversectomy[45]
3. Posterolateral approach (through a laminectomy, facetectomy, and pediculectomy)[46]

The procedure of choice should be capable of totally removing the protruded disk material within the canal, without manipulation of the cord.[39-41] Because the choice of decompression technique is dependent upon the type of disk herniation present, an accurate preoperative assessment of the gross pathological anatomy of the herniated disk is essential.

GROSS PATHOLOGICAL ANATOMY OF A HERNIATED THORACIC DISK

For surgical purposes a herniated thoracic disk resulting in nerve root or cord compression can be divided into soft and hard varieties.[39]

Soft disk herniations

1. Lateral soft herniation: A posterolateral approach through the lamina, facet, and pedicle is sufficient for safe removal. However, the anterolateral extrapleural

approach of Hulme[45] is also good (if not better). The transthoracic transpleural approach, despite affording the most direct exposure of the anterior aspect of the dura, may be too major a procedure for this situation.
2. Paramedian soft herniation: This lesion can be safely removed with an anterolateral (extrapleural) or transthoracic transpleural approach. The posterolateral is the least desirable.
3. Median soft herniation: This lesion may lie under the posterior longitudinal ligament, but it rarely extrudes past the ligament or penetrates the dura. The procedure of choice is a transthoracic transpleural approach. The anterolateral extrapleural approach is less suitable, and the posterolateral certainly the least suitable.

Hard disk herniations

For all varieties of hard disk herniation, except when there is associated posterolateral spondylosis, the procedure of choice is complete resection via a transthoracic transpleural route. This affords the most direct exposure of dura anteriorly and permits removal of the calcified material without manipulation of the cord. In addition, multiple levels can be approached with ease, and if fusion is deemed necessary it can be readily performed.

Posterolateral spondylosis with cord compression

Posterolateral spondylosis is an extremely rare pathological entity, with only a few reported cases.[47-51] In our series of 85 patients, 12 had this condition (Figs. 4-23 and 7-4). The procedure for the lesion is a posterolateral approach with bilateral removal of the lamina, the medial half of the diseased facet, and the buckled ligamentum flavum. Since by definition there is no anterior herniation of the disk, the cord does not have to be manipulated. In rare cases, when a significant herniation is present anteriorly, the transthoracic transpleural operation with interbody fusion should be done first. At a later date, a laminectomy can be performed and will result in decompression of the cord circumferentially.

Benjamin[40] prefers to open the chest on the right side in all patients for thoracic disk surgery, even though a left-sided exposure can be done and has been preferred by some authors. Benjamin reserves the left side for patients whose pulmonary status precludes opening the chest on the right. We believe this technique is suitable for lesions from T1 to T12. For lesions below T12, a left T9-10 thoracotomy with splitting of the diaphragm is best, to avoid mobilizing the liver. The operation is performed jointly with a thoracic and, if necessary, an abdominal surgeon.

We have used the transthoracic transpleural approach in 53 patients. The results, both in patients reported in the present series and in 93 cases collected from the literature, have been spectacular compared to those reported for laminectomy.

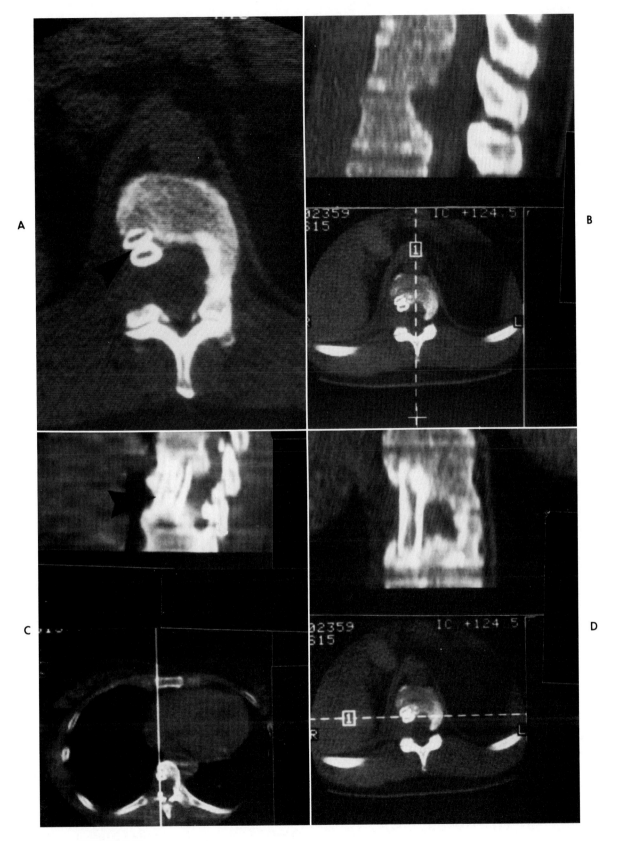

FIGURE 7-15

Postoperative thoracic spine. **A,** Status post—right transthoracic decompression of the canal and resection of a herniated disk at T9-10. The *arrowhead* points to the ribs used for interbody fusion. **B,** A midsagittal reformatted image shows the extent of resection of the T9 and T10 posterior surfaces. **C** is a right parasagittal reformatted image of the ribs used for fusion in A. (The *arrowhead* denotes the ribs.) **D,** A coronal reformatted image shows the extent of bone resection and the ribs used for the interbody fusion.

Laminectomy

The majority of devastating complications in surgery for thoracic disk herniation occur with attempted removal of a median or paramedian herniation via laminectomy, with or without opening of the dura. To reach and remove such a herniated disk, often calcified, in the anterior canal via laminectomy, the surgeon must manipulate the cord significantly. This, unfortunately, leads to cord injury, with resultant worsening of the neurological deficit or creation of a new one in a previously intact patient. Several series[52-55] have reported a new neurological deficit, including paraplegia, in more than half the patients treated by laminectomy.

The first reference in the literature to an anterior approach, rather than laminectomy, for decompression of the thoracic spinal cord is to the work of Capener in 1933. Alexander,[56] reporting in 1946 on work done by Norman Dott and himself, described an anterior approach for decompression of the thoracic canal in patients with Pott's disease and compression of the cord, pointing out the similarity of his technique to that of Capener. Interestingly, in 7 of his patients at surgery one or more calcified herniated thoracic disks were found at the apex of the gibbus. All these were removed through the anterior decompression technique. Capener and Alexander both stated that lateral decompression is obviously ineffective for removal of lesions producing compression of the cord in the anterior canal and they abandoned it after a poor experience in one patient.

Laminectomy, however, has for decades been the standard procedure in patients with thoracic disk herniation, until Hulme[45] reported having had disappointing results with it and deciding to abandon it in favor of the anterolateral approach (with which, in five of six patients, he had a satisfactory outcome).

Crafoord et al.,[42] likewise, reported successfully using an anterolateral approach (fenestration of the disk) to treat thoracic protrusions, and Perot and Munro[43] and Ransohoff, Spencer, et al.[44] described the transthoracic approach for this purpose in separate series, with successful results.

As stated by Maiman et al.,[57] several factors may account for the poor results associated with laminectomy: It is difficult to remove a mass anterior to the spinal cord without manipulating it, at least moderately, and this may be sufficient to cause mechanical injury and interference with blood supply to the cord. In addition, even minor kyphotic deformities initiated by laminectomy can cause a neurological deficit in the presence of inadequately removed disks or osteophytes.

POSTOPERATIVE FOLLOW-UP

When postoperative evaluation is desirable, computed tomography with reformatting is helpful for ascertaining the status of the bony canal as well as the interbody bone graft (Fig. 7-15). MRI examination will delineate the status of the cord. MRI is particularly useful in follow-up of patients in whom an increased signal on T2-weighted cross sections has been noted within the cord. Patients suffering from long-standing cord compression may show focal areas of increased signal on T2-weighted MRI cross sections. Although long-term follow-up is still not available, we believe that these areas may represent zones of edema or myelomalacia. If the high signal is due solely to edema, it may disappear following decompression (along with improvement in the clinical condition). If it is secondary to myelomalacia, a precursor of cavitation, there will usually be no improvement in the patient's condition and an intramedullary cyst may be noted on subsequent MRI examinations.

REFERENCES

1. Fineschi G: Patologia e clinica dell'ernia posteriore del disco intervertebrale. Florence, Edizioni Scientifiche del Istituto Ortopedico Toscano, pp 293-299, 1955.
2. Love JG, Kiefer EJ: Root pain and paraplegia due to protrusions of thoracic intervertebral discs. J Neurosurg 1950;7:62-69.
3. Arseni C, Nash F: Protrusion of thoracic intervertebral disc. Acta Neurochirurg 1963;11:1-33.
4. Kite WC, Whitfield RD, Campbell E: The thoracic herniated intervertebral disc syndrome. J Neurosurg 1957;14:61-67.
5. Schönbauer L: Einige bemerkenswerte Fälle von Bandscheibenvorfall. Arch Klin Chir 1952;271:297-301.
6. O'Connell JEA: Involvement of the spinal cord by intervertebral disc protrusions. Br J Surg 1955;43:225-247.
7. Logue V: Thoracic intervertebral disc prolapse with spinal cord compression. J Neurol Neurosurg Psychiatry 1952;15:227-241.
8. Kroll FW, Reiss E. Der thorakale Bandscheibenprolaps. Dtsh Med Wochenschr 1951;76:600-603.
9. Abbott KH, Retter RH: Protrusions of thoracic intervertebral discs. Neurology 1956;6:1-10.
10. Carson J, Gumpert J, Jefferson A: Diagnosis and treatment of thoracic intervertebral disc protrusions. J Neurol Neurosurg Psychiatry 1971;34:68-77.
11. Haley JC, Perry JH. Protrusions of intervertebral discs. Study of their distribution, characteristics and effects on the nervous system. Am J Surg 1950;80:394-404.
12. Fisher RG: Protrusions of thoracic disc. The factor of herniation through the dura mater. J Neurosurg 1965;22:591-593.
13. Love JG, Schorn VG. Thoracic-disc protrusions. JAMA 1965;191:627-631.
14. Arumugasamy N: Perforation of the spinal cord by a herniated thoracic intervertebral disc: report of a case. Med J Malaya 1969;23:(4)250-252.
15. Feiring EH: Extruded thoracic intervertebral disc. Arch Surg 1967;95:135-137.
16. Alberico AM: High thoracic disc herniation. Neurosurg 1986;19:(3)449-451.
17. Benson MK, Byrnes DP: The clinical syndromes and surgical treatment of thoracic intervertebral disc prolapse. J Bone Joint Surg 1975;57(4):471-477.
18. Gelch MM: Herniated thoracic disc at T1-2 level associated with Horner's syndrome: Case report. J Neurosurg 1978;48(1):128-130.
19. Kretschmer R, Gustorf R: Zur problematik der thorakalen bandscheibenvorfalle. Neurochirurgia 1979;22:41-47.
20. Taveras MJ, Wood EH: Herniated thoracic disks. In Taveras MJ, Wood EH (eds): Diagnostic neuroradiology. Baltimore, Williams & Wilkins, 1964, p 195.
21. Paajanen H, Alanen A, Erkintalo M, et al: Disc degeneration in Scheuermann disease. Skeletal Radiol 1989;18:523-526.
22. Alexander CJ: Scheuermann's disease. A traumatic spondylodystrophy? Skeletal Radiol 1977;1:209-221.

23. Aufdermaur M: Juvenile kyphosis (Scheuermann's disease): radiography, histology, and pathogenesis. Clin Orthop 1981; 154:166-174.

24. Blumenthal SL, Roach J, Herring JA: Lumbar Scheuermann's. A clinical series and classification. Spine 1987;12:929-932.

25. Greene TL, Hensinger RN, Hunter LY: Back pain and vertebral changes simulating Scheuermann's disease. J Pediatr Orthop 1985;5:1-7.

26. Horne J, Cockshott WP, Shannon HS: Spinal column damage from water ski jumping. Skeletal Radiol 1987;16:612-616.

27. McCall IW, Park WM, O'Brien JP, Seal V: Acute traumatic intraosseous disc herniation. Spine 1985;10:134-137.

28. Stoddard A, Osborn JF: Scheuermann's disease or spinal osteochondrosis. J Bone Joint Surg (Br) 1979;61:56-58.

29. Hilton RC, Ball J, Benn RT: Vertebral end-plate lesions (Schmorl's nodes) in the dorsolumbar spine. Ann Rheum Dis 1976;35:127-132.

30. Quinnell RC, Stockdale HR: The significance of osteophytes on lumbar vertebral bodies in relation to discographic findings. Clin Radiol 1982;33:197-203.

31. Murphey F, Simmons JCH, Brunson B: Ruptured cervical discs 1939 to 1972. Clin Neurosurg 1973;20:9-17.

32. Epstein JA: The syndrome of herniation of the lower thoracic intervertebral discs with nerve root and spinal cord compression. A presentation of four cases with a review of the literature, methods of diagnosis and treatment. J Neurosurg 1954;11:525-538.

33. Tovi D, Strang RR: Thoracic intervertebral disc protrusions. Acta Chir Scand (suppl) 1960;267:1-41.

34. Baker HL Jr, Love JC, Uhlein A: Roentgenologic features of protruded thoracic intervertebral discs. Radiology 1965; 84:1059-1065.

35. Firooznia H, Ahn JH, Rafii MR, Ragnarsson KT: Sudden quadriplegia after a minor trauma. The role of preexisting spinal stenosis. Surg Neurol 1985;23:165-168.

36. Arseni C, Nash F: Thoracic intervertebral disc protrusions. A clinical study. J Neurosurg 1960;17:418-430.

37. Terracciano S, Ambrosio A: Contributo allo studio delle ernie discali torciche. Rass Int Clin Ter 1960;40:1028-1043.

38. Ross JS, Perez-Reyes N, Masaryk TJ, et al: Thoracic disk herniation: MR imaging. Radiology 1987;165:511-515.

39. Benjamin V: Diagnosis and management of thoracic disc disease. Clin Neurosurg 1983;30:577-605.

40. Benjamin V: Anterior removal of thoracic disc protrusions. In Ransohoff J (ed): Modern techniques in surgery. Neurosurgery. Mt Kisco NY, Futura, 1979, Chap 18.

41. Benjamin BV, Ransohoff J: Thoracic disc disease. Spine 1975; 1:500-507.

42. Crafoord C, Hiertonn T, Lindblom K, et al: Spinal cord compression caused by a protruded thoracic disc. Report of a case treated with antero-lateral fenestration of the disc. Acta Orthop Scand 1958;28:103-107.

43. Perot PL Jr, Munro DD: Transthoracic removal of midline thoracic disc protrusions causing spinal cord compression. J Neurosurg 1969;31:452-458.

44. Ransohoff J, Spencer F, Siew F, et al: Transthoracic removal of thoracic disc. Report of three cases. J Neurosurg 1969;31: 459-461.

45. Hulme A: The surgical approach to thoracic intervertebral disc protrusions. J Neurol Neurosurg Psychiatry 1960;23:133-137.

46. Patterson RH Jr, Arbit E: A surgical approach through the pedicle to protruded thoracic discs. J Neurosurg 1978;48:768-772.

47. Barnett GH, Russell W, Little JR, et al: Thoracic spinal canal stenosis. J Neurosurg 1987;66:338-344.

48. Govoni AF: Developmental stenosis of a thoracic vertebra resulting in narrowing of the spinal canal. AJR 1971;112: 401-404.

49. Kodama T, Okubo K, Matsukado Y: Myelopathy due to ossified ligamenta flava in lower thoracic region (author's translation). No Shinkei Geka 1979;7:867-873.

50. Marzluff JM, Hungerford DG, Kempe LG, et al: Thoracic myelopathy caused by osteophytes of the articular process. Thoracic spondylosis. J Neurosurg 1979;50:779-783.

51. Yamamoto I, Matsumae M, Ikeda A, et al: Thoracic spinal stenosis: experience with 7 cases. J Neurosurg 1988;68:37-40.

52. Mixter WJ, Barr JS: Rupture of the intervertebral disc with involvement of the spinal canal. N Engl J Med 1934;211: 210-215.

53. Hawk WA: Spinal compression caused by ecchondrosis of the intervertebral fibrocartilage: with a review of the recent literature. Brain 1936;59:204-224.

54. Young S, Karr G, O'Laoire SA: Spinal cord compression due to thoracic disc herniation: results of microsurgical posterolateral costotransversectomy. Br J Neurosurg 1989;3:31-38.

55. Müller R: Protrusion of thoracic intervertebral disks with compression of the spinal cord. Acta Med Scand 1951;139: 99-104.

56. Alexander GL: Neurological complications of spinal tuberculosis. Proc R Soc Med 1946;39:730-732.

57. Maiman DJ, Larson SJ, Luck E, El-Ghatit A: Lateral extracavitary approach to the spine for thoracic disc herniation: report of 23 cases. Neurosurgery 1984;14:178-182.

8 Degenerative Disease of the Cervical Spine

ANDREW W. LITT
IRVIN I. KRICHEFF

Degenerative disease of the cervical spine, presenting as either spondylosis or a discrete disk herniation, is an extremely common condition. It is often asymptomatic, but when symptoms occur they are protean. The evaluation of patients with symptoms of radiculopathy and/or myelopathy related to the cervical spine and the discrimination of which patients will benefit from surgical intervention rather than conservative therapy are challenges to the neurologist and neurosurgeon. Both computed tomography, either alone or in conjunction with myelography, and magnetic resonance imaging have significantly increased the radiologist's ability to define precisely the anatomical disturbance produced by a spondylosis or disk herniation and the compression of neural structures that results. However, it should be stated at the outset that our ability to define a functional correlate of this anatomical disturbance is often limited.

PATHOPHYSIOLOGY

The description of degenerative changes in the intervertebral disks of the cervical spine with resultant "osteo-arthritis" began with Bailey and Casamajor[1] in 1911. They suggested that the primary pathological change is thinning of the disk with secondary trauma to the vertebral endplates and osteophyte formation. Brain et al.[2] and Brain and Wilkinson[3] distinguished two types of cervical disk disease, "spondylosis" and disk herniation.

Spondylosis is related to degenerative changes within the substance of the nucleus pulposus. These changes cause bulging of the annulus as well as increased mobility at the affected disk level. The two factors then induce formation of lamellar bone as osteophytes. The disk protrusion causing these osteophytes does not contain nuclear material, and there is no evidence to show prior disk herniations in cases of spondylosis.[3] Evidence of increased osteophyte formation at the levels above and below a vertebral body fusion supports the hypothesis that increased mobility caused by loosing of the annular fibers plays a role in the induction of bony outgrowths.[3,4] As a complicating factor, when the cervical vertebral bodies come together, the laminae also become more closely approximated. This may cause shortening and infolding of the ligamenta flava, with perhaps degeneration and swelling of these ligaments. The overall effect is to narrow the diameter and cross-sectional area of the spinal canal at the affected level.[4]

Herniation, the second form of cervical disk disease, is a discrete protrusion of disk material, similar to that seen in the lumbar region. In these patients the annulus tears and a localized mass is formed. This may go on to calcification if left untreated. The herniation may be either traumatic or degenerative and is said often to produce radicular rather than myelopathic symptoms.[2,3]

McRae[5] and Friedenberg and Miller[6] reviewed the conventional radiographic studies of large samples of patients both with and without symptoms referable to cervical spondylosis. In McRae's series only 28% of asymptomatic individuals between the ages of 40 and 49 had a completely normal x-ray study whereas by age 60

Table 8-1 Signs and symptoms of radiculopathy by involved disk level[9]

Disk level	Nerve root	Signs and symptoms
C2-3	C3	Pain and numbness in back of neck; no upper extremity weakness or reflex changes
C3-4	C4	Pain and numbness in back of neck radiating along levator scapulae; no upper extremity weakness or reflex changes
C4-5	C5	Pain radiating from side of neck to top of shoulder; numbness over mid-deltoideus; weakness of arm and shoulder extension; atrophy of deltoideus; no reflex changes
C5-6	C6	Pain radiating down lateral side of arm and forearm, often into thumb and index fingers; numbness in tip of thumb or over first dorsal interosseous muscle; weakness of biceps, with depression of biceps reflex
C6-7	C7	Pain radiating down medial aspect of forearm, usually to middle finger; weakness of triceps muscle with depression of triceps reflex
C7-T1	C8	Pain down medial aspect of forearm to ring and small fingers with numbness in those fingers; weakness of triceps and small muscles of hand; no reflex changes

From Simeone FA, Dillin WA: Contemp Neurosurg 1986; 8:1.

and over none did. Friedenberg's data are not quite as demonstrative (75% of 40-to-49-year-olds had a normal x-ray study and only 25% were normal above age 60), but again they show the large number of people in whom this degenerative process occurs. The two authors do concur on the common locations of cervical disk pathology. In populations with and without symptoms the most common levels for degenerative changes are C5-6 and C6-7, although at C5-6 the percentage of patients with demonstrable pathology is significantly greater. Similar data also are present for neural foraminal narrowing in both groups.

The presenting manifestations of patients with cervical spondylosis are divided into radiculopathic and myelopathic. Radiculopathic symptoms and signs usually are pain, paresthesia, and weakness and/or hyporeflexia in one or more nerve root distributions (Table 8-1). Myelopathic manifestations consist of weakness (usually symmetrical) of both lower extremities, spasticity of the lower limbs with hyperreflexia in the knees and ankles, pain and numbness in the upper limbs and neck, and some loss of vibration sense in the lower limbs. Radiculopathy and myelopathy often occur in the same individual, the myelopathy tending to be of more insidious onset with a longer history and more subtle symptoms, although the advanced clinical picture may involve paraplegia or quadriplegia with loss of sensation and sphincter control.[3]

How the bony, diskal, and ligamentous changes of spondylosis or disk herniation produce symptoms is still not clearly understood. The radiculopathy is thought to occur from direct compression or stretching of nerve roots in the lateral recess of the canal or in the foramen.[7] The production of myelopathic symptoms is less well understood. Simple compression of the cord, with resultant degenerative changes, undoubtedly plays a part. However, because most of this compression is directly anterior, it does not explain the oft-seen motor weakness, which should be related to the lateral corticospinal tract. Breig et al.[8] have shown pathological evidence that the degenerative effects are secondary to compression of intramedullary arteries, often on a temporary basis, producing repeated episodes of ischemia. These investigators also demonstrated the cord's inability to move a significant amount in flexion and extension; rather it is stretched and lengthened in flexion, adopting the length of the canal. This causes stretching of the axons, and if these axons are compressed at the same time they may be more susceptible to ischemic damage.

Regardless of the mechanism of cervical cord injury or degeneration, the radiologist must be able to document the size and location of potential spondylotic lesions as well as the amount of cord compression or atrophy. Moreover, the ability of the tomographic techniques to define accurately the location of true disk herniations is essential to the surgeon in planning the operative approach.[9]

COMPUTED TOMOGRAPHY

Although the diagnosis of spondylosis and disk herniation by CT had been reported in the cervical spine as early as 1976-1977,[10,11] it was not until the development of third- and fourth-generation scanners in the late 1970s and early 1980s that a routine detailed examination of the cervical spine for these conditions was possible.

Technique

The patient is examined in the supine position. A lateral projection digital radiographic scout is obtained (Fig. 8-1). Thin axial sections (usually 1.5 to 3 mm) are

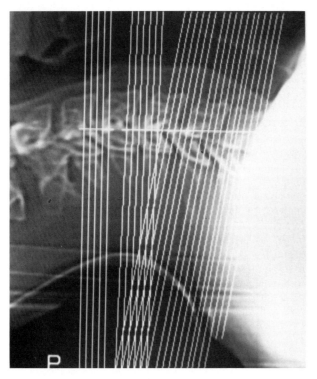

FIGURE 8-1
A digital scout radiograph obtained prior to axial CT scanning. The *lines* indicate planned slices. Note the change in angulation to remain parallel to the disk spaces.

FIGURE 8-2
Normal cervical spinal anatomy on CT. Soft tissue and bone windows at the junction of the inferior endplate of a vertebral body and the disk space, **A** and **B**, the center of the disk space, **C** and **D**, and the center of the vertebral body, **E** and **F**. The cord is seen on all soft tissue images (*straight arrow* in **A**, **C**, and **F**). The neural foramina are not narrowed (*open arrows* in **A** and **B**). There is a small amount of epidural fat lateral to the spinal canal (*small white arrows* in **C**). The foramen transversarium is seen within the vertebral body (*curved open arrow* in **B**, **E**, and **F**). On the bone window images the disk is seen as an area of decreased intensity *(D)*, the uncovertebral joint is well visualized on the left side (*curved solid arrow* in **B**), and the facet joints are seen bilaterally (*arrowheads* in **B**).

obtained at each disk space from C2-3 through C7-T1. The slices must be angled parallel to the individual disk spaces. Angulation should be continually adjusted by the technician to keep the slices parallel to the axis of the disk. Both the bone window and the soft tissue window must be imaged for each slice. Reformatted images may be useful in individual cases, but need not be obtained in every patient, nor is intravenous contrast routinely administered to every patient at our institution.

The imaging field of view should be matched to the size of the patient's neck by use of appropriate calibration files. Since a small field of view will most likely be utilized, noise may become an imaging problem if the milliamperage of the scanner is not increased. To minimize artifacts from the shoulders over the lower cervical spine, the patient should be instructed to attempt to lower his shoulders as much as possible during scans of this area. To help the patient keep the shoulders down, arm holds or straps that extend from the arms down around the feet may be useful. In addition, the patient should also be instructed not to swallow or breath during each scan slice.

Normal anatomy

Regardless of the level of section, the spinal canal is normally seen as a rounded triangle[12] with its transverse diameter greater than its anteroposterior diameter. Within the canal the spinal cord itself can often be detected (usually down to the C4 level) as an area of

slightly higher attenuation relative to the surrounding cerebrospinal fluid (Fig. 8-2). The extradural soft tissues, comprising both ligaments and venous plexus, are often seen as thin linear regions of increased attenuation bounding the subarachnoid space. Posteriorly the ligamenta flava are barely seen along the anterior margin of the lamina.

The disk space level can be identified either by seeing the lower-attenuation disk in place of the vertebral body or by noting the uncovertebral joints on each side (Fig. 8-2, *B* and *D*). The neural foramina are also present at this level and are usually filled with a fairly uniform soft tissue density, which represents both the exiting nerve root and the epidural venous plexus. In some cases the nerve roots can be distinguished as linear areas of slightly increased attenuation in the decreased-attenuation fat of the foramen.[13] The ganglion may be seen as a rounded area of increased attenuation laterally. The vertebral arteries can always be identified by their position within the foramina transversaria bilaterally (Fig. 8-2 *E* and *F*) and as discrete round soft tissue densities in the lateral and distal fat of the neural foramina at the disk space level.

The facet joints on each side consist of two semilunar-appearing facets, with the superior articulating facet of the vertebral body below being anterior to the inferior articulating facet of the body above. The combined appearance of the two facets and the joints should approximate a circle or slight oval without lateral or medial osteophyte extension (Fig. 8-2, *B* and *D*).

Spondylotic disease

Osteophytic ridges (''hard disks'') are easily detected on routine CT as areas of irregularly increased attenuation, corresponding to bone projecting posteriorly from the vertebral body at the disk space level, continuous with the vertebral body itself. They often are seen to be laterally placed, extending from the uncinate process as well as the vertebral body (Figs. 8-3 to 8-5), and often are accompanied by an abnormal soft tissue density within the canal that has a higher attenuation than the CSF. This most commonly represents fibrocartilage or a bulging annulus and is directly related to the etiology of the spur[12] (Fig. 8-4). A frank disk herniation may also be present (Fig. 8-5).

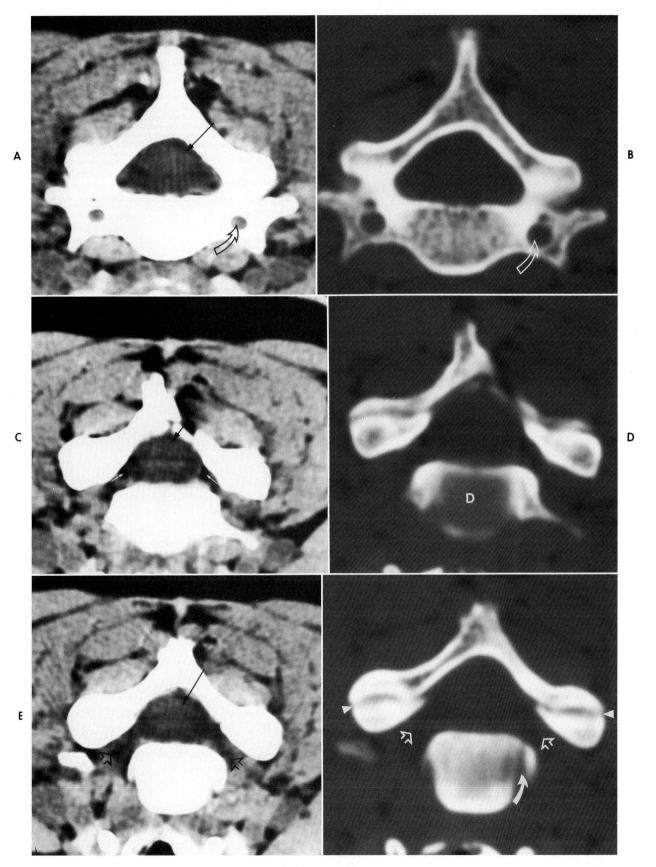

FIGURE 8-2
For legend see opposite page.

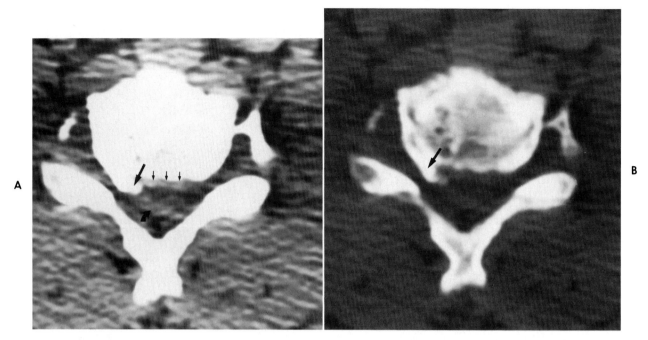

FIGURE 8-3
Soft tissue, **A,** and, bone window, **B,** images at the level of the disk space with a right-sided osteophytic ridge *(large arrow* in **A** and **B**) that is narrowing the neural foramen. There is a small amount of abnormal soft tissue density just behind the vertebral body that is likely related to a bulging annulus *(small arrows* in **A**). The cord, faintly visualized here, is atrophic *(curved arrow* in **A**).

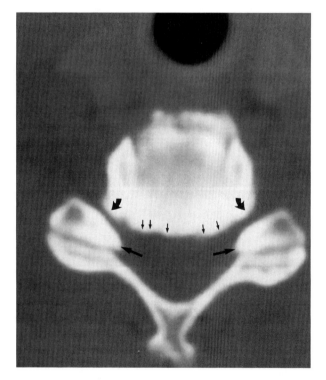

FIGURE 8-4
Bone window image at the level of the disk space. Note the ridge extending across the posterior surface of the vertebral body *(small arrows)* and the lateral ridges related to the uncovertebral joints bilaterally *(curved arrows).* Also there is slight facet joint hypertrophy *(straight arrows),* adding to the foraminal narrowing.

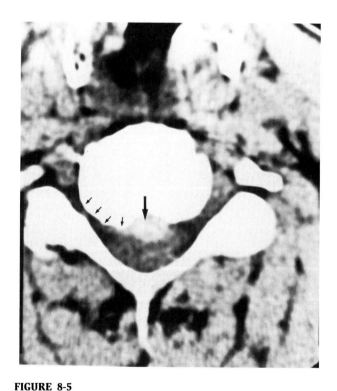

FIGURE 8-5
Soft tissue window image at the level of the disk space. There is a right-sided ridge present extending into the foramen *(small arrows).* In addition, a focal disk herniation is seen centrally *(straight arrow).* The spinal cord appears compressed.

If the cord can be delineated, abnormalities in its size and shape may be definable. These represent either compression by an osteophyte or atrophy of the cord due to repeated "trauma" from an osteophyte (Fig. 8-3). Even if the cord is not discernible, the overall size of the canal should be assessable on the bone window images. The anteroposterior diameter should exceed 12 mm[12]; otherwise, spinal stenosis is present.

Evaluation of the facet joints is important for detecting any hypertrophic changes that may have narrowed the canal at the lateral recess (Fig. 8-4) and caused nerve root or even lateral cord compression. In addition, the ligamenta flava often become prominent as part of the spondylotic process. This is not true thickening but infolding as a result of canal foreshortening. Nevertheless, it further reduces the overall size of the canal and may produce posterolateral cord compression.[12] The ligaments also become calcified in cases of prolonged degenerative disease.

The disk space itself in spondylosis often shows decreased height on the digital scout radiograph that is not detected on axial slices. There may be calcification within the disk, but this can be difficult to distinguish from degenerative changes at the endplates.[14] A vacuum phenomenon with gas in the intervertebral space is also occasionally seen.

Herniated disk

Frank disk herniations are seen as soft tissue with increased attenuation (Hounsfield units of approximately 100) surrounded by normal epidural fat and CSF, either centrally or laterally, anterior to the thecal sac[15] (Figs. 8-5 to 8-8). They are usually present at the disk space level and frequently extend inferiorly or superiorly by at least one slice (Fig. 8-6). Herniated disks tend to be irregular or lobulated and may be present independently or in association with spondylotic changes (Fig. 8-5). Calcification within the disk fragment is not uncommon (Fig. 8-8) and may be distinguished from osteophyte formation by its more punctate character (although differentiation is not always possible).

Because the difference in attenuation between a herniated fragment and the spinal canal soft tissues is small, careful attention to technique is important. Thin slices with sufficient milliamperage are essential to reduce the artifacts that can mimic or obscure a disk.[16] In addition, viewing of both the bone and the soft tissue window may improve the potential for diagnosis.

COMPUTED TOMOGRAPHY WITH INTRAVENOUS CONTRAST

Because of the limited contrast differences between the soft tissue density of a disk herniation and the CSF and cord within the canal, and because of frequent artifacts overlying the cervical canal from the lateral facet joints and the shoulders, several authors[17,18] have proposed using intravenous contrast to increase the sensitivity of CT for "soft" disk herniations in a relatively noninvasive manner. The contrast is utilized to enhance the normal basivertebral venous plexus, against which the nonenhancing disk material is more easily identified.

At each cervical level the venous drainage of the vertebral body is to the basivertebral vein, which drains into the retrocorporeal venous plexus just dorsal to the

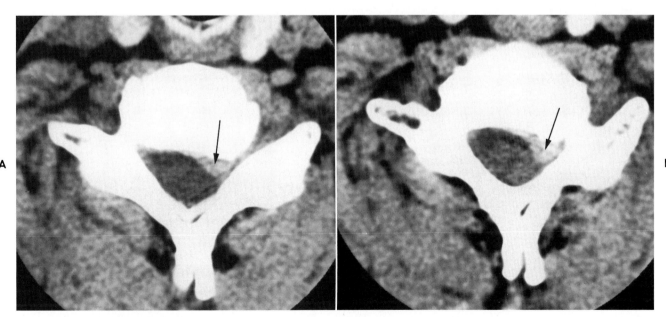

FIGURE 8-6
Soft tissue window images at the level of the disk space, **A,** and superiorly through the pedicle, **B.** There is a large left-sided herniation compressing the thecal sac and extending superiorly *(arrows).*

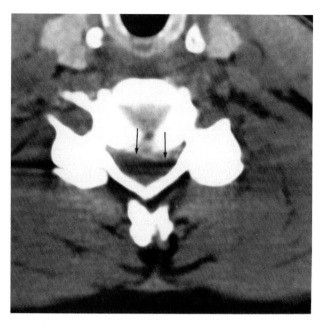

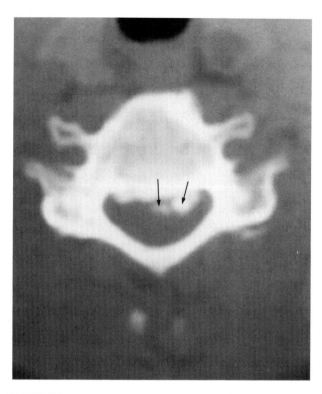

FIGURE 8-7
A diffuse herniated disk *(arrows)* extending across the midline on this bone window image. Although the cord is not well seen because of artifacts, it is likely compressed with such extensive herniation.

FIGURE 8-8
Bone window image demonstrating punctate foci of calcification *(arrows)* in a herniated disk.

A

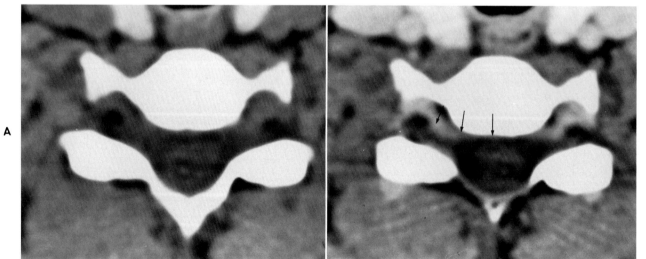

B

FIGURE 8-9
Images obtained, **A,** before and, **B,** after the administration of intravenous contrast in a normal patient. Note the enhancing retrocorporeal plexus extending laterally into the foramina (arrows in **B**). (Courtesy Eric Russell, M.D.)

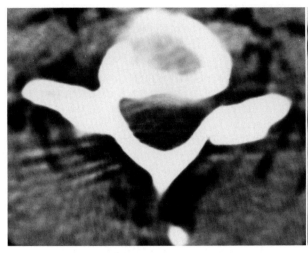
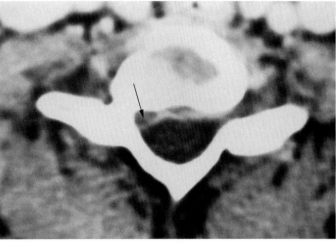

A

B

FIGURE 8-10
CT scans, **A**, before and, **B**, following intravenous contrast administration. The disk herniation is seen as an area of decreased attenuation with a rim of enhancement (*arrow* in **B**). This area is difficult to evaluate on the noncontrast study because of artifacts. (Courtesy Eric Russell, M.D. Reprinted with permission from Radiology 1984;152:703-712.)

posterior longitudinal ligament.[18] This plexus is transversely oriented and communicates on each side with the paired vertical anterior longitudinal epidural veins, which lie just medial to the foramina. These then communicate caudally with the epidural veins below and laterally with the foraminal veins extending to the plexus that surrounds the vertebral artery on each side.

In a normal individual, below the level of C2, the retrocorporeal plexus directly behind the vertebral body cannot be distinguished from the high-attenuation cortex itself. However, the anterior longitudinal epidural veins can be seen in the lateral recesses bilaterally, and the foraminal veins can be identified as linear enhancing structures within the foramina (Fig. 8-9).

If the retrocorporeal plexus is visualized, this implies that it has been posteriorly displaced and is pathognomonic of a disk herniation.[18] In addition, disk fragments can usually be seen as irregular areas of soft tissue attenuation within a rim of marginal enhancement (Fig. 8-10), the rim representing displaced plexus as well as local inflammatory reaction around the ruptured posterior longitudinal ligament caused by the herniation itself.[18]

The use of this technique is especially valuable in cases of localized radiculopathy when noncontrast CT has been equivocal. Moreover, specific delineation of the disk fragment can be important in planning the surgeon's anterior approach. The limitation of the technique comes in patients with extensive spondylotic disease, in whom the enhancing plexus may be confused with spondylotic ridges (both having high attenuation).[18]

COMPUTED TOMOGRAPHY FOLLOWING MYELOGRAPHY

Since its early description by DiChiro and Schellinger[19] in 1976, CT-myelography (CTM) has become the "gold standard" for imaging the cervical spine in disk disease and spondylosis. Because of the increased differential contrast provided by intrathecal metrizamide (formerly) or iopamidol and iohexol (now), better definition of a herniated disk or spondylotic ridge is possible than with either plain CT or plain film myelography alone. In addition, intrathecal contrast provides an accurate examination of the cord itself, allowing for determination of the effect of the herniation or ridge. Finally, the use of delayed CTM will often demonstrate pathology beyond the point of myelographic block as well as detect intramedullary changes (degeneration and syrinx formation) secondary to spondylosis.

Technique

At our institution, CTM is performed following a complete cervical myelogram. This consists of instilling 10 cc of 60% nonionic contrast agent suitable for myelography (iopamidol or iohexol) into the lumbar subarachnoid space in the usual fashion. By tilting the patient, contrast can be made to flow into the cervical theca; care must be taken, however, not to allow much contrast to pass cephalad of the foramen magnum. Routine myelographic images of the cervical spine are obtained and are used, along with the clinical history, in directing the CTM examination to the level of pathology. Optimal time for CT scanning following myelography is within 4 hours,[20] during which time the patient should be kept supine with the head slightly elevated to prevent contrast from passing intracranially. The patient is then rolled through 360 degrees at least once prior to being placed on the CT table. Contiguous 3 mm slices are obtained at each disk space level. Appropriate window width and level should be chosen for imaging to emphasize the contrast differences between bone, soft tissue, and the opacified subarachnoid space.

Rather than obtaining a full cervical myelogram, some institutions merely instill 4 to 6 cc of contrast into the subarachnoid space and keep the patient decubitus with the head slightly elevated for a time prior to scanning. Although this is effective for obtaining adequate contrast in CTM, it does not allow for tailoring of the examination.

If a myelographic block is noted on the plain film, CTM may be attempted within a short time following. Whereas a block may appear complete on the plain film, contrast often will be seen in the subarachnoid space beyond it on CT.[21] If this attempt is not successful, a C1-2 puncture with instillation of contrast can be employed or a delayed (4-to-6-hour) study may show some contrast passing beyond the point of the block.

When intramedullary degeneration or syrinx formation is suspected, either from the clinical history or because an expanded cord was discovered on conventional myelography or initial CTM, a delayed (4-to-6-hour) study should be obtained to detect abnormal contrast uptake within the cord itself.

Normal anatomy

The posterior surface of the vertebral body is separated from the opacified thecal sac by a 1 or 2 mm area of soft tissue attenuation representing the posterior longitudinal ligament and the epidural venous plexus (Fig. 8-11). The ligamenta flava are also seen as 1 to 2 mm curvilinear bands of soft tissue attenuation between the lamina and the sac dorsally.

The spinal cord itself is well visualized as an ovoid or round structure, with the most ovoid configuration at C4 and C5 and the most round at T1.[22] A minimal anterior median indentation is often present, corresponding to the anterior median fissure, but generally the right and left anterior portions should remain rounded and there should be no anterior, posterior, or posterolateral flattening. The anteroposterior diameter of the cord is smallest at C4 and C5, widening above and below, whereas the transverse diameter increases to a maximum at C4 and C5 and then becomes smallest at T1.[22] The

A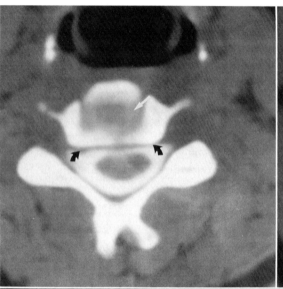

B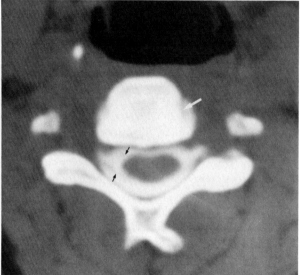

C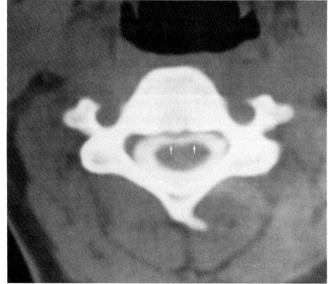

FIGURE 8-11
Normal CTM through the disk space, **A,** vertebral endplate, **B,** and midvertebral body, **C.** The disk is seen as an area of low attenuation (*arrow* in **A**) and the uncinate joint is evident at the level of the vertebral endplate laterally (*arrow* in **B**). The anterior margin of the cord on both the left and the right has a rounded appearance (*small white arrows* in **A** to **C**). The dorsal and ventral nerve roots are seen as linear filling defects in the increased attenuation of the CSF (*small black arrows* in **B**). The posterior longitudinal ligament and epidural venous plexus are the a thin area of soft tissue attenuation behind the vertebral body (*curved arrows* in **A**).

attenuation of the cord should remain uniform and at the level of the soft tissue attenuation.

The contrast-filled subarachnoid space is seen as a ring of increased attenuation around the cord. It is generally symmetrical and extends to the lateral recess adjacent to the medial portion of the facet joint. The dorsal and ventral roots may be seen as linear filling defects in the subarachnoid space, with contrast usually not extending out to the lateral recess.

Spondylotic disease

Ridges are seen as high-attenuation overgrowths adjacent to the vertebral endplate (Figs. 8-12 to 8-15). They

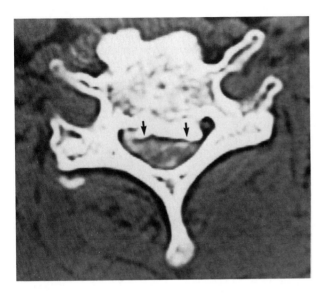

FIGURE 8-12
A large osteophytic ridge demonstrated on CTM *(arrows)*. The cord and thecal sac are not well visualized because of the amount of compression.

compress the dural sac, either narrowing or obliterating the soft tissue attenuation line of the posterior longitudinal ligament, and may be focal or diffuse, central or lateral. The sac itself is often deformed and posteriorly displaced. In fact, minimal thinning of the anterior rim of the subarachnoid space relative to the posterior rim is a subtle finding with small spurs.[21]

The spinal cord either may be flattened minimally or may demonstrate considerable loss of anteroposterior diameter (Fig. 8-12). Any diminution of the normal rounded margins of the anterolateral cord should be considered significant (Fig. 8-13). The cord may be rotated and/or displaced posteriorly or posterolaterally by large osteophytes. It is often small or flat, without significant anterior subarachnoid space narrowing. This may be explained by one of two mechanisms: either the cord is *atrophied* secondary to many years of compression or it is only *compressed* when the patient flexes or hyperextends his neck and does not completely return to normal during the CT examination (Figs. 8-14 and 8-15). This finding of a normal to increased ratio of cross-sectional areas between the cord and the subarachnoid space may have some prognostic value. Badami et al.[21] found that in patients with a cord to subarachnoid space ratio of greater than 50% (small subarachnoid space relative to cord size), good recovery of function occurred after surgical decompression. In those with a ratio less than 50% (large subarachnoid space relative to cord size), no recovery of function occurred. This finding makes intuitive sense, because one would not expect good recovery in patients with an atrophic cord; however, theirs was a small sample and the results have not been confirmed by other studies.

Intrinsic abnormalities of the spinal cord in the setting of spondylosis have also been demonstrated on delayed

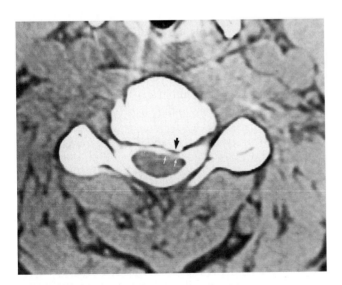

FIGURE 8-13
A small left-sided osteophytic ridge *(arrow)*. Note the mild flattening on the left side of the anterior cord *(small white arrows)*.

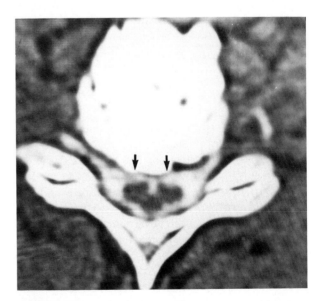

FIGURE 8-14
A large diffuse osteophyte with central focalization *(arrows)*. The cord is small and deformed, yet it does not appear compressed on this image. The implication here is cord atrophy.

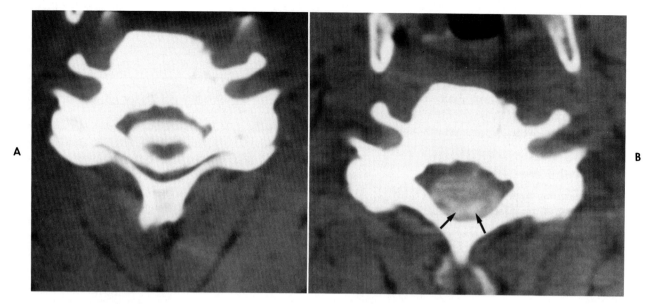

FIGURE 8-15
An immediate postmyelographic CT slice, **A**, and a 6-hour delayed slice, **B**, at the same level show the cord to be normally attenuated (on the immediate study) but of increased attenuation (later) due to either myelomalacia or syrinx formation (*arrows* in **B**).

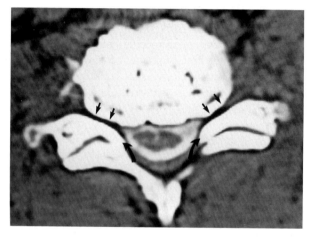

FIGURE 8-16
A large diffuse osteophyte with narrowing of the neural foramina bilaterally (*arrows*). There is also hypertrophy of the facet joints (*curved arrows*).

CTM (Fig. 8-15). Repeat scans are obtained from 4 to 6 hours following myelography with water-soluable contrast. The presence of local or remote areas of contrast enhancement within the spinal cord has been documented.[23] It is not clear in all cases, however, whether this enhancement represents a true syringomyelic cavity (similar to that seen in the posttraumatic state) or is an area of cystic necrosis or myelomalacia. Performing delayed CT scanning to search for these abnormalities is important in cases of spondylosis and clear-cut myelopathy, when the amount of cord compression on the initial CT following myelography is not impressive or there appears to be expansion of the cord.

Lateral spurring from the uncovertebral joints, causing either cord or nerve root compression, is readily demonstrated on CTM (Fig. 8-16). In fact, plain film myelography may miss them.[24] Degenerative changes of the facet joints lateral to the dural sac as well as thickening of the ligamenta flava posterolaterally can also be well appreciated on CTM. Flattening of the cord from these posterior and lateral "masses" may be clinically significant.

Herniated disk

The high contrast and spatial resolution of CTM are ideal for detecting and characterizing small fragments of herniated disk (Figs. 8-17 and 8-18), some of which may be missed on plain film myelography[25] and plain CT[26] (Fig. 8-18). This is especially true for central herniations, which were considered rare until the advent of CTM.[27] Many institutions now use conventional myelography as an adjunct to clinical history for directing the CT scan.[28]

The distinction between "soft" or noncalcified disk material and osteophytic spurs is easily made on CTM. The high-density subarachnoid space will be deformed by a soft tissue-density mass in the former and a high-density structure in the latter. One may not see the disk fragment as a discrete entity; but if the thecal sac is compressed or displaced and there are no osteophytes present at that level or at the levels above and below, one may assume that the compression is due to a soft herniation[26] (Fig. 8-18).

The presence of lateral disk herniations is also well shown on CTM. Detection of these lesions, especially in the setting of spondylotic changes at the same level, is important for the surgeon. In the anterior approach the surgeon's field of view is limited, especially on the side of entry, making knowledge of isolated lateral fragments paramount.

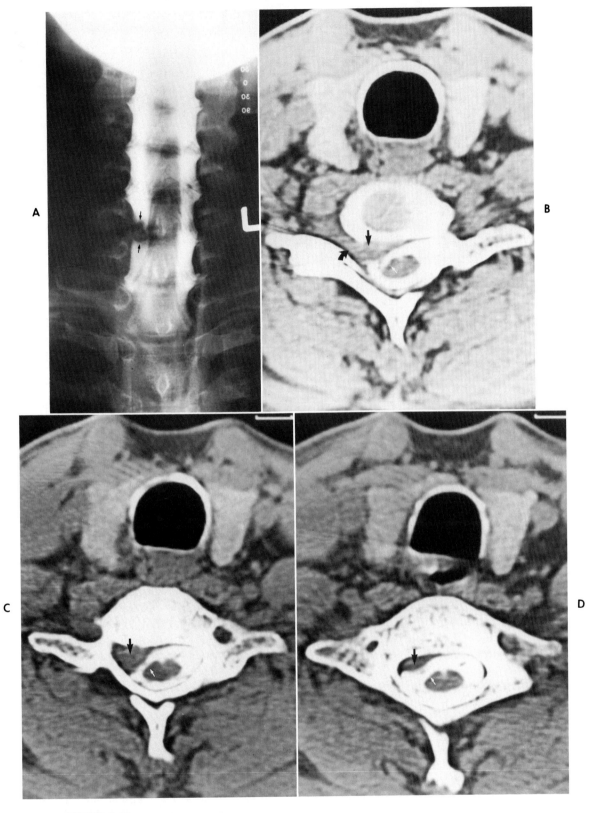

FIGURE 8-17
An AP film from a myelogram, **A**, shows a right-sided extradural defect *(arrows)* consistent with a herniation at C5-6. CT scans following the myelogram at the C5-6 level, **B**, and behind the C6 vertebral body, **C** and **D**, show the herniation *(arrows in **B** to **D**)* better, along with its extension behind the vertebral body and out into the neural foramen *(curved arrow in **B**)*. The cord is rotated and flattened on the right side *(white arrows in **B** to **D**)*.

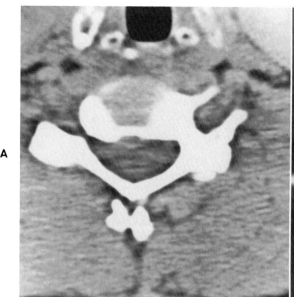

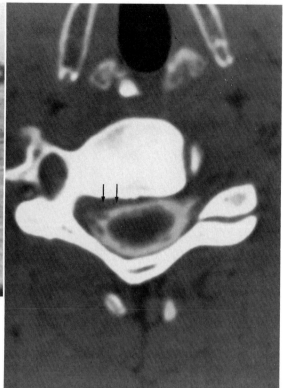

FIGURE 8-18
Premyelographic, **A**, and postmyelographic, **B**, CT scans at the same level in a patient with right-sided herniation. The disk, not clearly seen on the premyelographic study, is a diffuse area of soft tissue density anterior to the thecal sac. It extends into the lateral recess on the postmyelographic study (*arrows* in **B**).

MAGNETIC RESONANCE IMAGING

The advent of MRI has made it possible to examine patients for cervical disk and spondylotic disease without either ionizing radiation or contrast injection. However, although it has become the initial screening examination for these situations, it is still often not the definitive preoperative study. There are institutions where surgeons will operate on a patient with myelopathy and spondylotic cord compression visualized only on MRI, but many still request the CTM for confirmation prior to surgery. In a patient with radiculopathy, CTM is preferred over MRI because of better contrast, spatial resolution, and overall signal-to-noise. In addition, CTM can better determine whether the pathological entity is a disk or a ridge. Nevertheless, as the quality of MR imaging techniques improves, because of new hardware and new scan sequences, it will increasingly become the definitive study.

Technique

The utility of MRI arises from its multiplanar capability and its unique capacity to visualize differences between tissues in multiple ways. Therefore, the complete MR examination in a patient with myelopathy or radiculopathy should include a multiplanar and a multicontrast evaluation.

Sagittal T1-weighted images are used for the preliminary overview. Depending upon the capabilities of the machine and technical staff, a coronal scout sequence may be obtained first to ensure that the sagittal images are angled parallel to the cord. Thin sections (3 or 4 mm) should be used for the sagittal examination with a small (10% to 20%) interslice gap, and it is important to have one slice positioned precisely through the middle of the spinal cord. The precise scan parameters (TR, TE, number of acquisitions, field of view, etc.) depend upon the specific MR imaging device being used.

It is then often useful to obtain a T2-weighted (spin echo) or T2*-weighted (gradient echo) sequence in the sagittal plane. This will provide a "white CSF" appearance that mimics the myelographic image. Although the T1-weighted sagittal study is ideal for anatomical resolution, it provides minimal contrast between osteophytes (which are largely cortical bone and appear as low signal) and CSF (which also is of low signal). Contrast can be improved by using the T2-weighted study, in which ridges causing anterior epidural impression on the thecal sac are more easily visualized. Furthermore, the T2-weighted study allows for better detection of intrinsic cord abnormalities that are related to osteophyte formation or are independent (e.g., multiple sclerosis).

The availability of photoplethysmographic monitors, which perform cardiac gating of the MR data acquisition based on the capillary blush in the finger or toe, has proven quite useful in maximizing the signal-to-noise of these T2-weighted studies.[29] Gating can be coupled with flow compensation (gradient moment nulling) to further maximize both signal-to-noise and contrast. The other advantage of utilizing flow correction methods lies in their ability to reduce CSF pulsation artifacts. The motion of CSF protons along a gradient results in spin dephasing and signal loss, which may be confused with intradural pathology such as an arteriovenous malformation.

For further evaluation of findings seen on the sagittal studies, and for complete examination of the nerve roots in patients with radiculopathy, axial high-resolution T1-weighted and/or gradient-recalled echo images are required. The precise TR/TE and other sequence factors will depend upon the machine being used; but generally slices should be thin enough (preferably 3 to 5 mm), with sufficient acquisitions used to clearly delineate the structures within the spinal canal and the nerve roots within the lateral recesses and foramina. Interslice gaps of 20% to 40% are acceptable, and slices should be oriented parallel to the disk spaces. Axial slices should be acquired through levels that appear abnormal on sagittal images, and in patients with radiculopathy confined to one or more disk levels they should be obtained through these levels as well.

Many authors[30-32] have described various gradient echo techniques to provide myelographic-like images in a shorter time than required with the conventional T2-weighted studies. All these techniques utilize a relatively short TR (200 msec or less) and TE (10 to 25 msec) with a flip angle under 30 degrees. The studies provide good CSF/cord contrast and good CSF/disk/ridge contrast. In the axial plane they are capable of showing the course of the nerve roots in the lateral recesses and foramina. In fact, because of the slightly increased susceptibility effects generated by gradient echo studies, the conspicuity (though not necessarily the complete characterization of lesions) is felt to be increased with this type of examination.[32] The major limitation to the gradient echo technique has been in evaluating intradural and intramedullary pathology, for which the traditional spin echo technique is still favored.

Other MR techniques for evaluating the cervical spine in radiculopathy include postcontrast (gadolinium-DTPA) (gadopentetate) T1-weighted images, oblique imaging[33-35] (in which the plane of section is perpendicular to the neural foramina of interest), and thin section three-dimensional Fourier transform (3DFT) imaging (in which multiple [40 to 60] contiguous 3D gradient echo axial slices are obtained covering the entire cervical canal).[36] The advantages of the 3DFT technique are thinner slices (1.5 to 2 mm) with resolution similar to that of CT scanning, increased signal-to-noise, better depiction of the neural foramina, and enhanced CSF signal intensity due to the short TR employed. The disadvantages come from increased artifact in the presence of patient motion and the possibility of wrap-around artifact because of the use of a phase encoding gradient for slice selection.

Generally the exact MR protocol to be used for cervical spine imaging will depend not only on the preferences of the individual radiologist and referring clinician but also on the capabilities of the scanner and, in particular, its ability to perform rapid high resolution gradient echo scans.

Normal anatomy

On sagittal T1-weighted images the vertebrae should be of fairly uniform midintensity (Fig. 8-19, *A*). Small areas of increased or decreased signal within the bodies, especially adjacent to the endplates, may represent areas of degenerative change. The alignment should be examined and the presence (or absence) of subluxations noted. The disk spaces will have a moderately high-signal inner region surrounded by a low-signal rim, which represents the annulus and adjacent bony cortex. Depending upon the direction of the frequency-encoding gradient, this interface may be altered by chemical shift artifact (which can cause a black-and-white-stripe appearance). The posterior surfaces of the vertebral bodies also appear as rims of low signal merging with the low signal of the posterior longitudinal ligament. Behind this is the higher-signal "stripe" of the epidural venous plexus, which often appears thinner or even discontinuous at the disk space level. The overall thickness of this plexus in the sagittal plane is variable and, in fact, on midline sagittal images may not be clearly delineated at all.

Posterior to the vertebral column is the spinal canal and, on T1-weighted images, the CSF (which is of low signal and the cord of moderate signal). It is often difficult to define precisely the posterior vertebral body cortex/posterior longitudinal ligament / CSF interface. The posterior elements with associated fat and ligaments are situated behind the canal, but are also often difficult to evaluate on sagittal images.

The sagittal T2-weighted images are similar to T1-weighted images — except that the vertebral bodies have decreased signal, the disks somewhat increased signal, and the CSF significantly increased signal (Fig. 8-19, *B*). The cord, however, remains of moderate signal intensity. These characteristics are usually present whether the T2-weighted study is of the spin echo or gradient echo type. The epidural venous plexus is not well seen, although the interface between CSF and the posterior vertebral cortex/posterior longitudinal ligament is better delineated. In the lumbar spine the presence of decreased signal in the disk spaces on T2-weighted images correlates with degenerative changes, but in the cervical region this correlation is not as significant and decreased signal is often noted in young patients without other evidence of disk disease.

The axial sections will mimic the sagittal ones with regard to signal intensity depending upon the relative T1 or T2 weighting. On high-resolution examinations the ventral and dorsal nerve roots can be seen exiting the cord and heading toward the neural foramen (Fig. 8-19, *C*). These roots are often better seen on short TR/short TE gradient echo sequences or gadopentetate-enhanced T1-weighted sequences, in which the epidural venous plexus appears both anterior and posterior to the nerve roots in the lateral recess and in the foramen itself.

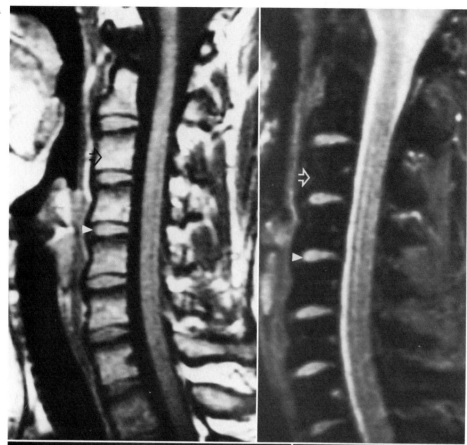

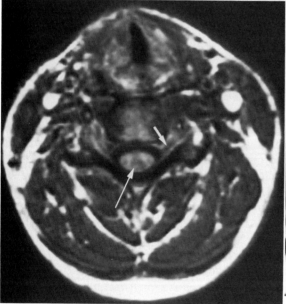

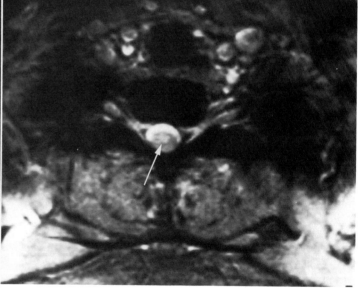

FIGURE 8-19
Normal anatomy on MR. Midline sagittal T1-weighted, **A**, and midline sagittal T2-weighted, **B**, images along with an axial T1-weighted image through the disk space, **C**, and an axial (gradient-echo) T2*-weighted through the disk space, **D**, show uniform signal intensity of the vertebral bodies (*open arrows* in **A** and **B**) and disk spaces (*arrowheads* in **A** and **B**) on the sagittal images. On the axial T1-weighted image the nerve root is seen in the foramen (*short white arrow* in **C**). Note also the normal heterogeneity of signal within the cord (*long white arrow* in **C** and **D**).

Although not routinely performed at most institutions, oblique sections parallel to the foramen may provide good depiction of the nerve root exiting the cord and extending through this area.[33,35] Images obtained perpendicular to the foramen are similar to lateral sagittal images in the lumbar spine and show the ventral and dorsal portions of the nerve root arranged vertically in the inferior portion of the foramen. The superior foraminal canal is filled with high-intensity fat and the epidural veins.

Spondylotic disease

Both sagittal T1- and sagittal T2-weighted images depict degenerative changes of the vertebral bodies and disk spaces. The disk spaces are usually narrowed, often with decreased signal and a poorly defined margin between the inner higher-signal region and the annulus.[37] As mentioned before, signal changes, whether increased or decreased in the vertebral body adjacent to the endplates, are also consistent with degenerative

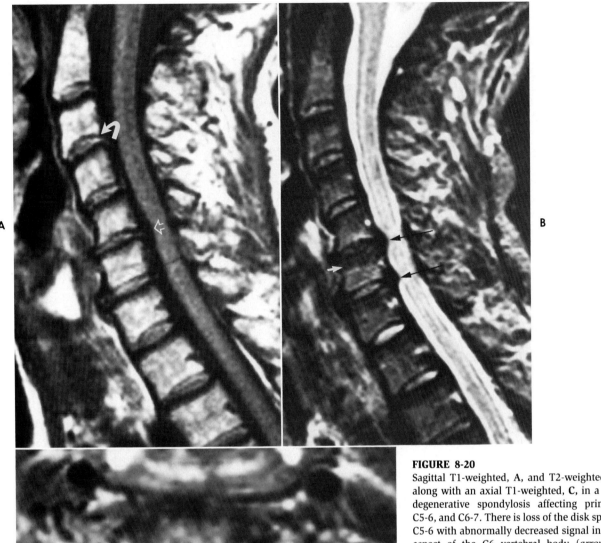

FIGURE 8-20
Sagittal T1-weighted, **A**, and T2-weighted, **B**, images along with an axial T1-weighted, **C**, in a patient with degenerative spondylosis affecting primarily C4-5, C5-6, and C6-7. There is loss of the disk space height at C5-6 with abnormally decreased signal in the superior aspect of the C6 vertebral body (*arrow* in **B**), all consistent with degenerative change. Note the anterior subluxation of C3 on C4 (*curved arrow* in **A**). The anterior epidural compressions of the thecal sac at C5-6 and C6-7 are best seen on the T2-weighted sagittal image (*long arrows* in **B**), but compression of the spinal cord is better visualized on the T1-weighted sagittal and axial studies (*open arrows* in **A** and **C**). However, on the sagittal T1-weighted image the osteophyte cannot be clearly differentiated from the CSF.

disease (Fig. 8-20). Subluxations which result from degenerative disease of the facets and ligamentous laxity are also occasionally present.

Osteophyte formation is seen on sagittal images as an extension of the vertebral body cortex in a triangular configuration either anteriorly or posteriorly.[37] On T1-weighted images these ridges have a low-signal margin, representing cortex, that may be difficult to differentiate from the low signal of CSF depending upon the exact scan parameters selected (Fig. 8-20). If the osteophyte is small, then only the low-signal cortex will be present; however, the larger the osteophyte grows, the more likely it is to have higher-signal marrow within it as an extension of the normal vertebral body marrow (Fig. 8-21). This higher-signal marrow provides a better contrast with the CSF on T1-weighted studies.

A T2-weighted study will better delineate the margin between an osteophytic ridge and the CSF (Fig. 8-20).

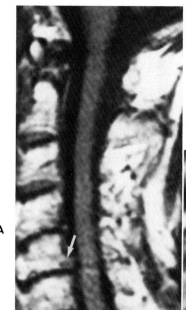

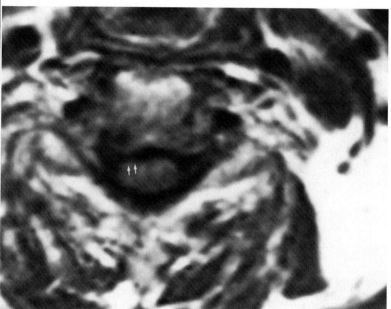

FIGURE 8-21
Sagittal, **A,** and axial, **B,** T1-weighted images of a patient with an osteophytic ridge at C5-6. Note the increased signal within the ridge consistent with marrow (*arrow* in **A**). There is subtle cord compression on the axial study (*small arrows* in **B**).

This may be particularly useful when the amount of epidural compression is small and the cord is not deformed. The size of the ridge and the amount of epidural compression may be exaggerated when gradient echo sequences are used because of the magnetic susceptibility effect produced at the cortex-CSF interface. The overestimation of osteophyte size may be reduced by shortening the echo time of the sequence, if possible.

Depending upon severity, deformity or compression of the cord can be seen on sagittal images, whether T1- or T2-weighted (Fig. 8-20). The cord may be locally indented by the extradural osteophyte and often will be displaced laterally over a longer segment. T1-weighted images better define the degree of indentation because of their higher signal-to-noise; however, subtle changes are more conspicuous on T2-weighted images (Fig. 8-20).

It is important to examine the laterally placed sagittal images for osteophytes extending into the neural foramina from the uncovertebral joints. Although they are often present with a central osteophyte (Fig. 8-22), they also may appear independently. The axial images should serve to confirm the presence of foraminal narrowing.

High signal may be noted within the cord on T2-weighted images in the area of compression. It is important to distinguish among three causes of increased signal.

The first is artifact related to truncation or to CSF pulsation, which in either case will be linear and extend along the entire length of the cord (Fig. 8-23). Truncation artifact can be recognized because it tends to be a very thin high-intensity line that may disappear in areas where the subarachnoid space is compressed. It can be reduced or eliminated by increasing the matrix size or changing the phase-encoding gradient direction. Flow-related artifact is usually present as multiple parallel curvilinear high-intensity bands that will disappear with gating or with changing the direction of the phase-encoding gradient. Neither of these artifacts will usually be associated with corresponding areas of low-signal abnormality on the T1-weighted study.

The second cause for increased intramedullary signal on T2-weighed images is syrinx formation. The formation of a syrinx in association with spondylotic changes and osteophytes is probably due to the multiple traumas of the ridge hitting the cord and is rare. The syrinx will usually be centered on the area of ridge formation and will also be present on the T1-weighted studies, both axial and sagittal, as an area of decreased signal. Septations may be present within the syrinx but will usually not be complete anatomically. The signal characteristics of the fluid within should match those of CSF on all pulse sequences.

The final cause for increased signal intensity within the cord in patients with spondylosis has not been confirmed, but is suspected to represent demyelination or myeloma-

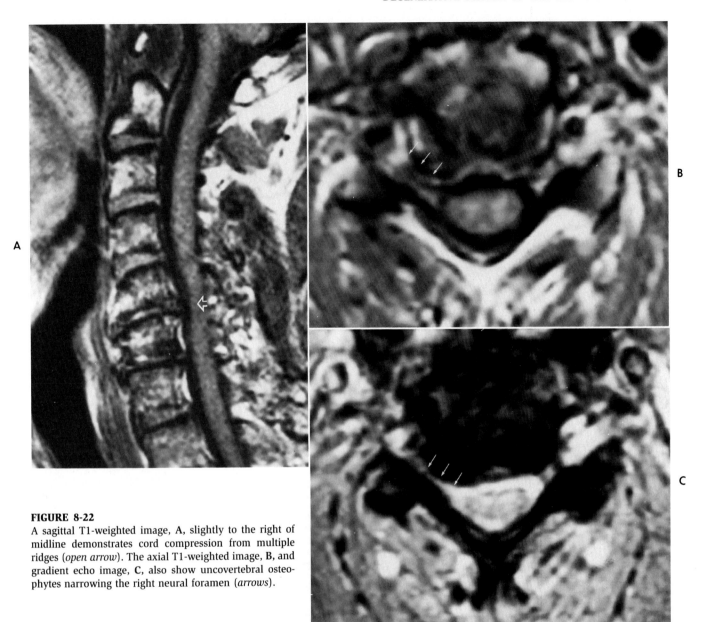

FIGURE 8-22
A sagittal T1-weighted image, **A**, slightly to the right of midline demonstrates cord compression from multiple ridges (*open arrow*). The axial T1-weighted image, **B**, and gradient echo image, **C**, also show uncovertebral osteophytes narrowing the right neural foramen (*arrows*).

lacia secondary to chronic compression[38] (Fig. 8-24). T1-weighted images may show slightly decreased or normal signal intensity in these areas. The high signal on T2-weighted images is similar to the cavitation or cystic necrosis seen on delayed postmyelographic CT. A recent study of over 600 patients with chronic cord compression[38] found this increased signal in 14.8%. Presence of the finding was correlated with the severity of clinical myelopathy and the degree of cord compression. Moreover, in 56% of patients with the high-signal area there was no or only poor improvement following decompression surgery compared to 15% of patients with no abnormal signal. Similar results were found with conservative therapy. Interestingly, in the three patients with increased T2-weighted cord signal, who improved following surgery and were studied with repeat MR, the high signal was not present on the postoperative examination.

Disk disease

Some disk material always accompanies the osteophytic ridges, although in a few cases there will be a frank disk herniation independent of other spondylotic changes. When the herniation is central or paracentral, it often can be recognized on sagittal images by the presence of an area of medium-intensity signal posterior to the disk space causing epidural compression (Figs. 8-25 to 8-27). Lateral herniations are more difficult to visualize on sagittal images and to separate from osteophytic ridges. On gradient echo or T1-weighted sequences disk material will often have a higher signal than the dense cortical bone of a ridge (Figs. 8-25 and 8-26), despite the fact that higher-signal marrow is present in many osteophytes. Often the distinction between ridge, ridge with accompanying disk, and disk herniation alone is difficult (Fig. 8-25). Some authors[31,36] believe that this may be easier on gradient echo sequences.

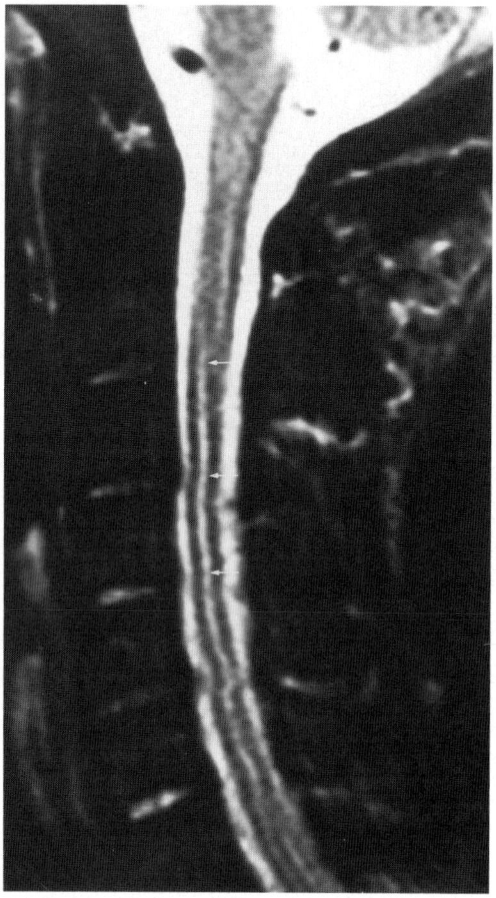

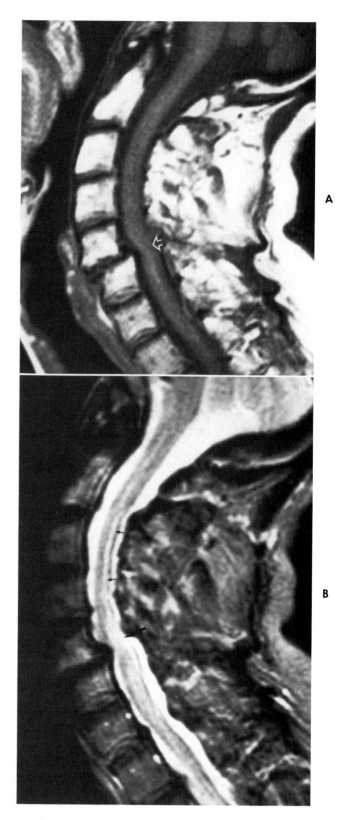

FIGURE 8-23
Truncation artifact on a T2-weighted sagittal image. The increased signal within the cord is a relatively thin line that extends over much of the visualized cord length *(arrows)*.

Much of the soft tissue within the epidural space may not represent disk material itself; rather it may be related to the inflammatory response to disk herniation. This can be demonstrated in some patients by performing T1-weighted scans after the administration of gadopentetate (Fig. 8-27).

Nevertheless, the most important information for the referring clinician, and especially for the surgeon, is not the distinction between ridge and disk but the identification of free fragments or sequestered fragments of disk material that may have migrated into a position that is difficult to see intraoperatively.

COMPARATIVE STUDIES

The question of which study, computed tomography, computed tomography following myelography, or magnetic resonance imaging, should be performed for the evaluation of patients with suspected cervical spinal degenerative disease has not been fully answered to date. In fact, the rapid continued evolution of MR imaging techniques makes a study to examine this issue problematic. However, experience, evaluation of the literature, and assessment of current state-of-the art techniques

FIGURE 8-24
Sagittal T1-weighted, A, and T2-weighted, B, images in a patient with anterior subluxation of C5 on C6 and cord compression *(open arrow in A)* at that level. The T2-weighted shows patchy signal in the cord at C5-6 *(large arrow in B)*, which is clearly different from the truncation artifact seen superiorly *(small arrows in B)*.

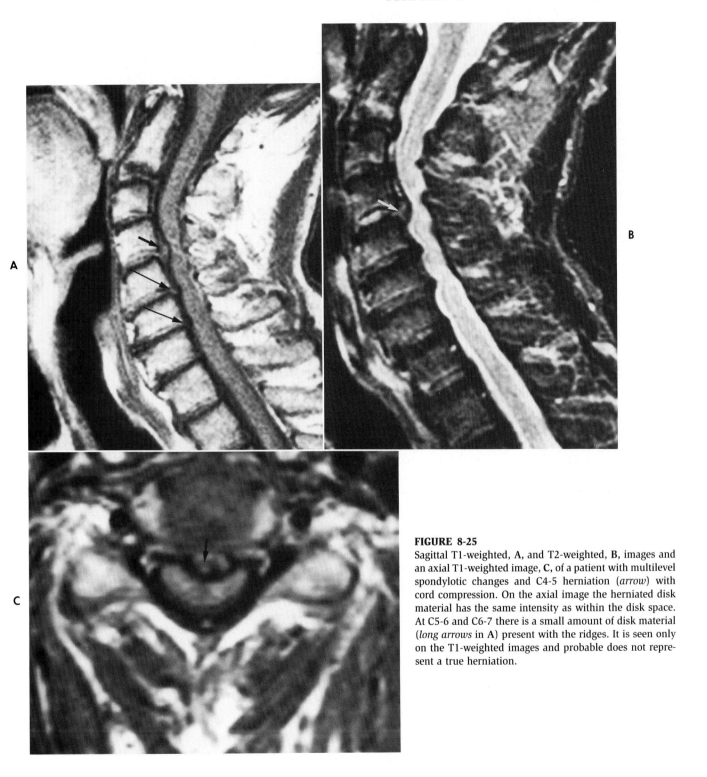

FIGURE 8-25
Sagittal T1-weighted, **A**, and T2-weighted, **B**, images and an axial T1-weighted image, **C**, of a patient with multilevel spondylotic changes and C4-5 herniation (*arrow*) with cord compression. On the axial image the herniated disk material has the same intensity as within the disk space. At C5-6 and C6-7 there is a small amount of disk material (*long arrows* in **A**) present with the ridges. It is seen only on the T1-weighted images and probable does not represent a true herniation.

allow for some conclusions to be drawn. Most important, the work-up of the patient must depend upon the initial working diagnosis based on clinical signs and symptoms.

Myelopathy

An early study of body-coil MR of the cervical spine in patients with myelopathy[39] found that MR was equal to or more informative than myelography in 75% of extradural lesions. The majority of these patients had degenerative disk disease and spondylosis. It was suggested that the ability of MR accurately to define the dimensions of the spinal canal as well as the cord itself might have significant value. Moreover, the ability of MR to detect other causes of myelopathy (e.g., intrinsic cord disease or syringohydromyelia) was considered an additional benefit. In some cases the T2-weighted image failed to depict accurately the epidural space narrowing at the site of osteophytes.

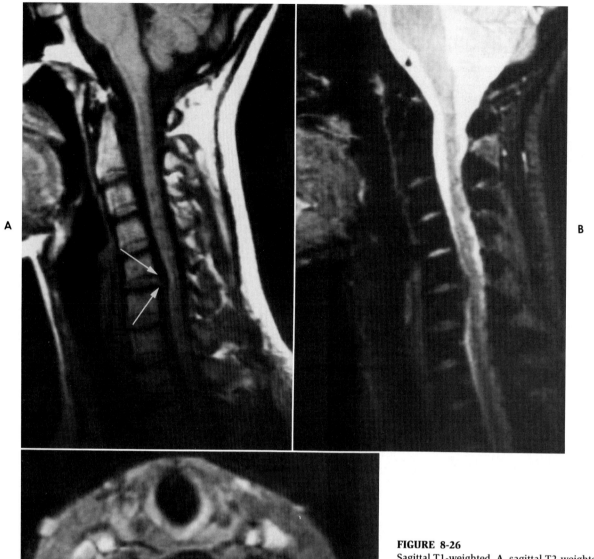

FIGURE 8-26
Sagittal T1-weighted, **A**, sagittal T2-weighted, **B**, and axial gradient echo, **C**, images of a patient with focal C5-6 herniation and cord compression. Disk material extends superior and inferior to the disk space itself behind the vertebral bodies (*arrows* in **A**). On the sagittal T2-weighted and axial images the disk has slightly lower signal than the rest of the disk space, except for a small central area on the axial (*open arrow* in **C**). This reduction in signal may represent dehydration of the disk fragment.

A more recent study of a small group of 26 patients,[40] eight of whom had myelopathic symptoms, demonstrated equivalent findings of cord compression on CTM and MR. Of the 32 disk-space levels examined overall for degree of narrowing, there was agreement between CTM and MR on all but two levels. This report also corroborated previous studies in stating that MR is less able to distinguish disk herniation from osteophyte formation; but, again, this would be of limited clinical significance.

We believe that MR is indicated as the initial screening examination for myelopathy, with CTM being reserved for difficult cases in which slightly better resolution is important for presurgical assessment.

Radiculopathy

Another early study of CTM versus MRI,[41] using surface coil technology, showed that in patients with radiculopathy the agreement between surgical findings

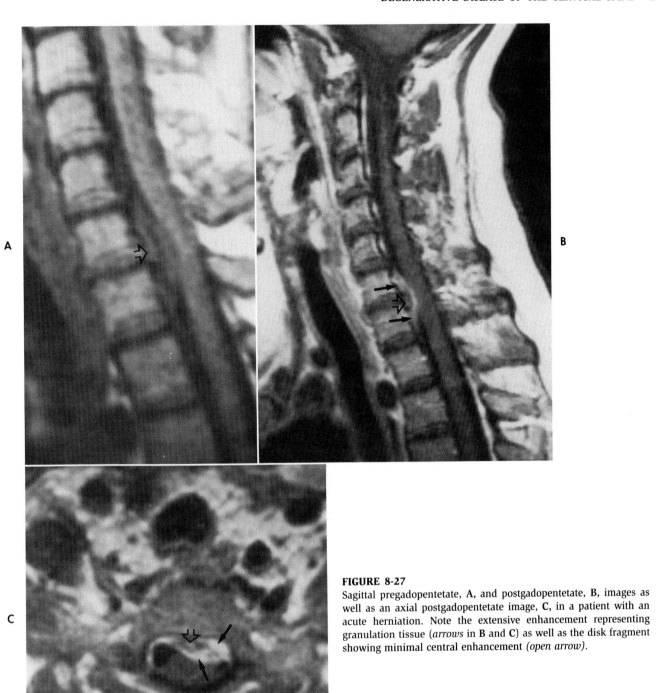

FIGURE 8-27
Sagittal pregadopentetate, **A**, and postgadopentetate, **B**, images as well as an axial postgadopentetate image, **C**, in a patient with an acute herniation. Note the extensive enhancement representing granulation tissue (*arrows* in **B** and **C**) as well as the disk fragment showing minimal central enhancement (*open arrow*).

and MRI was 74% compared to 85% for surgery and CTM. In general, CTM was not more sensitive than MRI but it provided better information as to the type of disease (disk vs. ridge). In addition, the higher resolution possible with thin-section CTM aided diagnostic accuracy. Furthermore, CTM provided greater accuracy in depicting the nerve roots themselves, showing the effect of compressive lesions better. Laterally placed disease was also better seen with CTM.

A more recent, though rather limited, study[40] had different results. It found the accuracy of CTM and MR using a dedicated cervical spine surface coil in the detection of nerve root sheath deformity to be 73% and 77% respectively. These authors also pointed out the difficulty of getting thin MR axial sections as well as the problems associated with gaps between the slices. The future widespread use of 3DFT gradient echo contiguous axial images with slice thickness of 1.5 to 2 mm may obviate some of these concerns.[36]

The evaluation of patients with radiculopathy is still somewhat difficult. MR is probably the best screening study available, particularly if accompanied by a good 3DFT gradient echo capability. Nevertheless, high-resolution CT may be preferable to thick-section MR in some cases. CTM often remains the study of choice in patients with radiculopathy, especially prior to surgery.

REFERENCES

1. Bailey P, Casamajor L: Osteoarthritis of the spine: a cause of compression of the spinal cord and its roots. J Nerv Ment Dis 1911;38:588.
2. Brain WR, Northfield D, Wilkinson M: The neurological manifestations of cervical spondylosis. Brain 1952;75:187-225.
3. Brain WR, Wilkinson M (eds): Cervical spondylosis and other disorders of the cervical spine. Philadelphia, Saunders, 1967.
4. McRae DL: The significance of abnormalities of the cervical spine. Am J Roentgenol 1960;84:3-25.
5. McRae DL: Asymptomatic intervertebral disk protrusions. Acta Radiol 1953;40:335-355.
6. Friedenberg ZR, Miller WT: Degenerative disk disease of the cervical spine. J Bone Joint Surg 1963;45A:1171-1178.
7. Wilkinson HA, LeMay ML, Ferris EJ: Clinical-radiographic correlations in cervical spondylosis. J Neurosurg 1969;30:213-218.
8. Brieg A, Turnbull I, Hassler O: Effects of mechanical stresses on the spinal cord in cervical spondylosis. J Neurosurg 1966;25:45-56.
9. Simeone FA, Dillin WA: Treatment of cervical disk disease: selection of operative approach. Contemp Neurosurg 1986;8:1-6.
10. Di Chiro G, Schellinger D: Computed tomography of spinal cord after lumbar intrathecal introduction of metrizamide (computer assisted myelography). Radiology 1976;120:101-104.
11. Coin CG, Chas YS, Keranen V, Pennink M: Computer assisted myelography in disk disease. J Comp Assist Tomogr 1977;1:398-404.
12. Miyasaka K, Isu T, Iwasaki Y, et al: High resolution computed tomography in the diagnosis of cervical disk disease. Neuroradiology 1983;24:253-257.
13. Pech P, Daniels DL, Williams AL, Haughton VM: The cervical neural foramina: correlation of microtomy and CT anatomy. Radiology 1985;155:143-146.
14. Matsuda T, Takahashi S: Latest developments in the evaluation of the spine with the Toshiba Transaxial Tomographic Unit. In Post MJD (ed): Radiographic evaluation of the spine. Current advances with emphasis on computed tomography. New York, Masson, 1980, pp 320-352.
15. Coin CG: Cervical disk degeneration and herniation: diagnosis by computerized tomography. South Med J 1984;77:979-982.
16. Coin CG, Coin JT: Computed tomography of cervical disk disease: technical considerations with representative case reports. J Comp Assist Tomogr 1981;5:275-280.
17. Balériaux D, Noterman J, Ticket L: Recognition of soft disk herniation by contrast-enhanced CT. AJNR 1983;4:607-608.
18. Russell EJ, D'Angelo CM, Zimmerman RD, et al: Cervical disk herniation: CT demonstration after contrast enhancement. Radiology 1984;152:703-712.
19. DiChiro G, Schellinger D: Ref 10.
20. Post MJD: CT update. The impact of time, metrizamide, and high resolution on the diagnosis of spinal pathology. In Post MJD (ed): Radiographic evaluation of the spine. Current advances with emphasis on computed tomography. New York, Masson, 1980, pp 259-294.
21. Badami JP, Norman D, Barbaro NM, et al: Metrizamide CT myelography in cervical myelopathy and radiculopathy: correlation with conventional myelography and surgical findings. AJR 1985;144:675-680.
22. Thijssen HOM, Keyser A, Horstink MWM, Meijer E: Morphlogy of the cervical spinal cord on computed myelography. Neuroradiology 1979;18:57-62.
23. Jinkins JR, Bashi R, Al-Mefty O, et al: Cystic necrosis of the spinal cord in compressive cervical myelopathy: demonstration by iopamidol CT-myelography. AJR 1986;147:767-775.
24. Fox AJ, Lin JP, Pinto RS, Kricheff II: Myelographic cervical nerve root deformities. Radiology 1975;116:335-361.
25. Landman JA, Hoffman JC Jr, Braun IF, Barrow DL: Value of computed tomographic myelography in the recognition of cervical herniated disk. AJNR 1984;5:391-394.
26. Scotti G, Scialfa G, Pieralli S, et al: Myelopathy and radiculopathy due to cervical spondylosis: myelographic-CT correlations. AJNR 1983;4:601-603.
27. Nakagawa H, Okumura T, Sugiyama T, Iwata K: Discrepancy between metrizamide CT and myelography in diagnosis of cervical disk protrusions. AJNR 1983;4:604-606.
28. Dublin AB, McGahan JP, Reid MH: The value of computed tomographic metrizamide myelography in the neuroradiological evaluation of the spine. Radiology 1983;146:79-86.
29. Enzmann DR, Rubin JB, Wright A: Cervical spine MR imaging: generating high-signal CSF in sagittal and axial images. Radiology 1987;163:233-238.
30. Enzmann DR, Rubin JB: Cervical spine: MR imaging with a partial flip angle, gradient-refocused pulse sequence. Radiology 1988;166:467-472.
31. Hedberg MC, Drayer BP, Flom RA, et al: Gradient echo (GRASS) MR imaging in cervical radiculopathy. AJR 1988;150:683-689.
32. VanDyke C, Ross JS, Tkach J, et al: Gradient-echo MR imaging of the cervical spine: evaluation of extradural disease. AJR 1989;153:393-398.
33. Modic MT, Masaryk TJ, Ross JS, et al: Cervical radiculopathy: value of oblique MR imaging. Radiology 1987;163:227-231.
34. Flannigan BD, Lufkin RB, McGlade CH, et al: MR imaging of the cervical spine: neurovascular anatomy. AJR 1987;148:785-790.
35. Czervionke LF, Daniels DL, Ho PSP, et al: Cervical neural foramina: correlative anatomic and MR imaging study. Radiology 1988;169:753-759.
36. Tsuruda JS, Norman D, Dillon W, et al: Three-dimensional gradient-recalled MR imaging as a screening tool for the diagnosis of cervical radiculopathy. AJNR 1989;10:1263-1271. AJR 1990;154:375-383.
37. Teresi LM, Lufkin RB, Reicher MA, et al: Asymptomatic degenerative disk disease and spondylosis of the cervical spine: MR imaging. Radiology 1987;164:83-88.
38. Takahashi M, Yamashita Y, Sakamoto Y, Kojima R: Chronic cervical cord compression: clinical significance of increased signal intensity on MR images. Radiology 1989;173:219-224.
39. Masaryk TJ, Modic MT, Geisinger MA, et al: Cervical myelopathy: a comparison of magnetic resonance and myelography. J Comp Assist Tomogr 1986;10:184-194.
40. Larsson EM, Holtås S, Cronqvist S, Brandt L: Comparison of myelography, CT myelography, and magnetic resonance imaging in cervical spondylosis and disk herniation. Pre- and postoperative findings. Acta Radiol 1989;30:233-239.
41. Modic MT, Masaryk TJ, Mulopulos GP, et al: Cervical radiculopathy: prospective evaluation with surface coil MR imaging, CT with metrizamide, and metrizamide myelography. Radiology 1986;161:753-759.

PART II SYSTEMIC DISORDERS

9 Bone and Soft Tissue Infection

CORNELIA N. GOLIMBU

Bone and soft tissue infections represent a category of diseases in which complete restoration of function and structure can be achieved only with early detection, followed by appropriate medical and surgical treatment. Because these processes are eminently curable, though at the same time often life threatening, due emphasis should be put on their early diagnosis.

OSTEOMYELITIS

The challenges that radiologists and clinicians face with osteomyelitis are early detection, characterization of the pathological process, and planning of therapy, all aimed at arresting the disease before significant loss of bone has taken place.

The clinical signs of the early stage of osteomyelitis are nonspecific: the pain may be localized or diffuse; fever may be high, low, or absent; soft tissue swelling may be undetectable at physical examination, particularly around the pelvis, shoulder, and spine. The laboratory data (leukocytosis, increased sedimentation rate) may be at times only moderately abnormal.

The clinical presentation of individual cases tends to follow several distinct patterns, or sometimes a combination of patterns:

1. First, is the patient, usually young, who presents with fever and acute onset of pain localized to an extremity. In this case the locus of involvement is known and it remains only to differentiate acute osteomyelitis from cellulitis and soft tissue abscess.

2. Second, is the patient, usually middle-aged or older, who presents with an insidious onset of pain in the back and pelvis, often without fever. In this case the locus of involvement in the spine or pelvis must be detected and a determination made as to whether the disease is tumor, arthritis, or bone infection.

3. Third, is the patient with recurrent symptoms at the site of an old osteomyelitis. In this case the locus of involvement is known and the process suspected; what must be determined is whether the patient has a reactivation of infection. This is accomplished by searching for sequestra, sinus tracks, and abscesses requiring drainage.

4. Yet another pattern occurs in the patient with soft tissue ulcers permitting access to the surface of a bone. This individual may present with one of the sequential stages of periostitis, osteitis, or osteomyelitis (assuming the infectious process has been allowed to continue), and in this case it is important to determine the exact depth of involvement of the soft tissue layers and bone.

In the diagnosis of osteomyelitis the role of the

radiologist is to detect, characterize, and differentiate the infection from other processes and to offer a "best route" approach for biopsy and surgical treatment. In many instances needle aspiration biopsy and drainage of periosseous abscesses will also be performed by the radiologist, with CT, sonographic, or fluoroscopic guidance.

Clinicopathological forms

Acute osteomyelitis, encountered in young patients, usually has an abrupt and suggestive clinical course: the child is febrile with intense pain and localized soft tissue swelling, usually in an extremity. The disease may follow an upper respiratory tract or skin infection.[1] In adults the onset is often insidious and symptoms may overlap those of conditions associated with bacteremia (e.g., diverticulitis, urinary tract infection, or endocarditis).[2-6]

Infectious material circulating in the bloodstream finds propitious conditions for its development in the sluggish blood flow of the metaphyseal sinusoids. Once lodged there, it induces formation of a nidus of infection with inflammatory exudate in the marrow. This increases the intraosseous pressure and leads to ischemia, which in turn facilitates the spread of infection in necrotic tissues.[7-8]

The marrow is contained within an unexpandable space limited by the cortical bone. This is conducive to a chain reaction—infectious nidus, exudate, ischemia, bone necrosis, advancement of infection—that eventually reaches the cortical bone and destroys it. In cases of extensive necrosis a segment of bone devoid of vascularity (sequestrum) forms; it appears denser than the surrounding viable bone, which becomes osteoporotic as a result of hyperemia.[9]

The destruction of cortical bone is initially linear, following the haversian channels; ultimately it appears as confluent areas of absent cortex.[9] When the process reaches the bone surface, a periosteal reaction occurs that initially is single layered; subsequent bouts of infection may give a multilayered aspect to the periostitis. At the same time the periosseous soft tissues are affected by hyperemia, an inflammatory reaction producing diffuse swelling, and (later) abscess collections contiguous with the subperiosteal pus and intracortical/intramedullary abscess. If they are left untreated, such abscesses may develop a sinus track, leading to spontaneous drainage through the skin surface.[9]

Chronic osteomyelitis is a continuing infection of bone usually characterized by relapses with exacerbation of symptoms. It can follow acute osteomyelitis left unhealed by poor response or insufficient treatment. Rarely it will take an indolent course from its onset, leading to localized forms such as Brodie's abscess and sclerosing osteomyelitis of Garré: the first is an intraosseous infection with well-defined sclerotic borders, the second a chronic infectious process manifesting as sclerosis with irregular thickening of the cortex in a long bone.[10,11]

With chronic osteomyelitis the long-standing inflammatory process causes a reactive bone sclerosis. Relapses of symptoms signal reactivation of the process, leading to new osteolysis and to formation of sequestra with fistulous tracks through the cortical bone into adjacent soft tissues. This intermingling of sequestration with bone destruction and sclerosis often makes the diagnosis of active osteomyelitis nearly impossible.[12]

The presence of a sequestrum is the most reliable sign that cure has not been accomplished. Pathogenic organisms lodged in the necrotic bone may intermittently reinfect adjacent areas, leading to relapse. The necrotic bone, devoid of vascular supply, cannot be reached by antibiotics and therefore is not sterilized in the healing phase; it remains a culture medium in which dormant populations of infective organisms may persist for years, ready to multiply at any reduction in the host's immune responses.

Radiological diagnosis
RADIONUCLIDE STUDIES

In the early stages of acute osteomyelitis there may be no abnormalities detectable by conventional radiography. In such instances radionuclide studies are used to determine whether skeletal involvement is present.

A three-phase technetium (medronate diphosphonate) bone scan will reveal the difference between osteomyelitis and cellulitis based upon the combination of increased blood flow and persistent osseous uptake on delayed images.[13] Although this sensitive examination is nonspecific, its value in diagnosing osteomyelitis can be increased by correlating with a positive gallium-67-citrate or indium-111–labeled leukocyte scan.[13-18] False-negative results have been reported in children with osteomyelitis,[19,20] presumably due to the peculiarities of vascularity in the epiphyses and metaphyses of young children (especially newborns).

In patients with chronic osteomyelitis, reactivation of the inflammatory process can be demonstrated when a localized area of increased uptake on gallium-67-citrate and indium-111–labeled leukocyte scans is detected.[15] However, the bone scans usually show persistent uptake at any site of old osteomyelitis and are therefore less helpful in diagnosing active infection.

All these nuclear studies are used either to detect bone involvement or to determine its activity; none has enough spatial resolution to establish morphological characteristics of the lesion. This can be accomplished by conventional radiography, CT, and MRI.

CONVENTIONAL ROENTGENOGRAPHY

Infections of the skeleton produce a limited number of roentgenographic abnormalities: soft tissue swelling, periosteal reaction, osteolysis, osteosclerosis, expansion of the cortex. These are nonspecific findings; infections, tumors, and trauma can have overlapping manifestations.[21]

Often in the early stages of acute osteomyelitis the only abnormality that will be seen is soft tissue swelling. *Periosseous soft tissue swelling* in acute osteomyelitis of a long bone can be best observed on roentgenograms when compared with the noninvolved side. In the axial skeleton the soft tissue manifestations of infection are often roentgenographically silent. Elevation of the periosteum produced by edema and inflammatory exudate is the roentgenographic sign of *periosteal reaction,* initially thin and single layered but subsequently becoming thick, dense, and occasionally multilayered. This can cause the "bone within a bone" pattern called involucrum, essentially a large cuff of periosteal new bone advancing centrally and replacing the necrotic or partially destroyed old cortex.

During the early phase of infection, when the site of involvement is limited to a small nidus in the spongy bone, roentgenograms may be negative. As the focus of bony destruction increases, a radiolucent area, usually with poorly defined margins, appears. Cortical invasion is signaled by a permeative *osteolysis* following the haversian and Volkman canals, which become visible as their walls are eroded.[9] Eventually large segments of bone are destroyed and cavities develop in the marrow space.

Chronic stages of infection are associated with *osteosclerosis,* manifested roentgenographically as increased density with focal or diffuse distribution around a nidus. The periosteal reaction becomes dense, blends with the original surface of bone, and causes expansion of the bone margin with increased thickness and density of the cortical layer.

On roentgenograms a *sequestrum* (a dense necrotic fragment of bone) stands out sharply against the radiolucent cavity of an intraosseous abscess. From this cavity *sinus tracks* are seen to penetrate the cortical bone, traverse the soft tissue, and ultimately drain through the skin. Positive contrast studies of these draining sinuses (sinography) can demonstrate their extent and ramifications. Small sequestra may be obscured by the surrounding sclerotic bone. Whereas in the past conventional tomography was used to detect these and the accompanying sinus tracks in cortical bone,[9] currently this is done with CT.[22]

COMPUTED TOMOGRAPHY

CT offers two major advantages: superior density resolution and axial display of anatomy. These facilitate the detection of subtle changes in the marrow, spongy and cortical bone, and surrounding soft tissues.[23-25] However, the spatial resolution of CT is less than that of conventional radiography and tomography.[26] A fine periosteal reaction in the early stages of osteomyelitis in a long bone may not be visible on CT images. Nevertheless, this is compensated by the improved density resolution, which makes small intraosseous erosions and subtle periosseous soft tissue swelling more clearly detectable.

TECHNIQUE

1. IV contrast is used for enhancement of the hyperemia present in tissues that are inflamed.
2. Whenever possible, slices should be oriented perpendicular to the long axis of the bone involved; (i.e., axial images for the spine, scapula, pelvis, and extremities; tilted coronal views for the dome of the talus or the sacral wing).
3. Slice thickness selection depends primarily upon the size of bone to be studied (i.e., 10 mm for the pelvis and long bones; 3 mm for the wrist, hand, ankle, and foot; 5 mm for most other segments, including the spine).
4. When feasible, the opposite extremity should also be scanned in a symmetrical position.

BONE ABNORMALITIES

Osteolysis limited to spongy bone is the earliest sign of infection that can be seen in the vertebral bodies, flat bones of the pelvis and shoulder, carpal and tarsal bones, and metaphyses of the long bones. CT reveals it as a localized area of diminished bone density (Fig. 9-1). Usually the margins of the lesion are irregular, and the center is occupied by a nonhomogeneous zone of low attenuation (representing pus) (Fig. 9-2). Occasionally the remaining trabecular bone, engulfed by the inflammatory process, is visualized as fragments with frayed margins (Fig. 9-3). Small areas of cortical bone destruction appear as interruptions in the dense envelope of compact cortex, usually contiguous with an intramedullary focus of osteolysis. Thin axial slices are particularly useful in detecting them (Fig. 9-4).

Bone marrow abnormalities demonstrated by CT vary in appearance according to their location. In the diaphy-

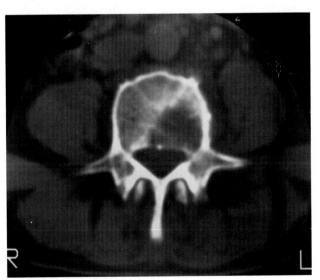

FIGURE 9-1
Early stage of osteomyelitis. A localized area of diminished bone density in the left side of the L4 vertebral body suggests a focus of infection detected before cortical erosion has taken place.

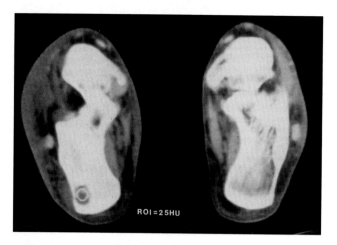

FIGURE 9-2
Marrow abscess. Osteomyelitis of the right os calcis presents as a zone of low attenuation in the bone suggestive of pus collection. (The cursor registers a mean density of 25 HU.)

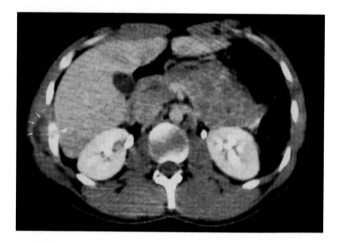

FIGURE 9-4
Osteomyelitis of the rib. CT image of the upper abdomen showing a soft tissue abscess (arrows) adjacent to an area of cortical and spongy bone erosion of the right eleventh rib (arrowhead).

ses of long bones, edema, pus, and granulation tissue can make the density higher than that of normal fatty marrow. Thus, on axial images obtained at identical levels in affected and normal extremities, the density of the marrow cavity of a long bone will change from negative to low-positive values as slices are obtained closer to the focus of osteomyelitis[27] (Fig. 9-5). In the metaphyses, where spongy bone and red marrow predominate, measurements of density will register in the opposite direction: decreasing at the pathological site (due to the destruction of bone trabeculae). This can usually be seen by adjusting the window and level settings. Exact density measurements (in Hounsfield units) are rarely necessary, especially within spongy bone (Fig. 9-6).

Bone sclerosis appears on CT images as thickening of the cortex and increased density of the affected bone (Fig. 9-7). With chronic osteomyelitis, demonstration of a *sequestrum* is important for planning treatment (its

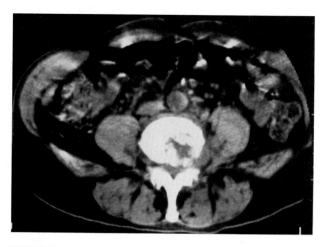

FIGURE 9-3
Advanced bony erosion in osteomyelitis. There is destruction of L3, with irregular margins. Fragments of bone engulfed by the inflammatory process protrude into the left neural foramen.

presence implies the need for surgical intervention). On CT images the sequestrum appears as a fragment of isolated dense bone surrounded by a low-density area representing pus[28] (Fig. 9-8). In cases in which the entire affected bone has become dense, it is necessary to use wide window (2000 to 4000 HU) and high level settings (400 to 600 HU) to facilitate detection of focal lesions such as cloacae and sequestra (Fig. 9-9).

Air (gas) in bone is seldom seen with hematogenous osteomyelitis, but when it is present a gas-forming organism is usually the cause.[29-31] Occasionally a fistulous track connecting the bowel lumen with a bone abscess in the pelvis will be responsible for gas accumulating in the marrow cavity; this has been described in Crohn's disease.[31] Sinus tracks draining through the skin or communicating with a decubitus ulcer (pressure sore) may also provide a route for air to reach the marrow cavity of bones affected by osteomyelitis (Fig. 9-10).

Fat-fluid levels have been found in patients with osteomyelitis of the epiphyses and metaphyses of long bones. They are produced when necrosis of the cell wall releases droplets of fat from the marrow cells into the cavity formed by an intraosseous abscess. When intraarticular cortical bony erosion is also present, this free fat may extend further into the synovial space[32] (Fig. 9-11).

SOFT TISSUE ABNORMALITIES

Swelling can be diffuse or localized to the tissues in the immediate vicinity of cortical bone destruction (Fig. 9-12).

Sinus tracks are visible on CT images as thin channels containing air[23] and can be outlined by positive contrast sinography. Their deep ramifications, often communicating with foci of intraosseous infection, are readily seen on CT images (CT-sinogram). The exact relationship between the abscess in the marrow cavity, a sequestrum, and the sinus track containing positive contrast is demonstrated best on CT axial images (Fig. 9-13).

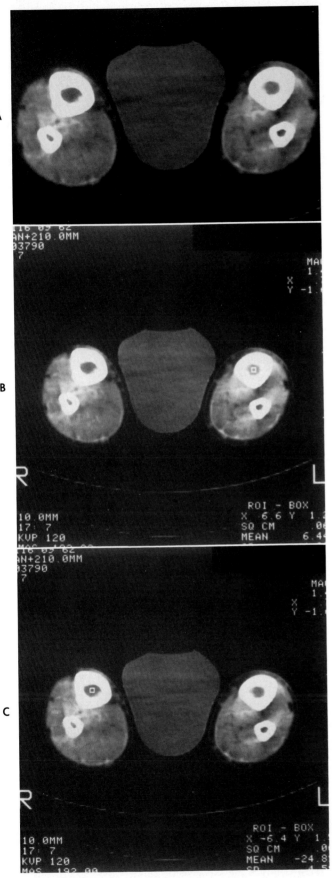

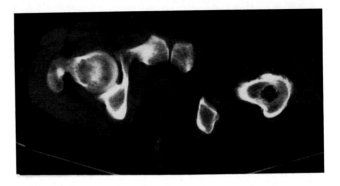

FIGURE 9-5
Osteomyelitis of the left tibia. **A,** CT image of the legs showing a soft tissue density in the medullary cavity of the left tibia (as opposed to fat on the right side). **B** and **C,** Same image with the density measured: *left,* +6 HU; *right,* −24 HU.

FIGURE 9-6
Osteomyelitis of the left femur. CT image of the hips showing an osteolytic zone in the intertrochanteric region of the left femur. It represents a focus of infection.

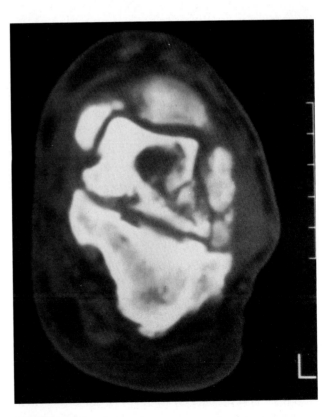

FIGURE 9-7
Chronic osteomyelitis of the talus and lateral malleolus. Increased density surrounding a central focus of osteolysis in the talus. The lateral cortex is fragmented, and there is soft tissue swelling.

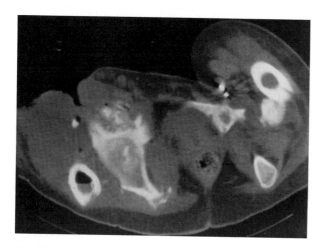

FIGURE 9-8
Sequestrum of chronic osteomyelitis. A CT image of the pelvis shows bony erosion of the right sacroiliac joint. A piece of bone detached from the adjacent structures represents the sequestrum. It is surrounded by a low-density collection of pus. A sinus track *(arrowheads)* originating in the focus of the infection traverses the soft tissue posteriorly.

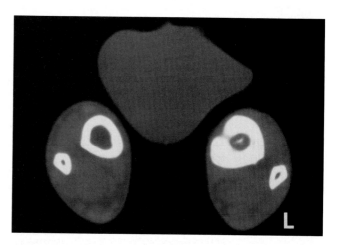

FIGURE 9-9
Chronic osteomyelitis of the left tibia. A CT image obtained with wide window and high level settings (3000/650) demonstrates a sinus track traversing the medial aspect of the thickened and sclerotic cortex. In the medullary cavity a sequestrum is present.

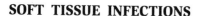

FIGURE 9-10
Chronic osteomyelitis secondary to decubitus ulcers. A sinus track provides access for air entering the marrow cavity of the femur, where an air-fluid level can be seen.

SOFT TISSUE INFECTIONS

Infections of soft tissues can take the form of cellulitis, phlegmon, or abscess:

Cellulitis is an inflammatory process of the superficial layer of soft tissues seen either as the only manifestation of disease or as part of an abscess. It appears on CT images as a reticular crisscrossing pattern of soft tissue densities, mostly linear, against the lower-density background of subcutaneous fat. The edematous skin appears thickened, and there is loss of definition between the fascial planes and the layers of fat separating muscle bundles (Fig. 9-14).

Phlegmon is an early stage of deep soft tissue infection that appears on CT images as an ill-defined mass blending imperceptibly with the surrounding layers. It may occupy a moderate to large volume and cause displacement of adjacent structures. The crisp separation between muscle bundles, fascial planes, and

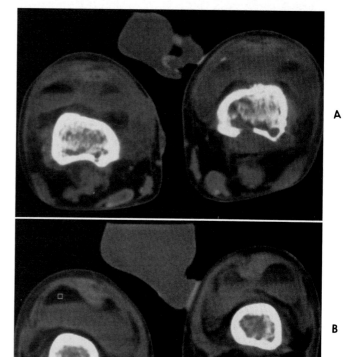

FIGURE 9-11
Fat-fluid level in the synovial space. The suprapatellar bursa contains a fat-fluid level secondary to the release of free fat into the synovial space of the knee from osteomyelitis foci in the marrow of both femurs. Culture of the aspirate grew *Klebsiella* and *Enterobacter* species. **A,** Nonenhanced CT of the supracondylar segments. The left femur has extensive cancellous and cortical bony destruction. **B,** Fat-fluid levels in the suprapatellar bursae. (The mean density is −94 HU.)

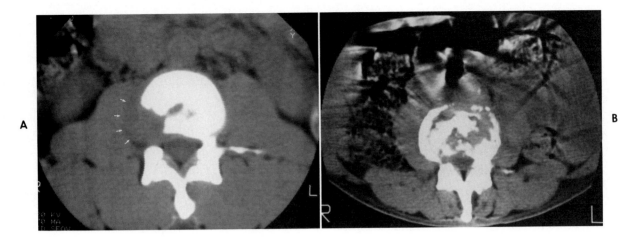

FIGURE 9-12
Soft tissue swelling around a focus of osteomyelitis. **A,** Localized and, **B,** diffuse.

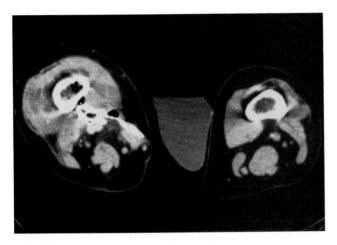

FIGURE 9-13
CT sinogram of chronic osteomyelitis. Contrast and air from the sinus track are visible inside the right femur and on its surface.

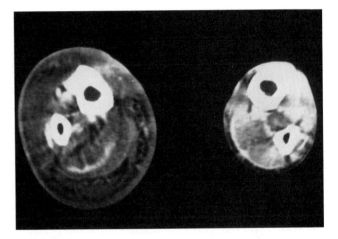

FIGURE 9-14
Cellulitis. Note the diffuse swelling and thickened skin. The subcutaneous fat of the right calf is traversed by a reticular pattern of lymphedema.

subcutaneous fat is lost; these boundaries are replaced by a continuum of nonhomogeneous soft tissue density with "shaggy" borders (Fig. 9-15). Tiny gas bubbles may be present in the lesion.

Soft tissue abscesses have fairly characteristic CT features,[33] consisting of a low-density center (the collection of pus) surrounded by a ring of higher density (representing the wall of the abscess) (Fig. 9-16). The high-density ring is composed of granulation tissue and/or fibrosis depending upon the duration of the process and in chronic abscesses is well defined (Fig. 9-17).

In all cases of infection with soft tissue involvement, iodinated contrast solutions should be administered intravenously at the time of CT scanning. We have obtained satisfactory results using a drip injection of 200 cc of iothalamate meglumine 43%. Scanning is started when half the dose is given; the intravenous drip is continued while the examination is performed. This method produces good opacification of the vascular system, and at the same time it shows an enhancement of density in

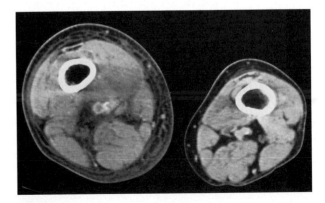

FIGURE 9-15
Phlegmon in the right thigh. A contrast-enhanced CT image shows diffuse swelling of the vastus medialis. An ill-defined area of lower density represents the inflammatory mass of the phlegmon. Lymphedema is present in the subcutaneous fat and between the muscle layers.

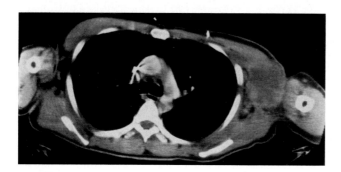

FIGURE 9-16
Acute abscess in the left axilla. A low-attenuation zone has irregular borders, with displacement and obliteration of the fat planes around it.

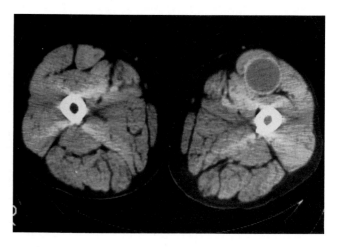

FIGURE 9-17
Chronic soft tissue abscess in the left thigh. Note the low-density collection surrounded by a well-defined fibrotic wall.

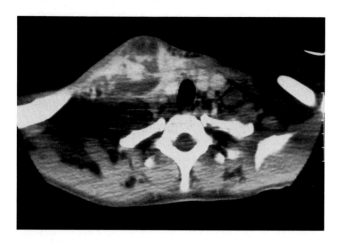

FIGURE 9-18
Acute abscess in the right supraclavicular fossa. A CT image obtained after intravenous contrast administration shows the walls of the abscess to be irregular and distinct from the low-density collections representing pus.

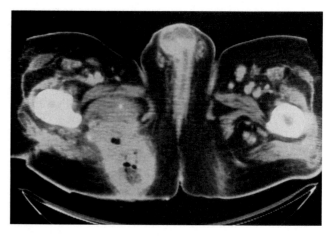

FIGURE 9-19
Sinus track. A CT image obtained after intravenous contrast administration shows a dense wall and air within the lumen of the track in the right buttock.

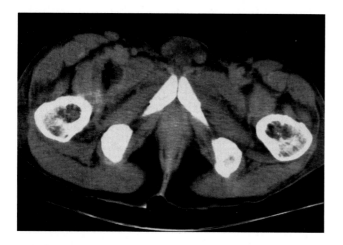

FIGURE 9-20
Soft tissue abscess containing gas. The low-attenuation zone represents necrosis and pus mixed with gas bubbles produced by a gas-forming microorganism *(E. coli)* in an abscess of the right groin.

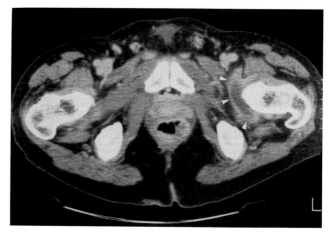

FIGURE 9-21
Early stage of a pyogenic arthritis. The synovium is thickened *(arrowheads)*, with a low-density area (fluid) around the medial aspect of the left femoral neck.

hyperemic areas, facilitating the differentiation of abscess wall from fluid content (Fig. 9-18). The same rationale applies when detecting a sinus track in the soft tissue: the wall becomes distinguishable from the surrounding tissue due to its increased density on postcontrast images (Fig. 9-19).

A most important finding in soft tissue abscesses is the presence of gas. This can be represented by a few small scattered bubbles, or by large collections intermingled with low-density necrotic tissue and pus (Fig. 9-20). The presence of air in an undrained abscess indicates infection by a gas-forming organism.[31]

INFECTIOUS ARTHRITIS

Infectious arthritis is recognized on standard roentgenograms when cortical erosion, joint effusion, and loss of the articular cartilage become apparent. Such abnormalities are seen in advanced stages of infection. The early signs of infectious arthritis (e.g., synovial thickning and minimal joint effusion) are better seen on CT (Fig. 9-21). These findings are nonspecific; they can be seen with any inflammatory process of the joints. The diagnosis of a septic joint becomes increasingly likely when articular cortical erosion appears early in patients with clinical signs of arthritis. In such cases CT shows small areas of bone destruction.[34] In joints with complex curvilinear and overlapping surfaces, CT can depict early and subtle abnormalities, because, unlike conventional radiography, it portrays the anatomy in axial planes and overcomes the overlapping of adjacent bone surfaces (Fig. 9-22).

There are no definite CT features characteristic of the type of pathogenic organisms that cause infection of the joints. In general, tuberculous arthritis tends to be associated with fairly profound juxtaarticular osteoporosis and minimal or no bony sclerosis around the erosions (Fig. 9-23). Pyogenic infections advance rapidly through articular cartilage and produce early bone erosions.

Sclerotic borders are seen at the margins of the erosions in both the subacute and the chronic phase of a pyogenic infection (Fig. 9-24).

DIFFERENTIAL DIAGNOSIS OF SOFT TISSUE AND BONE INFECTIONS

A *cellulitis* manifests with a reticular pattern of soft tissue density in the subcutaneous fat resembling that seen in lymphedema of elephantiasis or following lymph node dissection of the axilla and groin (Fig. 9-25). With

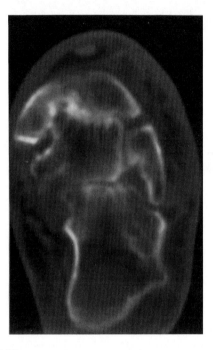

FIGURE 9-23
Tuberculous infection of the left ankle. There is a profound demineralization with erosion of the articular cortex and a loss of articular space in the tibiotalar and subtalar joints.

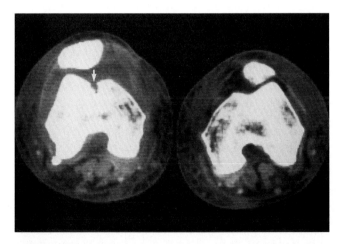

FIGURE 9-22
Pyogenic arthritis with articular cortical destruction. A CT image demonstrates erosion in the anterior aspect of the right femur *(arrow)*.

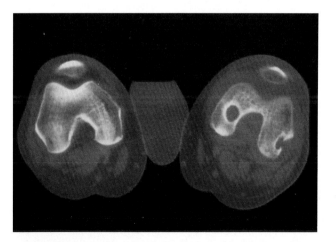

FIGURE 9-24
Chronic staphyloccocal infection. Bone erosions with a sclerotic border in the left femoral condyle.

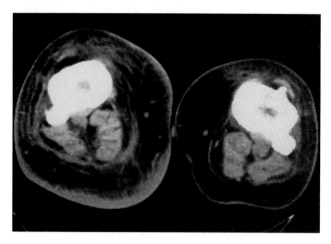

FIGURE 9-25
Chronic lymphedema secondary to lymphatic obstruction of the right leg. CT image of the calf showing thickened edematous skin and a reticular pattern of dilated lymphatics in the subcutaneous fat.

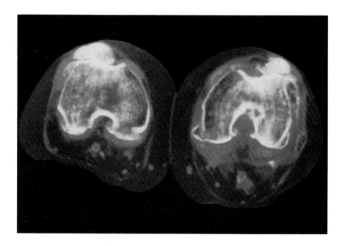

FIGURE 9-26
Joint infection complicating rheumatoid arthritis. There is asymmetrical patellar erosion with synovial swelling and effusion in the left knee. Cultures of the fluid grew *Staphylococcus aureus.*

soft tissue infection the process is more localized; with chronic obstructive lymphedema the abnormality affects the entire extremity.

A *soft tissue abscess* may be confused with necrotic soft tissue tumor, either primary or metastatic. However, tumor necrosis is usually of limited volume, central, and not likely to produce a homogeneous collection of fluid like that seen in the center of an abscess. A few reported cases have had massive necrosis of tumor, especially following chemotherapy, that produced tissue disintegration and gas accumulation[35]; but this is the exception rather than the rule, and gas in a nonhomogeneous space-occupying lesion is more likely to represent infection than tumor.[36] Another differentiating point between abscess and necrotic tumor is the proportion of solid tissue to central necrosis: in tumors the solid tissue component is usually predominant and the necrosis, represented by a nonhomogeneous low-density center, is smaller.

An *infectious arthritis* can easily be confused with rheumatoid or other noninfectious inflammatory arthritic processes, if CT appearance alone is considered. All show joint effusion, a thickened synovium, and articular bone erosion. It is the rate of progression that best differentiates an infectious from a noninfectious arthritis (rapid bone destruction suggesting a septic process).

In patients with *rheumatoid arthritis* the joints are usually affected in a symmetrical fashion and the articular cartilage and cortical bone erosions appear slowly, often over a period of months or years.[9] The clinical context is important in distinguishing noninfectious inflammatory arthritis from joint infection, especially when the two coexist. A most difficult radiological diagnosis is that of an infectious process complicating rheumatoid arthritis or kindred arthritides. Usually the infection appears in a large joint (shoulder or knee), often after a local steroid injection. The infected joint will manifest symptoms quite out of proportion to symptoms in other joints involved by

the underlying arthritis. The swelling, pain, and redness are more pronounced, and destruction of bone surfaces takes place more rapidly. On CT images these can resemble the manifestations of any aggressive erosive arthritis, whether infectious or not (Fig. 9-26). Therefore sequential studies and careful correlation with clinical findings are required to unravel the nature of the process.

The margin of error in differentiating between active noninfectious inflammatory arthritis and the same disease complicated by infection is very small. The ultimate step should always be tapping and culture of the joint fluid in any joint that shows unexpected or disproportionate inflammatory activity. In complex anatomical regions CT can be used to identify the nearest and safest location to obtain joint fluid for culture.

Osteomyelitis, with its diverse radiological features, has a relatively extensive differential diagnosis. Brodie's abscess has one outstanding feature in common with osteoid osteoma: a well-circumscribed lucent nidus surrounded by sclerotic bone reaction (Fig. 9-27 and 9-28). There are, however, subtle differences between them. The nidus of osteoid osteoma has smooth margins; that seen with osteomyelitis is irregular.[37] The sclerosis surrounding an osteoid osteoma nidus is eccentric in relation to the circumference of the bone; that with an infectious process may encircle the bone and involve the endosteal margin as well.

The sequestra characteristic of chronic relapsing osteomyelitis are not pathognomonic for it. Radiographically visible sequestra have been reported[28] with fibrosarcoma, desmoplastic fibroma, and eosinophilic granuloma. Even the central calcification in the nidus of an osteoid osteoma can be confused with a sequestrum.[37] With osteomyelitis, however, the sequestrum is usually much larger, eccentric, and of irregular contour and the soft tissues show a draining sinus, abscess, or diffuse swelling.

Sclerosing osteomyelitis of Garré, a rare form of chronic osteomyelitis, can be confused with Paget's disease of

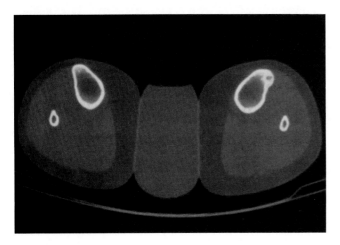

FIGURE 9-27
Osteoid osteoma of the left tibia. The nidus of infection (represented by a low-density center) is surrounded by sclerotic bone cortex. The remainder of the tibial cortex is normal.

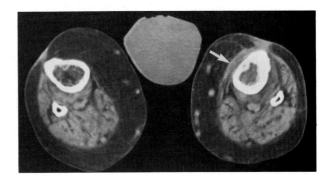

FIGURE 9-28
Brodie's abscess of the left tibia. The entire circumference of cortex is thickened, sclerotic, and irregular in its endosteal margin. Soft tissue swelling can be seen anterior to the abscess *(arrowhead).*

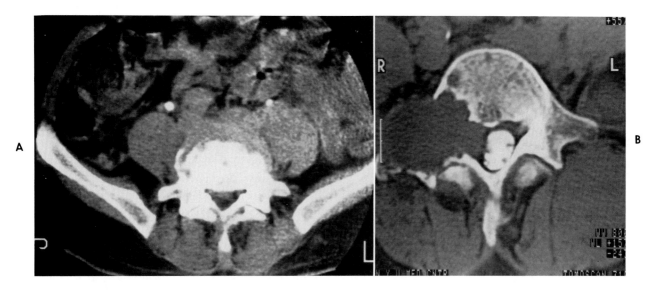

FIGURE 9-29
Soft tissue swelling of infection versus a soft tissue mass. **A,** Diffuse perivertebral swelling around pyogenic infection in L5. **B,** CT-myelogram. Neurofibroma (manifested as a localized soft tissue mass eroding the L4 vertebral body) is displacing the adjacent tissues, including the contrast-filled dural sac. The fat-muscle planes adjacent to the tumor are not obliterated.

bone. It presents with similar bony sclerosis and enlargement. The characteristic feature of Garré osteomyelitis is a focal cystic osteolysis, surrounded by bony sclerosis, that contrasts with the mixed form of Paget's disease (which progresses in an orderly fashion from the end of a long bone to the metaphysis and diaphysis, with a coarse trabecular pattern and uniform thickening of the cortex). Moreover, sclerosing osteomyelitis of Garré is seen mainly in young patients and thus confusion with Paget's disease is unlikely.[38]

An osteolytic malignant bone tumor must be distinguished from a bone abscess. With bone abscess the margins of the lesion on CT images are usually irregular and frayed whereas with most metastatic tumors the boundary is sharply defined. Infiltrative and permeative lesions, especially primary tumors, may have a wide zone of transition with irregular borders. Differentiation between these and infectious processes is dependent upon a number of factors: with tumors the soft tissue mass is exactly adjacent to the osteolytic area, centered around it, and there is minimal disturbance of the surrounding soft tissue other than displacement by the mere volume of the lesion (Fig. 9-29); by contrast, the soft tissue component of osteomyelitis is characteristically more diffuse, usually with a low-density center (representing the abscess), and the soft tissue planes are obliterated in concentric fashion.

• • •

The differentiation between tuberculous and pyogenic or other types of osteomyelitis has major implications in treatment planning, specifically in the selection of antibiotics. Unfortunately, there is a large overlap in the radiological appearances of these groups. No single feature is the exclusive indicator of a particular type of infectious agent.[39,40]

Tuberculous infections usually have a protracted clinical course, with minimal signs of disease. When first detected radiographically, the soft tissue abscess may be large and the bone destruction advanced; however, this could be more a reflection of the prolonged clinical course than a characteristic feature of the infectious process itself.[9,39] Extensive demineralization of bone surrounding a focus of tuberculous infection may be noted in the appendicular skeleton (Fig. 9-23).

Pyogenic infections have a dramatic clinical course, producing much more intense general and local signs, and as a consequence are diagnosed earlier. This may account for their (relatively) small soft tissue abscesses, diffuse swelling, and irregular frayed margins of bone destruction (which can sometimes engulf necrotic bone segments) (Fig. 9-30).

Frequently in the early stages of *brucellar osteomyelitis* the lumbar vertebrae are affected by a focal area of bony destruction limited to the endplates and disk cartilage. Infection may then extend to several vertebrae, as with advanced multilevel tuberculosis of the spine.[40]

Most of the musculoskeletal *fungal infections* have noncharacteristic CT features resembling those of other chronic infections[41] (Fig. 9-31).

When all criteria are taken into account, it is still extremely difficult to determine the causative agent of an

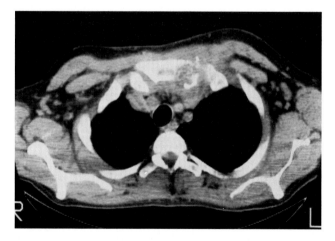

FIGURE 9-30
Acute *Pseudomonas* infection of the left sternoclavicular joint in an HIV positive patient. Note the diffuse soft tissue swelling, the necrotic bone in the center, and the irregular bone erosion.

infection if only the radiological features are considered. Percutaneous bone biopsy or aspiration of pus is essential for establishing a bacteriological diagnosis,[41,42] especially since antibiotic-resistant strains of the microbes commonly seen with osteomyelitis *(Staphyloccocus, Streptoccocus, Proteus, E. coli)* abound.[43]

CT guidance facilitates needle biopsy of infectious foci in soft tissue or bones and can reveal the most suitable site for pus aspiration as well as verify safe passage of the needle toward it[42,44-45] (Fig. 9-32).

MAGNETIC RESONANCE IMAGING

MRI has proven to be highly sensitive in detecting osteomyelitis and soft tissue infection,[46] surpassing radionuclide studies and conventional roentgenography in specificity and providing morphological details that make possible the precise localization of pathological processes. For instance, abscesses in the extremities are readily detected even when quite small, a situation in which CT may be hindered by streak artifacts generated by the beam hardening effect.[46] MRI can distinguish the inflammatory exudate from surrounding fatty marrow and thus reveal early stages of infection before cortical bony destruction appears.

A significant advantage of MRI is its ability to provide images in any plane. By selecting the appropriate plane the radiologist can visualize an entire involved segment. Longitudinal images are particularly useful for portraying extension of an abscess between layers of muscle following the planes of fascial compartments.[47] This is extremely helpful in planning surgery.

At the present stage of technical development, spatial resolution of MRI still lags behind that of CT. This and other factors can make subtle abnormalities in the cortex of bone relatively difficult to see, and a small sequestrum may be overlooked. However, in the case of osteomyelitis this is amply compensated by MRI's high sensitivity for intraosseous and periosseous abscesses.[48] Also the need for respiratory gating and the long period for data acquisition may create problems in examining the ribs, sternoclavicular joints, and sternum with MRI. (These structures are better seen on CT images.)

Technique

1. Ideally, the site to be studied should be preselected based on the abnormalities found at clinical, radiographic, or radionuclide examination. This permits tailored examinations, with adequate slice orientation, field of view, and pulse sequences.
2. T1-weighted images offer the best anatomical detail, providing excellent contrast between muscle and surrounding fat and between cortical bone and marrow. Any inflammatory process affecting the marrow will appear as a low or intermediate signal area, contrasting with the high signal of normal intramedullary fat.
3. T2-weighted images are especially helpful in detect-

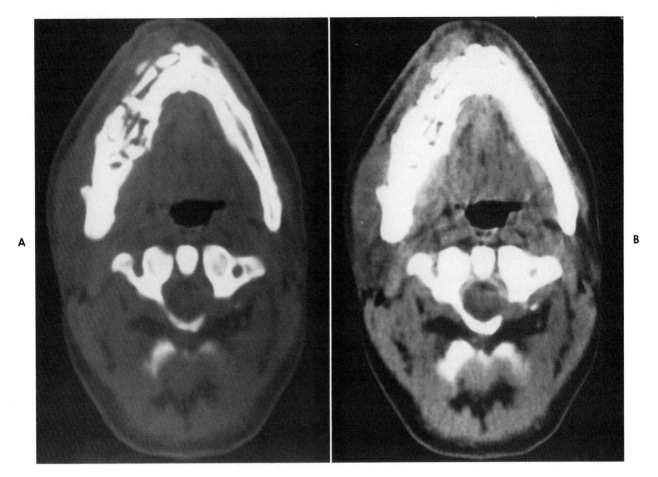

FIGURE 9-31
Actinomycosis of the right mandible. A CT image at bone window, A, and soft tissue window, B, shows
bone destruction, sequestration, and sclerosis along with moderate soft tissue swelling.

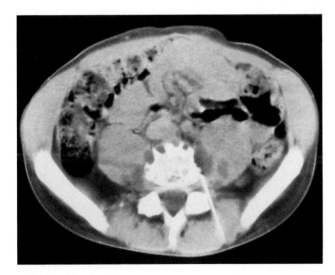

FIGURE 9-32
CT-guided percutaneous aspiration of an abscess. A needle has been
advanced toward the perivertebral soft tissue abscess, which is
contiguous with an L5 osteomyelitis. A separate loculated abscess is
visible in the left psoas.

ing abscesses. Collections of fluid (pus, hematoma,
synovial fluid) appear as high-signal zones, contrasting with the relatively low or intermediate
signal of most other tissues (including muscle, bone
marrow, and subcutaneous fat). The contrast between high signal in an abscess and signal void in
the cortical bone is particularly useful when looking
for sinus tracts traversing the bone. On the high-
signal background of an abscess the sequestra of
bone appear as dark zones of low signal.[49]

4. A short T1 inversion recovery (STIR) technique
   suppresses the signal from fat and creates better
   contrast between normal marrow (low signal) and a
   pathological process such as a focus of osteomyelitis
   (high signal). As opposed to T2-weighted images
   obtained with spin echo pulse sequences, STIR has
   the advantage of shorter scanning time and diminished artifacts.[50]

5. It is useful to obtain one set of T2-weighted images
   in an axial plane. This will eliminate most of the
   problems with partial volume visualization due to
   the slanting surfaces of metaphyses and diaphyses
   of long bones seen on coronal and sagittal images,

and it permits evaluation of the progression of infection from marrow through cortical bone into the soft tissues.[51]

T1-weighted images obtained after intravenous administration of gadopentetate show enhancement of the signal in hyperemic zones of inflammation, and thus allow distinction to be made between the wall of an abscess and the central necrotic area or pus.[52] This is in contradistinction to T2-weighted images, which portray both the hyperemic wall and the fluid center with similar high-signal intensities so that they are difficult to separate.

It is important to obtain T1-weighted images before and after Gadopentetate, because hyperemia diffusely involving the bone marrow appears high in signal on postinjection images and may blend with the normal marrow signal, thus obscuring the focus of infection.[52]

Gadopentetate-enhanced images are most useful in the detection of epidural abscesses. The inflammatory mass has high signal and can be easily separated from the compressed dural sac.[53]

MRI can detect progression toward healing, as manifested by transition from a high-signal to an intermediate- or low-signal zone, in the focus of osteomyelitis. This is a reflection of the ongoing repair of an abscess by replacement with fibrous tissue.[51,54]

MR diagnosis of infections

On T2-weighted images a *soft tissue abscess* appears as a zone of high signal (Fig. 9-33) whose margins may be smooth or irregular. If the abscess has been present long enough to become encapsulated, MR images will demonstrate a low-signal rim surrounding the high-signal pus collection. However, the presence of air in an abscess, a useful diagnostic sign clearly detected by CT, can be easily overlooked on MR images; the small bubbles may

have been volume averaged with surrounding structures and their signal void may not be apparent.

Cellulitis is characterized on T2-weighted images by diffusely increased signal in the soft tissues. The abnormality blends with the surrounding areas,[46] although in the subcutaneous fat a reticular pattern of abnormal signal may be noted (that usually represents the lymphedema commonly seen with cellulitis) (Fig. 9-34).

Synovitis manifests with fluid collections in the joints or synovial spaces of the tendon sheaths or bursae. On T2-weighted sequences it appears as high-signal collections, and on T1-weighted images as intermediate-signal collections, with an anatomical distribution conforming to the distended synovial space (Fig. 9-35). What distinguishes these accumulations from normal joint effusion is not the signal characteristics (which are identical in both cases) but the *abnormalities in adjacent tissues:* edema and inflammatory exudate in the muscles and fasciae resembling the pattern of diffusely increased signal on T2-weighted images seen with cellulitis. The acute phase of an inflammatory process in nonspecific bursitis can present the same MR features as an infection of the respective synovial space.[48] Clinical and laboratory data must be used to differentiate the two. Often culture of the fluid is the only way to provide a definitive answer.

Infectious arthritis presents a combination of joint effusion, articular cartilage erosion, and cellulitis surrounding the joint (Fig. 9-36). On T2-weighted images an area of signal hyperintensity can be seen in the soft tissues around the affected joint. The subcutaneous fat is traversed by a reticular pattern of lymphedema (low or intermediate signal on T1, high signal on T2), and erosion of the articular cartilage may be perceived as narrowing of the joint space. The fluid and superficial layers of articular cartilage have similar signal characteristics on both T1- and T2-weighted images. Therefore

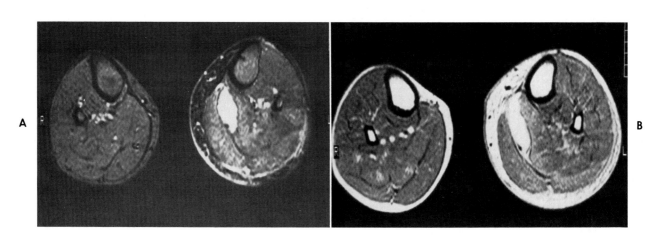

FIGURE 9-33
Soft tissue abscess. **A,** Axial T2-weighted image. The oval zone of high signal represents fluid (pus) in the medial aspect of the left calf. Edema of the subcutaneous soft tissue is manifested as diffuse signal hyperintensity. **B,** Axial proton density image. There is normal signal in the marrow. The reticular pattern of lymphangitis appears as a linear low-signal area against the background of high-signal subcutaneous fat.

cartilage loss is perceived only indirectly: the two opposing articular surfaces are closer, and the joint appears "etched in black" (Fig. 9-37). The articular cortex itself may become eroded, and zones of high signal may be seen traversing it. Once signal abnormalities involve the marrow adjacent to the destroyed articular cortex, a full transition to osteomyelitis has taken place. This is one of the most serious complications of infectious arthritis (Fig. 9-36).

Acute osteomyelitis is best seen on T2-weighted images as a focus of signal hyperintensity in the bone marrow (Fig. 9-38). A proton density type of image (long TR/short TE spin echo technique) is used mainly to provide a general anatomical map of the location. The signal pattern in this pulse sequence is usually not suitable for differentiating between normal and infected marrow.[55] The detection of an intramedullary abscess should be based upon the appearance of abnormalities in the long TR/long TE images (2000/80) or comparable gradient echo images. On T2-weighted images the periosteal reaction appears as a thin line of signal hyperintensity parallel to the cortex and marginated peripherally by low-signal lines representing the periosteum itself, often already calcified. The adjacent soft tissues may contain an abscess or be diffusely edematous (Fig. 9-39).

With *chronic osteomyelitis* bone sclerosis, whether

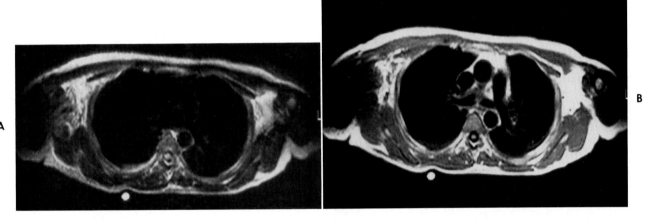

FIGURE 9-34
Cellulitis. **A,** T2-weighted axial image. Note the increased signal in the muscle bundles on the lateral aspect of the right axilla as well as the indistinct borders to axillary fat. **B,** Proton density sequence, same level. Here the reticular pattern of low signal and several enlarged lymph nodes can be seen in the fat of the right axilla. Compare with the normal left side.

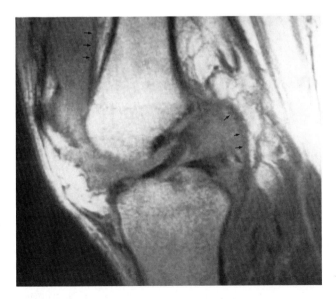

FIGURE 9-35
Synovitis as an early manifestation of infectious arthritis. A T1-weighted MR image of the knee shows joint effusion, thickening of the synovium *(arrows),* and inflammatory edema in the periarticular fat (the reticular pattern of low-signal lines).

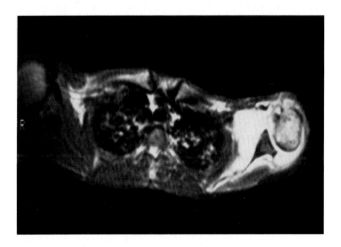

FIGURE 9-36
Tuberculous arthritis in the left shoulder. A T2-weighted axial image of the glenohumeral joint shows effusion with diffuse edema around the scapula and humerus represented by high-signal zones. Anterior to the humerus there is cellulitis of the subcutaneous fat layer. The medial cortex of the humerus is partially eroded. Increased signal in the marrow of the humeral head indicates edema and/or pus in the bone.

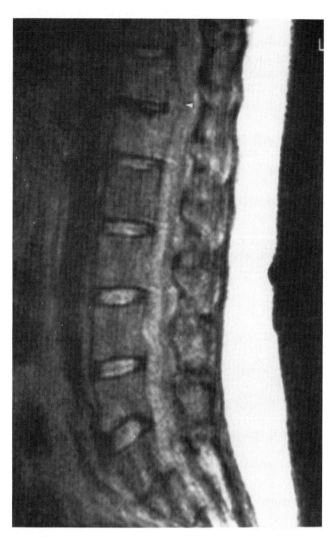

FIGURE 9-37
Infection causing loss of cartilage (joint "etched in black"). The T12-L1 disc space is narrowed and appears on this MR image to be marginated by a double low-signal line, representing the endplates of the vertebral bodies almost totally blended. The inflammatory mass bulges in the spinal canal *(arrowhead).*

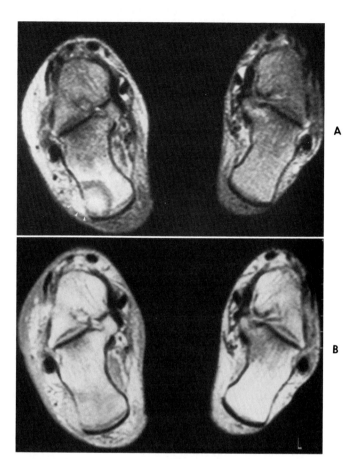

FIGURE 9-38
Acute osteomyelitis (demonstrating the usefulness of T2-weighted images). **A,** A spin echo T2-weighted axial image (TR/TE 1200/80) shows the high-signal zone surrounded by a low-signal rim in the posterolateral aspect of the right calcaneus. The adjacent soft tissues have an abscess *(arrowheads)* and diffuse swelling. **B,** Same level, proton density image (TR/TE 1200/30). Here the abnormalities are less obvious.

diffuse or limited to the periphery of the infection, will appear as a low-signal zone in the marrow. The signal void of cortex is usually irregular and thickened (Fig. 9-37). The most important feature, which MRI alone can demonstrate, is the presence of fluid in and around the bones, usually an indication of active infection. On long TR/long TE images it may appear as a hyperintense zone in the marrow cavity and periosseous soft tissues (Fig. 9-40). This sequence is particularly useful for detecting sinus tracts, which appear as high-signal bands traversing the layers of tissue. Sequestra are seen as hypointense zones of devitalized bone, contrasting with the surrounding hyperintense fluid and pus contained in the intramedullary abscess[49] (Fig. 9-40).

Caution should be exercised when interpreting MR images of comminuted fractures that may be harboring infection. The early stages of callus formation, before bone deposition, demonstrate a hyperintense signal on T2-weighted images. This should not be confused with pus accumulation at the site of osteomyelitis complicating a fracture. MRI probably cannot differentiate between early callus and early stages of infection[54]; but progressive enlargement of the fracture gap, resorption of the bone surface, and formation of cavities between the fragments are signs favoring infection.

Although a ferromagnetic orthopedic device usually degrades the MR image in its immediate vicinity,[51] often sufficient detail will remain to permit detection of an abscess in the medullary cavity or soft tissues. This is in contradistinction to CT images, on which artifacts generated by the presence of metallic implants interfere significantly with soft tissue and bone marrow visualization. The MRI artifacts around a ferromagnetic foreign body are more pronounced on scanners operating at high field strength (1.5 tesla and higher).[55]

FIGURE 9-39
Periosteal reaction in osteomyelitis. **A,** Coronal MR image (SE, TR 1000/TE 30). The reaction can be seen as a low-signal line parallel to the cortex of the distal femur on the right side. The surrounding soft tissue high-signal zone represents fluid or inflammatory edema. The marrow contains an abscess. **B,** Roentgenogram on the same day. Here the calcified periosteal reaction in the distal femoral diaphysis (*arrowheads*) is barely visible.

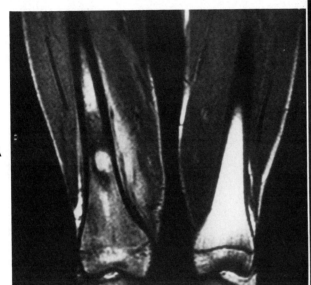

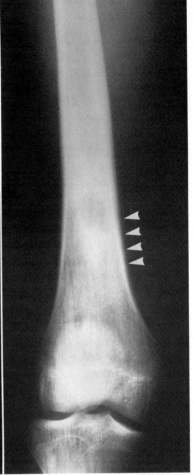

INFECTIOUS SPONDYLITIS

All segments of the skeleton involved by osteomyelitis may have impaired motion and weight-bearing function. In the spine anatomical peculiarities add the danger of cord or nerve compression, leading to radicular pain, paresis, or paralysis, with resulting morbidity and mortality. It is not surprising therefore to see the interest accorded early detection and diagnosis of osteomyelitis of the spine.[56-59]

In contrast to the decreased incidence of acute osteomyelitis in the extremities of children, the frequency of infectious spondylitis in adults has increased during the last two decades. This shift has undoubtedly come about because of the relatively larger proportion of elderly and debilitated patients in the general population as well as the increased incidence of infectious complications stemming from intravenous drug abuse and the acquired immunodeficiency syndrome.[6,60-62]

Pathogenesis

Usually infection reaches the vertebrae as septic emboli carried by the arterial blood.[63] Occasionally, however, emboli will travel from the pelvic organs through the veins of Batson to the perivertebral venous plexus and vertebral bodies.[64]

The metaphysis of a vertebra, the part immediately next to the endplate, is highly vascular. In adults most of the arterial branches in this region are end-arteries. Thus a septic embolus obliterating the lumen of such a small vessel can cause infarction of a portion of the metaphysis. Ordinarily only when there is simultaneous infarction of bone does a septic embolus develop into a focus of osteomyelitis. The initial site of bone infection corresponds to the infarcted wedge of the metaphysis. Further thrombosis of the metaphyseal arterial branches spreads the osteonecrosis and infection to the rest of the metaphysis. From here the infection can progress to destroy the endplate and invade the avascular disk cartilage (Fig. 9-41). Another route by which infection can spread is the intermetaphyseal anastomotic arteries, which permit sepsis to travel from the metaphysis of one vertebra to that of the next (skipping the intervening disk space)[65] (Fig. 9-42).

Age differences in intraosseous vascular anastomoses explain why infections of the vertebrae in children are rarely associated with marked bone destruction. Contrary

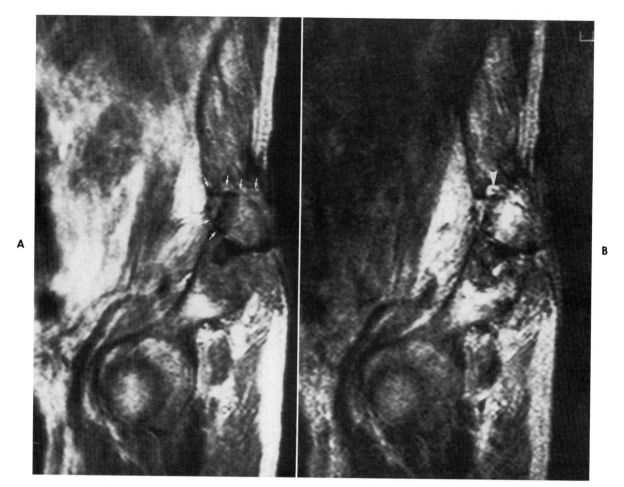

FIGURE 9-40
Chronic osteomyelitis with sequestration and draining sinuses. **A,** Sagittal T1-weighted image through the acetabulum. A sinus track extends from the skin into the iliac bone, where there is a cavity surrounded by low signal in the marrow. Superior to it another short sinus track is present *(arrows).* **B,** T2-weighted image, same level. In the superior sinus track, against the background of high signal representing fluid, there is a low-signal fragment signifying a sequestrum *(arrowhead).*

to adults, in whom the branches of the metaphyseal arteries are mostly terminal vessels, children have abundant anastomoses connecting the intraosseous metaphyseal arterioles. This makes infarction less likely in them and, when it does happen, proportionately smaller.[65] Although infection can spread to the disk cartilage as in adults, the initial focus of bone involvement is minor and remains undetected in most cases. The disk infection appears as the dominant process. It has been called *childhood diskitis* and it is distinguished from the infectious spondylitis seen in adults by its mild course and minimal bone destruction (often self limited).[66] There are transitional forms of spinal osteomyelitis bridging these two clinical forms. Intermediate stages, or transformation of diskitis into destructive osteomyelitis, can conceivably occur and have led to controversies regarding the definition of the disease process and the treatment of pediatric patients with vertebral infections.[66,67] In children with diskitis the modern radiological modalities, specifically

CT, can reveal even minor vertebral body erosions. Detection of these zones of bone destruction has strengthened the rationale for antibiotic therapy.[68]

Radiological diagnosis

The diagnosis of osteomyelitis by conventional radiography is often delayed because it is based on detection of obvious osteolysis and narrowing of the disk space. Technetium-99m and gallium scans are useful in detecting early stages of infection. However, these tests are nonspecific and occasionally misleading: false-negative results have been reported.[68]

COMPUTED TOMOGRAPHY

CT of the spine has proven to be a sensitive method for morphological characterization of vertebral infections. The focus of osteolysis representing the early stages of acute osteomyelitis is easily seen on CT images as a zone of decreased attenuation in the spongy bone of the

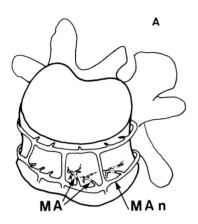
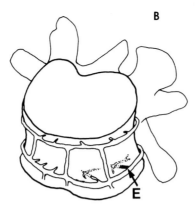
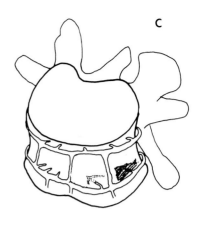

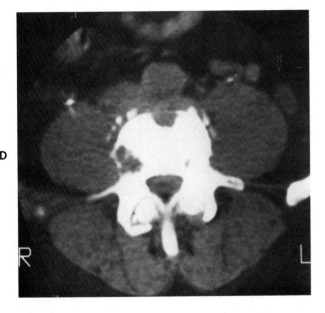

FIGURE 9-41

Pathogenesis of osteomyelitis related to the arterial supply of a lumbar vertebral body metaphysis. **A,** Normal metaphyseal arteries *(MA)* and their anastomoses *(MAn).* The intraosseous branches supply wedge-shaped zones of bone. **B,** Embolus *(E)* occluding one of the metaphyseal arteries. **C,** A wedge-shaped focus of osteomyelitis develops in the infarcted bone, corresponding to the zone supplied by the occluded artery. **D,** CT image of L3. Two distinct wedge-shaped zones of bony destruction caused by a pyogenic osteomyelitis correspond to the vascular distribution of two intraosseous branches of the metaphyseal artery.

vertebral body (Fig. 9-43, *A*). Axial images are particularly useful in detecting small areas of cortical bone destruction (Fig. 9-43, *B*). Invasion of the spinal canal is seen as an extension of the soft tissue inflammatory mass associated with the area of vertebral destruction. The dural sac appears compressed, and the epidural space may be occupied by inflammatory granulation tissue (which shows enhancement following intravenous injection of contrast) (Fig. 9-44). The dural sac compression is more evident after intrathecal injection of contrast. Partial or complete block of CSF flow can be detected at the level of osteomyelitis (Fig. 9-45) and directly influences the type of treatment selected; surgical decompression may be necessary in most of these patients.[69]

A decrease in the measured density of cartilage on CT has been reported[70] in the early stages of disk space infection. Presumably, this represents pus or other inflammatory exudate replacing the cartilage. Occasionally an accumulation of gas in the disk results from the activity of gas-forming bacteria. This, however, is a rare occurrence.[30] The most frequent cause of gas accumulation in the disk cartilage remains degenerative disease.[71]

Careful attention must be devoted to the lateral scout view of a CT examination. Any decrease in height of the disk may be important and should be noted. Although this finding is not always readily apparent on axial images, mostly because of the slice orientation, it can be seen when sagittal reformatted images are obtained from sequential axial slices.

CT can reveal a wealth of information about the perivertebral soft tissues: the contour and homogeneity of the psoas, the perivertebral fat layers, the aorta and venae cavae, the pleural surfaces, and the erector spinae group of muscles — all of which may become involved in the inflammatory process emanating from a focus of vertebral osteomyelitis.[57]

In the lumbar spine, one of the most frequently affected sites, osteomyelitis is often associated with a psoas abscess. This abnormality appears as a low-attenuation zone in the muscle sheaths surrounded by a dense irregular ring (representing the granulation tissue wall of the abscess)[33,58] (Fig. 9-46).

The inflammatory process may lift the paraspinal ligaments and take a preferential perivertebral route of spread, "jumping" the disk space and approaching an adjacent vertebral body from its anterolateral aspect, leaving the vertebral endplates intact. This is called the subligamentous form of vertebral osteomyelitis and has

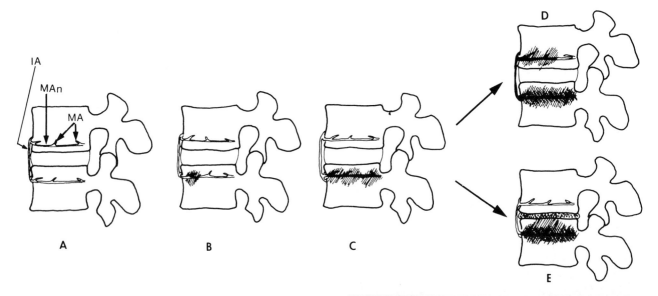

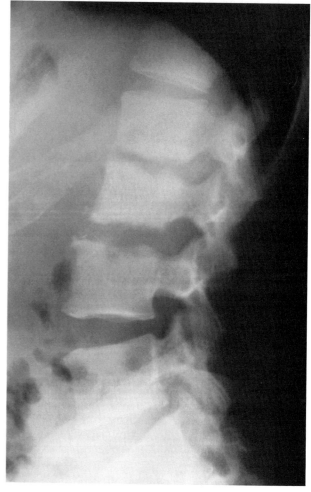

FIGURE 9-42

Spread of osteomyelitis related to arterial anastomoses of the lumbar vertebral bodies. **A,** Normal intraosseous branch of a metaphyseal artery *(MA)* with metaphyseal *(MAn)* and intermetaphyseal *(IA)* anastomoses uniting the arterial supply of two adjacent vertebral bodies. **B,** The focus of infection secondary to an embolus in one metaphyseal artery. **C,** A thrombus propagated in the metaphyseal anatomosis spreads the infarction and infection further in the same metaphysis. **D,** Through the intermetaphyseal artery the process spreads to the next vertebral body, skipping the disk cartilage. **E,** Contiguous spread of infection from the metaphysis to the endplate and disk cartilage (osteomyelitis and diskitis). **F,** Multilevel pyogenic infection of the spine. A lateral roentgenogram of the lumbar spine shows contiguous involvement of L2, L3, and the intervening disk cartilage. A lesion in the upper metaphysis of L4 has "skipped over" the L3-4 disk cartilage, which appears normal.

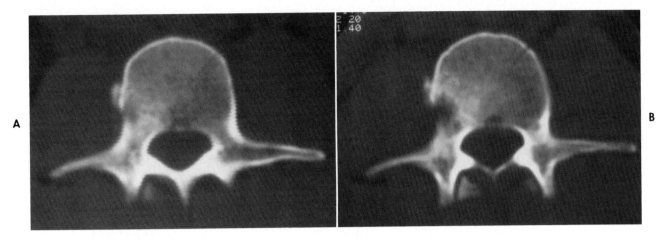

FIGURE 9-43
Early stages of vertebral osteomyelitis (staphyloccocal infection of L3). **A,** A CT scan obtained 1 week after the onset of symptoms shows osteolysis (barely visible) on the right side. **B,** A follow-up scan 10 days later shows the progression of osteolysis and cortical destruction.

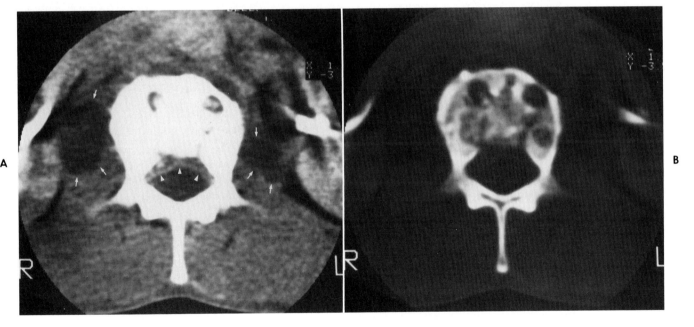

FIGURE 9-44
Tuberculous infection of L2 and a contiguous epidural abscess. **A,** A CT scan obtained after intravenous contrast injection (soft tissue window) shows the epidural abscess marginated by a dense ring of enhancement *(arrowheads)*. Two paravertebral abscesses *(arrows)* have less-defined borders. **B,** Same image (bone window). There are foci of destruction in the vertebral body, adjacent to the abscess.

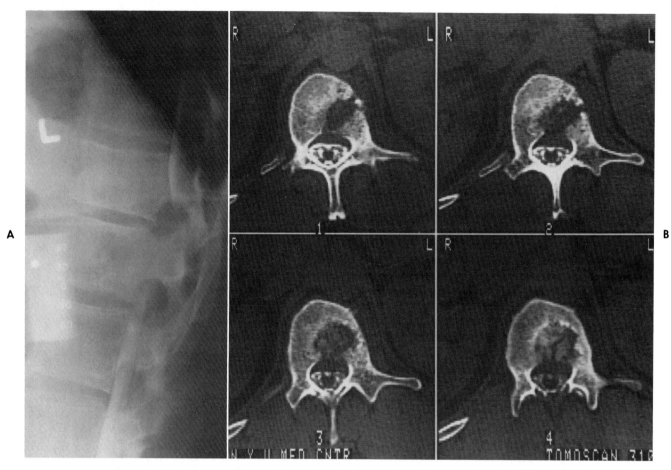

FIGURE 9-45
Osteomyelitis causing epidural block. **A,** Myelogram. Epidural compression is causing a partial block at L1. The barely visible lucency in L1 and decreased disk space of T12-L1 are subtle clues for infection. **B,** CT-myelogram. The focus of osteomyelitis has destroyed L1 and caused a partial block in the anterior epidural space.

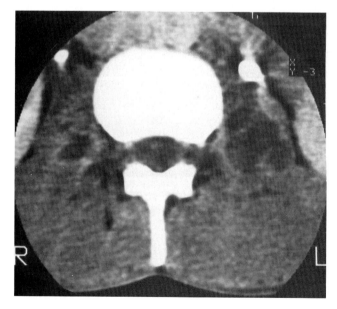

FIGURE 9-46
Bilateral psoas abscesses. CT after intravenous contrast injection. Note the low-density multilocular collection of fluid with a higher-density rim (representing granulation tissue walls of the abscesses).

been described in tuberculous infections[39] (Fig. 9-47). However, a similar manifestation may be seen in other types of infection.[40,41]

Chronic or subacute stages of infection show a sclerotic reaction at the margin of the destructive bone lesion (Fig. 9-48). Dense sclerosis of a vertebral body has been described in chronic osteomyelitis.[39] *Ivory vertebrae,* characterized by uniform osteoblastic reactions within the vertebral body, are occasionally seen in chronic osteomyelitis, although more often they appear with lymphoma or metastatic prostatic carcinoma. On CT images they appear as homogeneously increased vertebral densities with obliteration of the normal trabeculae and loss of endosteal cortical margins (Fig. 9-49).

In advanced stages of osteomyelitis there is marked destruction of spongy bone within the vertebrae. The osteolytic lesions have irregular margins and contain sequestra. When osteolysis involves mainly the anterior parts of the vertebrae, wedging can take place, with a resulting gibbus deformity (Fig. 9-50). This often leads to instability of the spine and compression of the neural elements. It is precisely these kinds of complications that are avoided by early diagnosis and prompt therapy.

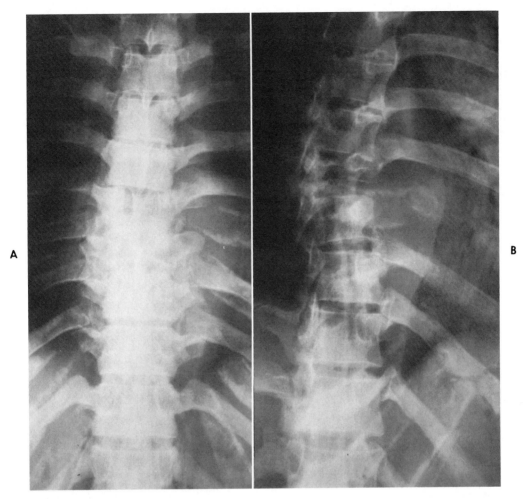

FIGURE 9-47
Subligamentous spread of infection. Tuberculous spondylitis of T7 has caused collapse of the vertebral body and destroyed the pedicle and rib on the left side. No disk pathology is visible, but fusiform soft tissue swelling can be seen. **A,** AP view of the thoracic spine. **B,** Left posterior oblique view showing lung pathology consistent with active pulmonary tuberculosis.

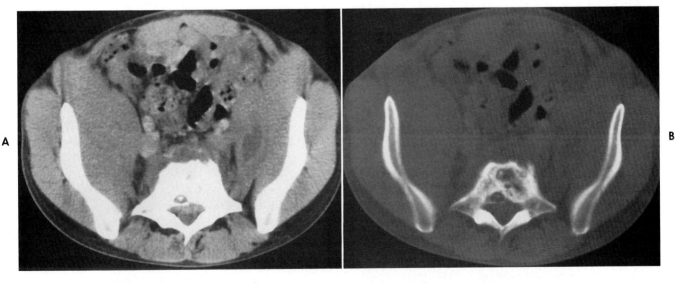

FIGURE 9-48
Chronic osteomyelitis: sequestra and psoas abscesses. **A,** Soft tissue window. There are perivertebral and left psoas abscesses. **B,** Bone window. Same images, showing the focus of bony destruction with a sclerotic border in L5. Sequestra are seen as two isolated fragments in the center of the intraosseous abscesses.

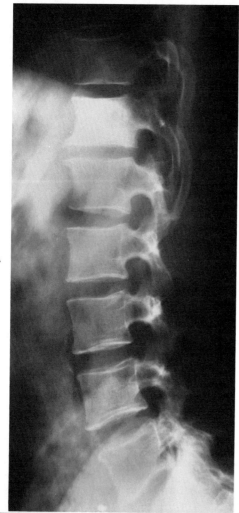

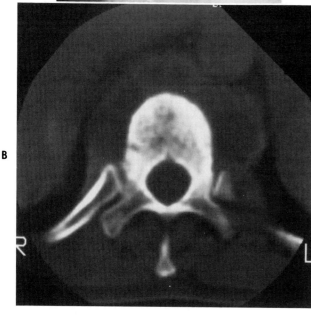

FIGURE 9-49

Ivory vertebrae due to a tuberculous infection. A, A lateral view of the spine shows osteosclerosis homogeneously involving the T12 vertebral body. A pair of reactive osteophytes and a minor decrease in the disk height at T12-L1 are subtle clues to the infection. B, A CT image through T12 (bone window) shows dense sclerosis of the vertebral body. A multiloculated perivertebral soft tissue abscess reveals the inflammatory nature of the process.

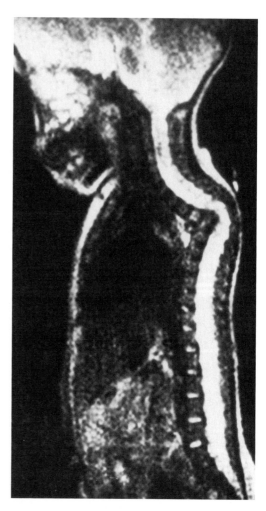

FIGURE 9-50

Gibbus. A sagittal T2-weighted image of the thoracic spine in a child with tuberculous spinal involvement shows the kyphosis with sharp angulation that resulted from destruction of T3 and T4 and an anterior wedge deformity.

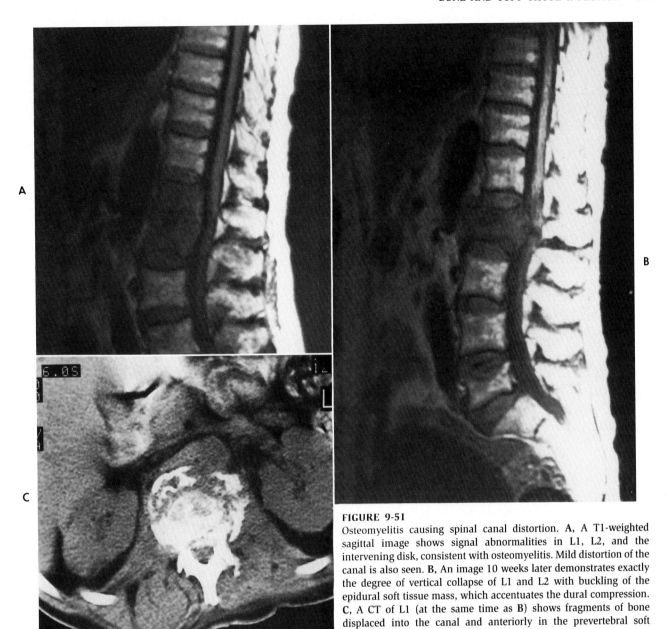

FIGURE 9-51
Osteomyelitis causing spinal canal distortion. **A,** A T1-weighted sagittal image shows signal abnormalities in L1, L2, and the intervening disk, consistent with osteomyelitis. Mild distortion of the canal is also seen. **B,** An image 10 weeks later demonstrates exactly the degree of vertical collapse of L1 and L2 with buckling of the epidural soft tissue mass, which accentuates the dural compression. **C,** A CT of L1 (at the same time as **B**) shows fragments of bone displaced into the canal and anteriorly in the prevertebral soft tissues.

Vertebral collapse, seen as a complication of advanced infections, results from the destruction of a large part of the vertebral body, which becomes unable to withstand the stresses of weight bearing. Normal motion and upright posture can bring about a fracture of the remaining shell of cortical and spongy bone, producing collapse of the vertebra, which may suddenly accentuate the degree of spinal cord compression by increasing the encroachment into the canal of the vertically compressed inflammatory mass. On CT images this is manifested as fragmentation of the endplate away from the infected disk with a centrifugal type of displacement of the fragments similar to that seen in a burst fracture (Fig. 9-51). The vertical compression and encroachment into the canal are better demonstrated on MR images (Fig. 9-51).

Rarely a vertebral osteomyelitis will affect primarily the pedicles, laminae, or spinous processes (Fig. 9-52). In patients with initial involvement of the vertebral arch, the inflammatory process frequently produces rapid invasion of the canal, with the resulting cord and nerve root compression leading to paraplegia.[72]

When progression of osteomyelitis is evaluated, consideration should be given to the usual and expected further osteolysis seen in the initial phases of healing.[73] This is due to the advancement of granulation tissue and the inflammatory process in devitalized necrotic bone at the margin of or engulfed by the infection. Bone that appears of normal density initially may, in fact, be avascular and histologically abnormal (devoid of osteocytes). Necrotic bone will be resorbed as the healing progresses and only later be replaced by new bone fusing the vertebrae in their deformed wedged shape.

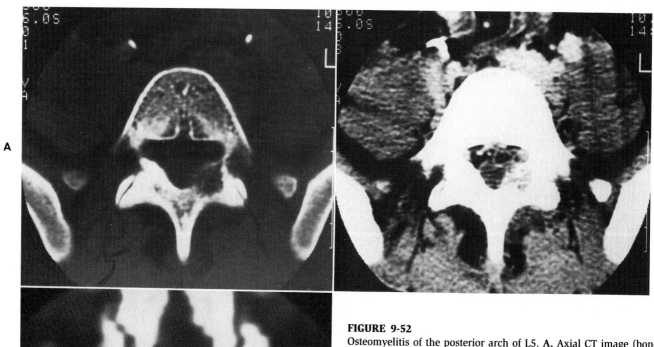

FIGURE 9-52
Osteomyelitis of the posterior arch of L5. **A,** Axial CT image (bone window). The focus of osteolysis in the left lamina is protruding into the canal as a soft tissue mass. **B,** Same image, soft tissue window. **C,** A coronal reformatted image demonstrates the vertical extent of the lesion in the left L5 lamina *(arrows)*.

The disk space itself continues to collapse during the early stage of successful therapy because the inflammatory exudate diminishes and the loss of substance in the disk cartilage is unmasked. This explains why in some cases, following appropriate antibiotic therapy, "the radiographs look worse" while the patient improves clinically. In such cases the most relevant radiological features of the follow-up examination are soft tissue characteristics at the site of vertebral infection. In patients with a favorable response to treatment the perivertebral soft tissue swelling diminishes, the abscesses decrease in size, and the amount of canal invasion is reduced (Fig. 9-53). These (rather than the bone changes, which can be

misleading in the initial period of recovery) are the more important elements demonstrating healing. Later, after the soft tissue component of the process has resolved, a slow progression toward rebuilding of bony margins takes place, ultimately leading to vertebral fusion (Fig. 9-54).

In the late phase of recovery, calcifications may be observed in the perivertebral soft tissues at the sites of previous abscesses. This is a characteristic of tuberculous infections and is similar to the calcifications seen with granulomatous lesions of the lungs, lymph nodes, spleen, and other tissues (Fig. 9-55).

MAGNETIC RESONANCE IMAGING

MR imaging of the vertebrae shows a characteristic pattern of signal abnormalities in the tissues affected by an infectious process. On T1-weighted images there is abnormally low signal in the marrow of affected vertebrae; this signal usually assumes an irregular bandlike configuration adjacent to and confluent with the involved disk cartilages. The cortical bone of the endplates loses its sharp definition as a line of signal void and blends with the adjacent abnormal signal zone of the vertebral marrow (Fig. 9-56). The disk cartilages lose their height and signal and the definition of their margins. On T2-weighted images a reversal of signal intensity is seen in a similar pattern of distribution (Fig. 9-57). The infected disk spaces have markedly bright signal and the involved vertebral endplates show increased signal; this

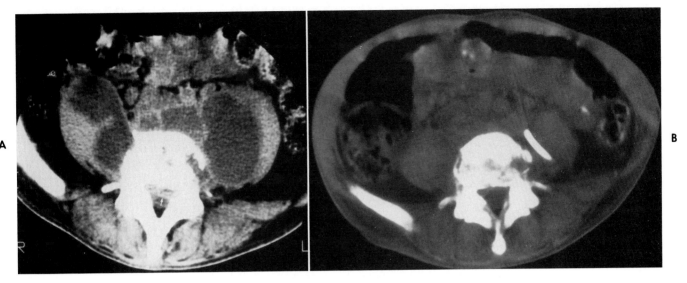

FIGURE 9-53
Healing phase of an L5 osteomyelitis with bilateral psoas abscesses. **A,** CT image. Multiloculated low-density collections in the psoas and prevertebral soft tissues. Focal area of bone destruction in the vertebral body. There is also epidural extension of the infectious process *(arrow)*. **B,** A CT image (same level) obtained 10 days later, after antibiotic therapy and percutaneous drainage of abscesses. The catheter is in the left psoas. There is now marked resolution of the abscesses; the bone destruction shows further advancement.

FIGURE 9-54
Healed infection of the lumbar spine. Lateral, **A,** and AP, **B,** roentgenograms demonstrate fusion of the L2-3 disk space.

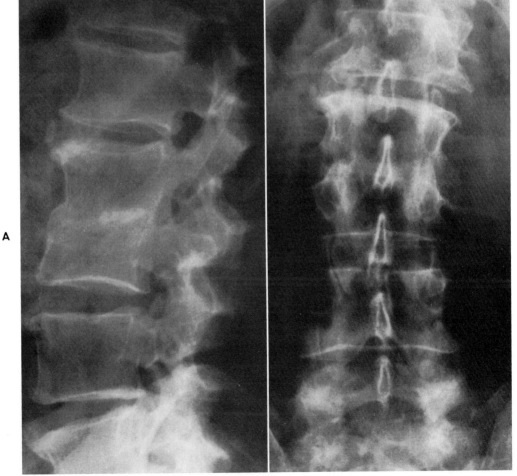

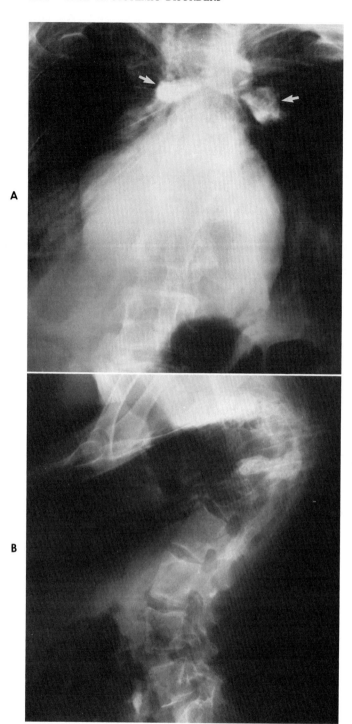

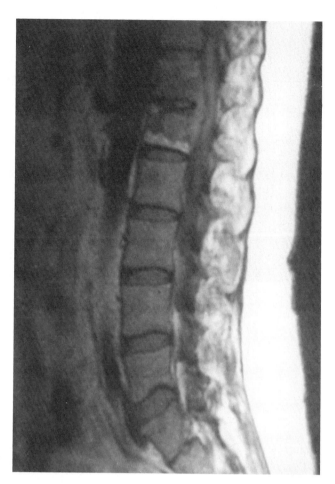

FIGURE 9-56
Osteomyelitis and infectious diskitis at T12-L1. A spin echo T1-weighted sagittal image (TR/TE 500/30) shows bands of low signal in the marrow of T12 and L1, with loss of disk height and a contiguous fusiform mass protruding into the canal.

FIGURE 9-55
Sequelae from Pott's disease. AP, **A**, and lateral, **B**, roentgenograms of the thoracic spine show calcifications in the paravertebral soft tissue *(arrows)* and a gibbus deformity secondary to multiple vertebral collapses with fusion.

contrasts with the normal marrow, which has low to medium signal at this pulse sequence.[74,75]

The most valuable information provided by MRI in patients with spinal osteomyelitis is the display of soft tissue abnormalities within the canal, specifically compression of the cord and dural sac by the inflammatory

mass[76] (Fig. 9-58). This makes CT-myelography unnecessary in most patients.

Axial images can demonstrate contiguous involvement of the bone and epidural or perivertebral soft tissues (Fig. 9-59). Fusiform psoas abscesses can be portrayed in their entirety on coronal and sagittal images,[47] which demonstrate the overall configuration of the abnormality and have an immediate impact, by conveying the extent of the process in a single image rather than demanding the effort of mental reconstruction based on a stack of axial images. They simplify the planning of needle aspiration or surgical approach for diagnostic or therapeutic purposes (Fig. 9-60).

Gadopentetate administered intravenously enhances the signal intensity of the hyperemic granulation tissue present in a focus of osteomyelitis (Fig. 9-61). It may also facilitate the diagnosis of epidural abscess by distinguishing the dural sac from the adjacent inflammatory mass.[53] In the healing phase of osteomyelitis the intensity of postgadopentetate enhancement gradually diminishes with time, reflecting a decrease in hyperemia.

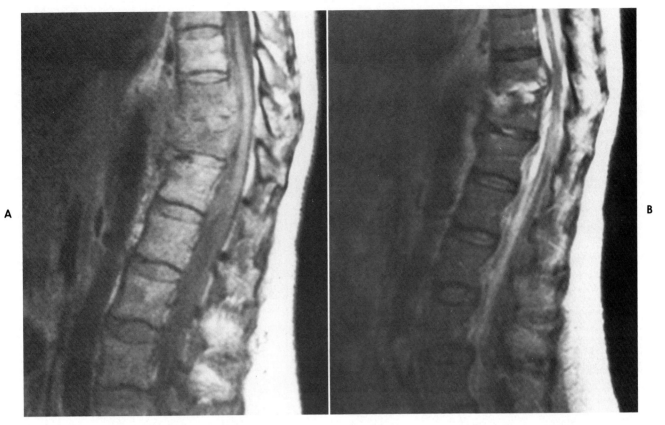

FIGURE 9-57
MRI of advanced osteomyelitis. **A,** T1-weighted midline sagittal image. There is decreased signal in the marrow of T11 and T12, and the T11-12 disk space is indistinct; the endplates, likewise, are ill defined. These vertebral abnormalities are contiguous with a fusiform epidural mass compressing the anterior surface of the cord. **B,** T2-weighted image, same level. The signal intensity in the pathological area is now the reverse of that in **A.** The disk and adjacent endplates appear bright. The epidural component of the inflammatory process is better seen at this pulse sequence.

Another advantage of enhancement studies is that they shorten the examination time; by obtaining T1-weighted images before and after gadopentetate injection, one can obviate the long scanning time characteristic of T2-weighted imaging. This becomes especially important in very sick or young patients who cannot remain immobile during scanning.

The signal abnormalities seen in the healing phase of osteomyelitis reflect the change from fluid (pus) and highly vascular inflammatory infiltrate to fibrosis. Thus, as the acute phase of infection subsides, the bright signal seen in the focus of osteomyelitis is replaced on T2-weighted images by a zone of intermediate signal and ultimately low signal, reflecting bony fusion.[51]

None of the signal changes described are pathognomonic for osteomyelitis. However, their distribution pattern makes this diagnosis likely: bandlike abnormality in the endplate confluent with a narrow disk cartilage with similar signal abnormality and a fusiform soft tissue mass. This is distinctly different from the pattern of signal characteristics of tumors, which usually spare the disk cartilage. Similarly, the presence of a normal disk carti-lage is a helpful sign in differentiating osteoporotic collapse from vertebral osteomyelitis and diskitis.

CASES

Five cases will be presented to exemplify the impact of CT and MRI on the clinical management of patients with infections of bone and soft tissues.

Case I. *Osteomyelitis of the cervical spine*
A 38-year-old woman was admitted to hospital for intense pain in the lower cervical spine. The only relevant factor in her medical history was a dental root abscess 3 months prior to admission. On physical examination there was limitation of motion in the cervicothoracic junction and tenderness on percussion of the lower cervical vertebrae. The neurological examination was negative.

AP and oblique roentgenograms of the cervical spine demonstrated erosion of the endplates and narrowing of the C6-7 disk (Fig. 9-62, *A* and *B*).

T1- and T2-weighted sagittal views were obtained (Fig. 9-62, *C* and *D*) as well as a T1 coronal view *(E)* and axial T1-weighted images before and after gadopentetate was injected intravenously *(F* and *G*). They demonstrated findings indicative of C6-7 infection manifested by erosion of adjacent endplates and

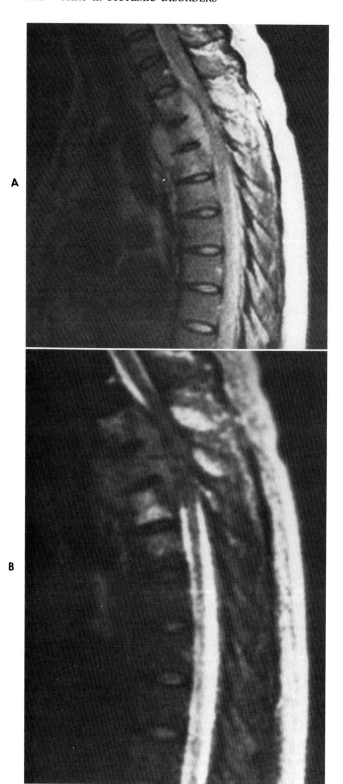

posterior surfaces of the vertebral bodies. On T2-weighted images a high signal zone in the disk and prevertebral soft tissues was interpreted as pus or granulation tissue. Posterior extension of this disk abnormality caused mild compression of the dural sac and cord.

Consecutive blood cultures were negative. This left aspiration of the C6-7 disk space as the only option for identifying the causative agent. Percutaneous aspiration was performed under CT guidance from a lateroanterior approach (Fig. 9-62, *H*). Through a 21-gauge spinal needle a few drops of turbid fluid were aspirated. Cultures of the aspirate grew *Staphylococcus aureus.* Intravenous antibiotic therapy was started immediately and continued for 6 weeks.

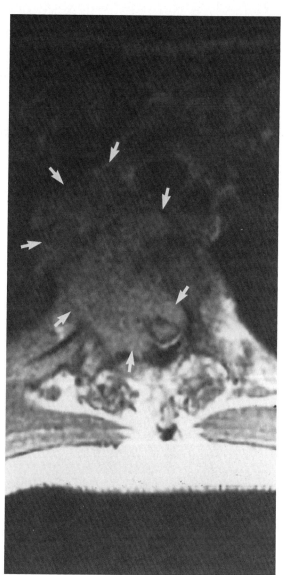

FIGURE 9-58

Cord compression caused by a tuberculous infection. **A,** T1-weighted. Note the fusiform soft tissue mass extending from T3 to T5. Disc cartilages T3-4 and T4-5 are narrowed and abnormally low in signal, and the cord also is compressed. **B,** A T2-weighted image better demonstrates the epidural compression and the bright signal representing edema and inflammatory exudate at the periphery of the vertebral involvement (upper aspect of T3 and lower T5).

FIGURE 9-59

Infection of T4 and the epidural and paravertebral soft tissues. An axial MR image (TR 900/TE 30) shows the intermediate-signal zone, representing inflammatory soft tissue that has replaced the right pedicle, lamina, and part of the vertebral body destroyed by infection. The process extends into the contiguous epidural space and paravertebral soft tissues *(arrows).*

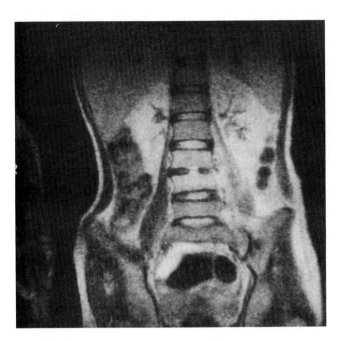

FIGURE 9-60
Psoas abscess, coronal MR image. The L3-4 disk cartilage is narrowed, and the cortex of the endplates and lateral margin of L4 are eroded. The contiguous signal abnormality and swelling of the left psoas indicate an abscess related to spinal osteomyelitis.

Surgical debridement and drainage of the soft tissue and epidural abscess were considered but held in reserve. The MR images were useful for defining the amount of cord compression and epidural disease, which were moderate. The absence of clinical signs of cord compression and the reassurance that MRI would immediately alert us to any further complications or progression of the infection were strong arguments in favor of nonsurgical treatment. The patient had a favorable clinical course on medical therapy alone.

Follow-up MRI at 6 weeks demonstrated a significant reduction in the perivertebral inflammatory mass, including the epidural component (Fig. 9-62, *K* and *L*).

Case II. Recurrent osteomyelitis
A 14-year-old boy was admitted to hospital for right knee pain that had persisted at least 2 weeks. At age 11 the child had had osteomyelitis of the right femur, treated with antibiotics and clinically healed.

On physical examination the only abnormality observed was a minimal soft tissue swelling in the distal portion of the right thigh, medial aspect. He was afebrile. The laboratory data showed normal WBC and sedimentation rate of 63 mm/hr. Blood cultures were negative.

Roentgenograms of the right femur revealed a zone of bony sclerosis in the medullary cavity of the distal diaphysis. The cortex was thick and moderately sclerotic. The knee joint was normal (Fig. 9-63, *A*).

CT examination with intravenous contrast enhancement showed sclerotic and thickened cortex with a central zone of low attenuation in the femur (Fig. 9-63, *B*). The significance of this finding was uncertain: a focus of active osteomyelitis or sequela of the old bone infection.

Coronal T2-weighted MR images demonstrated a zone of high

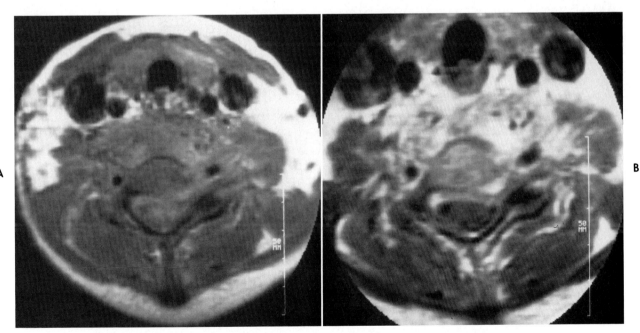

A   B

FIGURE 9-61
Use of gadopentetate in vertebral osteomyelitis. **A,** A T1-weighted axial image of C6 reveals the ill-defined prevertebral and epidural mass, of intermediate signal intensity, contiguous with a zone of bone erosion in the left side of the vertebra. **B,** Same level, same pulse sequence, postinjection. The increased signal of the inflammatory process produces better definition of the epidural disease, outlining its boundary with the dural sac. Mild epidural compression thus becomes clear.

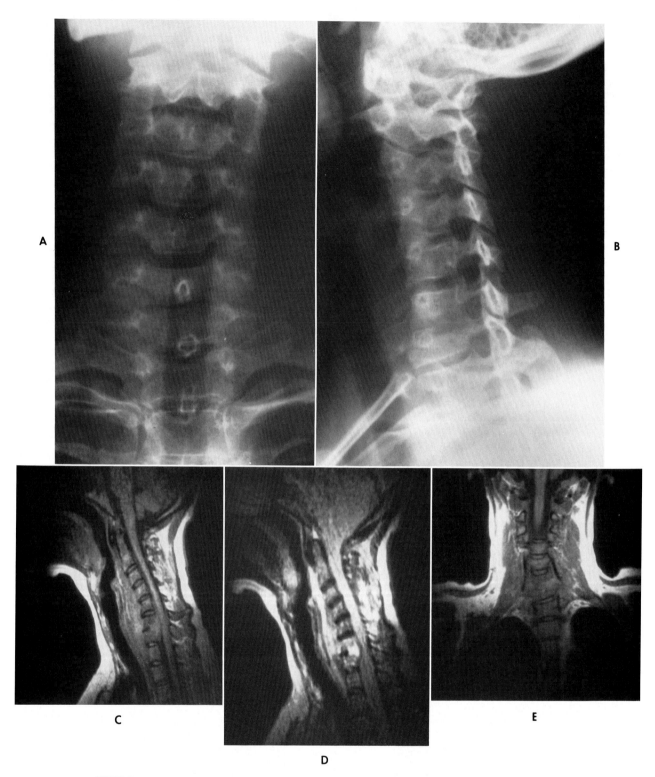

FIGURE 9-62

Staphylococcus aureus osteomyelitis of the cervical spine. Case I. Anteroposterior, **A,** and right posterior oblique, **B,** roentgenograms of the cervical spine demonstrate erosion of the endplates and narrowing of the C6-7 disk space. **C,** MRI, spin echo technique. A T1-weighted sagittal MR image (TR 530/TE 30) shows destruction of the posterior surfaces of C6 and C7, with a contiguous fusiform epidural process protruding 3 to 4 mm into the anterior aspect of the canal and causing mild compression of the dural tube. The only visible part of the disk space, seen anteriorly, is narrowed, with bulging of the prevertebral soft tissue. **D,** A T2-weighted sagittal (TR 2000/TE 80) reveals high-signal zones at the C6-7 disk and in the bulging soft tissue. These were regarded as signifying an abscess, with pus or granulation tissue. **E,** A T1-weighted coronal image (TR 585/TE 30) demonstrates abnormalities at the C6-7 level, similar to those in the sagittal image.

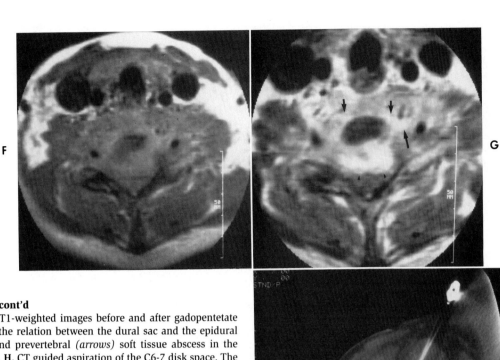

FIGURE 9-62, cont'd

F and **G,** Axial T1-weighted images before and after gadopentetate injection show the relation between the dural sac and the epidural *(arrowheads)* and prevertebral *(arrows)* soft tissue abscess in the C6-7 disk space. **H,** CT guided aspiration of the C6-7 disk space. The patient was positioned in a tilted right lateral decubitus, and a 21-gauge spinal needle was advanced from the lateroanterior approach until it reached the disk space. **I** and **J,** Follow-up examination 6 weeks later. Sagittal T1-weighted images before and after gadopentetate injection (TR 530/TE 30) show the prevertebral soft tissue swelling and epidural inflammatory mass to have decreased. The alignment of the vertebrae remains normal. The high-signal zone in the postinjection image signifies rich vascularity of the granulation tissue.

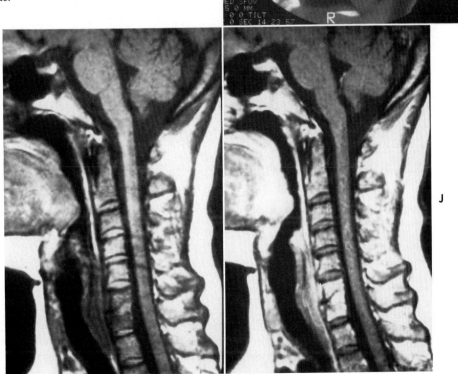

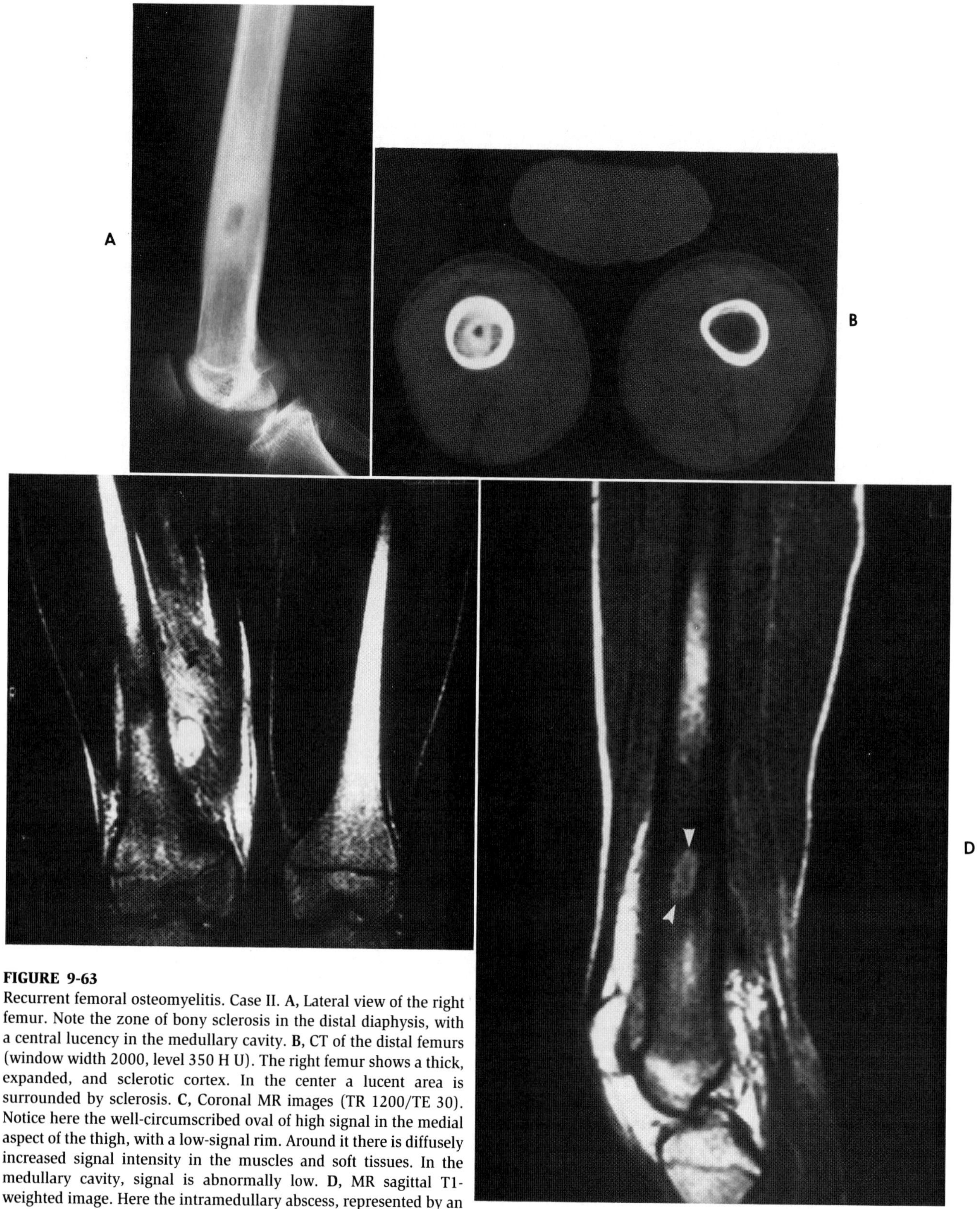

FIGURE 9-63
Recurrent femoral osteomyelitis. Case II. **A,** Lateral view of the right femur. Note the zone of bony sclerosis in the distal diaphysis, with a central lucency in the medullary cavity. **B,** CT of the distal femurs (window width 2000, level 350 H U). The right femur shows a thick, expanded, and sclerotic cortex. In the center a lucent area is surrounded by sclerosis. **C,** Coronal MR images (TR 1200/TE 30). Notice here the well-circumscribed oval of high signal in the medial aspect of the thigh, with a low-signal rim. Around it there is diffusely increased signal intensity in the muscles and soft tissues. In the medullary cavity, signal is abnormally low. **D,** MR sagittal T1-weighted image. Here the intramedullary abscess, represented by an intermediate-signal zone *(arrowheads),* is surrounded by low signal in the marrow.

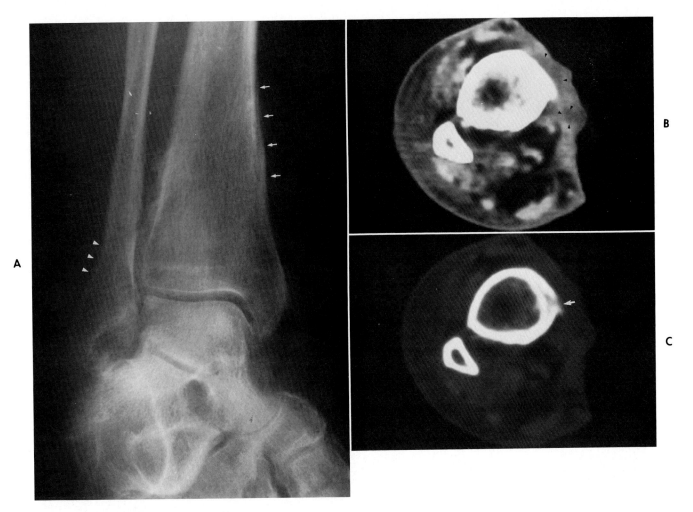

FIGURE 9-64

Chronic skin ulcer and bone infection. Case III. **A,** Oblique view of the right ankle. Periosteal reaction is seen along the medial aspect of the tibia *(arrows)*. A small line of reaction is also seen in the fibula *(arrowheads)*. The interosseous membrane is calcified. Periostitis is a nonspecific finding often seen in patients with chronic venous stasis. **B,** CT of the right ankle (contrast enhanced), soft tissue window, showing a large ulceration on the medial aspect. Two areas of low attenuation are compatible with pus accumulation beneath the crust covering the ulcer *(arrowheads)*. **C,** Same image, bone window, demonstrating a sinus tract traversing the outer cortical rim *(arrow)* and leading toward the pus collection in the adjacent soft tissue. This makes infection of bone a high probability. The diagnosis of periostitis secondary to venous stasis and edema at the bottom of the ulcer no longer applies.

signal with a sharp border located in the vastus medialis adjacent to the femoral cortex. A low-signal rim separated the high-signal area from a diffusely increased-signal zone in the surrounding soft tissues (Fig. 9-63, *C*). The sagittal T1-weighted (Fig. 9-63, *D*) showed an intramedullary intermediate-signal zone surrounded by signal void. These images were interpreted as demonstrating an intramedullary abscess with adjacent soft tissue abscess, signifying acute osteomyelitis.

Incision and drainage of the medial soft tissue abscess was performed. Fenestration of the cortex on the medial aspect of the femur was followed by curettage of the intramedullary cavity. The pus obtained was cultured and grew *Staphylococcus aureus*. The patient received 6 weeks of antibiotic therapy, and his recovery was both rapid and complete.

In this patient MRI established the existence of both an intramedullary and an adjacent soft tissue abscess. The exact location was determined preoperatively, and the incision and drainage targeted precisely, so that nonaffected tissues were spared.

Case III. *Chronic skin ulcer and bone infection*

A 53-year-old man with a long history of chronic venous stasis presented with a large ulcer on the medial aspect of his right ankle. Local debridement and skin grafting were planned. Preoperative roentgenograms demonstrated periosteal reaction on the medial aspect of the distal tibia (Fig. 9-64, *A*). Because this finding was considered nonspecific, a CT of the ankle was obtained and showed two distinct areas of low attenuation in the soft tissues suggestive of pus accumulation beneath the superficial crust covering the ulcer *(B)*. The cortex of the tibia appeared thickened and interrupted on the medial side by a sinus tract traversing the outer cortical rim *(C)*. This was regarded as indicating progression of infection from the ulcer to the periosseous soft tissue and further into the bone. It thus became clear that surgical treatment with skin grafting could not be performed until the underlying soft tissue and cortical bone infection had been eradicated. Local care of the ulcer and parenteral antibiotic therapy were required before skin grafting could be carried out.

Case IV. *Tuberculous infection of the sacroiliac joint*

A 27-year-old man presented with low back pain of several weeks' duration. Radiographs of the lumbosacral spine revealed an indistinct bone cortex in the right sacroiliac joint. The lumbar vertebrae appeared normal.

CT of the pelvis and sacroiliac joints was performed and showed a low-density collection anterior to the right sacroiliac joint with swelling of the iliacus (Fig. 9-65, *A*). The articular cortex was eroded, and the joint space was both enlarged and irregular *(B)*. These abnormalities were interpreted as consistent with infectious arthritis. Blood cultures were negative, and chest roentgenograms normal. A needle aspiration biopsy of the right sacroiliac joint was performed. The needle was advanced toward the anterior aspect of the joint and a small amount of fluid was

removed (*C* to *E*). A core of tissue representing a bone fragment from the medial wall of the joint was obtained. On histological examination it proved to contain caseating granulomas. Subsequently culture of the aspirated fluid grew *Mycobacterium tuberculosis*. The patient received triple drug antituberculous therapy and had a slow but progressive recovery.

In this patient CT demonstrated not only erosion of the cortex but also an abscess in the iliacus muscle, favoring the diagnosis of sacroiliac infection. Prompt search for the causative organism was undertaken. Placing the needle through the meandering course of the sacroiliac joint space was facilitated by CT guidance. In this manner the histological diagnosis of tuberculous infection was possible without the need for surgical intervention.

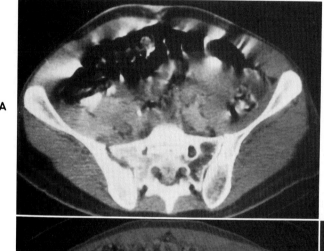

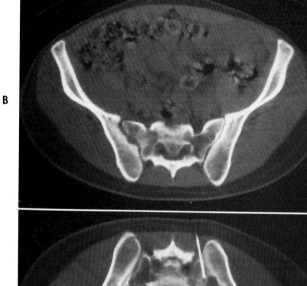

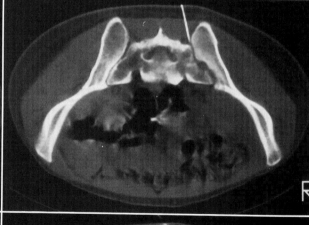

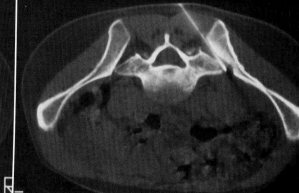

FIGURE 9-65

Tuberculous infection of the sacroiliac joint. Case IV. **A,** CT of the pelvis, soft tissue window. A low-density collection is present anterior to the right sacroiliac joint, with swelling of the iliacus. **B,** Same image, bone window, showing the joint space of the right sacroiliac joint enlarged and irregular. The articular cortex is eroded. **C to E,** CT-guided needle aspiration biopsy. The needle is advanced incrementally into the joint toward the fluid collection at the anterior margin.

Case V. *Soft tissue abscess.*

A 32-year-old man with acute immunodeficiency syndrome was hospitalized for several weeks with pneumonia. While in the hospital, he developed intense pain in the left calf and mild swelling. In view of his prolonged bed rest, it was thought that he might have deep venous thrombosis. However, infection of the soft tissues and osteomyelitis were also considered. Roentgenograms were normal, but CT (Fig. 9-66, *A*) demonstrated a zone of low attenuation with a dense rim in the soft tissues posterior to the tibia. The popliteal artery and vein were displaced posteriorly but were otherwise normal. The bones appeared normal on all CT images. The diagnosis of soft tissue abscess was established, and plans for therapy were made. A percutaneous drainage procedure was accomplished with CT guidance *(B)*. A total of 30 cc of pus was drained from the abscess. After placement of a radiopaque indwelling catheter, continuous closed irrigation was performed for 24 hours.

Cultures of the pus grew *Staphylococcus aureus,* for which the patient received appropriate antibiotics.

CT was important in this patient not only for the detection of an abscess but also for the facilitation of percutaneous drainage procedures essential to its local treatment.

CLINICAL UTILITY OF CT AND MRI IN THE MANAGEMENT OF BONE AND JOINT INFECTIONS

The MRI signs that suggest an infection of bone and soft tissues are nonspecific. Pus and noninfected synovial fluid have high signal on T2-weighted images[77,78] whereas an abscess of marrow has intermediate to low signal on T1-weighted images and high signal on T2-weighted images, features shared with many tumors, metastatic or primary. It is therefore most important to interpret the images in the context of the clinical history. MRI remains superior in delineating between various components of soft tissue, between normal structures and infection, and between hemorrhage and tumor. Thus the pathological process can be precisely located. Further characterization of the nature of an abnormality can be accomplished only to a certain degree. In many instances infections will mimic tumor. Certainly pyogenic, tuberculous, and fungal infections of bone and soft tissue all share common MR features, making differentiation among them difficult if not impossible.

A number of new questions have arisen in clinical practice since MRI was introduced into the armamentarium of radiological investigation. When is it better to perform MRI or CT? Do we really need both for certain patients? Some answers have emerged from the accumulation of experimental data and clinical practice with these modalities[79]:

1. CT can better show destruction of cortical bone as well as calcifications in the soft tissues and air bubbles in abscesses.
2. MRI is better for detecting subtle abnormalities of the soft tissues and marrow. The need to detect abscess collections in the soft tissues and bone makes MRI the modality of choice for patients with suspected infections of the musculoskeletal system.[80]
   a. Vertebral infections, in particular, are better studied by MRI, mainly due to its ability to define the contour of the spinal cord and dural and epidural structures while at the same time depicting changes in the water content of the disk cartilage and vertebral marrow. MRI can also portray in the same image the focus of osteomyelitis, its consequences on the neural structures, and any extension into the paravertebral soft tissue.
   b. The signal enhancement seen in the inflammatory tissue following intravenous administration of gadopentetate facilitates MR detection of even minor degrees of dural sac compression by depicting any epidural extension of the infection. Invasive procedures such as myelography are no longer routinely

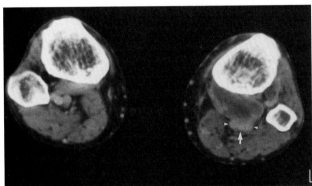

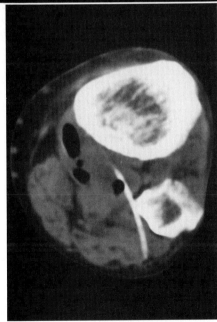

FIGURE 9-66
Soft tissue abscess. **A,** CT image of the inferior popliteal space. The abscess is represented by a low-attenuation zone with a dense rim at the periphery, posterior to the left tibia. The popliteal artery *(arrow)* and veins *(arrowheads)* are displaced posteriorly but otherwise appear normal. **B,** CT-guided aspiration of the abscess, radiopaque drainage catheter in place. The air bubbles were introduced during the drainage procedure.

necessary and will be replaced by MRI in the vast majority of patients with vertebral osteomyelitis.

3. MRI can also be used to document progression of healing in these patients. Follow-up examinations can be performed without the restraint implied by examinations necessitating irradiation of the patient (CT or CT-myelography).

4. Further technical improvements, specifically, better spatial resolution and shorter scanning time, together with lowering of the cost of the examination, will make MRI the modality of choice in radiological work-ups of patients suspected of having bony and soft tissue infections.

REFERENCES

1. Bobenchko WP: Infections of bones and joints. In Lowell WW, Winter RB (eds): Pediatric orthopedics. Philadelphia, Lippincott, 1986, pp 437-456.
2. Bonakdar-pour A, Gaines VD: The radiology of osteomyelitis. Orthop Clin North Am 1983;14:21-37.
3. David R, Barron BJ, Madewell JE: Osteomyelitis, acute and chronic. Radiol Clin North Am 1987;25:1171-1201.
4. Firooznia H, Golimbu C, Rafii M, Lichtman EA: Radiology of musculoskeletal complications of drug addiction. Semin Roentgenol 1983;18:198-206.
5. Waldvogel FA, Medoff G, Swartz MN: Osteomyelitis: a review of clinical features, therapeutic considerations, and unusual aspects. N Engl J Med 1970;282(4):198-206.
6. Waldvogel FA, Papageorgiou PS: Osteomyelitis: the past decade. N Engl J Med 1980;303:360-370.
7. Trueta J: The three types of acute haematogenous osteomyelitis: a clinical and vascular study. J Bone Joint Surg 1959;41(B):671-680.
8. Kahn DS, Pritzker KP: The pathophysiology of bone infection. Clin Orthop Rel Res 1973;96:12-19.
9. Resnick D, Niwayama G: Osteomyelitis, septic arthritis, and soft tissue infection: mechanisms and situations. In Resnick D, Niwayama G (eds): Diagnosis of bone and joint disorders. Philadelphia, Saunders, 1981, pp 2044-2129.
10. Miller WB Jr, Murphy WA, Gilula LA: Brodie abscess: reappraisal. Radiology 1979;132:15-23.
11. Collert S, Isacson J: Chronic sclerosing osteomyelitis (Garré). Clin Orthop Rel Res 1982;164:136-140.
12. Tumeh SS, Aliabadi P, Weissman BN, McNeil BJ: Disease activity in osteomyelitis: role of radiography. Radiology 1987;165:781-784.
13. Murray IP: Bone scanning in the child and young adult. II. Skeletal Radiol 1980;5:65-76.
14. Lisbona R, Rosenthall L: Observations on sequential use of 99mTc-phosphate complex and 67Ga imaging in osteomyelitis, cellulitis, and septic arthritis. Radiology 1977;123:123-129.
15. Merkel KD, Brown ML, Dewanjee MK, Fitzgerald RH Jr: Comparison of indium-labeled-leukocyte imaging with sequential technetium-gallium scanning in the diagnosis of low-grade musculoskeletal sepsis. J Bone Joint Surg (Am) 1985;67:465-476.
16. Gilday DL: Problems in the scintigraphic detection of osteomyelitis. Radiology 1980;135:791.
17. Bressler EL, Conway JJ, Weiss SC: Neonatal osteomyelitis examined by bone scintigraphy. Radiology 1984;152:685-688.
18. Seabold JE, Nepola JV, Conrad GR, et al: Detection of osteomyelitis at fracture nonunion sites: comparison of two scintigraphic methods. AJR 1989;152:1021-1027.
19. Garnett ES, Cockshott WP, Jacobs J: Classical acute osteomyelitis with a negative bone scan. Br J Radiol 1977;50:757-760.
20. Sullivan DC, Rosenfield NS, Ogden J, Gottschalk A: Problems in

the scintigraphic detection of osteomyelitis in children. Radiology 1980;135:731-736.
21. Cabanela ME, Sim FH, Beabout JW, Dahlin C: Osteomyelitis appearing as neoplasms. A diagnostic problem. Arch Surg 1974;109:68-72.
22. Wing VW, Jeffrey RB Jr, Federle MP, et al: Chronic osteomyelitis examined by CT. Radiology 1985;154:171-174.
23. Firooznia H, Rafii M, Golimbu C, Sokolow J: Computerized tomography of pelvic osteomyelitis in patients with spinal cord injuries. Clin Orthop 1983;181:126-131.
24. Azouz EM: Computed tomography in bone and joint infections. J Can Assoc Radiol 1981;32:102-106.
25. Rosenberg D, Baskies AM, Deckers PJ, Leiter BE, et al: Pyogenic sacroiliitis. An absolute indication for computerized tomographic scanning. Clin Orthop 1984;184:128-132.
26. Firooznia H, Golimbu C, Rafii M, et al: Computed tomography of the sacroiliac joints: comparison with complex motion tomography. J Comput Tomogr 1984;8:31-39.
27. Kuhn JP, Berger PE: Computed tomographic diagnosis of osteomyelitis. Radiology 1979;130:503-506.
28. Helms CA, Jeffrey RB, Wing VW: Computed tomography and plain film appearance of a bony sequestration. Significance and differential diagnosis. Skeletal Radiol 1987;16:117-120.
29. Ram PC, Martinez S, Korobkin M, et al: CT detection of intraosseous gas: a new sign of osteomyelitis. AJR 1981;137:721-723.
30. Bielecki DK, Sartoris D, Resnick D, et al: Intraosseous and intradiscal gas in association with spinal infection: report of three cases. AJR 1986;147:83-86.
31. Merine DS, Fishman EK, Magid D: CT detection of sacral osteomyelitis associated with pelvic abscesses. J Comput Assist Tomogr 1988;12:118-121.
32. Rafii M, Firooznia H, Golimbu C, McCauley DI: Hematogenous osteomyelitis with fat-fluid level shown by CT. Radiology 1984;153:493-494.
33. Jeffrey RB, Callen PW, Federle MP: Computed tomography of psoas abscesses. J Comput Assist Tomogr 1980;4:639-641.
34. Rafii M, Firooznia H, Golimbu C: Computed tomography of septic joints. J Comput Tomogr 1985;9:51-60.
35. Sarno RC, Carter BL, Bankoff MS: Computed tomographic demonstration of gas collections simulating infection. Comput Radiol 1984;8(3):171-174.
36. Ralls PW, Boswell W, Henderson R, et al: CT of inflammatory disease of the psoas muscle. AJR 1980;134:767-770.
37. Mahboubi S: CT appearance of nidus in osteoid osteoma versus sequestration in osteomyelitis. J Comput Assist Tomogr 1986;10:457-459.
38. Kopits SE, Debuskey M: Primary chronic sclerosing osteomyelitis. Johns Hopkins Med J 1977;140:241-247.
39. Chapman M, Murray RO, Stoker DJ: Tuberculosis of the bones and joints. Semin Roentgenol 1979;14:266-282.
40. Sharif HS, Aideyan OA, Clark DC, et al: Brucellar and tuberculous spondylitis: comparative imaging features. Radiology 1989;171:419-425.
41. Morgenlander JC, Rossitch E Jr, Rawlings CE 3rd: Aspergillus disc space infection: case report and review of the literature. Neurosurgery 1989;25:126-129.
42. Seltzer SE: Value of computed tomography in planning medical and surgical treatment of chronic osteomyelitis. J Comput Assist Tomogr 1984;8:482-487.
43. West WF, Kelly PJ, Martin WJ: Chronic osteomyelitis. I. Factors affecting the results of treatment in 186 patients. JAMA 1970;213:1837-1842.
44. Hardy DC, Murphy WA, Gilula LA: Computed tomography in planning percutaneous bone biopsy. Radiology 1980;134:447-450.
45. Adapon BD, Legada BD Jr, Lim EV, et al: CT-guided closed biopsy of the spine. J Comput Assist Tomogr 1981;5:73-78.
46. Beltran J, McGhee RB, Shaffer PB, et al: Experimental infections

of the musculoskeletal system: evaluation with MR imaging and Tc-99m MDP and Ga-67 scintigraphy. Radiology 1988;167: 167-172.

47. Weinreb JC, Cohen JM, Maravilla KR: Iliopsoas muscles: MR study of normal anatomy and disease. Radiology 1985;156: 435-440.

48. Beltran J, Noto AM, McGhee RB, et al: Infections of the musculoskeletal system: high-field-strength MR imaging. Radiology 1987;164:449-454.

49. Quinn SF, Murray W, Clark RA, Cochran C: MR imaging of chronic osteomyelitis. J Comput Assist Tomogr 1988;12: 113-117.

50. Bertino RE, Porter BA, Stimac GK, Tepper SJ: Imaging spinal osteomyelitis and epidural abscess with short T1 inversion recovery (STIR). AJNR 1988;9:563-564.

51. Modic MT, Pflanze W, Feiglin DH, Belhobek G: Magnetic resonance imaging of musculoskeletal infections. Radiol Clin North Am 1986;24:247-258.

52. Sharif HS, Clark DC, Aabed MY, et al: Granulomatous spinal infections: MR imaging. Radiology 1990;177:101-107.

53. Donovan Post MJ, Quencer RM, Eismont FJ, Green BA: Gadolinium-enhanced MR: its value in detection and diagnosis of spinal infection. Proceedings of the American Society of Neuroradiology. Twenty-seventh Annual Meeting, 1989. p 91.

54. Unger E, Moldofsky P, Gatenby R, et al: Diagnosis of osteomyelitis by MR imaging. AJR 1988;150:605-610.

55. Fletcher BD, Scoles PV, Nelson AD: Osteomyelitis in children: detection by magnetic resonance. Work in progress. Radiology 1984;150:57-60.

56. Allen EH, Cosgrove D, Millard FJ: The radiological changes in infections of the spine and their diagnostic value. Clin Radiol 1978;29:31-40.

57. Golimbu C, Firooznia H, Rafii M: CT of osteomyelitis of the spine. AJR 1984;142:159-163.

58. Whelan MA, Naidich DP, Post JD, Chase NE: Computed tomography of spinal tuberculosis. J Comput Assist Tomogr 1983;7:25-30.

59. Weaver P, Lifeso RM: The radiological diagnosis of tuberculosis of the adult spine. Skeletal Radiol 1984;12:178-186.

60. Messer HD, Litvinoff J: Pyogenic cervical osteomyelitis. Chondro-osteomyelitis of the cervical spine frequently associated with parenteral drug use. Arch Neurol 1976;33:571-576.

61. Musher DM, Thorsteinsson SB, Minuth JN, Luchi RJ: Vertebral osteomyelitis. Still a diagnostic pitfall. Arch Intern Med 1976;136:105-110.

62. Firooznia H, Seliger G, Abrams R, et al: Disseminated extrapulmonary tuberculosis in association with heroin addiction. Radiology 1973;109:291-296.

63. Wiley AM, Trueta J: The vascular anatomy of the spine and its relationship to pyogenic vertebral osteomyelitis. J Bone Joint Surg (Br) 1959;41:796-809.

64. Batson OV: The vertebral vein system. Am J Roentgenol 1957; 78:195-212.

65. Ratcliffe JF: Anatomic bases for the pathogenesis and radiologic features of vertebral osteomyelitis and its differentiation from childhood discitis. A microarteriographic investigation. Acta Radiol [Diagn] 1985;26:137-143.

66. Boston HC, Bianco AJ, Rhodes KH: Disc space infections in children. Orthop Clin North Am 1975;6:953-964.

67. Wenger DR, Bobechko WP, Gilday DL: The spectrum of intervertebral disc space infection in children. J Bone Joint Surg 1978;60A:100-108.

68. Sartoris DJ, Moskowitz PS, Kaufman RA, et al: Childhood diskitis: computed tomographic findings. Radiology 1983;149: 701-707.

69. Stone JL, Cybulski GR, Rodriguez J, et al: Anterior cervical debridement and strut-grafting for osteomyelitis of the cervical spine. J Neurosurg 1989;70:879-883.

70. Lardé E, Mathieu D, Frija J, et al: Vertebral osteomyelitis: disk hypodensity on CT. AJNR 1982;3:657-661. AJR 1982;139: 963-967.

71. Resnick D, Niwayama G, Guerra J, et al: Spinal vacuum phenomena: anatomical study and review. Radiology 1981;139:341-348.

72. Naim-ur-Rahman: Atypical forms of spinal tuberculosis. J Bone Joint Surg 1980;62B:162-165.

73. Golimbu C: Osteomyelitis of the spine: relative diagnostic value of radiographic radionuclide, CT, and MRI examinations. Contemp Diagn Radiol 1987;10:1-5.

74. Modic MT, Feiglin DH, Piraino DW, et al: Vertebral osteomyelitis: assessment using MR. Radiology 1985;157:157-166.

75. de Roos A, van Persijn van Meerten EL, Bloem JL, Bluemm RG: MRI of tuberculous spondylitis. AJR 1986;147:79-82.

76. Angtuaco EJ, McConnell JR, Chadduck WM, Flanigan S: MR imaging of spinal epidural sepsis. AJNR 1987;8:879-883. AJR 1987;149:1249-1253.

77. Kulkarni MV, Drolshagen LF, Kaye JJ, et al: MR imaging of hemophiliac arthropathy. J Comput Assist Tomogr 1986;10: 445-449.

78. Beltran J, Noto AM, Herman LJ, et al: Joint effusions: MR imaging. Radiology 1986;158:133-137.

79. Chandnani VP, Beltran J, Morris CS, et al: Acute experimental osteomyelitis and abscesses: detection with MR imaging versus CT. Radiology 1990;174:233-236.

80. Mason MD, Zlatkin MB, Esterhai JL, et al: Chronic complicated oseomyelitis of the lower extremity: evaluation with MR imaging. Radiology 1989;173:355-359.

10 MRI of Bone Marrow Diseases

MICHAEL M. AMBROSINO
NANCY B. GENIESER
MELVIN H. BECKER

Magnetic resonance imaging (MRI) is the first noninvasive means of evaluating medullary bone. Conventional roentgenography provides only indirect evidence of marrow disease, through changes in the bony cortex and trabeculae. Radionuclide scintigraphy has but limited spatial resolution capabilities and specificity. CT scanning does not adequately discriminate among the medullary soft tissues. The exquisite contrast resolution offered by MRI allows visualization of most elements of the marrow as well as identification of its nonmineralized components.

Medullary bone consists of three components: cancellous (trabecular) bone, hematopoietic (red) marrow, and fatty (yellow) marrow. The *trabeculae* are an integral part of the mechanical support structure of the skeleton and are organized for optimal distribution of the stresses of weight bearing. They constitute an osseous network, in a dynamic equilibrium, that is able to accommodate to new mechanical stresses (as occur with malaligned fractures) and respond metabolically to changes in hormonal balance (as occur during menopause). The *red marrow* consists of fat contained within adipocytes and water contained primarily within blood-forming cellular elements.[1] The ratio of fat to water in the hematopoietic marrow changes with age, physiological stresses, and hematological marrow disorders.[2] The *yellow marrow* consists solely of fat contained within adipocytes. The distribution of hematopoietic marrow throughout the skeletal system has been shown to change with age, gradually becoming more centrally distributed after childhood. The cellular precursors are replaced by adipose cells in the peripheral tubular bones and remain essentially in only the proximal humeri, femora, and axial skeleton by the third decade of life.

Neoplastic, infectious, or metabolic disease either replaces normal marrow or alters the normal balance between cellular and fatty elements. This altered composition is responsible for the changes in marrow signal intensity (SI) seen on spin echo (SE) images. Tumors and inflammatory tissue usually have relatively greater water content than red marrow and thus have lower intensity on short TR/short TE sequences and higher intensity on long TR/long TE sequences. Therefore the red marrow in infants and young children is often best evaluated for tumor or edema on T2-weighted images, which show the abnormal tissue as relatively bright (intense) regions against a less bright background. The red marrow of older patients has a greater fat content, and both T1- and T2-weighted images are helpful. Yellow marrow, because of its fat content, has short T1 and relatively long T2 relaxation times. Because of the relatively greater volume of trabeculae, marrow in the vertebral bodies and flat bones (e.g., the pelvis) has slightly lower signal than that in the long bones.

Evaluation for metabolic disease (including anemias) requires selecting the appropriate pulse sequence on the basis of the pathological entities to be imaged. For example, marrow containing reticuloendothelial cells laden with glucocerebroside has low intensity on both T1- and T2-weighted images; thus choosing the appropriate sequence depends upon whether yellow or red marrow is being evaluated; on the other hand, hematological marrow disorders are probably best evaluated using quantitative chemical shift MRI, which provides quantitative information about the cellular content of the marrow.[2]

More recently, short T1 inversion recovery (STIR) imaging sequences have gained popularity in imaging the musculoskeletal system. They can be designed to suppress the signal from fat (i.e., adipose tissue and yellow marrow) while allowing tissues with high water content to continue to appear as high-signal areas. (Muscle has medium to high signal.) The STIR sequence also better demonstrates soft tissue and marrow lesion margins.[3] The T1- and T2-weighted sequences are more sensitive for detecting cortical bone invasion by tumor. We now routinely supplement our T1- and T2-weighted scans with STIR images.

The use of contrast material is becoming routine for the MR evaluation of tumors. Gadopentetate (gadolinium-DTPA, Gd) is the most frequently used agent. It is a chelated paramagnetic material that markedly shortens T1 relaxation times, with relatively little effect on T2 relaxation times. Administered intravenously, it is rapidly distributed to the interstitial space. Highly vascular structures therefore show enhanced (increased or brighter) signal on short TR/TE sequences, maximum enhancement being attained approximately 15 minutes following the injection.

T1-weighted Gd scans may provide additional information with respect to tumor vascularity and often help in differentiating tumor from edema and compressed and/or atrophic muscle. Contrast-enhanced T1-weighted scan sequences, however, should not replace the routine long or short TR/TE sequences, since information that helps characterize tumors (e.g., detection of necrosis, fluid, or fat) may be lost. Current recommendations are that Gd scan sequences be added to the routine sequences to maximize the MR information obtained during initial evaluation. The T1-weighted Gd scans may obviate the need for long TR/TE sequences on follow-up studies.[4]

The uses of MR imaging to evaluate specific marrow disease are presented in this chapter. Although the SE signal behavior of marrow disease is largely nonspecific, MR is the imaging modality of choice for identifying the extent of medullary disease and visualizing extramedullary involvement. There is limited MR experience with many primary bone marrow disorders, however, since the technique is new and many of the entities of interest relatively uncommon.

PREPROCEDURE PREPARATION

CT and MRI studies require a *nonmoving* patient for optimal images. When an infant or child is scheduled for either examination, it is wise to explain the procedure for these studies to the parents and the child old enough to understand. This frequently achieves the desired cooperation. If the patient cannot comply, sedation will be needed.

The age and severity of the illness of the patient are factors to be considered when an infant or child is immobilized. If the patient routinely has a nap, the examination should be scheduled at that time. In general, infants under 1 year of age can be immobilized for the study by being wrapped in sheets or blankets after a feeding. Sedation is often needed for patients between the ages of 6 months and 6 years. Usually, after 6 years of age, cooperation can be obtained by reasoning with the child. If sedation will be required, the child should be brought to the examination area about 1 hour prior to the time scheduled for the study.

There is no standard method for sedating infants or children in the United States. Many different medications are in use, and there is continual debate as to which is best. An ideal method does not exist but would consist of a sedative or combination of medications that is safe and easy to administer, having consistent action, rapid onset, controllable duration and few or no side effects. Among the commonly used agents are barbituates, benzodiazepines, chloral hydrate, tricyclics, and combinations such as DPT (meperidine [Demerol]), promethazine (Phenergan), chlorpromazine (Thorazine), and AMPS (atropine, meperidine, promethazine, and secobarbital).

Respiratory depression and airway obstruction are the most serious adverse effects of sedation medications, it is therefore wise, when possible, to monitor the respiration, heartbeat, and oxygenation of the sedated patient. This can be done by observation, and may be supplemented with a pulse oximeter (monitors oxygen saturation and heart rate). However, at present we have not found a suitable pulse oximeter for use with magnetic imaging studies. Brachycardia may indicate respiratory depression. An agitated infant may be seen with airway obstruction or under sedation.

At many institutions, and in The New York University Medical Center pediatric angiocardiographic laboratories, DPT ("lytic" or "cardiac" cocktail) is used for sedating infants and children. The dosage is usually meperidine (2 mg/kg), promethazine (0.5 to 1 mg/kg), and chlorpromazine (0.5 to 1 mg/kg) given by intramuscular injection. Onset of sedation generally occurs in less than 30 minutes, and the duration ranges from 2 to 14 hours.

In the Radiology Department of The New York University Medical Center the preferred sedation regimen is chloral hydrate (Noctec syrup), probably the safest sedation regimen. It is given orally 75 mg/kg 30 minutes prior to the study, up to 2 g, with half the original dose repeated if the child is still awake. Chloral hydrate works best for children 6 months of age or less. The drawback is that it can take up to 1½ hours for the infant to fall asleep. Recovery time is between 1 and 2 hours.

Intramuscular pentobarbital (Nembutal) is useful if no IV line is available and no injection is to be given. The dose is 5 to 6 mg/kg; a supplemental 1 to 3 mg/kg can be given if needed. It takes slightly more than ½ hour for the child to fall asleep and over 1 hour to awaken. Parents should be told the child may be groggy and irritable.

IV pentobarbital is rapid acting and predictable. The dose is 2 to 6 mg/kg infused slowly in increments of a quarter to half the total dose. It takes 2 to 3 minutes to achieve full effect; an additional 1 to 3 mg/kg may be given, if necessary. Do not exceed 6 mg/kg total dose or 100 mg.

Following the study, the patient should be observed until sedation has worn off.

ANEMIA

Anemia, defined as a decrease in the circulating red cell mass, can be broadly organized into three categories: that caused by blood loss, that caused by inadequate production of mature erythrocytes, and that caused by excessive erythrocyte destruction. There are numerous etiologies in each of these groups, and MR imaging can be useful in studying them.

Myelofibrosis

Myelofibrosis is a disorder characterized by hepatosplenomegaly and associated general or patchy progressive marrow fibrosis. There is replacement of the normal medullary fat and cellular marrow elements (erythroid, granulocytic, and megakaryocytic), which causes varying degrees of leukoerythroblastic anemia. Myelofibrosis may result from any of the myeloproliferative syndromes or exposure to toxins (carbon tetrachloride, benzene, phosphorus) or radiation as well as from leukemia, lymphoma, tuberculosis, metastatic disease, or Gaucher's disease. Most affected patients are over 50 years of age. The clinical course is slow but progressive.[5]

MR scans obtained on adults with myelofibrosis show very low and primarily homogeneous marrow signal intensities on both T1- and T2-weighted SE sequences.[6] This is believed to be secondary to replacement of high-intensity fat by collagen, reticulin fibers, and cellular material. Some authors postulate that occasional areas of nonhomogeneity may be due to rests of preserved marrow. The low T1 and T2 signal intensity readily distinguishes myelofibrosis from most neoplastic processes. The marrow signal changes are not pathognomonic, however; similar marrow T1 and T2 changes can be seen in cells containing glucocerebroside (Gaucher's disease) and in patients with leukemia.

Aplastic anemia

Aplastic anemia is a disease of primary bone marrow failure in which hematopoietic marrow is replaced to varying degrees by fat, yielding either hypoplastic or aplastic marrow. Consequently there is a reduction in the number of circulating erythrocytes, platelets, and leukocytes. Although this entity is seen following exposure to medications, radiation, and viral infections, no etiology is identified in approximately 50% of the cases.[7] The large difference between the T1 and T2 relaxation times of protons in the overabundant fat and the presence of water molecules in the diminished red marrow make this entity particularly well suited for evaluation by MR.

Quantitative assessment of the ratio of fat to red marrow, and of the relative distribution of these components in the marrow, is optimally done on T1-weighted SE images.[8-10] The low-signal areas of marrow, usually sites of hematopoiesis, are replaced by high SI fat (yellow marrow). In adults, sites of hematopoiesis include the axial skeleton, pelvis, femoral neck, intertrochanteric region, and proximal humerus. The replacement by yellow marrow can be patchy, with persistently low SI areas representing nests of hematopoietic tissue. The number of low-signal areas does not, however, appear to correlate with the peripheral blood count.[11]

Evaluation of these scans requires knowledge of the normal sites of marrow blood production since the MR signal from *aplastic* yellow marrow does not appear to be significantly different from that of the "normal" yellow marrow. Despite this limitation, conventional SE images do provide a means of noninvasively distinguishing a clinically detected severe pancytopenia due to leukemia (low SI) from a primary aplastic anemia (high SI).[9] MR also provides a means of serially and noninvasively evaluating the aplastic marrow and the patient's response to therapy. A number of studies have shown that the marrow of treated adults developed multiple focal areas of low SI[11] while the marrow signal in children who had been adequately treated became homogeneously low in SI.[8] The decrease in SI seen in both pediatric and adult cases was attributed to the reconversion of aplastic marrow to hematopoietic tissue. Because different magnetic field strengths were used in these studies, it is not clear whether the differences in recovery pattern indicate differences in response to treatment, a spectrum of response to treatment regardless of age, or a difference in MR technique.

Whereas conventional SE images provide "bulk" signal intensity information reflecting the sum of signals from the primary marrow components (fat and water), routine SE images cannot quantify water and fat content. Therefore spin echo does not distinguish changes in the net (bulk) signal following relative alterations in fat and water content from changes due to altered relaxation times of the fat and/or water. Furthermore, there is an overlap of T1 values obtained as bulk marrow measurements between patients with aplastic anemia and those with normal marrow. This problem can be overcome with phase contrast chemical shift imaging, which provides quantitative evaluation of the bone marrow constituents.[2,12-14] Chemical shift imaging techniques exploit the presence of protons in fat and water in the cellular marrow to help distinguish the signals originating in fat from those originating in cellular components and to provide quantitative information about the fat content.[13,14]

Imaging parameters can be so arranged that known "water-dominant" structures (intervertebral disks) are displayed as a bright signal intensity and serve as an image "phase standard." With this standard, structures containing fat (180-degree phase shifted) are displayed as black and those containing water appear bright. For example, as one would expect, the signal from the vertebral bodies (marrow) in patients with aplastic anemia has intensities opposite those of the disk spaces, indicating a dominant fat fraction in the hypocellular marrow.[2] A quantitative marrow fat fraction can be calculated from the mean marrow signal intensities[2] and will serve to distinguish normal from hypoplastic marrow when this distinction cannot be made on the basis of indirect fat-content measurements from bulk T1-W SE images. It appears that the SI changes seen on T1-W SE images are indeed a result primarily of changes in the fat fraction signal following changes in lipid marrow concentration rather than in lipid relaxation times.[2]

Sickle cell disease

Sickle cell anemia is a chronic hemolytic disease in which erythrocytes lack HgA and assume a sickle or crescentic shape when deprived of oxygen. The disorder is characterized by painful "crises" due to trapping of sickled cells in small vessels, with erythrocytosis, vessel occlusion, and thrombosis causing bone and marrow infarction.[15] The bone pain often associated with these crises may be due to vascular engorgement and intramedullary cavity distension (edema); bone and marrow infarction are well known complications. Slow flow

through compensatory hyperplastic red marrow is believed to be an additional predisposing factor to sickling and marrow infarction.[16] These patients are also at increased risk for the development of osteomyelitis.

Radioiron has been used in evaluating the distribution of red cell precursors, and labeled colloids have been used to study the distribution of erythropoietic activity. The uptake of colloid by the reticuloendothelial system has been shown to parallel erythropoietic activity. Recent reports[17] indicate that all patients with sickle cell anemia have an increased uptake of radioisotope consistent with peripheral marrow expansion but, unfortunately, zones of both acute and chronic infarction appear as focal areas of decreased activity that cannot be individually identified; residual zones of yellow marrow may be mistaken for infarctions.

MR scans of asymptomatic sickle cell patients show diffusely decreased marrow signal on both long and short TR/TE images that correspond to radioisotope changes suggestive of red marrow hyperplasia. However, it is not clear to what degree the early deposition of hemosiderin contributes to this decreased marrow signal, which is attributable primarily to red marrow hyperplasia.

The MR criteria for distinguishing acute from chronic infarction have not been firmly established. Preliminary evaluation by Rao et al.[17] showed that areas of low signal

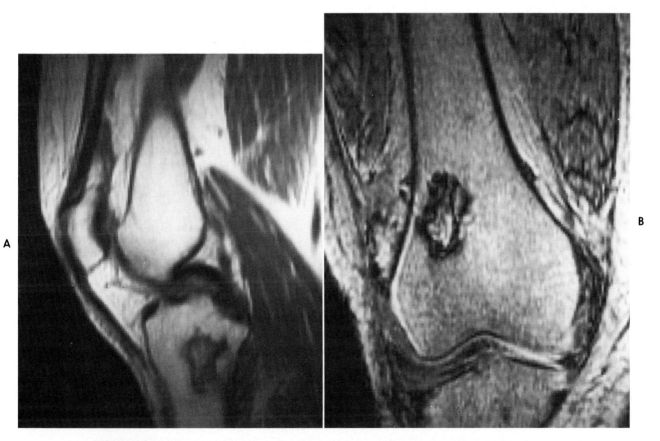

FIGURE 10-1
A, T1 and, **B,** T2-weighted scans of a 6-year-old boy with sickle cell disease and knee pain. Note the low-signal area in the proximal tibia. The distal femur shows a similar lesion, which becomes brighter with T2-weighting.

intensity on short TR/TE images, which became high intensity on long TR/TE sequences (probably representing edema), correlated well with pain and were considered consistent with acute infarction (Fig. 10-1). These authors further suggested that areas of low signal intensity on both long and short TR/TE sequences might represent areas of fibrosis or old infarction.

The increased water content found in areas of infection (as with acute infarction) is seen as decreased signal intensity on short TR/TE sequences and increased signal on long TR/TE sequences. MR visualization of the associated changes in cortical bone and periosteum can be difficult to identify. The distinction between early infarction and early osteomyelitis therefore often requires correlation with the clinical history, symptoms, and physical examination. The MR diagnosis of osteomyelitis in these patients is easier to make once the infection has extended through the cortex and periosteum to involve the adjacent soft tissues.

Thalassemia

Thalassemia is any of several genetic defects in hemoglobin production. Patients with homozygous beta-thalassemia (thalassemia major or Cooley's anemia) have deficient production of the hemoglobin beta chain that usually results in death during early adulthood. These patients are often managed with deferoxamine mesylate (Desferal)-hypertransfusion therapeutic regimens in an attempt to maintain hematocrits of approximately 37 with minimum soft tissue iron deposition (secondary hemochromatosis). Deferoxamine is an iron chelating agent that slows the soft tissue accumulation of iron. Several methods of monitoring soft tissue iron levels have been devised, but none is entirely satisfactory.[18] Dual energy CT scanning is an accurate but lengthy procedure requiring specialized equipment and calibration techniques.[19] The most accurate means of determining soft tissue iron stores is by the direct analysis of iron content in tissue biopsy specimens. However, serum ferritin levels are generally accepted as a noninvasive long-term means for estimating the total body iron load to monitor the efficacy of therapy.[20-22]

The paramagnetic effect of ferric ions in aqueous solution shortens both T1 and T2 relaxation times (Fig. 10-2). The in vivo effect observed with MR is complex and depends upon the major forms of tissue iron present and their concentrations within the tissues. It has recently been suggested that the T1 and T2 shortening seen with hepatic iron overload is due primarily to the presence of low-molecular weight cytosol iron and (to a lesser extent) ferritin, hemosiderin, and hemoproteins. Of the latter forms, ferritin (because of its iron core) appears to have the greatest effect.[23] Altered macromolecular binding of water secondary to changes in water content may also contribute to the shortened proton relaxation times produced by paramagnetic agents such as ferric compounds.[24] In vitro investigation[25] has shown that the proton relaxation enhancement observed predominantly on T2-weighted images occurs via cellular field gradients produced by intralysosomal granules of hemosiderin, and other in vitro work[26] has shown a linear relationship between 1/T1 and the iron content of human serum.[26]

In an effort to determine the efficacy of MR as a noninvasive means of estimating relative soft tissue iron depositions,[27] patients with Cooley's anemia have been evaluated to correlate in vivo organ signal intensities of the liver, vertebral marrow, myocardium, and skeletal muscle with serum ferritin levels. T1-weighted sequences provided quantitative in vivo information as to the relative soft tissue and marrow iron depositions, but T2 values were too small for reliable measurements. Of interest, however, was the fact that short TR/short TE regional myocardial SI values proved to correlate best with the clinical status of these patients when compared to serum ferritin levels, resting thallium scans, electrocardiograms, and echocardiography.[27]

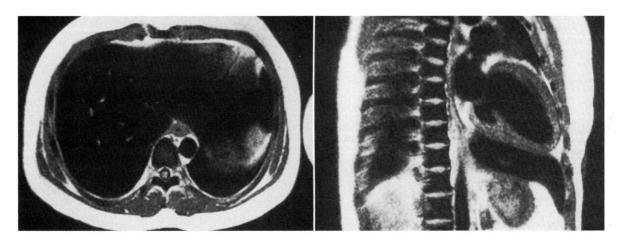

FIGURE 10-2
T1-weighted images from an MR scan of a 15-year-old boy with Cooley's anemia. Note the decreased signal arising from the marrow and the liver due to T1 relaxation time shortening.

BONE MARROW NEOPLASMS AND PRIMARY BONE TUMORS
General considerations

The MR signal characteristics of bone tumors are relatively nonspecific. The usual presentation of low signal intensity on short TR/TE sequences and high intensity on long TR/TE sequences can also be seen with nonneoplastic marrow entities such as inflammation. The diagnostic strength of MR lies in its unique ability to locate the soft tissue and marrow components of bone neoplasms by virtue of its high soft tissue–contrast resolution and multiplanar imaging capabilities. The presurgical definition of extraosseous and intramedullary tumor extent has become even more critical as treatment has shifted away from radical surgical procedures to more conservative regional resection techniques (including limb salvage and bone transplantation).[28,29]

Many studies have been performed comparing the diagnostic efficacy of MR with that of CT and nuclear scintigraphy in evaluating primary bone tumors. Current data indicate that MR is the most reliable modality for assessing the extent of marrow involvement[28] as well as differentiating between tumor and muscle, tumor and vessels, tumor and fat, tumor and joint, and tumor and bone.[30] In one study of 56 patients[29] the intraosseous tumor length predicted by MR correlated almost perfectly with the actual length measured in pathological specimens. MR has also been shown[30] to be better than CT and angiography at demonstrating the relationship between tumor mass and neurovascular bundles and at defining involvement of muscular compartments. Contrary to early reports, recent experience[29,30] shows that MR visualization of tumorous cortical involvement may be at least as good as that provided by CT. The cortex is best evaluated on transaxial views that avoid partial-volume artifacts between the medullary cavity signal and cortical bone signal. The ability of MR to demonstrate matrix mineralization, periosteal reaction, and tumor calcification is clearly inferior to that provided by CT.[31] However, these changes are adequately demonstrated with conventional roentgenography in the context of supplementing MR images.

There are no parameters unique to conventional SE MR that would be useful in differentiating benign from malignant disease. Calculated T1 and T2 relaxation times do not correlate well with histological tumor type, although one[32] study suggests that the numerical value of the ratio of calculated T1 to calculated T2 relaxation times (as well as the ratio of calculated T1 and T2 relaxation times of pathological marrow to homologous normal marrow) may help distinguish benign from malignant disease when scanning to evaluate for metastatic lesions. The classical signs used in other imaging modalities are usually helpful. Benign lesions often have well-defined margins and homogeneous intensities whereas malignant lesions commonly have poorly defined margins, nonhomogeneous intensities, and hazy intensity changes vis à vis the surrounding tissue. Lesions that do have a characteristic MR appearance include lipomas, which have the same signal characteristics as surrounding normal fat; fibrotic scars, which are of low signal on all sequences; and angiomas and angiolipomas, which are heterogeneous, with a high-and-low signal pattern.[30]

MR ^{31}P spectroscopy shows promise for tumor characterization. Preliminary results in a study of four patients with distal extremity tumors[33] showed that clinically active (malignant) neoplasms, with increased metabolism as demonstrated by bone scintigraphy, had relatively high adenosine triphosphate content and high levels of phosphodiester and inorganic phosphate with intermediate phosphodiester peaks. The MR spectrum of the unaffected contralateral extremity showed no well-resolved ^{31}P signal, as was expected in healthy bone. Limited experience indicates that there may be small changes in tumor metabolism following therapy, and that following the P-31 peaks may be useful in evaluating treatment efficacy.

MR imaging has also been useful in follow-up examinations of patients treated with radiation therapy and/or surgery. Frouge et al.[34] found that a low-signal lesion on long TR/TE sequences was 96% sensitive for indicating the absence of active disease. In patients treated with only surgery, high-intensity lesions were 100% accurate in detecting recurrent tumor. When studying patients treated only with radiation therapy, the authors decided that signal characterization of active tumor could not be differentiated from the signal of radiation-induced inflammation (low intensity on short TR/TE, high intensity on long TR/TE, sequences) and, they added, inflammatory changes were seen 1 month to 4 years after radiation therapy. The use of gadopentetate does not help in differentiating residual tumor from reactive change.[35]

Leukemia

Leukemia is the most common type of childhood cancer, representing approximately 35% of all pediatric malignancies. Acute lymphocytic leukemia (ALL) accounts for 85% of these. Although bone marrow is considered the originating site of ALL (as with all leukemias), the spleen, liver, lymph nodes, kidneys, testes, and thymus also can be involved. Symptoms are related to the replacement of normal marrow elements by proliferating leukemic blast cells, which causes decreased production of normal blood elements and results in anemia, thrombocytopenia, and granulocytopenia. Bone pain and arthralgia are due to bone marrow expansion. Combination chemotherapy, identification of leukemic "sanctuaries," central nervous system prophylaxis, and more aggressive treatment of bacterial and opportunistic infections, as well as the use of platelet and white blood cell transfusions, have vastly improved the prognosis of this disease.[36] Radionuclide bone marrow scanning correlated with repeat marrow biopsies has been the usual

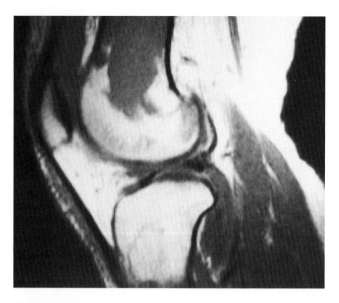

FIGURE 10-3
T1-weighted image of a 32-year-old man with leukemia. The high signal intensity from the normal marrow of the tibia contrasts with the low signal from the marrow cavity of the distal femur. The yellow marrow has been replaced by leukemic cells. Similar changes are seen in children.

means for evaluating posttherapeutic recovery following chemotherapy and/or radiation.

Early experience indicates that MRI may provide an alternative means of following these cases. Several authors[8,9] have reported that the marrow T1 signal intensity in untreated leukemic patients is decreased on short TR/TE images (Fig. 10-3) and becomes isointense on long TR/TE sequences. Of greater interest is the work of Moore et al.,[37] which has demonstrated that the lumbar marrow of children with newly diagnosed ALL, and of children with ALL in remission, has significantly longer calculated T1 relaxation times than normal. These calculated values were, in fact, found to be reliable in distinguishing children with newly diagnosed ALL (968 +/− 68 msec) from normal age-matched controls (441 +/− 82 msec) and from children with ALL in remission (404 +/− 135 msec). On the other hand, T2 relaxation times were not reliable in distinguishing among these groups. The authors suggested that prolongation of T1 was due to an increased intracellular water content, the inherently long T1 relaxation times of leukemic cells, or a change in the chemical environment of the marrow (e.g., pH) resulting from the increased metabolic activity of blast cells.

However, quantitative chemical phase-shift imaging has shown that the prolonged T1 relaxation times found on conventional SE images are due primarily to the decreased marrow fat fraction. Although there is no significant difference in their intrinsic lipid relaxation times, most leukemic patients have slight elevations in their water component T1 relaxation times. This latter finding is of uncertain significance, but it may be due to a complex interaction between abnormally high concentra-

tions of leukemic blast cells in the marrow (causing elevated T1 relaxation times), free triglyceride spectral components (shortening the relaxation times), and changes in the marrow iron content (causing a decrease in relaxation times with increased concentrations). As one would expect, phase-shift imaging is more sensitive than conventional SE techniques in evaluating leukemic changes of marrow because the lipid content is measured directly rather than inferred from its effect on total marrow (bulk) T1 relaxation times.

Multiple myeloma

Multiple myeloma is the most common of the plasma cell dyscrasias in which neoplastic plasma cells infiltrate the marrow. Although a significant number of patients with myeloma have no apparent bone lesions at the time of diagnosis, bone marrow needle aspiration studies[38] usually demonstrate widespread infiltration of marrow by malignant plasmacytes.

In patients strongly suspected of having myeloma, but with normal conventional radiographic studies, CT is often helpful. We obtain two 5 mm thick slices, spaced 5 mm apart, through the bodies of eight to ten thoracic and five lumbar vertebrae. In patients with early phases of myeloma, numerous small lytic lesions are noted in the vertebrae (Figs. 10-4 and 10-5). One may follow the course of these patients with serial CT studies. A favorable response is shown by stabilization of the size of the lesions and osteosclerosis.

The later stages of the disease are characterized by diffuse osteoporosis and widespread lysis of bone. Although the traditional imaging modalities are relatively insensitive at detecting the involvement of marrow by myeloma, MRI has been shown to be very sensitive. As with other neoplastic diseases of marrow, replacement of medullary fat by tumor causes decreased T1 signal and prolongation of T2 relaxation times (Figs. 10-6 and 10-7). Fatty replacement of vertebral marrow can be seen in some patients with myeloma, affecting practically all the vertebrae, long bones, and flat bones. The vertebral marrow of these patients is prominently bright on T1-weighted images.

Daffner et al.,[39] reporting on 30 myeloma patients, 24 of whom had negative bone scans and all of whom had abnormalities demonstrated by MR, found that, although generally the signal characteristics were nonspecific, MRI successfully located areas of abnormal marrow and thus provided the needed information for directed needle aspiration biopsies to achieve early tissue diagnosis. This was a particularly important discovery, since bone scans (the most sensitive "conventional" imaging modality) are known to serve poorly in this respect.

Occasionally a pathological fracture due to myeloma will resemble a nonpathological osteoporotic fracture. It is also helpful to keep in mind that patients with myeloma may present with profound osteoporosis and compression fractures. Therefore one should always look for evidence

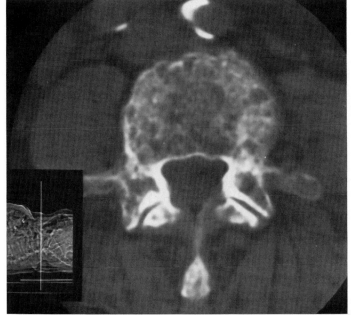

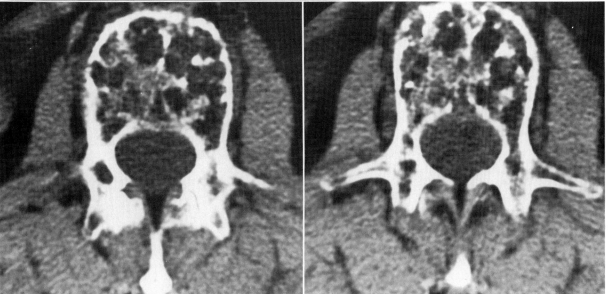

FIGURE 10-4
A, CT scan through L5 of a patient suspected clinically of having myeloma, but with negative plain films. Note the multiple small lytic lesions throughout the vertebral body. **B** and **C,** CT images from another patient with more severe disease. Although the lytic lesions are quite obvious on CT, this patient's plain films were normal.

of neoplastic involvement to exclude the possibility of malignancy in any patient presenting with profound osteoporosis and compression fractures.

Ewing's sarcoma

Ewing's sarcoma is a primary round cell tumor believed to be derived from immature reticular cells of the bone marrow. It is the second most common (after osteogenic sarcoma) bony tumor of children and young adults. The femur and pelvis are most commonly involved, but any bone can be affected.

The classical roentgenographic pattern of Ewing's sarcoma in the long bones is a mottled moth-eaten appearance (Fig. 10-8, A and B). As the tumor extends through the cortex, it stimulates periosteal new bone

formation, which can have a layered (onionskin) appearance or, less commonly, a radial spiculated (sunburst) appearance. In the flat bones the tumor is usually lytic, sclerotic, or mixed. Conventional roentgenograms provide the best basis for developing a differential diagnosis.

CT is helpful for evaluating questionable or poorly visualized lesions. In the past both CT and nuclear scintigraphy were used for estimating the intramedullary and soft tissue components of known tumors. Currently MRI is the imaging modality of choice.

The MR appearance of Ewing's sarcoma is relatively nonspecific, with low signal on T1-weighted images and increased brightness on T2 weighting. MRI provides more information than CT with respect to soft tissue involvement, extension into the medullary cavity,[35] and invasion

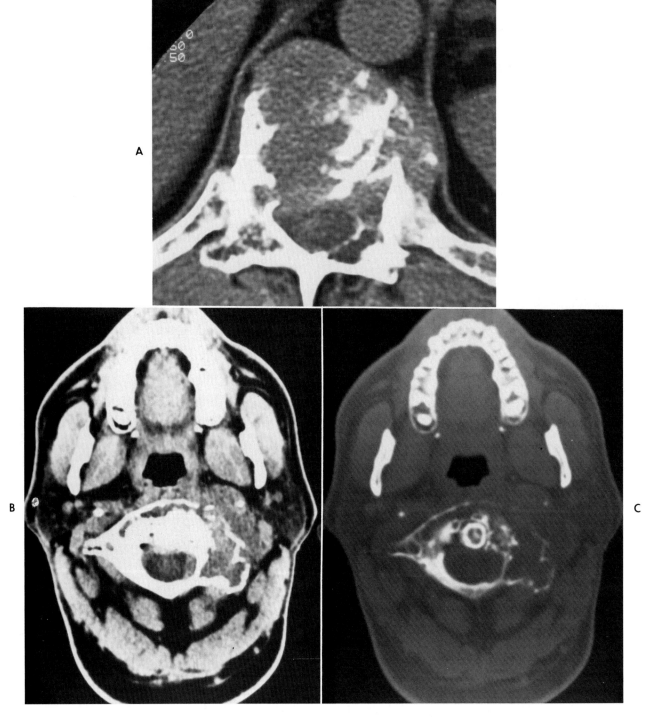

FIGURE 10-5
A, Marked vertebral marrow replacement by myeloma cells with extension into the spinal canal and paraspinal soft tissues at the level of T10. Pathological changes were seen on the plain films. **B** and **C,** A destructive expansile mass at the level of C1. Note the extension into the neural canal and paraspinal soft tissues.

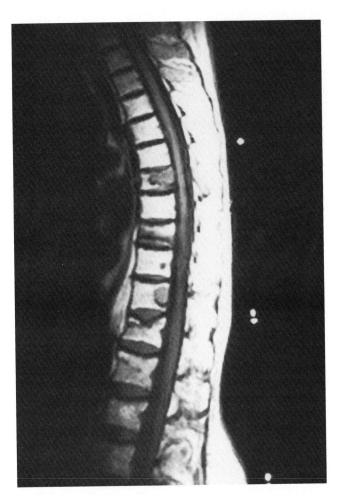

FIGURE 10-6
Areas of marrow replacement by myeloma are seen as regions of decreased signal on this short TR/short TE sequence image. Note the collapse of two midthoracic and one upper lumbar vertebral bodies.

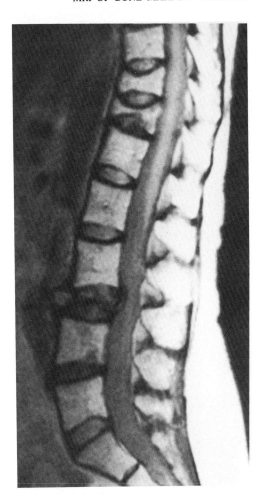

FIGURE 10-7
T1-weighted spine MR scan from a 44-year-old woman with multiple myeloma. The relatively bright signal indicates fat replacement of the marrow. There is a complete collapse of L3 with significant loss of height in T10 and T11.

through the physis into the epiphysis (Figs. 10-8, *C* to *F*, to 10-10).

Lymphoma

Primary non-Hodgkin's lymphoma of bone is much less common than the skeletal lymphomatous dissemination seen in with advanced Hodgkin's or non-Hodgkin's lymphoma. The lesion may remain confined to the skeletal area originally involved or may affect the associated regional lymph nodes and become a generalized lymphoma. On plain film studies it appears as a patchy radiolucency that may or may not be associated with new bone formation. Cortical involvement is seen as thinning along with focal areas of thickening. There are usually minimal changes in the contour of the bone.

CT was the traditional modality for estimating the degree of marrow invasion and tumor extension through the cortex (Fig. 10-11). As with Ewing's sarcoma, the MR appearance of lymphoma is relatively nonspecific, appearing as low signal areas on short TR/TE sequences and becoming brighter with T2-weighting (Fig. 10-12). MR has replaced CT as the imaging modality of choice for staging.

Reticulum cell sarcoma

Reticulum cell sarcoma of bone, derived from the primitive mesenchyme in the marrow, usually involves long tubular bones, especially the femur, tibia, and humerus in patients 20 to 30 years of age. It is an infiltrative tumor that first appears on plain films as irregular patchy osteolysis with focal areas of sclerosis, usually arising in the diaphysis and often extending into cortical bone to cause destruction with variable degrees of reactive periostosis.

No reports of MR experience with this tumor have been published. Presumably, it has the same signal characteristics as the neoplasms discussed above, low intensity on short TR/TE sequences and appearing bright on long sequences.

GAUCHER'S DISEASE

Gaucher's disease is a metabolic disorder in which a deficiency of glucocerebrosidase causes the accumulation of glucocerebrosides in the reticuloendothelial cells (Gaucher cells) of the liver, spleen, and bone marrow. The marrow replacement is seen on plain films indirectly as

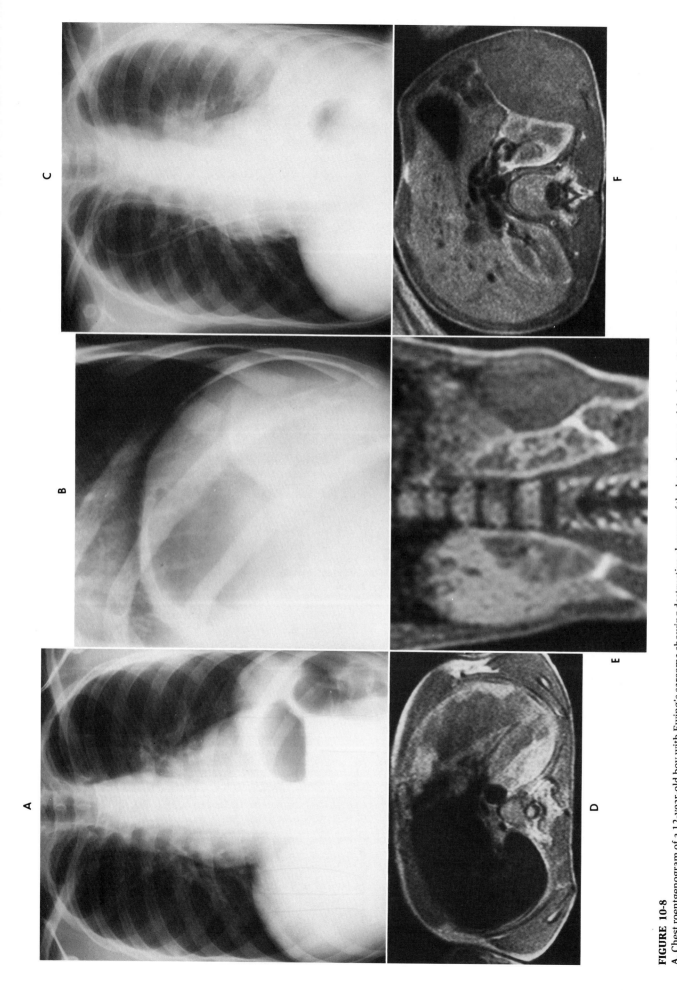

FIGURE 10-8

A, Chest roentgenogram of a 12-year-old boy with Ewing's sarcoma showing destructive changes of the lateral aspect of the left tenth rib. **B,** A coned view shows the typical destructive permeative changes. An MR scan was not done at this time. **C,** A follow-up roentgenogram several months later shows left lower lobe atelectasis and an apparent pleural effusion or pleural thickening. **D,** A transaxial T1-weighted image of the lower chest clearly shows the nodular nature of the pleural thickening, representing tumor extending into the thoracic cavity. Note the relatively bright signal from the atelectatic lung. Coronal, **E,** and transaxial, **F,** T1-weighted images show the tumor mass extending into the abdomen and superficially to distort the usual body contours. The lateral tumor margins are not sharp.

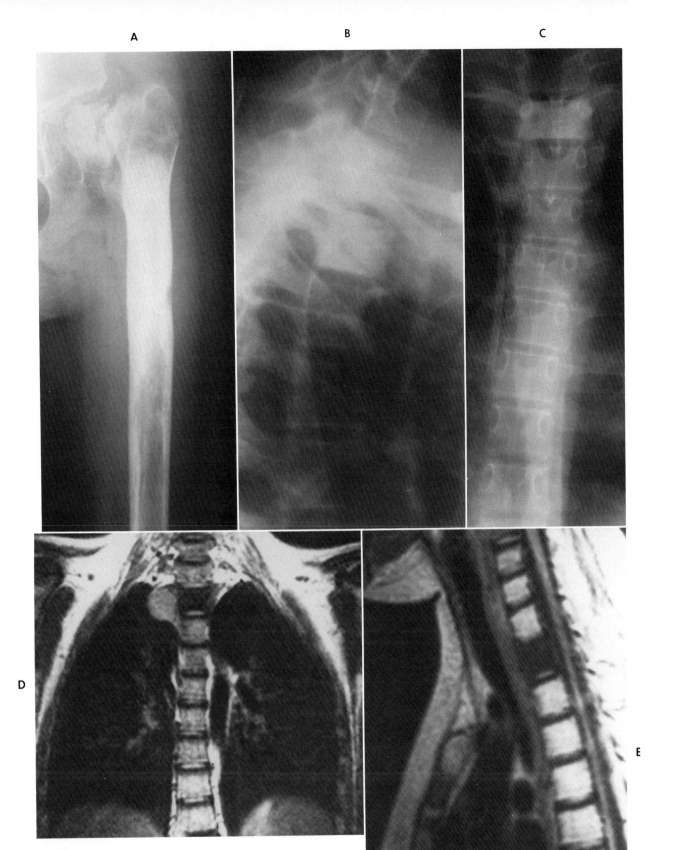

FIGURE 10-9
A 15-year-old girl who presented with left leg pain. **A,** Conventional roentgenogram showing sclerotic changes of the proximal femur, with some lytic areas more distally, suggestive of sclerosing Ewing's sarcoma (the defect seen laterally represents a biopsy site). Note also the pathological fracture through the femoral neck. While under treatment this patient experienced upper back pain. **B** and **C** show sclerosis of T3. The T1-weighted MR images, **D** and **E,** clearly illustrate decreased signal and an associated soft tissue mass, compatible with metastatic disease.

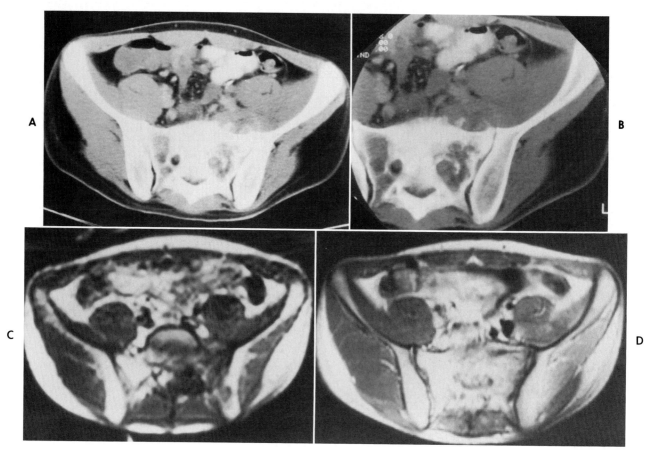

FIGURE 10-10

A and B, CT scans of a patient with Ewing's sarcoma involving the pelvis. Note the destructive changes of the medullary components and the extension of tumor into the soft tissues on the left side. C and D, Short and long TR/TE sequences obtained after radiation therapy. The decreased signal on the T1-weighted image becomes brighter with T2-weighting. Although the possibility of residual tumor cannot be excluded, the component of the tumor that extended into the soft tissues is no longer seen.

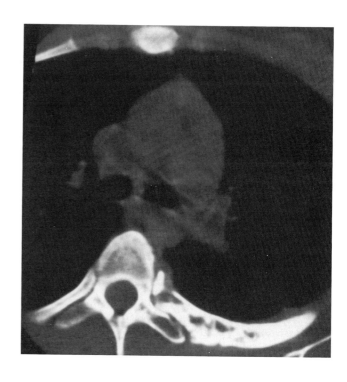

FIGURE 10-11

CT scan of a 26-year-old woman with Hodgkin's lymphoma of the rib showing the typical expansile changes with associated cortical thinning and thickening often seen.

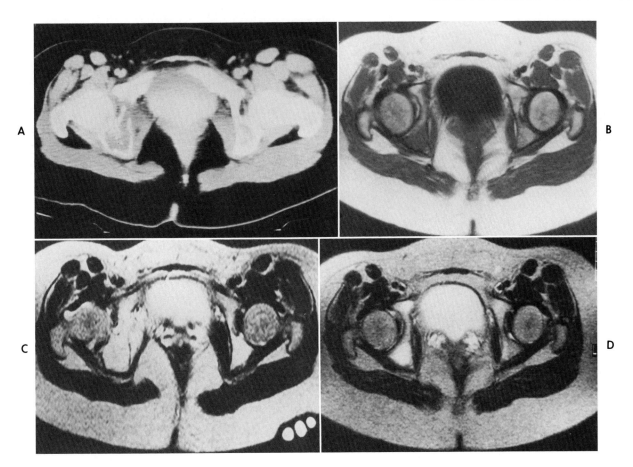

FIGURE 10-12

A, CT scan of a 14-year-old girl with primary lymphoma of the pelvis. Destructive changes of the medullary cavity and contour expansion are present bilaterally, though more prominent on the right. It is difficult to identify the tumor, which has extended into the adjacent soft tissues. **B** and **C,** Pretreatment T1-weighted and T2-weighted MR images show an abnormally low marrow signal on the T1-weighted image, clearly indicative of involvement by neoplastic cells. This area becomes brighter with T2-weighting. Distinguishing normal marrow from tumor is difficult, but soft tissue involvement on the right side is obvious. **D,** A postchemotherapy T2-weighted image shows partial regression of the tumor on the left but continued abnormally bright signal on the right. The soft tissue component has resolved. The bright signal area seen on the pretreatment scans now has the expected low signal intensity.

osteoporosis and as focal cortical bone destruction. Additional bone changes include ischemic necrosis and sclerosis.

Conventional plain film roentgenography and technetium-99m methylene diphosphonate (99m TcMDP) bone scintigrams have been shown to be useful primarily as screening procedures in evaluating the general extent of bony involvement or investigating bone pain and possible avascular necrosis.[40] CT and techetium-99m sulfur colloid are more effective imaging modalities. In a study by Hermann et al.,[40] 99mTcSC scans were found to demonstrate clearly the distribution of reticuloendothelial cells in the bone marrow. The abnormal scans in these patients showed varying degrees of decreased uptake consistent with the extent of marrow replacement. In the more advanced stages of the disease there was total absence of uptake or only isolated instances of uptake of sulfur

colloid by the marrow with associated retained activity in the vascular pool, indicating compromised marrow-reticuloendothelial function.

The CT scans of patients with Gaucher's disease show abnormally high bone marrow attenuation coefficients, usually ranging from +15 to +80 Houndsfield units. The most effective evaluation of bone is achieved through the use of both CT and 99mTcSC scanning: the extent of localized marrow and specific skeletal regional involvement being defined by CT, the more general regional and total skeletal involvement demonstrated by 99mTcSC scans. Furthermore, the areas of abnormal marrow identified by CT correlate well with abnormalities on the bone scans. CT reveals particularly useful information for measuring and fitting a prosthesis.[40]

Early experience using MR to evaluate the marrow in patients with Gaucher's disease is promising.[6] The re-

FIGURE 10-13
A, Gaucher's disease in a 63-year-old man. B, Note the patchy decreased signal from the marrow of the distal femur and proximal tibia on T1-weighted images.

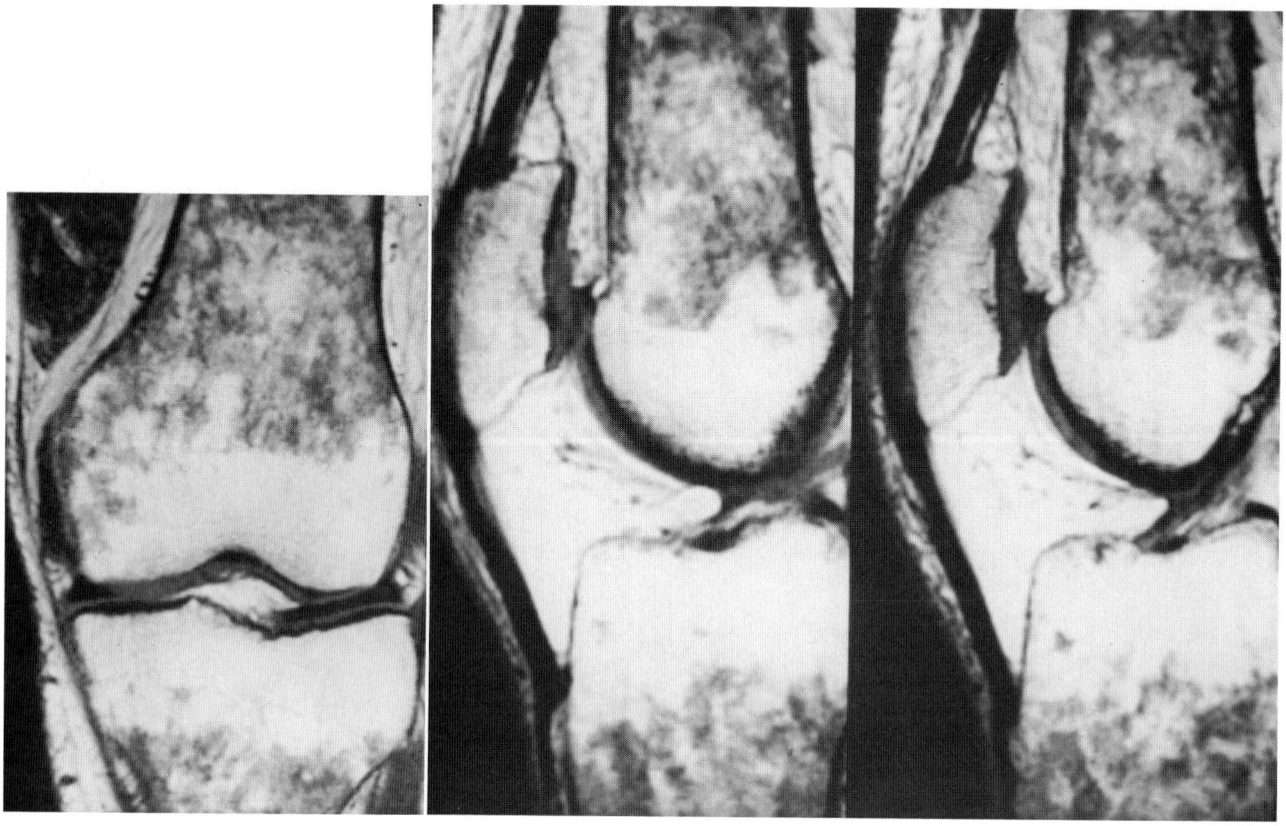

placement of marrow fat by Gaucher cells causes T1 shortening and T2 prolongation relative to matched control marrow signals. These changes, seen reasonably well in the vertebral bodies, are most pronounced in the long bones, especially around the hip, femoral head, acetabulum, and ilium (Fig. 10-13). Similar changes have been described in patients with myelofibrosis and leukemia.

MR has also been helpful in detecting avascular necrosis. The areas of involved marrow demonstrate MR signal changes in areas of acute bone pain, suggesting increased fluid and/or blood within the medullary cavity. The signal change is believed due to either reperfusion following a vascular insult or avascular necrosis caused by venous obstruction.

REFERENCES

1. Christy M: Active bone marrow distribution as a function of age in humans. Phys Med Biol 1981;26:389-400.
2. Rosen BR, Flemming DM, Kushner DC, et al: Hematologic bone marrow disorders: quantitative chemical shift MR imaging. Radiology 1988;169:799-804.
3. Graif M, Pennock JM, Pringle J, et al: Magnetic resonance imaging: comparison of four pulse sequences in assessing primary bone tumors. Skeletal Radiol 1989;18(6):439-444.
4. Pettersson H, Eliasson J, Egund N, et al: Gadolinuim-DTPA enhancement of soft tissue tumors in magnetic resonance imaging — preliminary clinical experience in five patients. Skeletal Radiol 1988;17:319-323.
5. Braunwald E, Isselbacher KJ, Petersdorf RG, et al: Harrison's Principles of internal medicine. 11th ed, New York, McGraw-Hill, 1987, pp 1531-1532.
6. Lanir A, Aghai E, Simon JS, et al: MR imaging in myelofibrosis. J Comput Assist Tomogr 1986;10(4):634-636.
7. Braunwald E, et al: Ref. 5, pp 1533-1536.
8. Kangarloo H, Dietrich RB, Taira RT, et al: MR imaging of bone marrow in children. J Comput Assist Tomogr 1986;10(2):205-209.
9. Cohen MD, Klatte EC, Baehner R, et al: Magnetic resosnace imaging of bone marrow disease in children. Radiology 1984;151:715-718.
10. Olson DO, Shields AF, Scheurich CJ, et al: Magnetic resonance imaging of the bone marrow in patients with leukemia, aplastic anemia, and lymphoma. Invest Radiol 1986;21:540-546.
11. Kaplan PA, Asleson RJ, Klassen LW, Duggan MJ: Bone marrow patterns in aplastic anemia: observations with 1.5-T MR imaging. Radiology 1987;164:441-444.
12. McKinstry CS, Steiner RE, Young AT, et al: Bone marrow in leukemia and aplastic anemia: MR imaging before, during, and after treatment. Radiology 1987;162:701-707.
13. Rosen BR, Carter EA, Pykett IL, et al: Proton chemical shift imaging: an evaluation of its chemical potential using an in vivo fatty liver model. Radiology 1985;154:469-472.
14. Buxton RB, Wismer GL, Brady TJ, Rosen BR: Quantitative proton chemical-shift imaging. Magn Reson Med 1986;3: 881-900.
15. Braunwald E, et al: Ref. 5, pp 1520-1522.
16. Alvavi A: Scintigraphic detection of bone and marrow infarction

in sickle cell disorders. In Bohrer SP, Green WH (eds): Bone ischemia and infarction in sickle cell disease. St Louis, Green, 1981.

17. Rao VM, Fishman M, Mitchell DG, et al: Painful sickle crisis: bone marrow patterns observed with MR imaging. Radiology 1986;161:211-215.

18. Long JA, Doppman JL, Nienhaus AW, Mills SR: Computed tomographic analysis of beta-thalassemic syndrome with hemochromatosis: pathologic findings with clinical and laboratory correlation. J Comput Assist Tomogr 1980;4:159-165.

19. Goldburg HI, Cann CE, Moss AA, et al: Noninvasive quantitation in dogs with hemochromatosis using dual energy CT scanning. Invest Radiol 1982;17:375-380.

20. Halliday JW, Russo AM, Cowlishaw JL, Powell LW: Serum-ferritin in diagnosis of haemochromatosis. A study of 43 families. Lancet 1977;2:621-624.

21. Bassett ML, Halliday JW, Powell LW, et al: Early detection of idiopathic haemochromatosis: relative value of serum-ferritin in HLA typing. Lancet 1979;2:4-7.

22. Braunwald E, et al: Ref 5, pp 1494-1495.

23. Stark DD, Moseley ME, Bacon BR, et al: Magnetic resonance imaging and spectroscopy of hepatic iron overload. Radiology 1985;154:137-142.

24. Brasch RC, Wesbey BE, Gooding CA, Koerper MA: Magnetic resonance imaging of transfusional hemosiderosis complicating thalassemia major. Radiology 1984;152:767-771.

25. Gomori JM, Grossman RI, Drott HR: MR relaxation times and iron content of thalassemic spleens: an in vitro study. AJR 1988;150:567-569.

26. Yilmaz A, Chu SC, Osmanoglu S: Dependence of the solvent proton on the iron content in normal human serum. Magn Reson Med 1988;7:337-339.

27. Ambrosino MM, Hernanz-Schulman M, Rumancik WM, et al: In vivo correlation between MR signal intensity values and serum ferritin levels in patients with Cooley's anemia. Radiology 1987;165(P):137.

28. Ehman RL: MR imaging of medullary bone. Radiology 1988;167:867-868.

29. Bloem JL, Taminiau AH, Eulderink F, et al: Radiologic staging of primary bone sarcoma: MR imaging, scintigraphy, angiography, and CT correlated with pathologic examination. Radiology 1988;169:805-810.

30. Pettersson H, Gillespy T 3rd, Hamlin DJ, et al: Primary musculoskeletal tumors: examination with MR imaging compared with conventional modalities. Radiology 1987;164:237-241.

31. Boyko OB, Cory DA, Cohen MD, et al: MR imaging of osteogenic and Ewing's sarcoma. AJR 1987;148:317-322.

32. Sugimura K, Yamasaki K, Kitagaki H, et al: Bone marrow diseases of the spine: differentiation with T1 and T2 relaxation times in MR imaging. Radiology 1987;165:541-544.

33. Nidecker AC, Müller S, Aue WP, et al: Extremity bone tumors: evaluation with P-31 spectroscopy. Radiology 1985;157:167-174.

34. Frouge C, Vanel D, Coffre C, et al: The role of magnetic resonance imaging in the evaluation of Ewing sarcoma. Skeletal Radiol 1988;17:387-392.

35. Vanel D, Lacombe MJ, Couanet D, et al: Musculoskeletal tumors: follow-up with MR imaging after treatment with surgery and radiation therapy. Radiology 1987;167:243-245.

36. Miller JH, White L (eds): Imaging in pediatric oncology. Baltimore, Williams & Wilkins, 1985, pp 406-407.

37. Moore SG, Gooding CA, Brasch RC, et al: Bone marrow in children with acute lymphocytic leukemia: MR relaxation times. Radiology 1986;160:237-240.

38. Petersdorf RG, Adams RD, Braunwald E, et al (eds): Harrison's Principles of internal medicine, 10th ed, New York, McGraw Hill 1985, pp 363-365.

39. Daffner RH, Lupetin AR, Dash N, et al: MRI in the detection of malignant infiltration of bone marrow. AJR 1986;146:353-358.

40. Hermann G, Goldblatt J, Levy RN, et al: Gaucher's disease type 1: assessment of bone involvement by CT and scintigraphy. AJR 1986;147:943-948.

11 Solitary Bone Lesions

MICHAEL M. AMBROSINO
NANCY B. GENIESER
MELVIN H. BECKER

Tumors arising from or forming fibrous connective tissue
  Fibrous metaphyseal defects
  Juxtacortical desmoid
  Desmoplastic fibroma
  Fibrosarcoma
Cartilage-forming tumors
  Chondromyxoid fibroma
Chondromas
  Enchondromas
  Periosteal chondromas
  Maffucci's syndrome and Ollier's disease
  Osteochondroma
  Chondroblastoma
  Hereditary multiple exostosis
  Chondrosarcoma
Bone-forming tumors

Osteoid osteoma
Osteoblastoma
Ossifying fibroma
Osteogenic sarcoma
  Central (classic) osteosarcoma
  Surface oseosarcoma
Tumors of histiocytic or fibrocystic origin
  Giant cell tumor
  Malignant fibrous histiocytoma
  Lipoma
Chordomas
Tumorlike lesions of unknown origin
  Unicameral bone cyst
  Aneurysmal bone cyst
  Soft tissue neoplasms
  Synovial sarcoma

The primary considerations for evaluating bone neoplasms with MR scanning are presented in Chapter 10. Briefly, the conclusions of a number of studies comparing the efficacies of MR and CT have shown the diagnostic capabilities of MR imaging to be superior for the following: definition of the intramedullary component of a tumor; evaluation of soft tissue extension into specific muscle compartments, especially in the extremities, where fat planes are poorly defined by CT; and identification of neurovascular and joint involvement by tumor.[1] MR is as effective as CT in detecting tumoral cortical invasion, but it provides poorer visualization of calcification and ossification (although these details are usually adequately evaluated by conventional roentgenography).

To utilize MR most effectively, one must select the correct imaging sequences to optimize the different MR properties of the structures in question. The extraosseous soft tissue component of tumors is best visualized on T2-weighted images, in which neoplastic tissue is seen as a bright-signal region against the dark lower signal of adjacent normal muscles. The preferred imaging sequence for estimating the intramedullary extension of tumor depends upon whether red or yellow marrow is being evaluated. Areas of pathology in the red marrow of infants and young children are visualized on T2-weighted images as regions of bright signal against the less bright background of normal red marrow. On the other hand, the red marrow in older children and adults, as well as the yellow marrow in all patients, is often best evaluated on T1-weighted or STIR imaging sequences.

Neoplastic tissue is seen as a low-signal area against the high-signal background of fat. It is important to keep in mind, however, that the MR appearance of solitary bone tumors may be more variable than that of either primary marrow neoplasms or soft tissue lesions. Tumors with a large ossific (sclerosing) and fibrous component, for example, will have low MR signal intensity (SI) on all imaging sequences because of the intrinsically long T1 and short T2 relaxation times and/or the relatively low proton densities. In these cases, conventional roentgenography serves as a useful and perhaps essential adjunct in interpreting MR images.

As clinical experience with MR grows, it is becoming more apparent that the primary role of MRI in evaluating bone tumors is usually one not of narrowing a differential diagnosis formulated on the basis of plain film or CT findings but rather of better defining the extent of known lesions when planning surgery. Conventional roentgenography and CT are, in fact, superior to MRI for characterizing lesions. Long bone lesions can almost always be better characterized on plain films whereas lesions of the flat bones such as the scapula and pelvis (in which plain film diagnosis is difficult) can be better characterized with CT. MRI is done when further or more accurate staging is required.[2] Precise staging of malignant bone tumors is of increasing importance as the current emphasis in treating many bone tumors has shifted to the use of relatively conservative surgery and limb salvaging techniques.

TUMORS ARISING FROM OR FORMING FIBROUS CONNECTIVE TISSUE
Fibrous metaphseal defects

Fibrous cortical defects and nonossifying fibromas are similar lesions distinguished on the basis of size and the age of the patient. The most common benign tumors occurring in children after 2 years of age, they share a common histological appearance of whorled bundles of connective tissue cells. Radiographically they appear as oval lytic cortical defects in the metaphyses of long bones, usually the femur and tibia. The distance from the physis varies depending on age, becoming more diaphyseal as the patient grows. Fibrous cortical defects (fibrous metaphyseal lesion less than 2 cm in size) rarely cause symptoms; nonossifying fibromas (fibrous metaphyseal lesions 2 cm or larger) may be detected first following a pathological fracture from relatively minor trauma. Although their etiology is uncertain, they appear to be related to subjacent inserting ligaments or tendons and an additional (unknown) pathological factor.[3]

These lesions have varying radiological appearances (Fig. 11-1) as they evolve,[4] and they have been classified as follows[3]:

Stage A: Located near the epiphyseal plate, with a round to oval shape and fine sclerotic margin

Stage B: Expansile polycystic defects with distinct sclerotic margins

Stage C: Representing initial healing, with early mineralization, usually located near the diaphysis

Stage D: Completely sclerotic

Not surprisingly, the MR signal characteristics also change as the lesion matures. Stage A lesions appear as homogeneous areas of variable intensity (fat to muscle intensity on short TR/TE sequences) with smooth borders and containing thin linear structures of very low intensity. Stage B lesions are heterogeneous, with increased numbers of low-signal linear structures defining many small round areas of varying signal intensity (best seen on long TR/TE sequences). The margins enhance with gadopentetate, suggesting the presence of peripheral hypervascular zones. The more diaphyseal areas show multiple 1 to 5 mm areas having intermediate to low signal on long and short TR/TE sequences. Stage C maturity lesions have MR findings similar to those of Stage B but differing in that they are more prominent and

there is a lower overall T1-weighted intensity. These lesions have low-signal margins that appear to correspond to the sclerotic margin seen on plain films. In the region closer to the diaphysis, small areas with signal characteristics of normal marrow are occasionally identified. Stage D lesions can appear as an area either of homogeneous low signal intensity (sclerotic lesion on plain films) or of increasingly homogeneous "normal marrow" signal that in time becomes indistinct from the signal of surrounding bone; it represents the final phase of healing.

The progression of the MR appearances correlates well with the known histology of these lesions. During the early stages the lesion consists of fibrous tissue with varying amounts of fat-storing foam cells and intracellular stromal hemosiderin. The linear areas of decreased signal are believed to represent fibrous septa or osseous pseudosepta. As the lesion matures, the signal intensity decreases due to progressive mineralization and assumes the appearance of normal marrow once healing is complete.[2]

It must be emphasized that the appearance on plain roentgenograms is practically diagnostic and rarely if ever requires further investigation.

Juxtacortical desmoid

Periosteal desmoids are benign fibrous lesions that arise beneath the periosteum and are associated with erosive changes of the subjacent cortex. They have been described as a variant of nonossifying fibroma, periosteal fibromatosis, or periosteal desmoplastic fibroma,[6] and as essentially a chronic traumatic lesion of weakened cortical bone (microavulsions) causing accelerated cortical resorption and fibroblastic healing. They usually are seen in teenage men, occurring in the area of the adductor tendon insertion on the posteromedial femoral cortex adjacent to the medial condyle, along the linea aspera.

Periosteal desmoids characteristically appear on conventional roentgenograms as sharply marginated saucer-like defects in the cortex. Associated periosteal new bone may be markedly regular, appearing simply as cortical thickening, or as irregular ossification with a lamellated appearance. Soft tissue swelling is often present. The differential diagnosis of lesions with this type of exuberant periostosis includes infection and osteosarcoma. CT scanning can help narrow the possibilities and eliminate malignancy by demonstrating the desmoid soft tissue mass without matrix calcification and without typical expansile cortical changes.

The MR appearance of desmoids has not been reported. The greater sensitivity of MR in evaluating tumor marrow invasion and soft tissue extension is particularly helpful for definitively excluding the possibility of malignancy.

Desmoplastic fibroma

Desmoplastic fibromas are rare benign lesions consisting of fibroblasts separated by collagenous stroma. They

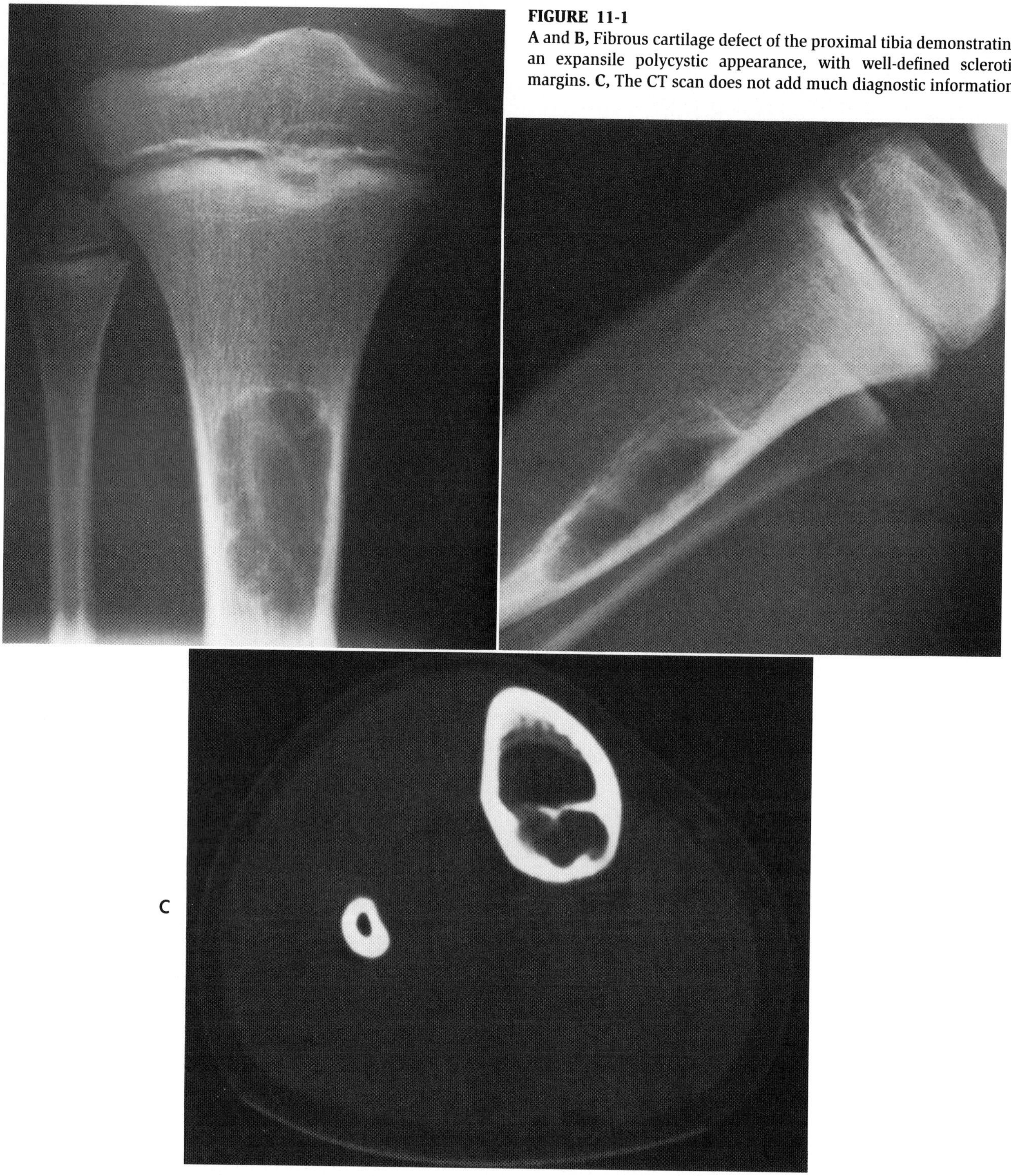

FIGURE 11-1
A and B, Fibrous cartilage defect of the proximal tibia demonstrating an expansile polycystic appearance, with well-defined sclerotic margins. C, The CT scan does not add much diagnostic information.

generally appear during the second or third decade of life and usually affect the flat bones and metaphyses of long bones. Conventional roentgenograms show them as homogeneously lytic, honeycombed, or trabeculated, with an associated mild cortical expansion and thinning. Occasionally a thin circumferential sclerosis will be present. Large desmoplastic fibromas can have an aggressive appearance suggesting the presence of malignancy (e.g., fibrosarcoma or metastatic disease).[5] Although their MR appearance has not been reported, it would probably be a useful diagnostic adjunct when plain film findings suggest a malignant lesion.

The lesions are benign, but nevertheless may be locally invasive, and histologically resemble soft tissue desmoid tumors (aggressive fibromatosis), consisting of fibroblasts separated by collagenous stroma. They usually occur in 10-to-20-year-old patients, who present with acute or chronic pain and, less frequently, pathological fractures.

On plain roentgenograms they appear as centrally located lesions with sclerotic borders, most often in the metaphyses of long bones (though not infrequently also in the mandible and ilium). They can expand the bone diameter through endosteal erosion and concomitant periosteal new bone formation, with residual columns of normal bone creating the trabeculated, soap-bubble, or honeycombed appearance. Their differential diagnosis includes nonossifying fibroma, giant cell tumor, aneurysmal bone cyst, and unicameral bone cyst. Although desmoplastic fibromas grow slowly, they can attain massive size and radiographically appear aggressive, with cortical erosion, permeative changes, coarse trabeculation, and associated soft tissue extension. It is this last appearance that resembles fibrosarcoma and metastatic renal or thyroid carcinoma.

CT scanning and MR imaging are helpful in narrowing the differential diagnosis: the scans show a well-defined lytic lesion with lobulated margins and marked cortical bone loss[7]; the MR images demonstrate a well-defined soft tissue component in addition to intramedullary extension.[6] Presurgical knowledge of the tumor margins is especially important, since its locally aggressive behavior predisposes to recurrence if fairly wide surgical margins are not obtained. Desmoplastic fibromas occur too infrequently for an ascertainment to be made of whether the better soft tissue visualization afforded by MR allows significantly better surgical planning than with CT, although one would expect better medullary visualization to be an advantage. Unfortunately, neither modality helps in further delineating the often difficult histological distinction between a desmoplastic fibroma and a low-grade fibrosarcoma.

Fibrosarcoma

Fibrosarcomas are rare fibroblastic malignancies affecting a wide age range of patients but occurring slightly more frequently in young adults. The patient presents with swelling and pain localized to the involved area. The better-differentiated tumors tend to be less painful. They may be central (arising within the medullary cavity) or peripheral (arising on the periosteal surface).

Periosteal fibrosarcomas are radiographically characterized by a large soft tissue mass and poorly defined areas of osteolysis consistent with invasion of the cortex and extension into the medullary cavity. The tumors produce no osteoid or chondroid matrix and, except for occasional small calcific foci in areas of necrosis, contain no areas of ossification or calcification. They occur most often in the pelvis, and less commonly in the femoral neck, scapula, and ribs. A central fibrosarcoma will usually originate in the medullary cavity and arise at the diaphyseal-metaphyseal junction in a long bone. It grows axially to involve remote areas of the medullary cavity (although involvement may not be contiguous) and radially to cause endosteal erosion, cortical thinning, symmetrical expansion, and eventually cortical destruc-

tion with periostosis. In contradistinction to periosteal fibrosarcomas, an associated extraosseous soft tissue mass may be evident only in long-standing lesions. The development of osseous sequestrations is a fairly characteristic finding.[8] It is important to note that slow-growing fibrosarcomas can sometimes have fairly well-defined margins.[9]

The usual absence of prominent tumoral calcifications makes fibrosarcoma ideally suited for evaluation with MR. Although clinical experience thus far is limited, extrapolation from experience with other bone tumors suggests that MR will probably be the best imaging modality for demonstration of medullary involvement and soft tissue extension. The current generation of MR scanners is capable of showing cortical invasion of many tumors as accurately as CT scanners can, obviating the need to perform CT examinations in most cases.

CARTILAGE-FORMING TUMORS

The MR appearance of cartilage-forming tumors can vary considerably depending upon the lesion's histology. A better understanding of the MR presentation is gained by recalling that hyaline cartilage consists of chrondrocytes (cellular component) dispersed in an acellular (water-trapping) matrix of mucopolysaccharides and collagen fibers. The parenchymal components of each cartilage-forming tumor varies with respect to the relative water, myxoid, and cellular composition.

Tumors composed primarily of hyaline cartilage demonstrate high signal intensities on long TR/long TE spin echo sequences, apparently due to the relatively high water content of the cartilage. Neoplasms that are cartilaginous derivatives but have a greater relative cellular or myxoid composition (i.e., essentially nonchondroid tumors) have signal intensities that are hypointense or isointense relative to muscle on both T1- and T2-weighted sequences.

Cartilaginous lesions have a well-defined lobular configuration on long TR/TE sequences that corresponds to the lobular morphology defined by fibrous septa seen histologically (Fig. 11-2). Tumors that do not contain well-differentiated hyaline cartilage do not have this lobular pattern.[10]

Chondromyxoid fibroma

Chondromyxoid fibroma is the least common benign tumor of cartilage and is composed of varying proportions of chondroidal, myxomatous, and fibrous tissue. It is slow growing and usually seen in the long bones of adolescents and young adults, appearing as well-defined and elongated radiolucencies with coarse trabeculation located eccentrically in the metaphysis.

The MR appearance of this lesion has not been described. One would anticipate, however, a heterogeneous tumor whose precise characteristics depended upon the histological organization and relative amounts of chondroidal, myxomatous, and fibrous tissue.

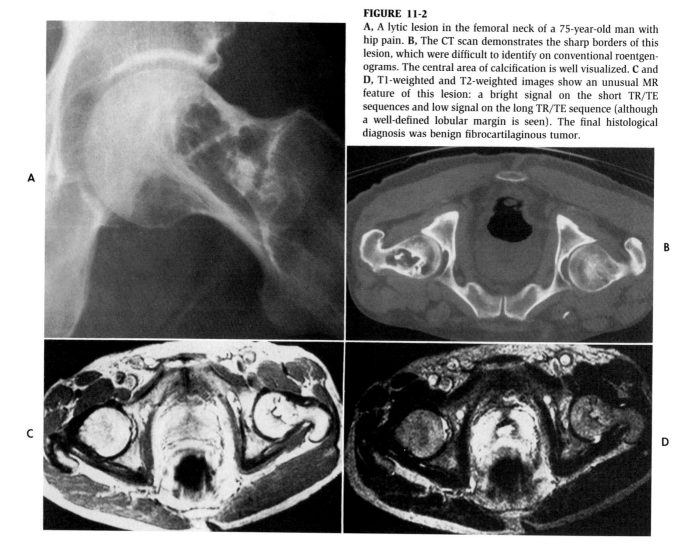

FIGURE 11-2

A, A lytic lesion in the femoral neck of a 75-year-old man with hip pain. **B,** The CT scan demonstrates the sharp borders of this lesion, which were difficult to identify on conventional roentgenograms. The central area of calcification is well visualized. **C** and **D,** T1-weighted and T2-weighted images show an unusual MR feature of this lesion: a bright signal on the short TR/TE sequences and low signal on the long TR/TE sequence (although a well-defined lobular margin is seen). The final histological diagnosis was benign fibrocartilaginous tumor.

CHONDROMAS

Chondromas are most often solitary lesions that can be classified on the basis of where they occur in bone. Those that arise within the medullary cavity are called enchondromas, and those arising between the bony cortex and periosteum are periosteal chondromas.

Enchondromas

The solitary enchondroma is a common benign tumor thought to arise from misplaced cartilaginous cells in the medullary cavity, adjacent to the metaphysis, that is usually seen in patients 10 to 30 years of age, and most often occurs in the short tubular bones of the hands and feet. Patients with enchondromas are generally free of symptoms, although some will present with painless swelling. Pathological fractures can follow minor trauma.

In the short tubular bones enchondromas are seen on conventional roentgenograms as well-defined round or oval medullary radiolucencies, usually in the metaphyses, that cause endosteal erosion and may lead to bony expansion. Calcifications are sometimes seen. Long bone enchondromas are often centrally or eccentrally located, with lobulated endosteal erosions and/or bony expansion, and frequently contain multiple punctate calcifications without an associated radiolucency.

No review of the MRI appearance of enchondromas has been published. The appearance of a single enchondroma was reported as part of a study investigating tumors of cartilaginous origin[10] that had very high signal on long TR/long TE sequences (because of its relatively high water content, which was organized in lobules separated completely or partially by lamellar bone and marrow fat). Noncartilaginous lesions do not have this lobulated morphology and usually do not have such short T2 relaxation times, which are characteristic more of chondroid lesions.

Periosteal chondromas

Periosteal chondromas are most commonly found adjacent to the metaphysis of a long tubular bone, especially the humerus and femur. Patients usually present with localized swelling and mild to moderate pain.

Periosteal chondromas have the same MR appearance as other benign cartilaginous tumors.[10] A definitive radiological diagnosis requires consideration of tumor location along with information probably better obtained from plain roentgenograms (e.g., surface cortical erosions and calcification). The fairly specific MR characteristics of hyaline cartilage do, however, serve to narrow the differential diagnosis of an extracortical mass causing cortical erosion with or without periostosis (e.g., tendon sheath giant cell tumor or soft tissue abscess) to only extramedullary cartilaginous lesions. MR may prove useful in distinguishing the soft tissue chondromas from periosteal malignancies such as chondrosarcoma.

Maffucci's syndrome and Ollier's disease

Maffucci's syndrome is defined as the association of enchondromatosis with soft tissue hemangiomas. Multiple enchondromatosis, with predominantly unilateral distribution, is known as Ollier's disease. Malignant transformation of an enchondroma to a chondrosarcoma is the most common serious complication of these syndromes. The malignancy rate has been reported[9,11] to be as high as 40% to 51% for Maffucci's syndrome and 20% to 40% for Ollier's disease.

The radiographic distinction between benign enchondroma and chondrosarcoma can be difficult. Unfortunately, there are no definitive MR signal characteristics that allow differentiation between benign and malignant disease. One must rely on the conventional radiographic signs of malignancy (e.g., extension through the physis or growth into the surrounding soft tissue) to suggest confidently the presence of malignancy. The advantage of MR over CT[10] is its greater sensitivity in detecting and defining tumoral extension. Experience with a single case of Marfucci's syndrome[12] indicates that the calculated T2 relaxation time of chondrosarcoma is significantly longer than that of enchondroma. It will be interesting to see whether this type of quantitative data proves reliable as a means of detecting malignancy in these patients.

Osteochondroma

Osteochondromas are benign lesions arising from the surface of a bone near the metaphysis. They consist of a cortex and medullary cavity that are contiguous with those of the host bone and they are covered by a hyaline cartilage cap. The presence of a small cartilaginous cap is usually considered an indication of benign growth. The signs of malignant transformation include enlargement of the cap, irregular cartilaginous calcifications, and poorly defined margins. The lesion in younger children is composed primarily of cartilage, and it ossifies as the patient grows older.

Osteochondromas generally are detected in children and adolescents as a painless slow-growing mass. Complications include fracture, pressure injury to adjacent vessels and nerves, osseous deformity (limiting full range of motion), and malignant transformation of the cartilag-

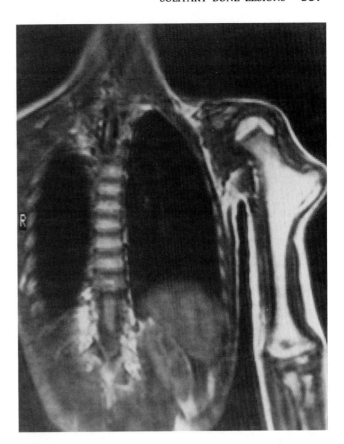

FIGURE 11-3
This T1-weighted scan beautifully demonstrates the continuity of the signal void cortex and relatively high signal meduallary cavity. The cartilaginous cap is well visualized.

inous cap to chondrosarcoma. A bursa can develop over an osteochondroma and become inflamed (bursitis) or develop synovial chondromatosis. The soft tissue mass and calcification of the secondary chondromatosis are sometimes confused with malignant transformation.

An osteochondroma usually appears roentgenographically as an osseous outgrowth arising from the external surface of a long bone. The continuity of the cortex and medullary cavity is evident radiographically. The lesion may be sessile (broad based) or pediculated (narrow stalk and bulbous tip). It usually occurs near the metaphysis and areas of tendinous or ligamentous attachment and commonly points away from the adjacent joint.

MRI provides an excellent means of visualizing the components of an osteochondroma (Fig. 11-3). The continuity of the exostotic cortex and medullary cavity with those of the parent bone can be beautifully demonstrated and distinguishes osteochondroma from other juxtacortical lesions, including chondroma. The superficial cartilaginous cap is easily identified and seen as a high signal region on long TR/long TE sequences.[12] The lobulation characteristic of hyaline cartilage is usually less prominent, probably due to the relatively small volume of cartilage being imaged.

The thickness of the cartilaginous cap, as measured on

CT, has been used as a criterion for predicting malignant transformation of hyaline cartilage to chondrosarcoma. The threshold thickness varies from 2 cm[13] to 2.5 cm.[14] MR allows visualization of a cap as small as 3 mm. Unfortunately, the accuracy of MR estimates of cap thickness probably depends upon the degree of cartilaginous calcification, being less reliable in the more calcified lesions.[12]

The visualization of perichondrium afforded by MR imaging is of great clinical importance, because surgical resection of an osteochondroma requires that the lesion be excised with the perichondrium intact. The outer perichondrium is seen on long TR/TE sequences as a smooth low-signal area adjacent to the cartilaginous cap. Defining the relationship of the perichondrium to the surrounding soft tissue structures helps in presurgical planning. This low-signal region also facilitates checking that the cartilaginous cap has a smooth border, another indication that no malignancy exists.[15]

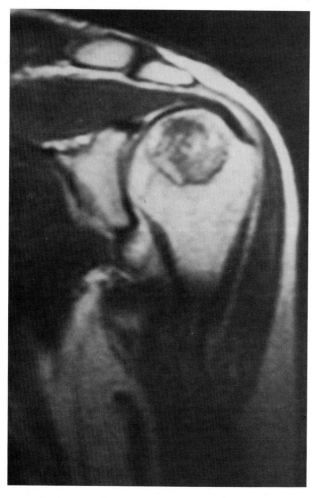

FIGURE 11-4
Coronal MR scan of a chondroblastoma in the humeral epiphysis of an 18-year-old boy. On this T1-weighted image the lesion has a generally lower signal intensity than the uninvolved portion of the (cartilaginous) epiphysis, suggesting a primarily cellular lesion.

Chondroblastoma

Chondroblastomas are benign, essentially cellular, cartilaginous tumors that usually occur before the physis closes. They arise in the epiphysis or apophysis of a long bone, especially the femur, humerus, and tibia. Men are more frequently affected than women, and the patient usually presents with local pain, swelling, and tenderness. Joint symptoms may mimic those of a primary synovial disease.

Chondroblastomas appear radiographically as a well-marginated, ovoid or round, lytic epiphyseal (or apophyseal) lesion extending into the subarticular bone or into the metaphysis. Calcifications are seen in 25% to 50% of cases.

A chondroblastoma does not have the characteristic high signal intensity or lobular configuration of other cartilaginous lesions. It is isointense with muscle on short TR/TE sequences, isointense to hypointense on long TR/TE sequences, and more homogeneous appearing or amorphous in general (Fig. 11-4). These findings are consistent with its predominantly (70%) cellular, rather than cartilaginous, composition.[6] MR studies are probably not necessary for differentiating chondroblastomas from giant cell tumors or chondromyxoid fibromas since this distinction can usually be made on the basis of roentgenographic findings. MRI does serve, however, to better define the intraosseous tumoral extension.

Hereditary multiple exostosis

Hereditary multiple exostosis is an autosomal dominant disorder characterized by numerous exostoses throughout the skeleton (Fig. 11-5). The condition is associated with shortening and bowing of bones, defects of normal modeling, joint restriction, and a greater tendency toward flat bone involvement. There is a much higher risk for malignant transformation (up to 25%) compared to solitary lesions.

The role of MRI in evaluating these patients has not been described in the literature, although its greater soft tissue contrast and multiplanar imaging capability would appear to offer clear advantages over CT.

Chondrosarcoma

Chondrosarcomas are a relatively common chondroid-producing malignancy of the skeletal system found in any bone that develops by enchondral formation. They are classified as either central (arising from the medullary cavity) or peripheral (arising from the bone surface). Either type can result from the malignant transformation of a chondroma or osteochondroma.

Central chondrosarcoma is a tumor of middle-aged adults, who usually present with a chronic dull aching pain. There are two apparently discrepant roentgenographic appearances:

1. One is a well-defined osteolytic lesion with small irregular areas of calcification and sclerotic margins. Tumors with this radiographically benign appear-

ance most often occur in the neck of the femur, pubic rami, and the proximal metaphysis of the humerus. As the lesion grows, a more aggressive, malignant radiographic appearance develops.

2. The other is an expansile, osteolytic, medullary lesion with endosteal scalloping, a wide zone of transition, and "snowflake" or irregularly focal areas of calcification. Lesions with this appearance most often occur in the pelvis, distal or proximal femur, proximal humerus, and proximal tibia. Although some authors believe that the set of lesions with the more aggressive initial appearance actually represents a later radiographic manifestation of the more benign appearing central tumors, lesions that initially have a malignant appearance can subsequently develop well-defined margins.[16]

Peripheral chondrosarcoma is usually found in the pelvis, scapula, sternum, ribs, or metaphyseal regions of the humerus and femur. Most of these lesions probably represent secondary malignancies arising from osteochondromas. They can become quite large without causing pain and often present as painless soft tissue masses.

On plain film roentgenography they initially appear as large soft tissue masses with "snowflakelike" calcifications and cortical thickening in areas of osseous attachment. Changes of extensive underlying bony destruction are seen later.

It is evident that both the central and the peripheral tumor may have a relatively benign plain film appearance despite its highly malignant biological behavior. For this reason, many authors[15] emphasize the importance of completely evaluating all benign-appearing cartilaginous tumors, especially when found in the diaphysis of a long bones and/or when associated with pain. The plain film findings usually suffice to establish the diagnosis. MRI is the imaging modality of choice for determining the soft tissue and medullary extension of these tumors (Fig. 11-6). As noted earlier, there are no MR imaging characteristics that can help distinguish reliably between benign and malignant disease. The superior soft tissue contrast of MR, however, enables the radiologist to determine the extent of marrow, cortical, transphyseal, and soft tissue invasion by tumor in estimating biological activity.[10]

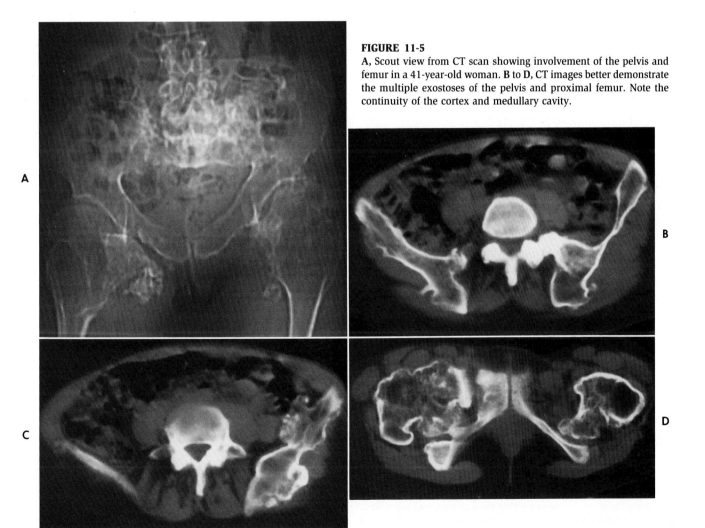

FIGURE 11-5

A, Scout view from CT scan showing involvement of the pelvis and femur in a 41-year-old woman. **B** to **D,** CT images better demonstrate the multiple exostoses of the pelvis and proximal femur. Note the continuity of the cortex and medullary cavity.

BONE-FORMING TUMORS
Osteoid osteoma

Osteoid osteomas are benign lesions occurring throughout the skeleton that consist of a central vascular osteoid core surrounded by sclerotic bone. Patients generally are adolescents or young adults who present with pain becoming worse at night that is characteristically relieved by aspirin. Osteoid osteomas have a predeliction for the diaphyses of long bones, especially the femur and tibia. Reduced range of motion and synovitis can occur with lesions that are either near or within joint capsules. Lesions of the spine usually occur in the neural arches and present with torticollis, stiffness, and scoliosis. The goal of surgical therapy is to remove the central nidus; the circumferential sclerosis subsequently resolves spontaneously.

The radiographic appearance of osteoid osteoma varies depending upon the bone involved and whether the lesion is located in the cortical bone, a subperiosteal or endosteal area, or the marrow. The classic long bone osteoid osteoma is seen on conventional roentgenograms as a central, well-defined, oval or round, lytic lesion with varying degrees of uniform circumferential sclerosis. Lesions of the carpus, tarsus, and epiphysis appear as either partially or completely calcified well-circumscribed areas of lysis that usually lack associated reactive sclerosis. Spinal lesions are seen as an area of sclerosis in one of the posterior elements (e.g., pedicle or lamina) at the concave aspect of a scoliotic curve.[17] The radiographic diagnosis of osteoid osteoma can, however, be difficult when the classic findings are not present. For example, femoral neck lesions are intraarticular and present with synovitis rather than cortical thickening, and vertebral lesions can present with unremarkable roentgenographic findings.

Osteoid osteomas take up bone-mimicking radiotracer agents avidly, and nuclear scintigraphy can be used for determining their preoperative and intraoperative location. Once they are identified, CT provides important supplemental information for more precise location of the tumor nidus. CT has, in fact, become the key imaging modality in evaluating lesions of the spine, pelvis, and femoral neck, helping to avoid unnecessary or misdirected resection. CT scaning performed with thin cuts and close spacing demonstrates a smoothly marginated, radiolucent, and central nidus (Fig. 11-7). If the lesion occurs in the cortex, associated circumferential reactive sclerosis is often much larger than in the central nidus.[18] When nidus calcification is present, it is usually centrally situated and has smooth borders, helping to distinguish osteoid osteoma from osteomyelitis (which has irregular margins) and associated sequestration (which is eccentric and has irregular margins).[19]

The MR appearance of osteoid osteoma in the proximal femoral metaphysis has been described on short TR/short TE sequences as a low-intensity ring with a surrounding irregular thin area of high signal intensity, surrounded by

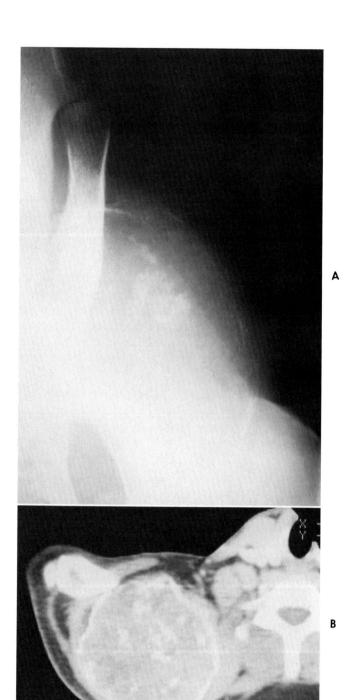

A

B

FIGURE 11-6
For legend see opposite page.

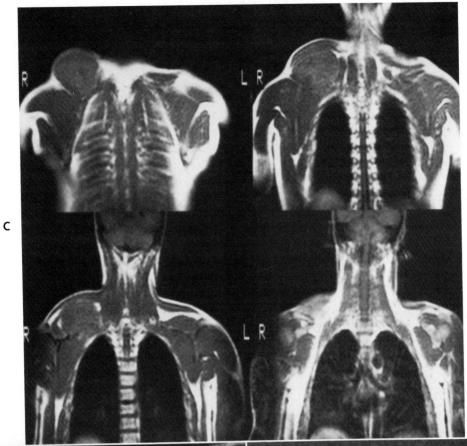

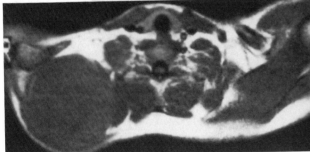

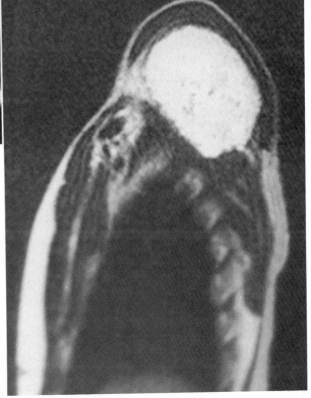

FIGURE 11-6
A, Chondrosarcoma arising from the scapula of a 28-year-old man. This is a well-defined osteolytic lesion with numerous small irregular areas of calcification and a sclerotic margin. B, The margin and calcifications are better appreciated on CT. C and D, The short TR/TE sequences show the tumor as a low signal area. E, The lesion appears bright and somewhat heterogeneous on the long TR/TE sequences.

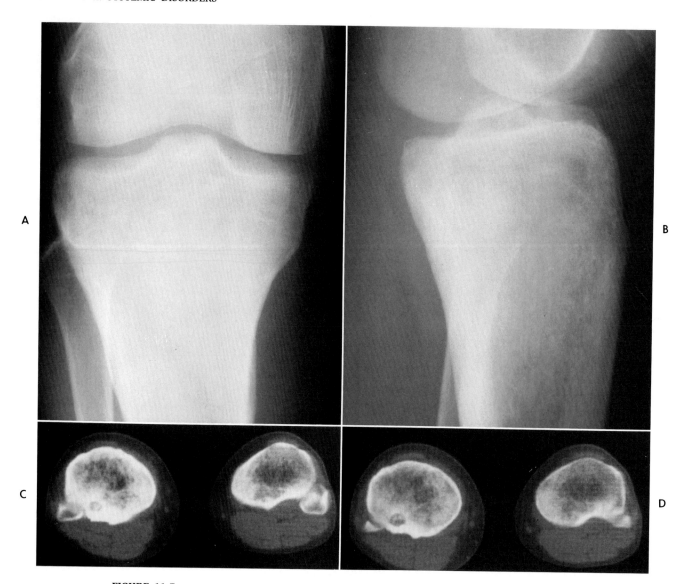

FIGURE 11-7
A and B, Roentgenograms of a 19-year-old boy showing a sclerotic area of the proximal tibia with a central lucency suggesting the diagnosis of osteoid osteoma. C and D, CT scan demonstrating the smoothly marginated lucency with a calcific nidus. The circumferential cortical sclerosis is clearly seen.

a rim of low signal. This appearance is believed to correlate with the presence of centrally calcified osteoid tissue and an associated rim of sclerosis (Fig. 11-8). The signal intensity of the lesion does not change with long TR/long TE sequences.[20] Whether MRI offers any diagnostic advantages over CT is not clear.

The CT appearance of vertebral body osteoid osteomas is essentially the same as for osteomas found in the tubular long bones.

Osteoblastoma

Osteoblastomas are rare benign bone tumors that resemble osteoid osteoma but have a larger nidus and cause greater bone expansion. They usually present in adolescents and young adults with dull aching, tender-

ness, and soft tissue swelling. The pain does not worsen at night and is not relieved by aspirin. They most often occur in the neural arches of the vertebrae (35% to 40%) and are a cause of scoliosis (Fig. 11-9). Less commonly they are encountered in the long bones of the lower extremities, and rarely in the long bones of the upper extremities.

Long bone osteoblastomas usually occur in metadiaphyseal areas and have a varied radiological appearance. They are usually seen as expansile lesions that may be completely lucent or contain either generalized or focal flecks of calcification. These lesions can expand through the cortex and appear as soft tissue masses, sharply marginated by a thin rim of periosteal new bone. Generally no central nidus is evident. Some lesions have associated surrounding zones of sclerosis.

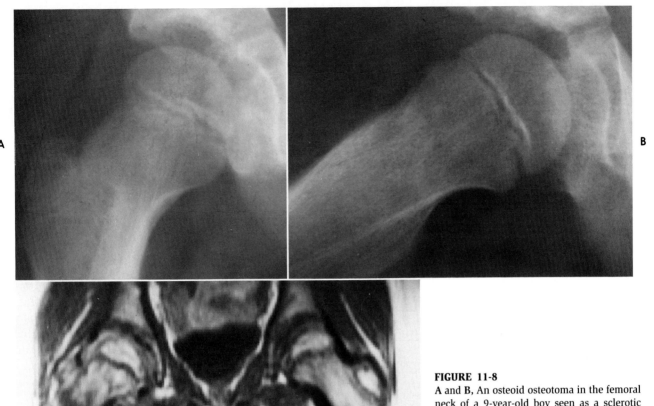

FIGURE 11-8
A and B, An osteoid osteotoma in the femoral neck of a 9-year-old boy seen as a sclerotic area with a central lucency. C, An early-generation MR scan shows the central low-signal region, circumferential high-signal ring, and part of the low-signal rim.

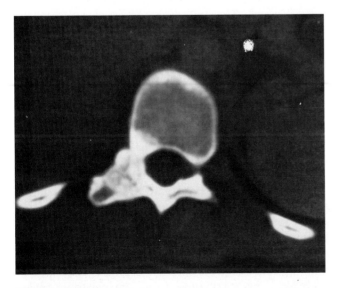

FIGURE 11-9
A CT scan through a lower thoracic vertebral body of an osteoblastoma shows a smoothly marginated lesion in the right neural arch.

The CT appearance of osteoblastoma has been described in a single case report.[21] In this instance the scan was helpful in that it confirmed the roentgenographic characterization of an intraosseous and expansile lesion. It also provided better definition of the tumor margins, as well as visualization and characterization of matrix calcifications. The MR appearance of these lesions has not been described.

Ossifying fibroma

Ossifying fibromas are benign fibroosseous neoplasms of bone pathologically and radiographically related to fibrous dysplasia. They most often occur in the facial bones (mandible and maxilla), less commonly in the tubular bones (especially the tibia).

Facial bone ossifying fibromas consist of woven and lamellar trabeculae in a fibroblastic stroma that may contain areas of dystrophic calcification. They present in adolescents or young adults as a painless expansion of tooth-bearing areas. Radiographically they appear as well-circumscribed unilocular or multiloculated areas of osteolysis, with varying degrees of calcification and/or ossification, causing cortical expansion and displacement of teeth.

Tubular bone ossifying fibromas (osteofibrous dysplasia) consist of vascular fibrous tissue containing trabeculae of new bone and circumferential osteoblasts. They are most often seen on the anteromedial surface of the tibia and are commonly associated with anterior tibial bowing. Ossifying fibromas appear radiographically as expansile, lytic, cortical lesions with a thin, almost imperceptible, periosteal border and a sclerotic medullary border. They can be single, coalesced and multiple (bubbly), or multiple and separate. The most common complication is incomplete pathological fracture. Pseudoarthrosis is an infrequent complication.

CT is helpful in further defining the precise anatomical nature of facial bone lesions. The MR appearance has not been described. Although the radiographic appearance of tubular bone lesions is fairly characteristic, MR may help when better definition of medullary involvement is required.

Osteogenic sarcoma

Osteosarcoma represents a group of related connective tissue tumors with varying degrees of malignant potential. A distinguishing feature is the production of bone or osteoid by neoplastic cells. The tumors usually present in adolescents who have a history of pain, swelling, and/or fracture following relatively insignificant trauma. The metaphyseal regions of the long bones around the knee (distal femur, proximal tibia) and the proximal humerus are most often affected. Osteosarcomas can occur within the medullary cavity (classic form) or arise from the bone surface (periosteal and juxtacortical forms).

Central (classic) osteosarcoma

Central osteosarcomas can appear radiographically as poorly defined lytic, sclerotic, or mixed-density lesions with associated cortical destruction and marked periosteal reaction. A soft tissue mass that may contain tumoral bone is often seen. Much less common variants[9] include telangiectatic osteosarcoma (aggressive, expansile, lytic lesion simulating an aneurysmal bone cyst), small cell osteosarcoma (histologically similar to Ewing's sarcoma with less sclerosis than a central osteosarcoma), fibrohistiocytic osteosarcoma (resembling a malignant fibrous histiocytoma but with small cloudlike areas of increased density), and low-grade central osteosarcoma (with either a radiographically benign appearance or an appearance of central osteosarcoma, but lacking massive bone destruction).

MRI has essentially replaced CT for the localized staging of conventional osteosarcoma. The tumor has low signal intensity on short TR/short TE sequences, clearly demonstrating the demarcation between tumor and yellow marrow. Long TR/long TE sequences reveal that the intramedullary tumor component has areas of relatively high intensity (equal to, or slightly greater than, that of normal marrow). This imaging sequence is useful for defining the tumor's extension in red marrow (Fig. 11-10). Primarily osteoblastic lesions have mixed signal intensity, the low-signal regions correlating with areas of sclerosis[22] (Figs. 11-11 and 11-12). The extraosseous component of these tumors is difficult to define on short TR/TE sequences since the tumor signal intensity is similar to that of normal adjacent muscle. Long TR/TE sequences allow ready differentiation of the soft tissue component, seen as a high-intensity region distinct from the normal low-intensity muscle. Areas of calcification appear as signal voids.

Coronal and/or sagittal T1-weighted images are preferred by many investigators for evaluating intramedullary tumor extension. However, great care must be exercised to ensure that full section slices are obtained so there is no partial volume averaging of marrow (tumor) signal with low-intensity cortex and the subsequent creation of an artifactually foreshortened lesion. Supplementary T1-weighted axial images are often helpful in avoiding this pitfall, and axial T2-weighted scans provide the best advantage for establishing the relationship of the tumor to muscle groups and/or neurovascular bundles.[22-25]

Surface osteosarcoma

Surface osteosarcomas can be further classified[26] as parosteal sarcoma, periosteal sarcoma, high-grade surface osteosarcoma, and dedifferentiated parosteal osteosarcoma.

Parosteal osteosarcoma is an indolent malignant bone tumor with a better prognosis than the classic central osteosarcoma. Most are found in 40-to-50-year-old patients and arise on the posterior aspect of the distal femur. The conventional roentgenographic appearance is a dense, broad-based, lobular mass blending with the normal cortex. The base often appears denser than the rest of the tumor. Early tumors may have only a small attachment to the cortex and a lucent zone separating the tumor bulk from the cortex. The tumor can circumferentially envelop the host bone.[27] The outer (soft tissue) margin may be irregular and poorly defined or sharply marginated. Although some authors[26] contend that a true parosteal sarcoma cannot be in continuity with the host bone medullary cavity, most[27] emphasize that a key anatomical feature to be analyzed for adequate staging is the presence of medullary involvement.[27]

CT imaging demonstrates parosteal sarcomas as homogeneously dense tumors, showing their true size and extent to better advantage as well as the cortical and/or medullary invasion and the relationship of the tumor to adjacent neurovascular bundles.[27,28] These tumors can also appear on CT scans as heterogeneously dense lesions with focal low-attenuation areas. The relatively lucent areas are believed to represent fibrous or cartilaginous tissue, enveloped benign soft tissues, or focal areas of dedifferentiated sarcoma.[29] Localization of these focal

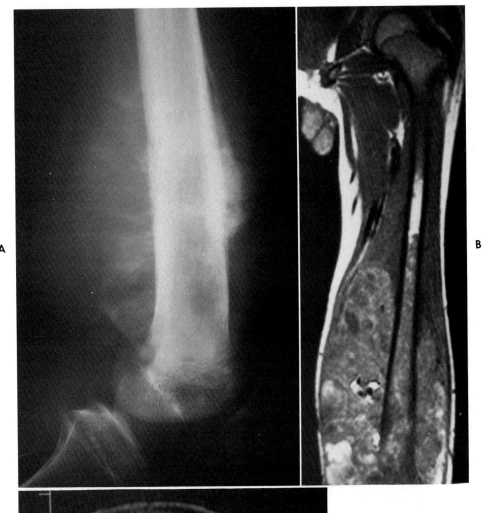

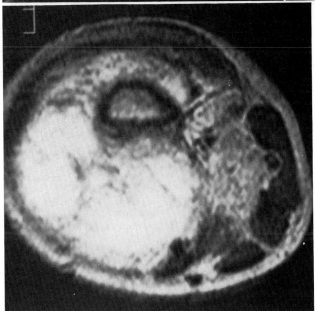

FIGURE 11-10

Characteristic appearance of osteosarcoma in the distal femur of a 15-year-old boy. **A,** The involved portion of bone has a mixed sclerotic and lytic appearance with periostosis and a soft tissue mass. Note the "sunburst" appearance caused by radially oriented linear ossification. **B,** A coronal T1-weighted image demonstrates the relatively low-signal tumor extending to the middiaphysis. The signal intensity of the tumor contrasts well with the normal bright signal of the yellow marrow. The rather low signal from the proximal diaphysis is caused by partial volume averaging of the cortical and medullary signal. The low signal in the proximal metaphysis is secondary to the presence of normal red marrow. Note the loss of signal void of the distal femoral cortex due to destruction (and replacement) by tumor. The signal intensity of the tumor is only marginally different than the normal skeletal muscle. The bright signal areas represent areas of hemorrhage. **C,** This T2-weighted image better defines the high signal intensity of the tumor from the surrounding low-signal muscle vessels.

lucent areas (with CT guidance) can therefore be of utmost importance when attempting to grade a lesion on the basis of tissue obtained through needle biopsies.[28]

Only one report of the use of MR to evaluate parosteal osteosarcoma[28] has appeared in the literature. Although one might anticipate that MR would allow better evalua-

tion of soft tissue and medullary involvement, the authors reported that it did not add any information to that obtained from the CT scan, apart from sagittal imaging (which allowed for the demonstration of cortical invasion and the depiction of tumor bulk). Of note, however, was the fact that this lesion had no significant medullary

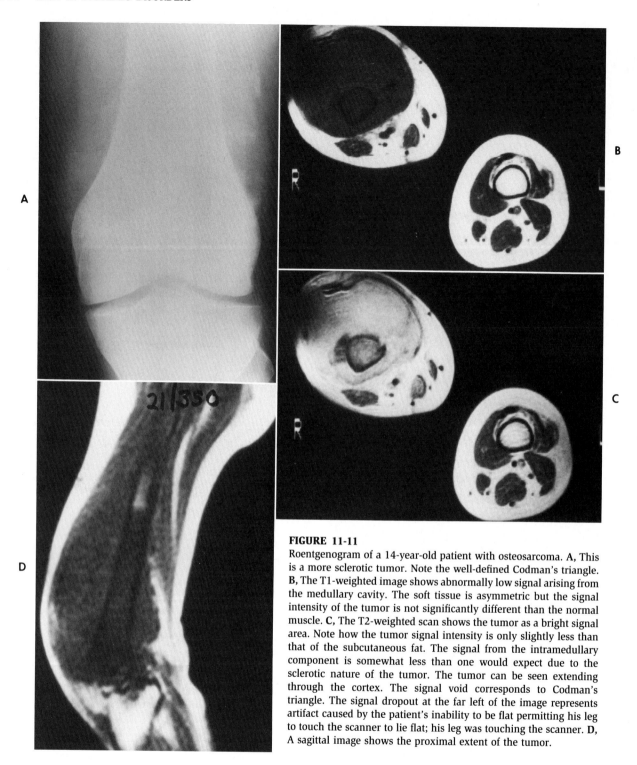

FIGURE 11-11
Roentgenogram of a 14-year-old patient with osteosarcoma. **A,** This is a more sclerotic tumor. Note the well-defined Codman's triangle. **B,** The T1-weighted image shows abnormally low signal arising from the medullary cavity. The soft tissue is asymmetric but the signal intensity of the tumor is not significantly different than the normal muscle. **C,** The T2-weighted scan shows the tumor as a bright signal area. Note how the tumor signal intensity is only slightly less than that of the subcutaneous fat. The signal from the intramedullary component is somewhat less than one would expect due to the sclerotic nature of the tumor. The tumor can be seen extending through the cortex. The signal void corresponds to Codman's triangle. The signal dropout at the far left of the image represents artifact caused by the patient's inability to be flat permitting his leg to touch the scanner to lie flat; his leg was touching the scanner. **D,** A sagittal image shows the proximal extent of the tumor.

extension, an aspect of staging wherein MRI would have had a clear advantage over CT.

Periosteal osteosarcoma is an uncommon tumor that arises from the surface of a long bone and usually affects adolescents. The characteristic histological feature is the presence of malignant cartilaginous tissue; the tumor can, in fact, mimic chondrosarcoma both radiographically and histologically. Its prognosis is significantly worse than that of parosteal osteosarcoma but remains better than that of central osteosarcoma.[26]

The CT and MR considerations are similar to those presented above.

TUMORS OF HISTIOCYTIC OR FIBROCYSTIC ORIGIN
Giant cell tumor

Giant cell tumors can be benign or malignant neoplasms consisting of multinucleated giant cells in a fibrous stroma. They usually affect 20-to-35-year-old patients (i.e., after the physis closes), who present with a

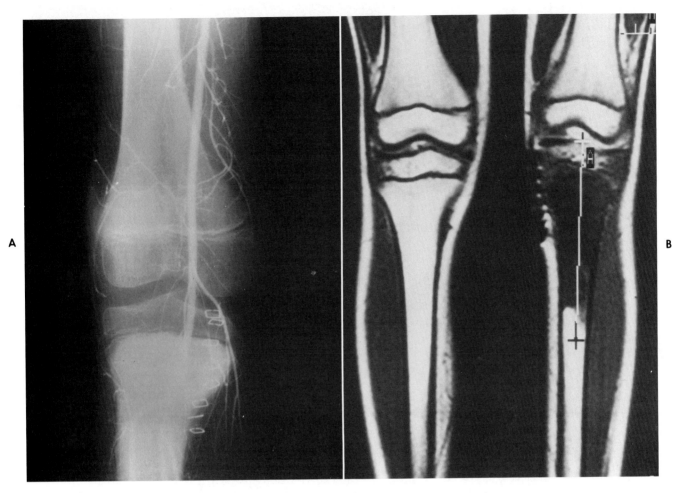

FIGURE 11-12
A, This angiogram was used to provide a vascular map for limb salvage in a patient with sclerosing osteosarcoma of the proximal tibia. Note the surgical clips from a biopsy procedure. B, These T1-weighted coronal images demonstrate the intramedullary extension of tumor. Note the contrasting bright signal from the yellow marrow and the loss of signal due to a ferromagnetic effect of the surgical clips.

dull aching, painful or restricted motion of an adjacent joint, or a pathological fracture. The tumors grow slowly and are usually fairly large when first diagnosed. Most occur in the metaphysis of the distal femur or proximal tibia, although not infrequently the patella, spine, and acetabulum are involved.

On conventional roentgenograms giant cell tumors appear as well-defined lucent, expansile, and eccentrically located metaphyseal lesions that usually extend through the region of the physis to the epiphysis. They often grow into the subchondral area of adjacent joints and can even extend through the articular surface to involve the joint space directly. Subchondral and articular space involvement, with a gradual transition zone in cancellous bone and/or disruption of the bony cortex, can be seen with both benign and malignant forms of giant cell tumor and serve to indicate the unreliability of radiological findings in predicting histological grades. Giant cell tumors have a high rate of recurrence following treatment.

The MR signal characteristics of a giant cell tumor are similar to those of any other nonossifying bony neoplasm (low signal on short TR/TE, high signal on long TR/TE sequences). MR is currently the preferred imaging modality for evaluating a giant cell tumor, since it is best able to define tumoral extension into the medullary cavity and soft tissues.[30,31] It may also offer advantages in identifying joint space involvement.[31] The role of MR in evaluating recurrence has not yet been defined, but one would anticipate the same limitations imposed by postsurgical inflammatory changes experienced with other neoplasms (Figs. 11-13 and 11-14).

Malignant fibrous histiocytoma

Malignant fibrous histiocytoma is a high-grade sarcoma of middle-aged adults, most often affecting the pelvis and the long bone metaphyses of the lower extremities. Patients usually present with pain, a slowly enlarging mass, or pathological fracture.

On conventional roentgenograms the tumor is clearly

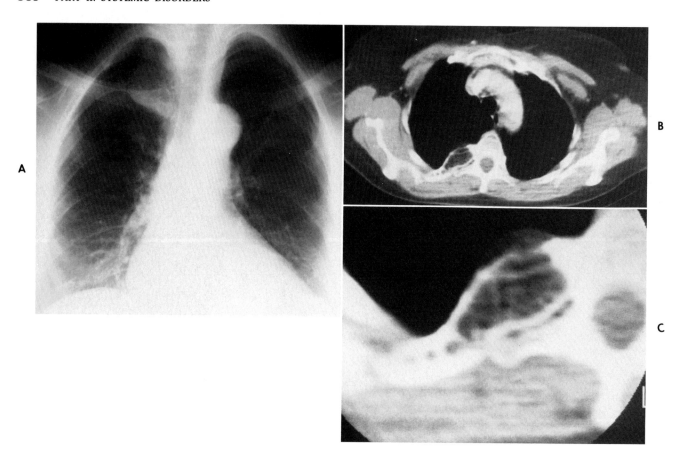

FIGURE 11-13
A, Chest roentgenogram of a 60-year-old woman with a giant cell tumor showing expansile changes in the medial aspect of the right fourth rib. **B** and **C,** The CT scan demonstrates the expansile nature and cortical thinning to better advantage. Note the small associated soft tissue mass anteriorly.

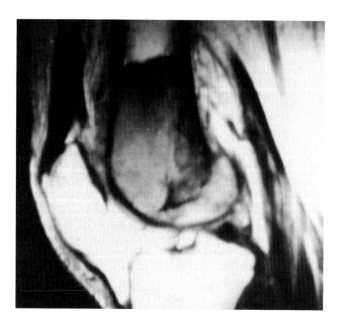

FIGURE 11-14
Giant cell tumor in a 52-year-old man. A T1-weighted image shows abnormally low signal in the distal femur.

osteolytic, having a permeative pattern of destruction and often showing evidence of an associated soft tissue mass. It may demonstrate extensive mineralization or focal areas of calcification. Malignant fibrous histiocytoma may have concomitant roentgenographic changes of benign disease such as infarction and osteitis deformans (Paget's).[6]

As with other malignancies, MRI best demonstrates the medullary involvement and soft tissue extension. These tumors do not appear to have any unique MR features.[6]

Lipoma

Intraosseous lipomas are rare benign lesions consisting of abnormal accumulations of fat.[32] They are usually discovered incidentally in young to middle-aged adults, affecting both the axial and the appendicular skeleton; the proximal femur appears to be the most commonly involved single site, although lipomas do not occur in the epiphysis. The location of the lesion within the bone (diaphyseal/metaphyseal) is not generally a useful diagnostic criterion.

The radiological appearance depends upon the degree of histological involution. Stage 1 lesions consist of viable

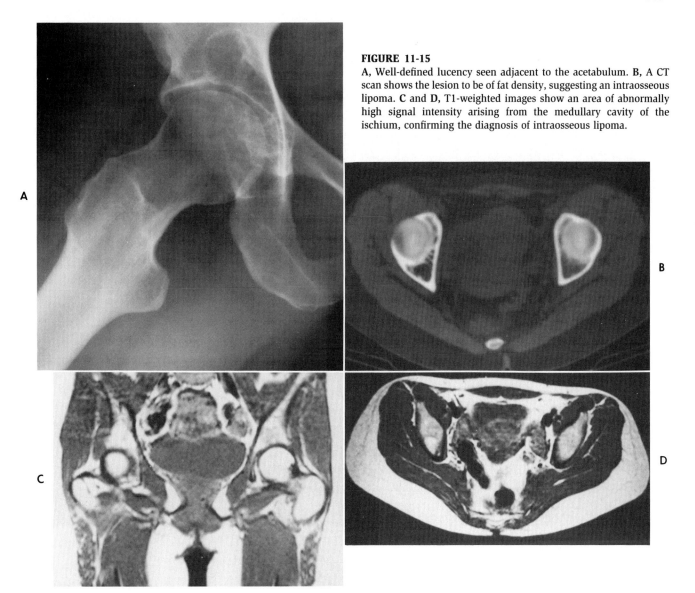

FIGURE 11-15
A, Well-defined lucency seen adjacent to the acetabulum. **B,** A CT scan shows the lesion to be of fat density, suggesting an intraosseous lipoma. **C** and **D,** T1-weighted images show an area of abnormally high signal intensity arising from the medullary cavity of the ischium, confirming the diagnosis of intraosseous lipoma.

fat cells. Roentgenographically they appear as lytic lesions, consistent with resorption of the trabecular architecture, and often have associated expansion due to periosteal bone formation. Small residua of trabeculae are not infrequently seen (Fig. 11-15). Stage 2 lesions contain focal areas of necrosis. They have sclerotic margins and focal areas of calcification. Stage 3 lesions are a terminal, involutional stage and have more diffuse calcific fat necrosis. Roentgenographically they have more pronounced sclerotic margins with central and peripheral diffuse marked radiodensity. The differential diagnosis of Stage 3 lesions includes bone infarction and enchondroma.

An atypical appearance of Stage 1 lesions (i.e., Stage 1 variant or ossifying lipomas) demonstrates extensive reactive bone within a region of viable lipocytes and no histological evidence of involution.

CT and MR would probably be useful in establishing the diagnosis of these lesions. Both modalities would

correctly identify the fatty nature of the Stage 1, Stage 1 variant, and Stage 2 lesions. Stage 3 lesions would probably be best evaluated with CT because of their extensive calcification and reactive bone formation. However, many authors emphasize the need for histological evaluation to make a definitive differentiation of lipoma from enchondroma, bone cyst, chondromyxoid fibroma, and fibrous dysplasia.

CHORDOMAS

Chordomas are slow-growing locally invasive malignancies of the axial skeleton (sacrum, clivus, vertebral column), believed to arise from heterotopic notochordal remnants, that grow slowly and relentlessly as a soft tissue mass and cause progressive destruction of bone. They generally are detected during middle age. Tumors of the clivus tend to present at a younger age, since even small masses in this area can produce significant symptoms. Chordomas tend to encase and eventually invade

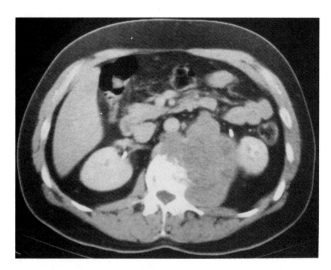

FIGURE 11-16
Chordoma arising from an upper lumbar vertebral body. This lesion is essentially lytic. There is a large soft tissue component, which tends to favor chordoma over metastatic disease.

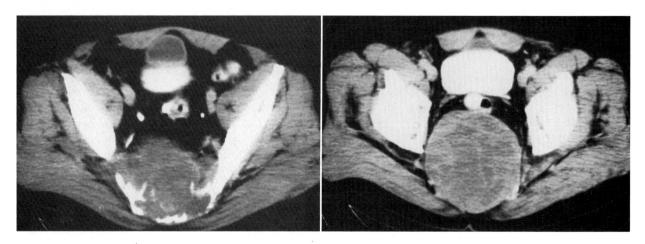

FIGURE 11-17
Contrast-enhanced CT demonstrating a lytic sacral chordoma with a relatively heterogeneous soft tissue mass.

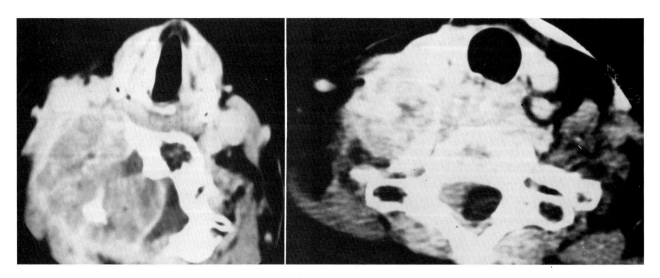

FIGURE 11-18
Contrast-enhanced CT scan showing a recurrent cervical chordoma with extension into the epidural space. The cord is displaced to the contralateral side.

adjacent structures. The presenting symptoms reflect the insidious nature of the growth, specific symptoms being related to the site of involvement, which explains the often vague and varied initial manifestations. A specific diagnosis is usually not made until the tumor is fairly large and neurological impairment is present.

The classic roentgenographic findings are of a solitary midline lesion; approximately two thirds are sclerotic, the rest lytic. Most show evidence of an associated soft tissue mass. Vertebral body lesions can grow across disk spaces to affect two or more vertebrae.

CT demonstrates the tumor to be of either lytic or mixed lytic and sclerotic appearance (Fig. 11-16). Sacral chordomas often contain calcifications. Intravenous contrast shows an essentially homogeneous soft tissue mass that enhances heterogeneously with multiple areas of decreased attenuation[33] (Figs. 11-17 and 11-18). The CT demonstration of epidural invasion is improved with CT-myelographic examination.

MRI appears equal to CT in the detection of chordomas, but it is superior in showing the cystic soft tissue components and defining the tumor margins. Chordomas appear isointense or hypointense on short TR / short TE sequences and moderately to markedly intense on long TR/long TE sequences. They also have septa of low signal that separate the lobulated areas of higher signal with a circumferential low-intensity band[37] (Fig. 11-19). The ability of MR to define these greatly facilitates

therapeutic decisionmaking. As with other tumors, MR is inferior to CT in demonstrating bone destruction and tumoral calcification, features that aid the establishment of a radiological diagnosis.[34,35]

TUMORLIKE LESIONS OF UNKNOWN ORIGIN
Unicameral bone cyst

Unicameral bone cysts are benign lesions that appear to be more of developmental than of neoplastic origin. They have a single cavity filled with synoviallike fluid, most often found in the proximal end of the femur or humerus. Children in their first or second decade are usually affected.

Radiographically, simple bone cysts appear as oval metaphyseal lesions lying close to the physis, their long axes paralleling the long axis of the bone. The increase in bone length originating from the physis causes apparent migration of these cysts to the diaphysis. Pathological fracture (fallen fragment sign) appears to be the only significant complication. The lesions have an involutional nature. Surgical intervention, when required, consists of curettage and bone grafting. Roentgenograms show findings so characteristic that further evaluation of uncomplicated cases with CT or MR is usually not warranted. A solitary cyst complicated by a healing pathological fracture can, however, resemble fibrous dysplasia radiographically. In such cases the use of MR (or CT) to identify the

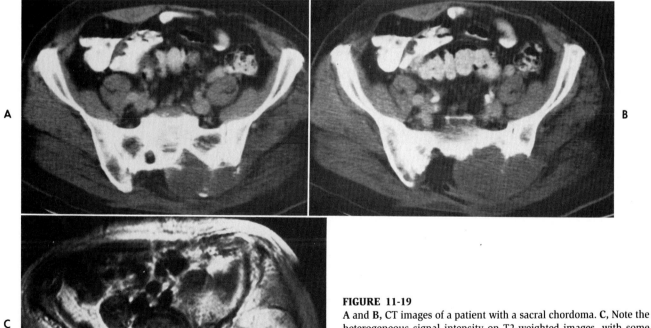

FIGURE 11-19
A and B, CT images of a patient with a sacral chordoma. C, Note the heterogeneous signal intensity on T2-weighted images, with some areas having low signal and others markedly intense signal intensity.

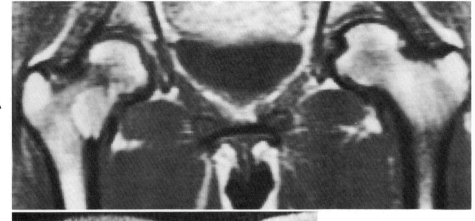

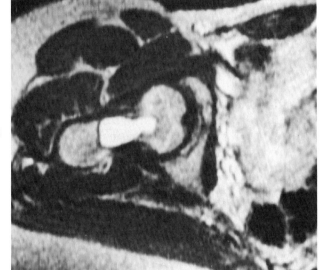

FIGURE 11-20

A T1-weighted MR image shows relatively bright signal from the femoral neck in this 13-year-old girl. The low signal from the neck and metaphysis is expected from red marrow. **B,** This T2 weighted shows the expected increased signal from the cyst, which better contrasts the lesion from adjacent normal red marrow.

presence of water signal (or attenuation) helps exclude the possibility of dysplasia (Fig. 11-20).

Aneurysmal bone cyst

Aneurysmal bone cysts are benign blood-filled lesions that affect older children and young adults. Patients present with painful swelling, limited range of motion, or pathological fracture. The tumors consists of multiloculated spaces lined by granulation tissue or osteoid; numerous associated giant cells are often seen. The cellular component can be a predominant feature, forming substantial areas of solid tissue. The etiology of aneurysmal bone cysts is not clear. Some authors[9] suggest that they are secondary to acute occlusion of segmental osseous venous drainage, resulting in the formation of arteriovenous shunts. Others[36] emphasize that they may arise from preexisting benign or malignant bone lesions that are rather small and missed both radiographically and pathologically. Some 30% to 40% of the cysts are found to be associated with another lesion.

Aneurysmal bone cysts appear on plain roentgenograms as well-defined, expansile, multichambered lucencies in the metaphysis of a long bone, in the neural arches

of a vertebra, or in the flat bones. Spinal lesions compromise the canal and compress the cord. CT demonstrates the expected findings of an expanded and thinned cortex with adjacent calcified or noncalcified periosteal membrane and thick trabeculations crossing the lesion. Fluid levels (sedimentation of erythrocytes and serum) are usually detected in patients who are scanned after being immobilized for approximately 10 minutes, appearing as a lower-attenuation component in the less dependent and a denser component in the more dependent areas. These levels do not enhance with contrast. The solid components of the tumors, however, do enhance following contrast administration.[37] The differential diagnosis of fluid levels includes telangiectatic osteosarcoma.[38]

MR scans of aneurysmal bone cysts show a circumferential rim of low intensity with multiple fluid levels contained within well-defined cystic cavities. A wide range of signal intensities is seen; there are both long and short TR/TE sequences, consistent with the various relaxation times expected in patients with intracystic hemorrhages of different ages. The prolonged T1 relaxation time for fresh blood causes low signal intensity (Fig.

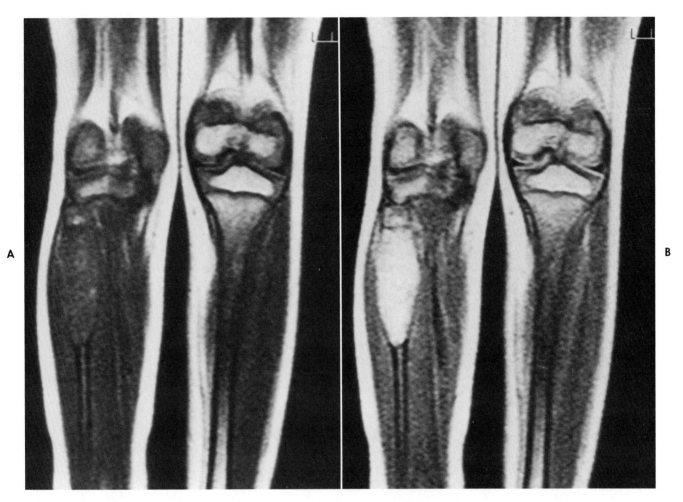

FIGURE 11-21
Roentgenograms of a pediatric patient that suggest aneurysmal bone cyst. **A,** The T1-weighted MR image shows an expansile area of the proximal right fibula giving a low signal. **B,** The signal from this lesion becomes brighter with T2 weighting. These signal characteristics can change as the lesion matures.

11-21). After several days methemoglobin is present in significant concentrations, which shortens the T1 relaxation time and causes increased signal on both long and short TR/TE sequences. Diverticulumlike projections arising from the walls of the larger cysts are a fairly specific MR feature. This constellation of findings is, in fact, more specific than both plain roentgenographic and CT findings.[37]

Soft tissue neoplasms

Soft tissue neoplasms have traditionally been difficult to evaluate radiographically. The advent of contrast-enhanced CT proved to be a quantum leap in advancing radiologists' abilities to identify and locate these tumors. MRI has all but replaced CT in this capacity. The advantages that MRI offers include multiplanar imaging and exquisite soft tissue contrast, which can be optimized through selection of the appropriate imaging (pulse sequence) parameters. The MR signal behavior of soft tissue tumors is similar to that of marrow and solitary

bone tumors. Soft tissue tumors are usually isointense or hypointense relative to normal adjacent muscle on short TR/TE sequences, and hyperintense and somewhat heterogeneous on long TR/TE sequences. Since calcification is seen as signal void on MR, CT remains the preferred means of studying highly calcified or ossified lesions.

It must be emphasized that SE MRI does not provide unique information to distinguish benign from malignant disease. It does, however, enable radiologists to apply conventional criteria to estimate biological activity with a greater degree of sensitivity. Definitive characterization usually requires histological examination. It is also imperative that MR studies be interpreted within the context of the clinical setting that prompted the examination. An extreme example, perhaps, is the rather benign appearance of many rhabdomyosarcomas, which contrasts with the infiltrative and aggressive appearance of most acute hematomas.

The real diagnostic utility of MR lies in its more precise staging, afforded by an improved ability to locate tumor

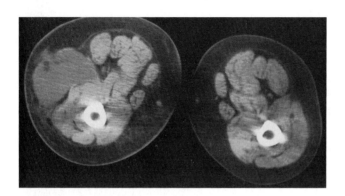

FIGURE 11-22

A CT scan demonstrating an acute hematoma in the lateral aspect of the right thigh of a 52-year-old woman. Note the poorly defined margins anterolaterally, posterolaterally, and medially, which suggest the presence of malignancy. The heterogeneity of the posterolateral aspect suggests an aggressive lesion with necrosis.

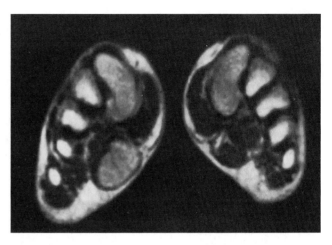

FIGURE 11-24

T2-weighted images showing a well-circumscribed soft tissue mass that gives an intermediate signal. The patient, an 11-year-old girl, presented with an insect bite on the plantar surface that had failed to resolve after 6 to 8 weeks. The pathological diagnosis was rhabdomyosarcoma.

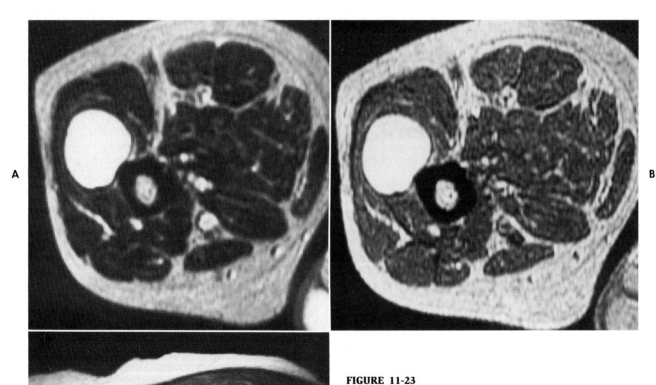

FIGURE 11-23

An MR scan of an organizing hematoma in the thigh. **A,** The initial T2-weighted image demonstrates a homogeneously bright lesion with sharp margins. **B** and **C,** Delayed images show layering (seen as different signal intensities due to separation of the organizing hematoma blood elements).

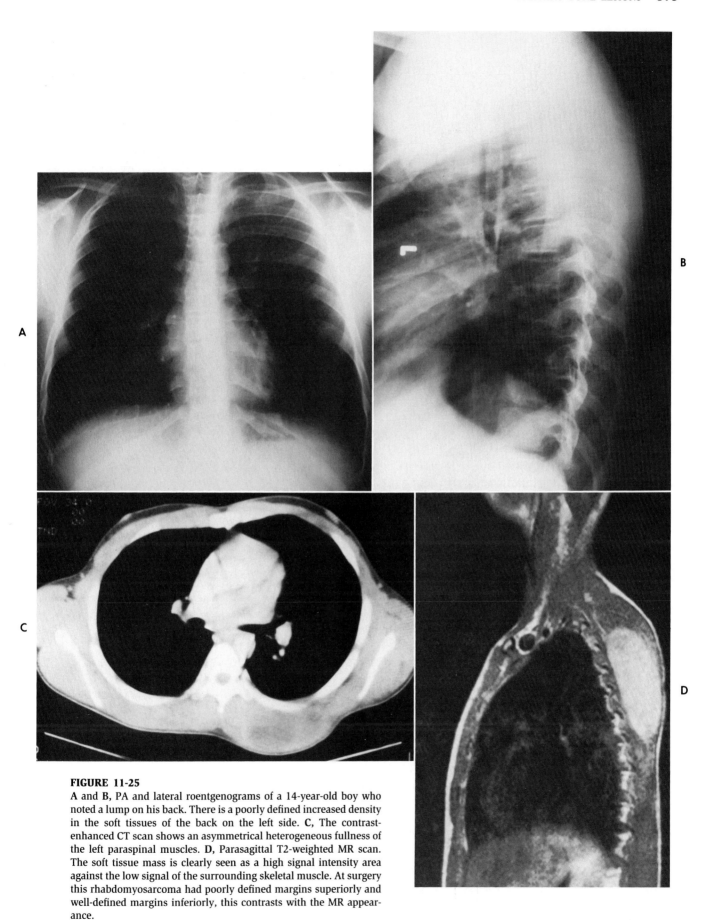

FIGURE 11-25

A and B, PA and lateral roentgenograms of a 14-year-old boy who noted a lump on his back. There is a poorly defined increased density in the soft tissues of the back on the left side. C, The contrast-enhanced CT scan shows an asymmetrical heterogeneous fullness of the left paraspinal muscles. D, Parasagittal T2-weighted MR scan. The soft tissue mass is clearly seen as a high signal intensity area against the low signal of the surrounding skeletal muscle. At surgery this rhabdomyosarcoma had poorly defined margins superiorly and well-defined margins inferiorly, this contrasts with the MR appearance.

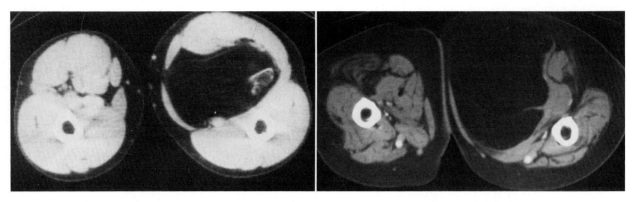

FIGURE 11-26
Lipomas are one of the few soft tissue lesions that can be diagnosed confidently using radiographic analysis alone. Masses with fat tissue attenuation are characteristic of lipoma. When high-attenuation areas are seen within the lesion, the radiologist cannot exclude the possibility of liposarcoma.

margins, identify involvement of specific muscle compartments, and define the relationships of tumor mass to neurovascular bundles (Figs. 11-22 to 11-26). This high degree of local staging has grown in clinical significance with the current emphasis on more conservative surgical procedures designed to salvage limbs and preserve function.

Synovial sarcoma

Synovial sarcomas are soft tissue malignancies that affect children and adults (most commonly young adults) and occur in the extraarticular soft tissues (tendons, tendon sheaths, bursal structures, and ligaments). Most are found in the extremities, especially around the knee and less commonly in the hands and feet. Patients often present with a painless slowly enlarging mass that becomes painful as the lesion grows.

Plain roentgenography demonstrates a soft tissue mass that may have either punctate or relatively large dense calcifications (25% to 30% of cases). Bone invasion occurs in almost 20% of cases, but extensive bone destruction is rare. Synovial sarcomas metastasize primarily to the lungs, although metastatic skeletal and nodal disease does occur. The rate of local recurrence is high (up to 60%).[39]

MR is the best imaging modality for evaluating both soft tissue (muscular) invasion and extension of tumor through the cortex into the medullary cavity. Soft tissue and red marrow involvement is best seen on long TR/long TE sequences, and yellow marrow on short TR/short TE sequences. It is interesting to note that these tumors may not be reliably demonstrated on CT. In one series of 10 patients,[39] half the lesions were not adequately visualized.

REFERENCES

1. Bloem JL, Bluemm RG, Taminian AHM, et al: Magnetic resonance imaging of primary malignant bone tumors. Radio-Graphics 1987;7(3):425-445.

2. Sundaram M, McGuire MH: Computed tomography or magnetic resonance for evaluating the solitary tumor or tumor-like lesions of bone? Skeletal Radiol 1988;17:393-401.

3. Ritschl P, Hajek PC, Pechmann U: Fibrous metaphyseal defects. Magnetic resonance imaging appearances. Skeletal Radiol 1989;18:253-259.

4. Ritschl P, Karnel F, Hajek P: Fibrous metaphyseal defects: determination of their origin and natural history using a radiomorphological study. Skeletal Radiol 1988;17:8-15.

5. Resnick DR: Bone and joint imaging. Philadelphia, Saunders, 1989, p 1145.

6. Marks KE, Bauer TW: Fibrous tumors of bone. Orthop Clin North Am 1989;20(3):377-393.

7. Young WRJ, Aisner SC, Levine AM, et al: Computed tomography of desmoid tumors of bone: desmoplastic fibroma. Skeletal Radiol 1988;17:333-337.

8. Edeiken J: Roentgen diagnosis of diseases of bone. Vol I, 3rd ed. Baltimore, Williams & Williams, 1981, p 257.

9. Ghelman B: Radiology of bone tumors. Orthop Clin North Am 1989;20(3):287-312.

10. Cohen EK, Kressel HY, Frank TS, et al: Hyaline cartilage-origin of bone and soft tissue neoplasms: MR appearance and histologic correlation. Radiology 1988;167:477-481.

11. Schwartz HS, Zimmerman NB, Simon MA, et al: The malignant potential of enchondromatosis. J Bone Joint Surg. [Am] 1987;69:269-274.

12. Lee JK, Yao L, Wirth CR: MR imaging of solitary osteochondromas: report of eight cases. AJR 1987;149:557-560.

13. O'Neal LW, Ackerman LV: Chondrosarcoma of bone. Cancer 1952;5:551-577.

14. Hudson TM, Springfield DS, Spanier SS, et al: Benign exostoses and exostotic chondrosarcomas: Evaluation of cartilage thickness by CT. Radiology 1984;152:595-599.

15. Greenspan A: Tumors of cartilage origin. Orthop Clin North Am 1989;20(3):347-366.

16. Edeiken J: Ref 8, pp 225-236.

17. Resnick DR: Bone and joint imaging. Philadelphia, Saunders, 1989, pp 1107-1114.

18. Aisen AM, Glazer GM: Diagnosis of osteoid osteoma using computed tomography. J Comput Tomogr 1984;8:175-178.

19. Mahboubi S: CT appearance of nidus in osteoid osteoma versus sequestration in osteomyelitis. J Comput Assist Tomogr 1986;10(3):457-459.

20. Glass RBJ, Poznanski AK, Fisher MR, et al: MR imaging of osteoid osteoma. J Comput Assist Tomogr 1986;10(6):1065-1067.

21. Farmlett EJ, Magid D, Fishman EK: Osteoblastoma of the tibia: CT demonstration. J Comput Assist Tomogr 1986;10(6):1068-1070.

22. Sundaram M, McGuire MH, Herbold DR: Magnetic resonance imaging of osteosarcoma. Skeletal Radiol 1987;16(1):23-29.

23. Gillespy T, Manfrini M, Ruggieri P, et al: Staging of intraosseous extent of osteosarcoma: correlation of preoperative CT and MR imaging with pathologic macroslides. Radiology 1988;167:765-767.

24. Bloem JL, Taminian AHM, Eulderink F, et al: Radiologic staging of primary bone sarcoma: MR imaging, scintigraphy, angiography, and CT correlated with pathologic examination. Radiology 1988;169:805-810.

25. Boyko OB, Cory DA, Cohen MD, et al: MR imaging of osteogenic and Ewing's sarcoma. AJR 1987;148:317-322.

26. Klein MJ, Kenan S, Lewis MM: Osteosarcoma, clinical and pathological considerations. Orthop Clin North Am 1989;20(3):327-345.

27. Hudson TM, Springfield DS, Benjamin M, et al: Computed tomography of parosteal osteosarcoma. AJR 1985;144:961-965.

28. Lindell MM, Shirkhoda A, Raymond AK, et al: Paraosteal osteosarcoma: radiologic-pathologic correlation with emphasis on CT. AJR 1987;148:323-328.

29. Stevens GM, Pugh DG, Dablin DC: Roentgenographic recognition and differentiation of parosteal osteogenic sarcoma. Am J Roentgenol 1957;78:1-12.

30. Brady TJ, Gebhardt MC, Pykett IL, et al: NMR imaging of forearms in healthy volunteers and patients with giant-cell tumor of bone. Radiology 1982;144:549-552.

31. Herman SD, Mesgarzadeh M, Bonakdarpour A, et al. The role of magnetic resonance imaging in giant cell tumor of bone. Skeletal Radiol 1987;16:635-643.

32. Milgram JW: Intraosseous lipomas: radiologic and pathologic manifestations. Radiology 1988;167:155-160.

33. Firooznia H, Golimbu C, Rafii M, et al: Computed tomography of spinal chordomas. J Comput Tomogr 1986;10:45-50.

34. Sze G, Uichanco LS, Brant-Zawadzki MN, et al: Chordomas: MR imaging. Radiology 1988;166:187-191.

35. Schweder BA, Wells RG, Starshak RJ, Sty JR: Clivus chordoma in a child with tuberous sclerosis: CT and MR demonstration. J Comput Assist Tomogr 1987;11(1):195-196.

36. Edeiken J: Ref 8, p 293.

37. Beltran J, Simon DC, Levy M, et al: Aneurysmal bone cysts: MR imaging at 1.5 T. Radiology 1986;158:689-690.

38. Hudson TM: Fluid levels in anurysmal bone cysts: a CT feature. AJR 1984;142:1001-1004.

39. Waag KL, Gerein V, Kornhüber B, et al: Synovial sarcoma in childhood. (English summary.) Z Kinderchir 1984;39(suppl I):48-50.

12 Skeletal Metastases

MAHVASH RAFII

After the lungs and the liver, the skeletal system is the most common site of involvement by metastatic disease. Lesions generally arise, in descending order of frequency, from primary malignancies in the lung, breast, prostate, kidney, and thyroid.[1] Metastatic foci generally are in the marrow and are transmitted to bone by the vascular system. Most involve, in descending order, the spine, ribs, pelvis, proximal ends of the long bones, sternum, and skull,[2] following the pattern of persistence of red marrow into adult life and with the possibility of direct extension through Batson's venous plexus to the spine.[1] Spinal metastases involve mainly the bodies of the vertebrae, usually in the lumbar region but also in the thoracic, cervical, and sacral vertebrae.[3] Compression fractures of the vertebrae and spinal cord compression are frequent complications.[4]

The detection of skeletal metastases plays an important role in the ultimate treatment of patients with extraosseous primary cancers. At the initial staging of a primary extraosseous lesion, detection of a metastatic bony focus can drastically alter the mode of treatment in favor of palliation rather than attempted cure by surgery. The development of a metastatic lesion after the primary cancer has been treated may also alter the treatment protocol, often necessitating aggressive irradiation or chemotherapy. Evaluation of the skeletal system, as part of the initial staging process or following treatment of the primary cancer, is often routinely done for malignancies with a high incidence of skeletal metastasis. It is imperative that various imaging modalities be efficiently utilized so the most accurate results will be obtained in a reasonable amount of time and with the least discomfort to the patient.

RADIOGRAPHIC APPROACH TO THE DIAGNOSIS OF SKELETAL METASTASES

Numerous studies[5-11] have evaluated and compared the sensitivity and specificity of various radiographic modalities used in the evaluation of skeletal metastases. Conventional roentgenography[5-7] has a high false-negative rate; experimental studies[8] have shown that 30% to 75% destruction of spongy bone of a vertebral body must occur before a lesion becomes visible roentgenographically; cortical involvement is readily detected with a lesser amount of bone destruction, but this is a delayed roentgenographic finding; intracortical lesions also are readily detected; however, they occur less frequently. Consequently a roentgenographic evaluation of the skeletal system or a "skeletal survey" as the primary mode of investigation in the staging of extraskeletal primary malignancies is inadequate. Radionuclide bone scanning[9-11] has proven a most efficient method for initially imaging skeletal metastases and is very sensitive in detecting areas of abnormal bone turnover, including both benign and malignant processes. The exceptions are instances when active bone formation is not encountered (e.g., plasmacytoma, multiple myeloma, or metastatic lesions from certain primaries in the thyroid, lung, and breast). A routine skeletal survey is prudent when such lesions are suspected. Although certain patterns of radioisotope uptake, such as multiple abnormal foci of bone-seeking radiopharmaceutical, are highly indicative of involvement by metastatic disease, a significant false-positive rate exists.[5,12] Further evaluation is therefore needed to determine the exact nature of a lesion detected by bone scanning—when a specific treatment for the primary is being considered or when the extent of the focus is uncertain.[11,12]

378

A radiographic correlation of the abnormal regions of isotope accumulation is often adequate for this purpose, although in certain instances computed tomography (CT) and magnetic resonance imaging (MRI) will be needed for further evaluation.

Computed tomography

Various publications[13-21] have investigated the role of CT in the evaluation of skeletal and spinal metastases. The value of CT is greatest in detecting lesions of the spinal column (Fig. 12-1) and pelvis (Fig. 12-2), reflecting both the high incidence of metastases to the axial skeleton and the complex anatomy of these regions. Lynn et al.,[22] comparing various modalities in a group of patients with metastatic pheochromocytoma, showed a sensitivity of 27% for roentgenography, 71% for CT, and 74% for bone scanning in detecting skeletal lesions. In another study Kido et al.[10] compared the sensitivity of roentgenograms (55%), CT (84%), and bone scans (90%) in detecting a variety of metastatic lesions to the calvarium. Still others[14,19,20,23] have used CT, with no false-positive or false-negative results, to evaluate suspected lesions detected by bone scan. However, there are no extensive and documented studies comparing radionuclide bone scanning and CT scanning. Considering the different mechanisms by which pathological processes can result in osseous alterations detected by these modalities, it would appear then that bone scanning is more sensitive than CT, but only a few cases have been reported. Mink et al.[24] described one in which the bone scan was positive but CT was negative for a metastatic lesion from the breast proved at biopsy. We have not seen such a case, but we suspect that there is a small percentage of false-negative CT examinations, probably more if CT is performed and reviewed without knowledge of the bone scan or MRI findings.

Subtle lesions may be recognized and detected by CT scanning when (1) the study is appropriately tailored for the suspected region, (2) a high-resolution scanning technique is utilized, and (3) the window settings are properly adjusted (Fig. 12-3). We have had several true-negative CT examinations with positive bone scan proven at biopsy and/or follow-up, as have others.[14,20]

INDICATIONS

1. When the bone scan is positive but a correlative roentgenogram is negative: In a study of 100 patients with known or suspected metastases,[20] we have concurred with Muindi et al.[14] that CT is most helpful in evaluating a normal or inconclusive roentgenogram obtained from the site of an abnormal isotope uptake on bone scan (Fig. 12-4). With a single focus of abnormal radioactive uptake there is an approximately 50% possibility that a metastatic lesion is present.[12,25] With multiple regions the probability of metastatic disease is even higher.

2. When the nature of a lesion detected by bone scanning and/or roentgenography is not clear: In these cases CT is often helpful for differentiating benign from malignant lesions (Fig. 12-5).

3. When the existence of a lesion is known but its extent must be determined, either because of proximity to a vital organ or for investigation of a possible pathological fracture[13,15,26] (Fig. 12-6): Detailed visualization of a lesion is necessary when a percutaneous aspiration biopsy is contemplated, particularly in the thoracic and cervical regions. It is also important to determine the integrity of the neural arch and to investigate for possible tumor extension into the epidural space (Figs. 12-7 and 12-8). CT-myelography has been extensively utilized in patients with manifestations of spinal cord compression but its use is gradually diminishing as MRI becomes more widely available.[23]

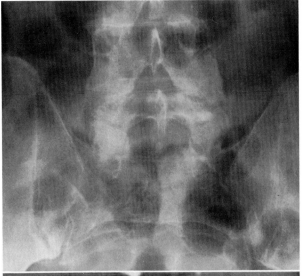

A

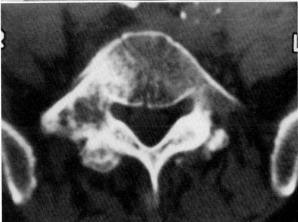

B

FIGURE 12-1
Metastatic adrenal adenocarcinoma to the lumbar spine. A radionuclide bone scan showed focal abnormal uptake to the right of L5. **A,** An AP roentgenogram of the region shows slightly increased density of the right L5-S1 apophyeal joint. **B,** CT scan at the level of L5. A mixed lytic/blastic lesion of the right pedicle and transverse process is visible.

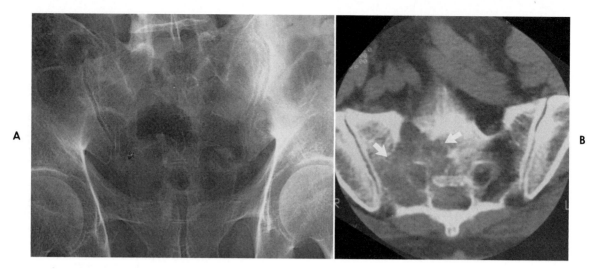

FIGURE 12-2
Metastatic renal tubular adenocarcinoma to the sacrum. **A,** AP roentgenogram. No abnormality is visible. **B,** CT scan at the level of S1-2. An ill-defined lytic lesion is present on the right side *(arrows),* and the S1 and S2 foramina are partly eroded.

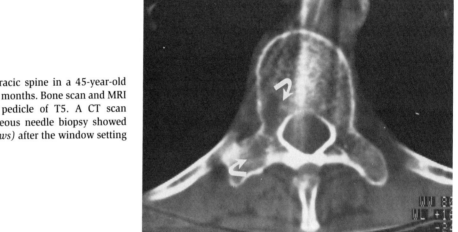

FIGURE 12-3
Primary osseous lymphoma of the thoracic spine in a 45-year-old woman with a history of back pain for 6 months. Bone scan and MRI showed an abnormality in the right pedicle of T5. A CT scan performed in preparation for percutaneous needle biopsy showed subtle destruction of spongy bone *(arrows)* after the window setting was properly adjusted.

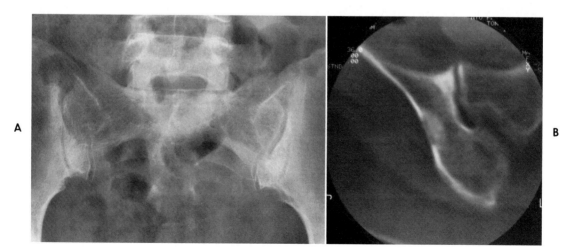

FIGURE 12-4
Metastatic lung carcinoma. A single focus of abnormal uptake was noted in the right sacroiliac joint region on bone scan. An AP roentgenogram, **A,** was inconclusive, but a CT scan, **B,** showed a predominantly blastic lesion in the posterior right ilium. Benign sclerosis of the iliac aspect of the sacroiliac joint is also present at the same level.

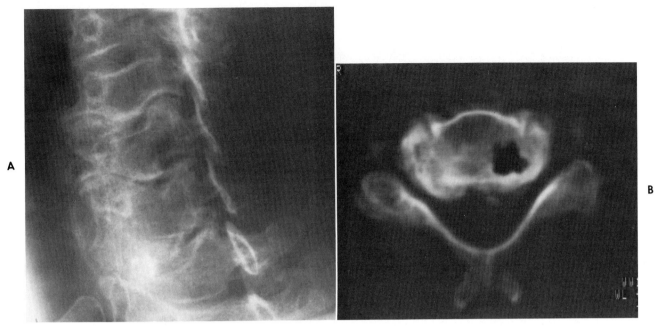

FIGURE 12-5
Benign degenerative intraosseous cyst of the cervical spine in a patient with carcinoma of the prostate. Bone scan showed a focus of abnormal uptake at C5 on the left side. **A,** An oblique roentgenogram of the cervical spine shows a cystic lesion posterolaterally. **B,** A CT scan at this level shows an air-containing cyst (attenuation coefficient, −450), apparently originating from the markedly degenerated Luschka joint. (From Rafii M, et al: J Comput Tomogr 1988;12:19-24.)

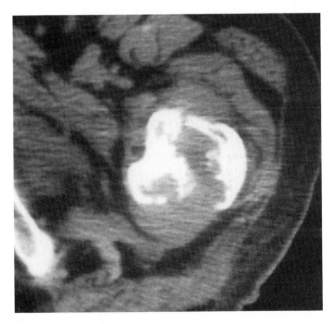

FIGURE 12-6
Metastatic breast carcinoma causing a pathological femoral fracture. A destructive lesion of the proximal left femur at the subtrochanteric level was detected on roentgenograms. The CT scan *(above)* shows extensive cortical bony destruction posteriorly, with a pathological fracture anteriorly. Extraosseous extension of the tumor is visible at both sites.

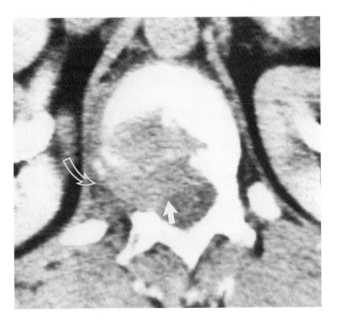

FIGURE 12-7
Metastatic lung carcinoma to the thoracic spine with epidural extension. A contrast-enhanced CT section shows the epidural *(solid arrow)* and paravertebral *(hollow arrow)* extension.

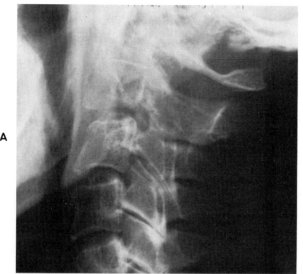

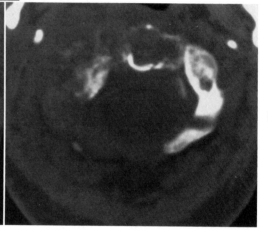

FIGURE 12-8
Metastatic breast carcinoma to the occipitoatlantoaxial region. **A**, Lateral view of the cervical spine. A destructive lesion of C2, with paravertebral soft tissue swelling, is present. **B** and **C**, CT sections at the level of the base of the skull and C2 show extensive destruction with involvement of the base of the skull and C1-2 on the right side. Spinal instability is also evident.

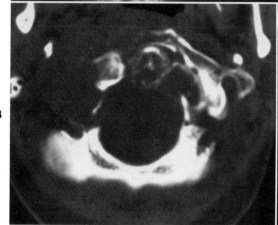

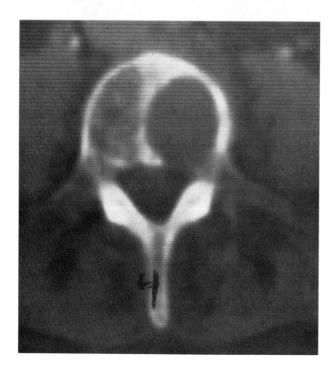

FIGURE 12-9
CT examination in a patient with known metastatic ovarian cancer and a recent onset of unremitting back pain. Several lytic lesions of the lumbar spine (including one seen at L4) were detected.

4. When the clinical presentation is highly suspicious for osseous metastases: CT or MRI may be employed primarily (Fig. 12-9). Also a CT or MRI examination should be obtained whenever a negative radionuclide bone scan does not explain the patient's persistent pain or neurological deficit.[27]
5. Following local or systemic treatment of skeletal metastases: The extent of tumor regression and the healing response, or lack thereof, can be determined by repeat CT examination[28,29] (Fig. 12-10).

DIAGNOSTIC FEATURES

Lytic lesions. Most metastatic lesions are lytic in nature and are therefore manifested by destruction of spongy and cortical bone.

Early bony destruction is seen on CT as focal or mottled areas of resorption (Fig. 12-11). In medullary regions the replacement of fatty marrow by tumor infiltration, resulting in loss of fatty marrow, is indicated by an increased attenuation coefficient of the medullary cavity (Fig. 12-12). Myeloproliferative disorders (e.g., multiple myeloma or early lymphoma) may result in only a generalized osteoporosis (due to the release of osteoclast activat-

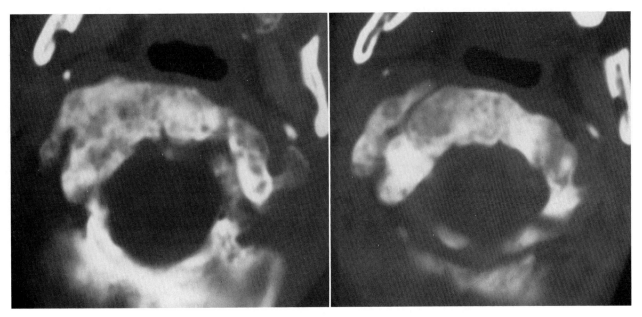

FIGURE 12-10
Metastatic breast carcinoma to the cervical spine following local irradiation (same patient as in Fig. 12-8). Three months after the completion of treatment there is complete reossification of the lesion, whose expansile nature is now more precisely demonstrated. Some normal anatomical boundaries are no longer present.

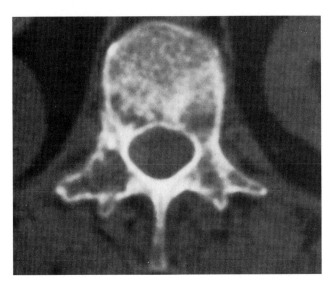

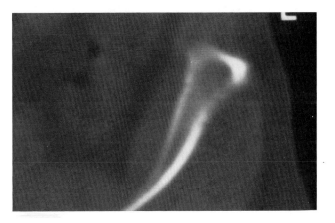

FIGURE 12-12
Metastatic lung carcinoma to the ilium. Mottled destruction of the cortical bone and increased density of the adjacent marrow cavity is demonstrated.

FIGURE 12-11
Metastatic breast carcinoma to the spine. Involvement of the right transverse process is indicated by destruction and loss of the trabecular bone and has resulted in a relative increased lucency of this region. A cortical interruption of the right pedicle is also visible.

ing factor).[30] Lytic metastases are often well delineated from the adjacent normal bone, and the presence of a sclerotic margin is occasionally demonstrated (Fig. 12-9). Tumor infiltration beyond cortical bone also may be well differentiated from adjacent soft tissue structures (Fig. 12-6). Calcification or ossification of the soft tissue component is a rare phenomenon, encountered with metastatic carcinoma of the colon or other gastrointestinal primaries. We have also seen this finding with metastatic lesions from the breast and lung. Lytic expansile lesions, a generally uncommon feature of skeletal metastases, are associated mostly with hypervascular primary cancers of the kidney, thyroid, and occasionally breast (Fig. 12-13), although they may also be seen with metastatic hepatoma.[31]

Cortical or *periosteal metastases* in the long bones are infrequently observed on CT, constituting only about 10%

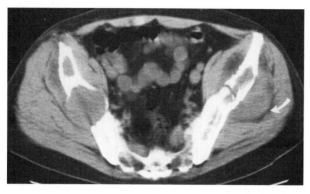

FIGURE 12-13
Metastatic renal cell carcinoma to the pelvis. Multiple lytic lesions, with a characteristically expansile one on the right, are visible. The lesion of the left ilium is associated with a pathological fracture and a large extraosseous soft tissue component *(arrow)*.

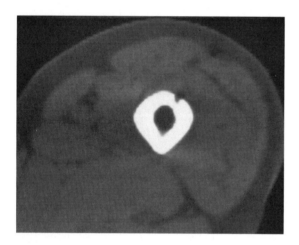

FIGURE 12-14
Metastatic lung carcinoma to the left femur. A subperiosteal intracortical lesion is visible. Note that it is sharply marginated.

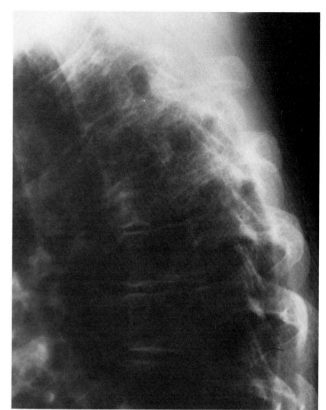

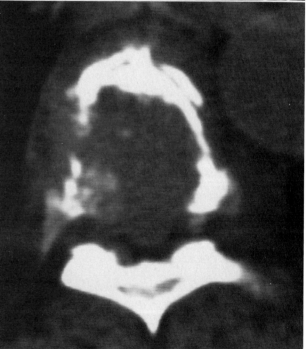

FIGURE 12-15
Metastatic lung carcinoma to the thoracic spine causing a pathological compression fracture. **A,** The initial roentgenographic examination in this patient with back pain shows a compression fracture of T6. The mottled appearance of the collapsed vertebra is suggestive of malignancy. **B,** A CT section confirms the presence of a large destructive lesion.

of all metastatic lesions.[32] When they occur, however, they may be sharply delineated (Fig. 12-14). Periosteal reaction is rarely encountered (being, as a rule, more easily detectable on conventional roentgenograms). Similarly, CT does not play much of a role in the investigation of hypertrophic pulmonary osteoarthropathy.

Pathological fractures are a not infrequent complication of skeletal metastases investigated by CT. In the spine vertebral collapse may be the initial presentation of a metastatic lesion (Fig. 12-15). A pathological fracture may involve the pelvis or long tubular bones (Figs. 12-6 and 12-13), most frequently in the proximal femur (Fig. 12-6). It has been suggested that pathological fractures in the long tubular bones occur when more than 50% of the cortical surface has been destroyed.[33]

Blastic lesions. Purely blastic lesions are characteristically associated with metastatic prostate cancer and, on conventional roentgenograms, are manifested by dense reactive bone formation (Fig. 12-16). Although as a rule they are more readily visualized by roentgenography,

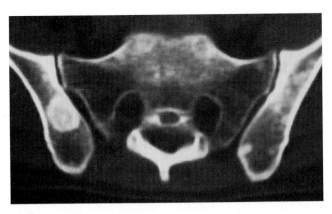

FIGURE 12-16
Metastatic prostate carcinoma to the pelvis. A large blastic lesion of the right ilium plus multiple small lesions of the left ilium and sacrum are visible. The large lesion shows variable density at its center and margin.

nevertheless CT plays a critical role in confirming their presence in the early stages (Fig. 12-17).

Blastic lesions are formed either as a reactive process to bony destruction or through the direct biochemical influence of tumor cells on osteoblasts.[34] Reactive bone may be deposited over preexisting trabeculae and result in trabecular thickening. More often, however, new bone is deposited as spicules extending from trabecular surfaces, with formation of a lacy network in the intratrabecular spaces, and this causes silhouetting of trabecular margins and a loss of the normal trabecular pattern. In more advanced stages new bone can occupy the entire marrow space, causing a homogeneously dense and sclerotic lesion. Then the periphery of the lesion is often indistinct and/or spiculated (Fig. 12-17), allowing differentiation from benign sclerotic lesions (which usually have well-demarcated margins) (see Fig. 12-29, *B*).

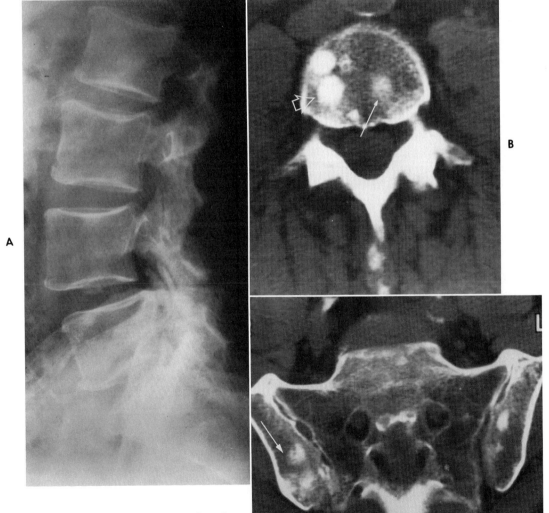

FIGURE 12-17
Metastatic prostatic carcinoma to the spine and pelvis. **A,** A lateral view of the lumbar spine shows ill-defined and subtle areas of increased density. **B** and **C** are CT sections at L4 and S2. Note the multiple blastic lesions. Several are relatively ill-defined and show loss of trabecular bone definition *(long arrows)*. Others are homogeneously dense and sclerotic but show a spiculated margin *(hollow arrow)*.

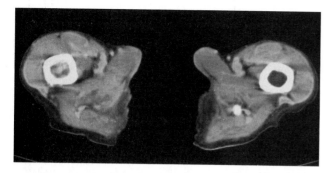

FIGURE 12-18
Metastatic adenocarcinoma of unknown origin to the right femoral medulla. In this patient with multiple lytic lesions of the spine and pelvis a bone scan showed increased uptake in the right femur. A CT scan reveals loss of marrow fat and a nonhomogeneous increased density of the medullary cavity, presumed to be tumor infiltration.

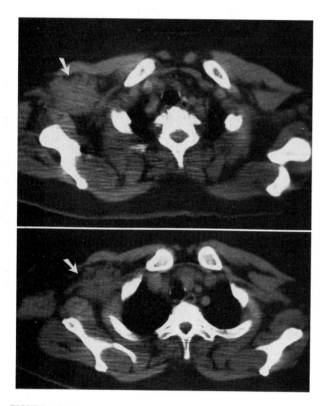

FIGURE 12-19
Metastatic laryngeal carcinoma to the lymph nodes. Nodal involvement and entrapment of the brachial plexus and subclavian vessels are evident *(arrows)*. (Courtesy D. McCauley, M.D.)

Involvement of an entire vertebral body results in a homogeneously dense pattern, the so-called "ivory vertebra," that is frequently seen with metastatic prostate cancer, often at more than one level, but also may occur with lymphoma and less frequently chordoma, plasmacytoma, and Paget's disease.[33] Stimulation of the periosteum in large lesions can cause osseous enlargement, a finding that simulates one manifestation of Paget's.[35] The CT demonstration of these details allows most blastic lesions to be accurately diagnosed, but the multiplicity of blastic metastases is additionally helpful (Fig. 12-17).

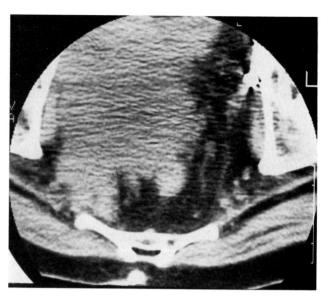

FIGURE 12-20
Carcinoma of the prostate with local invasion. Extension of tumor to the presacral space and into the greater sciatic notch has caused entrapment of the sacral plexus and sciatic nerve.

Nevertheless, in some cases, particularly if the lesion is small and isolated, differentiation may not be possible.

Mixed blastic and lytic lesions. These lesions (or metastases) are encountered more often than purely blastic lesions. They show variations of each pathological process and are usually readily recognizable.

Infiltration of the marrow. Infiltration of marrow by metastatic disease without destructive changes of bone is occasionally seen[36] (Fig. 12-18). Although totally undetectable by conventional roentgenography, marrow infiltration may be demonstrated by bone scanning, bone marrow scanning, and CT scanning. On CT, marrow infiltration is characterized by a loss of medullary fat (manifested as an increased attenuation coefficient).[21] When long bones are studied for this purpose, comparison with the opposite side is most helpful in confirming marrow involvement. An increase of 20 Hounsefield units compared to the contralateral medullary space is considered abnormal. This finding, however, is nonspecific and may be associated with a variety of benign disorders, including hematogenous osteomyelitis.[21]

Soft tissue metastases. These are rare unless manifested as lymph node involvement (Fig. 12-19). More frequently, local extension of an extraosseous primary cancer (Fig. 12-20) or recurrence of a previously treated lesion (Fig. 12-21) is investigated. Direct extension of an extraosseous malignancy to bones is usually seen with lung carcinoma metastatic to the chest wall or genitourinary or lymph node malignancies in the pelvis (Fig. 12-22). Paravertebral or epidural lymphoma is frequently associated with vertebral body involvement.

Healing of metastases. Regression and/or reossification of a destructive lesion following local or systemic treatment of metastases indicate a favorable healing response. Although these changes may be observed

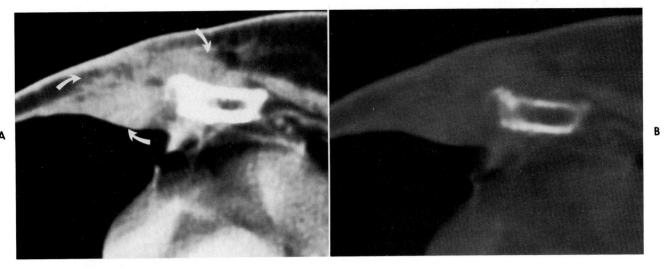

FIGURE 12-21
Carcinoma of the breast, local recurrence 6 months after mastectomy. **A,** A CT section shows a soft tissue mass in the anterior parasternal region with extension anteriorly to the sternum and into the subcutaneous tissue *(arrows)*. Also the skin is thickened. **B,** Same level, wide window settings. Note the eroded right sternal margin.

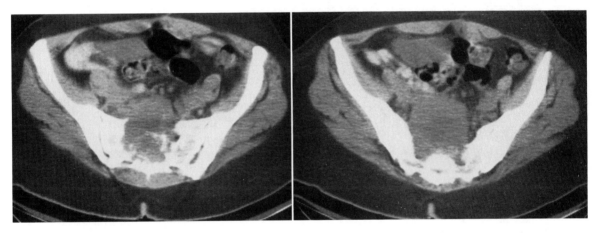

FIGURE 12-22
Uterine cervical cancer with local invasion. In this patient with advanced cervical cancer, local invasion of the tumor to the sacrum has resulted in a large destructive lesion.

roentgenographically as early as 6 weeks after the initiation of therapy, they are best assessed by CT[29,37] (Fig. 12-23).

However, it should be noted that a sclerotic healing response can induce apparent enlargement of a lytic or blastic lesion or result in the roentgenographic visualization of a previously unnoticed lesion.[14,38] Such changes should not be mistaken for progression of disease or the appearance of a new lesion (Fig. 12-24).

TECHNIQUE

1. Spine and pelvis: CT examination is usually limited to the area of suspected abnormality, based on either an abnormal radioisotope uptake or various physical and neurological manifestations. The examination should be targeted for bone with a field of view appropriate for the spine. The scanning parameters consist of 5 mm contiguous slices of the selected region, as determined on a lateral or AP scout image of the spine, with sections paralleling the endplate of the vertebral body. If reconstruction in orthogonal planes is desired, slices should overlap. Larger lesions are adequately visualized by 10 mm contiguous slices. Intravenous contrast enhancement is needed when epidural extension or vascularity of the tumor is to be evaluated. CT-myelography is often performed when neurological changes are present, with imaging directed to the region of epidural/intradural abnormality or myelographic block as visualized on myelography.

2. Thorax, excluding the spine
   a. Rib cage: Occasionally verification of a rib lesion will require examination by CT, which may prove difficult if the lesion is small or no radiographic

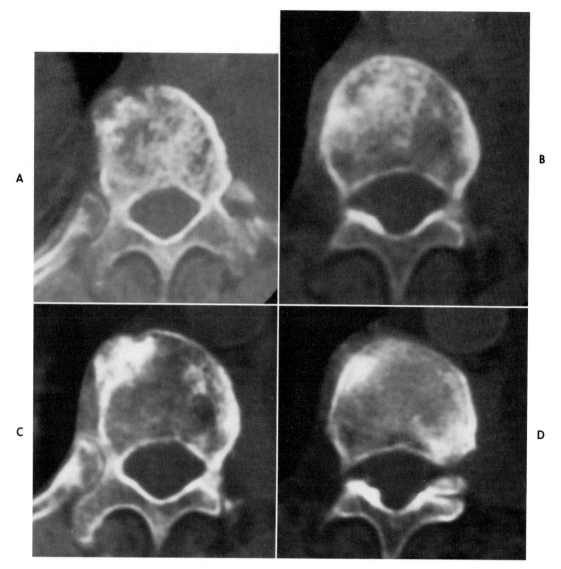

FIGURE 12-23
Healing response of a metastatic breast carcinoma. **A** and **B**, A mostly lytic lesion of T11. **C** and **D**, Ten weeks after systemic chemotherapy the lytic component has resolved. The anterior sclerotic component is now more prominent and confluent.

abnormalities are present. It is helpful to use a skin localizer based on either the bone scan or clinical findings. The lead marker should be removed after the scout view has been obtained and prior to scanning. Scanning techniques important in evaluating this region include bone targeting and thin slices (3 mm or less).

b. Sternum: Obtaining thin slices (5 mm) and an appropriately small field of view are necessary when searching for small lesions. Some irregularity of the posterior manubrial cortex is normally seen and should not be considered pathological.

c. Scapula: Examination of the scapula requires meticulous attention to normal regional anat-

omy. The upper aspect of the scapula — superior margin, scapular spine, and acromial and coracoid processes — on CT images may appear eroded due to their oblique and curved surfaces. It is again beneficial to employ thin slice imaging technique and also to use the normal side for comparison.

3. Extremities: Scanning parameters are dependent upon the extent of the suspected lesion. When possible, both extremities are examined and imaged, which helps in evaluating bony margins with thinning or irregularities due to a partial volume effect as well as in comparing the marrow density.

Intravenous contrast enhancement. Contrast enhancement is desirable when investigating a lytic lesion

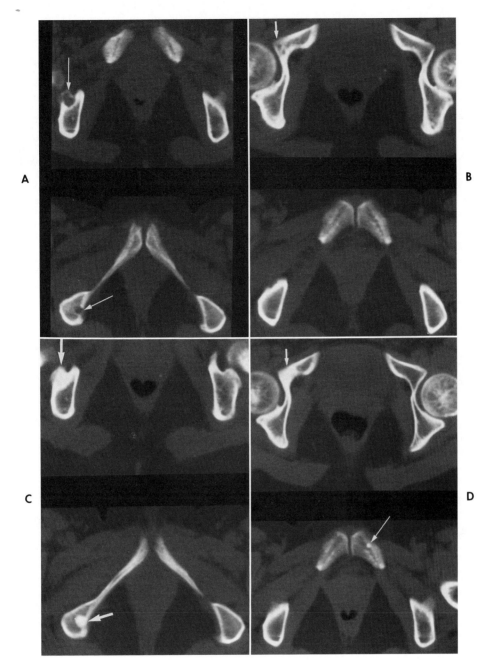

FIGURE 12-24

Healing metastatic lesions with a blastic response. **A,** CT images show lytic lesions of the posterior right acetabulum and ischium *(arrows)* detected by bone scan and also visualized on correlative roentgenograms (not shown). **B,** Another lesion in the anterior wall of the right acetabulum *(arrow)* was not visualized on roentgenograms. No abnormality is seen in the left pubic bone. **C** and **D,** CT images following chemotherapy (12 weeks after the initial examination). (The posterior acetabulum and ischial lesions, **C,** have healed and are completely ossified *[arrows].* Healing of the small anterior acetabular lytic lesion, **D,** has resulted in an apparently much larger sclerotic lesion [short arrow].) Also, a small sclerotic lesion is now visualized in the left pubis where no lesion was previously visible.

with suspected soft tissue component, particularly in the spine, for improved delineation of its epidural extension (Fig. 12-7). The degree of enhancement is a good indicator of tumor vascularity; a nonhomogeneous pattern, with region(s) of low attenuation, indicates areas of low vascularity or possible tumor necrosis (Fig. 12-24).

DIFFERENTIAL DIAGNOSIS

Osteomyelitis. Pyogenic and nonpyogenic infections of bone, particularly in the elderly, may mimic malignancy.

In the *spine* involvement of the disk and two or more adjacent vertebrae is characteristic. There is also usually an associated soft tissue inflammatory process obliterat-

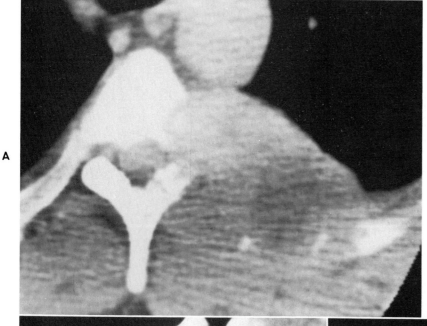

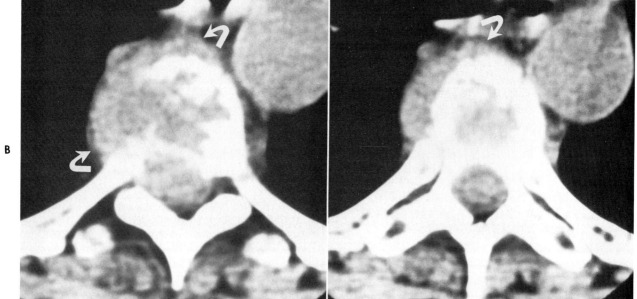

FIGURE 12-25
Contrast-enhanced CT. **A,** Metastatic renal cell carcinoma to the chest wall. Note the lytic lesion of T5 and the adjacent rib with a large soft tissue component. Enhancement at the medial aspect of the mass reveals a soft tissue density similar to the aorta. Laterally and centrally a low-density region is present. At biopsy necrotic material was aspirated. **B** and **C,** Metastatic lung carcinoma to the spine in another patient. The paraspinal extension is sharply demarcated, with preservation of the soft tissue planes *(arrows)*.

ing the normal paravertebral soft tissue planes and, at times, forming a paraspinal abscess (Chapter 9). Again, tumor infiltration is usually limited to one vertebral segment, with bony destruction often extending to the posterior neural arch. Paravertebral extension of tumor, if present, is usually focal, displacing the normal soft tissue planes rather than obliterating them[39] (Fig. 12-25). Intravenous contrast is most helpful for optimal delineation of a paraspinal abscess with characteristically enhanced margins and low-density center. Extension of an adequately vascular tumor shows a generalized homogeneous enhancement. Nonhomogeneous enhancement is seen when necrotic regions are present (Fig. 12-25, *A*).

More challenging is the occasional case of spinal osteomyelitis with focal involvement of only a vertebral body or when the neural arch is affected. These patterns often indicate tuberculous or fungal infections. In either case osseous changes of spinal osteomyelitis (e.g., erosion of bone adjacent to and including the vertebral endplate, with marginal reactive sclerosis) are helpful for making a differential diagnosis. Percutaneous aspiration biopsy is invariably needed to establish or confirm the diagnosis.

In the *pelvis* and *long bones* a focus of osteomyelitis may appear as an ill-defined lytic area or a mottled destructive lesion simulating metastases. In elderly and immunosuppressed individuals the osseous changes may be muted and, most important, periosteal reaction may be lacking. Periosseous soft tissue swelling, cellulitis, the loss of sharp fascial planes, all helpful signs in favor of osteomyelitis, are not usually seen with metastases (Fig. 12-25). The simultaneous presence of a primary extraosseous malignancy and an opportunistic infection,

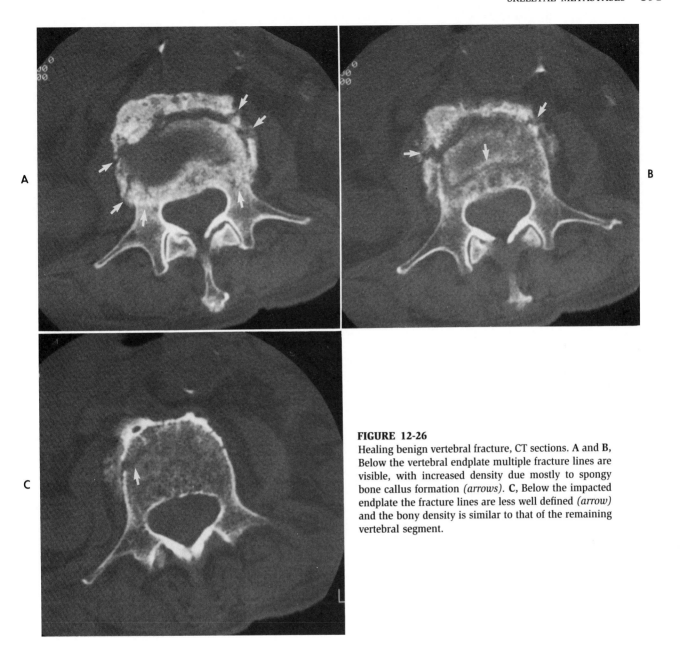

FIGURE 12-26
Healing benign vertebral fracture, CT sections. **A** and **B**, Below the vertebral endplate multiple fracture lines are visible, with increased density due mostly to spongy bone callus formation *(arrows)*. **C**, Below the impacted endplate the fracture lines are less well defined *(arrow)* and the bony density is similar to that of the remaining vertebral segment.

commonly noted in patients with acquired immune deficiency syndrome, further complicates the evaluation of skeletal (axial or peripheral) lesions. Aspiration of such lesions is required for either cytological verification or identification of the infectious agent.

Benign vertebral compression fracture. The accurate diagnosis of a pathological vertebral fracture and its differentiation from an acute or chronic osteoporotic or traumatic fracture are usually possible by CT,[40] based on visualization of a destructive lesion (usually lytic or mixed lytic/blastic) and its differentiation from (1) impacted spongy bone and callus in the subacute stage of a fracture (Fig. 12-26) or (2) a deformed but remodeled vertebral body in the chronic stage of a fracture (Fig. 12-27).

(1) Impacted spongy bone or endosteal callus in the subacute stage of a fracture characteristically forms a band of increased density in the vicinity of the impacted (usually superior) endplate (Fig. 12-27).
(2) A typical burst fracture of the spine indicates trauma and has been reported with osteoporotic fracture.[41]

Whereas compression of the superior endplate is often due to benign causes, depression of the inferior endplate raises the suspicion of an underlying malignancy. An acute fracture, either spontaneous in an osteoporotic individual or of traumatic origin, is usually accompanied by a rim of paravertebral and/or epidural soft tissue density due to hemorrhage that may mimic tumor infiltration. Recognition of the fracture pattern and, more

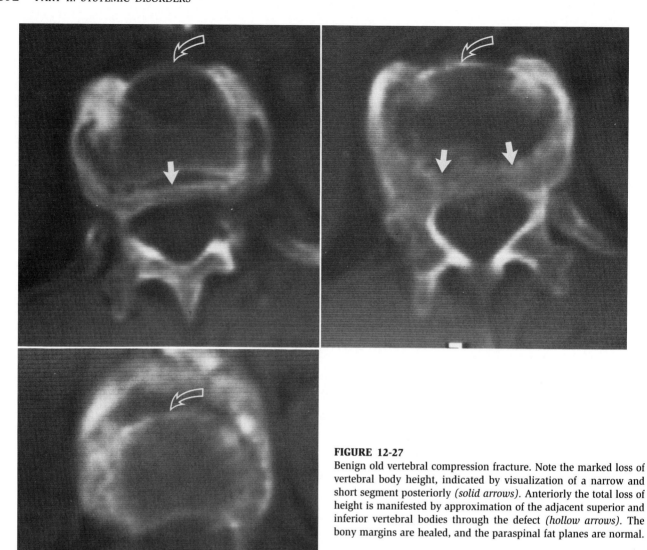

FIGURE 12-27
Benign old vertebral compression fracture. Note the marked loss of vertebral body height, indicated by visualization of a narrow and short segment posteriorly *(solid arrows)*. Anteriorly the total loss of height is manifested by approximation of the adjacent superior and inferior vertebral bodies through the defect *(hollow arrows)*. The bony margins are healed, and the paraspinal fat planes are normal.

important, failure to visualize a destructive lesion within the vertebral body are the important elements in differentiating the two conditions.

Degenerative disease. Degenerative disease of the intervertebral disks and apophyseal and costovertebral joints, along with large or small Schmorl nodes accompanying a disk herniation (Fig. 12-28) and focal sclerotic regions (similar to bone islands) in the spine or near the sacroiliac joints (Fig. 12-29), is frequently detected in patients under investigation for skeletal metastases. All these lesions generate an abnormal uptake on bone scan and can simulate malignancy.[42-44] A metastatic lesion may coexist with and be masked by such benign conditions on initial inspection of the plain film or CT, and this possibility should be borne in mind when the abnormality on bone scan does not appropriately correspond to a "benign" abnormality on plain film or to the patient's symptoms.

Resnick and Niwama,[33] in a study on cadavers, showed that erosion of the vertebral endplate due to an adjacent metastatic focus within the vertebral body could lead to intravertebral disk herniation and formation of a Schmorl node (Fig. 12-30). In addition, they suggested that extension of tumor to the endplate might interfere with proper nutrition of the disk, leading to degeneration of the disk cartilage.

Benign intravertebral disk herniation is best recognized by continuity of the vertebral body defect with the disk space and by a sclerotic margin with normal bone in the periphery (Fig. 12-28).

Radiation-induced osteonecrosis. Radiation-induced osteonecrosis or the late sequelae of medullary necrosis of

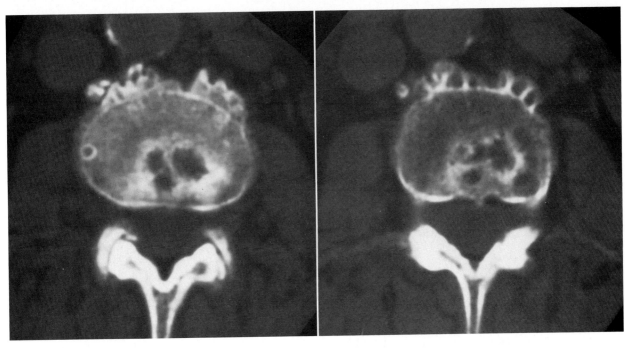

FIGURE 12-28
Large Schmorl nodes in a patient with prostate cancer and an abnormal bone scan. CT sections at the superior endplates of L2 and L3 show lobulated defects with well-defined sclerotic margins. These are indicative of Schmorl nodes and intravertebral disk herniation. The surrounding trabecular bone is otherwise normal.

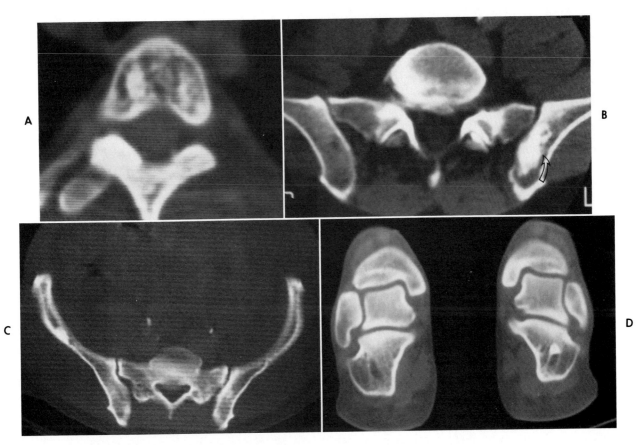

FIGURE 12-29
Bone islands (enostosis) of the spine, pelvis, and calcaneus. **A** is the thoracic spine, **B**, the left ilium, **C**, the right ilium, and, **D**, the left calcaneus. Well-demarcated and homogeneously dense sclerotic foci are visible within the spongy bone. These lesions are usually round or ovoid but, particularly in the vicinity of sacroiliac joint, may show a lobulated or geographic margin (*arrow* in **B**).

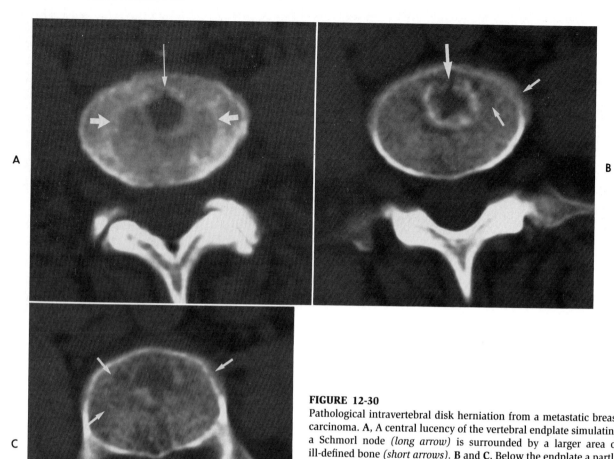

FIGURE 12-30
Pathological intravertebral disk herniation from a metastatic breast carcinoma. **A**, A central lucency of the vertebral endplate simulating a Schmorl node *(long arrow)* is surrounded by a larger area of ill-defined bone *(short arrows)*. **B** and **C**, Below the endplate a partly eroded sclerotic ring surrounds the Schmorl node *(thick arrow)*. There is also a permeative destruction of the spongy and cortical bone *(thin arrows)*.

bone as a result of systemic disorders may lead to an abnormality on bone scans and roentgenograms. Irradiation of bone with 4000 rads or more can cause significant alterations in osteoblastic activity and subsequent radiographically detectable changes. In mild forms a generalized type of bony atrophy is detected whereas in more severe cases there is osteonecrosis. CT scanning usually confirms the benign nature of the lesions by showing marked atrophy of bone or interspersed areas of cystic and sclerotic change limited to the irradiated region. Dystrophic soft tissue or medullary calcification may accompany the osseous change (Fig. 12-31).

In patients who have received prior pelvic irradiation a spontaneous fracture of the sacrum can develop as a complication of radiation-induced osteonecrosis or as a result of combined radiation-induced bone atrophy and postmenopausal osteoporosis.[45-47] These fractures, which may be suggested by radionuclide bone scanning and/or conventional roentgenography, are well demonstrated by CT scanning and can be differentiated from malignancy by their typical fracture patterns (Fig. 12-32). Inclusion of the hip region within the field of radiation when treatment is directed to the pelvic wall may result in avascular necrosis of the femoral head and/or insufficiency fracture of the femoral neck.

In contrast to the late sequelae of radiation osteitis, which are usually asymptomatic and discovered incidentally, fractures due to bony atrophy induce pain and the

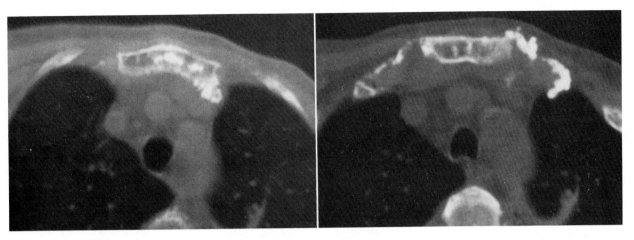

FIGURE 12-31
Postradiation calcinosis in the sternum and costal cartilage. Several years after left mastectomy and chest wall irradiation this patient presented with palpable hard nodules. Note the dense and well-defined calcific deposits.

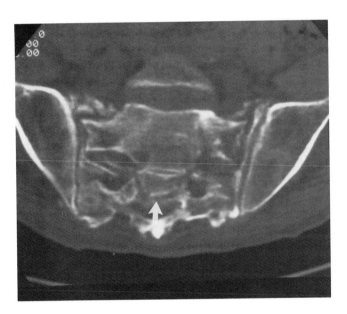

FIGURE 12-32
Postradiation insufficiency sacral fracture. Six months after a complete course of pelvic irradiation for invasive cervical carcinoma there are bilateral fractures with areas of bony resorption. The fractures, characteristically parallel to the sacral articular surfaces, have a transverse component (arrow).

patient seeks medical attention. Naturally the possibility of metastatic disease and, at times, further irradiation of the region is strongly entertained. Recognition of this relatively early complication of radiation-induced bone atrophy is important for preventing further weakening of the bone by unneeded irradiation and in providing the proper treatment.

Another late sequela of medullary necrosis in long bones due to a variety of systemic disorders is irregular but dense calcification within the medullary space. A diffusely increased density caused by fibrosis of the marrow is often present. No erosive process of either the spongy bone or the endosteal surface of the bone is seen with these lesions.

Posttraumatic sequelae. One sequela of musculoskeletal injury may be the abnormal accumulation of radioisotope up to several months or years after treatment. Often

a history of prior trauma exists and the roentgenographic examination is conclusive. When it is not, CT may be helpful in recognizing a traumatic lesion. The difficulty in daily practice arises when a radionuclide bone scan discloses an abnormality of the rib cage, a common site for metastases and fracture as well as other benign lesions (e.g., fibrous dysplasia). A CT examination may be required for delineation of existing pathology (Figs. 12-33 and 12-34). Also an abnormal accumulation of radiopharmaceutical at an old muscle injury site, with calcium deposition, may cause confusion as to the exact location of the uptake as well as suspicion regarding adjacent bony structures. When small, the calcific deposits may not be visualized on plain films, but they usually show up well on CT, often associated with atrophic changes of the surrounding tissue or a specific muscle bundle.

Paget's disease. Paget's disease frequently involves the spine and pelvis and is a rather common cause of abnormality on bone scan. The characteristic radiographic findings (coarsening and disorganization of the bony architecture, cortical thickening and overall enlargement of the bone) usually allow accurate recognition by conventional roentgenography. CT is helpful for differentiating Paget's disease from a malignancy in specific cases (e.g., during the blastic phase of the disease or when a compression deformity is present). Spinal stenosis due to

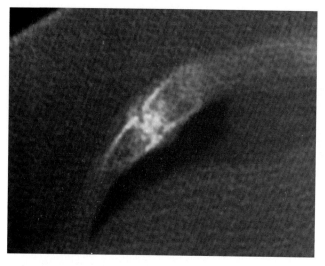

FIGURE 12-33
Rib fracture. Two months after mastectomy for breast cancer, this patient presents with pain, an abnormal bone scan, and an inconclusive roentgenogram. CT shows a benign healing rib fracture.

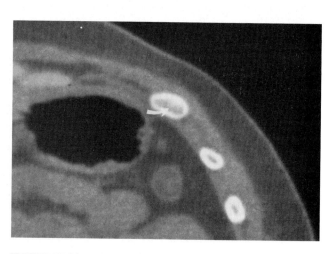

FIGURE 12-34
Metastatic squamous cell lung carcinoma to the rib. There was no roentgenogram abnormality at the site of abnormal uptake on bone scan. CT disclosed a small blastic lesion (biopsy proven) in this region *(arrow)*.

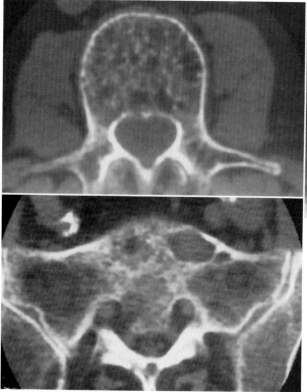

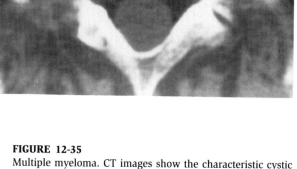

FIGURE 12-35
Multiple myeloma. CT images show the characteristic cystic lesions of spongy bone at L2, L5, and S1. The cortical bone is thin and irregular. There is also variable density of the lesions, probably representing the extent of cellular hyperplasia.

modeling abnormality and, less often, pagetoid facet arthropathy result in back pain[48] and may also raise the question of possible malignancy. In rare cases areas of pagetoid bone and marrow will extend beyond the cortical margin and into the paravertebral or epidural spaces, resulting in cord compression.

Benign primary tumors of bone. A benign skeletal hemangioma is most often seen in the spine, with either complete or focal involvement of a vertebra. It is readily recognized by the characteristic vertical trabecular thickening on conventional roentgenography and a "polka-dot" appearance on CT. The latter modality is particularly helpful in identification of a focal hemangioma that is causing an abnormal bone scan but is not visualized on roentgenograms. Although ordinarily hemangiomas do not expand the bone or extend beyond the cortical

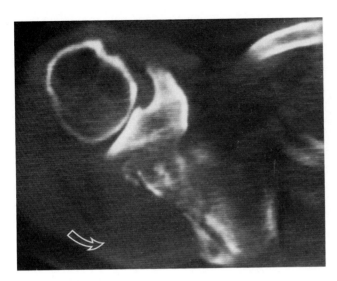

FIGURE 12-36
Malignant lymphoma in the right scapula. The destructive lesion was associated with a large extraosseous soft tissue component (*arrow*).

margin, a more aggressive one may manifest such findings.

In younger patients *primary tumors* of the spine are most often benign and include osteoblastoma, osteoid osteoma, and aneurysmal bone cyst. The characteristic features of these lesions are best demonstrated by CT. Paraspinal *neurofibromas* appear as soft tissue tumors extending into the spinal canal through the neural foramina. They are of low attenuation due to their high fat content, and they enhance well on contrast studies.

Other malignant lesions. Primary malignant tumors of bone or marrow may simulate metastases. *Solitary plasmacytomas* usually present as expansile, septated, lytic lesions of the spine or pelvis. However, they are highly vascular and cannot therefore be reliably differentiated from kidney or thyroid metastases. The metastases, furthermore, may be solitary at presentation, necessitating percutaneous biopsy for their histological documentation. *Multiple myeloma* is manifested by diffuse osteopenia at its onset followed by generalized small cystic areas of bone resorption (Fig. 12-35). These lesions are best demonstrated by CT scanning in their early stage.[49] *Chordomas* are generally readily recognizable by their predilection for the sacrum and upper cervical region, along with other characteristic roentgenographic features (including a large and often calcified soft tissue component).[50]

Osseous lymphoma may induce bone destruction or a blastic reaction indistinguishable from that caused by metastases. A permeative osteolysis of the appendicular skeleton is often seen with primary non-Hodgkin's lymphoma of bone,[28,51] frequently accompanied by a large soft tissue component (Fig. 12-36). In the spine epidural spread of lymphoma, with subsequent cord compression, is infrequent.[52] On roentgenograms 30% of epidural

lymphomas show osseous involvement.[53] Although there are no findings pathognomonic for spinal epidural lymphoma, lengthy involvement, coexistent bony lesions, and abnormal paravertebral soft tissue are quite common.

Magnetic resonance imaging

Our own experience and that of numerous investigators[54-60] have shown a definitive role for MR in the diagnosis of skeletal metastases. MR has proven to be as sensitive as, if not more sensitive than, radionuclide bone scanning. It is also more specific than the scan, exhibiting greater precision in the anatomical location and demonstration of osseous and soft tissue lesions. Its major role, however, is in the detection of known or suspected spinal metastases and cord compression. Although radionuclide scanning remains the modality of choice for screening the entire skeleton, certainly specific indications exist for MR imaging in the pelvis and appendicular skeleton (i.e., to search for early suspected bone involvement or to evaluate the extent of a known lesion).

DIAGNOSTIC FEATURES: SIGNAL ALTERATIONS AND PATTERNS IN SKELETAL METASTASES

The signal alteration generated by metastatic foci in bone is nonspecific. Tumor infiltration of marrow causes prolongation of T1 and T2 values, so these lesions generally appear as low signal on T1-weighted and high signal on T2-weighted images[61] (Fig. 12-37).

Signal changes in osteoblastic lesions are similar to those in osteolytic lesions on a T1-weighted sequence

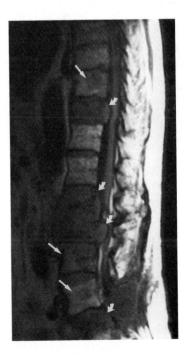

FIGURE 12-37
Metastatic renal cell carcinoma to the spine. A midsagittal T1-weighted (550/30) MR image of the thoracolumbosacral spine shows low-signal metastatic lesions of T9, L3, and L4 (*straight arrows*) and pathological compression fractures of T10, L1, L2, and L5 (*curved arrows*).

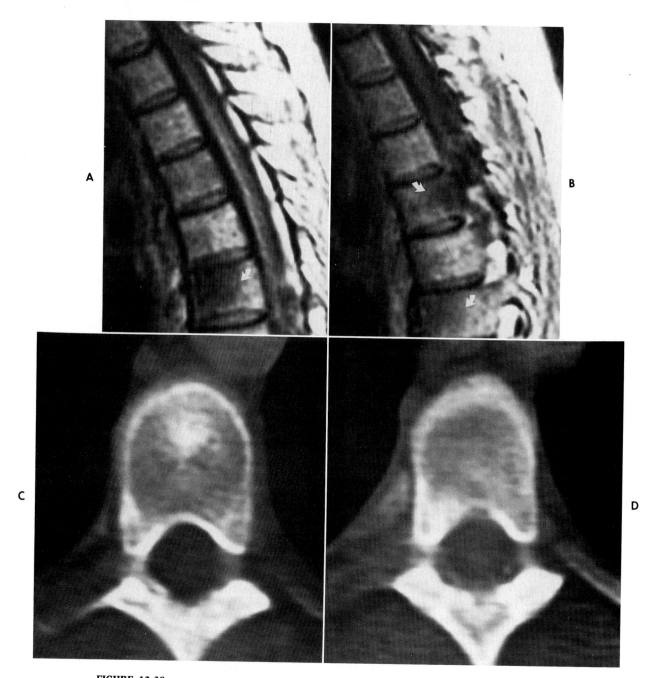

FIGURE 12-38
Osteoblastic metastatic squamous cell carcinoma of the lung. **A** and **B**, Sagittal T1-weighted images (470/30) of the thoracic spine. There are areas of low signal within T5 and T7 *(arrows)*. **C** and **D**, Corresponding CT images demonstrate blastic metastases in these regions.

with focal or diffusely reduced signal intensity (Fig. 12-38). Unless the metastatic lesions are entirely osteoblastic, at least some increased signal is seen on a T2-weighted pulse sequence (Fig. 12-39). Ordinarily, metastatic lesions are well seen on T1-weighted images as areas of low signal against a background of high-signal fatty marrow. However, nonneoplastic lesions may create a similar pattern, with only mixed- or high-signal lesions having a lower probability of representing malignancy.[62] Furthermore, in younger individuals with normal hyper-

cellularity of bone marrow, the signal intensity of metastatic deposits may not be significantly different from the background signal of normal marrow.

Rarely a metastatic lesion may show intermediate signal on T1-weighted imaging (Fig. 12-40), probably due to intramural bleeding. Plasmacytoma is also observed without significant loss of bone marrow signal, or with only slightly increased signal, especially of the extraosseous component of the lesion (Fig. 12-41). This observation has also been made with other metastases. Its

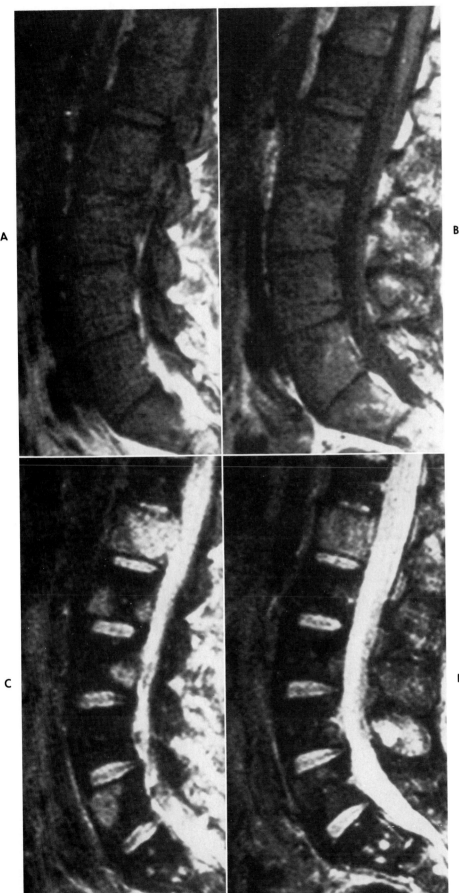

FIGURE 12-39
Generalized metastatic prostate carcinoma to the lumbar spine. **A** and **B,** Sagittal T1-weighted images (505/20) of the lumbar spine show a generalized decreased signal intensity due to widespread metastases. **C** and **D,** Corresponding sagittal T2-weighted images (2100/75) reveal several regions of high signal indicative of tumor cellularity and the absence of osteosclerosis.

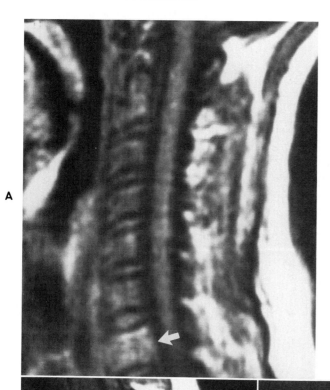

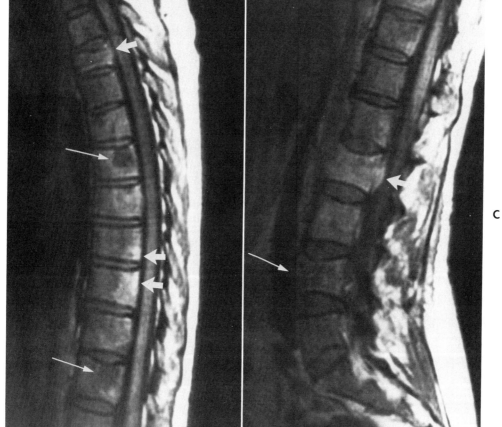

FIGURE 12-40
Metastatic melanoma to the spine with variable signal intensity. T1-weighted midsagittal MR images of the cervical, **A,** thoracic, **B,** and lumbar, **C,** spine (550/30) show widespread metastases with increased signal intensity of C7, T3, and L2 *(short arrows)* low-signal lesions at T6, T11, and L3 *(long arrows).* Note the epidural extension of tumor at L2 *(short arrow* in **C).**

nature is not clear, although it may be related to the lack of residual spongy bone trabeculae in the extraosseous soft tissue component.

Despite the limitations inherent in nonspecificity of the low-signal pattern on T1 weighted images, this sequence is considered adequate for routine evaluation of spinal metastases. Several abnormal patterns are frequently seen, and when present they strongly favor this diagnosis:

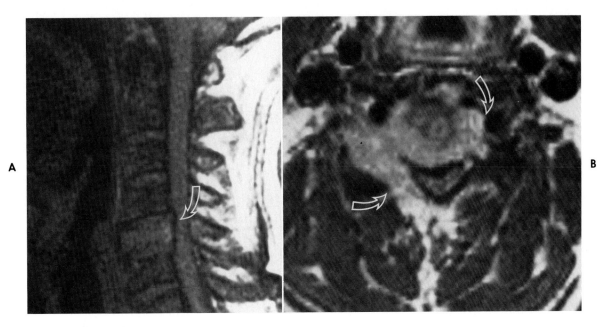

FIGURE 12-41
Solitary plasmacytoma of the cervical spine. **A,** Sagittal T1-weighted (550/30) MR image of the cervical spine. There is a pathological compression fracture with cord compression at C5 *(arrow)*. The signal intensity, compared to that in adjacent segments, is slightly increased. **B,** An axial density-weighted (1000/30) image shows destruction of the lateral mass and the lamina on the right side and epidural infiltration by moderate-intensity tumor *(arrows)*.

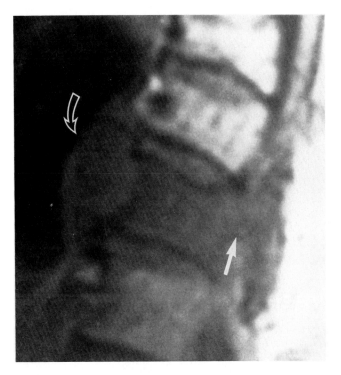

FIGURE 12-42
Metastatic carcinoma of the breast to T10, sagittal T1-weighted (470/20). Total infiltration of the vertebral body is indicated by low signal intensity. The pedicle is also involved *(solid arrow)*, and a paraspinal soft mass is present *(hollow arrow)*.

1. Multiple focal low-signal regions (Figs. 12-37 and 12-38)
2. Total involvement of one or more vertebral bodies with or without pathological compression fracture (Figs. 12-37 and 12-40)
3. Associated paravertebral or epidural soft tissue masses (Figs. 12-37 and 12-40 to 12-42)
4. Involvement of the pedicles and neural arches (Fig. 12-42)
5. MR evidence of cortical bony destruction (Figs. 12-37 and 12-40)

Improvement in signal abnormality, or a return to normal, is seen after local or systemic treatment of some metastatic lesions and constitutes an accurate indication of regression or total remission of the lesion (Fig. 12-43).

The *short T1 inversion recovery (STIR)* sequence dramatically enhances neoplastic tissue without administration of gadopentetate (Fig. 12-44). It suppresses fat and depicts normal marrow as low intensity. The relatively higher signal of tumor infiltration is well demonstrated against this low-intensity background; and it is done with a shorter imaging time than on T2-weighted sequences as well as with greater contrast.[63-65] In addition, paraspinal tumor infiltation (not adjacent to CSF) is optimally enhanced and delineated. However, false-positive findings may occur after radiation therapy or with benign marrow disorders[63] (p. 410).

After local or systemic treatment of spinal metastases, a change in signal, with decreased intensity on STIR sequences, has been reported as a reliable indicator of tumor regression.[63]

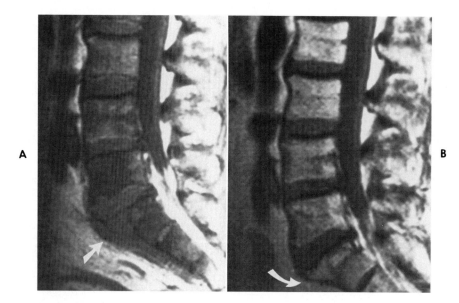

FIGURE 12-43

Malignant lymphoma, lumbar spine, pre- and posttherapy. **A,** Midsagittal MR image of the lumbar spine (600/20). There are multiple regions of low signal intensity (T12, L2, L5, S1) in this patient with a history of lymphoma. The S1 lesion is associated with cortical bony destruction and a paraspinal soft tissue mass *(arrow)*. **B,** Six months after systemic chemotherapy, midsagittal MR image (600/20). There is almost complete resolution of the lesions observed on the previous study. The presacral mass is diminished, and the cortical bone has reformed *(arrow)*.

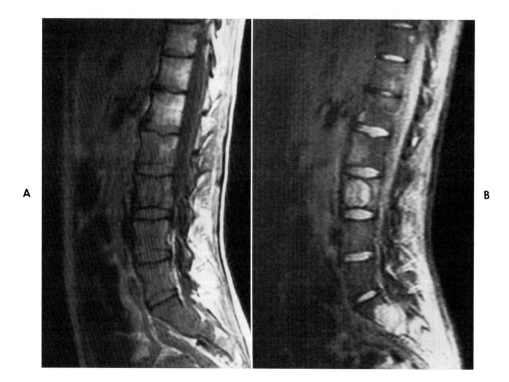

FIGURE 12-44

Metastatic melanoma to the lumbar spine. **A,** A sagittal T1-weighted (550/30) sequence shows variable signal intensity of the vertebral bodies. **B,** A sagittal STIR image (TR/TI/TE 1400/100/30) discloses enhanced metastatic foci in L2, L3, and L5.

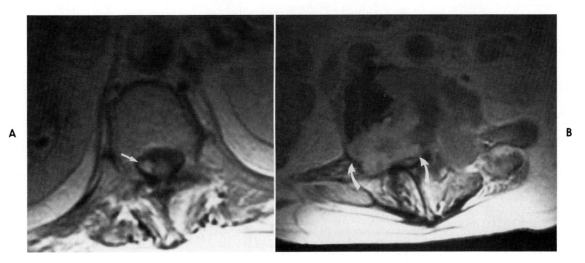

FIGURE 12-45
Metastatic renal cell carcinoma to the spine, same patient as in Fig. 12-37, post–Gd enhancement. Axial T1-weighted (850/30) images of T11, **A**, and L2, **B**, 5 minutes after injection demonstrate enhancement of a T11 intradural lesion *(single arrow)* and a large L2 epidural component *(arrows)*.

Gadopentetate enhancement of spinal metastases. The use of gadopentetate (gadolinium-DTPA) has markedly improved visualization of the soft tissue components of spinal metastasis[66] (Fig. 12-45). Gadopentetate shortens T1 and T2 values and therefore affects both T1- and T2-weighted spin echo, as well as STIR, images.

The greatest enhancement is seen on T1-weighted spin echo sequences.[64] These images are superior to T2-weighted in delineating tumor infiltration and are infrequently degraded by motion artifacts (often encountered with T2-weighted imaging); thus they are most helpful in evaluating intradural lesions.[64,67]

Generally, *epidural* extension of spinal tumors is well visualized without contrast enhancement.[68] In selected cases administration of gadopentetate helps in tumor location for biopsy and in differentiating tumor from herniated disk (Fig. 12-46). *Intramedullary* lesions are also usually well seen on T1-weighted spin echo imaging; however, gadopentetate enhancement better delineates and characterizes these lesions and should be routinely utilized when they are detected on unenhanced images[69,70] (Fig. 12-46).

Intradural/extramedullary metastases occasionally originate from primary tumors such as lung and breast or in the form of drop metastases from CNS tumors. They form nodules or sheaths of tumor along the meninges and, for a variety of reasons (including their small size and motion artifacts on T2-weighted images), may not be detected without enhancement. Also high-signal CSF may mask some intradural lesions on T2-weighted images. A T1-weighted gadopentetate-enhanced sequence is extremely effective in depicting these lesions, at times even better than on myelography and CT-myelography,[71] as high-signal regions on the background of low signal CSF (Fig. 12-47).

The difficulty in using gadopentetate is that the possibility exists of obscuring lesions that are situated against or surrounded by fat. An enhanced intradural lesion may be obscured by the high signal of epidural fat against which it is situated. Similarly, gadopentetate enhancement of a vertebral body that is infiltrated by tumor[64,71] or a medullary lesion of long bones may result in a high signal that mimics the signal from normal marrow fat (Figs. 12-48 and 12-49). Also enhancement of the basivertebral and lumbar perivertebral venous plexuses can cause confusion.[69] Another pitfall is that gadopentetate enhancement may be seen in various benign conditions with marrow edema or hyperemia, such as compression fractures or vertebral changes related to degenerative disk disease. To prevent all these, a precontrast T1-weighted study is needed.

Gadopentetate enhancement is an accurate indicator of tissue cellularity and can therefore be used in evaluating disease activity after treatment has been completed (Fig. 12-50). Residual tumor after surgery or recurrence may also be accurately evaluated. Serial examinations and comparison with a baseline study are needed.[64,68] In one reported study[67] low levels of enhancement at follow-up examination of treated myeloma and metastases from prostate and breast cancers may have reflected inactive or effectively treated disease with low cellularity and vascularity.

TECHNIQUE
Spine

1. The use of a dedicated surface coil is mandatory for obtaining optimal images of the entire spine.
2. We concur with other investigators[57,60,66,69] who maintain that the entire spine should be examined-

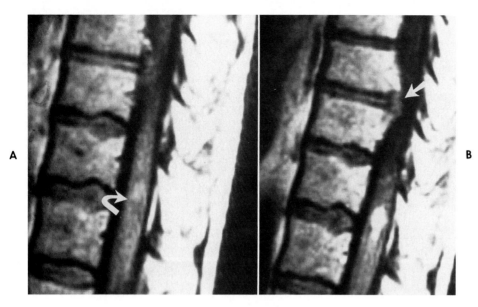

FIGURE 12-46
Metastatic renal cell carcinoma to the spinal cord. **A,** A sagittal T1-weighted (520/30) image of the thoracolumbar spine shows an area of mixed signal within the cord, representing a metastatic deposit *(arrow)*. **B,** Comparable image, 5 minutes post-Gd. Note the enhancement, resulting in improved delineation of the intramedullary lesion. Incidentally, a non-enhancing herniated thoracic disk is also visible *(arrow)*.

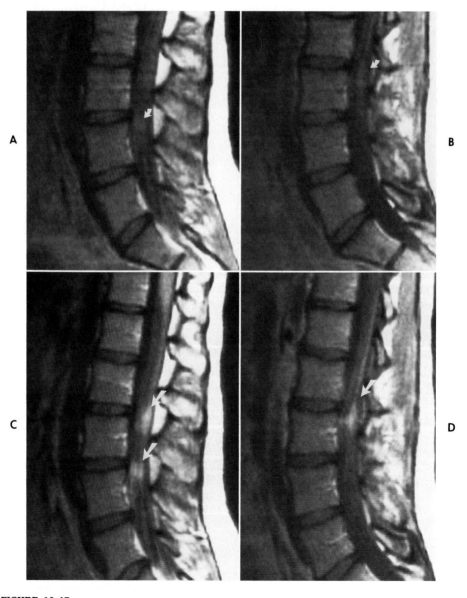

FIGURE 12-47
Intradural/extramedullary metastatic lesions. **A** and **B,** Sagittal T1-weighted images (550/30). Subtle intradural foci of increased signal are seen *(arrows)*. **C** and **D,** Same parameters, 3 minutes post−Gd injection. Note the marked enhancement of several intradural lesions *(arrows)*.

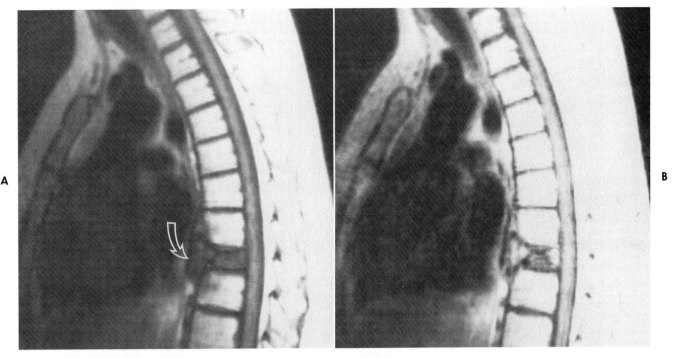

FIGURE 12-48
Gadopentetate enhancement of a T7-metastatic breast carcinoma. **A,** A midsagittal T1-weighted image (466/19) shows pathological compression fracture of T7 with a paraspinal mass *(arrow)*. **B,** Same level 1 minute post–Gd injection (466/19). There is now enhancement of the lesion, but its signal intensity is similar to that of normal vertebral bodies, which also show slight enhancement.

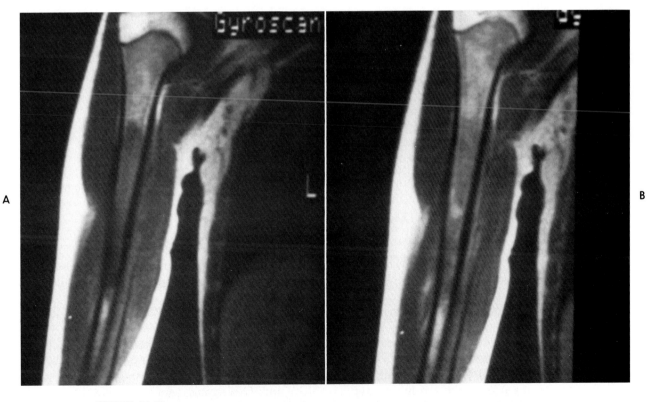

FIGURE 12-49
Metastatic nasopharyngeal carcinoma to the humeral shaft, gadopentetate enhancement. **A,** T1-weighted coronal image of the right humerus. Note the large segment of decreased signal due to an infiltrating process. **B,** Same level 3 minutes after injection. The lesion has a signal intensity approaching that of the normal adjacent marrow, and thus there is poor delineation of the lesion.

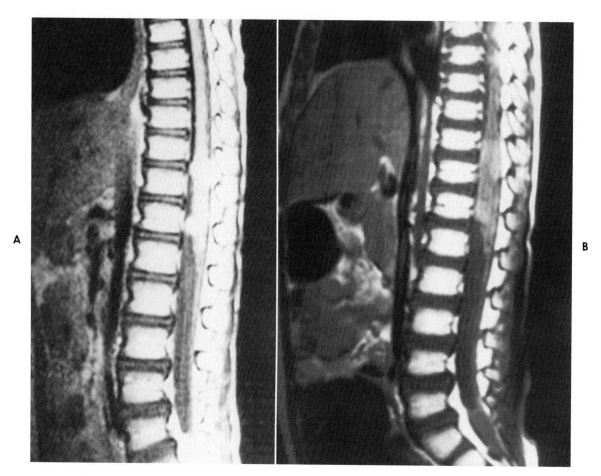

FIGURE 12-50
Intradural drop metastasis from a medulloblastoma, gadopentetate enhancement before and after therapy. **A**, A sagittal T1-weighted (550/30) image of the thoracolumbar spine, 5 minutes post–Gd injection, shows markedly enhancing lesions. **B**, Another sagittal T1-weighted image (516/20) 5 minutes postinjection. Note the overall reduction in tumor enhancement.

first in the sagittal plane with a T1-weighted pulse sequence.

3. Regions of abnormality may then be routinely examined in the axial plane with a T1-weighted pulse sequence. When the symptoms are localized and the pathology is not identified in the sagittal plane, orthogonal T1- or T2-weighted images are obtained. This is helpful for recognizing possible subtle subarachnoid or paraspinal lesions.[66] Sagittal images of the entire spine and axial images of regions of abnormality can be obtained in less than 1 hour.

4. Although T2-weighted images were initially used for better delineation of spinal neoplastic disease, with gadopentetate and newer pulse sequences (i.e., STIR) the utility of T2-weighted imaging has been drastically curtailed. Instead, STIR or a fat-suppression sequence is utilized for improved delineation of osseous lesions and paraspinal extension of tumor.[64,65,72,73]

In conclusion, a combination of nonenhanced T1-weighted and STIR sequences appears to be most effective for evaluating spinal metastases and diffuse bone marrow infiltration by tumor. Gadopentetate-enhanced T1-weighted spin echo and enhanced STIR sequences are used mostly for suspected intradural lesions, with T2-weighted spin echo reserved for occasional cases when differentiation from other disorders (e.g., herniated disk) is needed. Other pulse sequences (gradient recalled echo) do not play a significant role in the imaging of metastases. However, a single-slice multiecho sequence may be used for characterizing a signal abnormality rather than a lesion's morphology.

Pelvis and long bones

1. The examination is tailored according to the site or nature of the expected lesion.
2. Imaging in at least two orthogonal planes with T1- and T2-weighted spin echo or STIR sequence is needed for a thorough evaluation and delineation of intraosseous and soft tissue components of tumors (Figs. 12-51 and 12-52).

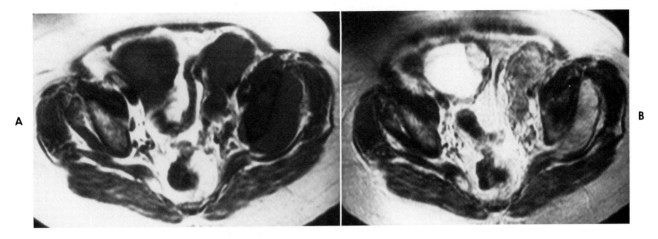

FIGURE 12-51
Metastatic malignant fibrous histiocytoma to the pelvis. **A,** Axial T1-weighted (550/30) image at the acetabular dome. The left dome shows decreased signal as a result of tumor infiltration. A large soft tissue mass and nodal involvement are also visible. **B,** A relatively T2-weighted (1600/60) image shows moderate enhancement of the soft tissue and nodal component, with only slight enhancement of the bone. This is indicative of a sclerotic lesion. Incidentally discovered was a cystic and solid pelvic mass arising from one of the ovaries.

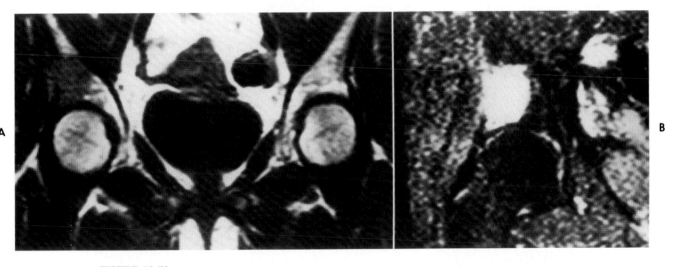

FIGURE 12-52
Metastatic lung carcinoma to the right acetabular dome. **A,** Coronal T1-weighted image. The lesion is identified as a low-signal region. The peripheral cortex is interrupted. No apparent invasion of the hip joint is seen. **B,** STIR sequence. Note the enhanced lesion, allowing better delineation of the articular cortex, which is confirmed to be intact.

PITFALLS AND DIFFERENTIAL DIAGNOSIS

Spinal osteomyelitis. Isolated vertebral involvement may be difficult to differentiate from a malignant lesion. Most often spinal osteomyelitis is manifested by involvement of two or more adjacent vertebral bodies and the intervening disks. On short TR pulse sequences the involved regions show low signal that may extend well beyond the areas of spongy bone erosion within the vertebral body detected by other imaging modalities (e.g., CT scanning). Low signal paravertebral or epidural abscesses often accompany vertebral osteomyelitis. On T2-weighted pulse sequences areas of acute inflammatory reaction and abscess, including the involved disk, are manifested by high signal intensity. The surrounding bone often retains low signal due to sclerotic and fibrotic reaction.

Benign vertebral fractures. Chronic benign fractures, either osteoporotic (spontaneous) or traumatic, characteristically show preservation of normal fatty marrow and appear isointense with other normal vertebral bodies on all pulse sequences (Fig. 12-53). They are readily distinguished from malignant compression fractures caused by tumor infiltration (which exhibit total replacement of the fatty marrow [Fig. 12-54], as manifested by a homoge-

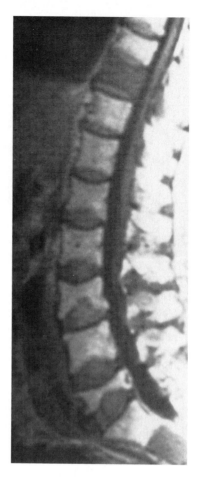

FIGURE 12-53
Metastatic breast carcinoma to T10 and S2 and old osteoporotic fractures of L3 and L5. A midsagittal T1-weighted (550/20) MR image shows total decreased signal intensity of T10 and S2 due to tumor infiltration. L3 and L5, however, despite a marked compression deformity, exhibit signal intensity similar to other normal vertebrae, indicative of old and remodeled fractures. L1, L2, and L4 show mild deformity.

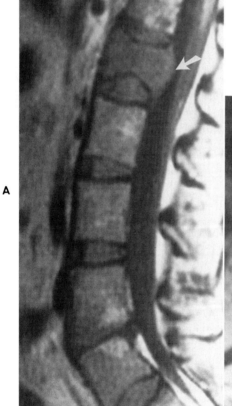

A

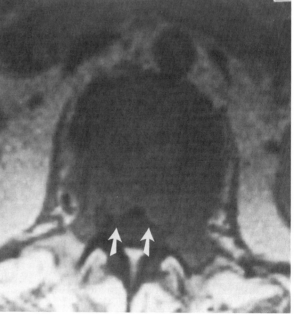

B

FIGURE 12-54
Malignant compression fracture with metastatic carcinoma of the breast. **A** and **B,** Sagittal and axial T1-weighted (550/30) images show the deformity of L1, with complete replacement of the marrow in the vertebral body and pedicles. The convex posterior vertebral surface is due to epidural extension of the tumor *(arrows)*.

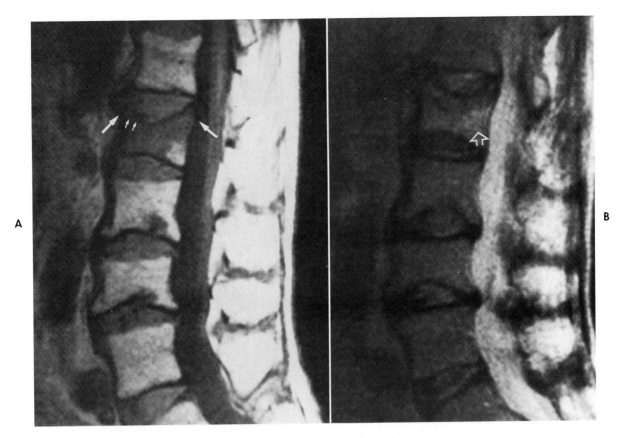

FIGURE 12-55

Benign compression fracture of L2 (same patient as in Fig. 12-27). **A,** A sagittal T1-weighted (550/30) image of the lumbar spine shows marked compression of L2, with mostly decreased signal intensity and preservation of a small region of normal marrow signal. Fragmentation of the superior endplate *(small arrows)* and angulation of the posterior and anterior cortical fragments *(large arrows)* are visible. L3 and L4 show old compression deformities with focal low-signal regions adjacent to the inferior endplate due to Schmorl nodes. **B,** A sagittal image relatively T2-weighted (900/150) discloses some increase in signal intensity *(arrow)*. Persistence of the low-signal region is due to callus formation.

neous low signal on T1-weighted images and a homogeneous high signal on T2-weighted and STIR images).[65,74] By contrast, acute or subacute benign vertebral body fractures show nonhomogeneous signal alterations (with some preservation of normal marrow signal, usually posteriorly) on various pulse sequences, particularly T2-weighted and STIR[65] (Fig. 12-55). Often there is a band or wide region of low signal adjacent to the collapsed endplate, with preservation of normal fatty marrow inferiorly (Fig. 12-56).

This band or wide region of low signal may reflect one or a combination of changes—including edema, old hemorrhage, impaction of spongy bone, and ensuing reactive bone (callus) formation.

At times there is difficulty with the MRI differentiation of benign and pathological vertebral body fractures. Occasionally an acute traumatic fracture will demonstrate low signal intensity of the entire vertebral body on T1-weighted images resembling that of tumor infiltration.[74,75] This pattern may also be observed with osteoporotic fractures (Fig. 12-57). A STIR sequence or a T1-weighted fat-suppression or T1-weighted gadopen-

tetate-enhanced sequence may, likewise, be misleading because edema and hemorrhage can also show high signal intensity.[68] However, generally this pattern is nonhomogeneous (Figs. 12-58 and 12-59), as opposed to the homogeneous increased signal with pathological fractures (Fig. 12-48).

Some secondary MR findings are helpful in differentiating acute traumatic from malignant vertebral fractures[74]:

Reversal to normal signal intensity is expected with an adequate time interval (Fig. 12-59, *C*).

Disk disruption, vertebral body fragmentation, and angulation of fragments strongly favor the diagnosis of traumatic nonmalignant fracture (Fig. 12-55).

Conversely, a vertebral body with a pathological fracture tends to have margins that are convex outward[65] (Fig. 12-54).

A paraspinal or epidural soft tissue mass may be seen in both instances, although more prominently with pathological fractures.

Visualization of other metastatic foci favors a diagnosis of malignant fracture.

Abnormal pedicle bone marrow is more frequently observed with malignant fractures but may be seen with traumatic fractures (Figs. 12-54 and 12-56).

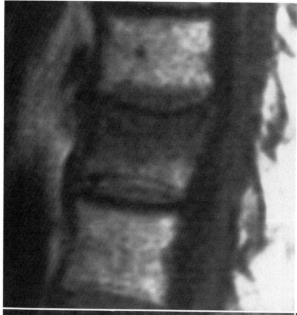

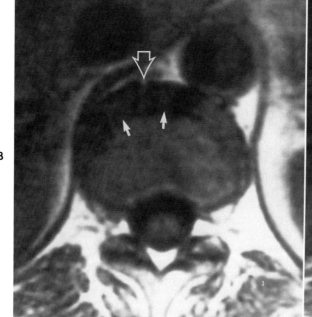

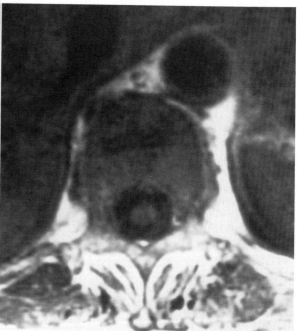

FIGURE 12-56

A, T1-weighted (612/20) sagittal image. There is signal depression of the superior endplate with partial decreased intensity of the marrow. The inferior region remains normal. **B,** T1-weighted (490/20) axial image at the superior aspect. The impacted cortical bone is manifested by low signal anteriorly *(solid arrows).* The interrupted anterior cortex represents a fracture line *(hollow arrow).* **C,** The low-signal abnormality extends below the impacted bone and into the vertebral pedicles.

Occasionally foci of high signal on T1-weighted images are noted with benign fractures; these have been attributed to degenerative yellow fat replacement, although they may also represent acute hemorrhage (Fig. 12-58).

Degenerative disease. On T1-weighted images characteristic changes related to degenerative disk disease at the endplate level consist of low-intensity regions (sclerosis) with or without high-intensity regions (fatty replacement). On T2-weighted images increased vertebral body signal in association with disk degeneration has also been reported.[76] This may be due to edema and hemorrhage. Focal fat deposition within the marrow occurs with aging, spondylitis, and kyphoscoliosis.[77]

Radiation-induced bony atrophy. Increased signal intensity of the vertebral marrow on short TR sequences has been shown 2 months to 10 years after radiation exposure.[78] These signal alterations concur with the effect of radiation on bone and eventual fatty replacement of the marrow (Fig. 12-60).

Benign hemangioma. A hemangioma is manifested by mottled increased signal on both T1 and T2 pulse sequences.[79]

Multiple myeloma. This myeloproliferative disorder is manifested by decreased bone marrow signal on T1-weighted images. The signal alteration is often patchy and generalized, but it may be focal[57,80] (Fig. 12-61). Al-

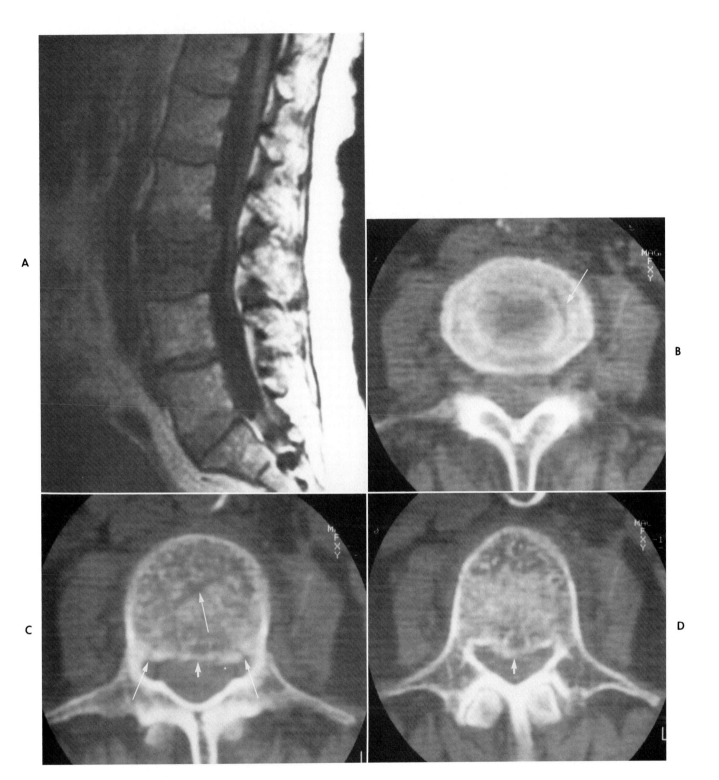

FIGURE 12-57
Subacute osteoporotic L2 compression fractures in an elderly woman with a history of extraosseous lymphoma who presented with acute-onset back pain. **A**, T1-weighted midsagittal. Note the homogeneously decreased signal intensity of the entire vertebral body suspected of harboring malignancy. **B** to **D**, CT sections show no destructive lesion. Fracture of the superior endplate and posterior cortex *(long arrows)* and a retropulsed fragment *(short arrows)* are visible. Needle biopsy showed only normal marrow elements; no malignancy was detected.

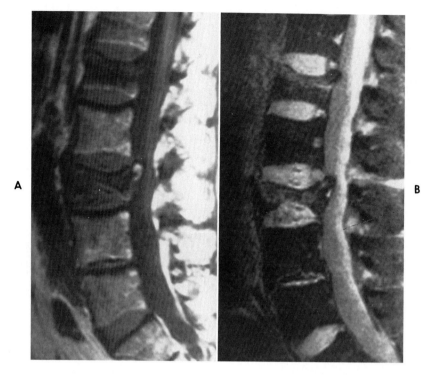

FIGURE 12-58
Subacute osteoporotic compression fractures (same patient as in Fig. 12-57, 2 months later). **A,** Sagittal T1-weighted image (505/20). Compression fractures of L1 and L3, with heterogeneously decreased signal intensity, are present. **B,** A sagittal TI-weighted fat-suppression (450/30) image shows heterogeneous increase in signal intensity at the fracture sites.

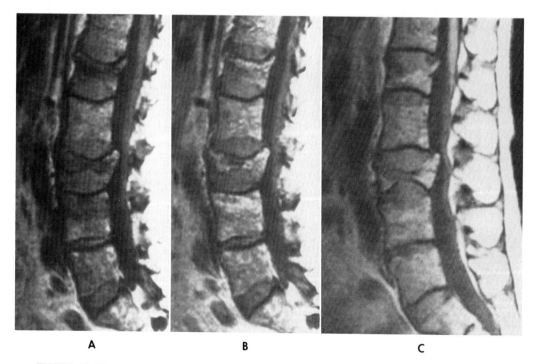

FIGURE 12-59
Benign compression fractures of L3, L1, and L4 (same patient as in Figs. 12-57 and 12-58) detected (in chronological order) following blackout spells and collapse. **A,** A midsagittal T1-weighted (550/30) image of the lumbar spine shows low-signal compression fractures of L3 and L1. Note the nonhomogeneous decreased signal of L4 without compression deformity. **B,** Another slice 3 minutes post-Gd, same parameters. There is some enhancement, although nonhomogeneous, in the regions of low signal intensity. **C,** Some 6 months later a T1-weighted study (550/30 shows residual deformity with reversal to normal signal intensity.

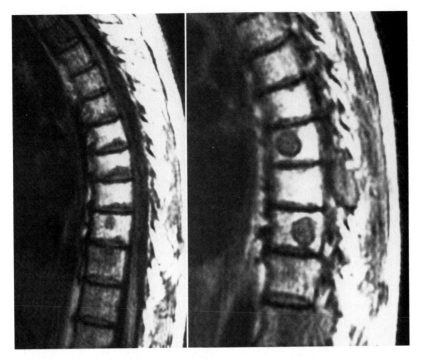

FIGURE 12-60
Metastatic lung carcinoma to the thoracic spine 2 months after radiation treatment. Sagittal T1-weighted images show increased signal intensity of the midthoracic vertebral bodies. Metastatic lesions with low-signal margins indicate reactive sclerosis.

though differentiating the focal pattern from metastases is not always possible, MRI may be helpful in locating a biopsy site (Fig. 12-62).

Plasmacytoma. This focal neoplasm also has a nonspecific pattern on MRI, except occasionally, when it may demonstrate moderate signal on T1-weighted images (Fig. 12-41).

Lymphoma. The permeative growth of lymphomas often results in more widespread tumor infiltration (soft tissue or marrow) than generally expected from other metastases. Certain features of a spinal lymphoma (e.g., invasion of the canal through the neuroforamina) are best detected by MR and may suggest the diagnosis.[81] On MRI bone marrow involvement with lymphoma, unlike that with leukemia, is often focal, patchy, or discrete[71] (Fig. 12-63).

COMPARISON OF IMAGING MODALITIES
Magnetic resonance versus computed tomography

Extensive comparative studies of MRI and CT in the evaluation of spinal or skeletal metastases are lacking. The foremost advantage of MRI is its suitability as a screening procedure for suspected spinal metastases. Its higher sensitivity in delineating the intraosseous extent and soft tissue components of skeletal tumors and in detecting early metastatic infiltration of bone marrow is well appreciated.[84] Marrow infiltration in patients with lymphoma, focal or diffuse, is also more readily demonstrated on MRI (Fig. 12-64).

Conversely, trabecular bone is not well visualized on MRI and erosive changes may not be detected. Destruction of cortical bone, mostly in advanced stages, is visualized on MRI (Fig. 12-65); but the details of normal cortical and spongy bone architecture and their abnormalities are better delineated by CT. Therefore, shown to a greater advantage by CT are the following[85,86]: cortical bony erosions, disruptive changes of trabecular bone, pathological fractures, and calcific deposits. As a result, CT provides a more specific image of skeletal lesions and should be utilized when other diagnostic modalities, including MR examination, have produced nonspecific or conflicting data. Perhaps the most important indication for utilizing CT is an acute or subacute vertebral compression fracture in an individual with suspected malignancy. Based on detailed visualization of cortical and trabecular architecture, CT is more specific and more reliable in demonstrating the specific patterns of traumatic or osteoporotic spinal fractures, and in detecting the underlying lesions of pathological compression fractures. Also CT is more specific in the diagnosis of other benign vertebral body conditions, with or without compression fractures, such as hemangioma and Paget's disease (Fig. 12-66).

Spontaneous sacral fractures in elderly persons (osteoporotic or radiation induced) appear as abnormal low-signal regions on MRI and may resemble malignancy. Although the characteristic distribution of these fracture lines (bilateral sacral wings) should be conducive to their clear demonstration on high-resolution axial MR

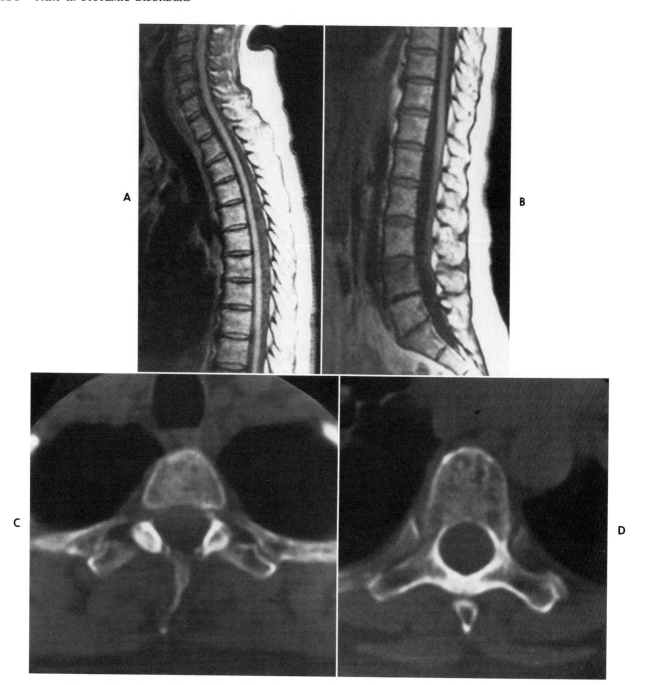

FIGURE 12-61
Multiple myeloma, early stage. Relatively T1-weighted (900/30) sagittal MR images of the thoracic, **A,** and lumbar, **B,** spine show generalized patchy and nonhomogeneous signal intensity of the vertebral bodies. At L4 a compression fracture of the superior endplate causes more prominent low signal of the vertebra. CT images at T3 and T5, **C** and **D,** reveal small lucencies and cystic lesions within the vertebral body, characteristic of myeloma.

images, CT provides a more definitive picture (Fig. 12-67). However, the higher sensitivity of MRI compared to other modalities in detecting early metastatic lesions should be reemphasized. When there is a strong suspicion of metastasis, based on clinical presentation or the nature of the MRI abnormality, such lesions should be subjected to percutaneous biopsy for conclusive diagnosis.

In the search for peripheral skeletal metastatic lesions

(e.g., bone marrow metastases suspected by radionuclide scanning, medullary extension of a known lesion, or a skip lesion), MR is considered beneficial. In addition, the ability of MR to scan in axial, sagittal, and coronal planes enhances visualization of an anatomical extension and improves visualization of its proximal and distal aspects.

Following local or systemic treatment of skeletal metastases, both MRI and CT may provide helpful information regarding the healing process or the progression of

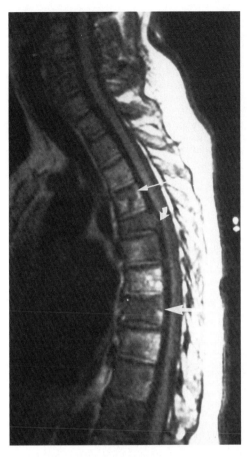

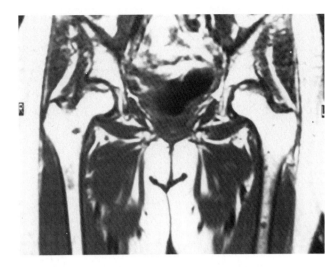

FIGURE 12-63

Lymphoma. A T1-weighted coronal image of the pelvis and proximal femora shows multiple focal low-signal lesions. Note the incidentally discovered bilateral avascular necrosis of the femoral heads.

FIGURE 12-62

Multiple myeloma, advanced stage. A sagittal T1-weighted (600/20) MR image of the cervical and thoracic spine shows a predominantly low-signal focal lesion *(thin arrow)* or total replacement of the vertebral marrow without pathological fracture *(thick arrow)* or with pathological fracture and an epidural mass *(curved arrow)*.

A   B   C

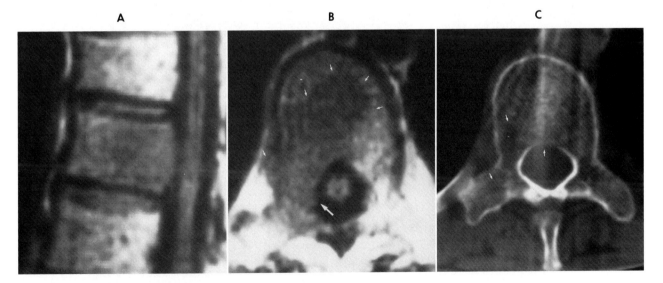

FIGURE 12-64

Primary osseous lymphoma of the thoracic spine (same patient as in Fig. 12-3). **A,** Sagittal T1-weighted (470/30) image. Note that the posterior vertebral surface has a convex contour, with partial low-signal alteration of marrow. **B,** Axial T1-weighted image (550/30). The low signal of the vertebral body and right pedicle is demonstrated *(small arrows)*. Epidural extension of the lesion is evident with no apparent cord compression *(large arrow)*. **C,** CT image at the same level. Only subtle loss of the spongy bone of the pedicle and transverse process with focal thinning of the anterior aspect of the spinal canal is demonstrated *(small arrows)*.

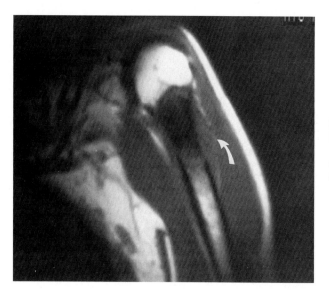

FIGURE 12-65
Metastatic pheochromocytoma to the humerus. A T1-weighted (440/30) coronal image of the proximal left humerus shows circumferential cortical bony destruction, along with extraosseous extension of the tumor *(arrow)*.

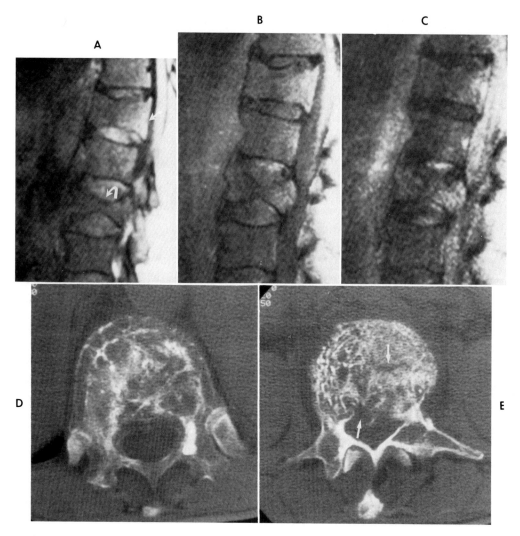

FIGURE 12-66
Paget's disease with pathological fracture. **A,** A sagittal T1-weighted image (470/30) of the thoracolumbar spine shows mild compression of T12 with increased signal *(straight arrow)* and a marked compression deformity of L2 that is isointense with adjacent segments *(curved arrow)*. **B** and **C,** Multiecho sagittal sections (900/60 and 900/120) disclose persistence of the high signal at T12 and increased signal at L2. A pathological fracture cannot be excluded. **D** and **E,** CT sections at T12 and L2 reveal the characteristic changes of Paget's disease. In addition, there is a compression fracture at L2 *(arrows)*.

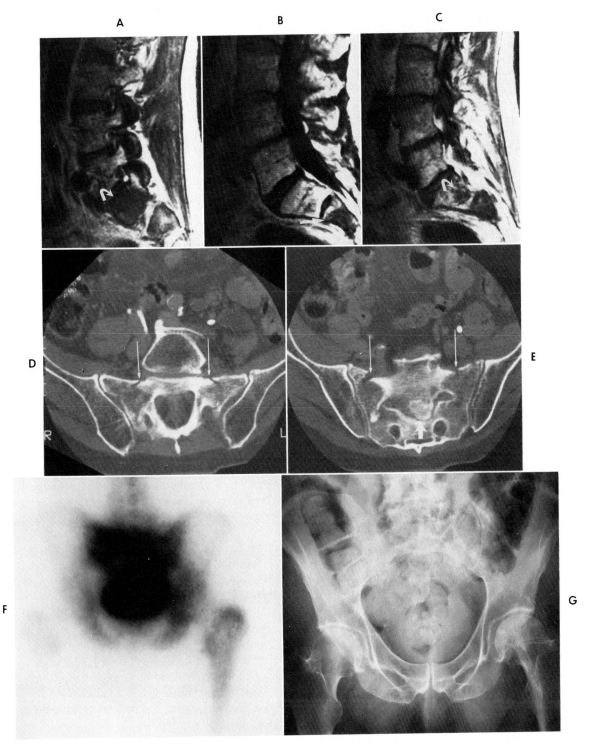

FIGURE 12-67
Osteoporotic sacral fracture in an elderly man who presented with persistent low back pain. **A** to **C,** Sagittal T1-weighted images of the lumbosacral spine show low-signal alteration at S1 *(curved arrow)* and S2 *(straight arrow)*. **D** and **E,** CT images demonstrating benign fractures of the sacral alae *(long arrows)* and a transverse fracture of S2 at the midline *(short arrow)*. **F,** A radionuclide bone scan shows markedly abnormal uptake in the sacrum. **G,** An anteroposterior roentgenogram of the pelvis discloses no abnormality.

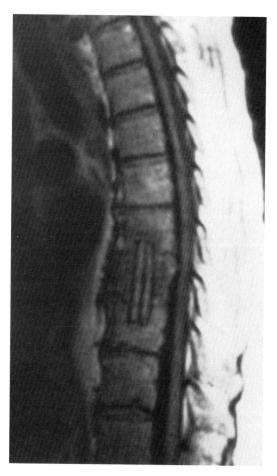

FIGURE 12-68
After spinal fusion at T10 for metastatic renal cell carcinoma. The sagittal T1-weighted (550/30) image shows bone grafts extending from T9 to T11, with preservation of the vertebral alignment.

disease. However, MRI more accurately projects disease activity in the early stages, after treatment has begun, and is therefore more suitable in this respect. After operative intervention and spinal fusion for metastatic disease, in addition to the evaluation of disease activity, MRI can aid the investigation of bone graft status and the alignment of vertebral bodies (Fig. 12-68).

Magnetic resonance versus myelography and CT-myelography

Before MR imaging, CT-myelography was the procedure of choice for evaluating patients with suspected spinal cord compression. Despite some earlier doubts,[75] MRI is now regarded as the optimum modality in the evaluation of epidural and spinal cord metastases[51,56,61,74] and its efficacy has been proven by numerous investigations. Technical advances have greatly lessened certain of its limitations (cited in earlier reports) such as the inability to detect small lesions and nerve root compression.[86] MRI lacks the potential for side effects from water-soluble contrast media and other complications related to myelography, especially rapid neurological deterioration following lumbar puncture.[66]

Its ability to screen the entire spine is another advantage of MR "myelography," and allows detection of additional osseous lesions as well as paravertebral extension of a tumor without cord compression. Also areas of cord compression not amenable to routine myelography, such as those between blocked regions, can be visualized.

Despite its high sensitivity in detecting both intramedullary and extradural lesions, however, MR has been less effective than myelography in assessments of intradural/ extramedullary lesions. There are a variety of reasons for this.[71-88] The nature of subarachnoid extension of tumor results in the formation of delicate and lacy tumoral "sheaths" along the nerve roots, usually without mass effect on the spinal cord, and with these even extensive spread of tumor may be poorly delineated on MRI. Also tumor nodules are usually small, and a partial volume effect can prevent their being visualized. In addition, their relaxation characteristics may be similar to those of the surrounding abnormal CSF, which usually has a high protein content due to underlying malignancy. Further difficulty arises with artifactual CSF nonhomogeneities (which may simulate small lesions) due to CSF pulsation and other motion artifacts. However, gadopentetate enhancement has been most effective at improving visualization of these abnormalities.

INTEGRATED APPROACH TO THE IMAGING OF SKELETAL METASTASES

Skeletal metastases are frequently found in patients with extraosseous primary cancer, most often associated with lesions of the lung, prostate, and breast, but virtually every other malignancy (including primary osseous cancers) also metastasizes to bone. Skeletal metastases may cause serious complications; they are painful, and they often lead to pathological fractures, cord compression, and a variety of other complications. Their diagnosis is important not only for purposes of palliation but also in the selection of treatment for the primary lesion (i.e., with metastases a radical surgical resection of the primary tumor is usually not done). When metastases are discovered after the initial treatment, a change in treatment protocol may be indicated.

There are certain clear choices to be made in approaching the diagnostic work-up of these patients. Except for patients in whom a lesion is discovered incidentally, in the routine search for skeletal metastases it is best to begin with a radionuclide bone scan. Although the majority of skeletal metastases are found in the axial skeleton, and MRI can effect their disclosure, radionuclide bone scanning provides for evaluation of the entire skeletal system. A roentgenographic correlation of abnormal regions is, in most instances, adequate for identification of malignant lesions. When in doubt, we use a CT scan for clarification. Perhaps CT is not as sensitive as MR in detecting osseous lesions; but it is more specific, permitting a more precise identification of osseous lesions. The role of MR, as has been stated, is mainly in the evaluation of a patient with known or suspected spinal metastases, particularly when cord compression is suspected. The role of myelography in this respect is secondary and limited to patients in whom an MRI cannot be obtained. MR also is the modality of choice for evaluating the effect of therapy and/or the progression of disease.

REFERENCES

1. Galasko CSB: The anatomy and pathways of skeletal metastases. In Weiss L, Gilbert H (eds): Bone metastasis. Boston, GK Hall, 1981, pp 49-63.
2. Berrettoni BA, Carter JR: Current concept reviews. Mechanisms of cancer metastasis to bone. J Bone Joint Surg (Am) 1986; 68:308-312.
3. Willis RA: Secondary tumors of bones. In Willis RA (ed): The spread of tumors in the human body. 3rd ed, London, Butterworth, 1973, pp 229-250.
4. Gilbert RW, Kim JH, Posner JB: Epidural spinal cord compression from metastatic tumor: diagnosis and treatment. Ann Neurol 1978;3:40-51.
5. Galasko CS: The significance of occult skeletal metastases, detected by skeletal scintigraphy, in patients with otherwise apparently "early" mammary carcinoma. Br J Surg 1975; 62:694-696.
6. McNeil BJ: Value of bone scanning in neoplastic disease. Semin Nucl Med 1984;4:277.
7. Citrin DL, Bessent RG, Greig WR: A comparison of the sensitivity and accuracy of the TC-99 phosphate bone scan and skeletal radiograph in the diagnosis of bone metastases. Clin Radiol 1977;28:107-117.
8. Edelstyn GA, Gillespie PJ, Grebbel PS: The radiological demonstration of osseous metastases: experimental observations. Clin Radiol 1967;18:158-162.
9. Mall JC, Beckerman C, Hoffer PB, Gottschalk H: A unified radiological approach to the detection of skeletal metastases. Radiology 1976;118:323-328.
10. Kido DK, Gould R, Taati F, et al: Comparative sensitivity of CT scans, radiographs, and radionuclide bone scans in detecting metastatic calvarial lesions. Radiology 1978;128:371-375.
11. Pagani JJ, Libshitz HI: Imaging bone metastases. Radiol Clin North Am 1982;20(3):545-560.
12. Corcoran RJ, Thrall JH, Kyle RW, et al: Solitary abnormalities in bone scans of patients with extraosseous malignancies. Radiology 1976;121:663-667.
13. Levine E, Lee KR, Neff JR, et al: Comparison of computed tomography and other imaging modalities in the evaluation of musculoskeletal tumors. Radiology 1979;131:431-437.
14. Muindi J, Coombes RC, Golding S, et al: The role of computed tomography in the detection of bone metastases in breast cancer patients. Br J Radiol 1983;56:233-236.
15. Cacayorin ED, Kieffer SA: Applications and limitations of computed tomography of the spine. Radiol Clin North Am 1982;20(1):185-206.
16. Green BA, Diaz RD, Post MJD: The diagnosis of spinal column and spinal cord tumors with emphasis on the value of computed tomography. In Post MJD (ed): Computed tomography of the spine. Baltimore, Williams & Wilkins, 1984, pp 659-695.
17. Kori SH: Computed tomographic evaluation of bone and soft tissue metastases. In Weiss L, Gilbert H (eds): Bone metastasis. Boston, GK Hall, 1981, pp 245-257.
18. Braunstein EM, Kuhns LR: Computed tomographic demonstration of spinal metastases. Spine 1983;8:912-915.
19. Redmond J 3rd, Spring DB, Munderloh SH, et al: Spinal computed tomography scanning in the evaluation of metastatic disease. Cancer 1984;54:253-258.
20. Rafii M, Firoozia H, Kramer E, et al: The role of computed tomography in evaluation of skeletal metastases. J Comput Tomogr 1988;12:19-24.
21. Helms CA, Cann CE, Brunelle FO, et al: Detection of bone-marrow metastases using quantitative computed tomography. Radiology 1981;140:745-750.
22. Lynn DM, Braunstein EB, Wahl RL, et al: Bone metastases in pheochromocytoma: comparative studies of efficacy of imaging. Radiology 1986;160:701-706.
23. O'Rourke T, George CB, Redmond J III, et al: Spinal computed tomography and computed tomographic metrizamide myelography in the early diagnosis of metastatic disease. J Clin Oncol 1986;4:576-583.
24. Mink JH, Weitz I, Kagan AR, Stekel RJ: Bone scan–positive and radiograph- and CT-negative vertebral lesion in a woman with locally advanced breast cancer. AJR 1987;148:341-343.
25. Tumeh SS, Beadle G, Kaplan WD: Clinical significance of solitary rib lesions in patients with extraskeletal malignancy. J Nucl Med 1985;26:1140-1143.
26. Keene JS, Sellinger DS, McBeth AA, Engber WD: Metastatic breast cancer in the femur. A search for the lesion at risk of fracture. Clin Orthop Rel Res 1986;203:282-288.
27. Van Zanten TE, Teule GJ, Golding RP, Heidendal GA: CT and nuclear medicine imaging in vertebral metastases. Clin Nucl Med 1986;11:334-336.
28. Ginaldi S, DeSantos LA: Computed tomography in the evaluation of small round cell tumors of bone. Radiology 1980; 134:441-446.
29. Bellamy EA, Nicholas D, Ward M, et al: Comparison of computed tomography and conventional radiology in the assessment of treatment response of lytic bony metastases in patients with carcinoma of the breast. Clin Radiol 1987;38: 351-355.
30. Mundy GR, Spiro TP: The mechanisms of bone metastasis and bone destruction by tumor cells. In Weis L, Gilbert H (eds): Bone metastasis. Boston, GK Hall, 1981, pp 64-82.
31. Golimbu C, Firoozria H, Rafii M: Hepatocellular carcinoma with skeletal metastasis. Radiology 1978;128:89-94.
32. Coerkamp EG, Kroon HM: Cortical bone metastases. Radiology 1988;169:525-528.
33. Resnick D, Niwayama G: Skeletal metastases. In Resnick D, Niwayama G (eds): Diagnosis of bone and joint disorders. 2nd ed, Philadelphia, Saunders, 1988, pp 3944-4010.
34. Aoki J, Yamamoto I, Hino M, et al: Sclerotic bone metastasis: radiologic-pathologic correlation. Radiology 1986;159:127-132.
35. Schreiber RR: The radiologist and the diagnosis of bone metastasis. In Weis L, Gilbert H (eds): Bone metastasis, Boston, GK Hall, 1981, pp 190-230.
36. DiSteffano A, Tashima CK, Yong Yap H, Hortobagyi GN: Bone marrow metastases without cortical bone involvement in breast cancer patients. Cancer 1979;44:196-198.
37. deSantos LA, Goldstein HM, Murray JA, Wallace S: Computed tomography in the evaluation of musculoskeletal neoplasms. Radiology 1978;128:89-94.
38. Lisbona R, Palayew MJ: Misleading skeletal surveys in prostatic carcinoma. J Can Assoc Radiol 1979;30:159-161.
39. Van Lom KJ, Kellerhouse LE, Pathria MN: Infection versus tumor in the spine: criteria for distinction with CT. Radiology 1988;166:851-855.
40. Rafii M, Firoozia H, Golimbu C, Beranbaum E: CT of skeletal metastasis. Semin Ultrasound CT MR 1986;7:371-379.
41. Kaplan PA, Orton DF, Asleson R: Osteoporosis with vertebral compression fractures, retropulsed fragments and neurologic compromise. Radiology 1987;165:533-535.
42. Resnick D, Nemcek AA Jr, Haghighi P: Spinal enostosis (bone island). Radiology 1983;147:373-376.
43. Williams AL, Haughton VM: Computed tomographic evaluation of lumbar and thoracic degenerative disc disease. In Post MJD (ed): Computed tomography of the spine. Baltimore, Williams & Wilkins, 1984, pp 307-321.
44. Kagen S, Rafii M, Kramer EL: Focal uptake on bone imaging in an asymptomatic Schmorl's node. Clin Nucl Med 1988;13:615-616.

45. Cooper KL, Beabout JW, Swee RG: Insufficiency fractures of the sacrum. Radiology 1985;156:15-20.

46. DeSmet AA, Neff JR: Pubic and sacral insufficiency fractures: clinical course and radiologic findings. AJR 1985;145:601-606.

47. Rafii M, Firooznia H, Golimbu C, Horner N: Radiation induced fractures of sacrum: CT diagnosis. J Comput Assist Tomogr 1988;12(2):231-235.

48. Zlatkin MB, Lander PH, Hadjipavlou AG, Levine JS. Paget disease of the spine: CT with clinical correlation. Radiology 1986;160:155-159.

49. Schreiman JS, McLeod R, Kyle R, et al. Multiple myeloma: evaluation by CT. Radiology 1985;154:483-486.

50. Firooznia H, Golimbu C, Rafii M, et al: Computed tomography of spinal chordomas. J Comput Tomogr 1986;10:45-50.

51. Bragg DG, Colby TV, Ward JH: New concepts in the non-Hodgkin lymphomas: radiologic applications. Radiology 1986;159:289-304.

52. Mikhael MA, Paige ML: Hodgkin's disease of spine: computed tomography and magnetic resonance imaging. J Comput Tomogr 1987;11:174-177.

53. Beres J, Pech P, Berns T, et al: Spinal epidural lymphomas: CT features in seven patients. AJNR 1986;7:327-328.

54. Ling A, Horvath K, et al: Comparison of radionuclide scintigraphy with MR imaging in evaluation of bone neoplasia. Radiology 1987;165(P):275.

55. Weaver GR, Sandler MP: Increased sensitivity of magnetic resonance imaging compared to radionuclide bone scintigraphy in the detection of lymphoma of the spine. Clin Nucl Med 1987;12:333-334.

56. Emory TH, Albuquerque NM, Orrison WW, et al: Comparison of Gd-DTPA MR imaging and radionuclide bone scans. Radiology 1987;165(P):342.

57. Daffner RH, Lupetin AR, Dash N, et al: MRI in the detection of malignant infiltration of bone marrow. AJR 1986;146:353-358.

58. Sarpel S, Sarpel G, Yu E, et al: Early diagnosis of spinal-epidural metastasis by magnetic resonance imaging. Cancer 1987;59:1112-1116.

59. Kattapuram S, Khurana J, Scott JA, El-Khoury GY. Negative scintigraphy with positive magnetic resonance imaging in bone metastases. Skeletal Radiology 1990;19:113-116.

60. Dooms GC, Maldague B, Malghem J, et al: Prospective comparison of nuclear medicine studies and MR imaging regarding the detection of vertebral and pelvic metastases. Radiology 1988;165(P):275.

61. Paushter DM, Modic MT, Masaryk TJ: Magnetic resonance imaging of the spine: applications and limitations. Radiol Clin North Am 1985;23(3):551-562.

62. Sugimura K, Yamasaki K, Kitagaki H, et al: Bone marrow diseases of the spine: differentiation with T1 and T2 relaxation times in MR imaging. Radiology 1987;165:541-544.

63. Porter BA, Olson DO, Stimac GK, et al: Low-field STIR imaging of marrow malignancies. Radiology 1988;165(P):275.

64. Stimac GK, Porter BA, Olson DO, et al: Gadolinium-DTPA–enhanced MR imaging of spinal neoplasms: preliminary investigation and comparison with unenhanced spin-echo and STIR sequences. AJR 1988;151:1185-1192.

65. Baker LL, Goodman SB, Perkash I, et al: Benign versus pathologic compression fractures of vertebral bodies: assessment with conventional spin-echo, chemical shift, and STIR MR imaging. Radiology 1990;174:495-502.

66. Smoker WR, Godersky JC, Knutzon RK, et al: The role of MR imaging in evaluating metastatic spinal disease. AJR 1987;149:1241-1248.

67. Berry I, Manelfe C, Chastin I: Gd-DTPA enhancement of cerebral and spinal tumors on MR imaging. Radiology 1988;165(P):38.

68. Sze G, Krol G, Zimmerman RD, Deck MD: Malignant extradural spinal tumors. MR imaging with Gd-DTPA. Radiology 1988;167:217-223.

69. Sze G, Krol G, Zimmerman RD, Deck MD: Intramedullary disease of the spine: diagnosis using gadolinium DTPA–enhanced MR imaging. AJR 1988;151:1193-1204.

70. Volk J. Gd-DTPA in MR of spinal lesions. AJR 1988;150:1163-1168.

71. Sze G, Abramson A, Krol G, Liu D, et al: Gadolinium-DTPA in the evaluation of intradural extramedullary spinal disease. AJNR 1988;9:153-163. AJR 1988;150:911-921.

72. Bydder GM, Young IR: MR imaging: clinical use of the inversion recovery sequence. J Comput Assist Tomogr 1985;9:659-675.

73. Porter BA, Olson DO, Stimac GK, et al: STIR imaging of marrow malignancies. In Proceedings of the annual meeting of the Society of Magnetic Resonance Medicine, Vol. 1. New York City, August 1987, p 146.

74. Yuh WTC, Zacher CK, Barloon T, et al: Vertebral compression fractures: distinction between benign and malignant causes with MR imaging. Radiology 1989;172:215-218.

75. Frager D, Eline, Swerdlow M, Bloch S: Subacute osteoporotic compression fractures: misleading magnetic resonance appearance. Skeletal Radiol 1988;17:123-126.

76. Sobel F, Zyroff J, Thorne RP: Diskogenic vertebral sclerosis: MR imaging. J Comput Assist Tomogr 1987;11:855-858.

77. Hajek PC, Baker LL, Goobar JE, Sartosis D: Focal fat deposition in axial bone marrow: MR characteristics. Radiology 1987;162:245-249.

78. Ramsey RG, Zacharias CE: MR imaging of the spine after radiation therapy: easily recognizable effects. AJR 1985;144:1131-1135.

79. Ross JS, Masaryk TJ, Modic MT, et al: Vertebral hemangiomas: MR imaging. Radiology 1987;165:165-167.

80. Fruehwald FX, Tscholakoff D, Schwaighofer B, et al: Magnetic resonance imaging of the lower vertebral column in patients with multiple myeloma. Invest Radiol 1988;23:193-199.

81. Holtas SL, Kido DK, Simon J: MR imaging of spinal lymphoma. J Comput Assist Tomogr 1986;10:111-115.

82. Shields AF, Porter BA, Churchley S, et al: The detection of bone marrow involvement by lymphoma using magnetic resonance imaging. J Clin Oncol 1987;5:225-230.

83. Coleman LK, Porter BA, Redmond J, et al: Early diagnosis of spinal metastases by CT and MR studies. J Comput Assist Tomogr 1988;12:423-426.

84. Lukas P, Stepan R, Bauer R, et al: MR imaging of skeletal metastases: evaluation of the therapeutic impact (WIP). Radiology 1969;173(P):397.

85. Zimmer WD, Berquist TH, McLeod RA, et al: Bone tumors: magnetic resonance imaging versus computed tomography. Radiology 1985;155:709-718.

86. Beltran J, Noto AM, Chakeres DW, Christoforidis AJ: Tumors of the osseous spine: staging with MR imaging versus CT. Radiology 1987;162:565-569.

87. Hagenan C, Grosh W, Currie M, Wiley RG: Comparison of spinal magnetic resonance imaging and myelography in cancer patients. J Clin Oncol 1987;5:1663-1669.

88. Carmody RF, Yang PJ, Seeley GW, et al: Spinal cord compression due to metastatic disease: diagnosis with MR imaging versus myelography. Radiology 1989;173:225-229.

13 CT-Guided Percutaneous Needle Biopsy of Skeletal Lesions

MAHVASH RAFII

In 1930 Martin and Ellis[1] first reported utilizing percutaneous needle aspiration biopsy in the histological diagnosis of soft tissue and bony tumors. Their 65 patients included 8 who had bone tumors. Subsequently, Coley et al.[2] reported 91% accuracy in a group of 35 patients with a variety of lesions diagnosed by percutaneous aspiration. These authors cited safety, expediency, and lower cost to the patient as advantages. As possible disadvantages they cited inadequate sampling of tissue, the potential for seeding malignant cells along the needle track, and the possibility of distant metastases caused by needle separation and entrance into the bloodstream of malignant cells as a result of intramural hemorrhage. In their cases, the biopsy site was selected on the basis of roentgenographic appearance and the procedure was performed under local anesthesia using an 18-gauge needle. In 1947 Ellis[3] introduced the drill biopsy technique, which provided a core of tissue for histopathological examination. Subsequently, other trephine needles were designed[4-6] that permitted sampling of osteoblastic lesions and of lesions embedded within normal bone. A review of the literature in 1981 by Murphy et al.[7] indicated that both aspiration and trephine techniques were rather widely utilized, mostly by surgeons, yielding clinically useful information in more than 75% of aspiration biopsies and more than 80% of core biopsies. In series combining aspiration and trephine the accuracy was 94%. A high accuracy of 95.4% was also reported by Mink[8] using a trephine technique, and of 80% and 90% by El-Khoury et al.[9] and Alder and Rosenberger[10] using fine needle aspiration of osteolytic lesions.

The techniques of aspiration and trephine biopsy were further refined and supported by radiological advances.

As early as 1939, image intensifiers were used for biopsy guidance.[11] In reporting the largest experience with spinal biopsy, including that of the thoracic spine, Ottolenghi[12] stressed the significance of roentgenographic control for its successful completion. In 1967 Rabinov et al.[13] and in 1970 Lalli[14] advocated the use of fluoroscopic guidance and, along with later authors (Debnam and Staple[15] in 1975 and Murphy et al.[7] in 1981), promoted it as a procedure that should be performed primarily by radiologists. Radionuclide bone scanning was used for selecting and locating the biopsy site when no radiographic abnormalities were detectable.[8] Finally, CT was introduced for the precise location of a lesion and as an aid in proper placement of the needle.[16-18] These techniques, along with advances in cytopathology, have enhanced the utilization of percutaneous biopsy in recent years.

CT VERSUS FLUOROSCOPY FOR PERCUTANEOUS BONE BIOPSY

Although fluoroscopic guidance for percutaneous bone biopsy is adequate when the lesion can be readily visualized and is accessible, there are numerous benefits to utilizing CT when a percutaneous biopsy is planned. In bone-scan-positive/radiograph-negative cases, CT can reveal an osseous abnormality anywhere in the skeletal system and thus avert a blind procedure.[8] CT may also demonstrate inaccessibility of a lesion and influence the choice of needle to be used.[17] It also allows the needle to be located precisely within the lesion, thereby improving results through appropriate tissue sampling. More important, it improves the safety of the procedure by allowing the radiologist to avoid vital organs in the path of the

421

needle. Finally, CT enables the operator to reach a deep-seated lesion in an area with complex anatomy.

However, the use of CT instead of fluoroscopy for percutaneous biopsy is not recommended by all, even for small lesions. This probably reflects individuals' prior good experiences with the fluoroscopy-guided biopsy technique.[9] Nevertheless, certain small or bone-scan-positive/radiograph-negative lesions may not be considered suitable for percutaneous biopsy with fluoroscopy. There are certain disadvantages in using CT for guidance because of difficulty visualizing the needle and the lesion in the same axial plane (e.g., at L5-S1), because of added radiation, and because the procedure is more time consuming.[19] A suitable alternative might be to use CT selectively for small or bone-scan-positive/radiograph-negative lesions and for lesions located deeply or in complex anatomic regions.[8,20] In one series[21] the lower accuracy rate reported for biopsies of flat bones and peripheral skeletal lesions compared to spinal lesions (66% vs. 84%) may have reflected difficulty in positioning the needle, a situation that could be positively affected by the use of CT guidance.

Thus the choice of fluoroscopy or CT for percutaneous bone biopsy appears to depend on a variety of factors — prior experience and personal preference of the radiologist, availability of the modality, the support personnel, and the type of lesion selected. In spite of several disadvantages, CT guidance for percutaneous bone biopsy is the preferred choice in most instances. Advances in imaging techniques (i.e., radionuclide bone scanning, CT scanning, MRI) have increasingly improved the early detection of osseous lesions when they are not readily visualized by conventional roentgenography and may not be satisfactorily located by fluoroscopy. Routine utilization of CT guidance, with the attendant increased familiarity in its use, can lead to expediency, reduced duration of the procedure, and lessened radiation exposure.

Indications

1. Percutaneous bone biopsy is most widely used for confirmation and histological verification of suspected skeletal metastatic lesions,[8,21-23] which may be discovered (a) during the investigation and staging of an extraosseous primary cancer, (b) after the initial treatment of a primary cancer, or (c) without a known primary malignancy. In each of these instances, and when two primaries are present simultaneously, histological documentation of the osseous lesion usually plays a significant role in proper treatment planning.

2. Occasionally other benign lesions or systemic disorders of bone will be subjected to percutaneous biopsy[7,25] — sarcoidosis, Paget's disease, fibrous dysplasia, histiocytosis. In most of these instances the purpose is to verify the radiographic diagnosis and exclude a malignant lesion.

3. When musculoskeletal or articular infection is suspected, aspiration is performed to obtain culture material and drain abscesses. It is used most widely in patients with suspected spinal osteomyelitis.[24]

Primary tumors of bone other than myeloma and round cell tumors comprise a small percentage of percutaneous biopsies reported in the literature, due in part to their significantly lower incidence than that of metastatic bony lesions. Also, although closed biopsy of primary bony tumors has been done with an accuracy as high as 93%[22,26] and recommended by some radiologists,[25,27] a lower success rate has been reported by others.[7,21] Certain investigators[28] do not recommend percutaneous techniques for obtaining tissue in suspected primary bone tumors. This variability of opinion may be related to the preferred needle biopsy techniques, some of which do not yield adequate amounts of tissue for a histological diagnosis (i.e., fine needle aspiration), or the preference of the pathologist who examines the biopsy material. Due to our skewed patient population, we have had less experience with percutaneous biopsy of primary bone tumors, but we have generally been successful. Although it seems logical that an aggressive approach to suspected primary musculoskeletal tumors with trephine needles and multiple sampling of the lesion should provide adequate tissue for a definitive histological diagnosis, nevertheless in many medical centers primary tumors of bone remain the concern of orthopedic surgeons who consider open biopsy a more definitive procedure without the risk of false-negative or false-positive results.[25]

Selection of the biopsy site

The biopsy procedure is usually requested by an orthopedist or oncologist who has been consulted to evaluate the patient for suspected skeletal malignancy or infection. Review of the patient's clinical history and available pertinent radiographic studies is mandatory for determining the feasibility of the procedure and selecting the site. The proposed site of a biopsy is most often based on an abnormality seen on roentgenograms, with or without a prior radionuclide bone scan. When a single focus of abnormal uptake appears on the bone scan, there is an approximately 50% chance of malignancy.[29] Collins et al.[30] detected malignancy in 41% of patients with a solitary focus on bone scan but no apparent roentgenographic abnormality at percutaneous biopsy of the suspected site. Nevertheless, any bone scan abnormality should be thoroughly evaluated by conventional roentgenography and/or CT before biopsy is planned. When multiple lesions are present, the most accessible one is chosen. Due to relative lack of specificity, lesions detected by MRI should be correlated with conventional roentgenographic and/or CT findings prior to biopsy.

Most lesions biopsied are suspected metastases and most involve the spine and pelvis. However, in one series[31] the majority of aspirated spinal lesions were suspected osteomyelitis; and in another[25] the number of peripheral skeletal lesions biopsied approached that of spinal lesions biopsied (probably indicative of either a skewed patient population or a personal preference by the radiologist or orthopedic surgeon). In the spine, the lumbar region is the most common site for biopsy (followed by the thoracic and cervical regions), because of the lower incidences of solitary thoracic and cervical involvement without simultaneous lumbar involvement and because a percutaneous biopsy in these regions is more difficult. Fluoroscopic guidance is particularly difficult because of the proximity to vital organs. CT guidance is most helpful in selecting a safe approach.[17,18]

The ribs and sternum, also common sites for metastases, are readily amenable to percutaneous biopsy with CT guidance. Aspiration of superficial or deep joints is frequently performed for diagnosis of infection. Deep joints, such as the sacroiliac, are best aspirated with CT guidance to ensure proper needle location, but the shoulder and hip may also be aspirated with fluoroscopic guidance unless the suspected lesion is primarily osseous and the procedure intended for tissue sampling.

Patient preparation

Unless there is a considerable risk for complications or the patient is in extreme discomfort and must be heavily sedated, percutaneous biopsy can be performed on an outpatient basis. At most, an overnight stay is all that is required. The patient should be fasting for several hours, and a moderate degree of sedation is generally recommended[21]: a dose of 10 mg diazepam PO, 50 to 75 mg meperidine IM, or 10 mg morphine IM. We use 50 mg of meperidine and 5 to 10 mg of diazepam PO. In some young children, depending at least in part upon the location of the lesion, general anesthesia (instead of heavy sedation) is unavoidable.

Choice of biopsy needle

A variety of needles can be used for aspiration or trephine biopsy dependent upon the type of lesion, the specific information needed, and the expertise of the pathologist. A core of tissue obtained by a trephine needle (with organization of the tissue maintained) permits histological evaluation of the lesion. Aspiration causes distortion of tissue, and the diagnosis relies mostly on cell morphology.

1. Aspiration biopsy: An 18- to 20-gauge spinal needle is used. Recently fine needles (21 to 22 gauge) have been proposed[9] for biopsy of the soft parts of osseous lesions. Chiba needles are used mostly for biopsy of the viscera but may be similarly employed to sample osteolytic lesions.[22]
2. Trephine biopsy: Various needles have been designed for obtaining cores of tissue from bone or soft tissue components of osseous lesions.[4–6,32] The set we most often utilize is a 12-gauge *Ackerman* (Fig. 13-1), which is available in two lengths for superficial and deep lesions. It has a cannula with a gauge diameter of 2.5 mm and a cutting trocar with a bore of 1.5 mm. The specimens obtained are 1.2 mm in diameter. The

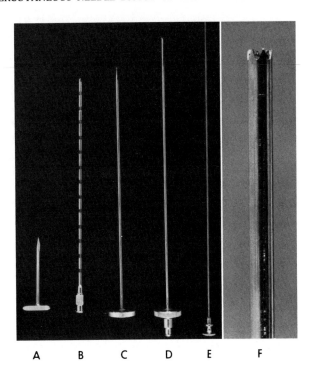

FIGURE 13-1
An unassembled Ackerman needle set for trephine bone biopsy. *A* is the perforator; *B*, the cannula (graded); *C*, the guide (pointed trocar); *D*, the cutting trocar; *E*, the blunt trocar; and, *F*, the magnified serrated tip of the cutting trocar. After preparation of the skin, the assembled cannula and guide are advanced to the lesion. The cannula is held in place while the guide is removed and replaced by the cutting trocar.

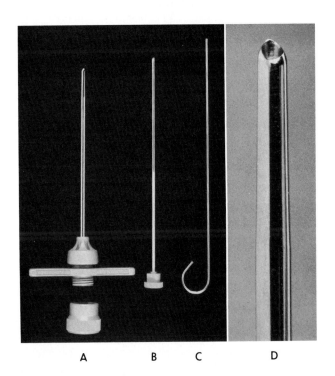

FIGURE 13-2
An unassembled Jamshidi needle set. *A* is the needle with rotating handle and detached screw top. This is assembled when the guide is in place. *B* is the guide (stylet). *C* is the blunt trocar and, *D*, the magnified tip of the needle.

Craig needle has a gauge diameter of 3.5 mm. Both these sets consist of a pointed trocar (locator), a cannula (or trephine guide), usually two cutting trocars with serrated ends, and a blunt trocar. The cutting trocar, when in place, projects 2.5 cm beyond the cannula, the maximum extent that the needle can be advanced into the lesion. The Craig set also includes a rotating handle. Variations of these needles with a rigid guidewire have been introduced.[33,34] The *Jamshidi needle* set (Fig. 13-2), originally introduced for marrow biopsy, consists of a cutting needle with a smooth tapered distal end (1 cm) and a stylet.[32,35] It is designed to produce less crush artifacts within the specimen.

Several types of needles are available for obtaining a core of tissue from osteolytic or soft tissue tumors. The *Westerman-Jensen* and *Vim-Silverman* have blades that grasp the tissue.[15] The *Vim Tru-Cut* includes a bayonet-shaped inner core[22] and features an unbeveled smooth cutting end. A variation of this needle, the Sur-Cut, includes an assembled syringe whose plunger attaches to a stylet. The plunger, when withdrawn, can be hooked to the top of the syringe to maintain negative pressure. The Vacu-Cut needle uses the same principle without a syringe.

TECHNIQUE

The procedure is performed under sterile conditions. The skin and subcutaneous tissue, down to and including the periosteum, are infiltrated with local anesthetic (usually 2% xylocaine). The anesthetic needle is then replaced by the appropriate aspiration needle. When possible, the anesthetic needle may be advanced into the lesion and an aspiration attempted. It may also be left in place, as a guide for the biopsy needle, which is then advanced alongside it.

Aspiration and trephine biopsy of osteolytic lesions

When a spinal needle is being used for aspiration, the combination needle and stylet is advanced to the surface of the lesion and the stylet is removed. First, a 10 ml syringe is firmly attached to the needle, and the combination is advanced into the lesion and pulled back several times while negative pressure is applied. Then the needle and syringe are removed together while the negative pressure is slowly released. Since some lesions have necrotic centers, it is best to direct the needle toward the periphery of the lesion.[9] With CT for guidance such necrotic foci are visualized and can be avoided.

To obtain a core of tissue from an osteolytic lesion, first the assembled needle is advanced to the periphery of the lesion; then, after the stylet or the attached syringe has been partially withdrawn, the needle is further advanced into the lesion once and withdrawn.

Trephine biopsy of osteoblastic lesions

When the *Ackerman* needle is used for trephine biopsy, the following technique is employed: After local anesthesia a small incision is made in the skin and the subcutaneous tissue is separated with the perforator device. The assembled cannula and guide (pointed trocar) are then advanced to the surface of the bone. At this point the guide is removed and additional anesthetic is applied to the periosteum. An attempt can be made to perforate the intact cortex with the guide. Otherwise, while the cannula is held in place, the guide is removed and replaced by the cutting trocar, which is advanced through the cortical bone and into the lesion with a rotating motion.

Before the cutting trocar is removed, a side-to-side motion will help separate the core from the surrounding bone. The cannula is held in place while the cutting trocar is pulled and the specimen is removed. If necessary, the sampling can be repeated at a slightly different orientation.

Occasionally a deep-seated lesion will be surrounded by normal bone and not be reachable by the cutting trocar (which extends only 2.5 cm beyond the tip of the cannula). If possible, the cutting trocar from the long set may be coupled with the short cannula; but extreme care must be exercised not to advance the cutting needle beyond the lesion.

When the *Jamshidi* needle is used, the needle and guide are advanced to the periphery of the lesion. Then the guide is removed and the needle is further advanced into the lesion with a rotary motion (NOTE: The handle can be attached to the needle at this point.)

Repeated sampling up to four to five times has been recommended[8]; but with CT for guidance and appropriate location of the needle within the lesion, it is usually not required (unless tissue is needed for additional histological or bacteriological studies). To optimize results, a combination of aspiration and core biopsy for nearly all lesions is recommended.[7]

Our preference is to aspirate osteolytic lesions first. The aspirated material is prepared on site by an experienced cytology technologist in the form of a smear. If it is considered adequately cellular and concurs with the clinical diagnosis, the study is terminated. Aspiration is repeated when the first attempt fails to obtain adequate tissue or when additional tissue for special staining is needed. The remaining aspirated material within the needle and syringe is flushed into a container of Hank's solution for cell block preparation.

In more complex situations, as when the lesion is obscure or unknown, a trephine biopsy is also obtained with (at most) two cores for histopathological examination. The aspirated osseous blood (clot and smear) is valuable for revealing the morphology of malignant cells and should not be discarded.[36] With suspected infection additional aspirated material is collected in sterile con-

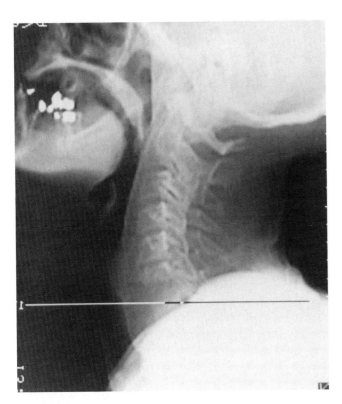

FIGURE 13-3
Locating a suitable site for needle biopsy. The digital scout view of the cervical spine clearly shows an abnormality (osteomyelitis). A single axial section is planned for biopsy.

tainers. If aspiration does not yield material for culture, a small amount of sterile saline (not containing bacteriostatic agents) is introduced and reaspirated. In approximately 50% of spinal osteomyelitis cases aspiration does not lead to positive identification of the infecting organism.[31] Then the availability of tissue for histological evaluation is helpful and for this reason an additional core biopsy is recommended.

Patient positioning and approach

Spine. The patient is placed prone. It has been suggested[33,34] that elevating to a prone oblique position will orient the lesion in the vertical path of the needle. This is helpful when fluoroscopic guidance is being used or the lesion is adjacent to a curved surface, such as the anterior aspect of the vertebral body, but otherwise it is cumbersome and unnecessary.

The region is first scanned to locate the lesion. Next, the images are viewed and the most suitable level for biopsy is selected and a trajectory formed. When the lesion is identifiable on the scout view (Fig. 13-3), it may be generally located by selection of the level on the digital scout. Then, with the available software the point of needle entry and the path of insertion are mapped on the image. Finally, the distance from the midline (based on an anatomical landmark [e.g., the spinous process] or the "grid localizer"), the depth of the lesion, and the angle of insertion are determined (Fig. 13-4).

A

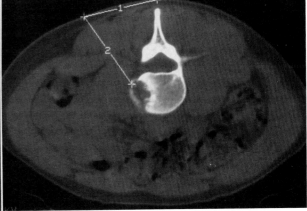

B

C

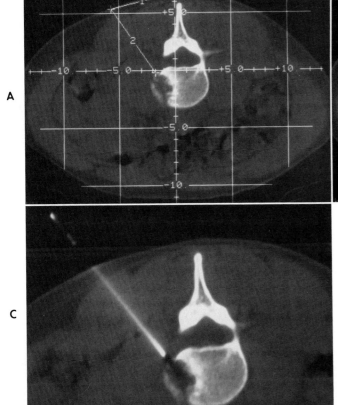

FIGURE 13-4
CT-guided spinal biopsy at L3. **A,** The selected level with grid displayed. The appropriate needle entry point is determined. The distances from the grid midline *(1)* and the surface of the lesion *(2)* are measured. **B,** The distance from the midline may also be measured using the spinous process as the point of reference. **C,** The orientation of the needle approximates that of line *2*, with the needle at the surface of the lesion. At this point the stylet is removed and the needle is advanced into the lesion while negative pressure is applied.

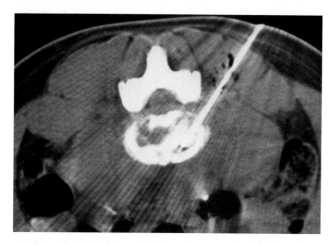

FIGURE 13-5
Percutaneous needle biopsy at L3-4 for spinal osteomyelitis. The needle is directed into the eroded vertebral endplate through the posterolateral vertebral surface.

The orientation of the needle and its distance from the midline are based on two critical factors: the shortest possible route and the proper needle-to-cortex angle. To prevent the needle tip from slipping off the bone surface, a perpendicular orientation (or close to it) is desirable. However, in approaching vertebral body lesions, an oblique orientation may be unavoidable unless the needle can be placed directly against the posterolateral vertebral or diskal surface (Fig. 13-5). Achieving proper orientation relative to the vertebral surface is particularly desired when the lesion is entirely blastic or surrounded by intact cortical bone, because an oblique orientation proves more challenging in these instances (Fig. 13-6). Passage of the needle peripheral to a lumbar neural foramen can produce radicular pain (which, though intense, fortunately, is only transient). Flexibility of the nerve root allows safe passage of the needle and avoids damage.

After mapping of the biopsy route and appropriate measurements, a laser localizer is used and a trajectory is formed by marking the site of needle entry on the skin with an indelible marker. Marking on the skin surface both the axial plane of the biopsy and the point of entry of the needle helps keep the needle within the biopsy plane while it is being advanced. Depending upon the complexity of the biopsy site, one or more images are obtained during needle advancement to ensure proper orientation with respect to the lesion. The needle must remain within the predetermined plane so its tip can be visualized during scanning. A thicker axial image is therefore more practical, although in the cervical and thoracic regions we routinely employ 5 mm sections during a biopsy procedure.

With solid-appearing lesions the needle may be conveniently angled in any direction. With lesions that contain low-density regions due to necrosis, the needle should be angled toward solid tumor or (as a rule) toward the periphery of the lesion (Fig. 13-7). Aspiration biopsy in spinal osteomyelitis may simply involve tapping a

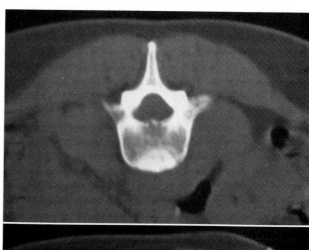

A

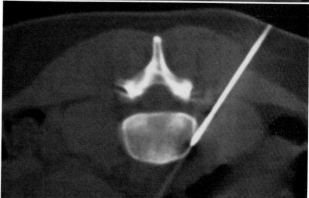

B

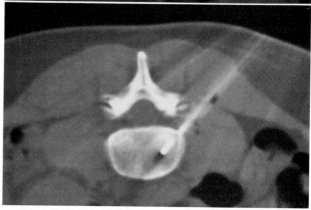

C

FIGURE 13-6
Trephine needle biopsy, lumbar spine, showing the position of the needle. **A,** This patient with carcinoma of the breast has a blastic lesion on the anterior aspect of L3. **B,** The cutting needle would not "hook" into the bone. This image confirms its poor alignment. **C,** It was withdrawn and repositioned relatively vertical to the posterolateral surface of the vertebra. Tissue recovered was consistent with metastatic breast carcinoma. Another option would have been to position the needle further from the midline with a steeper angle. However, this would have entailed a longer track through soft tissues.

paraspinal abscess, if one is present. Otherwise, the needle should be angled into the involved and eroded bone (Fig. 13-5). MRI may be utilized for identifying regions of acute inflammatory reaction or fluid collection prior to aspiration biopsy.

In approaching a *thoracic lesion* the same principles are followed, although certain deviations may become necessary:

FIGURE 13-7
Metastatic renal cell carcinoma (same lesion as in Fig. 12-25, *A*). The biopsy needle is appropriately directed to the vertebral aspect of the lesion, where solid tissue is present.

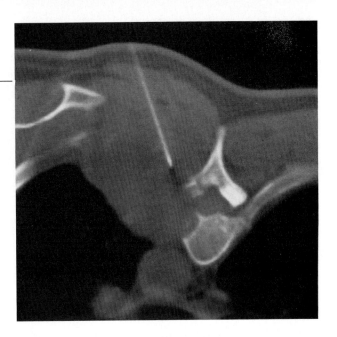

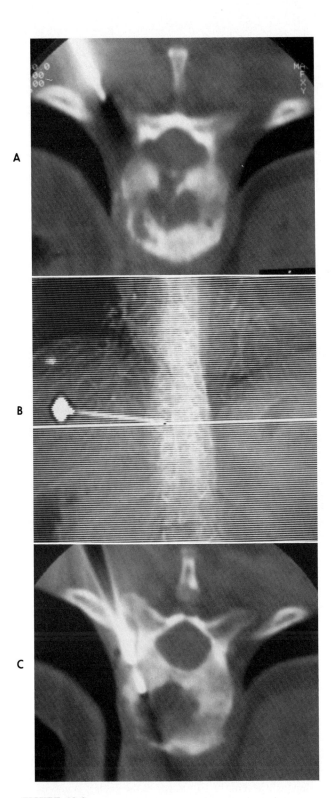

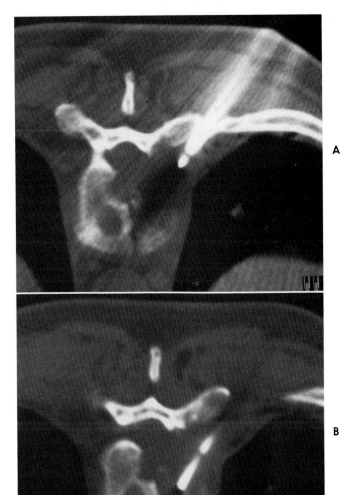

FIGURE 13-8
Biopsy needle location in the thoracic spine. **A,** In this patient the needle had to be maneuvered over the costotransverse junction. Its oblique orientation is suggested by the fact that its proximal end was seen in this section. Its distal end falsely resembles its tip. **B,** A scout view shows the tilted needle. **C,** An axial image at the level of the tip discloses that it is well within the lesion.

FIGURE 13-9
Biopsy needle location in the thoracic spine. In this patient the needle was tilted over the costotransverse junction. Two consecutive images — **A,** at the level of needle entry and, **B,** 5 mm above that level — were acquired. Notice the tip of the needle within the lesion (in **B**).

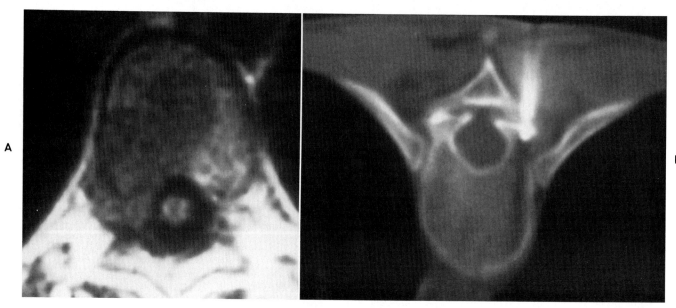

FIGURE 13-10
Trephine biopsy, thoracic spine. **A** shows a destructive lesion, primarily of the anterocentral aspect of T12, with erosion and extension into the spinal canal. The pedicles are intact. **B,** Steep angulation of the needle was required for a lateral approach, but this could not easily be done into the space between the rib and kidney. A posterolateral approach at the base of the pedicle was selected as a shorter and safer alternative. Due to the distance of the lesion from the cortical surface, the long cutting trocar was used through a short cannula.

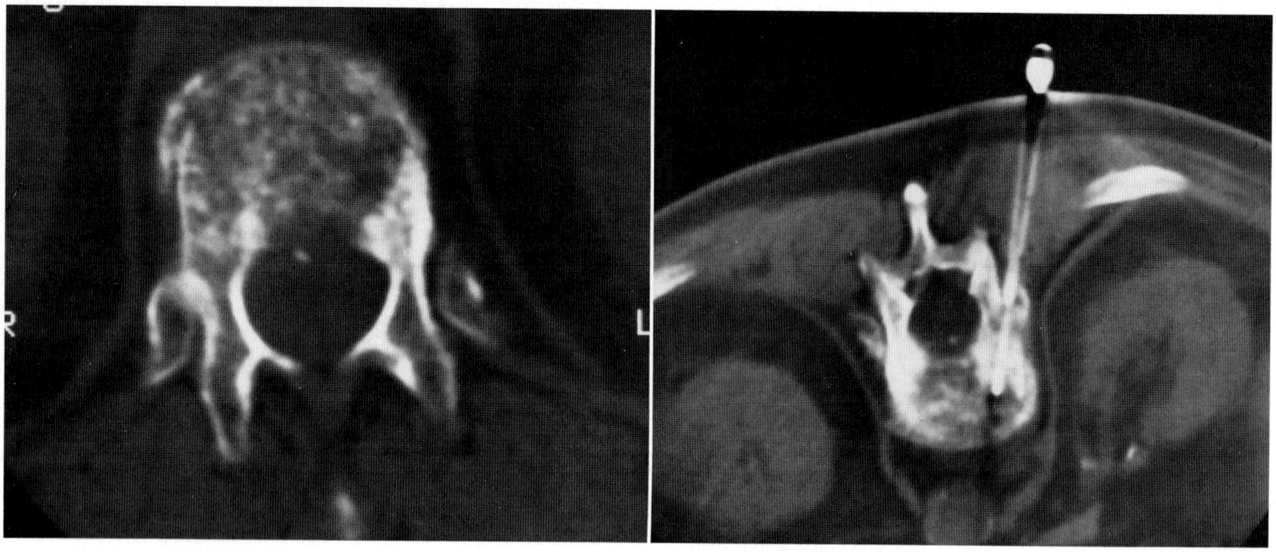

FIGURE 13-11
Trephine biopsy, thoracic spine, showing the approach to a single osseous lesion detected by bone scan at T7. **A,** The axial T1-weighted image (550/30) shows extension of the lesion into the body and pedicle of T7 and no paraspinal soft tissue mass. **B,** The needle could be advanced into the lesion only through the pedicle. The diagnosis was malignant lymphoma.

Often an oblique orientation of the needle relative to the axial plane will be unavoidable when maneuvering under a rib or transverse process. In these instances the location of the needle tip is determined by obtaining a scout view and scanning at the level where the tip is visualized (Fig. 13-8). An alternative is to obtain several (possibly three) consecutive axial images (Fig. 13-9).

A lateral approach to thoracic lesions may not be possible when little or no paraspinal soft tissue is present or there is an abnormal spinal curvature. In these instances the needle may be advanced, slowly and with great caution, through the pedicle (Fig. 13-10), provided the pedicle is normal or shows no signs of imminent pathological fracture (Fig. 13-11).

In approaching a *cervical lesion* the principles vary depending upon the level and the site of the lesion.

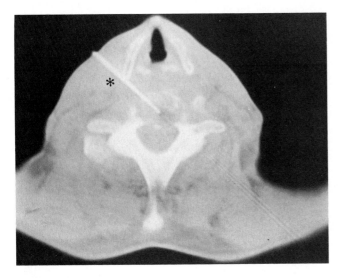

FIGURE 13-12
Needle aspiration biopsy at C5-6 for spinal osteomyelitis. The needle is passed immediately anterior to the carotid sheath *(asterisk)*. With this orientation it safely extends to the center of the lesion. (Courtesy Wendy Cohen, M.D.)

A posterior approach is best for lesions in the posterior arch at all levels, and the patient is positioned prone.[37,38]

An anterior pharyngeal approach, through the open mouth, to the upper cervical vertebral bodies has been described by Ottolenghi et al.[37]; however, it requires general anesthesia and cannot be performed in the CT suite.

An anterior or anterolateral approach may be used for lateral masses of C4 to C7. With the *anterior* approach the needle is passed between the trachea and the carotid artery[38]; however, despite its having been done safely under CT guidance, this is somewhat risky due to the possibility of passage through the thyroid. With the *anterolateral* (or *lateral*) approach the needle passes through or posterior to the sternocleidomastoideus respectively. (Ottolenghi et al.[37] have advocated the lateral approach to avoid entering the spinal canal through a neuroforamen. By using CT guidance it is possible to avoid this and other undesirable complications.)

The most suitable approach to cervical spinal lesions for a CT-guided biopsy is determined by precisely locating the lesion through a prebiopsy CT scan. Any approach (anterior, anterolateral, or lateral) can be safely utilized, and the patient is (accordingly) placed supine, elevated to an anterior oblique position, or simply turned to face the opposite side. Locating the

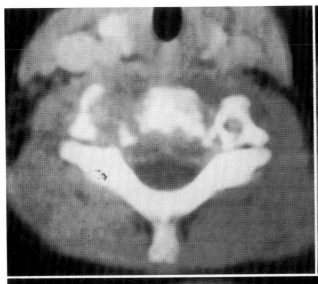

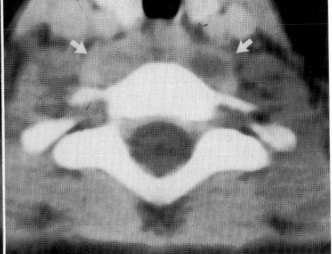

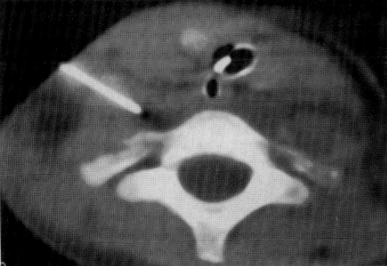

FIGURE 13-13
Cervical spinal biopsy, lateral approach, in a 6-year-old girl with a destructive lesion at C7. **A,** Contrast-enhanced CT shows the lesion with paraspinal and epidural extension. **B,** The paraspinal mass extends inferiorly to T1 *(arrows)*. This level was considered more accessible and was selected for biopsy. **C,** CT image for needle location. With the patient's head tilted to the left, the needle was placed at the lateral aspect of the sternocleidomastoideus and posterior to the carotid vessels. The tip, visible at the surface of the mass in this image, was then advanced and aspiration was performed. Recovered tissue indicated eosinophilic granuloma.

lesion and mapping the area are done as previously described. The needle path is planned to pass immediately in front of or behind the carotid sheath, with varying shifts for a vertebral body (or paravertebral soft tissues) or a lateral mass lesion (Figs. 13-12 to 13-15). This technique, with some reservations and the exercise of caution, may be applied to both the upper cervical spine (Fig. 13-16) and the occipital region (Fig. 13-17).

After the lesion is located and the area mapped, the anesthetic needle is advanced immediately posterior (or anterior) to the carotid sheath (which should be palpated and displaced away from the needle). Selection of a high-gauge (small) needle is prudent. An 18-gauge Seldinger needle, through which a 21-gauge needle can be passed, has been found useful for cervical spinal biopsies.[39] Similar to trephine needles (e.g., the Ackerman), it permits multiple samples to be obtained from the lesion after the Seldinger needle is properly placed. The

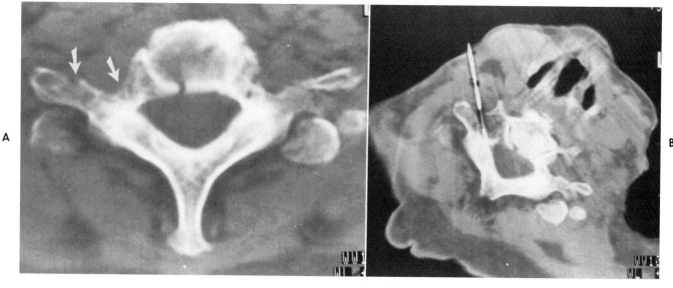

FIGURE 13-14
Cervical spinal biopsy, anterolateral approach, in a patient with no known primary multiple lesions of the liver but with a single permeative osseous lesion in the lateral body and transverse process of C7 (denoted by *arrows* in **A**). After two aspirations of liver lesions, a histological diagnosis had not been reached. **B,** The patient is supine, in an anterior oblique position with the head turned to the left. Aspiration produced material that was diagnosed as undifferentiated adenocarcinoma.

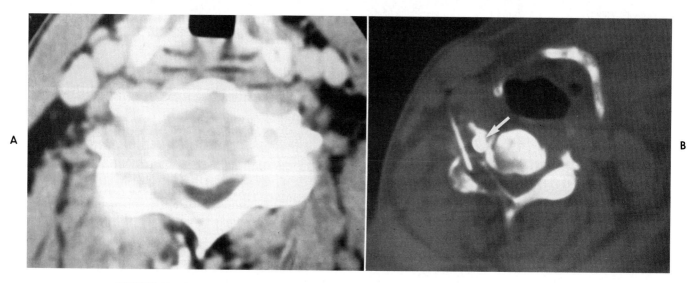

FIGURE 13-15
Cervical spinal biopsy, anterolateral approach. **A,** Contrast-enhanced CT shows a highly vascular expansile lesion in the right side and lamina of C5. It was embolized prior to biopsy and surgical stabilization was scheduled. **B,** With the needle safely directed posterolaterally through a cortical defect, material was obtained that indicated plasmacytoma. The *arrow* points to the cast of the embolized vertebral artery.

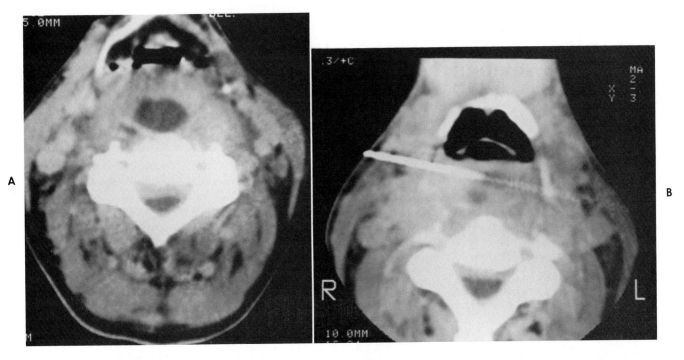

FIGURE 13-16
Aspiration and abscess drainage in a patient with C3-4 spinal osteomyelitis. **A,** Contrast-enhanced CT reveals a paraspinal abscess (3.5 × 1.5 cm) with a small epidural collection. **B,** Aspiration for bacteriological diagnosis was also intended as a simple drainage procedure. The needle was passed anterior to the carotid sheath and immediately above the thyroid cartilage into the abscess. Collection of pus amounted to 5 ml.

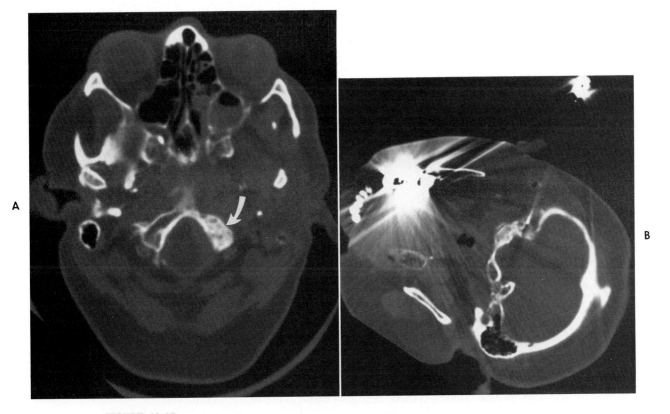

FIGURE 13-17
Aspiration biopsy, metastatic breast carcinoma to the occipital condyle. **A,** CT shows a mixed lytic/blastic lesion of the left occipital condyle *(arrow)*. **B,** With the patient in a steep anterior oblique position the lesion was cleared off the mastoid tip. A 20-gauge spinal needle readily penetrated the abnormal bone in this region. (**A** and **B** courtesy Roy Holliday, M.D.)

importance of thoroughly reviewing all radiographic examinations, particularly CT, and appropriately sedating the patient before the procedure cannot be overstated.

Pelvis. Positioning for pelvic lesions is variable and dependent upon the location of the lesion (Fig. 13-18). In flat bones (pelvis, scapula, and ribs) an oblique orientation of the needle relative to the lesion is desirable and the patient is accordingly positioned if possible. This is helpful in obtaining the maximum amount of tissue and avoiding penetration of underlying structures[22] (Fig. 13-19).

Shoulder and hip. Aspiration of the shoulder and hip for bacteriological investigation is routinely performed under fluoroscopic guidance and via an anterior ap-

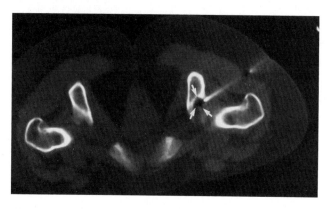

FIGURE 13-18
Aspiration biopsy for a lytic lesion of the posteroinferior acetabular margin. The patient is in an oblique prone position, and the needle is directed anteromedially into the lesion *(arrows).*

proach. Occasionally CT guidance will be needed (Fig. 13-20). A posterior approach may also be chosen for intraarticular osseous lesions (Fig. 13-21). Aspiration of the sacroiliac joint is considerably aided by CT guidance and is conveniently performed with the patient prone (Fig. 13-22).

Superficial joints and long bones. Other, more superficial, joints (sternoclavicular, knee, and ankle) can selectively undergo a CT-guided aspiration biopsy when sampling of a particular focus of infection or destructive lesion is intended (Fig. 13-23). Patient positioning in these cases, and in lesions of the long bones, may also be determined by a prebiopsy CT examination (Fig. 13-24).

PREPARATION OF TISSUE AND ASPIRATED MATERIAL

Tissue and aspirated material should be handled with care. Tissue cores are pushed out gently by the blunt instrument and placed in formalin (preparatory to histological examination) or glutaraldehyde solution (for electron microscopic examination). When lymphoma is suspected, additional tissue may be needed for determination of special lymphoma markers. This tissue is delivered to the laboratory in a separate container of normal saline or Hank's solution. Aspirated material for cytological examination is immediately smeared on glass slides and placed in alcohol. Material intended for bacteriological studies is placed in sterile test tubes or an appropriate culture medium and delivered to the laboratory. Proper handling and processing of biopsy material are as important as a meticulous biopsy technique.

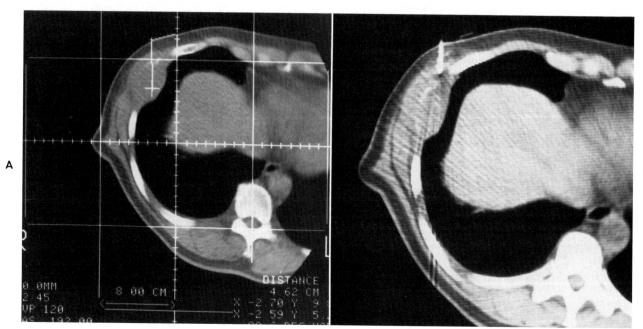

FIGURE 13-19
Percutaneous biopsy of the rib cage. **A,** The needle track is planned to extend obliquely, and the depth of the lesion is measured. **B,** The needle, appropriately oriented in the periphery of the lesion, is then advanced a predetermined amount and withdrawn.

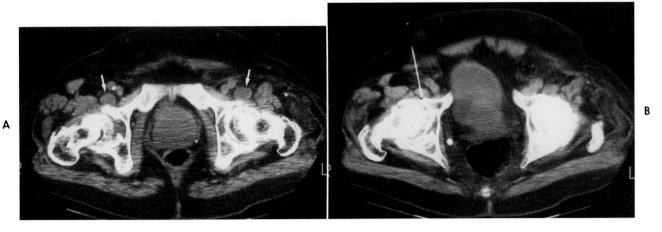

FIGURE 13-20
Needle aspiration of the right hip in an elderly patient with osteoarthritis. A recent episode of bacteremia and persistent hip pain prompted the aspiration by an orthopedist. No fluid was obtained. **A,** The postaspiration CT section shows synovial cysts in the hip joints *(arrows)*. **B,** Reaspiration under CT guidance yielded 2 ml of clear joint effusion.

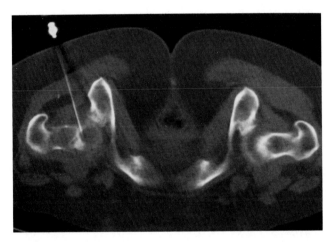

FIGURE 13-21
Percutaneous biopsy of a femoral head lesion. The posterior approach was selected based on proximity of the lesion to the cortical surface. A 20-gauge spinal needle, used for administering local anesthetic, was advanced into the lesion and aspiration was performed.

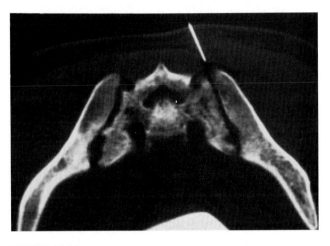

FIGURE 13-22
Needle aspiration for septic sacroiliitis in a patient with sickle cell anemia and a bilateral chronic sacroiliac infection. No abscess collections were present. The needle was advanced into the joint, and several drops of bloody fluid were obtained.

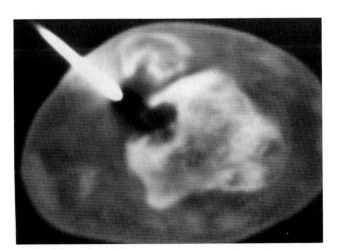

FIGURE 13-23
Trephine needle biopsy of the ankle in a patient with chronic inflammation and suspected septic arthritis. Focal erosive articular lesions of the talus and fibula were targeted for biopsy. The patient is supine, with the extremity rotated so that the medial aspect of the ankle and foot is on the table.

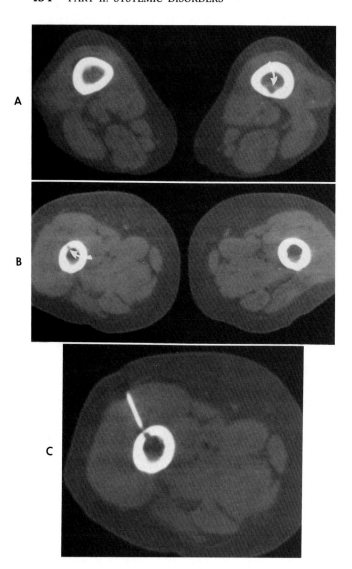

FIGURE 13-24
CT for selection of a biopsy site in a patient in whom two small cortical osteolytic lesions of the left femur were detected radiographically. **A,** The proximal lesion partially involves the cortical/ endosteal interface *(arrow).* **B,** The inferior lesion, which is larger, lies immediately beneath the periosteal/cortical interface. Also, in this region, no major vascular or nerve structures have to be bypassed. **C,** Aspiration was successfully carried out with a 20-gauge spinal needle.

POSTBIOPSY CARE

The care of the patient after biopsy generally depends upon the individual patient. Unless a lesion has invadedthe spinal canal or is found to be highly vascular, the patient may be discharged after a short period of observation. With largely destructive and vascular lesions of the spine or when postprocedure pain exists, the patient should remain under observation for several hours. Appropriate analgesics may be prescribed. After a rib biopsy, examination of the chest is prudent (a single PA view in expiration usually being adequate).

CONTRAINDICATIONS AND PRECAUTIONS

The only actual contraindication to percutaneous biopsy arises in patients with a known bleeding tendency or low platelet count.[25] Routine evaluation for such disorders has not generally been recommended, an opinion shared by us. We do not consider grossly destructive spinal lesions with penetration of the spinal canal a contraindication to percutaneous needle biopsy. Such lesions and those with a radiographic appearance suggesting hypervascularity can be safely aspirated with a 20-gauge spinal needle. Lesions located centrally within the vertebrae with erosion of the bony canal, but otherwise surrounded by normal bone, present a more serious problem in planning percutaneous biopsy (Fig. 13-11). A trephine needle must be used to reach the lesion, and the possibility of hemorrhage is therefore increased. This should be discussed with the referring physician and the patient. Compared to an open biopsy, which is more likely to result in extensive bleeding, fine needle aspiration of a hypervascular lesion (even a trephine biopsy) is a much safer procedure. In the great majority of cases the hemorrhage is contained within the lesion and is self-limiting. The needle (with stylet in place) may also be used as a means of applying pressure at the bleeding site.

Occasionally, a vascular lesion will be embolized prior to biopsy (Fig. 13-25). In addition to minimizing the possibility of hemorrhage, this eliminates or decreases the amount of blood in the aspirate (which improves the quality of smear for cytological preparation and evaluation); it also aids a planned surgical procedure by lowering lesional vascularity (particularly helpful in patients about to undergo tumor resection and/or spinal fusion).

FAILED PERCUTANEOUS BIOPSY

There are several causes for a failed needle biopsy. Faulty technique can lead to improper positioning of the needle, inadequate maneuvering within the lesion, or insufficient negative pressure applied. The consistency of lesions varies. Highly cellular ones generally yield adequate tissue when first attempted, but vascular or friable or necrotic ones may prove difficult and often require several aspirations.

Blastic lesions, particularly when small, may also prove challenging. Malignant cells may not be present within a sample that consists only of reactive bone. Nevertheless, immunohistochemistry tests will usually detect specific enzymes present within the specimens and identify the malignancy. Occasionally only fibrous tissue will be obtained. This totally nonspecific finding should not be accepted as a true-negative result. When the clinical and roentgenographic (or CT) findings are strongly suggestive of malignancy, a repeat core biopsy should be performed and occasionally an open biopsy will be needed to ensure an accurate result (Fig. 13-26).

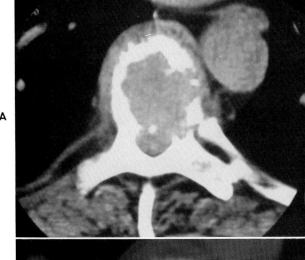

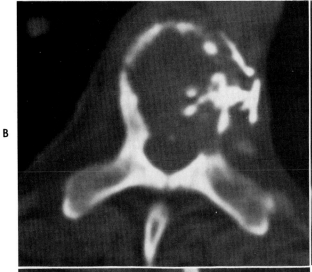

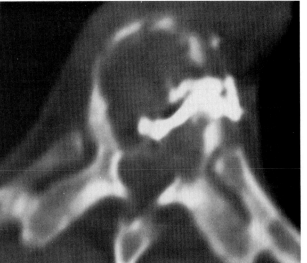

FIGURE 13-25
Prebiopsy embolization in metastatic hypernephroma. **A,** This CT slice depicts the highly vascular lytic lesion at T7. Hypervascularity was later confirmed by spinal angiography. **B** and **C,** Postembolization CT images reveal a large cast of feeding vessels. **D,** Postembolization aspiration biopsy was diagnostic for a hypernephroma.

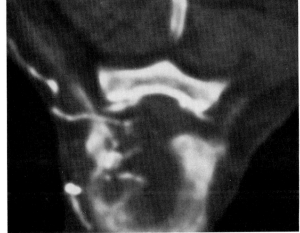

(controllable) hemorrhage. The overall rate of serious complications compiled from several studies has been estimated at 0.2%[7]—and included transient paresis, hemorrhage, infection, pneumothorax, and fracture. Two deaths have been reported, one following meningitis and another with paraplegia, both related to earliest experiences with the technique.

These data, it should be noted, were compiled *prior to* the utilization of CT guidance. Our complications during the past 10 years have consisted of one pneumothorax and one retroperitoneal hematoma. The small pneumothorax, which did not require placement of chest tubes, occurred during an attempt to biopsy a sclerotic benign-appearing lesion of a rib with an Ackerman needle. The retroperitoneal hematoma was due to slippage of the Ackerman pointed guide from the cortical surface of L3. The hematoma presumably resulted from injury to small vessels as the tip of the guide was visualized along the side and in between the aorta and the inferior vena cava. The patient was treated only by bed rest. We have not observed infection or seeding in the path of the needle.

COMPLICATIONS

Percutaneous biopsy of skeletal lesions is a simple and safe procedure. In our experience, and in that of most other investigators, no major complications have been encountered. The morbidity consists mainly of pain during, or less often following, the procedure and mild

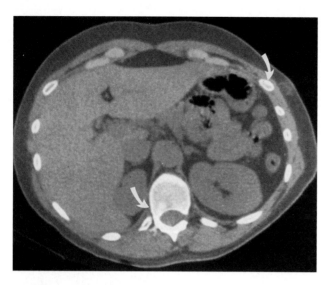

FIGURE 13-26
Blastic metastases from squamous cell carcinoma of the lung. A radionuclide bone scan prior to surgical resection of the primary lesion showed abnormal uptake in the thoracic spine and anterior left rib. No abnormality was detected on conventional roentgenograms, but CT disclosed small blastic lesions at the sites of abnormality on the scan (*arrows*). Needle biopsy of the rib lesion yielded only fibrous tissue. Due to the appearance and multiplicity of the lesions, however, the biopsy result was considered false negative and an open biopsy of the rib lesion was performed by resection of a small segment of rib. This confirmed the presence of metastases and led to the institution of chemotherapy rather than resection of the primary tumor.

REFERENCES

1. Martin HE, Ellis EB: Biopsy by needle puncture and aspiration. Ann Surg 1930;92:169-181.
2. Coley BL, Sharp GS, Ellis EB: Diagnosis of bone tumors by aspiration. Am J Surg 1931;13:215-224.
3. Ellis F: Needle biopsy in clinical diagnosis of tumours. Br J Surg 1947;34:240-261.
4. Turkel H, Bethell FH: Biopsy of bone marrow performed by a new and simple technique. J Lab Clin Med 1943;28:1246-1251.
5. Ackerman W: Vertebral trephine biopsy. Ann Surg 1956;143:373-385.
6. Craig FS: Vertebral-body biopsy. J Bone Joint Surg 1956;38(A):93-102.
7. Murphy WA, Destouet JM, Gilula LA: Percutaneous skeletal biopsy 1981: a procedure for radiologists. Results, review, and recommendations. Radiology 1981;139:545-549.
8. Mink J: Percutaneous bone biopsy in the patient with known or suspected osseous metastases. Radiology 1986;161:191-194.
9. El-Khoury GY, Terepka RH, Mickelson MR, et al: Fine needle aspiration biopsy of bone. J Bone Joint Surg 1983;65A:522-525.
10. Adler O, Rosenberger A: Fine needle aspiration biopsy of osteolytic metastatic lesions. AJR 1979;133:15-18.
11. Blady JV: Aspiration biopsy of tumors in obscure or difficult locations under roentgenoscopic guidance. Am J Roentgenol 1939;42:515-524.
12. Ottolenghi CE: Aspiration biopsy of the spine. J Bone Joint Surg 1969;51(A):1531-1544.
13. Rabinov K, Goldman H, Rosbash H, Simon M: The role of aspiration biopsy of focal lesions in lung and bone by simple needle and fluoroscopy. Am J Roentgenol 1967;101:932-938.
14. Lalli AF: Roentgen guided aspiration biopsies of skeletal lesions. J Can Assoc Radiol 1970;21:71-73.
15. Debnam JW, Staple TW: Trephine bone biopsy by radiologists. Radiology 1975;116:607-609.
16. Haaga JR, Alfidi R: Precise biopsy needle localization by computed tomography. Radiology 1976;118:603-607.
17. Hardy DC, Murphy WA, Gilula LA: Computed tomography in planning percutaneous bone biopsy. Radiology 1980;134:447-450.
18. Adapon BD, Legada BD Jr, Lin EV, et al: CT-guided closed biopsy of the spine. J Comput Assist Tomogr 1981;5:73-78.
19. Resnick D, Niwayama G: Needle biopsy of bone. In Resnick D, Niwayama G (eds): Diagnosis of bone and joint disorders. 2nd ed, Philadelphia, Saunders, 1988, pp 506-516.
20. Bernardino ME: Percutaneous biopsy. AJR 1984;142:41-45.
21. Tehranzadeh J, Freiberger RH, Ghelman B: Closed skeletal needle biopsy, review of 120 cases. AJR 1983;140:113-115.
22. de Santos LA, Lukeman JM, Wallace S, et al: Percutaneous needle biopsy of bone in the cancer patient. AJR 1978;130:641-649.
23. Golimbu C, Firooznia H, Rafii M: CT guided percutaneous bone biopsy in tumor staging of genitourinary malignancies. Urology 1983;22(2):322-325.
24. Cotty P, Fouquet B, Pleskof L, et al: Vertebral osteomyelitis: value of percutaneous biopsy. J Neuroradiol 1988;15:13-21.
25. Griffith HS: Interventional radiology. The musculoskeletal system. Radiol Clin North Am 1979;17:475-484.
26. Ayala AG, Zornosa J: Primary bone tumors: percutaneous needle biopsy. Radiologic-pathologic study of 222 biopsies. Radiology 1983;149:675-679.
27. Hajdu SI, Melamed MR: Needle biopsy of primary malignant tumors. Surg Gynecol Obstet 1971;133:829-832.
28. Debnam JW, Staple TW: Needle biopsy of bone. Radiol Clin North Am 1975;13:157-164.
29. Tumeh SS, Beadle G, Kaplan WD: Clinical significance of solitary rib lesions in patients with extraskeletal malignancy. J Nucl Med 1985;26:1140-1143.
30. Collins JD, Bassett L, Main GD, Kagan C: Percutaneous biopsy following positive bone scans. Radiology 1979;132:439-442.
31. Armstrong P, Chalmers AH, Green G, Irving JD: Needle aspiration/biopsy of the spine in suspected disc infection. Br J Radiol 1978;51:333-337.
32. Jamshidi K, Swaim WR: Bone marrow biopsy with unaltered architecture: a new biopsy device. J Lab Clin Med 1971;77:335-342.
33. Maclarnon JC: Biopsy of the spine using a needle with a rigid guide wire. Clin Radiol 1982;33:189-192.
34. Laredo JD, Bard M: Thoracic spine: percutaneous trephine biopsy. Radiology 1986;160:485-489.
35. Shaltot A, Michell PA, Betts JA, et al: Jamshidi needle biopsy of bone lesions. Clin Radiol 1982;33:193-196.
36. Hewes RC, Vigorita VJ, Freiberger RH: Percutaneous bone biopsy: the importance of aspirated osseous blood. Radiology 1983;148:69-72.
37. Ottolenghi CE, Schajowiez F, De Schant FA: Aspiration biopsy of cervical spine. J Bone Joint Surg 1964;46A:715-733.
38. Kattapuram SV, Rosenthal DI: Percutaneous biopsy of the cervical spine using CT guidance. AJR 1987;149:539-541.
39. Cohen W: Personal communication, 1990.

PART III JOINTS

14 Temporomandibular Joint

ROY A. HOLLIDAY

It has been estimated[1,2] that up to 28% of the United States adult population has some form of abnormality of the temporomandibular joints (TMJs). Patients with symptoms referrable to the TMJ (local pain, joint noises [clicking, popping, grinding], limited jaw motion, earache, headache) are seen by a variety of medical specialists. Although dentists and oral surgeons are most familiar with TMJ dysfunction, neurologists, neurosurgeons, otolaryngologists, and general practioners are often the first to see a patient so afflicted.

With the development of TMJ arthrography in the late 1970s came the discovery that many individuals previously diagnosed with "myofascial pain dysfunction syndrome" actually had internal derangement of the temporomandibular joint. Patients with "TMJ syndrome" could then be classified as having articular or nonarticular disease.[3] Whereas initially arthrography and conventional roentgenography concentrated on the morphology and function of the TMJs, more recently computer-assisted sectional imaging techniques (CT and MR) have provided a means for sophisticated and noninvasive investigation of joint morphology and function.[4-7] It is the purpose of this chapter to review the current status of CT and MR sectional imaging of the TMJs, with particular emphasis on the evaluation of joint anatomy and function.

NORMAL ANATOMY

An understanding of the gross and radiological anatomy of the TMJs is facilitated by separate analyses of their osseous and soft tissue components. The osseous components are maintained in position by the joint capsules, temporomandibular ligaments, and muscles of mastication. Each fibrous joint capsule, lined with synovium, is innervated by branches of the mandibular division of the trigeminal nerve and receives blood from branches of the superficial temporal and distal internal maxillary arteries.[8]

Osseous anatomy (Fig. 14-1, A)

The inferior osseous component of the TMJ is the head of the mandibular condyle (condylar process). There is wide variation in both size and shape of the condylar head; but regardless of its configuration (usually ellipsoid, ovoid, or cavoconvex), its transverse dimension is approximately twice its anteroposterior dimension.[9] It sits asymmetrically atop the condylar neck, two thirds of it medial to the neck, and only its lateral third is routinely visualized on conventional roentgenograms.

The superior osseous boundary of the TMJ is the articulating surface of the squamous temporal bone.

The glenoid (mandibular) fossa, a smoothly convex thin plate of bone separating the TMJ (inferiorly) from the middle cranial fossa (superiorly), is cleaved in the sagittal plane by the tympanosquamous suture laterally and by the petrotympanic fissure medially. The articulating portion of the glenoid fossa lies anterior to the fissure.[10]

Anterior to the glenoid fossa is the articular eminence (articular tubercle, glenoid tubercle). Because it

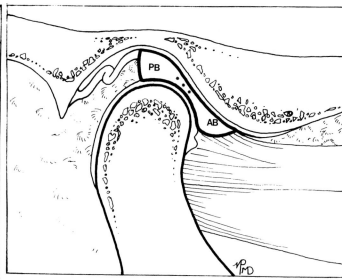

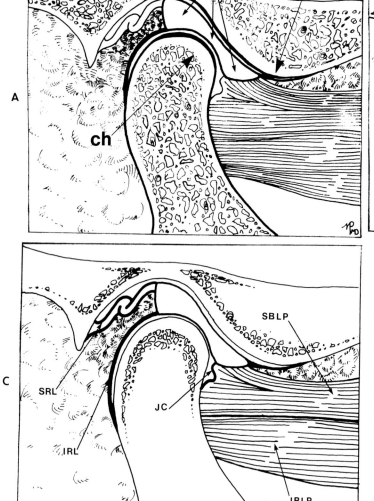

FIGURE 14-1

Sagittal diagram of the temporomandibular joint. **A,** Osseous anatomy. *ch,* Condylar head; *ae,* articular eminence; *double asterisks,* glenoid fossa; *ad,* articular disk. **B,** Discal anatomy. *PB,* Posterior band; *triple asterisks,* intermediae zone; *AB,* anterior band. **C,** Soft tissue anatomy. *SRL,* Superior retrodiscal lamina; *IRL,* inferior retrodiscal lamina; *SBLP,* superior belly of lateral pterygoid muscle; *IBLP,* inferior belly of lateral pterygoid muscle; *JC,* joint capsule (capsular ligament). (Adapted from Bell WE: Temporomandibular disorders, 2nd ed. Chicago, Year Book, 1986.)

must withstand greater physiological stress during TMJ motion than the glenoid fossa must, it is composed of thicker cortical bone than the fossa. However, only its posterior aspect represents an articulating surface within the joint and only this surface is concave.

The combination of glenoid fossa and articular eminence imparts an overall sigmoid curve appearance to the articulating portion of the temporal bone.[9] There is also some variation in the configuration of the articular eminence, and it has been suggested[11] that this may predispose certain individuals to TMJ dysfunction.

The articular eminence forms the anterior boundary of the TMJ. The posterior boundary is the tympanic portion of the temporal bone, and the lateral border is the anterior and posterior roots of the zygomatic arch.[9]

Soft tissue components (Figs. 14-1 and 14-2)

The key element to analyzing TMJ morphology and function is an assessment of the articular disk. The term *meniscus* has been used to describe the articular disk, but it is inaccurate since the structure and function of the disk are vastly different from those of a true meniscus (i.e., the knee).[12]

The normal articular disk has the shape of a biconcave lens, measuring approximately 20 × 22 mm in its greatest dimension (Fig. 14-1, *B*). Its posterior portion (also known as the posterior band) is the thickest segment, measuring some 3 mm, and in the normal closed-mouth position is directly interposed between the condylar head and the glenoid fossa (a relationship that has been termed the *12 o'clock position*[6]). Its thinner central portion (the intermediate zone), measuring roughly 1.5 mm in thickness, is in constant contact with the articulating surfaces of the joint. In the normal closed-mouth position this zone lies along the anterosuperior aspect of the condylar head, and in the normal open-mouth position directly between the condylar head and the articular eminence. Its most anterior portion (the anterior band), measuring some 2.5 mm in thickness, attaches directly to the anterior joint capsule.[9]

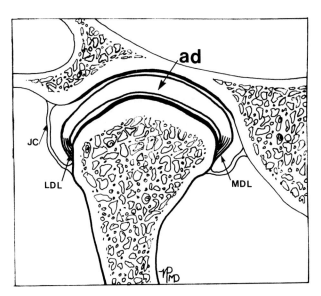

FIGURE 14-2
Coronal diagram of the temporomandibular joint. *LDL,* Lateral discal ligament; *MDL,* medial discal ligament; *ad,* articular disk, *JC,* joint capsule (capsular ligament). (Adapted from Okeson JP: Management of temporomandibular disorders and occlusion, 2nd ed. St Louis, Mosby, 1989.)

The articular disk in younger individuals is composed of avascular fibrous tissue, the interlacing fibers straight and tightly packed. With advancing age and stress on the disk, some of the fibroblasts develop into chondroid cells and later differentiate into true chondrocytes, forming islands of hyaline cartilage within the disk. Fibroblast differentiation can also result in deposition of hyaline ground substance within the disk.[13] The variable histological composition of the disk may be the source of mild variations in signal on MR.

The articular disk separates the joint space into distinct upper and lower synovium-lined compartments. The potential volume of the lower compartment (lower joint space) is larger than that of the upper. The disk is maintained in position within the joint by a number of ligaments. Collateral ligaments attach it medially and laterally to the condylar poles (Fig. 14-2), allowing for rotation during condylar movement. There are two retrodiscal laminae (Fig. 14-1, *C*), the superior attaching the posterior band to the tympanic plate, the inferior connecting the posterior band to the neck of the mandibular condyle. The superior retrodiscal lamina contains more elastin fibers whereas the inferior retroddiscal lamina contains a higher percentage of collagen fibers. Surrounding the laminae is a loose stroma of areolar tissue containing both nerves and vessels. The combination of the laminae and the areolar tissue has been termed the *bilaminar zone.*

The temporomandibular ligament reinforces the lateral aspect of the joint capsule. It consists of two portions, both arising from the articular eminence and zygomatic process of the temporal bone: the lateral oblique portion extends to the lateral surface of the condylar neck, the medial horizontal portion to the lateral pole of the condylar head and posterior aspect of the disk. The *oblique portion limits mouth opening.* As the mouth opens, the condylar head rotates around a fixed point in the articular fossa and the insertion of the oblique portion on the condylar neck moves posteriorly. The jaw can easily rotate until the teeth are 20 to 25 mm apart. At this point the temporomandibular ligament becomes taut and further mouth opening requires translation of the condylar head out of the articular fossa. The *horizontal portion limits posterior movement of the condyle and disk.* When force applied to the mandible displaces the condyle posteriorly, the horizontal portion of the ligament becomes taut, preventing the condyle from entering the posterior articular fossa. The temporomandibular ligament therefore serves to protect the retrodiscal laminae in cases of trauma.[14]

The lateral pterygoid muscle, although extracapsular in position, plays an important role in TMJ function since it is the muscle predominantly responsible for jaw opening. It originates from the lateral pterygoid plate of the sphenoid bone and has two distinct components — the inferior portion (belly), inserting on the neck of the condyle in the lower pterygoid fovea, and the superior portion, inserting on both the anteromedial joint capsule and the superior pterygoid fovea.[15]

NORMAL FUNCTION (Fig. 14-3)

The TMJ is a ginglymoarthrodial joint (i.e., it can both rotate and translate [slide]). The first 20 to 25 mm of mouth opening (as measured between the mandibular and maxillary incisors) is accomplished by rotation. Further opening requires translation.

The TMJ is also a compound joint. Its structure and function can be divided into two distinct components. The first is tissues that surround the lower joint space (the condyle and the disk). The disk is tightly bound to the condyle by the lateral and medial discal ligaments, with rotation as its only physiological movement. The second is tissues that surround the upper joint space (the glenoid fossa and the disk-condyle complex). The disk is not tightly bound to the fossa and therefore it is possible for a free translational movement to occur between the disk and fossa.

Normal translation of the TMJ occurs according to the following principles:

1. Ligaments do not actively participate in TMJ function. Their role is to restrict certain joint movements and permit others.
2. Ligaments do not stretch. If a traction force is applied, ligaments elongate; and once they are elongated, joint function is compromised.
3. The articular surfaces of the TMJ are maintained in constant contact.[14]

The normal functional movement of the TMJ is illustrated in Fig. 14-3. The first phase of mandibular opening

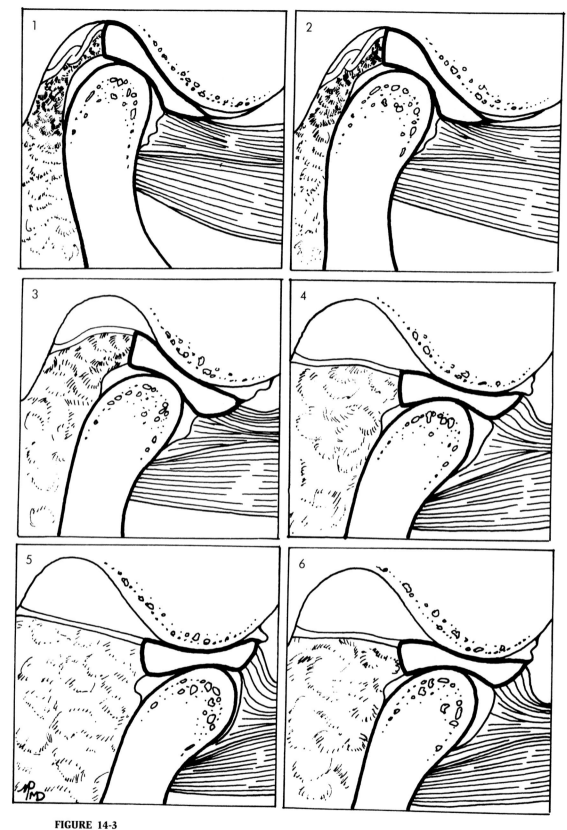

FIGURE 14-3
Normal function of the TMJ. *1,* Resting closed-mouth position; *2,* condylar rotation; *3* to *5,* sequential stages of anterior condylar translation (note that the disk rotates posteriorly as the superior retrodiscal lamina unfolds); *6* to *8,* closing motion. The return stroke is the exact opposite of opening. (Adapted from Okeson JP: Management of temporomandibular disorders and occlusion, 2nd ed. St Louis, Mosby, 1989.)

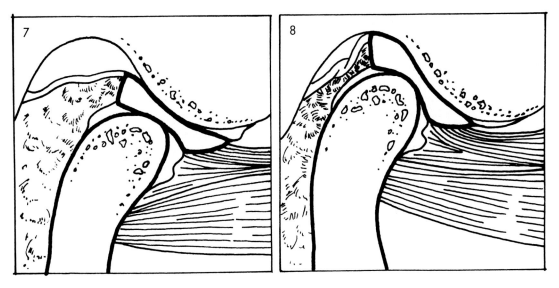

FIGURE 14-3 cont'd
For legend see opposite page.

occurs as the digastric and other assessory muscles of mastication contract, depressing the mandible. The condyle and articular disk rotate within the glenoid fossa. Rotation beyond 25 mm of interincisal distance is prevented by the temporomandibular ligament.

Further mouth opening requires translation of the mandible. The lateral pterygoid muscle contracts, protruding the mandible. Contrary to popular belief, only the inferior belly of the lateral pterygoid functions during mouth opening. The superior belly, although attached to the anterior aspect of the joint capsule, does not "pull" the disk anteriorly during mouth opening.

As the mandible protrudes, translational motion begins at the joint. During the initial phase of translation, pressure between the articular surfaces is increased. The upper and lower joint spaces narrow and the condylar head is more firmly seated on the apposing surface of intermediate zone. The increased intraarticular pressure, in combination with the shape of the articular disk, forces the disk to translate forward with the condyle, keeping the condylar head in constant contact with the intermediate zone and posterior band of the disk. The anterior capsular ligament and inferior retrodiscal laminae assist in maintaining the disk in normal position.

As further translation occurs, the superior retrodiscal lamina unfolds. When the retractive force of the elastic superior retrodiscal lamina is greater than the tonus of the superior belly of the lateral pterygoid, the disk rotates as far posteriorly as the width of the joint will allow. At complete mouth opening the superior retrodiscal lamina is tensed, the disk is rotated posteriorly on the condyle, and the condyle is translated anteriorly out of the glenoid fossa. As the condyle returns passively to the resting position (return stroke), the retractive force of the retrodiscal lamina diminishes and the disk is repositioned anteriorly due to tonus of the superior belly of the lateral pterygoid.

The superior belly of the lateral pterygoid plays an important role in maintaining normal disk position when the mandible encounters resistance during closure. When biting on hard food (power stroke), the force of closure is applied to the food, not the condyle, thereby decreasing the intraarticular pressure. With diminished intraarticular pressure and a wider joint space, the elastic force of the retrodiscal laminae would retract the disk away from its functional position, creating a posteriorly dislocated disk. To prevent this, the superior belly of the lateral pterygoid contracts during the power stroke, rotating the disk forward on the condyle so the disk maintains proper articular contact throughout the power stroke.[14]

IMAGING STRATEGIES

Cadaver studies[16-18] as well as extensive clinical experience[19-23] have established that MR is the modality of choice for noninvasive imaging of TMJ soft tissue components and CT is superior for analyzing the cortical margins of the osseous components. The medullary cavity of the mandibular condyle may be well assessed using both modalities.

The imaging plane of choice of the TMJ is the sagittal orientation. It is optimal for diagnosing most internal derangements of the articular disk and it closely reflects the appearance of the TMJ at surgery. The multiplanar capability of MR is ideal for obtaining direct sagittal images. Direct sagittal CT images may be obtained using special headholders or special positioning techniques.[24-26] Sagittal reformatted images, derived by manipulation of data obtained from axial and/or coronal images, are more commonly employed.

Computed tomography

MR has replaced CT in the diagnosis of internal derangement of the TMJ, and consequently the vast majority of images on CT are obtained only with the mouth closed. Intravenous contrast is not usually employed.

CT examination of the TMJ typically consists of contiguous or overlapping thin (1 to 2 mm) images in the coronal and axial planes. The kVp and mAS settings should be optimized to enhance bone detail. Retrospective images ("target reviews") may be successfully employed to enhance bony detail further (Fig. 14-4). The total examination time (risk of patient motion) can be decreased by using dynamic scanning. If sagittal reformatted images are to be obtained, overlapping of axial sections is recommended to optimize assessment of the thin bone comprising the glenoid fossa (Fig. 14-5). Three-dimensional reconstruction of CT images, originally described for use in craniofacial surgical planning and evaluation,[27] may be used to great advantage in preoperative evaluation of the TMJ, particularly in patients with congenital or traumatic abnormalities (Fig. 14-6).

Magnetic resonance

MR images may be obtained utilizing either medium strength or high field strength systems. Cadaver studies and clinical experience have demonstrated that images of higher diagnostic quality are obtained in a shorter period of time with the high field strength systems.[16,28] Regardless of field strength, the use of surface receiver coils is essential for adequate evaluation of the TMJ. A circular surface coil, typically 6 to 10 cm in diameter, is most commonly employed. Dual surface coil technology has been developed to allow for simultaneous acquisition of images from both TMJs, thereby decreasing scan time.[29]

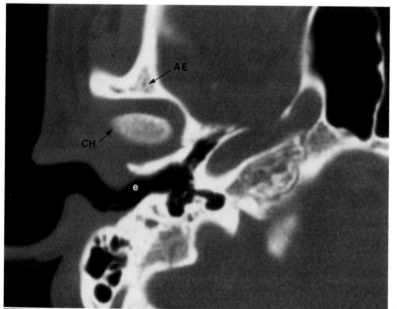

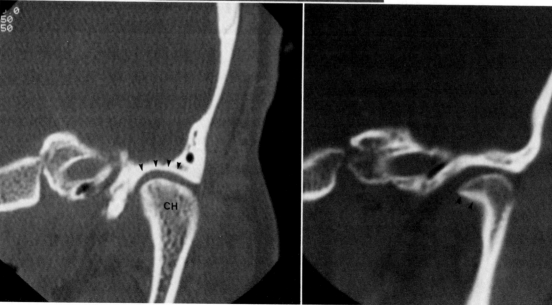

FIGURE 14-4

Normal TMJ on computed tomography. **A,** An axial 1.5 mm thick image of the superior aspect of the right temporomandibular joint shows the smooth contour of the articular eminence *(AE)* and the anterior (articulating) cortex of the condylar head *(CH)*. The external auditory canal *(e)* is also visible. **B,** A coronal 1.5 mm thick slice through the left joint demonstrates the condylar head contour and articulating surface of the glenoid fossa *(arrowheads)*. **C,** Another coronal 1.5 mm slice through the left joint in another volunteer reveals the variability in contour of the condyle and fossa. Most of the condylar head lies medial to the neck of the condyle *(arrowheads)*.

Proper positioning of the surface coil is essential for evaluation of the joint. One simple method to assure proper coil placement is for the imager to place his finger through the center of the coil. The position of the joint is then established by palpation while the patient opens and closes his mouth. The surface coil is then placed directly against the skin surface over the properly identified TMJ.

Most MR images are obtained using a two-dimensional Fourier transform (2DFT) spin-echo technique. Axial scout views are first obtained, using either the surface coil or the body coil as the receiver. With short TR/short TE sequences (T1-weighted images, T1-WI), the condylar head can be identified on axial images as an oval focus of hyperintense signal directly anterior to the signal void of air within the external auditory canal (Fig. 14-7). Scout views must always be carefully analyzed for the presence of masses involving the skull base, muscles of mastication, or parapharyngeal space (all of which can present with the symptoms of TMJ dysfunction)[30] (Fig. 14-8).

The long axis of the elliptical condylar head does not lie in an orthogonal plane. In most individuals it lies in a plane with an angle of 20 to 22 degrees to the perpendicular. Nonorthogonal sagittal images, oriented perpendicular to the long axis of the condylar head, should be employed when scanner software permits since they are best suited for diagnosing the majority of internal TMJ derangements.

The basic MR examination consists of sagittal T1-WI of the joint in the closed- and open-mouth positions (Fig. 14-9). Because of variations between manufacturers, it is impossible to describe in detail the "best" way to scan the TMJ on MR. The following recommendations are compiled from techniques used by leading investigators:

Slice thickness: 3 mm
Slice intervals: Less than or equal to 1 mm; true "contiguous" slices often increase scan time
Number of slices: It is essential that the entire transverse dimension of the condylar head be examined in the sagittal plane; when a slice thickness of 3 mm and a slice interval of 1 mm are utilized, most temporomandibular joints can be adequately scanned with 7 slices

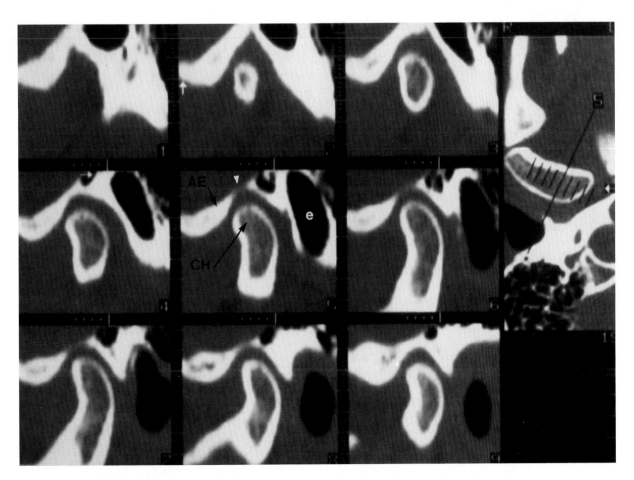

FIGURE 14-5
Sagittal CT of the TMJ. Reformatted sagittal images of the right TMJ in a symptom-free volunteer. The condylar head *(CH)* is centrally located within the joint space posterior to the articular eminence *(AE)*. Note the thin cortex of the glenoid fossa *(arrowhead)* in this case. These images were reformatted utilizing axial 1.5 mm thick images obtained at 1 mm intervals. The plane of reformatting parallels the long axis of the condylar head as shown. The distance between reformatted images is 2 mm. *e,* External auditory canal.

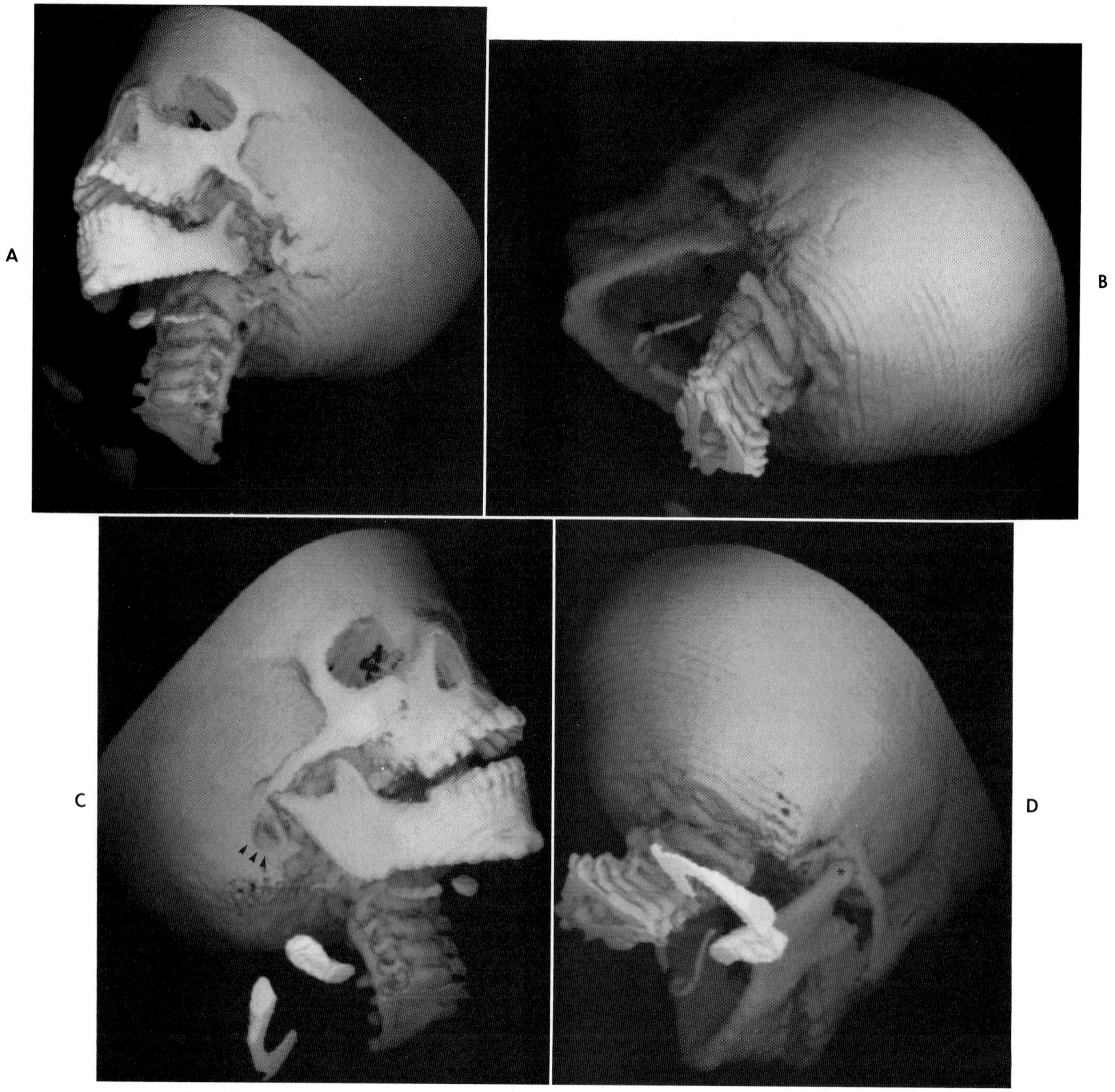

FIGURE 14-6
Three-dimensional CT images of the TMJ. **A** and **B,** In a patient with hemifacial microsomia, note the agenesis of the condylar head and atresia of the external auditory canal. **C** and **D,** Comparison images of the normal right TMJ. *Asterisk* in **D** is on the condylar head; *arrowheads* in **C,** on the external auditory canal.

Field of view: 12 to 16 cm

TR/TE: The minimum TR is limited by the number of slices to be acquired within one scan package; with single coil imaging a TR as short as 500 to 600 msec may be employed; dual-coil technology usually requires a TR in the range of 800 to 1000 msec; to optimize T1 weighting, TE must be kept under 30 msec; for dual surface coil imaging TE equal to 20 msec is preferable

Acquisition matrix and number of acquisitions: These two factors represent the source of widest variation between scanners and investigators.

Increasing the acquisition matrix and number of acquisitions will improve both signal-to-noise ratio and image resolution. However, these improvements require increased scan time, thereby increasing the risk of patient motion during the study. Images obtained on medium−field strength systems often require more acquisitions to achieve image quality comparable to that of high−field strength

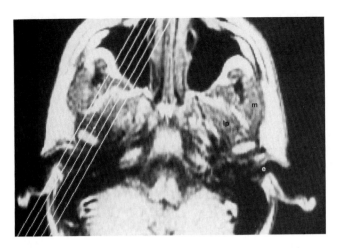

FIGURE 14-7
Axial scout view for an MR examination. Axial TR 350/TE 20 image through the condylar heads. Note the bright signal from the marrow directly anterior to the external auditory canal *(e)*. The proper orientation of sagittal images is demonstrated on the right TMJ. Signal-to-noise is decreased secondary to the use of a permanent body coil rather than a surface coil as the receiver. The muscles of mastication, including the lateral pterygoid *(lp)* and masseter *(m)*, are nevertheless well demonstrated.

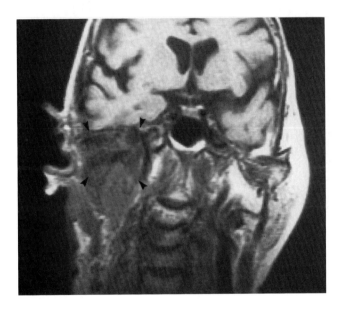

FIGURE 14-8
Metastatic disease to the TMJ. A preliminary coronal TR 450/TE 30 image through the temporomandibular joints demonstrates an abnormal mass encompassing the right joint and lateral pterygoid muscle, with erosion of the skull base *(arrowheads)*. The temporal lobe of the brain is displaced superiorly. The patient complained of pain on mouth opening (trismus), which was thought to be secondary to TMJ dysfunction. Biopsy revealed metastatic breast carcinoma.

systems. Lower-resolution matrices (256 × 128) are routinely used by experienced investigators[28] but may lack the resolution and anatomical detail necessary for easy interpretation by the novice imager.

Using the factors as listed above, most investigators report total scanning times of between 4 and 10 minutes.

It would be virtually impossible for even the most cooperative patient to remain motionless in the scanner if similar imaging parameters were used for open-mouth views. Patient cooperation during open-mouth views may be limited by local pain as well as by pooling of saliva in the posterior oropharynx. To facilitate imaging in the open-mouth position, either the number of acquisitions or the size of the acquisition matrix is usually reduced (Fig. 14-10). To compensate for decreased image resolution, increased slice thickness may be successfully employed. This will, in turn, decrease the number of slices necessary to study the joint and allow for a decrease in TR (further shortening the scan time).

A variety of devices can be used to maintain the mouth in a constant position during open-mouth imaging. The simplest of these bite blocks is a syringe wrapped with gauze. The size (diameter) of the syringe is selected to accommodate the degree of jaw opening attainable by the patient at the time of MR imaging. More sophisticated devices allowing for precise measurements of degree of mouth opening are also available.[31]

Additional imaging planes and pulse sequences may supplement the basic sagittal T1-weighted MR examination depending upon the patient's symptoms and the area of interest.

A coronal T1-WI is useful for detecting rotational internal derangements[32,33] (Figs. 14-11 and 14-12). However, it may be a technical challenge due to signal dropoff from a coil placed on the skin surface. Because of the relationship between surface coil radius and depth of penetration, a larger surface coil provides superior-quality images of the medial TMJ.

A long TR/long TE spin echo sequence (T2-WI) is useful for detecting fluid within either joint compartment (Figs. 14-12 and 14-13). It is more sensitive than T1-WI in the detection of pathological conditions involving the muscles of mastication.[30,34] It may also be useful for characterizing abnormalities of the marrow of the mandibular condyle.[35] The major limitations to T2-WI are its prolonged scan time, limiting its use to closed-mouth images.

Analysis of the condylar marrow cavity and joint space may also be obtained by means of gradient refocused imaging (gradient echo imaging, GRASS, FISP, FLASH). With single slice scan acquisition times as low as 6 to 25 seconds, this pulse sequence demonstrates to similar advantage the processes identified on the more time-consuming T2-WI.[36,37] Gradient echo imaging may be used to advantage in claustrophobic or other uncooperative patients and for reducing the chance of motion artifact in cooperative patients. An additional advantage of gradient echo imaging is the acquisition of multiple single slices of the joint in varying degrees of mouth opening (Fig. 14-14). These serial static images may then be displayed on a cine loop, allowing for a better analysis of TMJ function. Analysis of the cine loop allows for a more precise determination of the time of recapture of

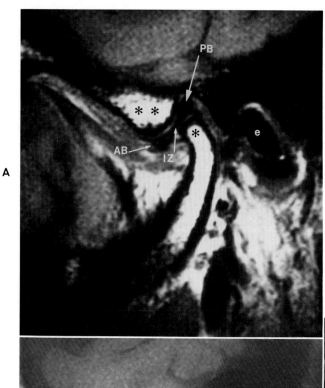

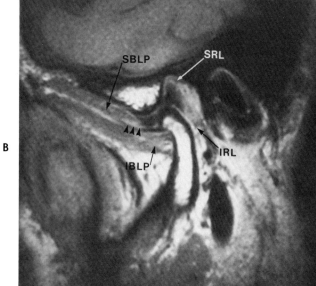

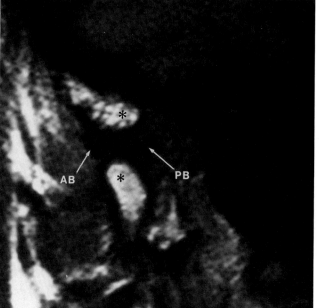

FIGURE 14-9

Normal TMJ on MR. **A,** A sagittal T1-WI in the closed-mouth position demonstrates the relationship of the posterior band of the articular disk *(PB)* to the superior aspect of the condylar head *(asterisk)*. The intermediate zone *(IZ)* and anterior band of the disk *(AB)* are readily identifiable. *Double asterisks,* articular eminence. **B,** Another sagittal T1-WI, this time in the partial open-mouth position (18 mm of interincisal distance), demonstrates the condylar head in contact with the intermediate zone of the disk. The superior belly of the lateral pterygoid *(SBLP)* inserts on the anterior band of the disk. The inferior belly *(IBLP)* inserts on both the head and the neck of the condyle. There is a hyperintense fat plane between the two portions of the muscle directly anterior to the disk *(arrowheads)*. Alteration of this plane is an indirect sign of anterior diskal displacement. The unfolded superior retrodiscal lamina *(SRL)* is also well shown. The inferior retrodiscal lamina *(IRL)* is intermittently visualized within the hyperintense fat of the bilaminar zone. **C** is another sagittal T1-WI, in the open-mouth position, demonstrating the intermediate zone directly between the articular eminence *(double asterisks)* superiorly and the condylar head *(asterisk)* inferiorly. The anterior *(AB)* and posterior *(PB)* bands produce a bow tie appearance of the disk.

internally deranged disks and may clarify discrepancies identified on static T1-WI. Although analysis of TMJ motion can suggest the presence of adhesions,[38] it must be remembered that these studies are a pseudodynamic evaluation of the TMJ. Optimal radiographic evaluation is provided by videofluoroscopy of the joint, usually following arthrography.[22,28]

Some investigators have proposed using a three dimensional Fourier transform (3DFT) technique to acquire images of the TMJ. This "multislice" and "multislab" study allows for the acquisition of overlapping or contiguous images, often with slice thicknesses smaller than those used in 2DFT imaging. Its main limitation is the increased sensitivity to patient motion.[39] The role of gadopentetate in TMJ imaging awaits further investigation.

The normal TMJ on MR

The normal temporomandibular joint as demonstrated by sagittal T1-W images in both closed- and open-mouth positions is demonstrated in Fig. 14-9. The articular disk has a normal biconcave lens shape. The larger posterior band is located directly superior to the condylar head. A sharp interface exists between the low-signal articular disk and the relatively high-signal areolar tissue of the bilaminar zone. The low-signal anterior band of the disk demonstrates a sharp interface with the medium-signal lateral pterygoid muscle as well as the bright signal from the fat present between the superior and inferior bellies of the lateral pterygoid. In some instances a small region of high signal intensity is identified within the posterior band (Fig. 14-15). The reason for this finding is not yet

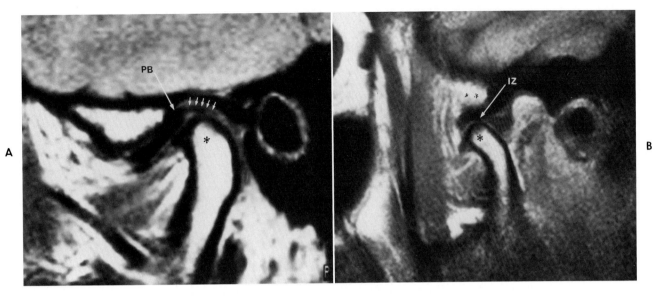

FIGURE 14-10
Anterior displacement with reduction. **A,** A sagittal T1-WI in the closed-mouth position demonstrates the posterior band *(PB)* rotated anterior to the condylar head *(asterisk)*. There is complete unfolding of the superior retrodiscal lamina *(white arrows)*. **B,** Another sagittal T1-WI, this time with the mouth open, shows a normal disk position with the intermediate zone *(IZ)* between the condylar head *(asterisk)* and articular eminence *(double asterisks)*. This image was obtained with a lower-resolution matrix and fewer acquisitions than in **A.**

determined, but it may well represent a variation in the histological or histochemical composition of the disk secondary to normal physiological stresses.

The dense cortical bone of the condylar head and articular eminence produces no signal on spin echo images. The position of the condylar head is usually identifiable by the high contrast between the bright-signal condylar marrow, the absent-signal cortical bone, and the low-signal joint space. The articular eminence can also be identified by its marrow signal. In a few cases, however, pneumatization of the articular eminence by the mastoid air cells limits efforts to locate the eminence (Figs. 14-16 and 14-17).

On open-mouth views the articular disk acquires its characteristic "bow tie" appearance, with the intermediate zone (the knot of the "bow tie") interposed between the condylar head and the articular eminence. On an open-mouth view the superior retrodiscal lamina may occasionally be identified as a thin band of relatively decreased signal within the brighter signal of the bilaminar zone areolar tissue.

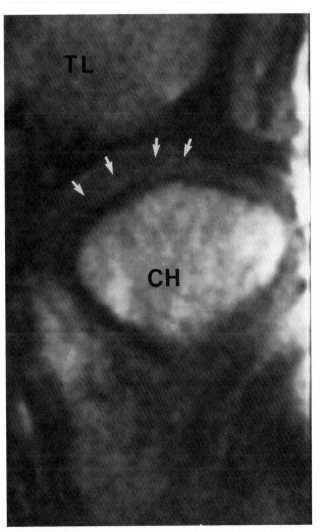

FIGURE 14-11
Normal TMJ on MR. A coronal T1-WI through the posterior band of the left disk *(arrows)* shows the position of the disk on the medial half of the condylar head *(CH)*. The posterior band appears slightly brighter in this projection than the sagittal. Minor variations in signal intensity are a normal finding on MR images. However, they are accentuated by the alterations of window and level settings necessary to compensate for the extremely bright signal of the subcutaneous fat lateral to the TMJ. Note the decreased signal/noise ("signal dropoff") in the medial aspect of the image. *TL,* Temporal lobe of the brain.

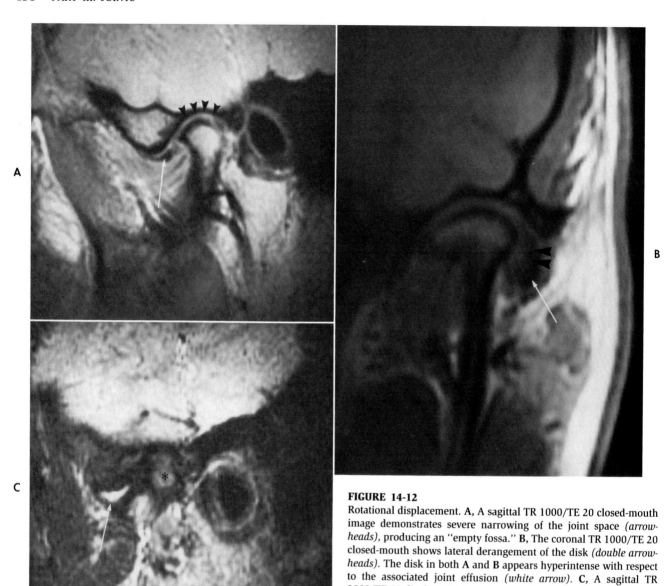

FIGURE 14-12
Rotational displacement. **A,** A sagittal TR 1000/TE 20 closed-mouth image demonstrates severe narrowing of the joint space *(arrowheads),* producing an "empty fossa." **B,** The coronal TR 1000/TE 20 closed-mouth shows lateral derangement of the disk *(double arrowheads).* The disk in both **A** and **B** appears hyperintense with respect to the associated joint effusion *(white arrow).* **C,** A sagittal TR 2000/TE 80 displays the hyperintense signal from the joint effusion *(arrow)* within the anterolateral joint space. Signal from the condylar head is diminished *(asterisk).* (Courtesy Per-Lennart Westesson, D.D.S. Ph.D.)

INTERNAL DERANGEMENTS

Internal derangement of the articular disk is defined as an abnormal positional and functional relationship between the disk, mandibular condyle, and articulating surfaces of the temporal bone.[28] It has a variety of predisposing factors — trauma, bruxism, malocclusion, and emotional stress being the most commonly cited.[1,2] The overwhelming majority of patients are women.

Internal derangements are classified according to the position of the displaced articular disk and the function of the joint, focusing on movement of the disk. One useful scheme describes the position of the disk as superior (normal), anterior, medial, or lateral. Two additional positional derangements, anteromedial and anterolateral, are considered as rotational displacements.

It is important to remember that internal derangements of the TMJ are part of a spectrum of functional joint disorders[40] (summarized in the box on p. 453). Only the later stages of this continuum can be reliably diagnosed with sectional imaging techniques. Drace[41] has identified a small population of patients with "minimal anterior displacements" on MR that may well represent functional displacements of the disk. Although thinning of the posterior band of the disk and/or elongation of the discal or retrodiscal laminae may be inferred from MR images, no correlative studies as yet exist to document the sensitivity of MR for these earlier changes. Current imaging strategies therefore concentrate on the diagnosis of internal derangements of the TMJ.

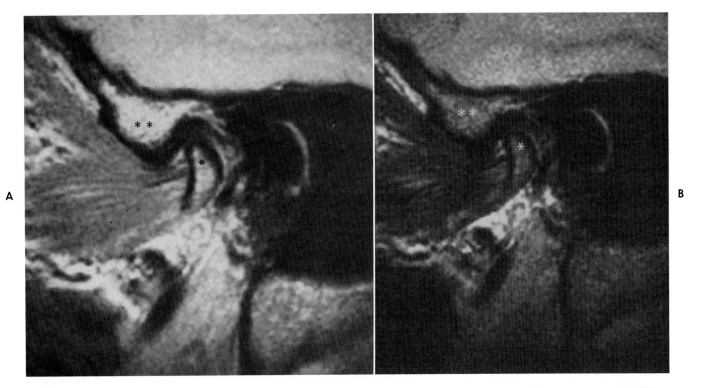

FIGURE 14-13

Normal TMJ on MR. The TR 2000/TE 20, **A**, and TR 2000/TE 80, **B**, demonstrate a loss of anatomical detail with progressive T2 weighting. Note the loss of signal from the marrow fat within the condylar head (*asterisk*) and articular eminence (*double asterisks*).

FIGURE 14-14

Normal TMJ on MR. **A**, Sagittal closed-mouth and, **B**, sagittal open-mouth views utilizing gradient echo imaging (TR 80/TE 20/flip angle 15 degrees) in a volunteer with no symptoms. The disk contrasts sharply with the surrounding tissues, producing a "pseudoarthrogram" effect. The posterior band *(PB)* may be difficult to identify on closed-mouth views, even in normal individuals. Partial open-mouth views may be useful for confirming disk position. (*single asterisk,* Condylar head; *double asterisks,* articular eminence.)

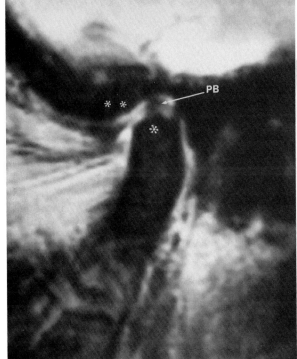

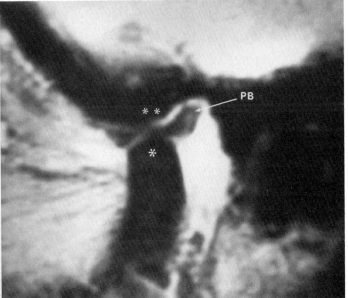

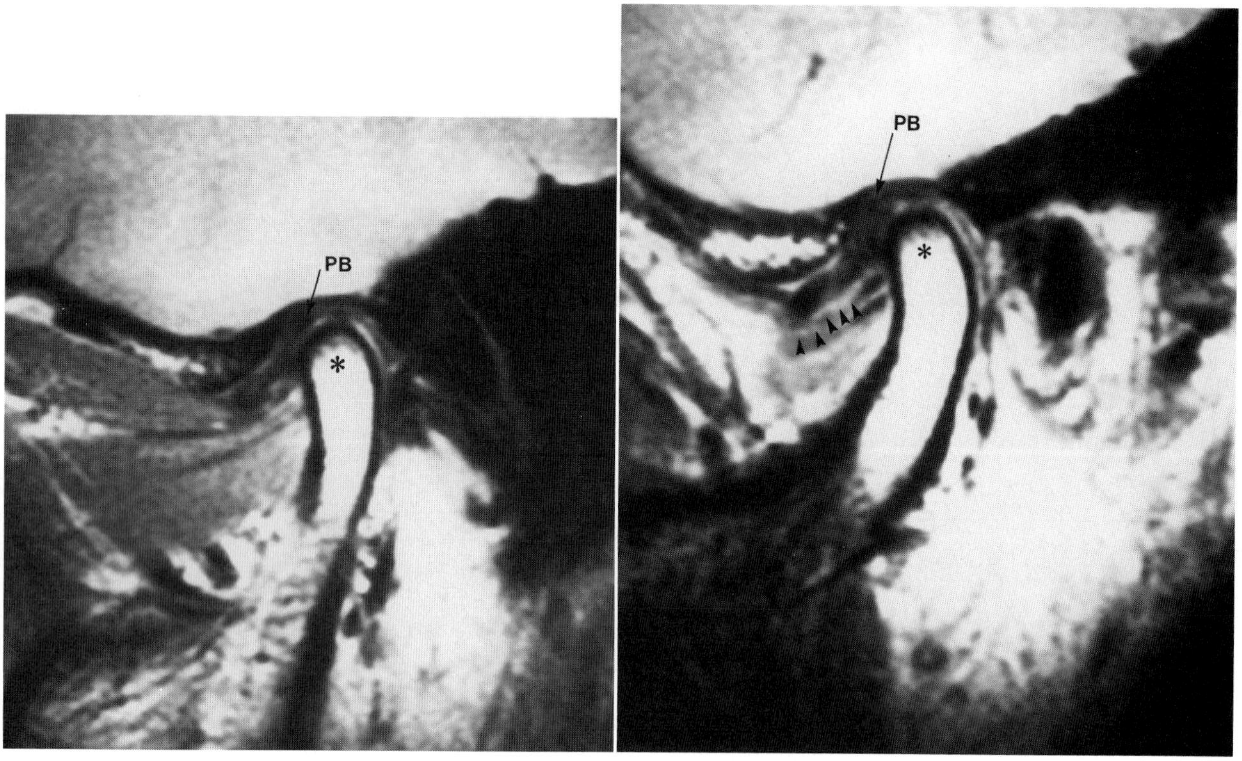

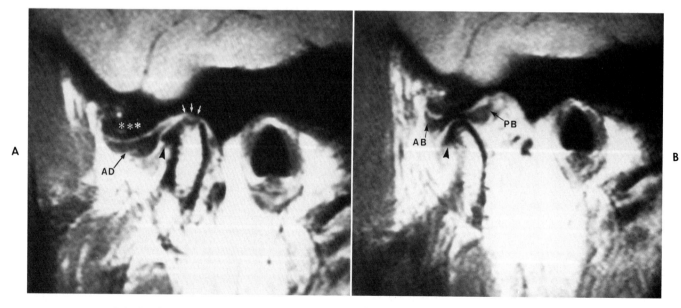

FIGURE 14-15
Anterior displacement of the articular disk. **A,** A sagittal T1-WI in the closed-mouth position demonstrates that the posterior band *(PB)* is anterior to the superior aspect of the condylar head *(asterisk).* **B,** A sagittal T1-WI closed-mouth in a second patient reveals anterior displacement of the disk, altering the contour of the fat plane *(arrowheads)* between the superior and inferior bellies of the lateral pterygoid. The signal from the posterior band of the disk *(PB)* is brighter than the anterior band. This is felt to be a normal variation.

FIGURE 14-16
Anterior displacement with reduction. **A,** A sagittal T1-WI in the closed-mouth position shows the entire articular disk *(AD)* rotated anteriorly under the articular eminence *(triple asterisks).* The lack of signal from the articular eminence is due to replacement of the marrow by mastoid air cells. The joint space *(white arrows)* is narrowed, and a triangular focus of signal void *(arrowhead)* is present along the anterior margin of the condylar head. This is the typical MR appearance of an oseophyte. **B,** Another sagittal T1-WI, in the open-mouth position, demonstrates the normal disk position. *AB,* Anterior band; *PB,* posterior band; *arrowhead,* osteophyte.

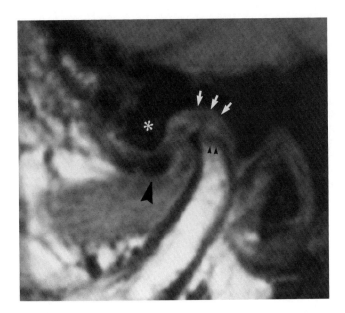

FIGURE 14-17

Rheumatoid arthritis and anterior disk displacement. A sagittal T1-WI closed-mouth view demonstrates anterior displacement of the articular disk *(arrowhead)* inferior to a pneumatized articular eminence *(asterisk)*. The retrodiscal tissues *(white arrows)* are markedly thickened, compatible with pannus formation. Nonhomogeneous signal replaces the normal signal void of the posterior condylar cortex *(double arrowheads)*, suggesting erosion of the juxtaarticular cortex by pannus.

Anterior displacement with reduction (Fig. 14-18)

In anterior displacements the posterior band of the disk is no longer present at the 12 o'clock position. The condylar head and glenoid fossa in the closed mouth position are now separated by only the retrodiscal laminae and areolar tissue of the bilaminar zone. The initial phase of mouth opening, condylar rotation, is usually normal. When the mouth is opened further, the condyle translates anteriorly under the posterior band, often producing an audible click. As condylar translation continues, the articular disk returns to a normal position so that, with full mouth opening, the intermediate zone is again interposed between the superior aspect of the condylar head and inferior aspect of the articular eminence.

During the return stroke the condylar head and articular disk do not move in unison, the condyle translating posterior to the disk; thus the articular disk is once again anteriorly displaced when the mouth is closed. It is not uncommon for an audible click to be produced as the articular disk slides both in and out of normal position. Such *reciprocal clicking* is a highly sensitive indicator of internal derangements with reduction. Clinically, it can be classified as early, intermediate, or late depending upon the relationship of the condyle to the fossa when the disk reassumes its normal position. The presence of a reciprocal click is a highly sensitive indicator of disk displacement with reduction.

Joint sounds (clicks, pops) identified only during

CONTINUUM OF TMJ DYSFUNCTION

1. Normal joint
2. Increased rotation of the disc on the condylar head
3. Hyperactivity of lateral pterygoid muscle, resulting in an anteromedial pull on the disc
4. Thinning of the posterior band of the disc
5. Elongation of the discal ligaments and retrodiscal laminae
6. Functional displacement of the disc
7. Functional dislocation of the disc
   a. Internal derangement with reduction
   b. Internal derangement without reduction
8. Perforation of the retrodiscal laminae or disc
9. Degenerative joint disease

Adapted from Okeson JP: Management of temporomandibular disorders and occlusion, 2nd ed. St Louis, Mosby, 1989.

mouth opening are a less sensitive indicator of changes in articular disk position. Joint clicks have been identified in association with intracapsular adhesions, loose joint bodies, jaw subluxation with or without disk displacement as well as degenerative change of articular surfaces.[28,42]

Anterior displacement without reduction (Fig. 14-19)

The nonreducing articular disk never returns to normal position despite all attempts at mouth opening. The displaced disk may serve as a mechanical block to mouth opening beyond initial condylar rotation. Such patients are described as having a "closed lock," and they can overcome it only by manually translating the condyle forward using force directed from behind the condylar neck. However, multiple attempts at mechanical decompression can also ultimately erode the articular surfaces of both the condylar head and the eminence and remodel the joint space.

As outlined in the box, additional anatomical changes may occur within the TMJ, thinning of the disk and fraying of the attachment of the retrodiscal laminae to the posterior band. These changes can ultimately lead to disk perforation, with resultant communication between the upper and lower joint spaces. Although perforations may occur anywhere within the joint space, they are most common at the junction of the posterior band with the retrodiscal laminae. Changes in the composition of the disk material itself may accompany changes in physiological stress. The most common of these is metaplastic transformation of fibrous tissue into fibrocartilage at the margins of the disk.[13,28]

Internal derangements on MR

Identification of the posterior band of the TMJ is the key to diagnosing internal derangements on MR. Identification of the posterior band anterior to the condyle is the

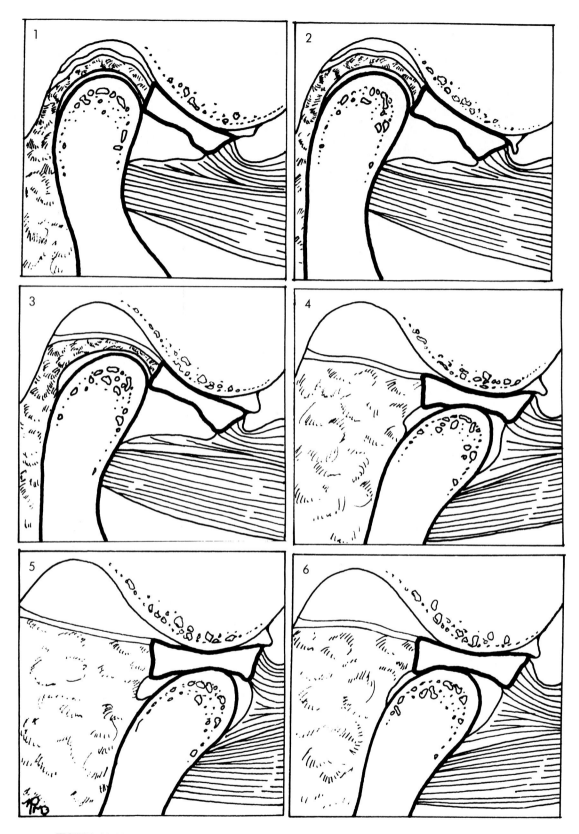

FIGURE 14-18
Anterior displacement with reduction. Condylar rotation *(2)* is normal. During anterior translation the condyle passes over the posterior band onto the intermediate zone *(4)*, often producing an audible click. During the return stroke the weakened retrodiscal laminae are unable to maintain the disk in articular position. The disk is displaced anteriorly, often producing a second audible click *(8)*. (Adapted from Okeson JP: Management of temporomandibular disorders and occlusion, 2nd ed. St Louis, Mosby, 1989.)

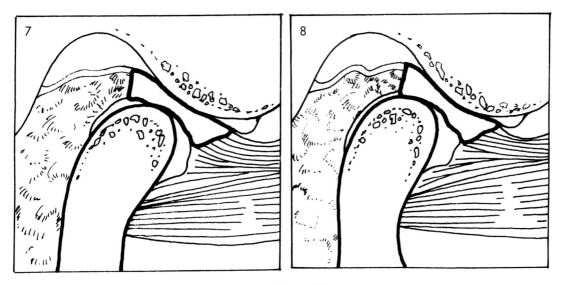

FIGURE 14-18 cont'd
For legend see opposite page.

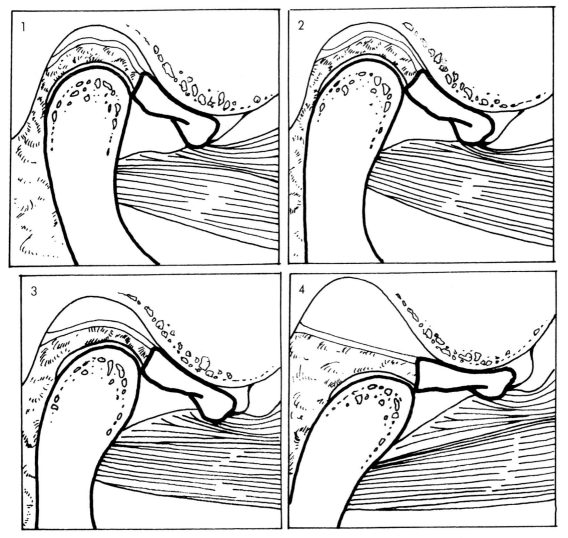

FIGURE 14-19
Anterior displacement without reduction. The condyle never assumes a normal relationship with the disk. The displaced disk acts as a mechanical obstruction to condylar translation ("closed lock"). (Adapted from Okeson JP: Management of temporomandibular disorders and occlusion, 2nd ed. St Louis, Mosby, 1989.)

Continued.

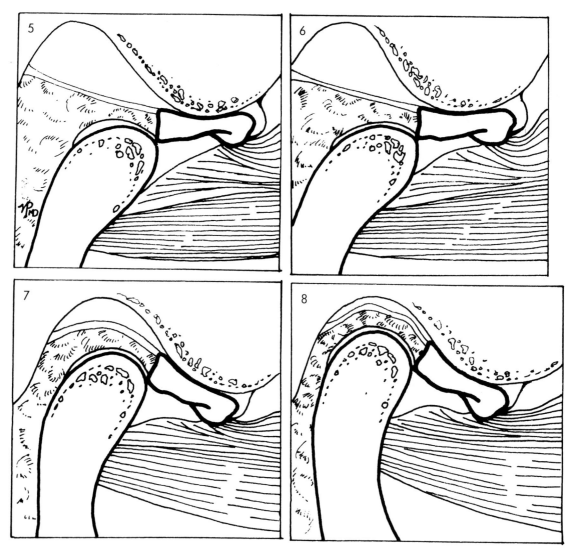

FIGURE 14-19 cont'd
For legend see opposite page.

most reliable indicator of derangement (Fig. 14-15). There are three factors that can limit identification of the posterior band on sagittal MR images: the band may be severely thinned as a result of degenerative changes; the internal derangement may be a pure medial or lateral event; or the band may be in normal position but crowded into the glenoid fossa and/or compressed between the condyle and articular eminence (Fig. 14-14). Helms et al.[43] advocate the use of partial open-mouth views to identify the posterior band when the last possibility is suspected.

Additional findings with internal derangement can assist in confirming the diagnosis, particularly when identification of the posterior band is limited. These include obliteration of the *pterygoid fat pad* by anterior displacement of the disk (Fig. 14-15, *B*) and a decrease in the distance between the condyle and the glenoid fossa (Fig. 14-16). This *empty fossa* appearance warrants careful analysis of serial sagittal views as well as coronal images to exclude the possibility of pure medial or lateral displacement of the disk (Fig. 14-12).

The MR diagnosis of reduction requires demonstration of the normal bow tie configuration of the articular disk on open-mouth views (Figs. 14-10 and 14-16). Nonreducing disks may have a variety of configurations on MR. In patients with long-standing symptoms the disk will often appear buckled anterior to the condyle (Fig. 14-20).

The degree of mouth opening should be noted at the time of study and included in the body of the report. Whenever possible, patients should be encouraged to open beyond the point when any clicking occurs.

The role of arthrography

Several investigators[22,23] have determined that MR is more accurate than dual joint space arthrography in the diagnosis of internal derangements of the TMJ. However, MR remains relatively insensitive for the detection of intracapsular adhesions or joint space perforations. Although the presence of adhesions within the joint space may be suggested by analyzing joint motion on serial gradient echo images displayed in a cine loop, the diagnosis of intraarticular adhesions is beyond the ability of available MR technology. Perforations of the joint may be diagnosed on MR only when the cortical signal void of the condylar head is directly continuous with the signal void of the glenoid fossa.[44] Arthrography remains the imaging modality of choice for diagnosing adhesions and

perforations. TMJ arthroscopy, which appears even more sensitive than arthrography, may ultimately limit the utility of TMJ arthrography. Thus, despite its limitations, MR should constitute the first line in imaging of the TMJ because it provides accurate information regarding disk position in a noninvasive manner. The information obtained is adequate for deciding whether to institute conservative or surgical management. In difficult cases triple correlation (MR, arthrography, arthroscopy) may be necessary.[22]

IMAGING OF TMJ ARTHRITIDES
Degenerative joint disease

Degenerative joint disease (DJD, osteoarthritis) is the result of long-standing alterations in the normal biomechanical stresses placed on the joint. Altered biomechanical stresses are usually the result of internal derangements or trauma to the joint. DJD of the TMJ is quite common. Up to 20% of patients with TMJ complaints will demonstrate the changes of DJD on initial transcranial roentgenograms.[45]

The roentgenographic manifestations of degenerative change in the TMJ are similar to those seen in other joints.[46] Joint space narrowing and subchondral sclerosis are common. Osteophyte formation typically occurs at the periphery of the articular surface and is demonstrated to best advantage along the anterior margin of the articular surface; in long-standing cases extensive joint space remodeling occurs.

The typical changes of DJD involving the TMJ are well demonstrated by computed tomography (Fig. 14-21),

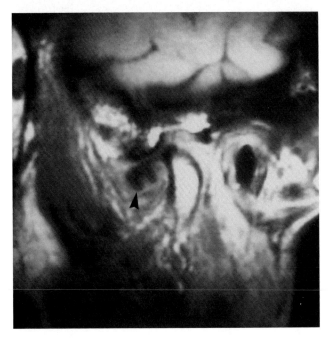

FIGURE 14-20
Anterior displacement without reduction. A sagittal T1-WI at the patient's maximum mouth opening (20 mm of interincisal distance) demonstrates a crumpled articular disk *(arrowhead)* anterior to the condylar head.

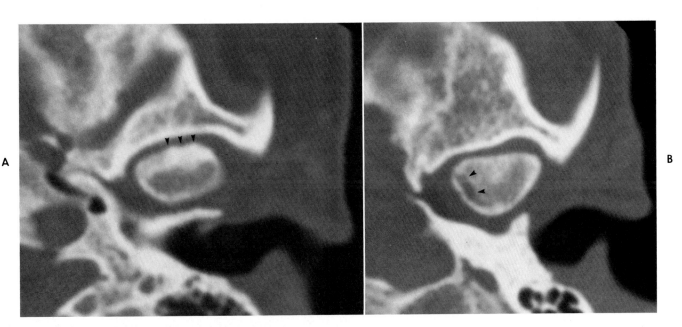

A

B

FIGURE 14-21
Degenerative joint disease. The initial transcranial roentgenograms in these two patients were interpreted as normal. **A,** An axial CT image of the left TMJ shows irregular hyperostosis along the anterior condylar head *(arrowheads).* **B,** An axial CT of the second patient demonstrates a well-circumscribed focus of subchondral cyst formation *(arrowheads).*

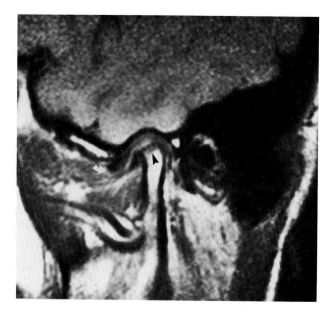

FIGURE 14-22
Degenerative joint disease. A sagittal T1-WI in the closed-mouth position demonstrates severe flattening of the articular portion of the condylar head *(arrowhead)*. The disk is displaced anteriorly *(curved arrow)*.

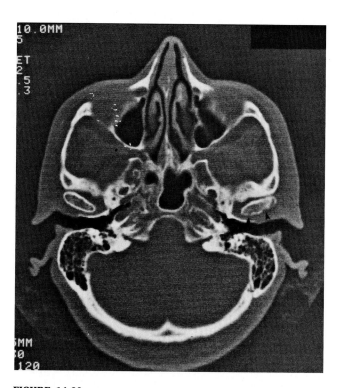

FIGURE 14-23
Rheumatoid arthritis. An axial CT image shows multiple erosions *(arrowheads)* on the posterior (juxtaarticular) surface of the left condylar head. (Courtesy Anton N. Hasso, M.D.).

which may reveal the erosive changes previously described as "osteoarthrosis."[46] Most, if not all, of the changes of late DJD can be identified on MR. The contour of the condyle may be assessed by analyzing the configuration of the cortical signal void (Fig. 14-22). Osteophytes may be identifiable as roughly triangular foci of absent signal along the anterior margin of the condylar head (Fig. 14-16). Joint space remodeling may be assessed by analyzing the configuration of the articular fossa signal void provided the articular eminence is not pneumatized. Recognition of the MR patterns of DJD is essential for accurate diagnosis of internal derangements. Identification of disk position in severe cases may be impossible due to extensive thinning of the disk.[43] Arthrography is usually necessary in these cases.

Inflammatory arthritis

As a synovium-lined joint, the TMJ is subject to any of the inflammatory or infectious arthritides that affect joints in the appendicular skeleton. Psoriatic arthritis, anklyosing spondylitis, and systemic lupus erythematosus may all affect the TMJ. However, involvement of the joint by these inflammatory arthritides may be clinically and radiographically indistinguishable. Analysis of other joints as well as careful evaluation of the clinical history is usually necessary to differentiate among them. In certain ethnic populations gout may involve the TMJ. Isolated cases of deposition of calcium hydrophosphate dihydrate in the TMJ (CPPD, "pseudogout") have also been reported.[47]

The most common inflammatory arthritis to affect the TMJ is rheumatoid arthritis (RA). As in other joints, inflammation of the synovial membrane (villous synovi-

tis) leads to formation of granulomatous tissue (pannus), which erodes into the fibrocartilaginous and osseous structures of the TMJ. CT may be used to identify the focal or diffuse cortical erosions seen in rheumatoid arthritis (Fig. 14-23).

A recent study by Larheim et al.[48] has documented the utility of MR imaging in patients with rheumatoid disease and symptoms of TMJ dysfunction. As in cases of DJD, areas of condylar deformation or destruction can be identified. MR can also portray destructive changes of the articular disk itself. In severely affected joints the joint space may be filled with intermediate signal on both T1W and T2W images (Fig. 14-17). This finding mimics the MR appearance of pannus and/or hyperplastic synovium as described in MR studies of RA involving other joints in the appendicular skeleton.[48] However, MR remains relatively insensitive to early synovial changes. The efficacy of MR contrast agents in detecting synovial abnormalities in the TMJ remains to be determined.

A surprisingly high incidence (12%) of internal derangements in otherwise normal-appearing joints was reported in Larheim's series,[48] which indicates that TMJ pain or dysfunction in a patient with known rheumatoid arthritis does not necessarily signify involvement by RA; radiographic investigation may be warranted (Fig. 14-17).

Pyogenic or granulomatous infections of the TMJ are uncommon but may be due to hematogenous seeding from a distant infection or, more commonly, may develop following TMJ surgery or as a direct extension of oral

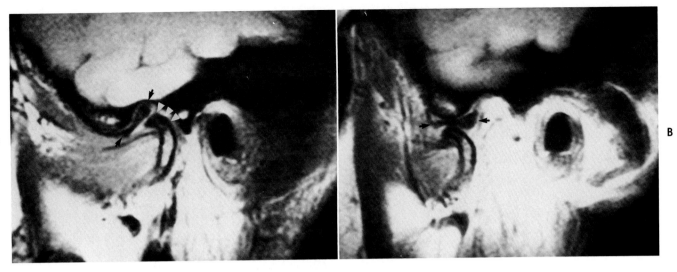

FIGURE 14-24
Avascular necrosis of the condylar head. **A,** Sagittal T1-WI closed-mouth. Note the complete loss of normal hyperintense marrow signal from the condylar head *(arrowheads).* Because of prior subcapital fracture, the condylar head is angled with respect to the condylar neck. The disk *(black arrows)* is in normal position. **B,** A sagittal T1-WI open-mouth confirms that it also is functioning normally *(black arrows).*

infections. The radiological findings are similar to those of rheumatoid arthritis, although the clinical course is much more rapid. History and physical examination should suggest the diagnosis. CT and MR may document the effectiveness of therapy or the various complications of infection.[48]

The MR and CT findings with avascular necrosis of the TMJ are similar to the changes identified in the femoral head. The primary manifestation of avascular necrosis is diminished signal in the condylar marrow on T1-WI (Fig. 14-24). The signal on T2-WI varies with the age of necrosis. These MR changes may be observed with internal derangement of the articular disk as well as with other well-known causes of aseptic necrosis (exogenous steroid administration, hematological disorders, trauma). It must be emphasized that the decreased marrow signal on T1-weighted images is not pathognomonic for avascular necrosis since hypointense marrow signal may be seen with a variety of pathological processes. Schellhas et al.[35] have described focal subcortical abnormalities of the condylar marrow in patients with osteochondritis dissecans.

Trauma

All the osseous components of the TMJ are subject to fracture.

The mandibular condyle is most commonly involved, usually from a direct blow to the chin. The majority of these fractures involve the condylar neck and are extracapsular. Depending upon the position of the fracture line relative to the point of insertion of the lateral pterygoid muscle, the condylar head either remains within the glenoid fossa or is displaced anteromedially. Although condylar neck fractures can be diagnosed with conventional roentgenography, CT best demonstrates the location of displaced fracture fragments.

Fractures involving the condylar head (intracapsular fractures) are much less common. CT studies are often invaluable in assessing the degree of comminution as well as delineating the intraarticular components of the fracture (Fig. 14-25).

Fractures of the articular eminence and glenoid fossa are usually the result of a direct lateral blow to the head. They often appear on CT with longitudinal fractures of the remainder of the temporal bone.

Trauma to the mandibular symphysis may injure the soft tissues of the TMJ without causing a fracture. The compressive force of a direct blow to the symphysis may be transmitted superiorly and posteriorly through the mandible, jamming the condylar head into the glenoid fossa and often eliciting an inflammatory response in the retrodiscal tissues (retrodiscitis), a traumatic joint effusion, and/or disruption of the attachment of the retrodiscal laminae to the posterior band. These soft tissue injuries are best evaluated with MR (Fig. 14-26).

The relationship between acceleration/deceleration (whiplash) injuries and TMJ dysfunction has not yet been thoroughly investigated. Whiplash injuries are theorized to produce direct injury to the retrodiscal laminae and anterior ligament of the TMJ. MR examinations, preferably obtained as soon after the injury as possible, are the only current imaging modality available for assessing the nature of any suspected injury to the TMJ following acceleration/deceleration trauma.[49]

Congenital abnormalities

The osseous and articular components of the TMJ are largely derived from the first branchial arch. Thus

FIGURE 14-25
Displaced fractures of the TMJ. **A,** Axial CT image in the closed-mouth position. Note the empty glenoid fossae bilaterally *(double asterisks)*. **B,** Coronal CT image. There is anterior and medial displacement of both condylar heads *(curved arrows)*. Note the fractured articulating surface of the left condylar head *(arrowhead)*.

FIGURE 14-26
Posttraumatic changes of the TMJ. **A,** Sagittal T1-WI in a patient complaining of TMJ pain following an auto accident. The anterior band *(white arrowhead)* is in normal position. There is marked thickening and irregularity to the retrodiscal tissues *(black arrowheads)* compatible with the traumatic retrodiscitis. **B,** Coronal T1-WI of the right TMJ in a second patient. The position of the articular disk *(white arrowheads)* appears normal. The medial discal ligament is thickened and irregular *(black arrowheads)*.

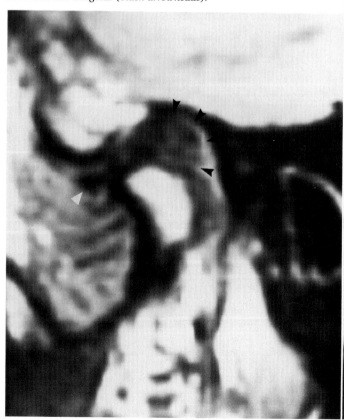
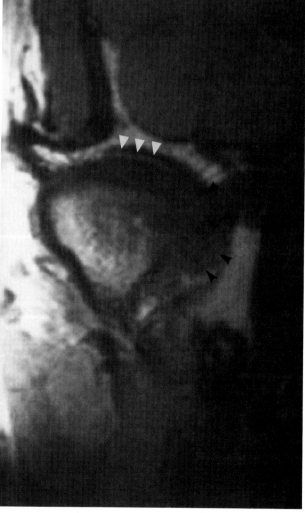

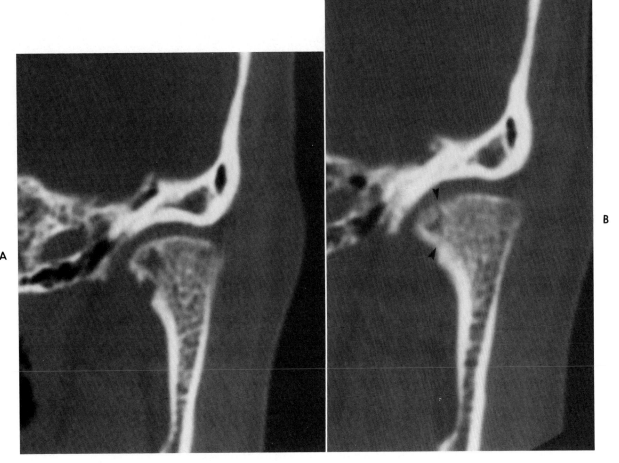

FIGURE 14-27
Metastatic disease involving the left TMJ. **A** and **B**, Coronal CT images in a child who complained of left ear pain. Multiple irregular lucencies are present in the cortex and medullary cavity of the condylar head. A pathological fracture (*arrowheads* in **B**) is present. The diagnosis was metastatic rhabdomyosarcoma.

congenital disorders (Treacher-Collins syndrome, Pierre Roban syndrome) are usually related to abnormal development of this arch.[47] Mandibular hypoplasia is a component of many craniofacial abnormalities, such as hemifacial microsomia. Because portions of the TMJ as well as the external and middle ear are derived from Meckel's cartilage, patients with developmental abnormalities of the ear (microtia or external auditory canal atresia) will often demonstrate concurrent abnormalities of the TMJ.

Hypoplasia and maldevelopment of the TMJ, as well as the rarer condylar head hyperplasia,[50] may be easily diagnosed using conventional radiography or polytomography. The role of CT is to acquire image data, which are then manipulated to create a three-dimensional image of the planned corrective surgery (Fig. 14-6). The role of MR in assessing patients with congenital abnormalities of the TMJ remains to be defined.

Neoplasms

Tumors of the TMJ are exceedingly rare. Most often they affect the joint secondarily by metastatic disease (Figs. 14-8 and 14-27) or extension of a primary mandibular tumor. As with the CT and MR manifestations of arthritides, the manifestations of primary TMJ neoplasms are similar to those identified in other joints of the appendicular skeleton. Osteochondroma (exostosis) is the most common benign tumor of the TMJ (Fig. 14-28), but osteomas and giant cell tumors have also been described. Primary sarcomas of the TMJ are very rare.

The recent radiographic literature includes several case reports of CT and MR in the diagnosis of synovial chondromatosis of the TMJ. The former is superior to conventional roentgenography in detecting intraarticular calcifications, but the latter is superior for identifying joint capsule enlargement as well as any potential intracranial extension.[51-53]

IMAGING THE TMJ FOLLOWING THERAPY

A complete description of the wide range of treatment options for internal derangements of the TMJ is beyond the scope of this chapter. The interested reader is referred to the comprehensive text by Okeson.[14] Medical therapy for TMJ symptoms includes oral analgesics, antiinflam-

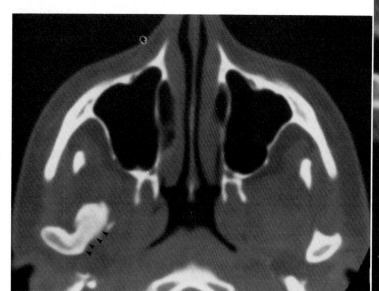

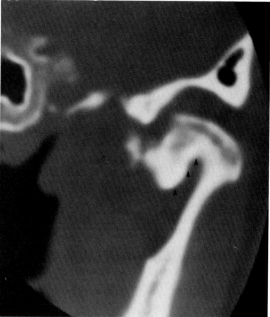

A

B

FIGURE 14-28
Osteoma of the condyle. **A,** Axial and, **B,** coronal CT images demonstrate a bony mass arising from the medial aspect of the right condylar head. The mass is continuous with the cortex and medullary cavity of the condyles *(arrowheads)*. These images were produced without the use of retrospective emphasis of bone detail.

matory agents, and muscle relaxants. Supportive therapies, including ultrasound, electrogalvanic stimulation, and topical moist heat, are directed at diminishing local pain and secondary muscle spasm. Relief of symptoms denotes success. Follow-up imaging studies are not routinely obtained.

Occlusal appliances are often used in the treatment of TMJ disorders. There are two broad categories, designed to provide relief of symptoms through different biomechanical principles. Occlusion splints (including flat splints and muscle relaxation appliances) alter the occlusal position and decrease masticator muscle spasm. Protrusive splints (also known as anterior repositioning appliances) alter the condylar position and reestablish a normal relationship between the condyle and the anteriorly displaced disk.

The end point of occlusal spint therapy, relief of local symptoms, is the same as that of medical and supportive management. Follow-up studies are not usually obtained. However, the goal of protrusive splint therapy is to reorient the TMJ into a more anatomical position. MR imaging may confirm successful repositioning of the joint prior to permanent orthodontic procedures.

Surgical repair of the TMJ is typically contemplated after failure of conservative (medical, supportive, and/or occlusive) therapy. The surgical procedure of choice is plication. During plication a portion of the retrodiskal laminae is removed. The intact articular disk is retracted to its correct position and secured with sutures. If it has been so damaged that it cannot be retained for use, it is removed (diskectomy, menicsectomy). Simple diskec-

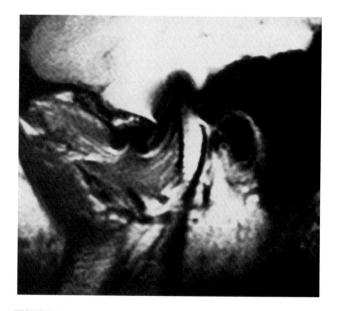

FIGURE 14-29
Warping artifact. Sagittal T1-WI in the closed-mouth position in a patient 1 year status post-meniscoplasty. Anatomical detail is completely obscured by the presence of ferromagnetic material within the joint.

tomy results in direct bone-to-bone contact between the articular surfaces of the condylar head and the temporal bone. To avoid the degenerative changes that usually follow, a variety of diskal implants as well as dermal grafts are utilized.

Imaging of postsurgical patients is typically performed only if there is recurrence or persistence of symptoms.

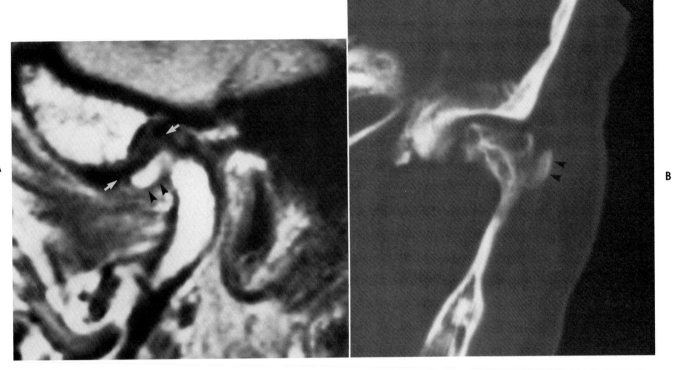

FIGURE 14-30
Myositis ossificans of the TMJ. **A,** Sagittal T1-WI closed-mouth demonstrating a mass of hyperintense signal anterior to the condylar head *(arrowheads)*. The articular disk *(White arrows)* is in normal position. **B,** Coronal CT image through the anterior condylar head. Note the mass with cortical and trabecular elements attached to the condylar head *(arrowheads)*.

Most studies to date have focused on the MR appearance of failed prosthetic disk implants, secondary either to implant fracture[54] or to destructive arthritis associated with Proplast implants.[55,56]

MR examinations in patients following diskectomy or disk plication may be hampered by field-warping artifacts, presumably due to minute foci of ferromagnetic material in the operative bed (Fig. 14-29). MR evaluation of the postplication patient is further hampered by the general lack of information on symptom-free postoperative patients. A recent study by Lieberman et al.[56] suggests that a "successful" disk plication may have a wide range of MR appearances. Of particular note is that over 50% of patients will demonstrate persistent anterior displacement of the disk following plication. Variations in the configuration and signal intensity of the plicated disk after dermal grafting may also be observed.[56]

Fig. 14-30 demonstrates a different reason for treatment failure. This patient complained of increasing local pain following a series of corticosteroid injections into the cortical space. CT studies demonstrated periarticular ossifications. The MR examination confirmed both a normal position of the disk and the presence of extensive periarticular ossifications, which were successfully resected.

REFERENCES

1. Guralnick W, Kaban LB, Merrill RG: Temporomandibular-joint afflictions. N Engl J Med 1978;299:123-129.

2. Solberg WK, Woo MW, Houston JB: Prevalence of mandibular dysfunction in young adults. J Am Dent Assoc 1979;98:25-34.

3. McNeill C, Danzig WM, Farrar WB, et al: Craniomandibular (TMJ) disorders: the state of the art. J Prosthet Dent 1980; 44:434-437.

4. Helms CA, Vogler JB, Morrish RB, et al: Temporomandibular joint internal derangements: CT diagnosis. Radiology 1984;152: 459-462.

5. Walter E, Huls A, Schmelzle R, et al: CT and MR imaging of the temporomandibular joint. Radiographics 1988;8:327-348.

6. Harms SE, Wilk RM, Wolford LM, et al: The temporomandibular joint: magnetic resonance imaging using surface coils. Radiology 1985;157:133-136.

7. Katzberg RW, Bessette RW, Tallents RH, et al: Normal and abnormal temporomandibular joint: MR imaging with surface coil. Radiology 1986;158:183-189.

8. Ten Cate A: The temporomandibular joint. In Ten Cate A (ed): Oral histology: development, structure, and function, 3rd ed. St Louis, Mosby, 1989.

9. Hasso AN, Christiansen EL, Alder ME: The temporomandibular joint. Radiol Clin North Am 1989;27:301-314.

10. Bergeron RT: The temporal bone. In Bergeron RT, Osborn AG, Som PM (eds): Head and neck imaging excluding the brain. St Louis, Mosby, 1984.

11. Bell, WE: Temporomandibular disorders, 2nd ed. Chicago, Year Book, 1986.

12. Harms SE: Temporomandibular joint imaging. In Kressel HY (ed): Magnetic resonance imaging annual, 1988, New York, Raven, 1988.

13. Sharawy M, Bhussry BR, Suarez FR: The temporomandibular joint. In Bhaskar SN (ed): Orban's oral histology, 11th ed. St Louis, Mosby, 1989.

14. Okeson JP: Management of temporomandibular disorders and occlusion. 2nd ed. St Louis, Mosby, 1989.

15. Carpentier P, Yung JP, Marguelles-Bonnet R, Meunissier M: Insertions of the lateral pterygoid muscle: an anatomic study of the human temporomandibular joint. J Oral Maxillofac Surg 1988;46:477-482.

16. Hansson LG, Westesson PL, Katzberg RW, et al: MR imaging of the temporomandibular joint: comparison of images of autopsy specimens made at 0.3 T and 1.5 T with anatomic cryosections. AJR 1989;152:1241-1244.

17. Westesson PL, Katzberg RW, Tallents RH, et al: CT and MR of the temporomandibular joint: comparison with autopsy specimens. AJR 1987;148:1165-1171.

18. Westesson PL, Katzberg RW, Tallents RH, et al: Temporomandibular joint: comparison of MR images with cryosectional anatomy. Radiology 1987;164:59-64.

19. Harms SE, Wilk RM: Magnetic resonance imaging of the temporal mandibular joint. Radiographics 1987;7:521-542.

20. Schellhas KP, Wilkes CH, Fritts HM, et al: Temporomandibular joint: MR imaging of internal derangements and postoperative changes. AJNR 1987;8:1093-1101.

21. Kaplan PA, Tu HK, Williams SM, Lydiatt DD: The normal temporomandibular joint: MR and arthographic correlation. Radiology 1987;165:177-178.

22. Rao VM, Farole A, Karasick D: Temporomandibular joint dysfunction: correlation of MR imaging, arthrography, and arthroscopy. Radiology 1990;174:663-667.

23. Schellhas KP, Wilkes CH, Omlie MR, et al: The diagnosis of temporomandibular joint disease: two-compartment arthrography and MR. AJR 1988;151:341-350.

24. Manzione JV, Seltzer SE, Katzberg RW, et al: Direct sagittal computed tomography of the temporomandibular joint. AJR 1983;140:165-167.

25. Sartoris DJ, Neumann CH, Riley RW: The temporomandibular joint: true sagittal computed tomography with meniscus visualization. Radiology 1984;150:250-254.

26. Simon DC, Hess ML, Smilak MS, Beltran J: Direct sagittal CT of the temporomandibular joint. Radiology 1985;157:545.

27. Vannier MW, Marsh JL, Warren JO: Three dimension CT reconstruction images for craniofacial surgical planning and evaluation. Radiology 1984;150:179-184.

28. Katzberg RW: Temporomandibular joint imaging. Radiology 1989;170:297-307.

29. Shellock FG, Pressman BD: Dual-surface-coil MR imaging of bilateral temporomandibular joints: improvements in the imaging protocol. AJNR 1989;10:595-598.

30. Schellhas KP: MR imaging of muscles of mastication. AJR 1989;153:847-855.

31. Burnettt KR, Davis CL, Read J: Dynamic display of the temporomandibular joint meniscus by using "fast-scan" MR imaging. AJR 1987;149:959-962.

32. Katzberg RW, Westesson PL, Tallents RH, et al: Temporomandibular joint: MR assessment of rotational and sideways disc displacements. Radiology 1988;169:741-748.

33. Schwaighofer BW, Tanaka TT, Klein MV, et al: MR imaging of the temporomandibular joint: a cadaver study of the value of coronal images. AJR 1990;154:1245-1249.

34. Beltran J, Noto AM, Herman LF, et al: Joint effusions: MR imaging. Radiology 1986;158:133-137.

35. Schellhas KP, Wilkes CH, Fritts HM, et al: MR of osteochondritis dissecans. Avascular necrosis of the mandibular condyle. AJNR 1989;10:3-12. AJR 1989;152:551-560.

36. Conway WF, Hayes CW, Campbell RL, Laskin DM: Temporomandibular joint motion: efficacy of fast low-angle shot MR imaging. Radiology 1989;172:821-826.

37. Schellhas KP, Wilkes CH: Temporomandibular joint inflammation: comparison of MR fast scanning with T1- and T2-weighted imaging techniques. AJNR 1889;10:589-594.

38. Harms SE: Correlation of cine spin-echo MR imaging with arthroscopy of the temporomandibular joint in the diagnosis of joint adhesions. Radiology 1989;173(P):100.

39. Wilk RM, Harms SE: Temporomandibular joint: multislab, three-dimensional Fourier transformation MR imaging. Radiology 1988;167:861-863.

40. Farrar WB, McCarty WL: A clinical outline of temporomandibular joint diagnosis and treatment. Montgomery Ala, Normandie Publications, 1982.

41. Drace JE: Natural history of minimal anterior displacements of the temporomandibular joint meniscus. Radiology 1988;169(P):98-99.

42. Miller TL, Katzberg RW, Tallents RH, et al: Temporomandibular joint clicking with nonreducing anterior displacement of the meniscus. Radiology 1985;154:121-124.

43. Helms CA, Kaban LB, McNeill C, Dodson T: Temporomandibular joint: morphology and signal intensity characteristics of the disk at MR imaging. Radiology 1989;172:817-820.

44. Nokes SR, Spritzer CE, Vogler JB, et al: Assessment of temporomandibular joint meniscus perforation with MR imaging. Radiology 1988;169(P):99.

45. Katzberg RW, Keith DA, Guralnick WC, et al: Internal derangements and arthritis of the temporomandibular joint. Radiology 1983;146:107-112.

46. Toller PA: Osteoarthrosis of the mandibular condyle. Br Dent J 1973;134:223-231.

47. Murphy WA: The temporomandibular joint. In Resnick D, Niwayama G (eds): Diagnosis of bone and joint disorders, 2nd ed. Philadelphia, Saunders, 1988.

48. Larheim TA, Smith HJ, Aspestrand F: Rheumatic disease of the temporomandibular joint: MR imaging and tomographic manifestations. Radiology 1990;175:527-531.

49. Schellhas KP: Temporomandibular joint injuries. Radiology 1989;173:211-216.

50. Munk PL, Helms CA: Coronoid process hyperplasia: CT studies. Radiology 1989;171:783-784.

51. Herzog S, Mafee M: Synovial chondromatosis of the TMJ: MR and CT findings. AJNR 1990;1:742-745.

52. Manco LG, DeLuke DM: CT diagnosis of synovial chondromatosis of the temporomandibular joint. AJR 148:574-576, 1987.

53. Nokes SR, King PS, Garcia R, et al: Temporomandibular joint chondromatosis with intracranial extension: MR and CT contributions. AJR 1987;148:1173-1174.

54. Kneeland JB, Ryan DE, Carrera GF, et al: Failed temporomandibular joint prostheses: MR imaging. Radiology 1987;165:179-181.

55. Schellhas KP, Wilkes CH, el Deeb M, et al: Permanent Proplast temporomandibular joint implants: MR imaging of destructive complications. AJR 1988;151:731-735.

56. Liberman JM, Bradrick JP, Indresano AT, et al: Dermal grafts of the temporomandibular joint: postoperative appearance on MR images. Radiology 1990;176:199-203.

15 Shoulder

MAHVASH RAFII

Although the shoulder is the most mobile joint in the body, its mobility is due to anatomical characteristics of the glenohumeral joint, which renders it inherently unstable. Stability is provided mostly by the soft tissue structures, consisting of the capsulolabral complex and the internal and external rotator muscles. These anatomical characteristics predispose the shoulder to a variety of disorders that are either uncommon or nonexistent in other joints.

Orthopedists deal with a myriad of painful and functional disabilities of the shoulder, some of which prove challenging in diagnosis and treatment. Radiographic evaluations, which in the past were limited to conventional roentgenograms, arthrograms, and sonograms, have traditionally been used for detection of arthritic processes, fractures, osseous lesions associated with shoulder instability, and the impingement syndrome, as well as in diagnosing rotator cuff tears. More recently imaging of the shoulder has been dramatically enhanced by the addition of computed tomography and by magnetic resonance imaging. Despite the fact that the accuracy of conventional arthrography in detection of rotator cuff tears has been undisputed, and CT arthrography has been found extremely reliable for evaluation of the capsulolabral complex of the glenohumeral joint, MRI is coming to be looked upon as the noninvasive modality capable of achieving these goals plus resolving the diagnostic difficulties associated with early stages of the impingement syndrome (i.e., rotator cuff tendinitis and partial noncommunicating rotator cuff tears). The exquisite soft tissue resolution and multiplanar imaging capability of MRI are the most important aspects of this modality, which may well become the singular diagnostic technique for evaluating all components of the shoulder in a noninvasive manner.

In this chapter the regional anatomy of the shoulder, primarily the glenohumeral joint region, techniques of CT, CT-arthrography, and MRI, and the normal planar anatomy as displayed by CT-arthrography and MRI are discussed. Disorders of the shoulder are included in two

465

ANATOMY OF THE SHOULDER MUSCLES

Scapulohumeral
    Subscapularis   Teres minor
    Supraspinatus   Teres major
    Infraspinatus   Deltoideus
Scapula to forearm
    Biceps and coracobrachialis
    Triceps
Axioscapular
    Trapezius
    Rhomboideus
    Serratus anterior
    Levator scapulae
Axiohumeral
    Pectoralis major
    Pectoralis minor
    Latissimus dorsi

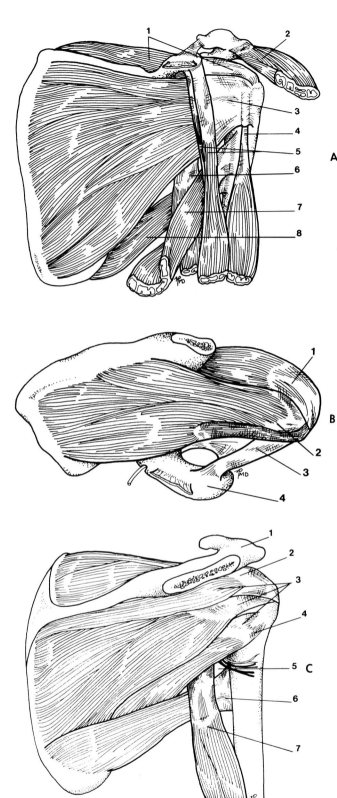

FIGURE 15-1
Muscular anatomy of the shoulder. **A,** Anterior view. *1,* Supraspinatus; *2,* deltoideus; *3,* subscapularis; *4,* biceps, long head; *5,* coracobrachialis and biceps, short head; *6,* triceps, long head; *7,* latissimus dorsi; *8,* teres major. **B,** Superior view. *1,* Infraspinatus; *2,* supraspinatus; *3,* coracohumeral ligament; *4,* coracoid process. **C,** Posterior view. *1,* Acromion; *2,* supraspinatus; *3,* infraspinatus; *4,* teres minor; *5,* quadrangular space; *6,* teres major; *7,* triceps, long head.

major categories — shoulder instability and impingement syndrome — with other topics discussed primarily as they relate to the relevant imaging modalities.

NORMAL REGIONAL ANATOMY

The shoulder girdle consists of four separate articulations — glenohumeral, scapulothoracic, acromioclavicular, and sternoclavicular — supported by several groups of strong muscles. Each plays an important role in coordinated movement of the arm.

The glenohumeral joint, complex yet highly mobile, consists of the relatively flat glenoid fossa and the round humeral head (whose articular surface is twice that of the glenoid).[1] Its wide range of motion is supported by a redundant fibrous joint capsule.[2] Also four strategically situated groups of muscles, acting together, provide stability as well as the wide range of motion afforded by this joint[3] (see box). The following discussion pertains primarily to the glenohumeral joint and the muscles in its immediate vicinity that are relevant to ensuing discussions in this chapter.

Muscular anatomy

Among the four groups of muscles listed above, the *scapulohumeral* group is the most significant in terms of function of the glenohumeral joint. This group—subscapularis, supraspinatus, infraspinatus, teres minor, teres major, and deltoideus—originates from the scapula and extends to the humerus. It holds the humerus against the glenoid and assists in medial (internal) and lateral (external) rotation as well as in elevation of the arm. The first four muscles, referred to as the "short rotators," form the tendinous rotator cuff and insert onto the humeral tuberosities.

Subscapularis. The subscapularis, a broad muscle with several components, arises from the medial two thirds of the costal surface of the scapula (Figs. 15-1, *A,* and 15-2).

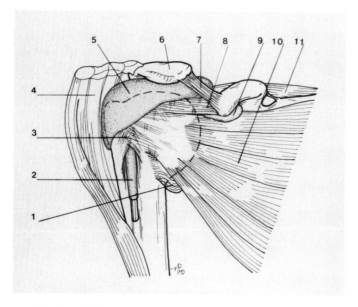

FIGURE 15-5
Anterior view of the glenohumeral joint. *1*, Joint capsule; *2*, bicipital tendon sheath; *3*, transverse humeral ligament; *4*, deltoideus; *5*, SA-SD bursa; *6*, acromion; *7*, coracoacromial ligament; *8*, coracohumeral ligament (joint capsule); *9*, subscapular bursa; *10*, subscapularis; *11*, supraspinatus.

Infraspinatus. The infraspinatus arises from the infraspinatus fossa of the scapula, crosses the glenohumeral joint posterosuperiorly, and inserts on the middle facet of the greater tuberosity (Figs. 15-1, *C*, and 15-2). It invariably is formed from several components whose tendons unite to make up the most prominent tendinous structure within the rotator cuff.[4] The infraspinatus is a lateral rotator and also holds the humeral head in the glenoid cavity.

Interrelations. The relationship between the spinati is worth some detailed discussion. Beyond the lateral margin of the scapular spine the two muscles gradually approximate and their tendons eventually blend. In this region (posteriorly) the supraspinatus tendon is comparatively thinner than its anterior component (it thins in an anteroposterior orientation) and thinner also than the infraspinatus tendon. As demonstrated in some anatomy texts and stressed by Neer,[5] the two tendons overlap just prior to their greater tuberosity insertion (Fig. 15-1, *B*). According to Skinner,[6] from childhood to adult life there is a progressive transformation of muscle to tendon at the supraspinatus musculotendinous junction, along with a progressive incorporation of tendon and joint capsule. In addition, the connective tissue interface between the spinatus tendons becomes more fibrous with advancing age. This latter observation may explain the varying distinguishability of the two tendons on MRI and the fact that overlapping of the tendons is seen better in some patients than in others.

Teres minor. The teres minor is a narrow muscle originating from the lateral border of the scapula (Figs. 15-1, *C*, and 15-2). It extends upward to insert on the lower facet of the greater tuberosity and the surgical neck

of the humerus. It is intimately associated with, and at times inseparable from, the infraspinatus. It acts as a lateral (external) rotator and an adductor of the arm.

Teres major. The teres major arises from the lateral border of the scapula near the inferior angle and forms a tendinous insertion onto the crest of the lesser tuberosity (Figs. 15-1, *C*, and 15-4). It is an adductor, medial rotator, and extensor of the arm.

Deltoideus. The deltoideus is a triangular muscle that arises from the lateral third of the clavicle, the lateral border of the acromion, and the adjacent scapular spine (Figs. 15-1, *A*, 15-3, and 15-4). It inserts on the deltoid tuberosity of the humerus. This muscle is the principal abductor of the humerus, with the supraspinatus participating up to 90 degrees of abduction.

• • •

Other muscles especially identified with the glenohumeral joint include the biceps brachii, coracobrachialis, triceps brachii, and latissimus dorsi.

Biceps brachii. The biceps brachii is the most prominent muscle in the anterior humeral area (Fig. 15-1, *A*). The long head of its tendon originates from the supraglenoid tubercle (Fig. 15-2) and exits the glenohumeral joint through an opening in the capsule above the bicipital groove (Fig. 15-4). Within the groove the tendon is secured by the rigid transverse humeral ligament, which bridges the humeral tuberosities at the upper aspect of the groove (Figs. 15-1, *A*, and 15-5). A synovial sheath covers the long head of the tendon from its origin and extends into the bicipital groove, forming the sleeve of the tendon (Fig. 15-5). Therefore the intraarticular component of the tendon, although intracapsular, is extrasynovial. The synovial cavity of the shoulder joint and the synovial sleeve of the biceps tendon freely communicate. The short head of this muscle arises from the tip of the coracoid process, in conjunction with the tendon of the coracobrachialis (Fig. 15-1, *A*).

Coracobrachialis. This relatively flat muscle arises from the tip of the coracoid process and inserts by a flat tendon on the medial surface of the humerus proximal to its midportion (Figs. 15-1, *A*, and 15-2).

Triceps brachii. The triceps brachii consists of three separate heads and occupies the entire posterior aspect of the arm. The long head arises by a broad tendon from the infraglenoid tubercle of the scapula and descends between the teres minor and teres major (Figs. 15-1, *A* and *B*, and 15-2). The lateral and medial heads originate from the humerus. The distal tendon inserts on the olecranon process.

Latissimus dorsi. The flat tendon of this large, triangular muscle inserts on the floor of the bicipital groove, ventral to the insertion of the teres major (Fig. 15-1, *A*).

Articular, bursal, and ligamentous anatomy
GLENOHUMERAL JOINT

The articulation of the glenohumeral joint consists of the humeral head, the glenoid fossa, and the capsular

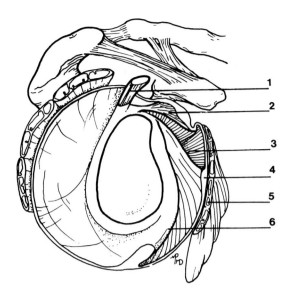

FIGURE 15-6
Glenohumeral capsular ligaments. *1*, Biceps tendon, long head; *2*, superior glenohumeral ligament; *3*, middle glenohumeral ligament; *4*, anterior joint capsule and inferior glenohumeral ligament; *5*, subscapularis; *6*, inferior fold of the inferior glenohumeral ligament.

structures. The spherical *humeral head* is situated against the relatively flat glenoid fossa. An indentation of its superior aspect between the articulating surface and the tuberosities forms the anatomical neck (Fig. 15-4). The *glenoid cavity* is wider in its inferior margin and relatively pointed superiorly, having the overall appearance of an inverted comma[7] (Fig. 15-2). The hyaline articular cartilage is thinner in the center, providing a slight degree of concavity for the flat articulating surface of the glenoid. The *capsular mechanism* of the joint consists of the fibrous capsule and the capsular ligaments, the synovial recesses, and the glenoid labrum, all of which are intimately associated with the rotator cuff tendons (Fig. 15-2). The long head of the biceps tendon superiorly and the long head of the triceps muscle inferiorly designate the division of the capsular mechanism into anterior and posterior components.

Joint capsule. The fibrous capsule is normally lax and redundant.[1] Anteriorly three capsular (glenohumeral) ligaments are recognized[1,2]: the superior, the middle, and the inferior (Fig. 15-6). They are thick fibrous bands formed within the capsule that act as reinforcing structures, limiting the external rotation of the humeral head.[2] Laterally the superior and middle glenohumeral ligaments are attached to the anterior anatomical neck adjacent to the lesser tuberosity (Fig. 15-4). Medially the superior ligament and the joint capsule extend to the glenoid margin, with attachments to the base of the coracoid process and supraglenoid tubercle. The glenoid insertion of the middle glenohumeral ligament extends from the insertion of the superior ligament to the junction of the middle and inferior thirds of the glenoid rim.[8] There is considerable variation in the development of the middle glenohumeral ligament, which may be associated with the formation of more than one subscapular bursa.[7]

The most constant synovial bursa, the superior subscapular, is formed through an opening in the capsule between the superior and middle glenohumeral ligaments[2,7] (Figs. 15-2 and 15-6). The inferior glenohumeral ligament is more constant and the most important of the glenohumeral ligaments in providing stability for the joint. It is a broad ligament with attachment to the anterior, inferior, and posterior glenoid margin near or continuous with the inferior glenoid labrum.[8]

Anteriorly below the subscapular bursa the joint capsule forms a smooth reflection over the scapular cortex while adhering to its periosteum. It extends toward the glenoid margin and blends with the labrum (Figs. 15-2 and 15-4).

Three types of anterior capsular insertions have been recognized, based on their proximity to the glenoid margin[2,9]: type I (near or on the labrum), type II (medial to it), and type III (near the scapular neck). Of the three, type I is considered most stable; types II and III are thought possibly to be prone to instability. The middle glenohumeral ligament is quite variable and, when present, may or may not have a labral attachment[2] (p. 474). Posteriorly the capsule is more intimately related to the glenoid labrum along the entire posterior glenoid margin. Laterally it inserts on the anatomical neck of the humerus, and it extends inferiorly and medially along the surgical neck.

Glenoid labrum. The glenoid labrum, a fold of articular capsule, is composed mostly of dense fibrous tissue.[2] A small amount of fibrocartilage is found at its base. Superiorly it blends with the long head of the biceps tendon (Figs. 15-2 and 15-6), anteriorly it is usually triangular, and posteriorly it is somewhat rounded. Peripherally its nonarticulating surface is contiguous with the capsule and may be covered by a layer of synovial tissue. Its articular surface is contiguous with, and loosely adherent to, the hyaline articular cartilage of the glenoid, which extends beneath the labrum to the osseous glenoid margin (Fig. 15-3).

SYNOVIAL BURSAE

Subscapular bursae. The superior subscapular bursa is the most constant of the synovial bursae, being encountered in 80% to 89% of individuals.[2] It is a fingerlike extension of synovium protruding through an anterior capsular opening between the superior and middle glenohumeral ligaments (Figs. 15-2, 15-5, and 15-6). Extending medially along the superior border of the subscapularis tendon toward the base of the coracoid process, it forms a "saddle" over the free margin of this tendon and provides a gliding mechanism between the tendon and the coracoid process. The larger component of the bursa, variable in size, is formed between the tendon and the scapular cortex (p. 474).

Based on the variable anatomy of the capsular ligaments, in particular that of the middle glenohumeral ligament, one or more inferior subscapular bursae may be present.[7]

Subacromial-subdeltoid bursa. The SA-SD bursa is a constant structure cushioning the rotator cuff tendons and the coracoacromial arch (Figs. 15-3 to 15-5). Laterally it extends between the greater tuberosity and the deltoideus, facilitating movement of the latter over the former. It is covered by an extrasynovial layer of fat 1 to 2 mm wide.[11] The floor of the bursa is firmly adherent to the greater tuberosity and musculotendinous cuff, and the roof is adherent to the undersurface of the acromion and the coracoacromial ligament. The lateral walls extend loosely downward under the deltoid muscle, backward, and outward under the acromion and medially beneath the coracoid process.[7]

Other bursae. A noncommunicating bursa, the *subcoracoid,* has been described situated at the ventral aspect of the subscapularis tendon. However, it is generally believed to be an extension of the subacromial bursa.[10] Occasionally another bursa is found posteriorly between the infraspinatus tendon and the joint capsule.

LIGAMENTS

The ligaments in the anterior shoulder include (1) the coracohumeral, which is an external thickening of the glenohumeral joint capsule (Fig. 15-5), (2) the coracoclavicular, which is a stabilizer of the clavicle to the scapula (Fig. 15-6), and (3) the transverse, which is an extension of the coracohumeral ligament and subscapularis tendon and forms the rigid roof of the bicipital groove (Fig. 15-5).

CORACOACROMIAL ARCH

This bony/ligamentous arch includes the acromion and coracoid processes as well as the coracoacromial ligament between them (Figs. 15-2 and 15-6). The acromion process is the flat termination of the scapular spine that protects, along with the coracoacromial ligament and coracoid process, the humeral head posteriorly, superiorly, and (to a lesser extent) anteriorly. The coracoacromial ligament is a triangular band of tissue extending from the anterior margin of the coracoid process to the inner border of the acromion, in front of the acromioclavicular joint.

ACROMIOCLAVICULAR JOINT

The acromioclavicular joint has a variable plane, from vertical to nearly horizontal.[12] Its synovium-lined articular capsule is supported by the superior and inferior acromioclavicular ligaments. It often contains a fibrocartilaginous disk, which is more pronounced in its superior aspect (Fig. 15-3).

IMAGING TECHNIQUES
Computed tomography

CT of the shoulder without intraarticular contrast enhancement is utilized when plain roentgenography has failed to substantiate adequately a suspected osseous or paraarticular abnormality. It is most beneficial in evaluating acute intraarticular fractures but is also helpful in recognition of etopic ossifications and fractures associated with glenohumeral instability. Less often, it is used when there is suspicion of an osseous or soft tissue tumor about the shoulder girdle. Intravenous contrast enhancement is required in the latter instances.

Technique. Routine imaging of the shoulder is performed with the patient supine and the arm alongside. In patients with a wide shoulder girdle the contralateral arm is elevated with the hand beneath the head. This reduces the width of the shoulder girdle and prevents formation of linear artifacts on axial images.

Slice thickness varies in accordance with the suspected pathology. Ordinarily 5 mm thick sections consecutively obtained will provide adequate bony detail and are suitable for evaluating traumatic lesions of the shoulder. The slice thickness can be increased to 10 mm when larger paraarticular lesions are suspected. However, when searching for smaller lesions or in restricted anatomical areas (e.g., the AC joint), 3 mm thick slices are necessary. Based on available computer software, reconstruction of these images can be limited prospectively or retrospectively to the shoulder, with an appropriate magnification factor. Reconstruction algorithms designated for bone or soft tissue enhancement are also utilized depending upon the nature of the suspected lesion. The hard copies are produced twice, first with a wide window setting (2000/200) and then with a narrow setting (500/50).

CT-arthrography

CT-arthrography was introduced primarily for evaluation of glenoid labral tears, most investigators[13-15] having recognized the limitations of conventional arthrography in this respect. Prior to the availability of CT, double-contrast arthrography and arthrotomography were advocated for these injuries.[16-19] Computed arthrotomography, however, tremendously improved visualization of the capsulolabral complex and became the modality of choice for detecting and quantifying lesions associated with shoulder instability.

Technique. A conventional double-contrast arthrogram is obtained using 3 to 4 ml of positive contrast agent, 0.33 ml of 1/1000 epinephrine, and 12 ml of room air.[20] The use of a lesser amount of positive contrast or air alone has also been reported.[14] Although adequate coating of the synovial surfaces and the glenoid labrum can be achieved by small amounts of contrast, and diagnostic images of the capsulolabral complex can be obtained with air alone, in some cases adequate visualization of partial or full-thickness cuff tears will not be accomplished. For this reason CT-arthrography with smaller amounts of positive contrast should be reserved strictly for patients suspected of having only capsulolabral pathology, bearing in mind that shoulder instability and rotator cuff disorders, including cuff tears, may coexist. Most investigators use 12 ml of air.

Roentgenographic examination is limited to AP views, with internal and external rotation, prior to and following the injection of contrast medium. If a rotator cuff tear is not visualized on postinjection views, the shoulder is exercised and similar views are again obtained. This underscores the need for a thorough and adequate arthrographic examination in detecting rotator cuff tears, despite the possibility that leakage of air through the capsule may occur (usually from the subscapular bursa); incidentally, however, leakage does not interfere with optimal visualization of the labrum.

The patient is then transferred to the CT suite. It is desirable that there be no delay in obtaining the CT examination, which is performed with the patient supine

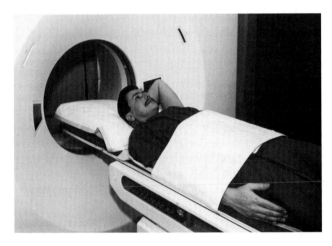

FIGURE 15-7
Patient position for CT-arthrography. Neutral rotation of the humerus is achieved by placing the arm alongside the supine patient, thumb pointing up. The contralateral arm is elevated and flexed at the elbow, hand under the head.

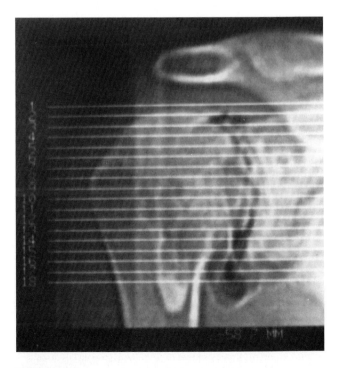

FIGURE 15-8
CT-arthrography, right shoulder. Posted "scout" view.

and the arm in neutral rotation (alongside, palm against the thigh). In patients with a wide shoulder girdle the contralateral arm is elevated and the hand placed behind the head (Fig. 15-7). With neutral rotation of the humerus, the anterior and posterior components of the joint capsule are similarly relaxed and the glenoid labrum can be adequately visualized. Additional sections with the arm in external rotation are obtained either routinely or when a posterior lesion is suspected.[14,15] Routine imaging, with the arm first internally and then externally rotated is, in our opinion, redundant.[21] Contiguous 3 mm thick slices of the glenohumeral joint region are obtained (Fig. 15-8). The acromioclavicular joint may be included in the field of examination. Enhanced and magnified images are reconstructed based on available software. The standard algorithm (General Electric 9800) is preferable to either soft tissue or bone algorithms, since the soft tissue and osseous structures and the dense contrast medium are equally enhanced. To resolve the capsulolabral complex against the osseous glenoid, wide window settings (window/level 3000/300) are used for producing hard copies. Narrow window settings of 1000/100 have also been suggested for evaluation of musculotendinous structures.

Direct sagittal computed arthrotomography can improve the visualization of cuff tears.[22] The patient is seated at the end of the scanner, side of interest next to the gantry, and leans into the gantry with the forearm resting on the table.

Some difficulty with interpretation can arise due to faulty injection of contrast. Extraarticular or intracapsular injection may result from inadequate advancement of the needle, with consequent loss of definition of the capsule. The needle tip may also lodge within the labrum, and forced injection of contrast may obscure a lesion or produce an artifact that simulates a labral tear.[23] These complications are best avoided by meticulous observation of the technique of arthrography.[20] Needle positioning should be guided by fluoroscopy. A test injection of a small amount of air or contrast medium should meet no resistance when the needle is in the joint, and the contrast should flow away from the tip of the needle rather than pool around it. In patients with suspected anterior pathology a posterior approach has been suggested,[24] but this is cumbersome and unnecessary.

Magnetic resonance

Although development of an MR technique for imaging the shoulder has proven challenging, the availability of flexible surface coils coupled with the advent of high-resolution scanning techniques, and particularly an off-center zoom technique, has provided a crucial incentive.[25-28] The early literature dealt with demonstrating the normal MR anatomy of the shoulder, including a description of the imaging planes suitable for evaluation of various disorders. Subsequently numerous investigators[29-40] have reported the findings associated with shoulder impingement syndrome, rotator cuff tears, and shoulder instability. With improvements in technique and increasing experience, it has become evident that MR imaging is highly accurate in detecting rotator cuff tears and other findings of the impingement syndrome (i.e., rotator cuff tendinitis, SA-SD bursitis, and osseous changes of the coracoacromial arch, AC joint, and humeral tuberosities). Also the glenohumeral joint and capsulolabral complex are concomitantly evaluated for manifestations of instability or arthritic processes.

Technique. The use of a surface coil is mandatory. Various types of coils are now available, either made specifically for shoulder imaging[36] or adaptable to the shoulder (Fig. 15-9). Patient positioning is similar to that for computed arthrography (i.e., supine with the arm in neutral rotation) (Fig. 15-10) and is favored because with the arm in neutral rotation the supraspinatus (muscle and tendon) assumes an orientation parallel to the anatomical

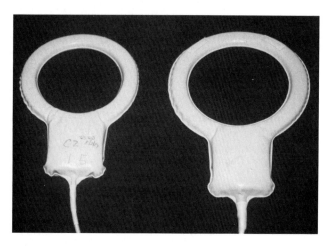

FIGURE 15-9
Adaptable circular surface coils for MR imaging of the shoulder. (Gyroscan, Philips Medical Systems North America, Shelton Conn, 06484.)

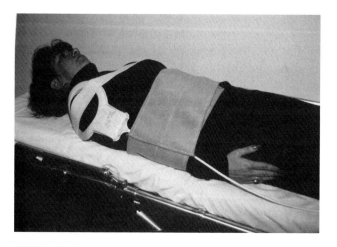

FIGURE 15-10
Patient position for MR imaging of the shoulder. The flexible surface coil is placed over the shoulder with a slight anterior tilt. Note the neutral rotation of the arm, with the palm against the thigh.

coronal plane of the shoulder. Also, in this position, the posterior and anterior components of the glenoid labrum are not adversely affected by the capsular tightening that occurs during internal or external rotation of the humerus. It is important that the patient be as comfortable as possible. Providing support for the arms and knees with sponges or specific holding devices is helpful. The patient should be positioned far to the side of the table, with the shoulder as close to the center of the magnet as possible, and should be instructed to breathe gently. Mild sedation may be used if deemed necessary.

A complete examination requires imaging in three planes: axial, oblique coronal, and oblique sagittal. In the axial and oblique coronal planes the bulk of information needed can be obtained. Oblique sagittal imaging provides complementary information regarding the rotator cuff and the coracoacromial arch.

Axial plane. Axial sections are obtained based on a series of coronal scout images ("plan-scan") that identify the glenohumeral joint (Fig. 15-11). A T1-weighted or intermediate (long TR/short TE) spin echo sequence provides adequate information about the glenoid labrum and glenohumeral joint. In patients with suspected shoulder instability and labral tear we use an intermediate sequence or a gradient-recalled echo sequence. Due to an increased signal arising from the hyaline articular cartilage, this latter sequence results in better visualization of the glenoid labrum. However, the signal from bone is diminished and the details of bony margins are not well seen. If possible, thinner slices (less than 5 mm) are preferred for evaluation of the glenoid labrum.

The use of a T2-weighted sequence has been advocated in patients with suspected instability for detection of labral tears.[40] However, this sequence may be more

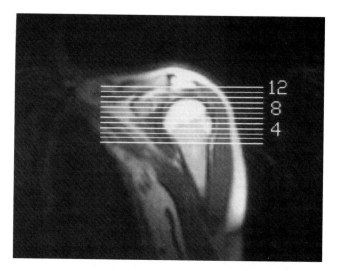

FIGURE 15-11
"Plan scan" for axial sequence, left shoulder. The image selected from a coronal "scout" sequence (Philips Gyroscan) is used as a locater for planning the axial sequence.

informative only when joint effusion is present. We have not found the T2-weighted sequence for axial imaging especially rewarding, unless examination is done after an acute episode of dislocation and/or subluxation. The use of a radial fast-imaging sequence has also been suggested for improved cross-sectional imaging of the glenoid labrum.[41] This sequence is technically more difficult, and resolution of images may be inferior compared to other routine imaging sequences.

Oblique coronal plane. This imaging plane is based on the orientation of the supraspinatus (muscle and tendon). Anatomically it represents the plane of the scapula and is perpendicular to the glenoid fossa when the arm is in neutral rotation. Nevertheless, it is best to use the axial image of the supraspinatus to determine its longitudinal axis as a guide (Fig. 15-12).

The normal anatomy of the rotator cuff in this plane, as well as other planes of imaging, is best evaluated using a T1-weighted pulse sequence.[25,27,28] However, although this sequence is adequate for detection of massive rotator cuff tears, a T2-weighted sequence is needed for identification of most other tears and for differentiation of these lesions from tendinitis.* A T1-weighted sequence has been advocated by some,[37] in addition to the proton density and T2-weighted sequence, for determining the integrity of the subacromial peribursal fat. However, the combination of proton density and T2-weighted sequences is adequate for this purpose, and the T1-weighted sequence could be eliminated. Smaller slice thicknesses (3 to 5 mm) are desirable. The time factor is an important consideration in choosing the parameters for this sequence and should be kept at a minimum without sacrificing image quality and loss of information. Otherwise, motion artifacts result in degradation of images.

Oblique sagittal plane. This imaging plane is based on the orientation of axial images and is parallel to the glenoid fossa or perpendicular to the long axis of the supraspinatus (Fig. 15-13). Although a T1-weighted sequence can be utilized, we prefer a T2-weighted for detection of small or partial cuff tears. In addition, the anteroposterior dimension of full-thickness tears is optimally visualized. The protocol we use for shoulder imaging is demonstrated in Table 15-1.

NORMAL PLANAR ANATOMY
Axial CT-arthrography

Four representative images are used to demonstrate the axial anatomy as seen on CT arthrography[15,42] (Fig. 15-14): (1) proximal aspect of the joint at the level of the superior glenoid margin (Fig. 15-8, slice *3*), (2) base of the coracoid process (Fig. 15-8, slice *7*), (3) midglenoid level (Fig. 15-8, slice *11*), and (4) inferior glenoid level (Fig. 15-8, slice *15*).

At the upper aspect of the joint (Fig. 15-14, *A*), the combined insertion of the long head of the biceps tendon and the superior glenoid labrum on the glenoid tubercle is demonstrated. The joint capsule above the biceps and glenoid extends slightly medially, forming the superior

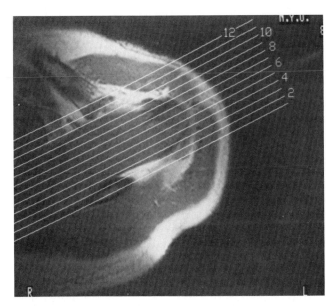

FIGURE 15-12
Oblique coronal sequence "plan scan," left shoulder. The image at the level of the supraspinatus, selected from the axial T1-weighted sequence (900/30), is used to locate the oblique coronal sequence.

*References 25, 26, 30, 32, 33, 37, 39.

Table 15-1   Shoulder MR Protocol

Sequence		TR	TE	No. of slices	Slice thickness	Slice gap	Matrix	No. of excitations	Field of view
Axial:	SE, T1-WI	800	30	12	3 to 5 mm	0.7 to 1 mm	256 × 180	2	160
	SE, PD	1400							
	GRE (70° FA)	480	20	12	5	1	256 × 256	4	160
Oblique coronal:	SE, T2-WI	2100	30/80	12	3.6	0.7	256 × 205	2	160
Oblique sagittal:	SE, T2-WI	1800	30/80	12	5	1	256 × 180	2	180

Code: PD, Proton density–weighted
GRE, Gradient-recalled echo
FA, Flip angle
SE, Spin echo

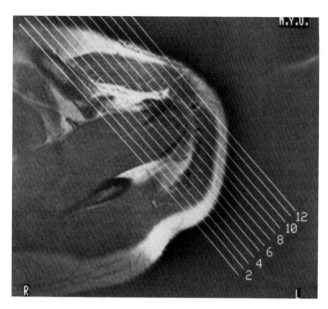

FIGURE 15-13
Oblique sagittal sequence, "plan scan," left shoulder. With the same axial image as in Fig. 15-12, the sagittal sequence is planned perpendicular to the supraspinatus. This plane roughly parallels the plane of the glenoid cavity.

recess. The superior glenohumeral ligament is often visualized as a vertical band at the base of the coracoid process.

At the level of the subscapular bursa (Fig. 15-14, *B*), this medial extension of synovial lining of the capsule is visualized over the scapular cortex and beneath the coracoid process. Within the bursa one or more thin folds of the capsule are often seen, representing normal divisions of this bursa. They should not be mistaken for adhesions. Another structure identified in the upper aspect of the bursa is the inferior portion of the superior glenohumeral ligament.[43] The middle glenohumeral ligament may also be visualized at this level. The superior free margin of the subscapularis tendon is seen as a horizontal band within the bursa, but more often its visualization is graduated on consecutive sections due to its oblique orientation in relation to the axial plane. The anterior labrum at this level is small and generally triangular in outline.

Below the subscapular bursa (Fig. 15-14, *C*), the smooth reflection of the anterior capsule over the glenoid and its continuity with the labrum are demonstrated. The extent and the depth of the furrow formed depends upon

normal variations of the capsule, the capsular ligaments, and the existence of other bursae. The anterior labrum at this level is usually triangular but may vary in size and configuration.[44]

At the inferior aspect of the joint (Fig. 15-14, *D*), the inferior glenohumeral ligament, though variable in thickness, is more consistently visualized and is characteristically contiguous with the inferior glenoid labrum. The labrum at this level is smaller and may be rounded or show a notched contour at its junction with the inferior glenohumeral ligament.

The posterior capsulolabral complex is more uniform in appearance, with a rounded contour of the labrum and a near-labral attachment of the capsule along the entire posterior glenoid margin.

Above the bicipital groove the long head of the biceps tendon may not be differentiated from the adjacent capsular and rotator cuff elements (Fig. 15-14, *B*). Within and beyond the groove it is seen surrounded by contrast medium in its distended synovial tendon sheath (Fig. 15-14, *C*).

The humeral head on axial images appears as a rounded surface covered by articular cartilage. However, the articular cartilage is not always adequately resolved.[44] Superiorly the indentation of the anatomical neck separates the articulating surface from the humeral tuberosities. Posteriorly this junction is rather flattened.

Variation of the anterior capsulolabral complex is frequently observed. The middle glenohumeral ligament may be variably visualized with a direct labral or near-labral insertion (Fig. 15-15, *A* to *C*). This ligament may also be visualized as a linear band parallel to the capsule (Fig. 15-15, *D* to *F*). In these instances another capsular bursa (the inferior subscapular) is also present. Variations in the inferior glenohumeral ligament and its continuity with the inferoanterior labrum may occasionally be seen as a prominent and elongated labrum (Fig. 15-16). This variation occurs at times in individuals with clicking of the joint. The variations in scapular insertion of the anterior capsule should be viewed with caution. Careful inspection of images and reference to the posted scout, when needed, should be done so the normal subscapular bursa is not considered a Type III capsule or, conceivably, a stripped capsule (Fig. 15-17, *A*). Deviations from neutral rotation of the humeral head may drastically change the appearance of the capsular furrow. Although external rotation improves visualization of the

FIGURE 15-14
Normal axial anatomy, CT-arthrography, right shoulder. (See the posted scout, Fig. 15-8.) **A** and **B**, Level 1, superior glenoid (slice *3*). *1*, Glenoid; *2*, humeral head; *3*, coracoid process; *5*, long head of the biceps tendon; *6*, anterior capsule (superior glenohumeral ligament); *7*, superior glenoid labrum. **C** and **D**, Level 2, subglenoid (slice *7*). *3*, Anterior glenoid labrum; *4*, long head of the biceps tendon; *5*, middle glenohumeral ligament; *9*, subscapularis tendon. **E** and **F**, Level 3, midglenoid (slice *11*). *1*, Glenoid; *2*, humeral head; *3*, anterior labrum; *4*, long head of the biceps tendon; *7*, scapular insertion, anterior capsule; *8*, posterior labrum. **G** and **H**, Level 4, inferior glenoid (slice *15*). *3*, Anteroinferior labrum; *5*, inferior glenohumeral ligament. (**A** from Rafii M, et al: AJR 1986:146:361-367. **B** to **H** from Rafii M, et al: Am J Sports Med 1988;16:352-361.)

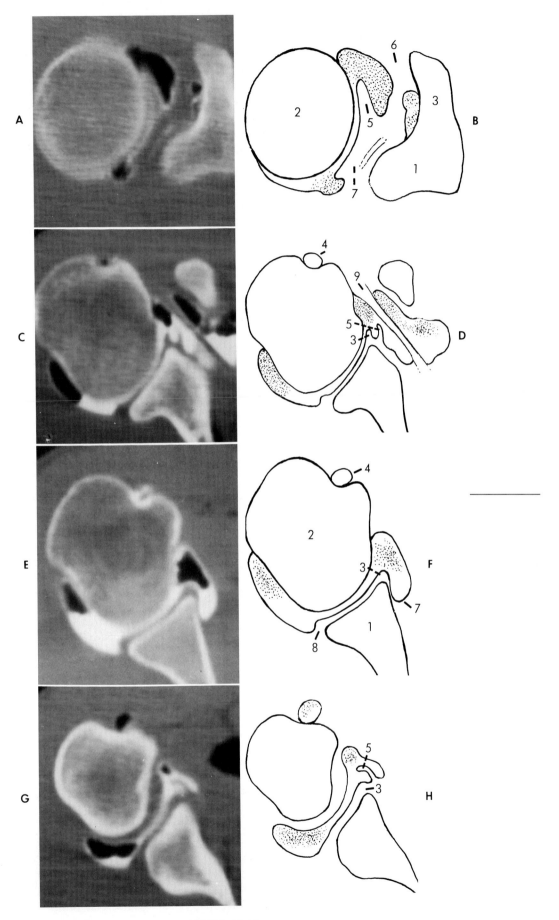

FIGURE 15-14
For legend see opposite page.

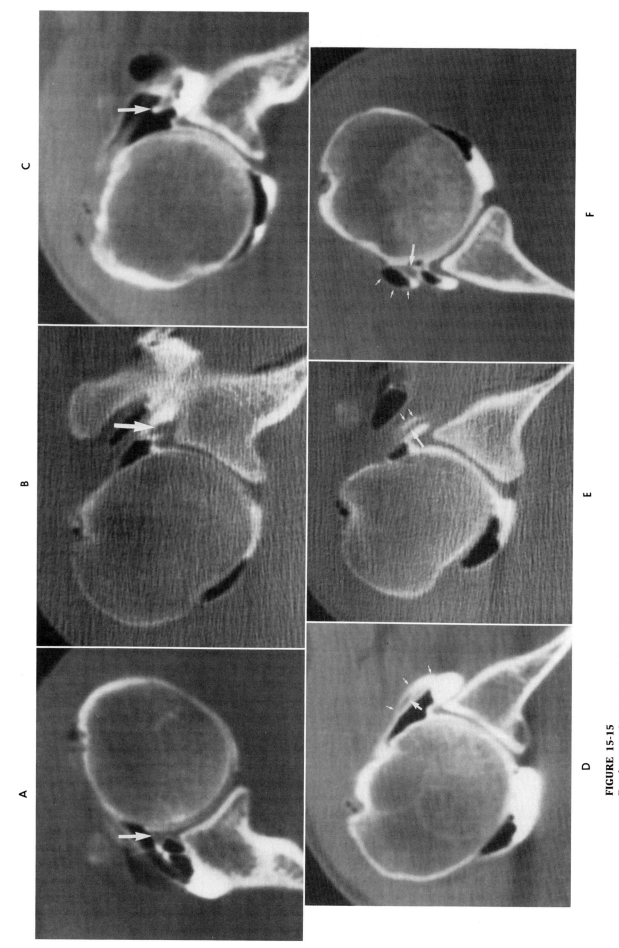

FIGURE 15-15
Developmental variations of the middle glenohumeral ligament. **A,** Labral attachment, at the level of the subscapular bursa *(arrow)* left shoulder. **B,** Near labral insertion of the middle glenohumeral ligament *(arrow)*, right shoulder. **C,** Capsular origin of the ligament close to the scapular insertion *(arrow)*, right shoulder. **D** and **E,** Right shoulder and, **F,** left shoulder at the midglenoid level demonstrating variations of the midglenohumeral ligament *(large arrow)* and the inferior subscapular bursa between them and the capsule *(small arrows)*. (**D** to **F** from Rafii M, et al: AJR 1986;146:361-367.)

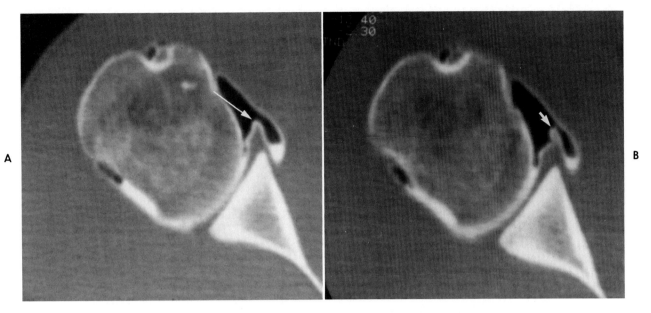

FIGURE 15-16
Developmental variation of the inferior glenohumeral ligament. A and B, Consecutive CT-arthrographic images at the distal aspect of the glenoid, right shoulder. The inferior glenohumeral ligament (*short arrow*, B) inserts directly and is combined with a rather prominent inferior glenoid labrum. This forms a prominent and elongated labrum (*long arrow*, A) extending along the anterior glenoid margin.

posterior labrum, it reduces or totally obliterates the anterior capsular space (Fig. 15-17, *B*). A normal labrum is smoothly outlined by contrast medium. Imbibition of contrast is an indication of labral substance abnormality, and most likely a tear exists. A faulty technique may also result in opacification of the labrum due to direct and forceful injection of contrast material into the labrum (Fig. 15-18).

Planar magnetic resonance

The normal MR anatomy of the shoulder has been the subject of several publications.[25-28]

Axial plane (Fig. 15-19). The supraspinatus and its tendon are visualized at the superior aspect of the joint. The infraspinatus is also observed at this level posteriorly behind the scapular spine, its tendon merging with the tendon of supraspinatus. Below this level the long head of the biceps tendon is often visualized extending from the superior glenoid margin anterior to the humeral head into the intertuberosity groove. Within the groove the cross section of the tendon is visualized. The glenoid labrum in young persons is seen as a signal void with a contour similar to that seen on computed arthrography. A fine line of medium signal between the labrum and the glenoid articular cortex, which is more pronounced with proton density and gradient echo sequences, represents normal extension of the hyaline articular cartilage beneath the labrum. Some signal alteration of the glenoid labrum may be seen with aging.

The low-signal articular capsule is identified against the medium-signal muscles of the rotator cuff, and its confluence with the scapular cortex is usually discernible. Otherwise, it is confluent with the rotator cuff tendons.

The glenohumeral ligaments are occasionally identifiable as low-signal bands at the capsular surface and are better seen when joint effusion is present (Figs. 15-20 and 15-21). The nondistended subscapular bursa beneath the coracoid process is perceived by virtue of the high signal intensity of fatty connective tissue in this region. The capsulolabral interface is identifiable either because of minute amounts of joint fluid or (as suggested by Seeger et al.[28]) due to synovial villi. The anterior rotator cuff tendon (i.e., the subscapularis) is seen as a thick broad band of signal void crossing anterior to the glenohumeral joint and humeral head, inserting on the lesser tuberosity. The thin posterior cuff elements (i.e., the infraspinatus and teres minor tendons) appear as a less conspicuous band of low signal and form within the immediate vicinity of the posterior aspect of the greater tuberosity.

Oblique cornal plane (Fig. 15-22). On anteromedial images, the subscapularis (muscle and tendon), acromioclavicular joint, coracoclavicular ligament, coracohumeral ligament, coracoacromial ligament, and intra- and extraarticular segments of the long head of the biceps tendon are visualized (Fig. 15-22, *A*). On anterior sections the more prominent anterior component of the supraspinatus tendon is seen, with a graduated musculotendinous junction, at approximately the level of the AC joint. More posteriorly muscle fibers extend further laterally (peripherally), blending with the infraspinatus and forming the musculotendinous junction above the center of the humeral head or about the peripheral margin of the acromion (Fig. 15-22, *C*). The midsuperior sections show the acromion, supraspinatus muscle and tendon, and glenohumeral joint in a craniocaudal orientation (Fig. 15-22, *E*).

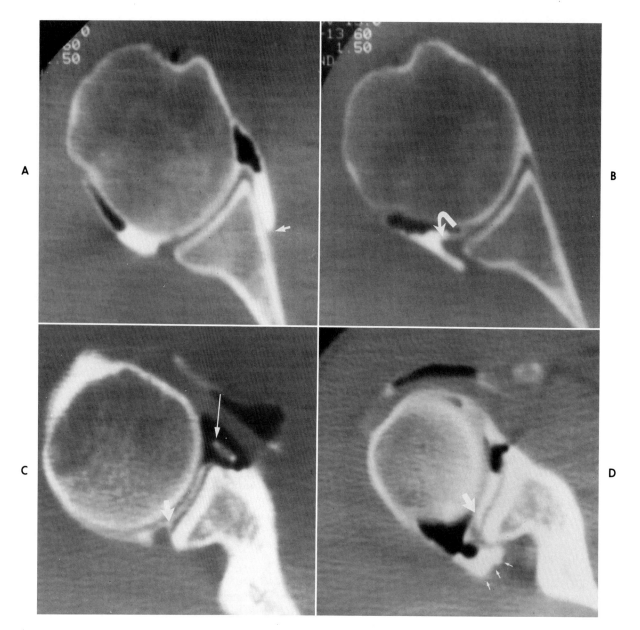

FIGURE 15-17
Normal-variation Type III capsule, variably visualized because of humeral external rotation, two cases. **A,** The CT-arthrographic image at the midglenoid level, right shoulder, neutral humeral rotation, shows the anterior capsule extending to the scapular neck *(arrow),* forming a smooth and narrow reflection over the scapular cortex. **B,** Same patient, same level, with external humeral rotation. The anterior capsular space is obliterated. Now the posterior capsule is relaxed and the posterior labrum optimally visualized *(arrow).* **C** and **D,** Another patient with known anterior instability, right shoulder. These CT-arthrographic images are at the level of the subscapular bursa. (The posterior capsule [C] is normal, and a small labral tear is barely visible *[short arrow].* Note the anterior labral tear *[long arrow].* With external humeral rotation [D] the posterior labral tear is better seen *[thick arrow].* Also the capsular outline near the scapular insertion shows some irregularity *[thin arrows].*) (A from Rafii M, et al: AJR 1986;146:361-367.)

FIGURE 15-18
Labral opacification due to faulty technique. The anterior glenoid labrum is opacified due to inadvertent placement of the needle tip in the labrum and forceful injection of contrast *(arrow).*

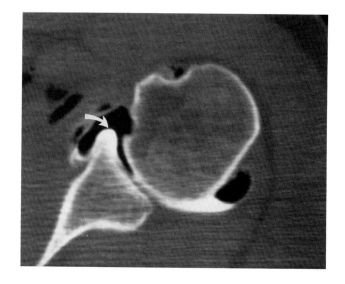

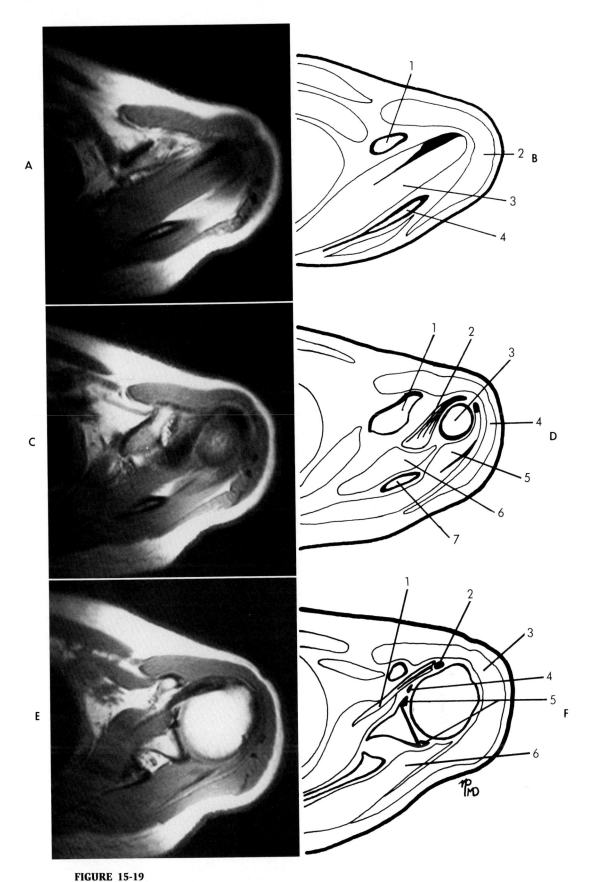

FIGURE 15-19

Normal MRI planar anatomy, axial plane, left shoulder. (See the plan scan, Fig. 15-11.) All images T1-weighted (900/30). **A** and **B,** At the level of the Subacromial space (slice *11,* Fig. 15-11). *1,* Coracoid process; *2,* deltoideus; *3,* supraspinatus; *4,* scapular spine. **C** and **D,** At the superior glenoid (slice *10,* Fig. 15-11). *1,* Coracoid; *2,* long head of the biceps tendon; *3,* humeral head; *4,* deltoideus; *5,* infraspinatus; *6,* supraspinatus; *7,* scapular spine. **E** and **F,** Below the coracoid (slice *8,* Fig. 15-11). *1,* Subscapularis; *2,* long head of the biceps tendon; *3,* deltoideus; *4,* capsule (glenohumeral ligament); *5,* anterior and posterior labrum; *6,* infraspinatus.

Continued.

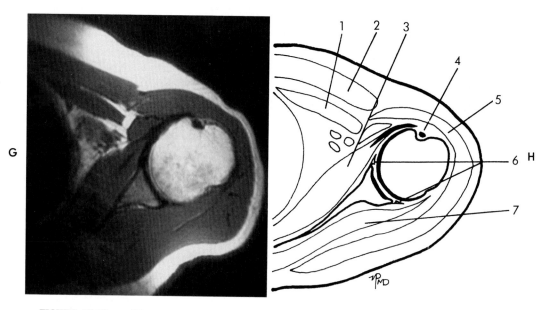

FIGURE 15-19 cont'd
G and **H**, Midglenoid (slice *6*, Fig. 15-11). *1*, Pectoralis minor; *2*, pectoralis major; *3*, subscapularis; *4*, long head of the biceps tendon; *5*, deltoideus; *6*, glenoid labrum; *7*, infraspinatus.

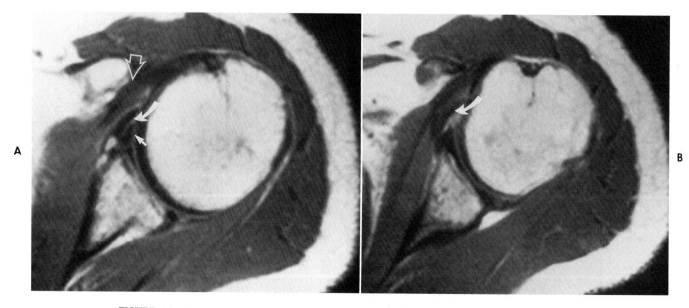

FIGURE 15-20
Midglenohumeral ligament, left shoulder. Axial proton density images (1400/30) at the levels of the coracoid tip and the midglenoid. **A,** Adjacent to the normal glenoid labrum *(straight arrow)*, the signal void middle glenohumeral ligament *(curved arrow)* is clearly visualized, distinct from both the labrum and the subscapularis tendon *(hollow arrow).* **B,** Inferior to **A,** the ligament *(arrow)* remains distinct from the subscapularis tendon by medium-signal tissue, which is most likely the less condensed aspect of the fibrous joint capsule.

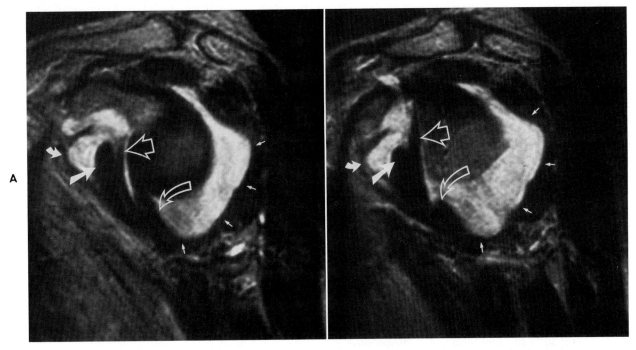

FIGURE 15-21
Anterior capsular ligaments. **A** and **B,** Oblique sagittal, T2-weighted (1800/80) images at the level of the glenoid, **A,** and glenohumeral joint, **B.** There is distention of the joint capsule *(small arrows)* and subscapular bursa *(curved solid arrows)* due to large effusion. The outline of rather prominent capsular ligaments (i.e., the mid- *[straight hollow arrows]* and inferior *[curved hollow arrows]* glenohumeral and their continuity with the glenoid labrum are optimally demonstrated. The normal anatomical position of the subscapular bursa *(curved arrows)* relative to the subscapularis tendon *(slanted arrows)* is evident.

On further posterior sections the infraspinatus (muscle and tendon) is visualized. Often on one image from medial to lateral (anterior to posterior), the supraspinatus, scapular spine, and emerging infraspinatus muscle and tendon are visualized (Fig. 15-22, *G*). Beyond the scapular spine the two muscles are separated by high-signal fat containing connective tissue; the infraspinatus gradually approximates and becomes confluent with the tendon of the supraspinatus. Occasionally a moderate-signal notch identifies this junction (Fig. 15-23). Not infrequently the overlapping tendons will be visualized, separated by a fine medium-signal tissue plane. The greater tuberosity insertion of the supraspinatus tendon begins in the vicinity of the anatomical neck and extends to the periphery of the tuberosity. The SA-SD bursa is not per se visualized, but the peribursal fat identifies the bursal region and separates the cuff tendons from the acromion and overlying deltoideus. This fat plane is contiguous with the fascia of the trapezius and deltoideus. In the oblique coronal plane the glenohumeral joint, superior and inferior glenoid labrum, and axillary pouch are also visualized. However, due to its contiguity with the joint capsule and inferior glenohumeral ligament, the inferior glenoid labrum may not be as clearly outlined.

Oblique sagittal plane (Fig. 15-24). In this plane the rotator cuff tendons, coracoacromial arch, and subacromial space are evaluated in a medial-to-lateral orienta-

tion, which is particularly helpful for visualizing the coracoacromial arch and the orientation of the acromial process. However, the coracoacromial ligament is usually not prominent and may not be well visualized. On the other hand, the intraarticular segment of the long head of the biceps tendon is well seen as a flat structure in front of the humeral head immediately beneath the anterior supraspinatus tendon. The variable thickness of the supraspinatus (which becomes thinner in an anteroposterior orientation) is also well appreciated on these images.

SHOULDER INSTABILITY AND LESIONS OF THE GLENOID LABRUM

Glenohumeral disorders are a major cause of shoulder disability, especially among athletes,[45] and can be divided into two major categories: those of traumatic and those of atraumatic origin. The atraumatic category includes congenital lesions (e.g., capsular laxity and glenoid hypoplasia).[7,46,47] Instabilities are also divided by the direction of the abnormal humeral head motion relative to the glenoid; it may be anterior, posterior, superior, or inferior and in simple or coupled (multidirectional) form. Anterior instability constitutes approximately 95% of all glenohumeral instabilities clinically observed.[46] More recently "functional instability" of the glenohumeral joint due to traumatic tears of the glenoid labrum has been described.[48]

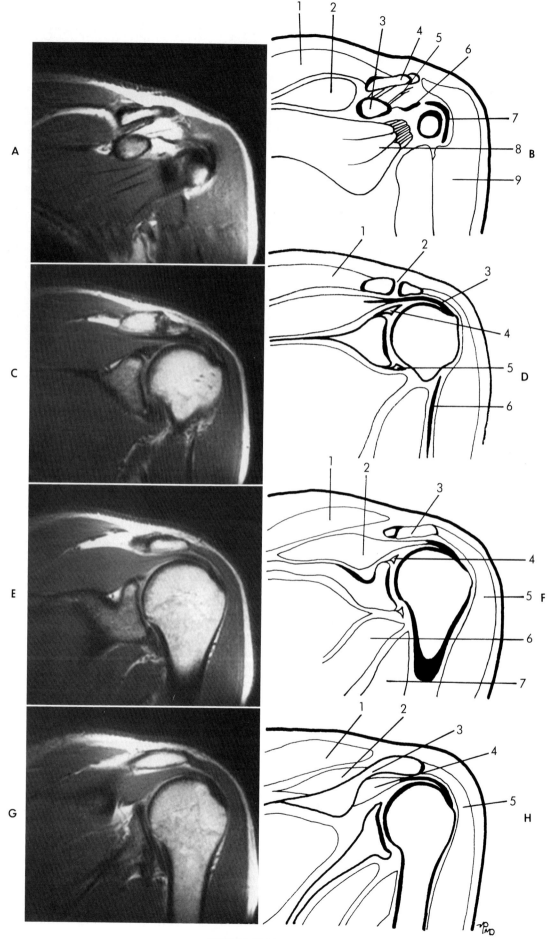

FIGURE 15-22
For legend see opposite page.

FIGURE 15-22
Normal MRI planar anatomy, oblique coronal plane, left shoulder. (See the plan scan, Fig. 15-12.) All images proton density (2100/30). A and B, Anterior to the glenohumeral joint (slice *11*, Fig. 15-12). *1*, Trapezius; *2*, supraspinatus; *3*, coracoid and coracoclavicular ligament; *4*, clavicle; *5*, coracoacromial ligament; *6*, coracohumeral ligament; *7*, long head of the biceps tendon; *8*, subscapularis; *9*, deltoideus. C and D, Anterior glenohumeral joint (slice *8*, Fig. 15-12). *1*, Trapezius; *2*, AC joint; *3*, supraspinatus; *4*, superior labrum; *5*, inferior labrum; *6*, long head of the biceps tendon. E and F, Midglenohumeral joint (slice *6*, Fig. 15-12). *1*, Trapezius; *2*, supraspinatus; *3*, acromion process; *4*, superior labrum; *5*, deltoideus; *6*, teres major; *7*, latissimus dorsi. G and H, Posterior glenohumeral joint (slice *2*, Fig. 15-12). *1*, Trapezius; *2*, supraspinatus; *3*, scapular spine; *4*, infraspinatus; *5*, deltoideus.

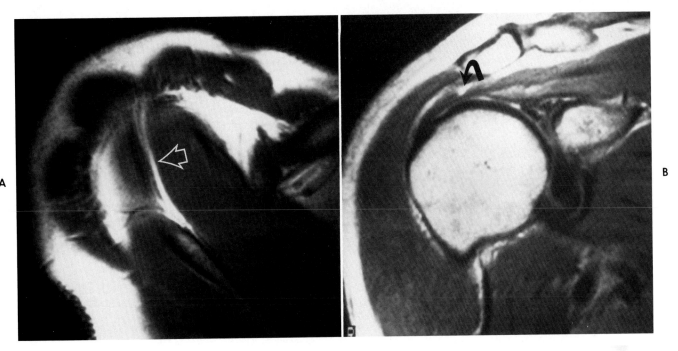

FIGURE 15-23
Normal prominent junctional line supraspinatus and infraspinatus, right shoulder. A, An axial T1-weighted (500/29) image at the level of the subacromial space shows the high-signal, fat-containing, fascial plane at the junction of the spinati tendons *(arrow)*. B, An oblique coronal proton density-weighted image (1600/60) shows the high-signal band as a notch-shaped defect at the bursal surface of the cuff *(arrow)*. At surgery the cuff was intact.

Mechanism and pathological findings

Anterior glenohumeral instability. Anterior dislocations, with ensuing recurrence, generally result from major traumatic events (a fall on an outstretched hand or a direct blow to the shoulder region).[49-51] Instabilities in the form of recurrent anterior subluxations can result from repeated microtrauma due to overuse of the arm in overhead sports activities.[52-58] The pathogenesis, prevalence, and pathological changes of anterior glenohumeral instability have been extensively investigated.* Experimental studies have challenged the role of the glenoid labrum in providing or enhancing stability, and have promoted the more vital role of the capsular mechanism of the glenohumeral joint in shoulder stability.[2,8,61]

The joint capsule and inferior glenohumeral ligament are the primary elements that keep the humeral head from displacing anteriorly during abduction and external rotation of the humerus.[8,50] This is accomplished by limiting the extent of external rotation of the humeral head. By forced abduction, however, the capsule can rupture (in an elderly person) or detach from the glenoid (in an adolescent), allowing subluxation or dislocation of the humeral head anteriorly.[50,61] The glenoid labrum may avulse along with the capsule, or secondarily sustain injury consequent to the displacing forces on the humeral head[50] (Fig. 15-25). It is this detachment of the capsulo-

*References 2, 49-51, 53-55, 58-60.

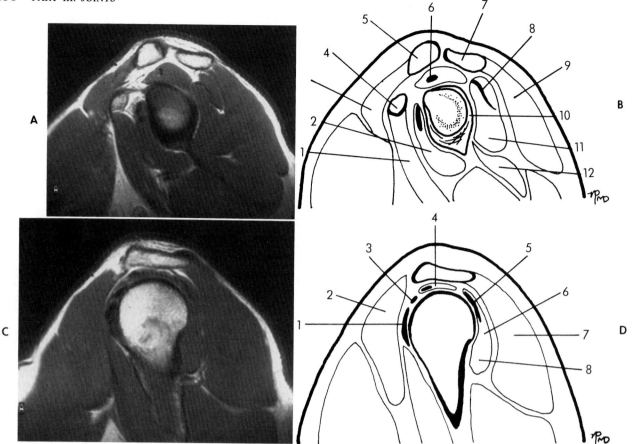

FIGURE 15-24

Normal MRI planar anatomy, oblique sagittal plane, left shoulder. (See the plan scan, Fig. 15-13.) All images proton density–weighted (1800/30). **A** and **B**, Level of the glenohumeral joint (slice *4*, Fig. 15-13). *1*, Coracobrachialis; *2*, subscapularis; *3*, deltoideus; *4*, coracoid process; *5*, clavicle; *6*, supraspinatus; *7*, acromion process; *8*, infraspinatus; *9*, deltoideus; *10*, labrum and capsule; *11*, teres minor; *12*, triceps, long head. **C** and **D**, Lateral to **A**, midhumeral head (slice *7*, Fig. 15-13). *1*, Subscapularis tendon; *2*, deltoideus; *3*, long head of the biceps tendon; *4*, supraspinatus tendon; *5*, infraspinatus tendon; *6*, teres minor; *7*, deltoideus; *8*, teres major.

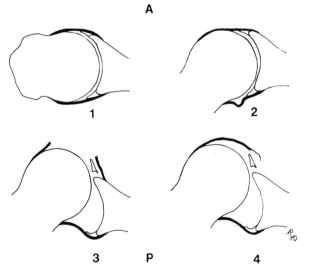

FIGURE 15-25

Mechanism of anterior glenohumeral dislocation. Normal alignment in neutral humeral head rotation *(1)*. With external rotation the anterior capsule is stretched around the head *(2)*. Dislocation (or subluxation) may occur if the anterior capsule is ruptured *(3)*, or stripped from the glenoid *(4)*. *A*, Anterior; *P*, posterior.

head[50] (Fig. 15-25). It is this detachment of the capsulolabral complex in younger individuals that fails to heal and gives rise to subsequent recurrence, with an incidence of up to 90%.[55,60] Capsular injury in athletes with recurring anterior subluxation may be mild, occurring mainly in the form of stretching of the capsule or glenohumeral ligaments rather than avulsion of the capsular complex,[48] and is probably due to the protective nature of the well-developed musculature in these individuals.

The characteristic pathological finding of anterior shoulder instability, first described by Bankart,[49,62] is tearing or detachment of the capsulolabral complex along the anteroinferior glenoid margin. This so-called "essential lesion" may consist of only soft tissue elements (i.e., the glenoid labrum and capsule) or may include a fractured glenoid margin (osseous Bankart lesion). A calcific ridge may also form along the scapular margin as a result of periosteal elevation at the site of capsular avulsion or recurrent stress to the region.[59,62]

The frequency of glenoid labral tears documented at surgery has been reported as high as 100% in various series.[50,59,60,63] An intact or only slightly deformed labrum is occasionally seen with instability.[7] However, the incidence of an intact labrum with anterior instability may be as high as 28%.[2,64] It should also be noted that subtle deformities of the glenoid labrum and osseous glenoid margin may not be visualized at surgery, especially when viewed without the benefit of arthroscopic magnification. In addition, the site of capsular insertion on the glenoid may be difficult to see at surgery.[49,50] A greater incidence of intact labra is observed in individuals with atraumatic shoulder instability and those with congenital joint laxity.[63]

Another frequent osseous abnormality seen following a single episode of anterior dislocation or in recurrent dislocation or subluxation is the Hill-Sachs compression fracture (of the posterosuperior humeral head, by impaction against the glenoid margin).[65] The incidence of this lesion is reported as high as 80% in recurrent dislocation and as low as 25% in recurrent subluxation.[66] The Hill-Sachs defect is variable in size, regardless of the chronicity of the disorder, and may involve only the articular cartilage.[67] The osseous Bankart and Hill-Sachs lesions are pathognomonic for recurrent anterior dislocation and/or subluxation. Their presence may be verified by routine roentgenography of the shoulder or, more precisely and definitively, by specialized views[68] and computed tomography.

Posterior instability. Traumatic posterior shoulder dislocations are uncommon. They result from a fall on outstretched hand with the arm in forward flexion, abduction, and internal rotation. Seizure disorders due to variety of etiological factors may, similarly, cause posterior dislocation. Although recurrent posterior dislocation is rare,[57,69] in recent years posterior instability in the form of recurrent subluxation has increasingly been recognized as a cause of pain and shoulder disability among young athletes.[57,66,69] The mechanism is the applied athletic force (swimming, throwing, punching) of the adducting, flexing, internally rotating humerus. Preexisting laxity of the capsule may play a role as a predisposing factor or constitute the main etiological factor.

Posterior instability constitutes only 2% to 4% of all shoulder instabilities, but it may present the clinician with a diagnostic and therapeutic dilemma. Its pathological changes parallel the severity of the disorder. A posterior glenoid labral tear and frank capsular tear are often present. Various deformities of the glenoid margin (erosion, sclerosis, or ectopic bone formation) also may be present.[66] However, a vertical impaction fracture of anterior humeral head ("reversed Hill-Sachs"), which may be encountered following posterior dislocation,[70] is not commonly seen with posterior subluxations, despite thinning and erosion of the articular cartilage and articular surfaces of the anterior humeral head and posterior glenoid.

Multidirectional instability. Shoulder instability may be present in more than one direction. It may exist anteriorly or posteriorly, and include an inferior component of laxity, or may be noted in all three directions. The shoulder may dislocate in one direction and subluxate in one or two others.[46] This type is usually atraumatic, but a violent injury to the shoulder and repeated microtrauma also are etiological factors.

Imaging of glenohumeral instability

Shoulder instability is most often evident by history and physical examination[45,48,55] and may frequently be documented by conventional roentgenography.[68,71] However, at times, diagnosis will be difficult.[45,48,72] In mild forms the patient may not feel the abnormal glide of the humeral head and may complain of or perceive pain only during certain motions of the arm (abduction and external rotation). Several factors, including pain and overdeveloped muscles, especially in athletes, can prevent a thorough physical examination, necessitating general anesthesia or arthroscopy for this purpose.[73,74] In these cases or when there is a need for more precise delineation of the suspected pathology for surgical planning, less invasive diagnostic procedures are favored.

The role of conventional arthrography in evaluating shoulder instability has been limited, with only the major abnormalities of the articular capsule demonstrated. Refinements in technique (introduction of the double-contrast method[19-20] and arthropneumotomography) have made possible visualization of the glenoid labrum and labral tears associated with shoulder instability.[16-18,63] Further improvements have come about with the introduction of CT-arthrography, which proved to be not only more accurate than arthropneumotomography but also technically easier to perform and became the procedure of choice for evaluating shoulder instability.* More recently, MR imaging has been used for this purpose.

CT-ARTHROGRAPHY

The high sensitivity (up to 100%) of CT arthrography in detecting labral and capsular lesions has been documented.[13-15,77] A less than 90% accuracy and 75% specificity for anterior labral lesions in one study[78] was probably the result of the imaging technique; all patients were scanned only with the arm in external rotation.

Anterior instability. Lesions of the capsulolabral complex cause a wide range of abnormal configurations of the glenoid labrum depending upon the severity of the initial injury and the frequency of dislocation or subluxation. Characteristically, the anteroinferior capsulolabral complex is torn and may, in fact, be totally detached from the glenoid margin (Figs. 15-26 and 15-27). The labrum may also be torn and shredded, or disintegrated and small, or even absent (Figs. 15-28 and 15-29). An intact labrum is less frequently seen (Fig. 15-30). The osseous glenoid

---

*References 13-15, 23, 42, 75-77.

FIGURE 15-26
Recurrent anterior dislocation, right shoulder. CT-arthrogram image at level of the inferior half of the glenoid. The anterior capsulolabral complex is partly detached and is grossly separated from the glenoid margin *(curved arrow)*. The anterior capsular space is expanded. The anterior glenoid margin is deformed and sclerotic. A linear band of periosteal new bone formation is present in continuity with the cortical bone *(straight arrow)* at the site of capsular elevation.

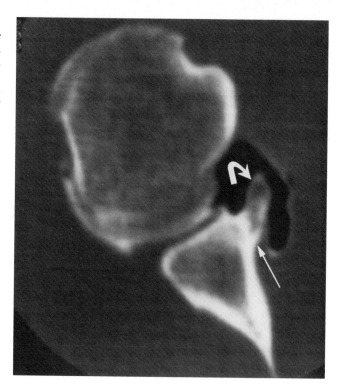

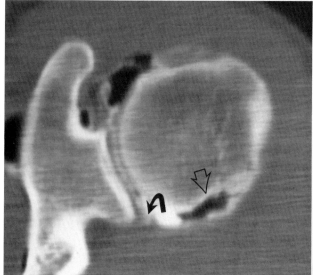

A

FIGURE 15-27
Recurrent anterior dislocation, left shoulder. **A,** CT-arthrogram image at the distal glenoid. The anterior glenoid labrum is torn and almost completely detached *(curved arrow)*. The anterior glenoid margin is fractured *(slanted arrow)*. **B** and **C,** CT-arthrogram images at the superior aspect of the glenoid. The posterosuperior labrum is torn, a companion lesion of anterior instability *(curved arrows)*. A Hill-Sachs lesion of the humeral head is visualized *(hollow arrows)*.

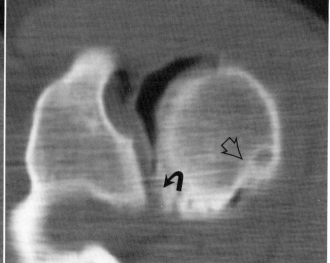

B

C

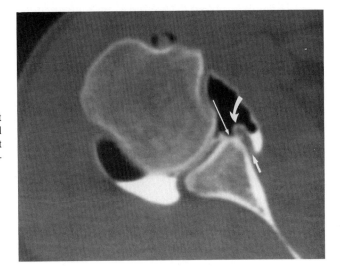

FIGURE 15-28
Recurrent anterior dislocation, right shoulder. A torn and deficient anterior labrum is visualized *(curved arrow)*. The osseous glenoid margin is exposed due to deficiency of the labrum and the adjacent articular cartilage *(long straight arrow)*. Thickened scapular insertion of the anterior capsule is present *(short straight arrow)*.

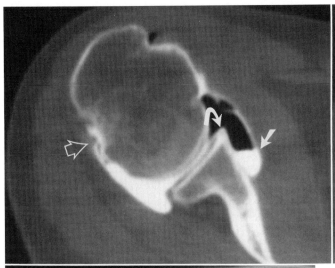

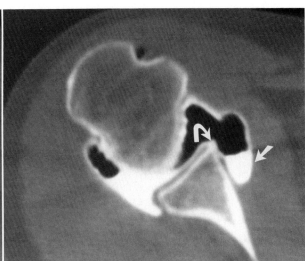

FIGURE 15-29
Recurrent anterior dislocation, right shoulder. CT-arthrogram images at the midglenoid, A, and distal half of the glenoid. **B,** The anterior labrum is mostly disintegrated *(curved arrows);* the small remnant (in **A**) shows imbibition of contrast material. There is stripping of the joint capsule forming a large furrow *(straight arrows)*. Focal ballooning of the capsule in **B** is an indication of weakening or actual tear of the capsular ligament in this region. Note the relatively flat Hill-Sachs lesion *(hollow arrow* in **A**). This extends along and to the proximity of posterior capsular-cuff insertion at the humeral neck, resulting in some irregularity of the cuff. **C,** Correlative conventional arthrogram in upright position and with internal rotation of humerus. The characteristic enlarged appearance of the anterior capsule with continuity of the subscapularis bursa and medial margin of the capsule is noted *(straight arrow)*. Hill-Sachs lesion *(curved arrow)*.

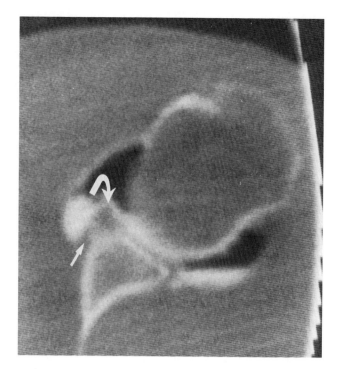

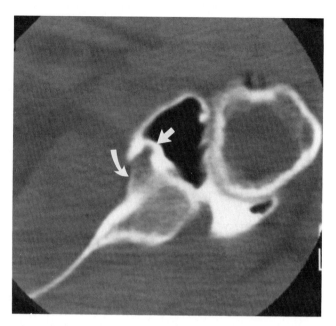

FIGURE 15-30
Anterior glenohumeral instability, intact labrum, left shoulder. CT-arthrogram image at inferior glenoid level. The anterior labrum is intact *(curved arrow)*. However, the capsular insertion is thickened and periosteal new formation is evident *(straight arrow)*. The anterior glenoid margin is flattened.

FIGURE 15-31
Recurrent anterior dislocation, left shoulder. CT-arthrogram image at the inferior glenoid level. A Bankart lesion is present *(straight arrow)*. There is a large ossification of the raised capsulolabral complex *(curved arrow)*.

margin may be irregular (Fig. 15-26), deformed (Figs. 15-28 and 15-30), or fractured (Fig. 15-27).

Along with glenoid labral tears, violation of the anterior scapular insertion of the capsule is also frequently demonstrated by CT-arthrography[15,75,77] and, when present, is a reliable indicator of shoulder instability. Changes include the following:

1. Irregularity or soft tissue thickening of the site of capsular insertion, indicative of swelling or a proliferative process of the periosteum and capsule (Figs. 15-28 and 15-30)
2. Stripping of the capsule away from the scapular surface, uncovering the cortex and/or creating a large furrow (Fig. 15-29)
3. Ectopic calcification or ossification at the site of capsular insertion due to chronic stress on the scapular periosteum (Figs. 15-26, 15-30, and 15-31)

Stripping and medial expansion of the anterior joint capsule about the glenoid result in a loss of the normal anatomical boundary between the anterior capsule and subscapular bursa, leading to the formation of one large cavity over the scapular neck. This continuity of the bursa and capsular space is readily recognized on conventional arthrography (Fig. 15-29, *C*); its recognition on CT-arthrography requires proper location of each image so the expected boundaries of the bursa and the capsular reflection (insertion) at the glenoid can be determined. This distinction is important, because a normal but

prominent subscapular bursa can simulate and be mistaken for a stripped anterior joint capsule (Fig. 15-34).

Other abnormalities of the capsule (e.g., redundancy and enlargement of the capsular recesses) have been associated with anterior shoulder instability.[2,79] However, because of considerable variation in the development of the anterior capsular ligaments and synovial recesses, these findings should be regarded with caution. An enlarged subscapular bursa has also been specifically described as a normal finding.[2,23,80] In addition, quantification of bursa size may be difficult. Congenital laxity of the glenohumeral joint with global (multidirectional) instability may be recognized by the generalized redundancy of the capsule as well as by nonvisualization of the glenohumeral ligaments, which are either nonexistent or underdeveloped[64] (Fig. 15-32).

The site of scapular insertion of the anterior joint capsule is another anatomical variation that has been related to instability[2,9]; but unless the insertion demonstrated by CT-arthrography was at the medial third of the scapular neck, correlations to instability have been low.[44] However, distinction between a normal, albeit remote, capsular insertion on the scapular neck (Fig. 15-17, *A*) and one induced by stripping of the capsule (Fig. 15-29) may be difficult. Regardless of the type of capsular insertion visualized on CT-arthrography, abnormalities of its insertion site (thickening, irregularity, or absence of the normal layer of soft tissue over the scapular cortex)

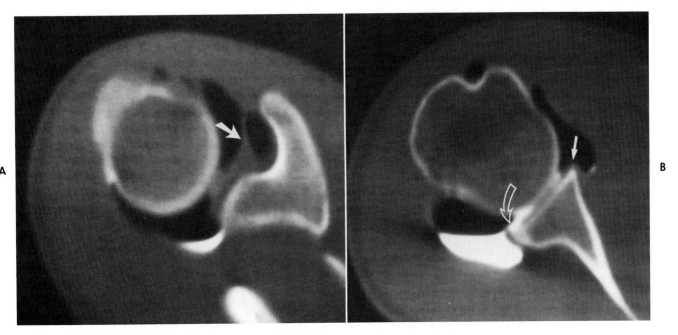

FIGURE 15-32
Congenital capsular laxity and multidirectional instability, right shoulder. CT-arthrogram images at the superior glenoid, **A**, and midglenoid, **B**, levels. Generalized laxity of the capsule is evidenced by the expanded and undulating appearance of the capsular outline. The superior glenohumeral ligament is thin *(slanted arrow)*. The middle and inferior glenohumeral ligaments are not visualized (underdeveloped). The anterior labrum is eroded *(straight arrow)*. The posterior labrum is torn and attenuated *(hollow arrow)*.

and/or associated tear of the glenoid labrum must be present for the diagnosis of anterior glenohumeral instability to be established.

Whereas stretching and laxity of the subscapularis tendon may be present and observed at gross inspection, their detection or quantification by CT-arthrography is difficult. A frank tear of the tendon with or without avulsion of the lesser tuberosity is rare in young individuals with traumatic recurrent anterior dislocation (Fig. 15-33).

The characteristic location and overall configuration of capsulolabral lesions in cases of glenohumeral subluxation resulting from sports-related injuries are similar to those observed in cases of traumatic recurrent dislocation[42,75,77] (Fig. 15-34). However, they will more likely be mild or even subtle (Fig. 15-35). A labral tear may not necessarily be present with occult forms of instability; the anteroinferior labrum may simply appear attenuated (see Fig. 16-6). The capsular lesions are generally less pronounced in the former group, even being limited to stretching or tearing of the glenohumeral ligaments.[43,75]

A Hill-Sachs compression fracture is variably seen on CT-arthrographic images depending upon the extent of the lesion. There may be mere flattening (Fig. 15-33), an actual depression (Figs. 15-29 and 15-35), or the formation of a groove in the posterosuperior humeral head (Figs. 15-27 and 15-34). Although it may not be difficult to recognize a depressed lesion, small or flat ones are likely to be overlooked. Subtle change in the perfectly

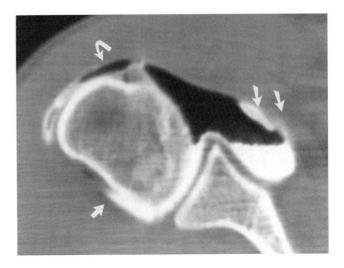

FIGURE 15-33
Anterior instability, right shoulder. CT-arthrogram image at the midglenoid level. Avulsion fracture of the lesser tuberosity and marked retraction of the avulsed fracture fragment, which includes the attached subscapularis tendon, are demonstrated *(slanted arrows)*. The labrum is normal. Communication with the subdeltoid bursa *(curved arrow)* was apparently established through an anterior capsular defect. The supraspinatus tendon was intact at arthrography and at surgery. The posterior contour of the humeral head is markedly flattened, consistent with a Hill Sachs lesion *(straight arrow)*.

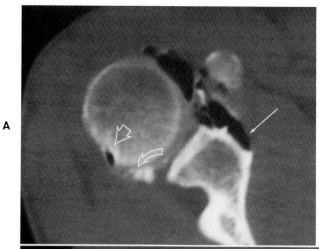

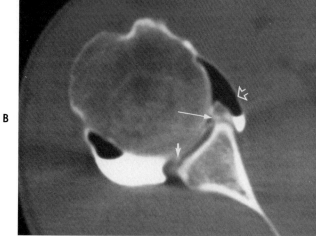

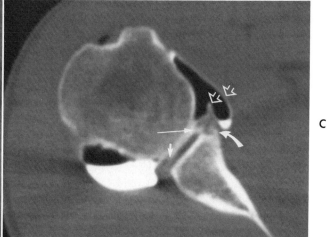

FIGURE 15-34

Recurrent anterior subluxation, right shoulder. **A,** A CT image below the coracoid process shows a Hill-Sachs defect *(short arrow)* and synovial tabs of the posterior capsule *(curved arrow)*. The subscapular bursa extends over to the scapular neck, a normal finding *(long arrow)*. **B** and **C,** At the distal aspect of the glenoid. The anterior labrum is torn. This is in the form of a bucket handle tear at the midglenoid and a partial tear inferiorly *(long arrows)*. The capsule and the inferior glenohumeral ligament *(hollow arrows)* show no abnormality other than slight expansion of the capsule. An anterior bony ridge of the capsule *(curved arrow)* and a posterior labrum tear *(small arrows)* are also present.

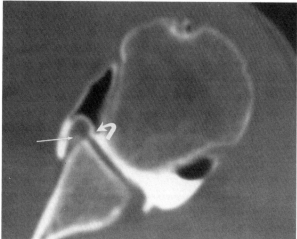

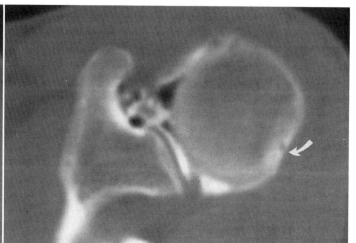

FIGURE 15-35

Anterior instability (recurrent subluxation), left shoulder. **A,** A notched configuration of the labrum *(curved arrow)* and a small avulsion fracture of the glenoid margin *(straight arrow)* are visible. The joint capsule is normal. **B,** A Hill-Sachs compression fracture in this patient *(arrow)* is confirmatory evidence for instability.

round contour of the humeral head may be the only finding (Fig. 15-36). Small and focal articular compressions along the anatomical neck are also a possible source of confusion, resembling degenerative expansion. Furthermore, CT-arthrography is not particularly sensitive in detection of purely cartilaginous Hill-Sachs lesions. Correlation with conventional arthrographic images in various degrees of internal rotation is helpful.

Posterior instability. On CT-arthrography the spectrum of tears in the posterior capsulolabral complex is diagnostic of posterior glenohumeral instability (Figs. 15-37 and 15-38). Findings include tearing, detachment or stripping, and shredding of the posterior glenoid labrum.

Capsular detachment or stripping, as seen with anterior instability, is not the norm; more often, in flagrant types of posterior subluxation, a capsular tear or subcapsular formation of a synovial recess is seen (Fig. 15-37). There may be deformity of the glenoid margin with heterotopic calcification and ossification along the glenoid margin (Figs. 15-37 and 15-38). Actual impaction of the anterior contour of the humeral head ("reversed Hill-Sachs") is often visualized following posterior dislocation (Fig.

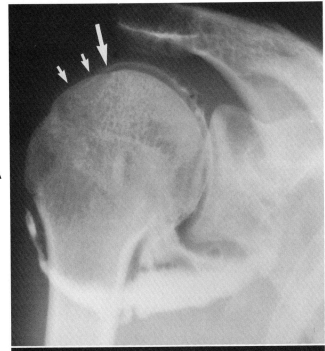

A

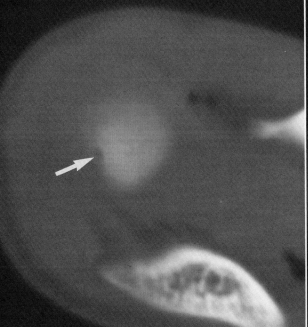

B

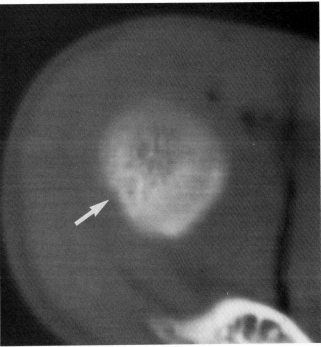

C

FIGURE 15-36
Hill-Sachs compression deformity, right shoulder. Same patient as in Fig. 15-33. **A,** Conventional arthrogram image. Slight loss of convexity of the superior aspect of the humeral head, as well as thinning of the articular cartilage *(small arrows),* is visualized. The junction with the normal aspect of the head forms a small notch *(large arrow).* **B** and **C,** CT-arthrogram images of the superior aspect of the humeral head show the small notch defect of the humeral head *(arrows).* Flattening of the posterior surface of the humeral head at this level is mild, but is more prominent on lower cuts. (See Fig. 15-33.)

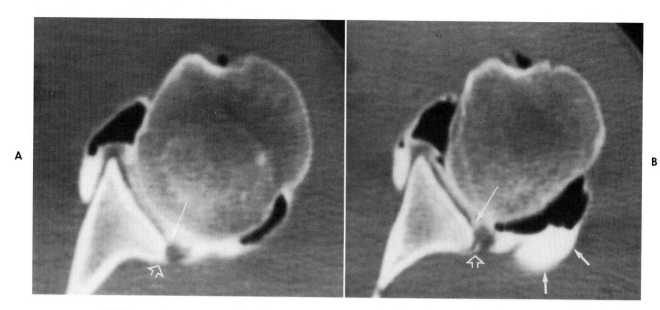

FIGURE 15-37
Posterior instability, left shoulder. **A,** CT-arthrogram image at the midglenoid. At this level a posterior labrum tear *(long white arrow)* and a small bony ridge *(hollow arrow)* are present. **B,** CT image at the junction of the middle and distal third of the glenoid. There is a posterior labrum tear *(long arrow)* associated with a capsular tear and subcapsular formation of a bursa *(short arrows)*. The calcific ridge is also visualized *(hollow arrow)*. (**B** reprinted with permission from Rafii M, et al: Am J Sports Med 1988;16:352-361.)

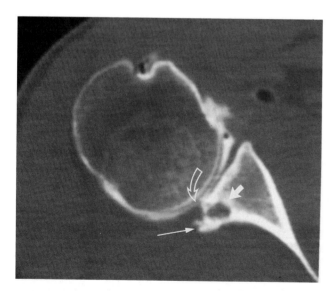

FIGURE 15-38
Posterior instability, right shoulder. The posterior glenoid margin is deformed, with a subcortical cyst *(short arrow)*. The labrum is detached and displaced peripherally over the deformed glenoid margin *(hollow arrow)*. Calcific ridges also are present *(long arrow)*.

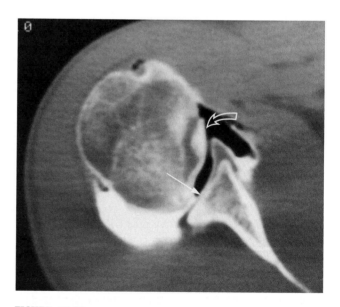

FIGURE 15-39
Reversed Hill-Sachs, right shoulder. Compression fracture of the anterior aspect of the humeral head following posterior dislocation is visualized *(hollow arrow)*. There is a cartilage defect of the glenoid *(long arrow)*, along with outward orientation of the posterior labrum, sclerosis of the posterior glenoid margin, and a small calcific ridge of the capsule.

15-39). With recurrent subluxation, articular cartilage erosion and subarticular sclerosis of the humeral head may be detected.

Multidirectional instability. With multidirectional instabilities alterations of both the posterior and the anterior component of the capsulolabral complex may be visualized (Fig. 15-40). Inferior subluxation is presumed to be present. Inferior instability may also be confirmed simply by use of a stress view (i.e., an upright projection of the shoulder with hand-held weights). Multidirectional instabilities usually have one direction that is predominant; and, accordingly, a predominance of either anterior or posterior lesions is noted on CT-arthrograms (Fig. 15-41).

Perhaps the most important aspect of CT-arthrography has been its usefulness in establishing the diagnosis of glenohumeral instability in clinically unsuspected or unproven cases or when it has not been possible to examine the shoulder except under general anesthesia (Figs. 15-41 and 15-42). This difficulty is more significant with posterior subluxations, but it is also important when surgical therapeutic choices are being considered in a patient with multidirectional instability. However, an abnormal configuration of the posterior glenoid labrum, or even a frank tear, not infrequently will also be seen in patients with CT-arthrographic manifestations of anterior shoulder instability (Fig. 15-27). These lesions involve mainly the posterosuperior segment of the labrum and must be distinguished from lesions indicative of multidirectional instability. The latter are usually more exten-

sive, involve more the entire posterior or posteroinferior labrum, and have associated capsular tears.

Isolated labral tears. Symptomatic tears of the glenoid labrum without associated shoulder instability have long been recognized as a source of shoulder dysfunction,

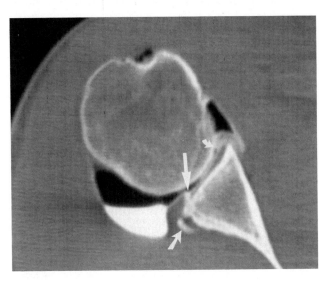

FIGURE 15-41
Multidirectional instability, posterior predominance, right shoulder. There is detachment of the posterior glenoid labrum, and the posterior glenoid margin is irregular *(straight arrow)*. The posterior capsule is distended and contains a calcific ridge along the site of glenoid insertion *(slanted arrow)*. There is also a tear of the anterior glenoid labrum present *(curved arrow)*. Global instability was confirmed with examination under anesthesia.

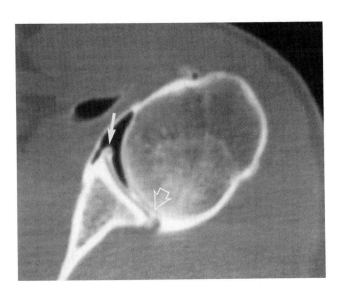

FIGURE 15-40
Multidirectional instability, left shoulder, in a patient with long standing global joint laxity. **A,** The anterior labrum is torn with an irregular remnant remaining *(solid arrow)*. The posterior labrum is also torn *(hollow arrow)*. Although there is no pronounced capsular laxity present, an abnormal posterior shift of the humeral head is visible and the anterior capsular reflexion over the glenoid is diminished. This finding indicates of stripping of the capsule. A small Hill-Sachs lesion was also present in this patient, with a more pronounced anterior slide of the glenohumeral joint.

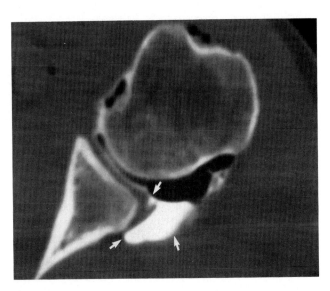

FIGURE 15-42
Posterior instability, left shoulder, in a patient with the sensation of uncertain directional instability not previously documented by radiographic means. Clinical evaluation was inconclusive. This CT arthrographic examination shows tearing of the posterior capsulolabral complex *(arrows)*. The anterior complex is normal.

particularly in the athletic population.[48,81-84] Isolated tears are most often associated with throwing-type injuries in athletes, but they may also be induced by any severe direct injury to the shoulder. The concept of "functional instability" is based on the sensation of joint laxity, with pain and clicking, created by a torn labral

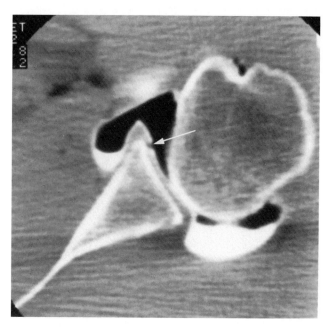

FIGURE 15-43
Anterior labral tear, left shoulder, in a patient with a history of pain and clicking following a weight-lifting accident. An anterior labral tear is visualized *(arrow)*. Although the capsular space is enlarged, there were no clinical manifestations of instability present in this patient, who was not examined under anesthesia.

fragment[48] (Fig. 15-43). Removal of such a fragment often results in marked improvement of joint function.

Labral tears related to throwing usually involve the superior and parasuperior or anterior segments of the glenoid and may assume various configurations.[81,84,85] Detachment of the conjoined superior labrum and long head of the biceps tendon from the supraglenoid tubercule has been suggested[81] to be due to forceful contraction of the biceps, pulling on the glenoid labrum during the last phase of the throwing motion (Fig. 15-44). Tears of the superior glenoid labrum with extension to the anterior or posterior segments (SLAP lesion [superior labrum, anterior and posterior]) have been postulated[86] to result from indirect injury to the shoulder. It has also been suggested[42,75] that the throwing act itself causes tearing of the midanterior glenoid labrum by pinching the labrum between the humeral head and superior free margin of the subscapularis tendon (Fig. 15-45). This last is probably due to translation of the humeral head over the glenoid margin.[47]

Similarly, a torn posterior glenoid labrum may be seen in athletes.[46,87-89] A calcific ridge at the outer margin of the glenoid often occurs, specifically in baseball pitchers,[87] either alone or with a posterior labral tear (Fig. 15-46), and is usually the result of capsular inflammation and fibrosis.

Therefore, it should be evident that these lesions can be differentiated from anatomical instabilities both by their configuration and by their location on the glenoid. The wider range of motion (especially external rotation) normally exerted by throwers may account for some degree of instability as an etiological factor,[46] but labral

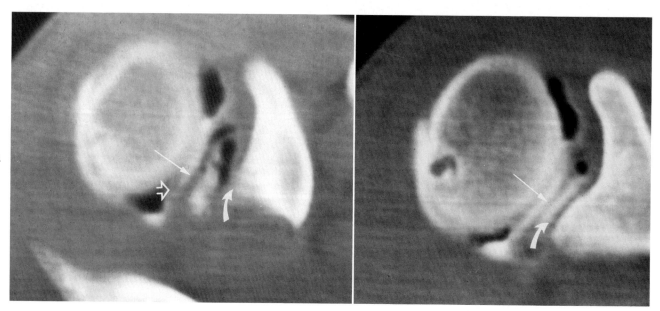

FIGURE 15-44
Superior labral tear, right shoulder, in a recreational tennis player. The superior labrum *(long arrows)* including the insertion of the long head of biceps *(hollow arrow* in **A**) is entirely detached and separated from the superior glenoid margin *(curved arrows)*. (**A** reprinted with permission from Rafii M, et al: Radiology 1987;162:559-564.)

tears discovered following a specific traumatic incident are most likely due to a transient subluxation that, in and of itself, does not necessarily cause recurrent instability. However, in our experience with several acute posttraumatic labral tears, documented by CT-arthrography, not infrequently they have been a harbinger of instability that becomes evident only at a later time. In these cases some alteration of the capsular insertion, subtle though it may be, is usually seen in addition to the tear detected by CT-arthrography (Figs. 15-47 and 15-48).

Aging and other variations of the glenoid labrum. Extensive studies by DePalma et al.[7] have revealed various pathological changes, progressive with advancing age, in the glenoid labrum and the articular and synovial surfaces of the glenohumeral joint.

> The articular aspect of the labrum is gradually detached from the glenoid articular cartilage, to which it is loosely adherent. This phenomenon is most marked in its superior aspect, at the site of attachment of the biceps tendon (Fig. 15-49).

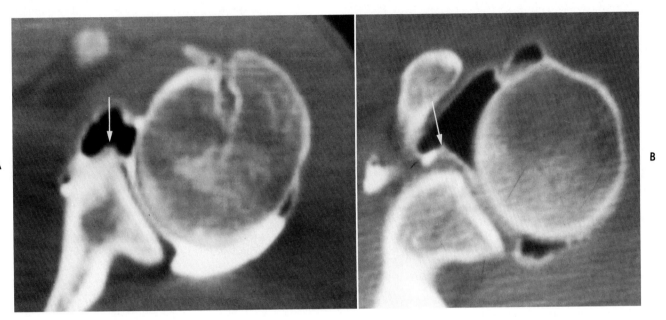

A **B**

FIGURE 15-45
Anterior labral tear in throwing athletes, two cases. **A,** Midanterior labral tear, left shoulder *(arrow).* The inferior labrum was normal. **B,** The midanterior labrum, right shoulder, is deformed and superficially torn *(arrow).* (Both figures reprinted with permission from Rafii M, et al: Am J Sports Med 1988;16:352-361.)

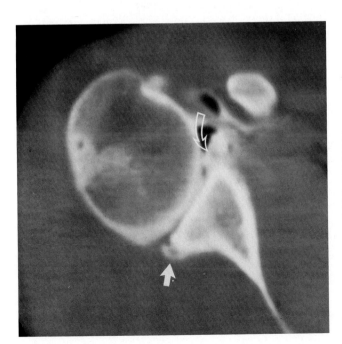

FIGURE 15-46
Labral tear and calcific ridge, right shoulder, in a veteran major league baseball player. A CT image at the midglenohumeral joint level demonstrates the torn anterior labrum *(hollow arrow).* A calcific ridge is formed at the expected site of capsular insertion and the base of the posterior glenoid labrum *(solid arrow).* (Reprinted with permission from Rafii M, et al: Radiology 1987;162:559-564.)

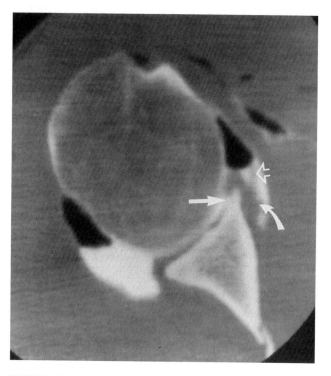

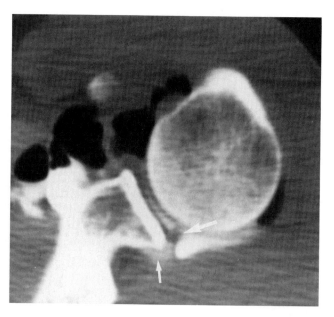

FIGURE 15-47
Acute anterior labral tear, right shoulder, in a major league hockey player following injury to the shoulder with forced abduction and external rotation. There is a tear of the anterior labrum along the lower glenoid margin *(straight arrow)*. Marked prominence of soft tissues at the peripheral aspect of the labrum and along anterior cortical margin of glenoid *(curved arrow)* is indicative of injury and swelling of the capsular and periosteal elements. The soft tissue band *(hollow arrow)* is the midglenohumeral ligament. (Reprinted from Rafii M, et al: In Nicholas JA, Hershman EB [eds]: The upper extremity in sports medicine. St Louis, Mosby, 1990.)

FIGURE 15-48
Acute posterior labral tear, left shoulder. Major league hockey player following injury with forced flexion and adduction. The posterior labrum is torn *(large arrow)*. Leakage of contrast material along the posterior glenoid margin *(small arrow)* is indicative of capsular injury.

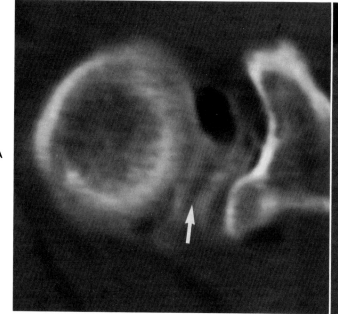

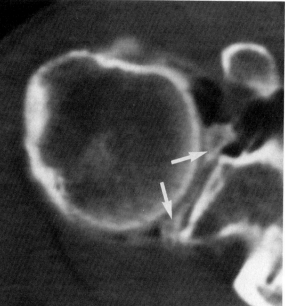

FIGURE 15-49
Degenerative process and aging of the superior labrum, right shoulder. The superior and parasuperior segment of the glenoid labrum is detached from the glenoid margin *(arrows)*.

There is also a gradual fissuring, attenuation, or at times apparent enlargement of the labrum due to extension of the hypertrophied synovium (Fig. 15-50). In these cases the similarity of the detachment to that seen in athletes of much younger age is noteworthy.

The clinical relevance of many labral lesions has been questioned, in part because of their unusually high incidence in cadavers and in part because they are commonly detected in patients without associated symptoms.[90,91] Nevertheless, athletic activity appears to promote them, which otherwise normally tend to occur later in life. However, in an athletic population such labral lesions may produce symptoms that are relieved by arthroscopic surgery.[76,84] This concept may also be considered when minor lesions (e.g., attenuation or notching of the labrum) are detected at CT-arthrography. These lesions have been suggested[78] as representing variations of the labrum, presumably nonpathological in nature.

We have observed similar lesions of the labrum specifically at the anteroinferior glenoid in association with mild shoulder instabilities. It bears reemphasizing that such findings must be correlated not only with the patient's symptoms but also with the expected level of joint function.

MAGNETIC RESONANCE

The experience with MRI in diagnosing glenohumeral instability is scanty, attention having been focused mostly on rotator cuff tears.[30,40,92,93] Comparison of MR with CT-arthrography in small groups of patients who have anterior recurrent dislocations has revealed a diagnostic accuracy for MRI similar to that for CT-arthrography.[92,93]

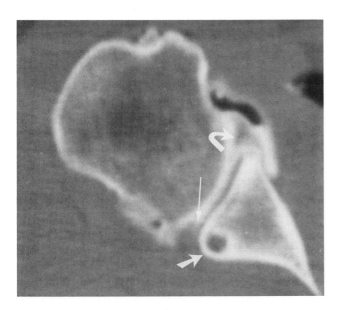

FIGURE 15-50
Degenerative process and aging of the glenoid labrum. The anterior labrum is enlarged and almost completely detached from the glenoid margin *(curved arrow)*. There is partial detachment of the posterior labrum *(thin arrow)*. A subcortical degenerative cyst of the glenoid is also present *(slanted arrow)*. (Reprinted with permission from Rafii M, et al: Am J Sports Med 1988;16:352-361.)

However, in an earlier study of two patients with chronic instability,[30] lesions of the labrum were not observed although, conversely, labral tears in other patients following acute trauma were visualized. This was presumed to be due to the presence of effusion in the latter group. In another larger study[40] no false-positive diagnoses were made by MRI in the diagnosis of labral pathology. All these studies showed a low sensitivity in outlining the capsular insertion and in detecting capsular abnormalities associated with shoulder instability, apparently related to the absence of joint effusion and lack of capsular distention.

Citing these difficulties in the accurate assessment of capsulolabral pathology on conventional MRI, Flanigan et al.[94] suggested MR arthrography (with intraarticular gadopentetate) as an alternative. Of 9 surgically proved labral tears in their series, 3 were missed on nonenhanced images but all were accurately detected on enhanced images. In an earlier study[95] experimentally induced labral lesions were accurately visualized in cadaver shoulders that had been distended and enhanced with intraarticular gadopentetate. The true accuracy of conventional MR imaging in detection of labral tears and the merits of MR-arthrography (which has the negative factors of relative invasiveness and added expense) must still be determined by studies of larger groups of patients and after the development of a learning curve for performance and interpretation of the technique.

MR patterns of labral tears. Since the early literature cited above, our experience has been that image resolution is considerably improved and increasing confidence in detecting lesions of the capsulolabral complex has followed. Utilizing high-resolution conventional MR imaging techniques, we have been able to show the various pathological changes associated with shoulder instability and have achieved a high degree of accuracy. The MR criteria for labral lesions vary in accordance with the concomitant pathology. Compared to what is seen on CT-arthrography, glenoid labral lesions on MRI may be manifested and detected by their configurational abnormalities (i.e., their irregular outline, attenuation, or total absence). A substance tear or detachment from the glenoid margin is seen as a region or band of increased signal intensity traversing the low-signal labral substance and a separation or elevation of the labrum from the glenoid by a zone of moderate signal intensity (Fig. 15-51).

Recognizing a labral substance tear or detachment from the glenoid on MRI involves entirely different principles from those used in recognizing configurational abnormalities. In the absence of joint effusion, signal change is most likely due to tissue alteration in the region of a tear or reactive changes at the site of a capsulolabral detachment and should be differentiated from the normal extension of medium-signal hyaline cartilage beneath the glenoid labrum (Fig. 15-51, A). This normal anatomical feature, not recognized on CT-arthrography, can be a

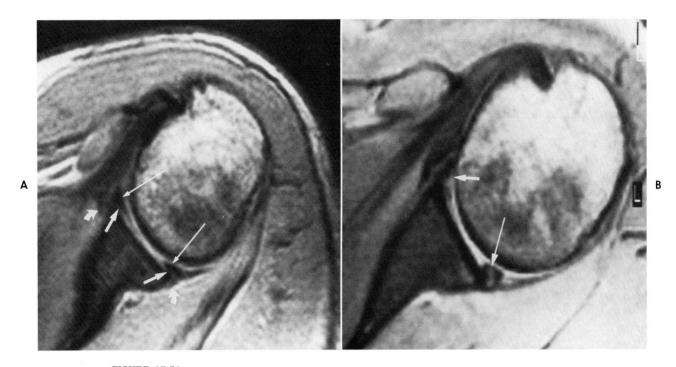

FIGURE 15-51
Normal glenoid labrum morphology and MR patterns of glenoid labral tears. **A,** Axial gradient echo sequence (400/191/65°). The anterior and posterior glenoid labrum is visualized as a signal void structure *(long arrows).* The medium-signal hyaline glenoid articular cartilage extends beneath the labrum to the glenoid margin *(short arrows).* Note the smooth contour of the capsule and the clearly visualized anterior and posterior glenoid insertions *(curved arrows).* **B,** Axial gradient echo sequence (400/19/65°). Tearing of the anterior labrum is evidenced by contour abnormality *(short arrow).* A linear tear of the posterior labrum is manifested by a band of medium signal through the labral substance *(long arrow).*

source of error on MRI. However, the normal extension of articular cartilage (which gradually becomes thinner toward the periphery) terminates at the angle of the osseous glenoid margin. Thickening or extension of the medium-signal band under the peripheral labrum and elevation of the capsule from cortical bone are to be considered pathological in nature. Joint effusion, when present, improves visualization of contour abnormalities and helps outline a torn or detached capsulolabral complex on T2-weighted sequences. Otherwise, contour abnormality and signal alterations of the torn glenoid labrum are best detected on proton density sequences.

Abnormal signal intensity may also result from degenerative changes within the glenoid labrum and should not be mistaken for instability lesions. The differentiation is based primarily on the characteristic location of instability lesions and the more generalized nature of degenerative changes.

Anterior shoulder instability. For an accurate assessment on MRI of shoulder instability, all aspects of expected pathological changes should be evaluated and considered in concert:

1. Capsulolabral complex: The hallmark of an anterior shoulder instability or "Bankart" lesion is the torn labrum, characteristically involving just the anteroinferior aspect with or without involvement of the osseous glenoid margin. The labrum may be clearly torn or detached from the glenoid (Figs. 15-52 and 15-53) or may be irregular (Fig. 15-54), small, or totally absent (Fig. 15-55). Capsular laxity or redundancy, when present, is shown as an undulation (Figs. 15-52, 15-54, and 15-55) or infolding of the anteroinferior capsule against the subscapularis tendon and into the joint. Stripping of the capsule, when prominent, is seen as a distant site of capsular merging with the glenoid relative to the glenoid margin (Fig. 15-55). Associated laxity of the capsule, indicated by irregularity of the capsular outline, helps in differentiating these pathological cases from the normal-variant type III capsular insertion. Following an acute episode of anterior dislocation, injury to the capsulolabral complex may be depicted by nonhomogeneity of soft tissues due to edema rather than an obvious stripping of the capsule or detachment of the glenoid labrum (Fig. 15-56). As demonstrated by the preceding examples, although joint effusion improves visualizing lesions of the capsulolabral complex, most instability lesions can be optimally visualized in the absence of joint effusion and with proper imaging techniques.

2. Subscapularis tendon: Retraction of the subscapularis musculotendinous junction due to stretching and laxity of the tendon with recurrent anterior dislocation has been reported.[40] Obviously, this

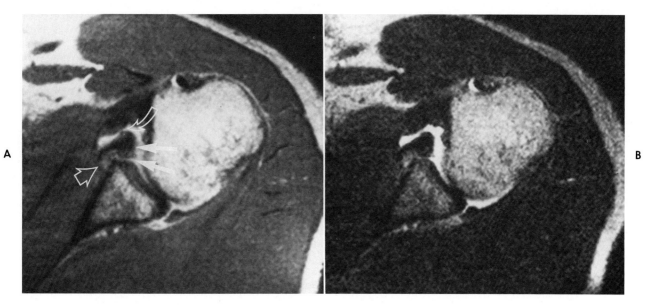

FIGURE 15-52
Recurrent anterior dislocation, right shoulder with a detached anterior capsulolabral complex. **A,** Axial MR image, proton density (2100/30), at the distal glenoid level. There is detachment of the anterior capsulolabral complex with erosion of the glenoid margin *(solid arrows)*. Thickening of the capsulolabral junction *(straight hollow arrow)* and a wavy contour of the capsule and subscapularis tendon *(curved hollow arrow)* are also demonstrated. Note the high-signal joint effusion, resulting in clear demarcation of the joint surfaces. **B,** Same level, T2-weighted image (2100/80). The intense signal of joint effusion does not add to the diagnostic capability of MR images in this case. Also there is a small posterior labral tear.

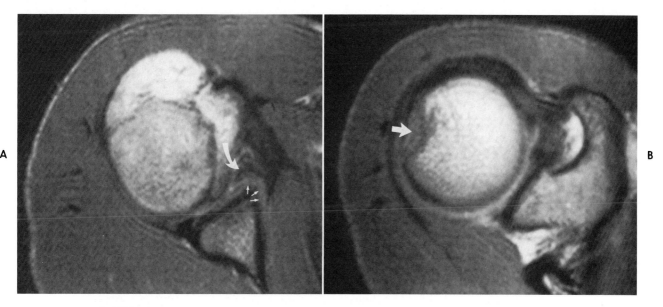

FIGURE 15-53
Anterior instability, right shoulder. **A,** MR axial image, proton density (2100/30) at the distal glenoid. There is a soft tissue Bankart lesion *(curved arrow)*. The capsulolabral complex is elevated from the glenoid, manifested by a thick band of medium-signal soft tissue *(small arrows)* similar to muscle and articular cartilage. The abnormal morphology is diagnostic in this case, even in the absence of joint effusion. **B,** Axial MR image, proton density (2100/30) at the superior aspect of the glenoid. A Hill-Sachs compression fracture is visible *(arrow)*.

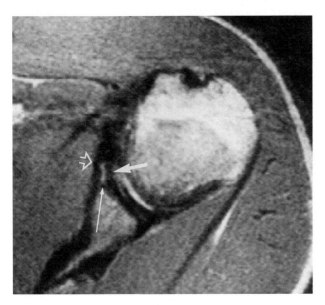

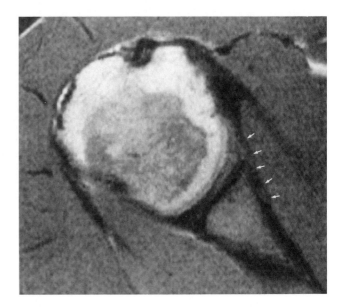

FIGURE 15-54
Anterior instability, left shoulder. Axial MR image, proton density (2100/30) at the distal aspect of the glenoid. Note the attenuated and irregular labral remnant *(solid arrow)*, eroded glenoid margin *(long arrow)*, and undulating wavy capsular outline *(hollow arrow)*.

FIGURE 15-55
Anterior instability, right shoulder. Axial proton density image (1100/29) at the distal glenoid. The anterior glenoid labrum is not visualized. Instead, a wavy capsular outline can be seen extending to the scapular neck region *(arrow)*. This is indicative of capsular stripping and laxity.

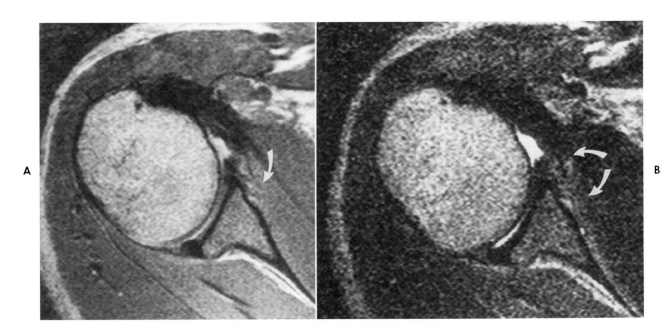

FIGURE 15-56
Acute anterior capsulolabral injury following anterior dislocation of the right shoulder in a young adult. **A** and **B**, Proton density and T2-weighted images (2100/30/80) at the middle glenohumeral joint level demonstrate an indistinct capsular reflection with nonhomogeneously increased signal due to edema *(arrows)*. The undulating outline of the capsule in both images indicates capsular laxity.

finding is evident with more flagrant and chronic instabilities and is usually not seen with mild subluxations. Nor are subscapularis tendon tears a common pathological feature with recurrent anterior dislocation or subluxation. However, they may be seen in elderly persons following a dislocation, with or without an associated tear of the supraspinatus tendon (Fig. 15-57).

3. Osseous lesions with anterior instability: One helpful adjunctive finding in the diagnosis of glenohumeral instability is the presence of a Bankart lesion, manifested as irregularity, erosion (Figs. 15-52 and 15-54), or fracture of the anterior glenoid margin (Fig. 15-58). In young persons with anterior glenohumeral laxity or recurrent subluxation a remodeled glenoid margin with elongation (not unlike marginal osteophyte formation) is occasionally demonstrated (Fig. 15-59). Ectopic bone formation at the site of capsular detachment may be suggested by its configuration, location, and signal void characteristics. However, ectopic bone, especially in the early state of evolution, is not always reliably detected by MRI. A Hill-Sachs compression deformity of the humeral head is well visualized, based

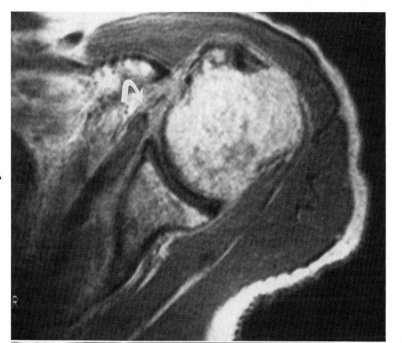

A

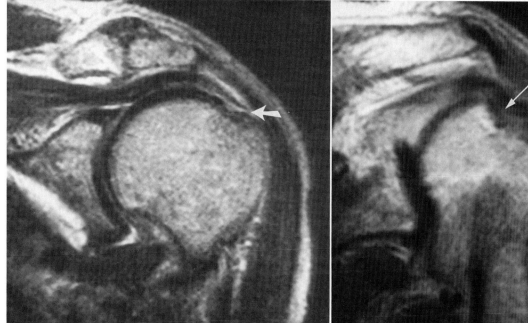

B

C

FIGURE 15-57
Rotator cuff tear with anterior dislocation of the left shoulder in an elderly man following reduction. **A,** Axial proton density–weighted (1600/30) image at the midglenoid level. The subscapularis tendon is torn from the lesser tuberosity and retracted to the level of the glenohumeral joint *(arrow).* The anterior labrum is not visualized, but the glenoid margin is normal. **B** and **C,** Oblique coronal proton density (2100/30) images at the anterior and posterior aspects of the joint show a nonretracted tear of the supraspinatus tendon *(slanted arrow)* and a Hill-Sachs compression fracture *(straight arrow).*

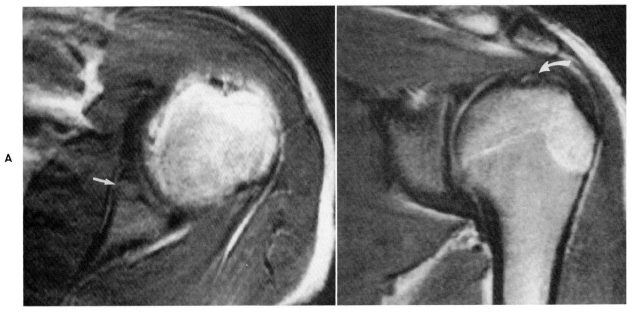

FIGURE 15-58

Osseous Bankart lesion, right shoulder. **A,** Axial proton density–weighted (1100/29) image at the distal glenoid level. A fracture of the anterior glenoid margin is visible *(arrow)*. **B,** Oblique coronal proton density (2100/30) image. A Hill-Sachs lesion, with thinning and mild depression of the superior aspect of the humeral head is also visualized in this patient *(arrow)*.

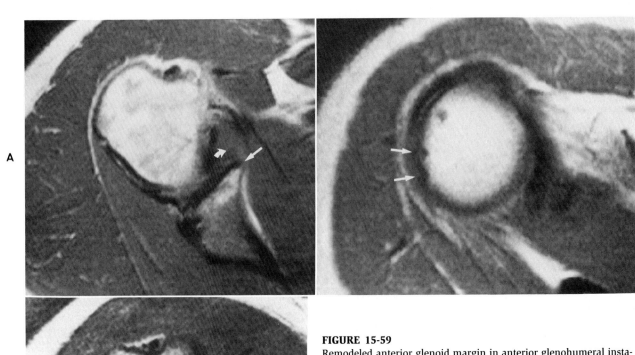

FIGURE 15-59

Remodeled anterior glenoid margin in anterior glenohumeral instability, two cases. Case 1, Axial proton density–weighted (1100/30) images at the inferior glenoid, **A,** and superior joint, **B,** levels, right glenohumeral joint. The glenoid margin is elongated *(straight arrow,* **A)**, with loss of the subcortical spongy bone and fatty replacement of marrow. The torn and attenuated labrum is barely seen *(curved arrow,* **B).** At the superior aspect of the joint a double notched Hill-Sachs lesion is visible *(arrows)*. Case 2, An axial T1-weighted (600/30) MR image, right glenohumeral joint at the distal aspect. The remodeled anterior glenoid with an elongated margin is seen *(long straight arrow,* **C).** The labral outline *(small straight arrows)* without a definite tear or detachment is notable. (**B** from Rafii M, et al: In Nicholas JA, Hershman EB [eds]: The upper extremity in sports medicine, St Louis, Mosby, 1990.)

on the extent and location of the lesion on one or all imaging planes[30] (Figs. 15-56, 15-58, and 15-59).

By virtue of its multiplanar capability, MRI is probably the most accurate modality for detecting Hill-Sachs lesions. This aspect of MR imaging and its inherent resolution of the articular cartilage allow recognition of the cartilaginous lesions with greater ease than is possible with CT-arthrography (Fig. 15-60). Various alterations of signal intensity from the immediate subcortical bone at the site of a Hill-Sachs lesion may be observed due to edema, sclerosis, or cystic rarefaction of the spongy bone (Figs. 15-60 and 15-61). Recognition of these changes is particularly important in the diagnosis of mild instabilities with subtle Bankart and Hill-Sachs lesions.

Posterior instability. Similar to lesions of anterior in-

stability, alterations of the posterior capsulolabral complex alone are visualized on MR with posterior instability (Fig. 15-62, *A*) or combined with anterior lesions in patients who have multidirectional instability (Fig. 15-62, *B*).

Choice of imaging modality

From our experience and based on our as yet unpublished data, it appears that shoulder instability or suspected labral tears can be evaluated by MRI with a high degree of accuracy. Additionally, patients with glenohumeral instability are simultaneously evaluated for manifestations of impingement syndrome, which may develop secondary to shoulder instability.[96] With the use of a proton density sequence and thin sectioning (approximately 3 mm), axial images are generally of good diagnostic quality for detection of capsulolabral lesions of

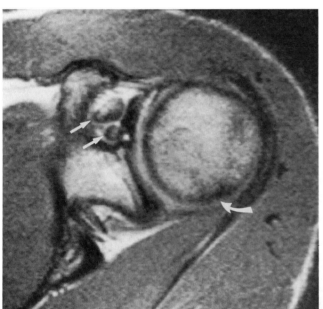

A

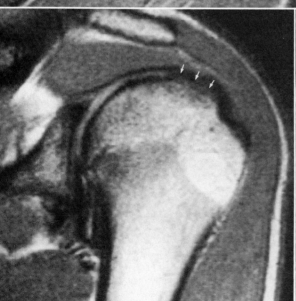

B

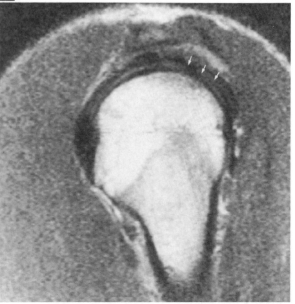

C

FIGURE 15-60
Shallow Hill-Sachs lesion with cartilaginous defect. (Same patient as in Fig. 15-54.) **A,** Axial proton density–weighted (1500/30) image at the superior aspect of the joint showing only slight flattening of the humeral articular cortex *(curved arrow).* Loose bodies are visible lodged in the anterior recess of the joint *(straight arrows).* **B,** Oblique coronal proton density–weighted (2100/30). Attenuation of the humeral head articular cartilage and underlying cortical bone is seen *(arrows).* **C,** Oblique sagittal T1-weighted (600/29) image showing obliteration of the humeral head articular cartilage and loss of definition of the cortical bone *(arrows).* The signal intensity of cortical bone marrow in all images is decreased.

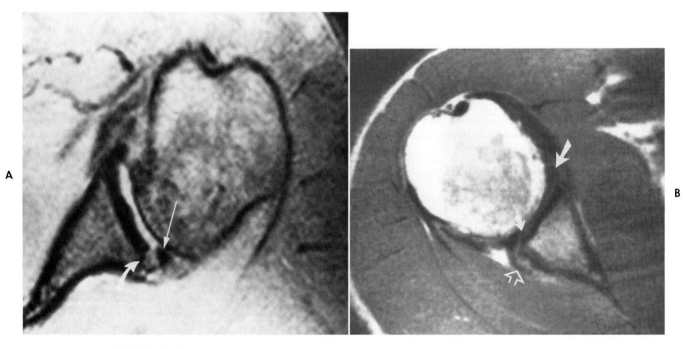

FIGURE 15-61
Subtle cortical Hill-Sachs lesion. (Same patient as in Fig. 15-55.) **A,** Oblique sagittal proton density–weighted (1800/30). This Hill-Sachs lesion is manifested by loss of cortical bone *(white arrow)* and rather extensive alteration of the subcortical marrow signal *(black arrows).* The articular cartilage is preserved. **B,** Axial proton density–weighted (1100/29). The subcortical cystic and sclerotic changes of the humeral head are notable *(arrows).* Normal articular cartilage and cortical bone exist at this level.

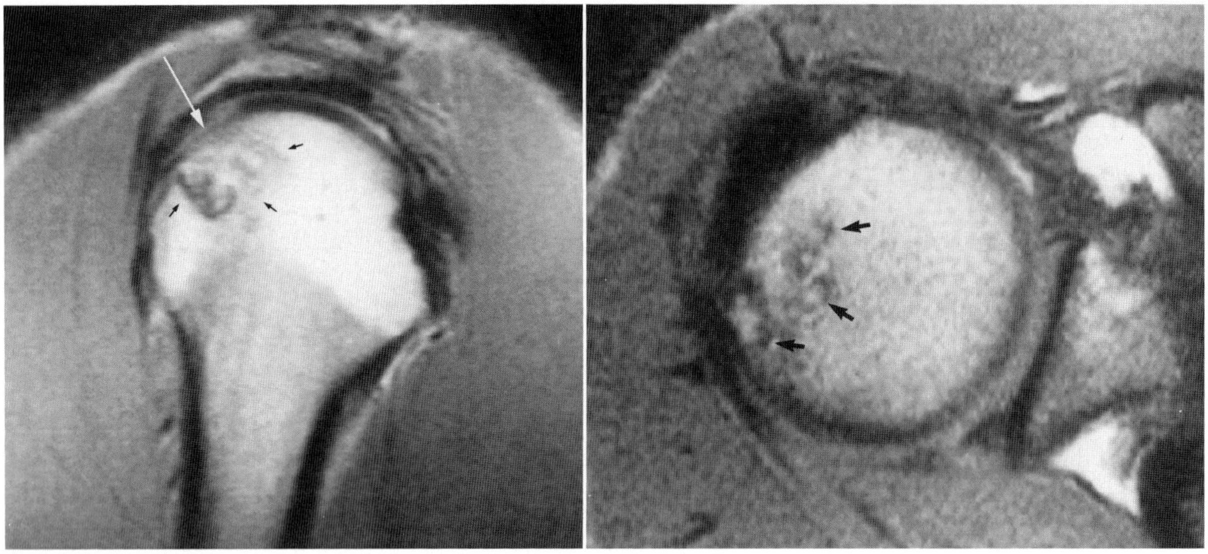

FIGURE 15-62
Posterior and multidirectional instabilities. **A,** Posterior instability, left shoulder. (Same patient as in Fig. 15-48, 2 years following injury and CT-arthrography.) Axial gradient echo (400/19/65°) MR image. Torn posterior labrum *(straight arrow)* and erosion of the glenoid margin *(curved arrow)* are visible. **B,** Multidirectional instability, right shoulder. (Same patient as in Fig. 15-41.) Axial T1-weighted (600/29) MR image obtained several days prior to CT-arthrogram (Fig. 15-41). The anterior labrum is torn, and an irregular remnant can be seen *(slanted arrow).* The posterior labrum is detached from the irregular glenoid margin *(curved arrow).* The curvilinear signal void density along the posterior glenoid margin is a calcific ridge of the capsule *(hollow arrow).*

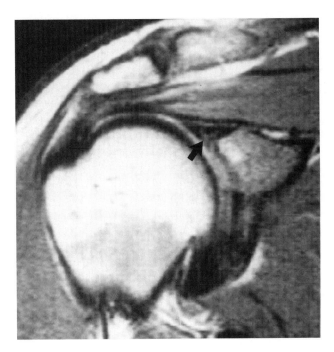

FIGURE 15-63
Superior glenoid labral tear, right shoulder. Oblique coronal proton density-weighted (2100/30) image. A complex tear of the superior labrum is present *(arrow)*. It was confirmed at and resected by arthroscopic surgery.

instability, comparable to that with CT-arthrography (Figs. 15-41 and 15-62, *B*). The multiplanar capability of MRI is more suitable for detecting superior labral tears (Fig. 15-63). In our experience capsular abnormalities (stripping, laxity, or sprain in acute lesions) are also well visualized on MR images, even without joint effusion. Nevertheless, the presence of effusion, even small amounts, undoubtedly help in outlining the configurational abnormalities of the capsulolabral elements, an important factor in the detection of more subtle lesions. Therefore the limitations of MRI in this aspect should be recognized. In these instances (i.e., when occult glenohumeral instability is suspected or there is uncertainty as to the direction of glenohumeral instability) CT-arthrography and gadopentetate MR-arthrography may be the preferred diagnostic modalities. One may also opt for MRI and consider CT-arthrography if the outcome does not answer all questions or does not concur with the clinical picture. MRI, however, with its ability to detect intrinsic soft tissue injuries, is the modality of choice for evaluating the shoulder following episodes of acute trauma (in general) and dislocations/subluxation (in particular).

IMPINGEMENT SYNDROME AND ROTATOR CUFF TEARS

Pain associated with the impingement syndrome and related disorders of the rotator cuff is the most common cause of shoulder disability in all age groups, including young athletes.[3,45,97-102] Although a traumatic incident (usually trivial) may be present in the history, most cuff tears are the result of chronic impingement.[53] Acute traumatic tears are believed to account for less than 5% of such lesions.[99]

Pathophysiology

A brief review of regional anatomy of the shoulder underscores the pathophysiology of rotator cuff disorders and explains the concentration of lesions within the supraspinatus tendon. The rotator cuff is surrounded by the partly osseous, partly ligamentous, coracoacromial arch. When the arm is in anatomical position, the supraspinatus tendon is mostly anterior (peripheral) to the acromion process.[5] When the arm is elevated, the central portion of the supraspinatus tendon first glides under the coracoacromial ligament, and with further elevation it passes beneath the acromion and the acromioclavicular joint. The movement of the supraspinatus tendon under the coracoacromial arch is cushioned by the subacromial bursa. Anatomical variations of the arch, pathological processes resulting in compromise of the subacromial space, and repeated microinjuries sustained as a result of athletic or occupational activities all may cause inflammation, degeneration, and eventual tearing of the tendon.[5,99] Early pathological changes of the subacromial soft tissues (e.g., inflammation of the subacromial bursa or hemorrhage and edema of the rotator cuff tendons) may further compromise the subacromial space, resulting in aggravation of the insult to the tendon.[66,103]

The great majority of cuff lesions involve the "critical zone" of the supraspinatus tendon, the area immediately proximal to its greater tuberosity insertion.[10,104] Several vascular studies point to hypovascularity[105] or the presence of vascular anastomoses[104] in this region. However, these concepts are not universally accepted. Another study has demonstrated normal vascularity of this region with the arm 90 degrees abducted but poor perfusion when the arm is held in anatomical position. This so-called "wring-out" phenomenon is hypothesized[106] to enhance degeneration of the supraspinatus tendon in the critical zone.

The concept of rotator cuff impingement as the source of cuff degeneration and tearing had been introduced by several investigators as early as 1906.[10] Neer[5] reintroduced it in 1972, and in 1977 he and Welsh[53] emphasized the role of the anterior acromion process and hypertrophic changes of the acromioclavicular joint in producing these lesions. Neer's clinical classification portrayed the onset of cuff tendinitis (Stage I) as the result of a combination of anatomical alterations in the arch and overuse of the arm, progressing gradually to cuff degeneration (Stage II) and eventually to tendon tear (Stage III).

A role for acromioclavicular osteophytes in rotator cuff impingement has also been propounded.[107] There is a high incidence of such spurs in patients with rotator cuff tears. Abnormalities of the acromioclavicular joint and other osseous alterations about the acromion process and greater tuberosity (including traction spurs of the anterior acromial margin, hypertrophy of the acromial undersurface, sclerosis of the greater tuberosity, and subcortical cysts in the vicinity of the anatomical neck of the humerus) are commonly seen in elderly persons.[108,109] These changes occur mostly late in the second or in the third stage of impingement.[108] Despite this frequent association, the cause-and-effect relation between these findings and the pathophysiology of rotator cuff lesions is not clearly understood.

Pathological changes of the cuff associated with the impingement syndrome are described as possible edema and hemorrhage in Stage I, fibrosis and degeneration in Stage II, and eventual tendon tearing in Stage III.[99] Necrosis and degeneration of the rotator cuff tendons due to hypovascularity are also postulated as the basic underlying pathological process promoting rotator cuff tendinitis and concurrent or ensuing disorders (e.g., bursitis, calcific tendinitis, tendon tears).[110] Strizak et al.[111] in a study of subacromial bursography described tendons as showing either hypocellularity and myxomatous changes or simply other unspecified manifestations of tendon degeneration. Brewer[112] considered aging of the rotator cuff tendons to be the single basic etiological factor in a variety of clinical entities, including impingement syndrome, rotator cuff tendinitis, supraspinatus tendinitis, and rotator cuff rupture. His histological evaluation underscored extensive descriptions by Skinner,[6] DePalma,[7] Codman,[10] Cotton and Rideour,[113] and Wilson[114] of a gradual and progressive tearing of the tendon fibers at the undersurface of the supraspinatus, with separation from the greater tuberosity, eventually forming the "rim rent" of Codman. Although these partial tears were seen as typically communicating with the joint through a gap in the synovial surface and superficial tendon fibers, other partial tears were also recognized as involving either the superior bursal surface of the tendon or the central tendon fibers (i.e., intratendinous tears).[7,10,115,116]

The various pathological processes begin usually in a person's teens or twenties and span several decades. Nevertheless, the onset of symptoms in a middle-aged individual is likely due to a single recreational or work-related activity. Except when the bursa is acutely traumatized, the associated subacromial bursitis is thought to be subsequent to a tendinitis.[53,100] Frequent involvement of the biceps tendon is observed, reflecting its proximity to the supraspinatus tendon (with simultaneous impingement by the coracoacromial ligament).[5,53,100] Gradual degeneration ultimately leads to a complete tear of the long head of the biceps tendon, with subluxation developing after a tear of the coracohumeral (transverse humeral) ligament.[53]

DISTRIBUTION AND MORPHOLOGY

The morphology of cuff tears has been extensively studied.[6,7,10,113,114] Most often a tear originates at the greater tuberosity insertion of the supraspinatus tendon, with the tendon retracting from the sulcus (anatomical

neck) of the humerus. These "rim rents"[10] or insertion tears characteristically involve the anterior component of the supraspinatus tendon and evolve from partial separation of the tendinous fibers at the synovial surface into complete detachments.[10] Another common site is the critical zone of the supraspinatus tendon. Partial tears, therefore, may involve the inferior synovial surface of the tendon. Partial intratendinous and bursal surface tears are also commonly encountered in cadaver studies. In one postmortem investigation[115] full-thickness and partial-thickness tears were observed in 7% and 13% respectively. Among the partial-thickness tears, intratendinous tearing was the most frequent type observed, twice as common as tears of the synovial side and three times as common as bursal side tears.[116]

By definition, a full-thickness rotator cuff tear is a defect that permits communication between the glenohumeral joint and the subacromial bursa. Full-thickness cuff tears are classified according to size[7]: small, less than 1 cm; medium, 1 to 2 cm; large, 2 to 4 cm; and massive, more than 5 cm. A more recent classification[117] has taken into consideration the anatomical location of the tear. An important aspect of this classification is its better correlation with patient symptoms and prognosis. Four groups are recognized: group one lesions comprise either partial-thickness or small full-thickness (less than 1 cm) tears of the supraspinatus and occasionally subscapularis tendons; group two lesions are full-thickness tears of the supraspinatus tendon measuring up to 2 cm; in group three, more than one tendon is involved, with the tear exceeding 2 cm (defects may be anterosuperior or posterosuperior); group four lesions comprise large defects in association with humeral head elevation (osteoarthritis of the joint is often present).

Recognition of the presence and the extent of full-thickness cuff tears is an important clinical determination in surgical treatment planning. Although not universally followed by more modern philosophies in shoulder surgery (which favor conservative treatment and/or arthroscopic decompression of the subacromial space in all stages of impingement, including those with cuff tears), the consensus appears to favor repair of the torn cuff along with an anterior acromioplasty as suggested by Neer.[5,118-120] Factors in surgical consideration include age, level of activity, and chronicity of the tear.

• • •

The role of conventional roentgenography in evaluating rotator cuff impingement is limited to visualization of the various osseous changes about the greater tuberosity, acromion, and AC joint.[97,108,109] Roentgenographic assessment of rotator cuff tears has traditionally and reliably been achieved by shoulder arthrography, despite its limitations in detecting partial intratendinous and superior surface tears.[20,121-124] The false-negative rate for full-thickness tears on arthrography has been debated as truly very small, or otherwise underestimated because of a tendency to refrain from surgery in patients in whom arthrography has failed to detect a tendon tear. False-negative arthrographic findings are believed due to adhesions, scar, or granulation tissue, which limit the flow of contrast medium from the joint to the subacromial bursa through the torn region. Another drawback of conventional arthrography is its limitation in the accurate assessment of tear size and the extent of cuff degeneration without the use of tomographic techniques.[22,125]

Although the role of ultrasonography as a noninvasive means of screening for rotator cuff lesions is well established,[126-128] this modality has not been widely utilized — due in part to its relatively low sensitivity and specificity in detection of cuff tears and in part to its inability to differentiate certain cuff tears from tendinitis. It is also technically difficult to perform, and its accuracy is greatly operator dependent.[76,127]

Ordinarily conventional arthrography performed for detection of cuff tears does not need to be complemented by CT. Occasionally, however, a small tear not detected by arthrography will be visualized on subsequent CT images.[44] This higher incidence of detection by CT-arthrography compared to arthrography preceding the CT probably reflects the limited nature of the particular arthrographic study performed.

The necessity of a CT examination, therefore, in patients with suspected rotator cuff tears may be debated. However, visualization of tear size is improved by CT and the margins of the torn tendon are better demonstrated (Fig. 15-64). Also the possible association of shoulder instability with cuff tears[66] (Fig. 15-65) may be shown by CT-arthrography, which would thus make it helpful in overall assessment of the patient.

Direct sagittal CT examination following arthrography has been recommended for improved visualization of cuff tears and for better demonstration of the quality of tendinous margins.[22] (See under *Technique,* p. 472.) CT-arthrography does not contribute to evaluation of the earlier manifestations of cuff pathology and other aspects of the impingement syndrome.

• • •

MR imaging of impingement lesions

The major contribution of MRI to shoulder imaging is in evaluation of the impingement syndrome and rotator cuff disorders.[29-39] At present, MRI is the most comprehensive, yet totally noninvasive, modality available for shoulder imaging. It can reveal not only cuff tears but also the array of pathological processes associated with the impingement syndrome, including rotator cuff tendinitis, subacromial bursitis, and AC joint arthritis. At the same time, the glenohumeral joint is adequately depicted for evaluation of possible instability and/or associated arthritic processes.

Diagnosis of rotator cuff lesions by MRI is based primarily on alterations in anatomical features and signal intensity of the involved tendons. The nuances of signal intensity are best visualized on T1-weighted or proton density sequences; the T2-weighted sequence, by detecting fluid, is more helpful in delineation of the cuff defect. (See under *Technique,* pp 472 and 473.) Other osseous and soft tissue changes visualized in the subacromial space (e.g., SA-SD bursal abnormalities and hypertrophic changes of the acromion on process and AC joint), when present, provide additional diagnostic information on the

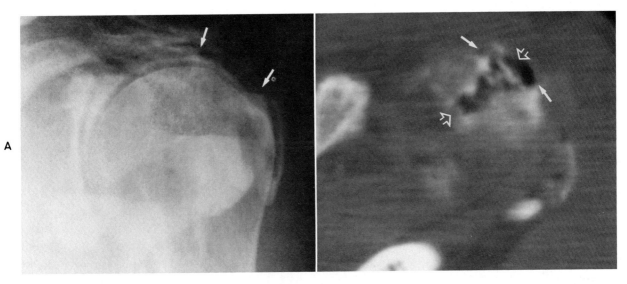

FIGURE 15-64
Rotator cuff tear visualized by CT-arthrography. **A,** A conventional double-contrast arthrogram of the left shoulder shows a full-thickness tear *(arrows).* **B,** A CT image following the arthrogram reveals the anteroposterior *(solid arrows)* and mediolateral *(hollow arrows)* extent of the defect. The irregular margin of the tear is well demonstrated. Pooling of contrast adjacent and proximal to the cuff defect indicates regions of partial thickness tearing.

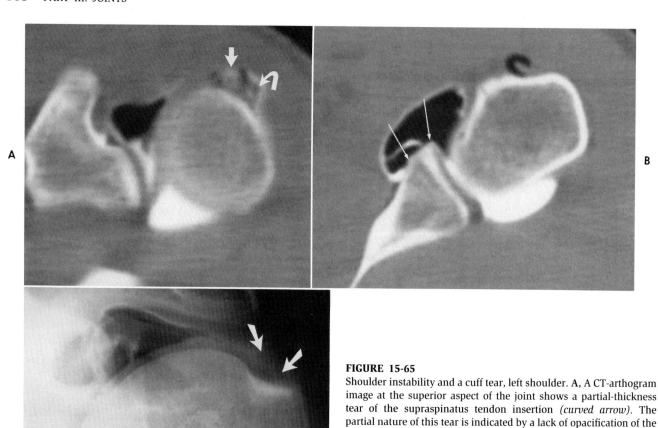

FIGURE 15-65

Shoulder instability and a cuff tear, left shoulder. **A,** A CT-arthogram image at the superior aspect of the joint shows a partial-thickness tear of the supraspinatus tendon insertion *(curved arrow)*. The partial nature of this tear is indicated by a lack of opacification of the subdeltoid bursa. The tear is focal and involves the anterior margin of the tendon. The biceps tendon is also visualized at this level *(straight arrow)*. **B,** A CT image at the lower aspect of the glenohumeral joint shows attenuation of the anterior labrum with stripping of the capsule, indicative of anterior instability *(arrows)*. **C,** Conventional arthrogram, external humeral rotation. The partial-thickness tear of the supraspinatus is visible *(arrows)*.

spectrum of the disease. A combination of MRI findings has been used for staging the impingement syndrome and for diagnosing and differentiating tendinitis from cuff tears.[37-39] Although various pathological changes may coexist or MRI findings may overlap, they are best discussed separately.

SUBACROMIAL-SUBDELTOID BURSITIS

MR manifestations of subacromial-subdeltoid (SA-SD) bursitis are based primarily on alterations in the peribursal fat, account being taken of variations in its presence and thickness.[11] This abnormality is in the form of a total or partial loss of the peribursal fat signal on T1-weighted or of decreased signal on T1-weighted and increased signal on T2-weighted sequences (Fig. 15-66). The bursa may contain fluid, demonstrated on T1-weighted and proton density sequences as loss of the peribursal fat signal. The characteristically intense signal of fluid may be observed on a T2-weighted sequence (Fig. 15-67). At times a layer of low-signal tissue element replacing the peribursal fat is clearly visualized with or without small

pockets of fluid (Fig. 15-68). The low-signal alteration represents a proliferative process, with thickening of the bursa in chronic bursitis commonly accompanying rotator cuff disorders. By contrast, accumulation of fluid within the bursa indicates an acute inflammatory response and/or may represent the flow of joint fluid through a cuff defect. This latter observation has lent itself to use as a criterion for diagnosing cuff tears.[32]

Inflammation of the SA-SD bursa, without manifestations of tendinitis or tendon tear, is an infrequent observation on MRI. This agrees with the existing surgical literature and findings in postmortem studies that imply inflammation and subsequent scarring of the SA-SD bursa are associated with and result from tendinitis.[10,53,110,111] Our experience with MR imaging has been that at this stage fluid pockets or a small amount of free fluid may be present within the bursa, which otherwise shows a proliferative process manifested by low signal alterations in the peribursal layer of fat (Figs. 15-66 and 15-68). A similar appearance, or actual distention of the bursa with fluid, may be seen with cuff tears. A distended bursa in

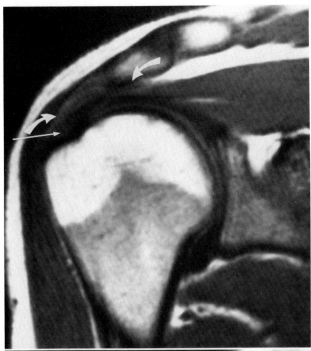

A

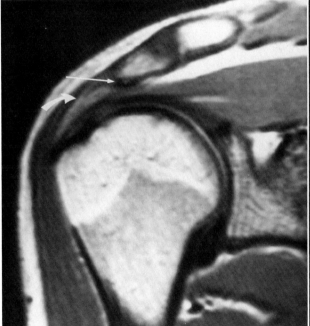

B

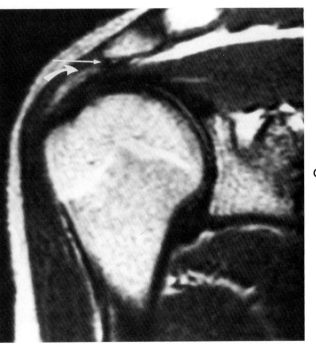

C

FIGURE 15-66

Impingement syndrome. SA-SD bursitis and tendinitis, right shoulder. **A,** Oblique coronal T1-weighted (600/29) image. There is obliteration of the peribursal fat, with a marked decrease in signal intensity *(curved arrows)*. Some increase in signal of the supraspinatus tendon *(long arrow)* indicates associated tendinitis. The tendinous morphology is normal. **B** and **C,** Same level, proton density and T2-weighted images (2100/30/80). Note the persistent abnormality of the peribursal fat signal, with progressive but nonhomogeneous increase in signal intensity *(curved arrows)*. This is indicative of an inflammatory and proliferative process of the bursa. Signal void beneath the acromion *(long arrows)* due to bony proliferation is visible. The abnormal signal intensity of the supraspinatus tendon is better seen in **B.**

the presence of normal morphology and normal signal intensity of the cuff is also infrequently encountered and may constitute merely an isolated incident of nonspecific synovitis or be just part of a systemic disorder (Fig. 15-69).

ROTATOR CUFF TENDINITIS

Tendinitis or tendon degeneration is recognized on MR when the tendons' signal void appearance changes and is replaced by mild to moderate signal intensity on T1-weighted and proton density sequences; the abnormal signal intensity is less evident or absent on a T2-weighted sequence (Fig. 15-66). It has been suggested[37] that the

peribursal fat signal remains normal, a differential criterion between tendinitis and cuff tear. However, our experience with a large group of patients[39] indicates that abnormality of the peribursal fat signal can be and often is an affiliated finding in tendinitis.

Increased signal intensity of the rotator cuff is an indication of chemical or histological alteration within the tendon and may reflect a variety of tendinous disorders, including degenerative, inflammatory, and posttraumatic reparative processes.[35,39,129] In a study of several cadaver tendons,[129] we found histological manifestations of degeneration in several supraspinatus tendons with increased signal intensity on MRI — including

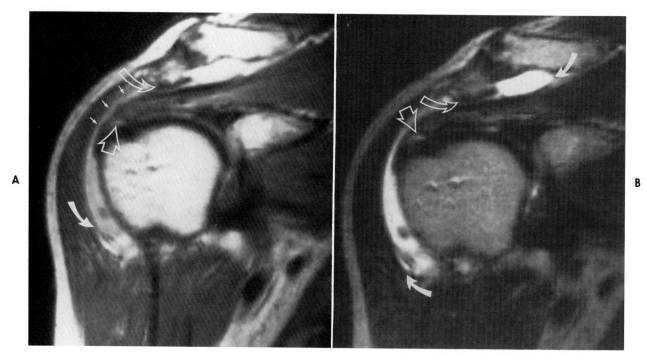

FIGURE 15-67

Distended subacromial-subdeltoid bursa, partial cuff tear. **A** and **B**, Oblique coronal proton density–weighted and T2-weighted (2100/30/80) MR images of the right shoulder. The SD peribursal fat is obliterated *(small arrows* in **A**). Note the marked distention of the bursa, with characteristic signal of fluid and containing low-signal debris *(solid curved arrows).* A large acromial spur *(hollow curved arrows)* and a partial thickness tear of the supraspinatus *(hollow arrows)* are also present. The "low-lying" position of the acromion is demonstrated.

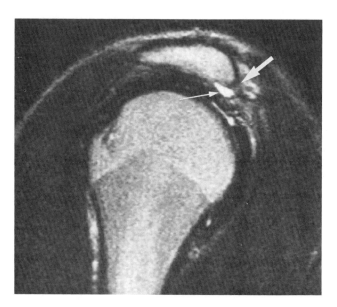

FIGURE 15-68

Subacromial bursitis. Oblique sagittal T2-weighted (1800/80) image. Note the small pocket of fluid in the SA bursa *(thin arrow).* This is in the vicinity of the anterior acromion and coracoacromial ligament *(thick arrow).* Increased signal intensity above the ligament is consistent with an inflammatory process in this region.

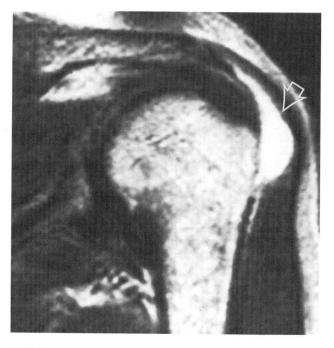

FIGURE 15-69

Subdeltoid bursitis, left shoulder. This middle-aged patient presented with a palpable mass and no clinical manifestations of the impingement syndrome. T2-weighted (2100/80) oblique coronal image. The distended SD bursa is visible *(arrow).* Otherwise, no cuff abnormality was present on MRI.

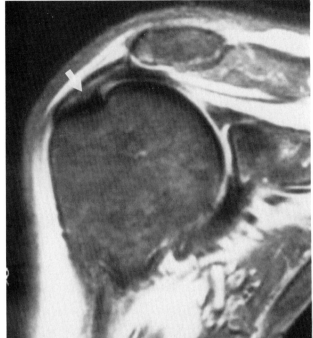

A

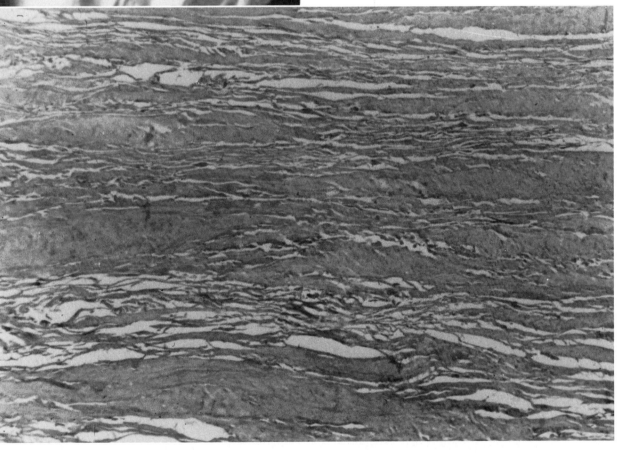

B

FIGURE 15-70
Degenerative process of the supraspinatus tendon in a cadaver shoulder. **A,** Oblique coronal T2-weighted (2100/80) image with the region of increased signal in the tendon *(arrow)*. **B,** Histological appearance of this tendon, showing disorganization of the fibers.

Continued.

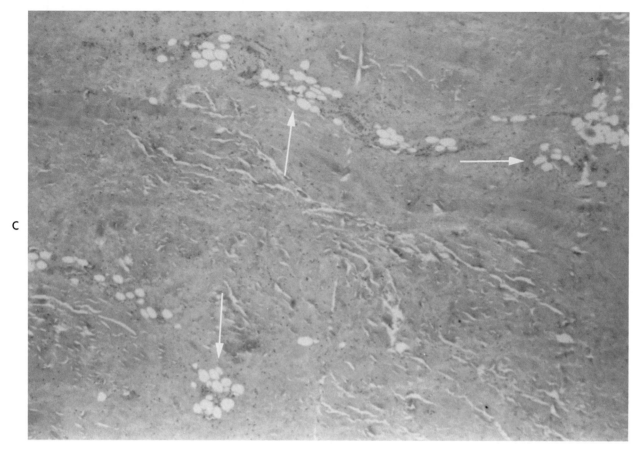

FIGURE 15-70 cont'd
C, Histological appearance of another supraspinatus tendon with increased signal intensity. In addition
to distortion of the tendinous fibers, regions of fatty infiltration are visible *(arrows).*

disorganization and separation of fibers and regions of fatty degeneration (Fig. 15-70). Other investigators[35] have reported finding myxoid degeneration and inflammatory changes of unspecified nature in three cases that underwent biopsy at the time of surgery. Based on these (limited) investigations, we feel that the abnormal signal intensity of the rotator cuff tendons is a nonspecific finding and it may not be possible to differentiate various pathological processes (edema, hemorrhage, inflammatory or degenerative changes) using signal intensity alone; This pertains in particular to tendinitis, tendon degeneration, and some small partial tears.

Our experience with MR imaging of asymptomatic shoulders, though limited, has shown mild and usually focal regions of increased signal on T1-weighted and proton density images, probably reflecting the degenerative process of aging. The peribursal fat signal is normal in these individuals, but the manifestations of bursitis not infrequently are associated with tendinitis (p. 508). In symptomatic shoulders without MR evidence of a tear, tendinitis is manifested by more diffuse increased signal intensity of variable extent. The increased signal may be homogeneous (focal, diffuse, or bandlike) or nonhomogeneous and associated with tendinous enlargement[39]

(Fig. 15-71). We have also observed increased signal in the proximity of partial or small full-thickness tears (Fig. 15-77). Based on the available data, though limited,[39,129] this finding (enlarged tendon with increased signal) likely represents the process of reparative change and healing in an interstitial tendon tear (p. 522).

Thus it appears that the MR findings with "tendinitis" and interstitial tears may overlap. These two entities, however, represent separate points in the spectrum of one pathological and clinical entity (an inflammatory or reparative process following repeated microinjury to the tendon, recognized in early stages of the impingement syndrome, prior to the development of a cuff tear).

Similarly tendinitis and tendon degeneration may not be distinguishable, based on MR findings, unless the tendinitis is diffuse or, in particular, is associated with a nonhomogenous signal pattern and/or tendinous enlargement. The presence of SA-SD bursitis is another indication that the process is tendinitis rather than asymptomatic tendinous degeneration. Degeneration of a tendon due to aging is manifested mostly by mild and focal regions of increased signal without apparent change in tendinous thickness. On the other hand, tendinous

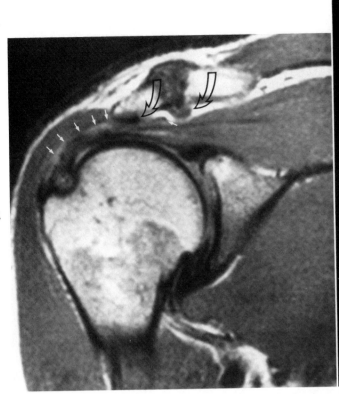
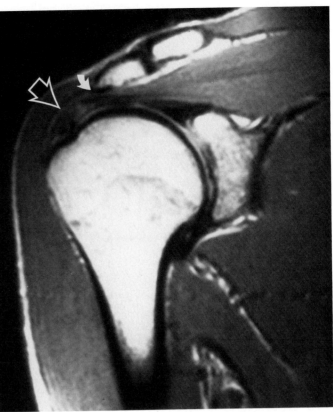

FIGURE 15-71

Supraspinatus tendinitis, two cases. **A,** Case 1. Oblique coronal proton density (2100/30) MR image of the right shoulder. There is nonhomogeneously increased signal intensity of the supraspinatus tendon. The SA-SD peribursal fat is irregular and generally diminished in signal *(white arrows).* The AC joint and acromial spurs impinge on the cuff *(hollow curved arrows).* **B,** Case 2. Oblique coronal proton density–weighted (2100/30) image of the right shoulder. In addition to increased signal intensity, the supraspinatus tendon is enlarged (thickened) *(hollow arrow).* There is only a small spur of the acromion visible *(solid arrow).* The AC joint is normal. The "low-lying" position of the acromion is demonstrated.

degeneration as a result of prior injury and/or long-standing tendinitis can be deduced when attenuation of the tendon is also present.

ROTATOR CUFF TEARS

Early investigators[30,31] faced unexpected difficulties in detecting rotator cuff tears by MRI, mostly due to the anatomical complexity of the cuff tendons and the poor distinguishability of the low-signal tendon from adjacent cortical bone. The difficulty was not so much in detecting large or massive tears as in recognizing small full-thickness and partial-thickness tears and differentiating them from one another or from other tendinous lesions without a tear.[32,33] Concomitant with further improvements in imaging techniques and the availability of specialized surface coils, and with the experience gathered, the detection and differentiation of small and partial tears have drastically improved.

The most characteristic and reliable criterion for diagnosing cuff tears (established early on) is visualization of a *tendinous defect.* This is indicated by an interruption of

the tendon's signal void, manifested by an area of increased signal on T1-weighted and proton density images and an intense or marked increase in signal on T2-weighted images (representing joint fluid or granulation tissue)[30-35] (Fig. 15-72). Large or massive cuff tears are also adequately visualized by T1-weighted imaging (Fig. 15-73), whose use for this purpose was suggested as early as 1987 and 1988,[30,32] along with retraction of the musculotendinous junction and atrophy of the supraspinatus muscle. These findings, however, are seen mostly with large or massive cuff tears of a chronic nature. Therefore, despite the fact that alterations in signal intensity of the rotator cuff tendons are best depicted on T1-weighted or proton density sequences, the sensitivity of these sequences in diagnosing cuff tears in general, and small or partial tears in particular, is limited.[33]

Secondary manifestations of rotator cuff tears are recognized with variable severity and may be helpful in diagnosing cuff tears.[33,37]

Retraction of the supraspinatus musculotendinous junc-

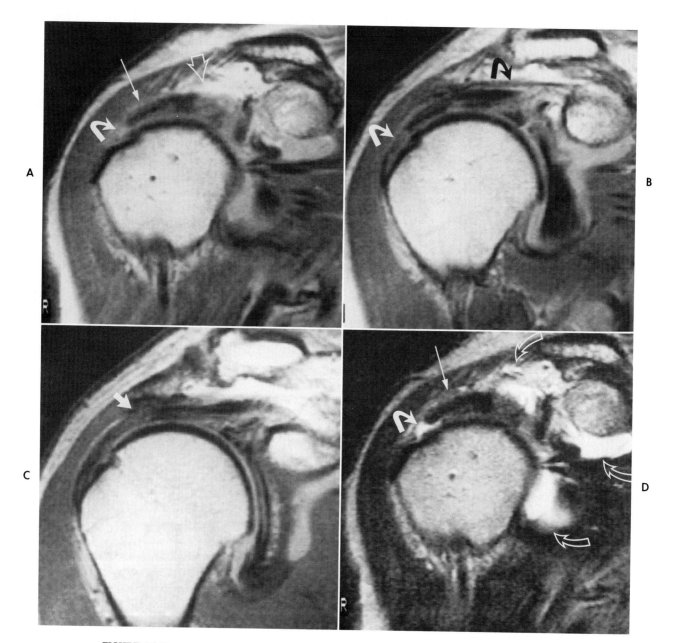

FIGURE 15-72

Full-thickness supraspinatus rotator cuff tear, right shoulder. **A**, Oblique coronal proton density–weighted (2100/30) image, anterior aspect of the joint. The supraspinatus tendon is interrupted by increased signal intensity near the tuberosity insertion *(curved arrow)*. The SD space has a heterogeneous signal, partly decreased *(straight arrow)* and partly increased *(hollow arrow)*, compared to subcutaneous fat. **B**, Same sequence, one slice posterior to **A**. The tendon is in continuity, but it shows marked irregularity and attenuation *(white arrow)*. The coracoacromial ligament is visible *(black arrow)*. **C**, Posterior to **B**. The tendon morphology is normal. Increased signal is noted in the immediate level of a large acromial spur *(arrow)*. **D**, Same plane as **A**, T2-weighted sequence (2100/80). The cuff defect is identified by an intense signal *(curved arrow)*. The SD fat plane remains low signal in the vicinity of the cuff defect *(straight arrow)*, indicating a proliferative bursitis. Fluid is present in various recesses of the glenohumeral joint and medial aspect of the subacromial bursa *(hollow arrows)*. T2-weighted images at the levels of **B** and **C** confirmed the continuity but also the focal thinning of the tendon (partial-thickness tear) in **B**. The signal change in **C** did not increase, indicating tendinitis or tendon degeneration.

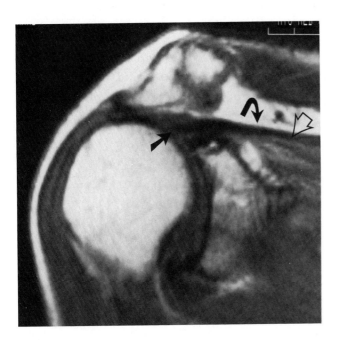

FIGURE 15-73
Massive and chronic supraspinatus rotator cuff tear, right shoulder. Oblique coronal T1-weighted (650/30) image. The tear is indicated by the absence of signal void tendon in the subacromial space, which is occupied by the superiorly displaced humeral head. The margin of the cuff defect is visualized medial to the humeral head *(slanted arrow)*. The musculotendinous junction is retracted *(curved arrow)*. Loss of muscle mass and fatty atrophy of the supraspinatus are present *(hollow arrow)*. Note the atrophy and loss of peribursal fat with this chronic cuff tear. Note also the prominent inferiorly pointing AC spur, and flattening of the greater tuberosity.

tion may be used as an associated criterion in the diagnosis of complete ruptures.[33] This finding is prominent with large or complete tears (Fig. 15-73) but absent or difficult to ascertain with small ones; in the former a globular configuration of the supraspinatus muscle may be observed.[36]

Atrophy of the rotator muscles is also often seen with large or complete ruptures of the rotator cuff tendons. This is manifested by generalized loss of muscle mass as well as areas of fatty replacement (Fig. 15-73). The severity of these changes is dependent upon the extent and chronicity of the cuff lesion.

Abnormality of SA-SD peribursal fat is a constant finding.[39] However, this is not always in the form of fluid accumulation within the bursa. In some cases the peribursal fat is either diminished (Fig. 15-73) or replaced by low-signal tissue (Fig. 15-72), indicating atrophy or granulation tissue and scar formation. These changes may be limited to the vicinity of the cuff tear.[39]

The presence of one or more secondary findings is particularly helpful and should be looked for when a suspected cuff tear is not readily visualized.

MR accuracy. Using the presence of intense signal on T2-weighted imaging, Seeger et al.[33] accurately diagnosed

18 complete rotator cuff ruptures. MRI, however, did not detect 3 small or partial tears, which were detected by arthrography or arthroscopy. In a study by Kneeland et al.,[31] MRI detected 20 tears accurately but 2 were missed. Analysis of these data shows 18 tears manifested by markedly increased signal in the region of cuff tear. The nature of the abnormality in 2 remaining cases (which were accurately diagnosed) and in 2 that were misdiagnosed was not clarified. Based on a visualized discontinuity of the tendon when significantly increased signal intensity on T2-weighted images was used, Evancho et al.[34] accurately diagnosed 8 of 10 full-thickness tears (sensitivity 80%) and 1 of 3 partial tears (overall sensitivity 69%). The false-negative cases consisted of small lesions without marked signal intensity and with apparent preservation of tendinous continuity. Burk et al.,[38] using similar criteria, detected 11 of 12 surgically proved tears (sensitivity 92%). In this study MRI and arthrography successfully identified lesions with equal accuracy. These investigators generally regarded full-thickness and partial-thickness tears as separate entities and attempted to differentiate them on the basis of their morphological appearance.

In a broader form of diagnostic rotator cuff grading, Zlatkin et al.[37] used a combination of abnormal signal intensity, abnormal tendon morphology (thinning, irregularity, disruption), and abnormal peribursal fat line. A cuff tear was diagnosed when the tendon demonstrated both an increase in signal intensity and an abnormal morphology and, in addition, was associated with an abnormal peribursal fat signal indicative of fluid. Such fluid within the bursa is presumed to originate from the glenohumeral joint. Based on these diagnostic criteria, an abnormal peribursal fat signal is affiliated with both partial- and small full-thickness tears. An additional scoring system devised by these authors was suggested for differentiating partial- and full-thickness tears. With this grading system, they demonstrated sensitivity of 100% in the diagnosis of 17 full-thickness and 91% in the diagnosis of 22 full- and partial-thickness tears of the inferior surface.[37]

Tabulation of our data[39] in 80 surgically documented cases has also yielded excellent results in the detection of cuff tears when a high-resolution technique and thin-slice imaging parameters were used in a high-field scanner. The criteria in our study were based primarily on changes in the tendon configuration and morphology as well as signal intensity on proton density and T2-weighted images. Of 37 documented full-thickness tears, 36 were accurately detected (sensitivity of 94%). Of 16 partial tears, 14 were accurately diagnosed (Table 15-2).

MR signal patterns in cuff tears. Most full-thickness tears are characterized by intense signal within the cuff defect on a T2-weighted sequence.[39] An intense or markedly increased signal may also optimally visualize small or linear nonretracted tears (Fig. 15-74). This specific finding, however, is not present in approximately

20% of cuff tears.[39] In these cases the defect is either obliterated by a severely degenerated tendinous remnant (Fig. 15-75) or filled with low- to medium-signal tissue, presumably representing scar formation (Fig. 15-76).

Obliteration of a cuff tear by scar or granulation tissue in the subacute stage is well recognized.[101] This phenomenon is a noted, though infrequent, cause of false-negative arthrograms.[124] The arthrographic diagnosis may be aided, however, by increasing the intraarticular pressure and exercising the joint during arthrography. These elements notwithstanding, the diagnosis of such tears on MRI is basically dependent upon recognition of the contour and signal abnormality of the torn tendon. Some observations that may be helpful in accurately

assessing such tears are that (1) there is often an abrupt change in signal character of the tendon at the boundary of the cuff defect (Figs. 15-75 and 15-76) and (2), depending upon the extent and chronicity of the lesion, secondary manifestations (e.g., retraction of the musculotendinous junction, atrophy of the supraspinatus muscle, or leakage of joint effusion into the subacromial bursa) may be present.

Although low-signal cuff tears, particularly when small, remain a difficult object for MR visualization, other small full-thickness tears that may skip detection by arthrography and surgery are usually well shown[37,39] (Fig. 15-77). Intact synovial and bursal surfaces often account for nonvisualization of these tears at arthrogra-

Table 15-2   Accuracy of MRI in Detection of Rotator Cuff Tears

	Full-thickness tears (n = 31)	Partial-thickness tears (n = 16)
Sensitivity	0.97	0.89
Specificity	0.94	0.84
Accuracy	0.95	0.85
Positive predictive value	0.94	0.73
Negative predictive value	0.97	0.94

From Rafii M, et al: Radiology 1990;177:817-823.

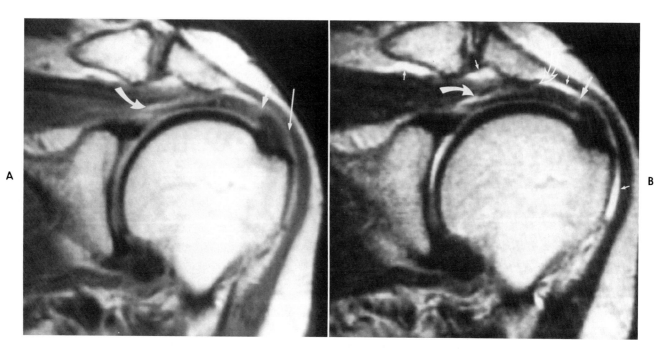

FIGURE 15-74
Linear full-thickness supraspinatus tear, left shoulder. **A,** Oblique coronal proton density–weighted (2100/30) image. The supraspinatus tendon is interrupted by an oblique band of increased signal intensity *(curved arrow)*. There is also a focal increase in signal near the tuberosity insertion *(short arrow)*. The SA-SD fat signal is partly decreased *(long arrow)*. **B,** Same level, T2-weighted sequence (2100/80). Visualization of the linear cuff tear is enhanced, in part by intense signal within the torn region *(curved solid arrow)*. The bursal aspect of this tear is confluent with the tip of the acromion and does not show intense signal *(curved hollow arrow)*. The focal configuration of the region of signal abnormality near the tuberosity insertion (and the nature of signal change) is indicative of a partial tear *(long arrow)*. There is fluid in the SA-SD bursa *(short arrows)*. Note the subacromial impingement by the prominent end of the clavicle and inferiorly pointed acromion.

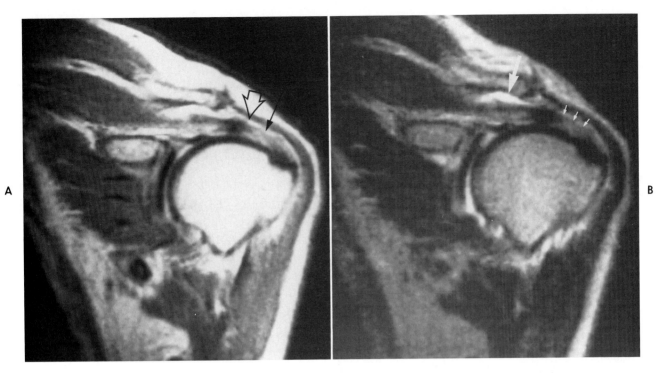

FIGURE 15-75
Full-thickness supraspinatus tear (severe tendon degeneration), left shoulder. **A,** Oblique coronal proton density–weighted sequence (2100/30) at the anterior aspect of the joint. There is marked attenuation with irregularity of the distal tendon *(solid arrow)*. This region is sharply defined from the more proximal normal tendon by an abrupt change in signal intensity and tendon width *(hollow arrow)*. **B,** Same level, T2-weighted sequence. The severely degenerated and torn tendon maintains continuity along the bursal surface *(short arrows)*. Note the small amount of fluid in SA bursa *(long arrow)*. At surgery the bursal surface appeared intact. However, gentle probing resulted in disintegration of the degenerated tendinous cuff remnant. Clinically, this was considered a full-thickness tear.

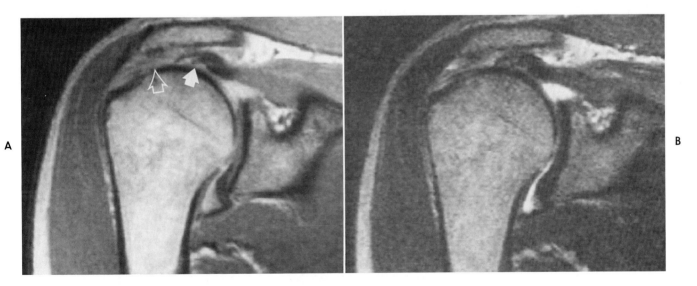

FIGURE 15-76
Full-thickness supraspinatus tear, right shoulder. **A,** Oblique coronal proton density (2100/30) image showing the torn and retracted tendon with an irregular margin *(solid arrow)*. The defect exhibits medium signal intensity *(hollow arrow)*. **B,** Same level, T2-weighted sequence (2100/80). The cuff defect remains low signal due to remnants of the degenerated tendon and scar tissue. The peribursal fat is obliterated in both sequences.

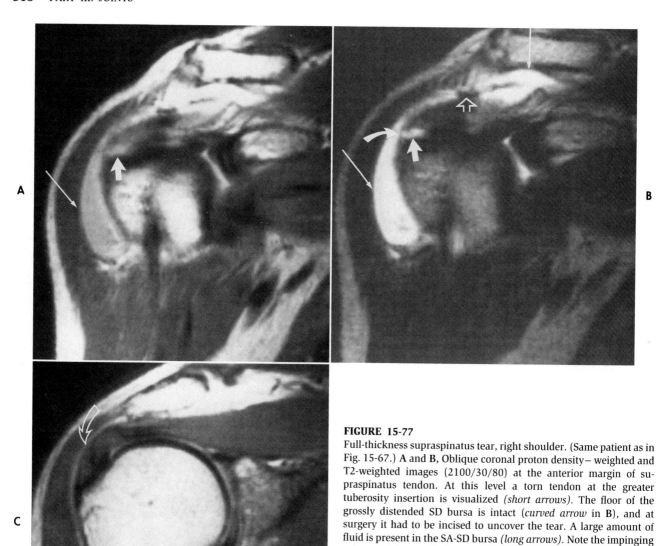

FIGURE 15-77

Full-thickness supraspinatus tear, right shoulder. (Same patient as in Fig. 15-67.) **A** and **B**, Oblique coronal proton density–weighted and T2-weighted images (2100/30/80) at the anterior margin of supraspinatus tendon. At this level a torn tendon at the greater tuberosity insertion is visualized *(short arrows)*. The floor of the grossly distended SD bursa is intact *(curved arrow* in **B**), and at surgery it had to be incised to uncover the tear. A large amount of fluid is present in the SA-SD bursa *(long arrows)*. Note the impinging subacromial spur *(hollow arrow* in **B**). **C**, Oblique coronal proton density–weighted (2100/30) image posterior to **A**, midsupraspinatus. There is marked thickening with heterogeneously increased signal intensity of the tendon *(arrow)* due to tendinitis or interstitial tendon tear in this region. (**B** reprinted with permission from Rafii M, et al: Radiology 1990;177:817-823.)

phy, which would be consistent with observations by Skinner[6] (in cadaver shoulders) of retracted supraspinatus tendons concealed by intact synovial and bursal surfaces.

Assessment of the torn cuff. There is considerable variation in the appearance of the remaining tendon and margins of the cuff defect. The retracted margin may be thickened as part of the attempted healing response.[7] In addition, traumatic tears demonstrate a more pronounced thickening (initially as a result of hemorrhage and edema and later due to the ensuing reparative process) (Fig. 15-78). Formation of a hematoma with characteristic high

signal on T1- and T2-weighted sequences is not seen unless an underlying bleeding disorder exists (Fig. 15-79). On the other hand, an attenuated margin indicates chronicity of the tear, with continued pinching of the tendon between the acromion and humeral head. The remaining tendon may be of normal morphology or signal intensity. More often, however, it will show various degrees of degeneration, partial thickness tear, or tendinitis (Fig. 15-80). An accurate display of the size and condition of the remaining tendon is an important attribute of MRI in surgical planning.

Distribution and size of cuff tears. An advantage of MRI

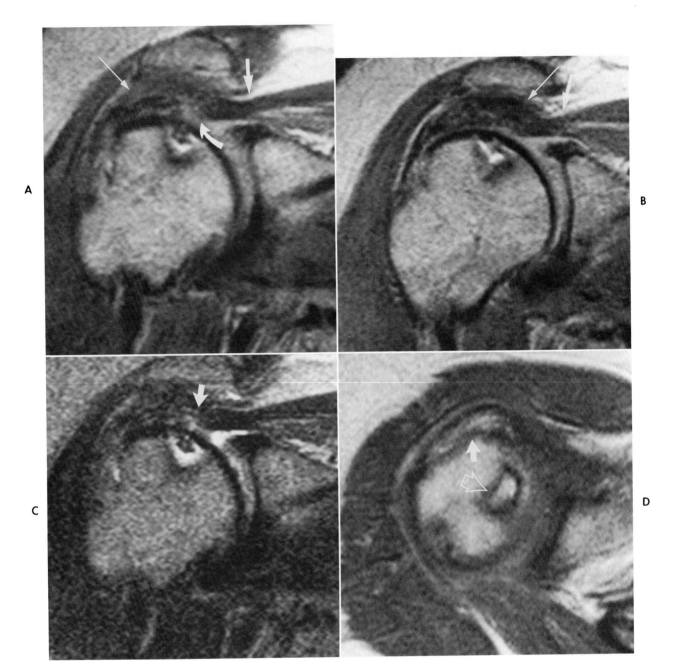

FIGURE 15-78
Subacute rupture of the supraspinatus tendon, right shoulder. Following trauma, a greater tuberosity fracture was detected several weeks prior to MRI. **A** and **B**, Adjacent oblique coronal proton density–weighted (2100/30) images (**A** anterior to **B**). Full-thickness tear of the tendon is manifested by a relatively abrupt change in the tendon's contour and signal intensity *(curved arrow)*. The ruptured tendon distal (**A**) and posterior to this region (**B**) is thickened and shows a heterogeneous signal change *(thin arrows)*. Complete rupture of the tendon is further indicated by the apparent retraction of the musculotendinous junction *(thick arrows)*. **C**, A T2-weighted image (2100/80) shows persistent increase in signal intensity and better delineation of the torn margin of the tendon *(arrow)*. An osteochondral fracture of the humeral head is also detected on all images. **D**, Axial T1-weighted image (700/30) at the superior aspect of the joint. The greater tuberosity fracture *(solid arrow)* and the osteochondral defect *(hollow arrow)* are visualized.

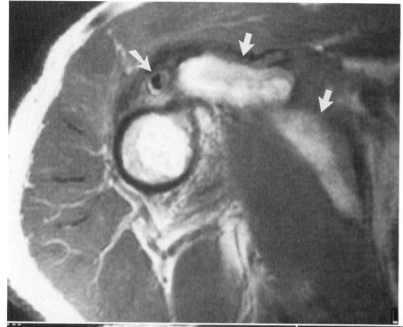

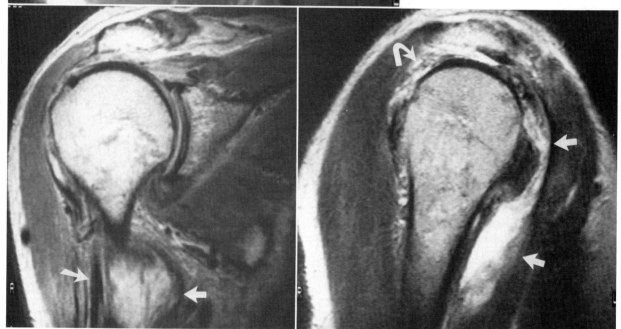

FIGURE 15-79
Traumatic rotator cuff tear, right shoulder, with large hematoma in a patient on anticoagulation therapy. **A,** Axial T1-weighted (600/30), **B,** oblique coronal proton density-weighted (2100/30), and **C,** oblique sagittal T2-weighted (1800/80) images of the right shoulder demonstrate a high-signal hematoma *(straight arrows)* extending in the anterior subdeltoid space and medial to the long head of the biceps tendon *(slanted arrows).* Note the presence of high-signal blood in the bicipital tendon sheath. The cuff tear is massive and includes the supraspinatus (**B** and **C**) and infraspinatus (*curved arrow* in **C**) tendons.

is its ability to demonstrate the exact location, the configuration, and extent of rotator cuff tears. Supraspinatus cuff defects are best seen on oblique coronal images, which show the medial and lateral extension of the tear. The anteroposterior dimension of the tear is visualized on oblique sagittal images. Tears of the subscapularis and posterior aspect of the cuff can be seen on both sagittal and axial sequences.

The distribution of cuff tears as depicted on MRI correlates closely with surgical and cadaveric observations.[37,39,129] By far, most involve the anterior component of the supraspinatus tendon (Figs. 15-72, 15-77, and 15-80). These tears are depicted either as a tendinous rent with retraction from the greater tuberosity or an involve-

ment of the critical zone with the remaining portion attached to the greater tuberosity. The cuff defect usually expands posteriorly and may eventually include the infraspinatus tendon. Less often the subscapularis tendon also is torn (Fig. 15-81). A subscapularis tendon tear with or without supraspinatus tendon tear may be observed in elderly persons following anterior dislocation of the glenohumeral joint (Fig. 15-57). A degenerative tear of the supraspinatus at the musculotendinous junction is unusual and often an indication of acute trauma (Fig. 15-82). The tear size on MRI is an accurate indicator of the actual size at surgery.[37] However, occasionally a discrepancy will be encountered and is usually due to underestimation of the extent of degeneration on MRI.

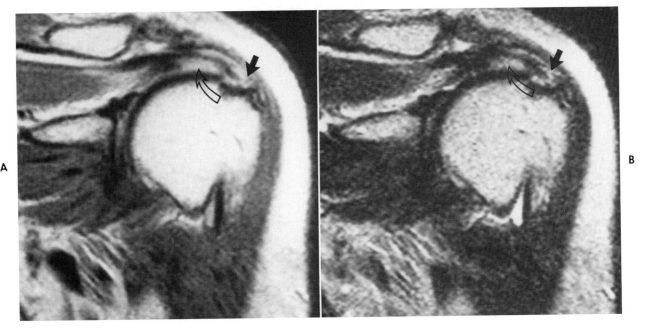

FIGURE 15-80
Full-thickness and partial-thickness tears, supraspinatus tendon, left shoulder. Oblique coronal, **A,** proton density–weighted and, **B,** T2-weighted (2100/30/80) images demonstrate a small full-thickness tear at the tuberosity insertion *(solid arrows)* and a large partial thickness tear of the synovial surface *(hollow arrows).*

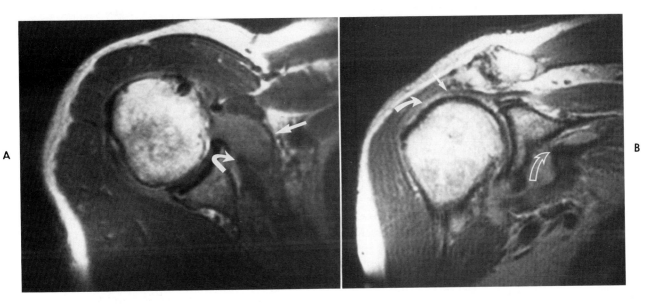

FIGURE 15-81
Supraspinatus and subscapularis cuff tear, right shoulder. **A,** Axial T1-weighted (600/29) image at the midglenohumeral joint. The torn and retracted subscapularis tendon is visualized medial to the glenoid margin *(curved arrow).* There is outward expansion of a distended capsule with effusion *(straight arrow).* **B,** Oblique coronal proton density–weighted (2100/30) image. A medium-sized tear of the supraspinatus tendon is visible *(curved arrow).* The supraspinatus is atrophied, with retraction of its musculotendinous junction. The torn margin is markedly attenuated *(straight arrow).* The retracted subscapularis tendon is seen medial to the glenoid *(hollow arrow).*

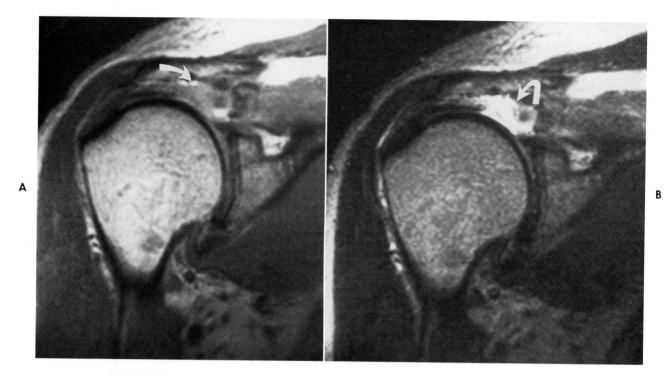

FIGURE 15-82
Traumatic tear of the supraspinatus musculotendinous junction, right shoulder. Oblique coronal proton density–weighted and T2-weighted (2100/30/80) images show a medium-sized tear of the musculotendinous junction *(arrows)*, with retraction of the supraspinatus muscle.

Conversely, a cuff tear may conceivably appear larger at arthroscopy because of the necessity for distention of the joint and traction on the arm during the procedure.

Partial-thickness tears. These are most accurately manifested by a region of intense signal on T2-weighted images. The specific pattern commonly seen is partial retraction of the anterior component of the supraspinatus tendon from the greater tuberosity (Fig. 15-83, *A*). This pattern correlates with the so-called "rim rent" described by Codman.[10] These insertion tears, even in later stages (Fig. 15-77), may skip detection by arthrography and/or surgery because of retained superficial tendon fibers at the synovial or bursal surfaces. Visualization is particularly difficult at arthroscopy.

Partial-thickness tears may also be manifested as focal or linear regions of increased but not intense signal on T1-weighted, proton density, and T2-weighted images. Among 16 surgically proven partial tears in our series, more than 50% lacked the specific finding of intense signal in the region of partial cuff tear. These included some superficial tears of either the inferior or the superior surface of the tendon or focal intratendinous tears. Superficial tears are seen as an irregularity or defect of the synovial or bursal surfaces (Fig. 15-83, *B* and *C*). Less advanced superficial tears are relatively shallow lesions and may be interpreted either as a partial-thickness tear or tendinous degeneration both on MRI and at gross inspection. Intratendinous tears may also be manifested as bands or focal regions of high or intense signal and communication with the superior or inferior surface may

be demonstrated (Fig. 15-83, *D*). Also shown by increased though not intense signal abnormality are interstitial tears of tendinous substance. These represent clefts or regions with torn or degenerated tendinous fibers infiltrated by connective tissue (Fig. 15-84). The correlative surgical data on these lesions are as yet scanty,[39] primarily because most are not surgically treated. In addition, interstitial and even small full-thickness tears may be overlooked at surgery.[100]

CALCIFIC TENDINITIS

The etiology of calcific tendinitis is unclear. A considered pathogenetic sequence includes initiation by mild trauma. The trauma produces slight injury with microtears of the poorly vascularized tendon, later followed by necrosis and then attempted healing.[7,10,110] This postulated format, however, does not solely involve the critical zone of the supraspinatus tendon, and does not usually coexist with cuff tears. Nevertheless, it has been suggested that the calcific foci may gradually resolve, leading to formation of a cuff defect at their site.[10] The pain associated with calcific tendinitis is due to the release of calcium particles, inducing an inflammatory reaction in the surrounding tendon and the subacromial bursa.

Although calcific deposits within the rotator cuff may be recognized easily on conventional radiography and computed tomography, they are not readily identifiable on MRI, due mainly to the fact that their signal void character simulates that of the host tendon. Only when

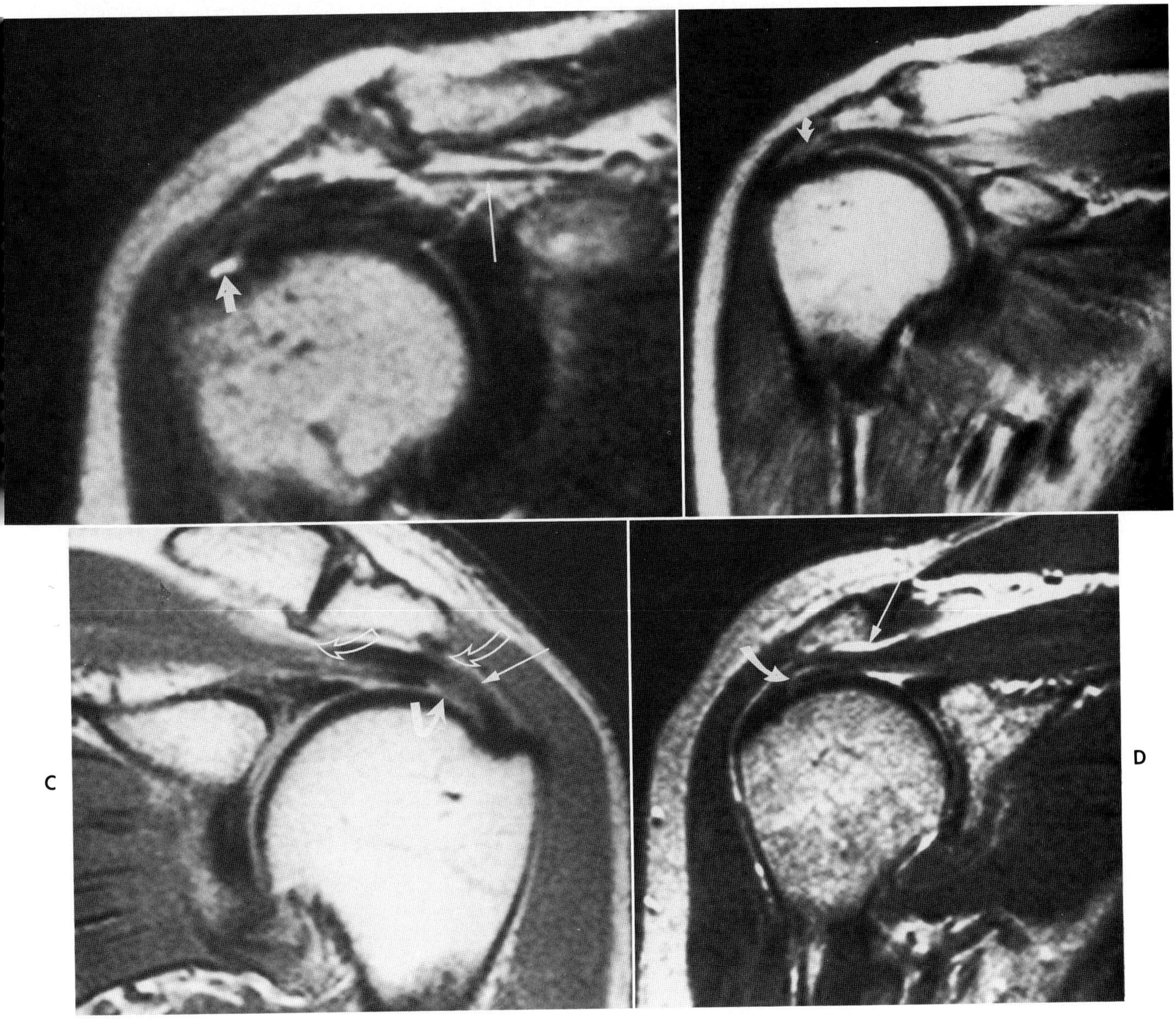

FIGURE 15-83

Supraspinatus partial-thickness tears. **A,** At the muscle insertion, right shoulder. An oblique coronal T2-weighted (2100/80) image at anterior aspect of the joint shows partial detachment of the tendon from the greater tuberosity *(short arrow)*. The bursal surface of the tendon (which itself demonstrates heterogeneous signal intensity) is obliterated due to bursitis. The coracoacromial ligament is visible *(long arrow)*. This tear was only retrospectively seen on arthrographic images, due to the confluence of positive contrast with cortical bone. **B,** At the bursal surface of the supraspinatus, right shoulder. An oblique coronal proton density (2100/30) image demonstrates a defect at the bursal surface of the tendon *(arrow)*. **C,** At the synovial surface of the supraspinatus tendon, left shoulder. Oblique coronal proton density (2100/30) image. A shallow defect of the inferior surface of the supraspinatus is visible *(solid curved arrow)*. Increased signal intensity of the remaining tendon is also visible in this region, indicative of tendon degeneration or tendinitis *(straight arrow)*, with impingement by the AC joint and acromial spurs *(hollow arrows)*. **D,** Intratendinous partial-thickness tear, right shoulder. Oblique coronal T2-weighted (2100/80) image. A longitudinal intratendinous tear is demonstrated, with markedly increased signal intensity *(curved arrow)*. There is a small amount of fluid in the subacromial bursa *(straight arrow)*. This tear was surgically exposed when the retained bursal surface was incised. The synovial surface was interrupted, allowing communication with the joint.

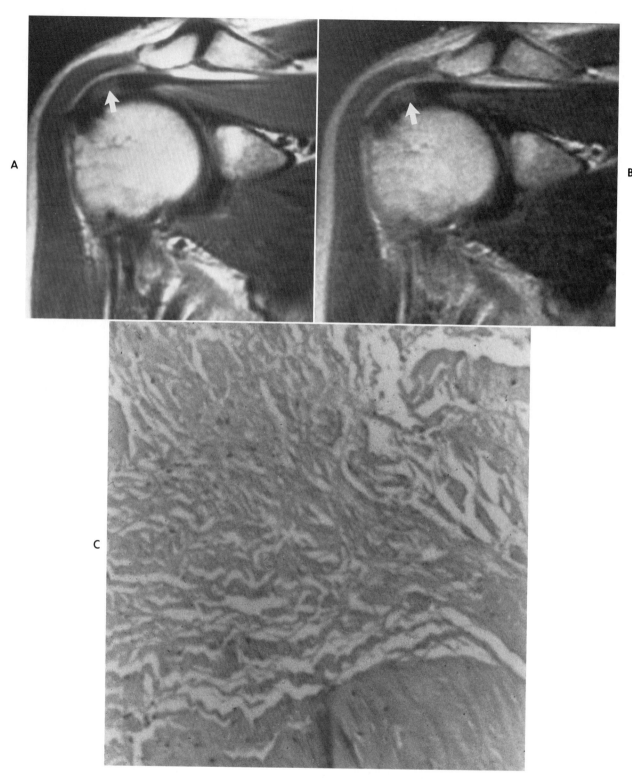

FIGURE 15-84
Interstitial partial-thickness supraspinatus tear, right shoulder. **A** and **B,** Oblique coronal proton density and T2-weighted (2100/80/30) images. There is a focal region of increased signal intensity extending to and including the synovial surface of the supraspinatus tendon *(arrows).* At surgery this region, which was exposed by incising the bursal surface, showed abnormal consistency and marked discoloration. It was debrided and repaired. **C,** Histological section of the abnormal tendon showing marked disorganization of the tendinous fibers and infiltration by loose connective tissue. (H & E; ×100.) (**A** to **C** reprinted with permission from Rafii M, et al: Radiology 1990;177:817-823.)

sizable or clearly outlined by the increased signal of the surrounding abnormal tendon are they suggested by MRI (Fig. 15-85). Otherwise, manifestations of tendinitis and bursitis may be the major findings. Due to the prevalence of calcific tendinitis in older persons, review of the patient's radiographs at the time of MR imaging is helpful for the appropriate interpretation of findings.

OSSEOUS AND ARTICULAR LESIONS IN THE IMPINGEMENT SYNDROME

A number of congenital and acquired osseous lesions can be associated with the impingement syndrome and rotator cuff disorders.

The contribution of the *coracoacromial arch* to rotator cuff impingement has been alluded to in preceding paragraphs. An anatomical variation of the arch (i.e., decreased slope of the acromion) is considered to play a role in producing impingement.[99] However, this finding has not been adequately investigated by imaging techniques. Orientation of the anterior acromion, on the other hand, has been evaluated relative to the incidence of cuff tears and impingement: an inferior orientation has increased incidence compared to a horizontal orientation in patients with a rotator cuff tear.[5,33,107,130] A low-lying acromion in relation to the distal end of the clavicle has been observed in patients with the impingement syndrome and MR manifestations of tendinitis[33] (Figs. 15-67 and 15-71, *B*). An anterior acromial spur or more

extensive proliferative changes of the undersurface of the acromion are seen as regions of low signal intensity, with the development of marrow fat, accordingly, showing high signal intensity.

Sclerosis of the *greater tuberosity,* an early finding in the impingement syndrome, is manifested by low signal alteration of the subcortical bone or proliferative changes of the cortical bone. In advanced stages the tuberosity will gradually reduce due to continuous impingement against the acromion (Fig. 15-73). The anatomical neck of the humerus becomes more pronounced (Fig. 15-71, *A*), and subcortical cysts (often with bright signal on T2-weighted images) are visualized.

An arthritic process of the *acromioclavicular joint,* with various degrees of soft tissue or osseous proliferation, is frequently observed and optimally visualized on both oblique coronal and oblique sagittal images (Figs. 15-71, *A,* 15-73, and 15-86). Impingement of the supraspinatus tendon or musculotendinous junction by spurs of the AC joint and acromion as demonstrated on MR images obtained with the arm at the side is less than with the arm in flexion and internal rotation or elevation and external rotation.

The secondary osseous changes described are not constant findings and are visualized mostly in later stages of the impingement syndrome, often with rotator cuff tears. Furthermore, acromioclavicular joint arthritis can be present independently, often as a result of direct injury to the joint. The diagnosis of rotator cuff tendinitis, bursitis, or cuff tears on MRI, therefore, should be established independent of the presence or absence of these osseous changes or actual impingement of the

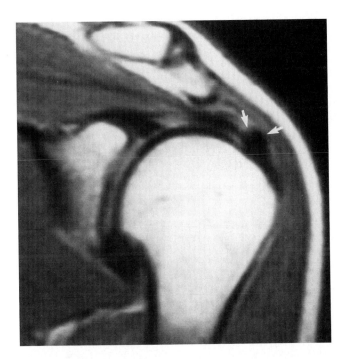

FIGURE 15-85
Calcific tendinitis, left shoulder. An oblique coronal proton density (1800/30) image shows the calcific deposit manifested by a globular signal void region near the tuberosity insertion of the supraspinatus tendon *(arrows).* It also reveals expansion into the subacromial bursal region and is demarcated proximally by increased signal within the tendon.

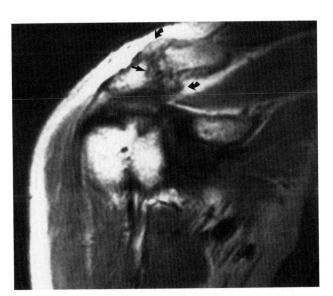

FIGURE 15-86
Posttraumatic acromioclavicular joint arthritis, right shoulder. Oblique coronal proton density (2100/30) image. There is irregularity of the articular surfaces of the AC joint *(straight arrow).* The joint cavity shows nonhomogeneous signal. Expansion of the capsule due to a proliferative process with impingement of the supraspinatus musculotendinous junction is also demonstrated *(curved arrows).*

supraspinatus apparatus demonstrated by MRI. However, visualization and accurate assessment of these osseous changes are important when surgical decompression of the subacromial space is contemplated.

Rotator cuff arthropathy. Abnormal alignment of the glenohumeral joint and elevation of the humeral head due to muscle imbalance are frequent findings with advanced and chronic cuff tears.[131] A pattern of degenerative joint disease referred to as "rotator cuff arthropathy" may then evolve, with the loss of articular cartilage, alteration of the articular surfaces, formation of osteophytes, and eventually advanced erosive process of all articular components[132] (Fig. 15-87). These changes are the result of upward migration of the humeral head or gross instability of the joint. Assessment of the glenohumeral joint is important in treating patients with rotator cuff tears; operative results are usually suboptimal after the onset of degenerative joint disease.[120]

CORACOACROMIAL LIGAMENT AND THE IMPINGEMENT SYNDROME

The coracoacromial ligament is visualized on oblique coronal or oblique sagittal images (Figs. 15-68 and 15-83, *A*). Thickening of this ligament is a frequent surgical observation in patients with clinical manifestations of the impingement syndrome. MR imaging does not help in evaluating the ligament's role in actual impingement of the rotator cuff, nor does it reliably detect its pathological alterations. Occasionally, inflammatory and proliferative process beneath and superficial to the ligament will be observed (Fig. 15-68).

DISORDERS OF THE LONG HEAD OF THE BICEPS TENDON

Congenital or acquired abnormalities of the bicipital groove may interfere with the function of the biceps tendon. A predisposition to displacement out of the groove may be due to the presence of a bony ridge at the proximal aspect of the groove or to abnormal obliquity of its medial wall.[7] Considerable variation exists in the degree of obliquity of the medial wall and may contribute to shoulder pain.[133] After 40 years of age, degenerative alterations of the long head of the biceps related to aging (thickening, fraying, and shredding) similar to those of the rotator cuff may be seen. Also bony ridges are frequently formed within the groove and interfere with the tendon's motion. The formation of adhesions and bony ridges may result in adherence of the tendon to the capsule or binding of the tendon to the groove and provides a new anchor for the tendon with a torn intraarticular segment. Progressive degeneration with complete tearing of the biceps tendon is usually an associated finding in cases of advanced impingement and rotator cuff tears. Acute traumatic rupture of the biceps tendon occurs in young individuals or as a result of vigorous physical activity.[98]

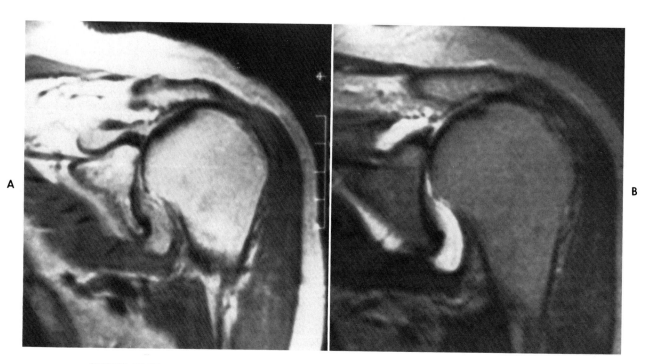

FIGURE 15-87
Rotator cuff arthropathy, left shoulder. A and B, Oblique coronal proton density and T2-weighted (2100/30/80) images in an elderly patient with a long-standing massive cuff tear and atrophy. There is superior migration of the humeral head, with remodeling of the undersurface of the acromion and osteochondral erosion of the humeral head. Note also flattening of the greater tuberosity, erosion of the glenoid articular cartilage, and joint effusion.

Bicipital tenosynovitis is uncommonly an isolated source of shoulder pain and is usually manifested on MRI with other components of subacromial impingement. Arthrographic findings, such as attenuation of the tendon, filling defects due to synovial villi, and elevation of the tendon from the groove or at its origin may be observed on MR imaging. Bicipital tenosynovitis may also be observed in earlier stages as an enlarged tendon exhibiting increased signal intensity with fluid accumulation in the bicipital tendon sheath (Fig. 15-88). It should be noted that a small amount of fluid within the tendon sheath is frequently seen on MR imaging and is considered normal. Degeneration of the long head of the biceps tendon is manifested as an attenuated tendon with irregular margins and increased signal intensity (Fig. 15-89). These findings are best demonstrated on oblique sagittal images. A complete tear and retraction of the tendon results in nonvisualization of the tendon and the groove. However, not infrequently the tendon will be anchored within the groove and be well visualized on axial images. Then dislocation or subluxation can occur with degeneration and tearing of the transverse humeral ligament, usually associated with rotator cuff tears (Fig. 15-90). An associated subscapularis tendon tear may cause the dislocated tendon to assume an intraarticular position (Fig. 15-91).

CT-arthrography is also effective in the detection of a torn or subluxated biceps tendon (Fig. 15-92). However, pathological changes of the intraarticular components of the biceps tendon long head are more effectively detected by MR imaging.

POSTOPERATIVE SHOULDER

Persistence or recurrence of shoulder pain or instability after a reconstructive or corrective surgical procedure may necessitate a diagnostic reevaluation. The choice of imaging modality, in part, depends upon the type of previous surgical procedure and the nature of the expected pathology. Conventional roentgenography and/or CT are helpful and may adequately demonstrate abnormal position or relocation of surgical pins and screws. When persistence or recurrence of soft tissue abnormality is suspected, CT arthrography and/or MRI should be considered.

Recurrent postoperative glenohumeral dislocation

The rate of recurrence of shoulder instability following reconstructive surgery has been reported[134] as varying from 1% to 8% depending upon the method of repair. Inadequate repair of the preexisting lesion or reinjury may lead to recurrence of instability after surgical reconstruction. Most often a Bankart lesion or excessive laxity of the capsule is found.[135,136] Other complications and the nature of the existing lesion may reflect the format of prior instability and the type of reconstructive procedure performed (Fig. 15-93). Tearing and shredding of the subscapularis tendon may be seen in failed bone block (Eden-Hybinette) and Bristow procedures.

These complications usually arise from faulty surgical techniques (e.g., a high position of the coracoid implant in Bristow procedure). In the modified Bristow the tip of the coracoid process, including its biceps and coracobra-

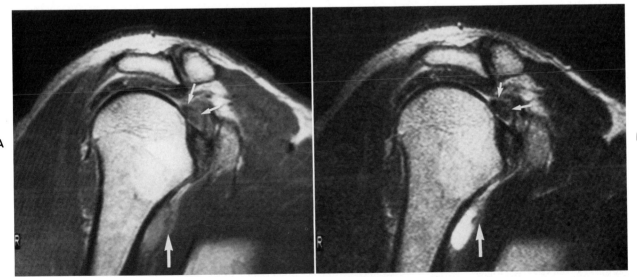

FIGURE 15-88
Tenosynovitis, long head of the biceps tendon, right shoulder. **A** and **B**, Oblique sagittal proton density–weighted and T2-weighted (1800/30/80) images at the level of the lesser tuberosity of the humeral head. The enlarged cross section of the long head of the biceps tendon, which also shows increased signal intensity, is demonstrated *(short arrows)*. Below the lesser tuberosity the medial expansion of the distended bicipital synovial tendon sheath, including low-signal synovial proliferative tissue can be seen *(long arrows)*.

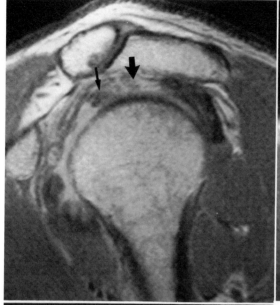

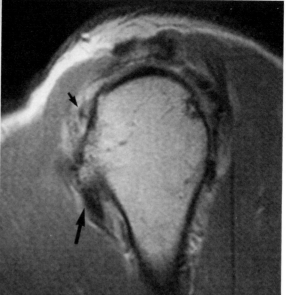

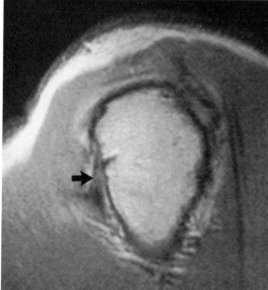

FIGURE 15-89

Degeneration and partial tear, long head of the biceps tendon, right shoulder. Oblique sagittal proton density–weighted (1800/30) MR images. **A,** At the level of the AC joint. The superior cuff is markedly degenerated and torn *(thick arrow)*. The proximal aspect of the long head of the biceps tendon shows increased signal intensity *(thin arrow)*. **B,** Lateral to A, at the level of the lesser tuberosity, bordering the bicipital groove. Above the tuberosity the degenerated (frayed) distal aspect of the intraarticular component of the tendon is visible *(small arrow)*. Below the groove the exiting tendon is of normal caliber and signal intensity *(large arrow)*. **C,** Lateral to **B,** at the level of the groove. The biceps tendon can be seen within the groove. The change in caliber of the tendon is demonstrated *(arrow)*. The tendon is probably anchored within the groove.

FIGURE 15-90

Subluxation of the long head of the biceps tendon, left shoulder. **A,** Axial T1-weighted image (600/30). The subluxated long head of the biceps is visualized *(curved arrow)* under a torn transverse ligament *(slanted arrow)*. Tearing, retraction, and atrophy of the subscapularis tendon *(straight arrows)* and a large effusion are observed. **B,** Oblique sagittal proton density–weighted (1800/30) image at the level of the lesser tuberosity. The biceps tendon is visualized extending over the lesser tuberosity *(arrow)*. Absence of the superior cuff tendons and superior migration of the humeral head is also observed.

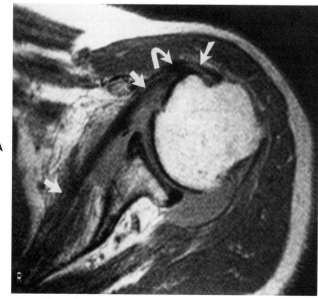

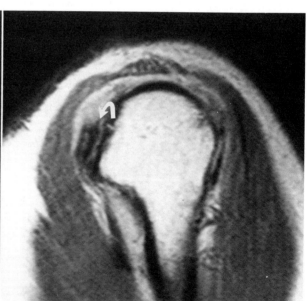

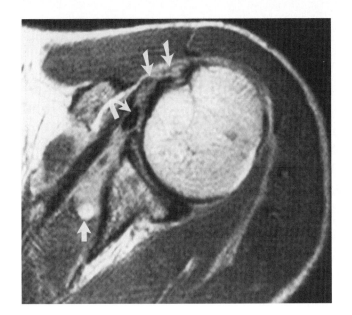

FIGURE 15-91

Dislocated biceps tendon, left shoulder. Axial proton density (1800/30) image. The long head of the biceps tendon *(curved arrow)* is displaced out of the bicipital groove and into the glenohumeral joint through the torn transverse ligament and subscapularis tendon *(slanted arrows)*. A high-signal loose body is visible in the distended subscapularis bursa *(straight arrow)*.

FIGURE 15-92

Subluxation and degenerative tear, long head of biceps tendon, two cases. **A,** Case 1. CT-arthrogram of the left shoulder at the midglenoid level. In this patient with adhesive capsulitis, the biceps tendon is displaced medially over the lesser tuberosity *(straight arrow)*. The empty tendon sheath is visualized within the bicipital groove *(curved arrow)*. **B** to **D,** Case 2. CT-arthrogram of the right shoulder in a patient with a massive cuff tear. (**B,** At the level of the superior glenoid the labrum is hypertrophied and irregular [*thick arrow*]. The insertion of the biceps tendon is not visualized. **C,** Below the coracoid process an irregular biceps tendon is seen anterior to the humeral head [*thick arrow*]. The tendon remains in this position and at the inferior aspect of the joint [**D**] is visualized out of the bicipital groove [*thick arrow*].) The SA-SD bursa is opacified in all images *(thin small arrows)*, and the torn margins of the supraspinatus *(slanted arrow in **A**)* and infraspinatus *(slanted arrow in **B**)* are visualized. The bony density in **C** *(slanted arrow)* is due to an old avulsion injury.

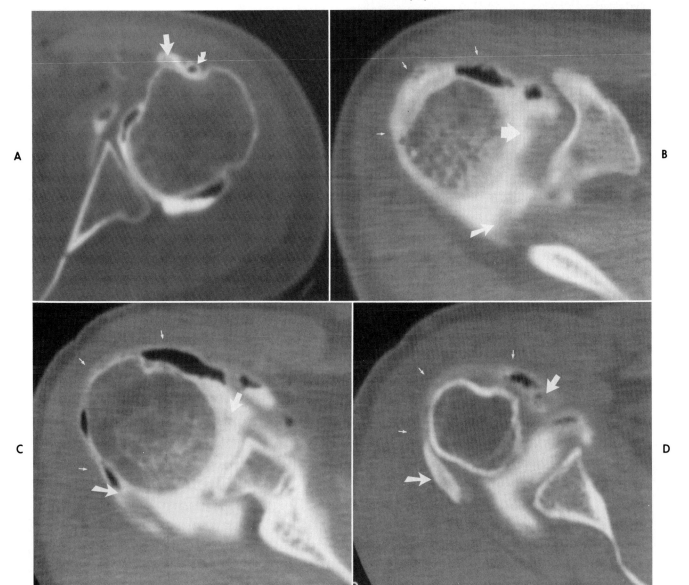

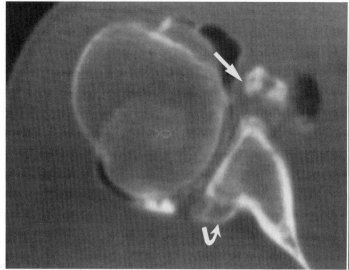

A

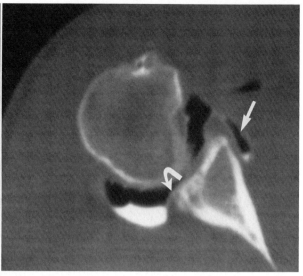

B

FIGURE 15-93

Postoperative Bristow reconstruction for anterior shoulder instability 8 years prior to the study. One year after surgery the fixating screw was removed due to pain. The graft was found to be stable at surgery, but the patient continued to have pain. CT-arthrographic images. **A,** At the midglenoid level the coracoid implant *(straight arrow)* shows no bony union with the glenoid. There is a prominent posterior capsular ossification *(curved arrow)*. **B,** Further inferiorly the anterior capsular reflection and the capsular space are normal *(straight arrow)*. Posteriorly a labral tear and detachment *(curved arrow)* are visualized. Both **A** and **B** show degenerative attenuation of the posterior glenoid articular cartilage. Despite a nonunited coracoid implant, CT-arthrographic findings indicate posterior instability as the cause of this patient's continuing symptoms. This was clinically confirmed.

FIGURE 15-94

Failed Bristow procedure, right shoulder. A loosened screw was suspected on roentgenograms. Consecutive CT-arthrographic images demonstrate the nonunited transplanted coracoid process *(straight arrows* in **A, B,** and **C**) displaced away from the glenoid margin, resulting in incongruity of the joint *(slanted arrows* in **A** and **C**). Loosening and backtracking of the screw are best visualized by the hollow and enlarged track within the glenoid *(curved arrow* in **C**). Incongruity of the glenoid has resulted in erosion of the anterior aspect of the humeral head *(hollow arrows* in **B** and **C**).

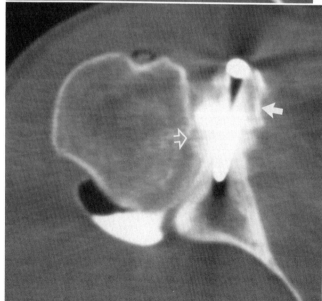

A

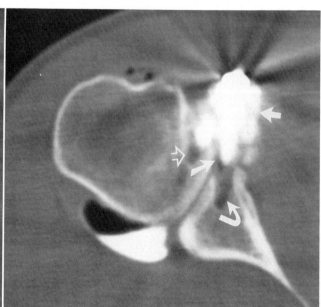

B

C

chialis tendon insertion, is transferred to the anterior glenoid margin. This fragment of bone may not properly heal (Fig. 15-94). Occasionally the metallic screw used for fixation of this fragment will protrude into the joint. It may also extend into the posterior soft tissue elements through the scapular cortex, disturbing the function of the posterior rotator cuff elements and resulting in tendinitis. Furthermore, screws used in the modified Bristow procedure can cause pain, restriction of motion, and erosion of the humeral articular surface when they are placed too close to the edge of the glenoid. Occasionally, loosening and backing out of the screw is observed, causing pain in the surrounding soft tissues[137] (Fig. 15-94). The exact position of such hardware about the shoulder can be investigated by CT when this determination is impossible by conventional roentgenography.[138] However, distortion of MR images by a metal artifact precludes the use of MRI for this purpose (Fig. 16-8). Other than in the immediate vicinity of the screw, the articular and periarticular soft tissue elements are adequately visualized on MRI.

After successful treatment of anterior instability a posterior subluxation may develop (Fig. 15-93), stemming from either progression of a previously unrecognized or development of a new posterior lesion.[134] Overcorrection of the anterior aspect of the joint immedi-ately following surgery is manifested by tightness and limitation of the joint (Fig. 15-95). Excessive tightening of the capsule can result in fixed posterior subluxation, which even when mild may lead to degenerative arthritis (Fig. 15-96).

In evaluation of the glenohumeral joint following arthroscopic surgery of the glenoid labrum the surgically altered anatomy should be recognized. Absence of the glenoid labrum in this setting cannot be considered pathological, and capsular abnormalities such as laxity or stripping from the glenoid should be sought in the search for instability. These changes are perhaps best evaluated by CT-arthrography.

Postoperative subacromial decompression and rotator cuff repair

After anterior acromioplasty with or without rotator cuff repair, persistence of symptoms may be due to reinjury of the cuff, inadequate decompression of the subacromial space, or improper repair of the cuff tear. Some difficulty exists in evaluation of the rotator cuff by MRI following a cuff repair due to scar tissue formation and signal alterations at the surgical site (Fig. 15-97). The confusion arises mostly in recognizing small tears. Larger defects with retraction of the tendinous margin are more readily recognized. However, persistence of small cuff

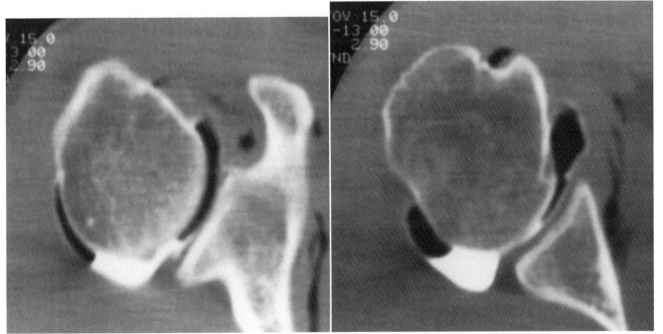

A   B

FIGURE 15-95
Overcorrected capsular shift procedure. Following surgery for anterior instability of right shoulder, this patient presented with limitation of motion. CT-arthrograms, **A,** at the superior and, **B,** at the midaspect of the joint demonstrate characteristic shortening of the anterior joint capsule and loss of the capsular space along the glenoid and peripheral aspect of the labrum. Slight malalignment of the glenohumeral joint and posterior shift of the humeral head are present. A capsular release procedure was subsequently performed.

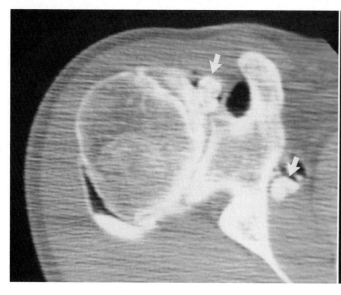
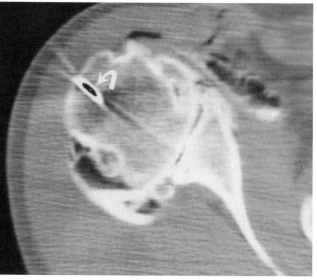

FIGURE 15-96

Degenerative arthritis 15 years following a Magnuson-Stack procedure for anterior instability, right shoulder. In this procedure the subscapularis tendon is separated from the lesser tuberosity and reimplanted over the greater tuberosity. CT-arthrographic images at the superior, **A**, and middle, **B**, aspects of the glenohumeral joint demonstrate posterior shift and flattening of the humeral head and deformity of the posterior glenoid margin. Note the marked irregularity of the posterior capsulolabral complex, osteophytes of the anterior joint margin, and multiple loose bodies *(straight arrows)*. The metallic pin, part of a surgical staple, designates the site of tendon implantation *(curved arrow in* **B***)*.

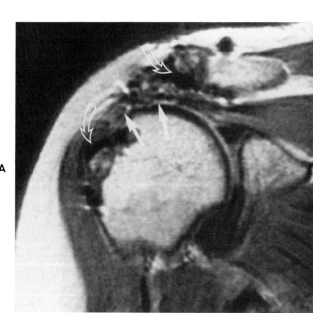
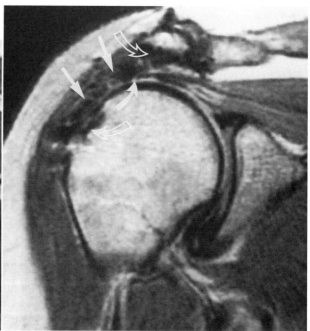

FIGURE 15-97

Postoperative acromioplasty and rotator cuff repair, right shoulder. Due to sustained injury and pain several months following an uneventful surgical procedure, MR examination was performed. Oblique coronal proton density (2100/30) images at the anterior aspect of the glenohumeral joint show the site of the repaired supraspinatus tendon manifested by markedly nonhomogeneous low signal intensity *(straight arrows)*. The peribursal fat signal is absent. Although some bright signal *(curved solid arrow,* **A***)* suggests interruption of the tendon, a tendon defect is not visualized. The presumed linear tear in this region may be a residual lesion or, conceivably, a new tear. The patient responded to conservative treatment. There is foreshortening of the acromion due to surgical resection and irregularity of the greater tuberosity, the site of tendon reattachment *(curved hollow arrows)*. Micrometallic artifacts are also evident.

defects without retraction of the tendinous margin or musculotendinous junction may not be incompatible with good surgical results. An arthrographic study of a group of patients following successful cuff repair[139] showed many such patients with persistent leakage of contrast through the cuff.

The acromion process (anterior margin and undersurface) and AC joint must be scrutinized to determine whether an accurate and adequate acromioplasty has been performed. Alterations in the normal anatomical landmarks on MRI do not necessarily indicate a pathological process. The most significant of these is obliteration of the normal peribursal fat. However, formation of excessive scar tissue and persistence of inflammation are abnormal (Fig. 15-98). Micrometallic artifacts on MRI following anterior acromioplasty (arthroscopic or open) or AC joint resection may be seen and, when present, are due *only* to the release of tiny metallic particles from the surgical instrument used for shaving bony spurs. Usually these are not radiographically visualized.

OTHER LOCAL AND SYSTEMIC DISORDERS OF THE SHOULDER
Trauma

Fracture-dislocations about the shoulder are routinely assessed by conventional roentgenography.[140] Assessment of reduction and healing is also adequately done with roentgenograms, although when the patient has a displaced fracture of the proximal humerus, roentgeno-grams alone may not demonstrate it sufficiently to permit realignment. The extent of displacement or angulation of the fragment and the degree of comminution, important factors in treatment planning and especially in selecting cases for surgical intervention,[141] are best evaluated by CT scanning.[142] Similarly, a displaced fracture of the greater tuberosity can best be assessed with CT for the possible need of surgical reduction. Also a lesser tuberosity avulsion fracture (not as common an injury) requires an axillary projection, and for this a CT scan optimally confirms the presence and demonstrates the extent of the fracture (Fig. 15-99).

The role of CT in evaluating a scapular fracture is somewhat different. This type of fracture is often not well visualized by conventional radiography, and thus CT scanning is needed for evaluation of its extent (with possible involvement of the glenoid fossa) and degree of comminution (Fig. 15-100). A displaced fracture of the scapula near the glenoid fossa and coracoid process may require surgical reduction, and detailed visualization is necessary for this (Fig. 15-101). Of particular importance, evaluation of an osteochondral fracture of the humeral head and glenoid articular surface (usually resulting from an impaction injury) requires CT-arthrography for detailed visualization of the articular abnormality (Figs. 15-102 and 15-103).

The role of CT scanning in evaluation of an acute glenohumeral dislocation is limited. However, occasionally a posterior dislocation, acute or chronic, will require

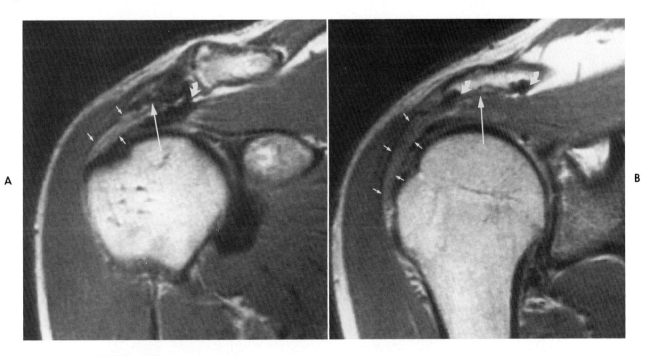

FIGURE 15-98
Postoperative arthroscopic subacromial decompression, right shoulder. Oblique coronal proton-density (2100/30) MR images at the anterior, **A**, and middle, **B**, aspects of the glenohumeral joint show irregularity and slight concavity of the acromion cortex (*long arrows*) as a result of bone debridement. The peribursal fat is somewhat expanded and replaced by a lower-signal tissue (*small arrows*), which remains low signal on T2-weighted images (not shown), indicative of fibrosis and scar tissue formation. Micrometallic artifacts are visualized (*curved arrows*).

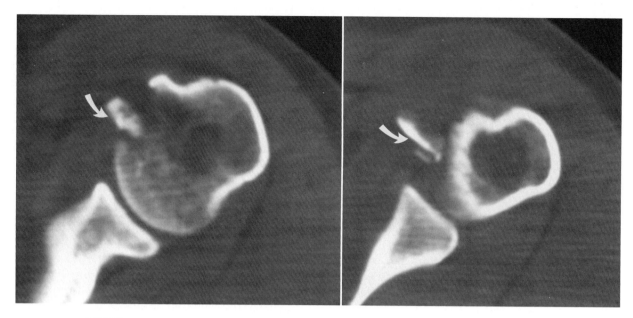

FIGURE 15-99
Avulsion fracture of the lesser tuberosity, left humerus. CT images at the inferior glenohumeral joint level show avulsion of the lesser tuberosity with displacement of the fracture fragment *(arrows)*.

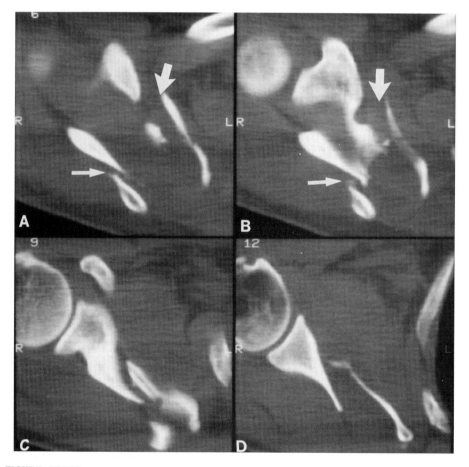

FIGURE 15-100
Scapular fracture. CT images demonstrate a vertical fracture extending from the superior scapular margin *(thick arrows)* and scapular spine *(thin arrows)* through the blade of the scapula. Overriding of the fracture fragments is also shown.

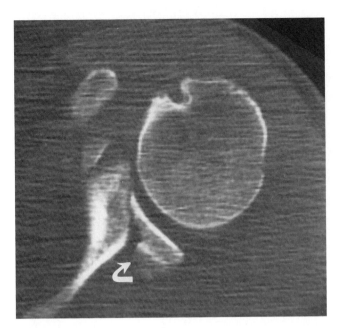

FIGURE 15-101
Comminuted and displaced glenoid fracture, left scapula. This CT image demonstrates marked displacement of a largely intact glenoid articular surface *(arrow)*. The fracture therefore is readily reducible.

CT for confirmation and evaluation. Following reduction of an anterior dislocation, the presence and severity of a Hill-Sachs or Bankart fracture are visualized by both CT and MRI. With an anterior glenohumeral instability, recurrent dislocation or subluxation is visualized, including deformity of the anterior glenoid margin, ectopic calcification at the site of anterior capsular insertion, and a Hill-Sachs compression fracture of the humeral head. With a posterior dislocation, impaction or a vertical linear compression of the humeral head may be seen as well as ectopic ossification along the posterior glenoid margin (pp. 488, 491, and 501).

Although MRI has no primary role in the investigation of a fracture-dislocation of the glenohumeral joint, a fracture in the vicinity of the humeral head, glenoid fossa, and AC joint is optimally visualized. The multiplanar capability of MR provides an advantage over CT in evaluating fragment displacement without requiring reformation. A nondisplaced fracture is also likely better visualized on MRI by virtue of the change in marrow signal intensity. Bone contusions are exclusively demonstrated by MR imaging. The greatest advantage of MR imaging with shoulder trauma, however, is in the assessment of associated ligament or muscle tears (Fig. 15-104). Follow-up examinations are helpful in the evaluation of healing and detection of sequelae.

Healing fractures. On CT a healing fracture is manifested by the formation of ossified callus bridging the fracture lines. CT scanning with multiplanar reformation is useful for detecting nonunion, when suspected. Fracture union can also be demonstrated by MR imaging.

Although the calcified callus is not specifically shown by an MR signal change, persistence of a low-signal

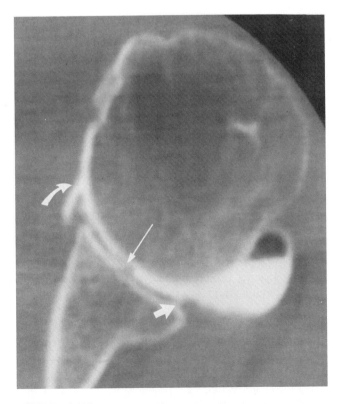

FIGURE 15-102
Glenoid osteochondral fracture, left shoulder. This CT-arthrogram shows a focal osteochondral fracture of the glenoid *(long arrow)*. A posterior labral tear *(short arrow)* with adhesive capsulitis of the anterior capsule (manifested by diminished capsular space, *curved arrow*) is also demonstrated. This patient had a history of prior trauma and persistent pain.

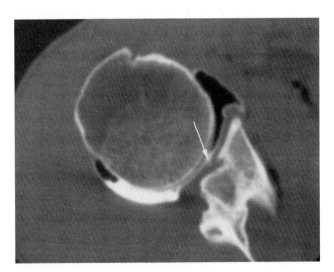

FIGURE 15-103
Posttraumatic glenoid deformity, right shoulder. This CT-arthrogram shows only a slight residual cartilage defect *(arrow)* at the site of an old depressed glenoid fossa fracture.

FIGURE 15-104
Nondisplaced greater tuberosity fracture and partial rotator cuff tear. **A,** Axial T1-weighted (600/30) MR image. The fracture is manifested as a low-signal band *(arrows)* with decreased bone marrow signal in the tuberosity. **B,** An oblique coronal, proton density (2100/30) image at the anterior glenohumeral joint shows, in addition to the nondisplaced greater tuberosity fracture *(straight arrow),* a partial tear of the supraspinatus tendon *(curved arrow).* Persistence of symptoms in this young person several weeks later was better explained by the partial tear of the rotator cuff.

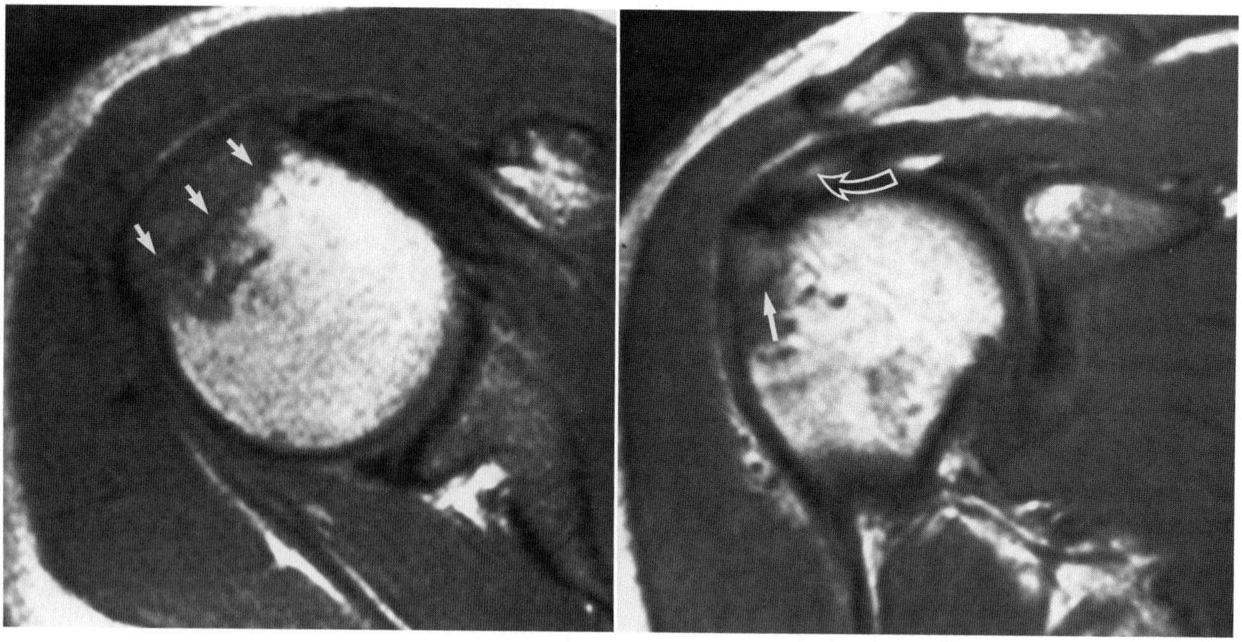

interface at the fracture site is suggestive of callus formation and early bony union. With complete remodeling at the fracture site medullary elements of the fracture fragments are revealed by the high signal intensity of bone marrow. Nonunion is manifested by medium- or low-signal tissue at the fracture site and persistence of a similar signal on T2-weighted sequences, indicating the presence of soft tissue elements. In this respect there is difficulty differentiating between old dense fibrous tissue and calcified osteoid tissue, both of which demonstrate low signal intensity on these sequences (Fig. 15-105). With pseudoarthrosis the medium signal intensity of fibrocartilage is well shown on T1- and T2-weighted sequences.

Tumors

Except for myeloproliferative disorders, primary tumors of bone are relatively uncommon in the shoulder region. Nevertheless, with varying frequency, benign or malignant bone tumors may involve the immediate vicinity of the glenohumeral joint, and for these conventional roentgenography is the primary modality. CT and MRI play complementary roles, mainly due to their greater sensitivity in depicting marrow and extraosseous extension. The multiplanar capability of MRI makes it especially useful with tumors of the shoulder girdle (Fig. 15-106). Of particular importance is the delineation of tumor extension through the articular components as well as involvement of the neurovascular bundle (Fig.

15-107). On the other hand, certain early tumor characteristics (calcified matrix, cortical erosion) are better demonstrated by CT. Periosteal elevation is also better shown by CT.

Both CT scanning and MRI play significant roles in the evaluation of soft tissue tumors. Although the nature and biological behavior of these lesions cannot be definitively demonstrated, the aggressive nature of some is revealed by an accurate portrayal of their margins (MRI providing a more detailed visualization than CT). However, in certain instances active tumor cannot be differentiated from necrotic tissue or surrounding edema using either modality. Also the signal intensity of a lesion on MRI and the attenuation coefficient on CT are relatively nonspecific as regards tumor histology. An exception is fatty tumors, which frequently occur in the shoulder girdle (Fig. 15-108).

Malignant lesions in the vicinity of the shoulder are frequently metastatic deposits, and CT scanning is specifically helpful when one of these is suspected and roentgenograms are nondiagnostic (Fig. 15-109). MR imaging is more helpful in evaluating the extent of a known lesion or determining marrow involvement. (See Chapter 12.)

Arthritides

Although the glenohumeral joint is frequently affected by inflammatory arthritides, its involvement is seldom isolated. Usually the diagnosis of a specific arthritis (e.g.,

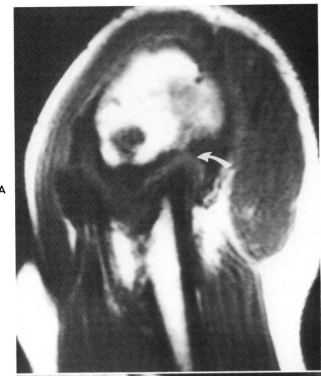

A

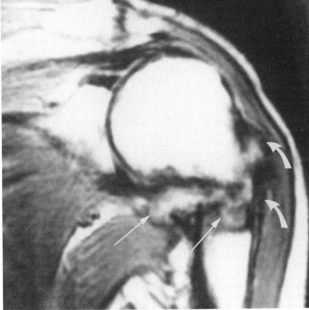

B

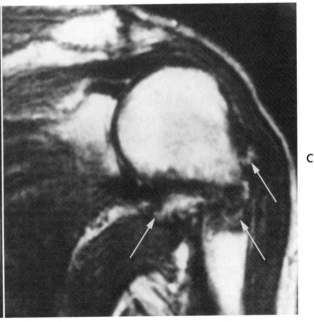

C

FIGURE 15-105

Fracture nonunion, surgial neck of the left humerus. **A,** An oblique sagittal T1-weighted (650/20) MR image demonstrates medium-signal tissue separating the humeral head and shaft segments *(curved arrow).* The signal-void bony margins indicate sclerosis of long duration. Findings suggest nonunion. **B** and **C,** Oblique coronal proton density and T2-weighted (2000/30/80) images showing marked angulation at the fracture site. Again no osseous continuity is present. A peripheral band of low signal extending between the two segments *(curved arrows,* **B**) is probably fibrous tissue. The fracture region is surrounded by high-intensity fluid (or granulation tissue), another indication of motion at the fracture site *(long arrows* in **B** and **C**).

rheumatoid) has been established by the clinical and laboratory data and by roentgenographic findings in various other joints. Nevertheless, the onset of disease in the glenohumeral joint may be insidious and its presence and extent difficult to determine by clinical and roentgenographic means. In more advanced cases the extent of synovial proliferation, the presence of articular cartilaginous or bony erosion, and the likelihood of associated deterioration in the surrounding musculotendinous structures may have to be evaluated; and for these MRI is the preferred modality.[143,144]

A synovial proliferative process (pannus) is manifested on MRI by low signal on T1-weighted and low or high signal on T2-weighted images.[143] This variation in signal on the latter sequences probably reflects acute and chronic phases of inflammation.[145] It may also be due to hemosiderin deposits within the hypertrophied synovium.[144] Although pannus and joint effusion show similar signal intensities on T2-weighted imaging sequences, with extreme T2-weighting pannus reveals a lower signal than effusion.[143]

Erosion of the hyaline articular cartilage appears as focal or generalized thinning; that of bone as defects at the surface of the articular cortex. Subcortical cysts are manifested as low signal on T1-weighted and low or high signal on T2-weighted imaging.

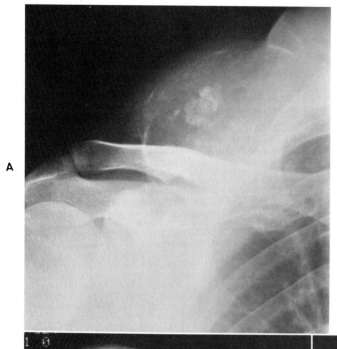

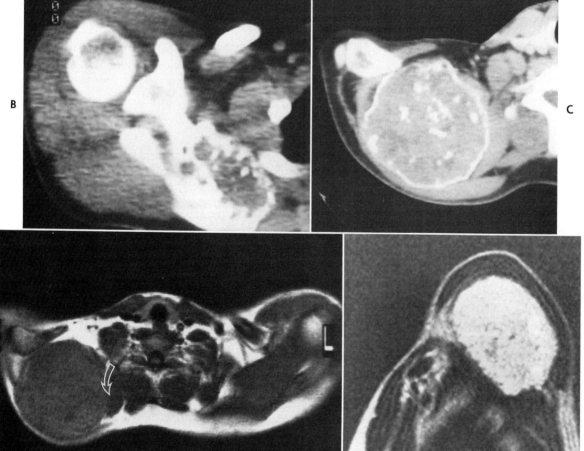

FIGURE 15-106

Chondrosarcoma, right scapula. **A,** An AP roentgenogram shows a mass with characteristic calcifications of a cartilaginous-type tumor arising from the right scapula. **B** and **C** are CT images. The lesion orginates from the superior aspect of the scapula **(B).** Its characteristic calcifications are well shown in the periphery and within the lesion. Although it is mostly well delineated, chest wall involvement could not be entirely excluded based on this study. **D,** An axial T1-weighted (500/29) MR image shows the lesion's nonhomogeneously low signal character. With this pulse sequence the interface between the lesion and skeletal muscle is indistinct *(arrow).* **E,** Sagittal T2-weighted (1800/80) image. Note the background of intense signal with irregular punctate low-signal foci, indicative of the calcified matrix. The boundary of the lesion is optimally visualized and well demarcated. In particular, the chest wall is cleared of tumor invasion.

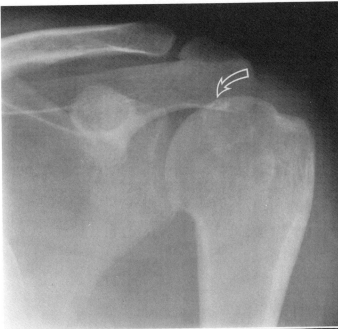

A

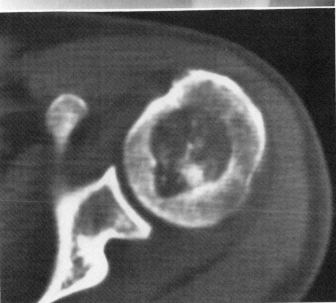

B

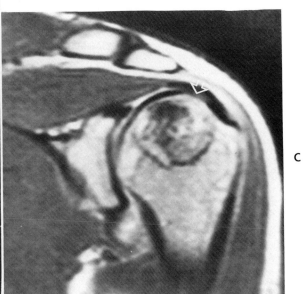

C

FIGURE 15-107
Chondroblastoma, left humeral head. **A,** An AP roentgenogram of the left shoulder shows the partly calcified lesion extending to the superior articular surface *(arrow)*. Its roentgenographic features are indicative of chondroblastoma. The exact size of the lesion and, more important, the integrity of the articular surface are not well demonstrated. **B,** CT optimally demonstrates the boundary of the lesion and its calcified matrix. **C,** An oblique coronal proton density (1600/30) MR image showing focal erosion of the articular cortex *(arrow)*. There is no extension of tumor beyond the articular surface. The boundary of the lesion *(arrow)* is also well demonstrated.

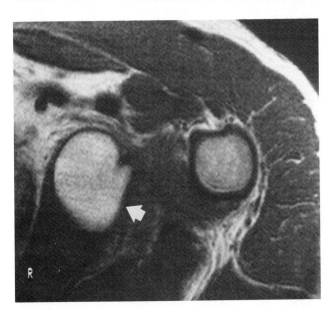

FIGURE 15-108
Benign intramuscular (subscapularis) lipoma, left shoulder, T1-weighted (900/30) MR image. This lesion *(arrow)* was an incidental finding in a patient being evaluated for rotator cuff pathology.

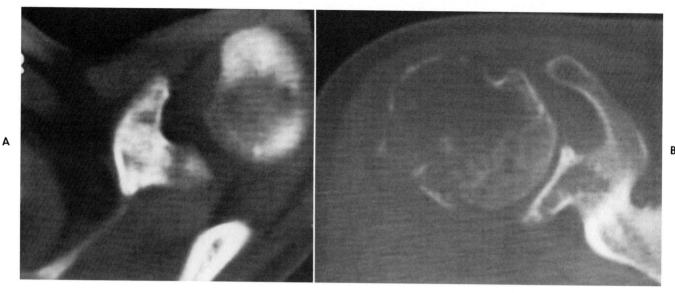

FIGURE 15-109
Metastatic lesions. **A,** Adenocarcinoma of the adrenal gland. A CT image demonstrates the mixed blastic character of this lesion in the coracoid process. It was one of two skeletal metastases detected by bone scan in this patient. Roentgenograms were not diagnostic. **B,** Metastatic hypernephroma. In this patient CT was performed to evaluate the extent of the lesion, originally detected by roentgenography.

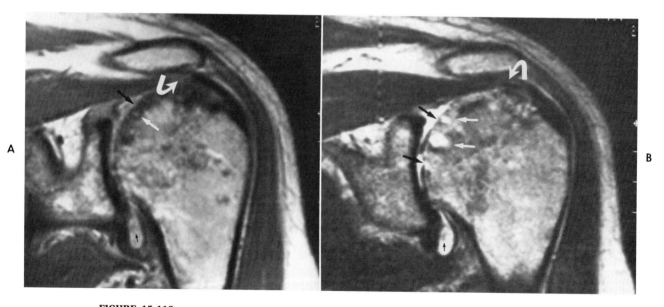

FIGURE 15-110
Calcium pyrophosphate arthropathy, left glenohumeral joint, in a patient with established pseudogout evaluated for cuff pathology due to persistent pain after a fall. Oblique coronal proton density–weighted and T2-weighted (2100/20/80) images. There is marked erosion of the humeral head articular surface *(large black arrows)* with subarticular cyst formation *(straight white arrows).* The glenoid fossa also shows cartilage loss. Note the joint effusion in the axillary pouch with low-signal tissue, most likely of synovial origin *(small black arrows).* An intense cuff defect is not visualized, but irregularity and thinning in central aspect of the tendon are due to partial tear or degeneration *(curved arrows).*

Other inflammatory arthritides, including calcium pyrophophate deposition (CPPD) disease, have not been extensively studied by MR imaging, but findings are not expected to be significantly different from those described above (Fig. 15-110). Calcium deposition in the hyaline articular cartilage or on synovial surfaces with CPPD disease may be visualized as linear low-signal bands on MRI (though they are best visualized by CT scanning).

Osteoarthritis. Osteoarthritis of the glenohumeral joint is relatively uncommon. However, an idiopathic or degenerative form exists in which loss of the articular cartilage, bony sclerosis, and osteophytes become apparent (Fig. 15-111). Similar changes may be observed secondary to a variety of underlying disorders, including CPPD disease, gout, ochronosis, acromegaly, and trauma.[146]

The association of rotator cuff tears with degenerative arthritis of the glenohumeral joint has been variably recorded. Some investigators[147] consider a full-thickness cuff tear to be a significant contributing factor, due primarily to leakage of joint fluid through the defect and the consequent reduced perfusion of nutrients through the cartilage. This concept has been disputed by others,[32] who report surgically verified advanced cases of degenerative arthritis of the glenohumeral joint without a full-thickness cuff tear. Neer et al.[132] described one type, resulting from advanced tears of the rotator cuff (the so-called "cuff arthropathy"), in which relatively rapid progression, with collapse of the humeral head, was related to the ensuing instability and superior migration of the humeral head (Fig. 15-87).

Degenerative disease of the glenohumeral joint is often asymptomatic or only mildly symptomatic even when considerable joint abnormality is discovered on radiographic studies. In persons who have symptoms the most important piece of information needed following the discovery of an arthritic process at conventional roentgenography is whether there is indeed pathology of the cuff present and, if so, its nature (Fig. 15-112). For this, MR imaging is the modality of choice.

Acromioclavicular joint arthritis. Degenerative disease of the AC joint is a frequent finding, but not necessarily the symptomatic focus, at routine radiography of the painful shoulder.[148] The AC joint is often involved in inflammatory arthritides, and pathological changes similar to those of the glenohumeral joint may be present and visualized by MR imaging. However, although it has been suggested that the sensitivity of conventional roentgenography in depicting AC joint erosion is greater than that of MR imaging,[143] this has not been substantiated by other studies. In our experience high-resolution MR imaging has generally been very accurate in the detection of articular erosion. Furthermore, various manifestations of AC joint derangement (loss of the articular disk, disruption of the capsular ligaments, the presence of inflammatory synovial reaction) are best detected by MR imaging (Fig. 15-113), which therefore is the most sensitive and discriminating technique for recognizing "symptomatic" AC joint disease.

Paraarticular synovial cysts. Synovial cysts in the vicinity of the glenohumeral and AC joints are formed in association with degenerative or inflammatory arthritides, as a result of capsular disruption and deterioration with disruption of the rotator cuff tendons. These cysts may assume considerable proportions, and their extent and site of origin are best determined by MRI (Fig. 15-114). Small synovial (ganglion) cysts are also observed, characteristically at the posterosuperior aspect of the glenoid (Fig. 15-115).

Infection. Infections within or surrounding the shoulder joint are optimally evaluated by MR imaging. The role

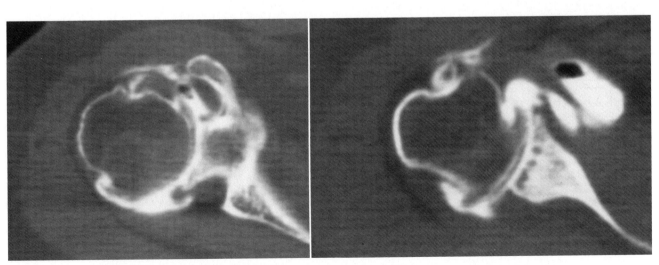

A   B

FIGURE 15-111
Glenohumeral osteoarthritis, right shoulder. CT-arthrographic images, **A,** at the level of the coracoid process and, **B,** at the midglenoid level. Large osteophytes of the humeral head, subcortical cysts of the glenoid fossa, and irregular loss of the articular cartilage are all visible. The posterior labrum in **A** is prominent and irregular, with posterior shifting of the humeral head.

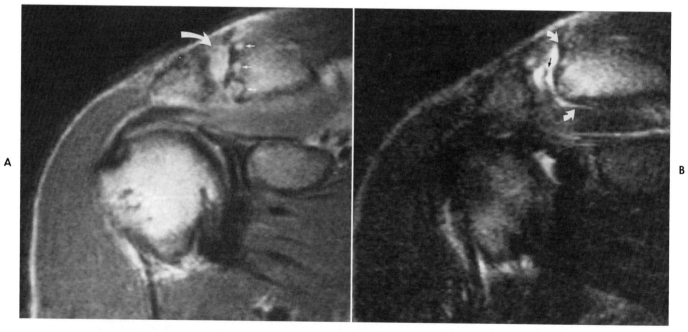

FIGURE 15-112
Glenohumeral, osteoarthritis, left shoulder in a 35-year-old man with pain and no history of prior trauma. **A,** Axial T1-weighted (800/30) image at middle glenohumeral joint. Note the prominent osteophytic process of the humeral head and glenoid margin *(arrows)*. **B,** An oblique coronal proton density (2100/30) MR image shows the prominent spur of the inferior humeral head *(solid arrows)* and loose bodies in the axillary pouch *(hollow arrow)*. The rotator cuff tendons are all normal. However, note the abnormal glenohumeral joint alignment with posterior shift **(A)** and superior migration **(B).** The cause of these is not entirely clear.

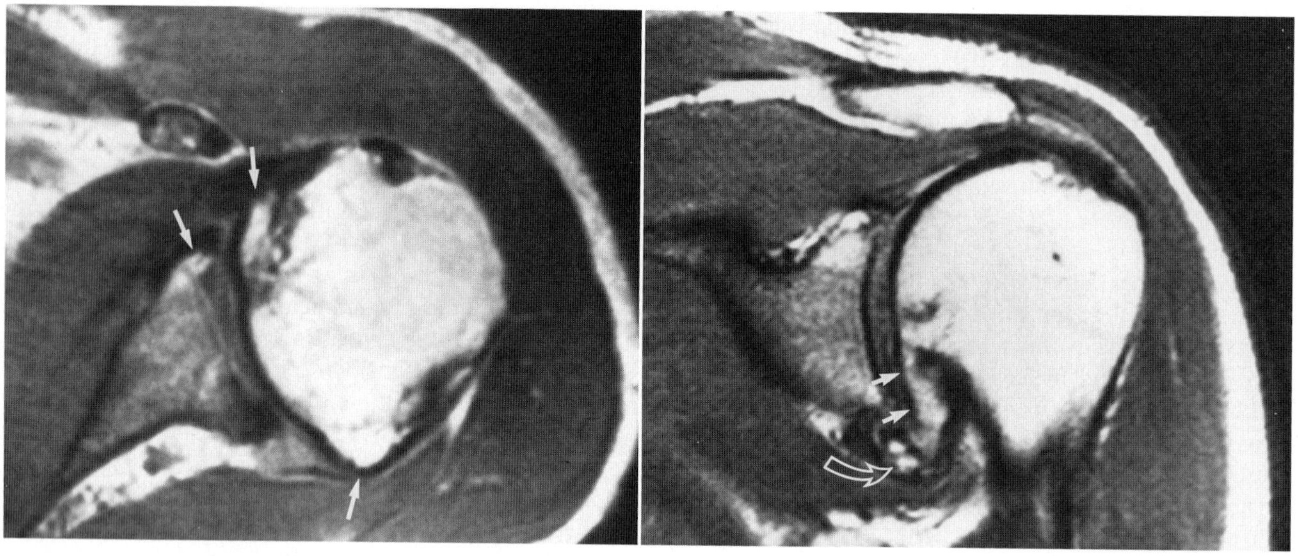

FIGURE 15-113
Posttraumatic AC joint derangement. Consecutive oblique coronal images, proton density–weighted and T2-weighted (2100/30/80), at the anterior aspect of the glenohumeral joint (**A** posterior to **B**). Marked widening of the AC joint space in **A** due to erosion of the articular surfaces *(curved arrow)* and subcortical cysts *(small arrows)* are visible. The capsule and supporting ligaments are no longer present. The low-signal character of the osseous margins indicates sclerotic response. The widened joint space in **B** is mostly filled with fluid, which extends above and below the osseous joint margins *(white arrows)*. The low-signal tissue within the widened joint is probably hyperplastic synovium *(black arrow)*. These changes all indicate persistent instability of the joint.

of MRI in detecting osteomyelitis and septic arthritis in various stages of the disease has been established. (See Chapter 9.) Early diagnosis of osteomyelitis and septic arthritis, with immediate initiation of treatment, is the most important factor in achieving optimal results. Roentgenographic findings are delayed in both conditions. Furthermore, soft tissue infections may not be readily differentiated from osteomyelitis or septic arthritis. Effusion in deep-seated joints is also difficult to detect by clinical and roentgenographic methods.

The pathological changes of septic arthritis, including joint effusion (or exudate) and cartilaginous and articular bone erosion, are optimally depicted by MR imaging. In the shoulder, with extension of infection through the joint capsule, paraarticular fluid collections or abscesses may

form, and these are visualized as low-density areas on CT or high-intensity masses on T2-weighted MR images. With chronic stages of septic arthritis low-signal tissue elements may be found in the joint effusion or synovial fluid collections and indicate the presence of debris. MR imaging is particularly helpful for differentiating these various components of infection in or about the shoulder joint[144] (Fig. 15-116).

The soft tissue and osseous pathological changes of septic arthritis and osteomyelitis in the shoulder are also detected by CT scanning. Intravenous contrast enhancement is useful in delineation of abscess collections or demonstration of areas with soft tissue inflammation. However, except for visualizing small sequestra and minute foci of gas, MRI has greater sensitivity than CT.[144]

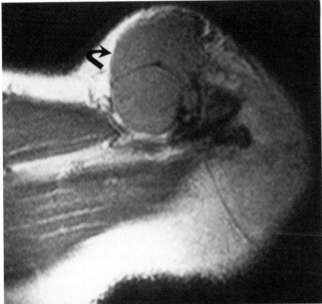

A

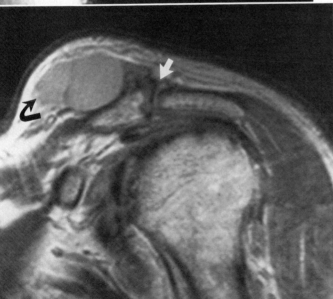

B

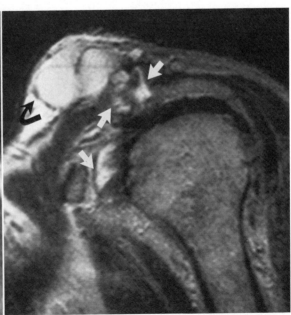

C

FIGURE 15-114

Paraarticular synovial cyst, degenerative arthritis, left shoulder. **A,** Axial T1-weighted (600/30) and, **B,** oblique sagittal proton density–weighted (1800/30) images. A multiloculated cyst with signal characteristics suggestive of fluid can be seen above and anterior to the distal clavicle *(black arrows)* and AC joint *(white arrow,* **B**). There is apparent soft tissue continuity between the cyst wall and the AC joint. **C,** Oblique sagittal T2-weighted image lateral to **B** (at the level of the acromion). The high-intensity fluid-filled cyst *(black arrow)* as well as other small collections anterior to the acromion (and AC joint) and within the glenohumeral joint *(white arrows)* are visualized. The humeral head is moderately arthritic. The origin of the cyst from the glenohumeral joint and extending through the AC joint was confirmed at surgery.

FIGURE 15-115
Pararticular synovial (ganglion) cyst. **A,** Axial T1-weighted (900/30) image at the superior aspect of the glenoid. A medium-signal lobulated mass is present in the space between scapular neck, posterior capsule, and infraspinatus *(arrows)*. **B,** An oblique coronal T2-weighted sequence (2100/80) image at the posterior aspect of the joint confirms this to be a cystic fluid-filled structure *(arrows)*.

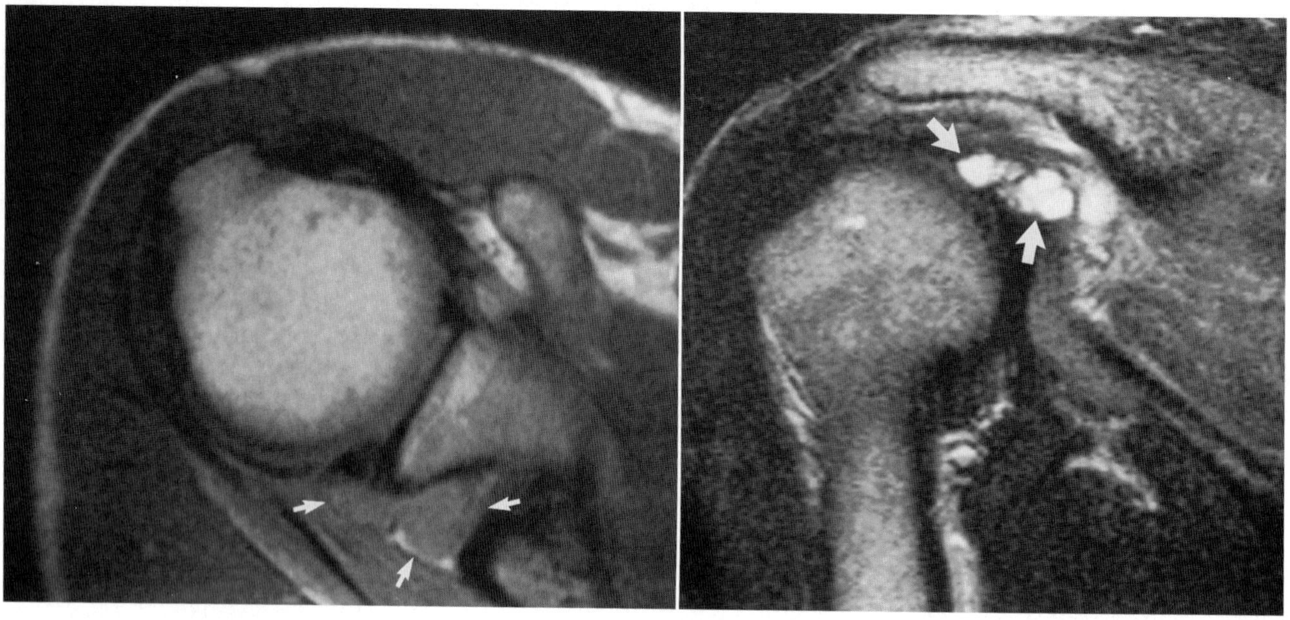

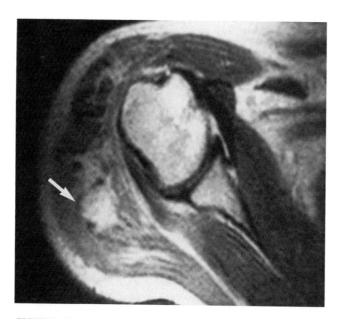

FIGURE 15-116
Deltoid abscess, right shoulder in a patient with suspected infection at an injection site on the posterior deltoideus. On this axial relatively T2-weighted (1500/60) image, note the high-intensity abscess collection *(arrow)*. The lateral aspect of the deltoideus shows nonhomogeneous signal intensity due to induration. The posterior cuff is normal, and the glenohumeral joint is not involved.

Synovial osteochondromatosis

In the diffuse form of this disease numerous cartilaginous bodies result from metaplasia of the synovium and may remain adherent to the synovial surface, gradually undergoing calcification or ossification.[149] If separated, they form loose bodies.

The disorder may involve a limited portion of the synovium or may arise from the synovial surface at extraarticular sites (i.e., *tenosynovial chondromatosis*). In this form isolated involvement of the bicipital synovial tendon sheath is sometimes present[150] (Fig. 15-117). Osteochondral fragments are also occasionally formed or become lodged within the subscapular bursa and may coalesce into a lobulated mass containing several small calcific or ossific densities. Histologically this form is similar to *benign chondroma*,[151] which may (rarely) originate from intraarticular soft tissues and become partially calcified, with resultant pressure erosion of the underlying cortical bone (Fig. 15-118). Its CT and MR characteristics reflect the basic histology described above.[152] *Loose bodies* within the glenohumeral joint may also result from traumatic events. They are usually few and may become lodged within the subscapular bursa (Fig. 15-60, *A*). Osteoarthritis is another etiological factor in the formation of loose bodies (Fig. 15-112).

Avascular necrosis

Avascular necrosis of the humeral head has variable causes, similar to those of the more frequently encountered and extensively studied avascular necrosis of the femoral head, including fracture at the anatomical neck (which disrupts blood flow to the humeral head), systemic disorders (e.g., sickle cell disease), alcoholism, collagen vascular disorders, and treatment with steroids.

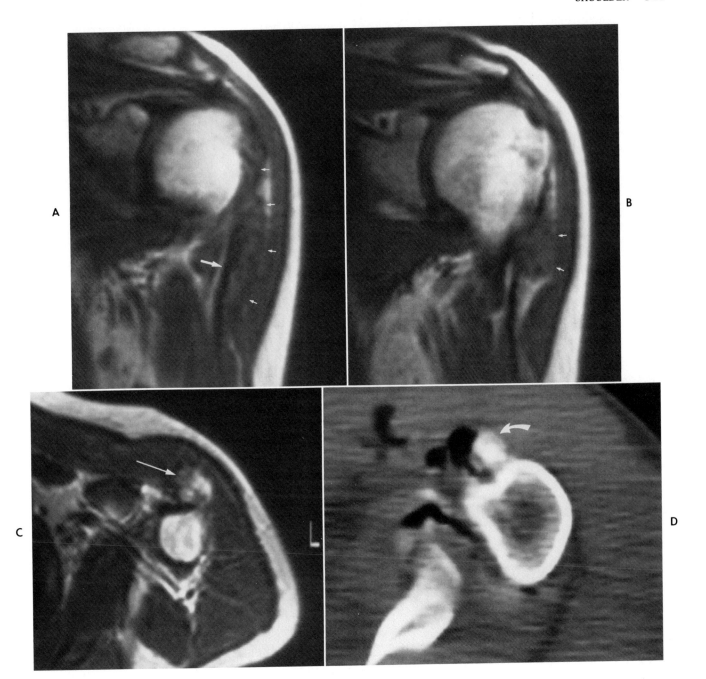

FIGURE 15-117

Bicipital tenosynovial osteochondromatosis, two cases. Case 1. **A** and **B**, Oblique coronal T1-weighted (600/30) and axial T2-weighted (1800/60) images of the left shoulder. There is distention of the bicipital tendon sheath *(small arrows)* lateral to the long head of the biceps tendon *(long arrow,* **A**). The signal intensity is low, with foci of signal void. **C**, The lobulated mass shows high-intensity signal (cartilaginous component) with foci of low signal (calcific component) *(arrow)*. Case 2, **D**, CT-arthrogram image, left shoulder. A lobulated, partly calcified mass is visualized in the distended bicipital sheath *(arrow)*. The long head of the biceps tendon is not identified. There is poor coating of the joint surfaces as a result of effusion.

As with other sites affected by avascular necrosis, in the early stages radiographs are normal. Although the radio-nuclide bone scan is usually abnormal early, more specific documentation is needed. With the development of resorptive changes in the necrotic bone and reactive sclerosis, high-resolution CT scanning is helpful in making the diagnosis; but for early detection of avascular necrosis in the hip, MR imaging is the most sensitive, and thus it is recommended for general evaluation of the various sites. (See Chapter 19.)

The evolution of pathological changes in avascular necrosis of the humeral head as depicted by MRI has not been extensively studied, but it should be similar to that of femoral head necrosis as well as to the appearances of

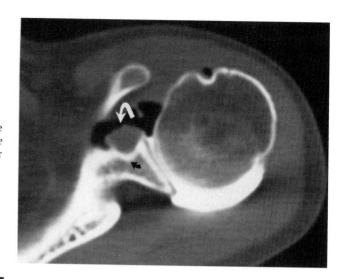

FIGURE 15-118
Synovial chondroma, left shoulder. A, CT-arthrogram shows the lobulated soft tissue mass at the anterior aspect of the joint (white arrow) against the scapular neck. The concavity in the scapular cortex (black arrow) is due to pressure erosion.

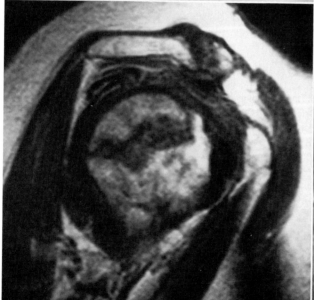

A

FIGURE 15-119
Avascular necrosis, right humeral head in a 65-year-old woman with a history of metastatic disease (treated by chemotherapy, including steroids) and shoulder pain. Metastatic disease was suspected clinically. A, An AP roentgenogram shows increased density and an apparent crescent sign of the humeral head. Although the radiographic pattern is that of avascular necrosis, MR examination was requested to support the findings. B, Oblique sagittal T2-weighted (1800/80) image. The characteristic low-signal band with geographic margin is present at the base of the humeral head. C, Oblique coronal T2-weighted (2100/80) image. The high-signal band in the subcortical region (straight arrow) and partly at the base of the humeral head (curved arrow) indicate regions of spongy bone infraction. These MR findings are characteristic of avascular necrosis.

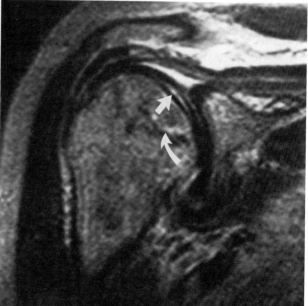

B

C

such conditions reported at other sites. Specifically, in the early stages signal from the humeral head marrow should be decreased on T1-weighted sequences (due to edema of the marrow) but with resolution of the edema and resorption of necrotic bone should show an increase (due to replacement by fatty or fibrotic tissue). The boundary of the vascular region should be manifested by a band of decreased signal intensity on T1- and T2-weighted images, indicating the area of active bone formation.

REFERENCES

1. Warwick R, Williams PL: Gray's anatomy, 36th ed. Philadelphia, Saunders, 1980, p 456.
2. Moseley HF, Overgaard B: The anterior capsular mechanism in recurrent anterior dislocation of shoulder. Morphological and clinical studies with special reference to the glenoid labrum and the gleno-humeral ligaments. J Bone Joint Surg (Br) 1962;44:913-927.
3. Bland JH, Merrit JA, Boushey DR: The painful shoulder. Semin Arthritis Rheum 1977;7(1):21-47.
4. Middleton WD, Kneeland JB, Carrera GF, et al: High-resolution MR imaging of the normal rotator cuff. AJR 1987;148:559-564.
5. Neer CS: Anterior acromioplasty for chronic impingement syndrome in the shoulder: a preliminary report. J Bone Joint Surg (Am) 1972;54:41-50.
6. Skinner HA: Anatomical considerations relative to rupture of the supraspinatus tendon. J Bone Joint Surg 1937;19:137-151.
7. DePalma AF: Surgery of the shoulder, 3d ed. Philadelphia, Lippincott, 1983, pp 51-63, 100-173, 211-241.
8. Turkel SJ, Panio MW, Marshal JL, Girgis FG: Stabilizing mechanisms preventing anterior dislocation of the glenohumeral joint. J Bone Joint Surg (Am) 1981;63:1208-1217.
9. Rothman RH, Marvel JP Jr, Heppenstall RB: Anatomic consideration in glenohumeral joint. Orthop Clin North Am 1974; 6:341-352.
10. Codman EA: The shoulder. Rupture of the supraspinatus tendon and other lesions in or about the subacromial space. Boston, Thomas Tod, 1934.
11. Mitchell MJ, Camsey G, Berthoty PD, et al: Peribursal fat plane of the shoulder: Anatomic study and clinical experience. Radiology 1988;168:699-704.
12. Neviaser RJ: Anatomic considerations and examination of the shoulder. Orthop Clin North Am 1980;11(2):187-195.
13. Shuman WP, Kilcoyne RF, Matsen FA, et al: Double-contrast computed tomography of the glenoid labrum. AJR 1983;141: 581-584.
14. Deutsch AL, Resnick D, Mink J, et al: Computed and conventional arthrotomography of the glenohumeral joint: normal anatomy and clinical experience. Radiology 1984;153:603-609.
15. Rafii M, Firooznia H, Golimbu C, et al: CT arthrography of capsular structures of the shoulder. AJR 1986;146:361-367.
16. El-Khoury GY, Albright JP, Abu-Yousef MM, et al: Arthrotomography of the glenoid labrum. Radiology 1979;131:333-337.
17. Braunstein EM, O'Connor G: Double contrast arthrotomography of the shoulder. J Bone Joint Surg (Am) 1982;64:192-195.
18. Kleinman PK, Kanzaria PK, Goss TP, Pappas AM: Axillary arthrotomography of the glenoid labrum. AJR 1984;141:993-999.
19. Mink JH, Richardson A, Grant TT: Evaluation of glenoid labrum by double-contrast shoulder arthrography. Radiology 1985;157:621-623.
20. Goldman AB, Ghelman B: The double contrast shoulder arthrogram. A review of 158 studies. Radiology 1978;127:655-663.
21. Pennes DR, Jonsson K, Buckwalter K, et al: Computed arthrotomography of the shoulder: comparison of examinations made with internal and external rotation of the humerus. AJR 1989:153:1017-1019.
22. Beltran J, Gray LA, Bools JC, et al: Rotator cuff lesions of the shoulder: evaluation by direct sagittal CT arthrography. Radiology 1986;160:161-165.
23. Randelli M, Odella R, Gambrioli PL: Clinical experience with double-contrast medium computerized tomography (arthro-CT) in instability of shoulder. Ital J Orthop Traumatol 1986;12(2):151-158.
24. Resch H, Helweg G, Zur Neddon D, Beck E: Double contrast computed tomographic examination techniques in habitual and recurrent shoulder dislocation. Eur J Radiol 1988;8:6-12.
25. Huber DJ, Sauter RS, Muller E, et al: MR imaging of the normal shoulder. Radiology 1986;158:405-408.
26. Middleton WD, Kneeland JB, Carrera GF: High resolution MR imaging of the normal rotator cuff. AJR 1987;148:559-564.
27. Kieft GJ, Bloem JL, Oberman WR: Normal shoulder: MR imaging. Radiology 1986;159(3):741-745.
28. Seeger LL, Ruszkowski JT, Bassett LW, et al: MR imaging of the normal shoulder: anatomic correlation. AJR 1987;148:83-91.
29. Kneeland JB, Carrera GF, Middleton WD, et al: Rotator cuff tears: preliminary application of high-resolution MR imaging with counter-rotating current loop-gap resonators. Radiology 1986;160:695-699.
30. Kieft GJ, Sartoris DJ, Bloem JL, et al: Magnetic resonance imaging of gleno-humeral joint diseases. Skeletal Radiol 1987;16:285-290.
31. Kneeland BJ, Middleton WD, Carrera GF, et al: MR imaging of the shoulder: diagnosis of rotator cuff tears. AJR 1987;149:333-337.
32. Zlatkin MB, Reicher MA, Kellerhouse LE, et al: The painful shoulder: MR imaging of the glenohumeral joint. J Comput Assist Tomogr 1988;12:995-1001.
33. Seeger LL, Gold RH, Bassett LW, Ellman H: Shoulder impingement syndrome. MR findings in 53 shoulders. AJR 1988; 150:343-347.
34. Evancho AM, Stiles RG, Fajman WA, et al: MR imaging diagnosis of rotator cuff tears. AJR 1988;151:751-754.
35. Kieft GJ, Bloem JL, Rozing PM, et al: Rotator cuff impingement syndrome: MR imaging. Radiology 1988;166:211-214.
36. Zlatkin MB, Dalinka MK, Kressel H: Magnetic resonance imaging of the shoulder. Magn Reson Q 1989;5:3-22.
37. Zlatkin MB, Ionnatti JP, Roberts MC, et al: Rotator cuff tears: diagnostic performance of MR imaging. Radiology 1989;172: 223-229.
38. Burk DL, Karasick DK, Kurtz AB, et al: Rotator cuff tears: prospective comparison of MR imaging with arthrography, sonography, and surgery. AJR 1989;153:87-92.
39. Rafii M, Firooznia H, Sherman O, et al: Rotator cuff lesions: signal patterns at MR imaging. Radiology 1990;177:817-823.
40. Seeger LL, Gold RH, Bassett LW: Shoulder instability: evaluation with MR imaging. Radiology 1988;168:695-697.
41. Munk PL, Holt GR, Helms CA, Genant HK: Glenoid labrum: preliminary work with use of radial-sequence MR imaging. Radiology 1989;173:751-753.
42. Rafii M, Minkoff J, Bonamo J, et al: CT arthrography of shoulder instabilities in athletes. Am J Sports Med 1988; 16:352-361.
43. Zlatkin MB, Bjorkengren AG, Gylys-Morin V, et al: Cross-sectional imaging of the capsular mechanism of the glenohumeral joint. AJR 1988;150:151-158.
44. Wilson AJ, Totty WG, Murphy WA, Hardy DC: Shoulder joint: arthrographic CT and long-term follow up, with surgical correlation. Radiology 1990;173:329-333.
45. Moseley HF: Athletic injuries to the shoulder region. Am J Surg 1959;98:401-422.
46. Skyhar MR, Warren RF, Altcheck DW: Instability of the shoulder. In Nicholas JA, Hershman EB (eds): The upper extremity in sports medicine. St Louis, Mosby, 1990, pp 181-212.

47. Cofield R, Irving JF: Evaluation and classification of shoulder instability. Clin Orthop Rel Res 1987;223:32-43.

48. Pappas AM, Goss TP, Kleinman PK: Symptomatic shoulder instability due to lesions of the glenoid labrum. Am J Sports Med 1983;11:279-288.

49. Bankart SB: The pathology and treatment of recurrent dislocation of the shoulder joint. Br J Surg 1938;26:23-29.

50. Townley CO: The capsular mechanism in recurrent dislocation of the shoulder. J Bone Joint Surg (Am) 1950;32:370-380.

51. Du Toit GT, Roux D: Recurrent dislocation of the shoulder. A twenty-four year study of the Johannesburg stapling operation. J Bone Joint Surg (Am) 1956;38:1-12.

52. Bateman JE: Athletic injuries about the shoulder in throwing and body contact sports. Clin Orthop Rel Res 1962;23:75-83.

53. Neer CS II, Welsh RP: The shoulder in sports. Orthop Clin North Am 1977;8:583-591.

54. Blazina E, Satzman JS: Recurrent anterior subluxation of the shoulder in athletes: a distinct entity. J Bone Joint Surg (Am) 1969;5:1037-1038.

55. Rowe CR, Zarins B: Recurrent transient subluxation of the shoulder. J Bone Joint Surg (Am) 1981;63:863-871.

56. Protzman RR: Anterior instability of shoulder. J Bone Joint Surg (Am) 1980;62:909-918.

57. O'Donoghue DH: Treatment of injuries to athletes, 4th ed. Philadelphia, Saunders, 1984, pp 118-220.

58. McLaughlin HL: Recurrent anterior dislocation of the shoulder. 1. Morbid anatomy. Am J Surg 1960;99:628-632.

59. Bost FC, Inman VT: The pathological changes in recurrent dislocation of the shoulder. A report of Bankart's operative procedure. J Bone Joint Surg 1942;15:595-613.

60. Rowe CR, Patel D: The Bankart procedure. A long-term end-result study. J Bone Joint Surg (Am) 1978;60:1-16.

61. Reeves B: Experiments on the tensile strength of the anterior capsular structures of the shoulder in man. J Bone Joint Surg (Br) 1968;50:858-865.

62. Bankart, ASB: Recurrent or habitual dislocation of the shoulder joint. Br Med J 1923;2:1132-1133.

63. Mizuno K, Hiorhata K: Diagnosis of recurrent traumatic anterior subluxation of the shoulder. Clin Orthop Rel Res 1983;179:160-167.

64. Uhthoff HK, Piscopo M: Anterior capsular redundancy of the shoulder: Congenital or traumatic. J Bone Joint Surg. 1985; 65B:363-366.

65. Hill HA, Sachs MD: The grooved defect of the humeral head. A frequently unrecognized complication of dislocation of the shoulder joint. Radiology 1940;35:690-700.

66. Warren RF: Instability of shoulder in throwing sports. Instructional course lectures. St Louis, Mosby, 1985. Vol 34, pp 337-348.

67. Danzig L, Greenway G, Resnick D: The Hill-Sachs lesion. Am J Sports Med 1980;8(5):328-331.

68. Pavlov H, Warren RF, Weiss CB Jr, et al: The roentgenographic evaluation of anterior shoulder instability. Clin Orthop Rel Res 1985;194:153-158.

69. Hawkins RJ, Koppert G, Johnston G: Recurrent posterior instability (subluxation) of the shoulder. J Bone Joint Surg (Am) 1984;66:169-174.

70. McLaughlin H: Posterior dislocation of the shoulder. J Bone Joint Surg (Am) 1952;34:584-590.

71. Norris TR: Diagnostic techniques for shoulder instability. Instructional course lectures. St Louis, Mosby, 1985. Vol 34, pp 239-257.

72. Neer CS II, Foster CR: Inferior capsular shift for involuntary inferior and multidirectional instability of the shoulder. A preliminary report. J Bone Joint Surg (Am) 1980;62:897-908.

73. Caspari RB: Shoulder arthroscopy: a review of the present state of the art. Contemp Orthop 1982;4:523-530.

74. Johnson LL: Arthroscopy of the shoulder. Orthop Clin North Am 1980;11:197-204.

75. Rafii M, Firooznia H, Bonamo JJ, et al: Athlete shoulder injuries: CT arthrographic findings. Radiology 1987;162:559-564.

76. Rafii M, Minkoff J, Destefano V: Diagnostic imaging of the shoulder. In Nicholas JA, Hershman EB (eds): The upper extremity in sports medicine. St Louis, Mosby, 1990, pp 91-158.

77. Singson RD, Feldman F, Bigliani L: CT arthrographic patterns in recurrent glenohumeral instability. AJR 1987;149:749-753.

78. McNiesh LM, Callaghan JJ: CT arthrography of the shoulder: variations of the glenoid labrum. AJR 1987;149:963-966.

79. Kummel BM: Arthrography in anterior capsular derangements of the shoulder. Clin Orthop Rel Res 1972;83:170-176.

80. Preston BJ, Jackson JP: Investigation of shoulder disability by arthography. Clin Radiol 1977;28:259-266.

81. Andrews JR, Carson WG, McLeod WD: Glenoid labrum tears related to the long head of the biceps. Am J Sports Med 1985;13:337-341.

82. Andrews JR, Carson WG, Ortega K: Arthroscopy of the shoulder: Technique and normal anatomy. Am J Sports Med 1984;12:1-7.

83. Mendoza FX, Nicholas JA, Reilly J: Anatomic patterns of glenoid labrum tears. Orthop Trans 1987;11:246.

84. Mendoza FX, Moskwa CA Jr: Shoulder arthroscopy. In Nicholas JA, Hershman EB (eds): The upper extremity in sports medicine. St Louis, Mosby, 1990, pp 159-168.

85. Zarins B, Matthews LS: Evaluation and treatment of glenoid labrum tears. In Jackson DW (ed): Shoulder surgery in the athlete. Rockville Md, Aspen Publications, 1985, pp 31-44.

86. Synder SJ, Karzel RP, Del Pizzo W, et al: SLAP lesions of the shoulder. Arthroscopy 1990;6(4):274-279.

87. Lombardo SJ, Jobe FW, Kerlan RK et al: Posterior shoulder lesions in throwing athletes. Am J Sports Med 1977;5:106-110.

88. Bennett GE: Shoulder and elbow lesions distinctive of baseball players. Ann Surg 1947;126:107-110.

89. Barnes O, Tullos HS: An analysis of 100 symptomatic baseball players. Am J Sports Med 1978;6:62-67.

90. Kohn D: The clinical relevance of glenoid labrum lesions. Arthroscopy 1987;3(4):223-230.

91. Kneisl JS, Sweeney HJ, Paige ML: Correlation of pathology observed in double contrast arthrotomography and arthroscopy of the shoulder. Arthroscopy 1988;4:21-24.

92. Kieft GJ, Bloem JL, Rozing PM, Obermann WR: MR imaging of anterior dislocation of the shoulder: comparison with CT arthrography. AJR 1988;150:1083-1087.

93. Habibian A, Staufer A, Resnick D, et al: Comparison of conventional and computed arthrotomography with MR imaging of shoulder. J Comput Axial Tomogr 1989;13:968-975.

94. Flannigan B, Kursunogla-Brahme S, Snyder S, et al: MR-arthrography of the shoulder: comparison with conventional MR imaging. AJR 1990;155:829-832.

95. Hajek PC, Baker LL, Sartoris D, et al: MR arthrography: Pathologic investigation. Radiology 1987;163:141-147.

96. Jobe FW et al: The relationship of anterior instability and rotator cuff impingement in the throwing athlete. Presented at the American Shoulder and Elbow Surgeons Annual Open Meeting, Las Vegas, February 21, 1989.

97. Rogers LF, Hendrix RW: The painful shoulder. Radiol Clin North Am 1988;26(6):1359-1371.

98. Leach RE, Schepsis AA: Shoulder pain. Clin Sports Med 1983;2:123-135.

99. Neer CS II: Impingement lesions. Clin Orthop Rel Res 1983;173:70-77.

100. Hawkins RJ, Kennedy JC: Impingement syndrome in athletes. Am J Sports Med 1980;8(3):151-158.

101. Jobe FW, Jobe CM: Painful athletic injuries of the shoulder. Clin Orthop Rel. Res. 1983;173:117-124.

102. Jackson DW: Chronic rotator cuff impingement in the throwing athlete. Am J Sports Med 1976;4(6):231-240.

103. Penny JN, Welsh MB: Shoulder impingement syndromes in athletes and their surgical management. Am J Sports Med 1981;9:11-15.

104. Moseley HF, Goldie I: The arterial patterns of the rotator cuff of the shoulder. J Bone Joint Surg (B) 1963;45:780-789.

105. Rothman RH, Parke WW: The vascular anatomy of the rotator cuff. Clin Orthop Rel Res 1965;41:176-186.

106. Rathbun JB, Macnab I: The microvascular pattern of the rotator cuff. J Bone Surg (B) 1970;52:540-553.

107. Kessel L, Watson M: The painful arc syndrome. J Bone Joint Surg (B) 1977;59:166-172.

108. Cone RO III, Resnick D, Danzig L: Shoulder impingment syndrome: radiographic evaluation. Radiology 1984;150:29-33.

109. Golding FC: The shoulder — the forgotten joint. Br J Radiol 1962;35:149-158.

110. Macnab I, Hastings D: Rotator cuff tendinitis. Can Med Assoc J 1968;99:91-98.

111. Strizak AM, Torrance LD, Jackson D, et al: Subacromial bursography: an anatomic and clinical study. J Bone Joint Surg (Am) 1982;64:196-201.

112. Brewer BJ: Aging of the rotator cuff. Am J Sports Med 1979;7:102-110.

113. Cotton RE, Rideout DF: Tears of the humeral rotator cuff. A radiological and pathological necropsy survey. J Bone Joint Surg (B) 1964;46:314-328.

114. Wilson CL: Lesions of the supraspinatus tendon: degeneration, rupture, and calcification. Arch Surg 1943;46:307-325.

115. Fukuda H, Mikasa M, Yamanaka K: Incomplete thickness rotator cuff tears diagnosed by subacromial bursography. Clin Orthop Rel Res 1987;223:51-58.

116. Tamai K, Ogawa K: Intratendinous tear of the supraspinatus tendon exhibiting winging of the scapula. Clin Orthop Rel Res 1985;194:159-163.

117. Gschwend N, Ivosevic-Radovanovic D, Patte D: Rotator cuff tear — relationship between clinical and anatomopathological findings. Arch Orthop Trauma Surg 1988;107:7-15.

118. Neviaser RJ: Tears of the rotator cuff. Orthop Clin North Am 1980;11:295-306.

119. Cofield RH: Tears of rotator cuff. Instructional course lectures. St Louis, Mosby, 1981. Vol 30, pp 258-273.

120. Post M, Silver R, Singh M: Rotator cuff tear. Diagnosis and treatment. Clin Orthop Rel Res 1983;173:78-91.

121. Lindblom K: Arthrography and roentgenography in ruptures of tendons of the shoulder joint. Acta Radiol [Diagn] 1939;20:548-562.

122. Killoran PJ, Marcove RC, Freiberger RH: Shoulder arthrography. AJR 1968;103:658-668.

123. Mink JH, Harris E, Rappaport M: Rotator cuff tears: evaluation using double contrast shoulder arthrography. Radiology 1985;157:621-623.

124. Resnick D: Arthrography, tenography, and bursography. In Resnick D, Niwayama G (eds): Diagnosis of bone and joint disorders. 2nd ed, Philadelphia, Saunders, 1989, pp 302-440.

125. Kilcoyne RF, Matsen FA: Rotator cuff tear measurement by arthropneumotomography. AJR 1983;140:315-318.

126. Middleton WD, Edelstein G, Reinus WR, et al: Sonographic detection of rotator cuff tears. AJR 1985;144:349-353.

127. Middleton WD, Reinus WR, Nelson GL, et al: Pitfalls of rotator cuff sonography. AJR 1986;146:555-560.

128. Farin PA, Jaroma H, Harju A, Soimakallio S: Shoulder impingement syndrome. Sonographic evaluation. Radiology 1990;176:845-849.

129. Zaslav K, Rafii, M, Sherman O, et al: Magnetic resonance imaging of rotator cuff. Anatomic and histologic correlations of alteration in signal intensity. Presented at the meeting of American Society of Sports Medicine. New Orleans, February 9, 1990.

130. Bigliani JA, Morrison DS, April EW: The morphology of the acromion and its relationship to cuff tears (abstr). Orthop Trans 1986;10:216.

131. Ellman H, Hanker G, Bayer M: Repair of the rotator cuff. J Bone Joint Surg (A) 1986;68:1136-1144.

132. Neer CS, Craig EV, Fukuda H: Cuff arthropathy. J Bone Joint Surg 1983;65A:1232-1244.

133. Ahovuo J: Radiographic anatomy of the intertubercular groove of the humerus. Europ J Radiol 1985;5:83-86.

134. Morrey BF, James JM: Recurrent anterior dislocation of the shoulder: long term follow up of the Putti-Platt and Bankart procedures. J Bone Joint Surg (Am) 1976;58:252-256.

135. Rowe CR, Zarins B, Ciullo JV: Recurrent anterior dislocation of the shoulder after surgical repair: apparent causes of failure and treatment. J Bone Joint Surg (Am) 1984;66:159-168.

136. Singson RD, Feldman F, Bigliani LU: Recurrent shoulder dislocation after surgical repair: double contrast CT-arthrography. Work in progress, Radiology 1987;164:425-428.

137. Zuckerman JD, Matsen FA III: Complications about the glenohumeral joint related to the use of screws and staples. J Bone Joint Surg (Am) 1984;66:175-180.

138. Lower RF, McNiesch LM, Callaghan JJ: Computed tomographic documentation of intra-articular penetration of a screw after operations on shoulder. J Bone Joint Surg (Am)1985:67:1120-1122.

139. Calvert PT, Packer NP, Stoker DJ, et al: Arthrography of the shoulder after operative repair of the torn rotator cuff. J Bone Joint Surg (Am) 1986;68:147-150.

140. Pavlov H, Freiberger RH: Fractures and dislocations about the shoulder. Semin Roentgenol 1978;13(2):85-96.

141. Neer CS: Displaced proximal humeral fractures. J Bone Joint Surg (Am) 1970;52:1077-1103.

142. Castagno AA, Shuman WP, Kilcoyne RF, et al: Complex fractures of the proximal humerus: role of CT in treatment. Radiology 1987;165:759-762.

143. Kieft G, Dijkman BAC, Bloem JL, Kroon HM: Magnetic resonance imaging of the shoulder in patients with rheumatoid arthritis. Ann Rheum Dis 1990;49:7-11.

144. Beltran J, Caudill L, Herman LA, et al: Rheumatoid arthritis. MR imaging manifestations. Radiology 1987;165:153-157.

145. Yullish BS, Lieberman JM, Newman AJ, et al: Juvenile rheumatoid arthritis. Assessment with MR imaging. Radiology 1987;165:149-152.

146. Kerr R, Resnick D, Pineda C, Haghighi P: Osteoarthritis of the glenohumeral joint: a radiologic-pathologic study. AJR 1985;144:967-972.

147. Peterson CJ: Degeneration of the glenohumeral joint: an anatomical study. Acta Orthop Scand 1983;54:277-283.

148. Zanca P: Shoulder pain. Involvement of the acromioclavicular joint. AJR 1971;112:493-506.

149. Madewell JE, Sweet DE: Tumors and tumor like lesions in or about joints. In Resnick D, Niwayama G. (eds): Diagnosis of bone and joint disorders. Philadelphia, Saunders, 1988, pp 3889-3943.

150. Small R, Jaffe W: Tenosynovial chondromatosis of the shoulder. Bull Hosp Jt Dis Orth Inst 1981;41:37-47.

151. Resnick D, Niwayama G: Soft tissues. In Resnick D, Niwayama G (eds): Diagnosis of bone and joint disorders. Philadelphia, Saunders, 1988, pp 4208-4224.

152. Tuckman G, Wirth CZ: Synovial osteochondromatosis of the shoulder: MR findings. J Comput Assist Tomogr 1989;13:360-361.

16 CT-Arthrography and MRI of the Shoulder in Diagnosis and Treatment by the Orthopedic Surgeon

JEFFREY MINKOFF
ORRIN SHERMAN
GARY GILYARD

Prior to 1980, diagnostic radiology of the shoulder consisted primarily of roentgenography and arthrography; exploratory and/or therapeutic surgery of the shoulder was accomplished mainly by open, rather than arthroscopic, approaches. Since 1980, however, the radiographic repertoire has been expanded to include CT arthrotomography[1-9] and, more recently, magnetic resonance imaging.[10-16] Cotemporally, orthopedic surgeons have been accumulating experience in, and developing facility with, arthroscopy for both diagnostic and therapeutic purposes. The horizons provided by these advances are proclaimed to be of significant and mutual value to radiologists and orthopedic practitioners.

To evaluate the absolute and relative values of these advances requires an awareness and consideration of numerous variables, which have a different import for the orthopedic surgeon (charged with the responsibility for treatment) from what they have for the radiologist. The latter has the unenviable task of providing an interpretation without a full knowledge of the clinical details and dilemmas of a given case. Furthermore, as technology has provided a means of achieving greater diagnostic specificity, an even greater responsibility has fallen on the radiologist to provide more detailed and less speculative information to the surgeon. The orthopedic surgeon may avail himself (or herself) of this radiological wisdom, but often remains ungratified.

The reason for this apparent paradox is that the surgeon is provided with valuable factual clues but not necessarily with a decision in choosing the appropriate therapeutic course for the individual case in point. In fact, the surgeon may even feel compelled to assail the radiologist, out of frustration, with an audible or telepathic interrogatory: Does this explain the pain? Is it the source of dysfunction? Is the cuff tear as small as the study reveals? Many such questions may fuel the exchange between surgeon and radiologist with respect to tests such as CT arthrography and magnetic resonance imaging. One major question stands out, to which this chapter is largely dedicated: Do these special test forms offer enough additional practical and/or academic information — over that acquired from physical examination, conventional roentgenography, arthrography, and arthroscopy — to justify their routine use?

In approaching afflictions of the shoulder, the orthopedic surgeon must assimilate historical, physical, and laboratory data (including roentgenography) and then compute the magnitude, severity, and urgency of the problem at hand. Obviously, the efficacy and appropriateness of the ensuing treatment are dependent upon the computation. The accuracy of the computation, in turn, is contingent upon a number of variables. The depth of historical information is one variable, and it must include not only a documentation of symptoms and chronology but also an assessment of patient goals, temporal exigencies, and the degree of actual disability. The physical must assess motion, strength, stability, tenderness, and neurovascular integrity. Once the history and physical examination have been completed, an impression of pathology has often already been formulated. The issue is whether the impression permits a conscionable therapeutic action or whether more objective and/or more specific data are necessary for a reliable computation. Today, the objectification and/or specificity are most customarily derived

550

from either surgery (particularly arthroscopy) or special radiography (which includes procedures such as CT arthrography and MRI).

These studies offer greater detailing of the pathology, a corroboration of the clinical impression, a type of second opinion for third party carriers, and solace to the patient (who may have doubted the magnitude of his affliction).

When contemplating the ordering of special radiographic procedures, the clinician should bear in mind a few questions:

1. What is the potential upside?
2. What is the potential downside?
3. How sure are you about the diagnosis without the tests?
4. May the test results alter your therapeutic approach?

Typically, patients with shoulder problems presenting to the orthopedic surgeon for treatment offer a varied palette of complaints: pain, instability, weakness, stiffness, cracking, locking.

It is unfortunate that no combination of these symptoms is pathognomonic for a given diagnosis, not even a complaint of instability. Instability can be experienced with a torn rotator cuff, loose bodies, a bucketed labrum, or a subluxating or dislocating glenohumeral joint.

Only when the patient reports that the ball comes out of the socket, or appears in the wrong place, and is then self- (or otherwise) reduced can the history be considered reliable for a specific diagnosis of glenohumeral instability. Even then, the magnitude of pathology and the direction(s) of the instability are not known and may not even be clear after the physical examination.

The symptoms listed above relate to pathology that may exist in any of the following structures: (1) labrum, (2) rotator cuff, (3) capsule, (4) joints, or (5) bones. The common clinical entities that derive from this pathology, either singly or in combination, are

1. Torn labrum
2. Torn rotator cuff
3. Impingement
4. Glenohumeral instability
5. Fracture
6. Arthritis (including the AC joint)

HISTORY AND PHYSICAL EXAMINATION

From the history and physical it is possible to deduce the presence of one or more of the above-listed clinical entities, with greater certainty for some than for others. However, only the presence of glenohumeral instability can be ascertained with relative certainty and only when pain or guarding is not prohibitive of an adequate examination. The direction(s) of the instability (single, multiple, anterior, posterior, etc.) is sometimes less evident than the knowledge that an instability exists. When examination under anesthesia is deferred until or unless surgery is undertaken, special radiography may help to discern the directions of instability[7-9,17,18] with reasonable though not necessarily unerring accuracy.

The clinical signs of "impingement" are so well established[14,15,18-24] that the examiner can usually diagnose this conglomerate entity with a high level of confidence.* In fact, the confidence level is usually sufficient to motivate the undertaking of a surgical decompression with no additional aids other than conventional roentgenography.[19] Nevertheless, physical examinations for impingement simply disclose the quantities of pain elicited with each posture or maneuver. They do not quantitate the magnitude of each contributing component: rotator cuff disease, acromial hypertrophy, bursal enlargement, acromioclavicular joint arthritis, coracoid and coracoacromial ligament strain. It is in the realm of impingement that special radiography in the form of magnetic resonance imaging demonstrates a unique and exclusive ability to illustrate the quantitative involvement of individual constituents.[18] This is a wonderful attribute of special imaging of the shoulder. Yet, it is not clear in what manner the detection of visually evident impingement findings correlates with the specific clinical complaints being registered (Fig. 16-1).

Hence, the findings on MR fail to predict with reasonable certainty whether surgery will produce substantial improvement or, for that matter (if it is undertaken), which structures must be attacked and to what quantitative extent. The findings of impingement on MRI have never been specifically correlated with those seen in physical examination or with symptoms. Furthermore, findings after a repeat MRI (after treatment) have not been correlated with changes in symptoms and signs on physical examination. In other words, after treatment and the subsidence of symptoms, MRI may show the same abnormalities as previously.

CONVENTIONAL ROENTGENOGRAPHY

Returning to the general subject of clinical entities of the shoulder, it is recognized that their diagnosis is often enhanced by conventional plain roentgenography but with some limitations.

It has been suggested to this point that the history, physical examination, and "plain x-rays" have limited ability to diagnose labral tears, many rotator cuff tears, and certain information about glenohumeral instability and impingement syndromes. Diagnostic and management approaches for each of these entities will vary with the magnitude of disability and the individual philosophies of the treating physicians.

PHILOSOPHY OF APPROACHING SHOULDER PATHOLOGY (THE ROTATOR CUFF)

It is difficult to extract and segregate rotator cuff pathology from the entity of impingement, but for this

---

*Impingement syndromes, as shall be pointed out later in the chapter, are not simply "subacromial compressions" of the variety described by Neer et al.[23,24] They may be as complex and variable as the patellofemoral syndromes.

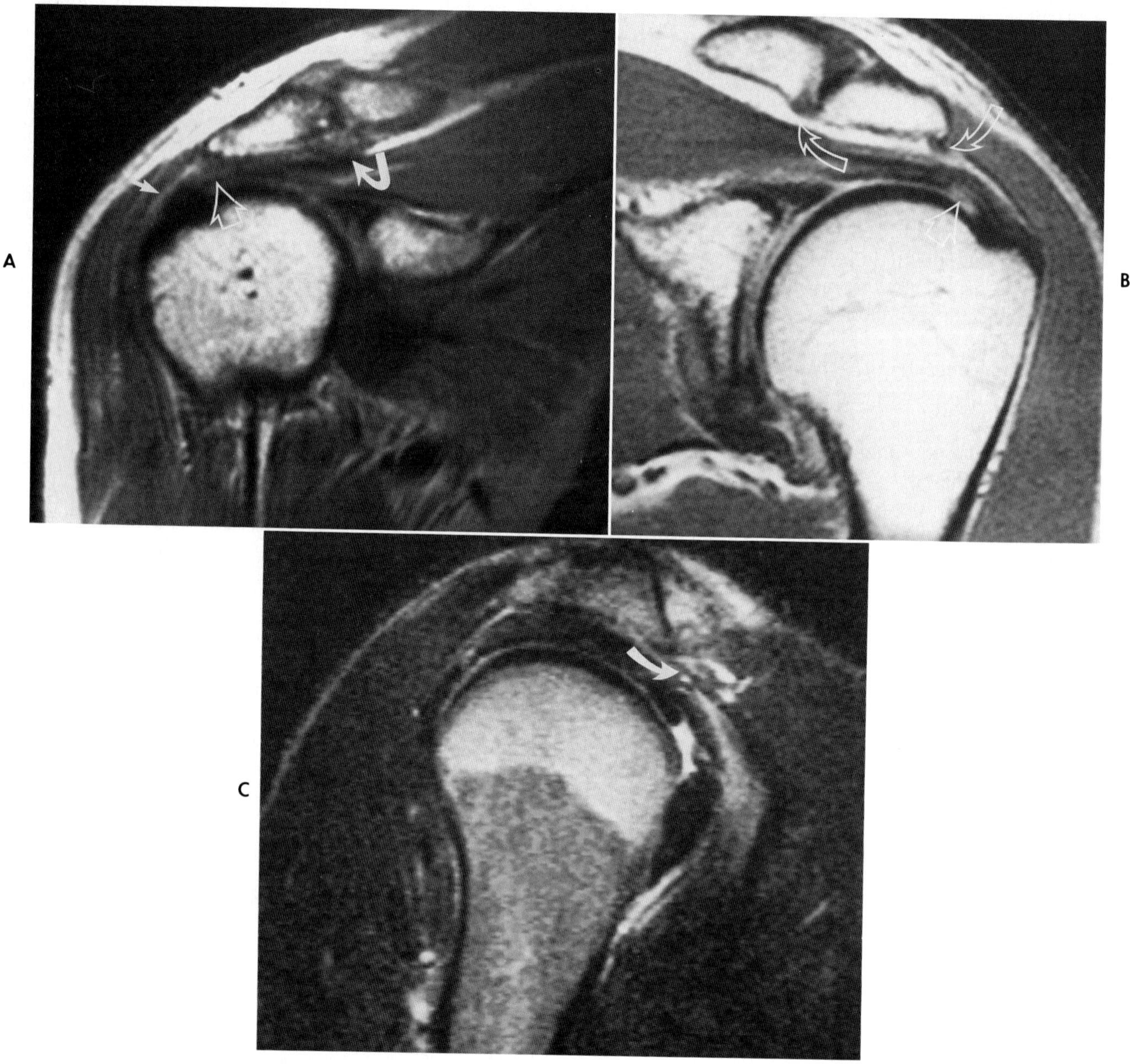

FIGURE 16-1

Subacromial impingements in conjunction with rotator cuff disease and/or acromioclavicular joint arthritis. **A**, Case 1: Oblique coronal proton density (2100/30) MR image, right shoulder. The AC joint is seen, with its articular surfaces indistinct and its capsule expanded (causing presumed impingement on the supraspinatus tendon *[solid curved arrow]*). Also evident is a diminution of the peribursal fat signal *(small solid arrow)*, indicating the presence of bursitis. Finally, a supraspinatus tendinitis is revealed by an increased signal intensity within the tendon *(hollow arrow)*. **B**, Case 2: Oblique coronal proton density (2100/30) image, left shoulder. Both acromial and AC joint downspurs are demonstrated *(hollow curved arrows)*. In addition, there is a partial synovial surface tear of the rotator cuff *(hollow straight arrow)*. **C**, Case 3: Oblique sagittal T2-weighted (1800/80) image, left shoulder. A high signal inflammatory process is visualized surrounding the coracoacromial ligament *(arrow)*.

This figure demonstrates a spectrum of impingement components: rotator cuff disease, acromial and acromioclavicular joint downspurs, bursitis, and inflammatory response about the coracoacromial ligament. The mere demonstration of these findings does not reveal the contribution, if any, of the individual components to symptoms. The expanded AC joint capsule appearing to compress the underlying tendon in **A** may be blameless with respect to symptoms or impingement. The inflammatory response about the coracoacromial ligament in **C** may not be the result of impingement by this ligament. Clinical correlations are a necessary adjunct to the interpretations of MRI significance.

See with plain x-rays	Don't see with plain x-rays
1. Fractures (most)	1. Labral tears
2. Arthritis	2. Capsular abnormalities
3. +/− Avascular necrosis	3. +/− Instability
4. +/− Instability (chronic)	4. Rotator cuff tear
5. +/− Cuff disease/impingement (moderate to advanced)	5. Impingement (early and mild to moderate)

discussion the cuff will be treated in isolation. The rotator cuff may manifest inflammation (as in tendinitis) or tears (acute, chronic, partial thickness, full thickness, small, large).

A torn and/or inflamed cuff may be suspected when the arm has been used with undue force at a time shortly (days to weeks) before the rapid onset of pain and weakness or when there is a history of repetitive shoulder use with a progression of pain and weakness. Often there is radiation of pain to the lateral aspect of the arm. Associated impingement signs, tenderness near the greater tuberosity, pain elicited when applying downward resistance to the forward flexed, internally rotated, slightly abducted arm (at chest level), and weakness in the mid-arc of abduction (and in other arcs as well) are physical signs suggesting a cuff tear. Plain roentgenograms are rarely of value unless the history is long-standing and arthritic periacromial spurs have formed, or the acromiohumeral interval has been significantly diminished.[18,23] The evidence alluded to thus far is clearly insufficient to justify a treatment decision, surgical or otherwise. There are more definite ways to diagnose a torn rotator cuff:

1. Arthrography
   a. Single contrast
   b. Double contrast
   c. With CT
2. Sonography
3. MRI
4. Arthroscopy

Arthrography, in one form or another, has for the past 20 years been the gold standard of shoulder imaging. Its efficacy in detecting rotator cuff tears is well documented.[25-27] Shortcomings include its invasive nature (contrast injection plus radiation), its failure to detect intrasubstance and superior substance tears (without bursography) as well as tears that have developed a tissue seal, and its inability effectively to reveal pathology of the labrum, capsule, and subacromial space. Without the addition of computerized tomography it has little if any predictive value in determining the size of an existing tear,[4] although it may attest to the quality and thickness of the cuff tear margins.

Sonography is a good screening tool with reasonable accuracy in the detection of rotator cuff tears.[28,29] It is entirely noninvasive and has an ability to reveal intrasubstance tears, a potential advantage over arthrography.

However, it is relatively valueless in detecting pathology of structures other than the rotator cuff, and there are few centers with sufficient expertise in sonographic interpretation to make the test as useful as it might be.

MRI is a reputedly expensive test for the shoulder, requiring a special coil for good resolution and an experienced radiologist to interpret the findings. However, it is noninvasive; it demonstrates tendinitis and rotator cuff tears; and, within reason, it can predict the magnitude of existing tears, albeit suggesting only the smallest possible size of tear. For some tears detected by MRI, subsequent arthroscopy has revealed them to be moderately larger than the MR prediction. It is speculated, though not yet proven, that distention of the joint during arthroscopy may spread the relaxed convoluted margins of somewhat puckered and collapsed tears seen on MRI. Nevertheless, Burk et al.[11] have indicated that MR provides an accurate assessment of cuff tear size and the quality of remaining tendon tissue, and Zlatkin et al.[16] revealed an excellent correlation between MR prediction of cuff tear size and tear sizes measured at surgery (r = 0.95 using a linear regression analysis in a double-blind study).

Unlike arthrography of sonography, MRI can demonstrate the contents of the subacromial space, labrum, and capsule as well as the rotator cuff, and therefore has more ubiquitous value.

Arthroscopy, of course, permits direct viewing of the rotator cuff, labrum, capsule, and subacromial space. Its disadvantages include its invasiveness and the inability to detect intrasubstance pathology. Its overwhelming advantage is its concurrent diagnostic and therapeutic capability.

The selection and sequencing of any of the above tests become a function of the philosophy of treatment, the availability and expertise of test administrators (an institutional or geographical factor), and expediency. The experience and expertise of the orthopedic surgeon in understanding the benefits of each diagnostic form, and in implementing possible treatment options, are of obvious importance.

WHAT DOES THE ORTHOPEDIC SURGEON WANT TO KNOW, AND WHY?

In the absence of evident instability or of special pathology (e.g., tumors), rotator cuff impingement and pathology are the most suspect causes of significant shoulder symptoms (particularly pain, weakness, and restricted motion). Of course, labral pathology (unassociated with instability) may be included in the group. Within this framework many orthopedic surgeons are content to advance directly to arthroscopy as a first-line diagnostic (and therapeutic) tool. In such instances they may warn the patient that the discovery of a full-thickness rotator cuff tear will sometimes necessitate addition of an arthrotomy and cuff repair. In terms of the high probability of success with this approach, a primary arthroscopy without preceding special radiography is an arguably reasonable choice of procedure.

Still the patient must be educated to the fact that a number of other diagnostic avenues are available before a surgical one is undertaken. Certainly, a primary arthroscopy is a very reasonable choice in many rural areas or Third World nations, where sophisticated diagnostic modalities are not available. Failure to perform expert diagnostics can lead to failure to diagnose important pathology, such as tumors (see Fig. 15-118). Patients obligated to arduous work schedules probably deserve to know in advance whether their operation will lead to prolonged disability (as with a cuff repair) prior to their submission to arthroscopy and possible arthrotomy.

With advances in arthroscopic technique and ability it has been possible to repair some rotator cuff tears when they are several millimeters to a few centimeters in size. Knowing the size of a cuff lesion in advance may help the patient and surgeon anticipate the need for an open

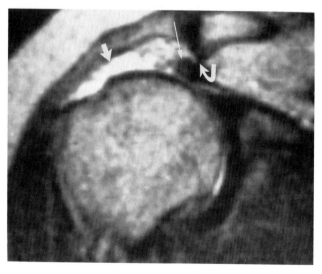

FIGURE 16-2
MRI as a diagnostic/prognostic tool. Oblique coronal T2-weighted (2100/80) image demonstrating a massive defect of the supraspinatus tendon (*straight thick arrow*). The remnant of the torn tendon (*straight thin arrow*) is visualized immediately beneath a large AC joint downspur (*curved arrow*). The magnitude of the tear indicates the likelihood of a protracted postsurgical recovery. A meaningless exploratory or decompressing arthroscopy is precluded by advanced knowledge of lesional size, information not provided by clinical examination or arthrography.

versus closed repair. In such instances the use of MRI or possibly CT-arthrography may be of benefit (Fig. 16-2). Admittedly, tears amenable to arthroscopic repair are relatively few and far between. Arthroscopic surgeons capable of doing arthroscopically assisted repair of cuff tears are increasing in number. However, the efficacy of such repairs, both in absolute terms and in relation to success with open repair techniques, is basically unknown as yet. Factors of potential import include tear size, quality of the remaining tendon tissue, and location of the tear. MR may disclose all of this information (in the event any of these factors correlate with repair success). There is little information relating to the success of special radiography (MRI) in ascertaining whether a cuff repair has been successful, and arthrographic evidence has likewise been meager.

Although much ado has been made over the determination of tear size,[4,12,18,28] for most cases the issue of its importance is controversial. The finding of a large tear may lead one to presume that symptoms are unlikely to resolve, or even to regress, especially in an active individual. Surgeons whose philosophy it is to repair basically all full-thickness tears need not avail themselves of special efforts to document the size of the lesion. Tear size has been related to length of recovery after repair and bears a prognostic implication. Surgeons who routinely repair only larger tears or who desire maximum of preoperative prognostic information would naturally be interested in knowing the dimensions of a tear. Perhaps the most elemental issue concerns the role of the cuff in producing symptoms and dysfunction. The presence of a cuff tear does not automate the production of significant symptoms or dysfunction. Associated tendinitis and impingement may be more direct sources of pain in the presence of associated cuff tears.

In this regard, the work of Calvert et al.[30] is of particular interest. They used double-contrast arthrography to study the efficacy of rotator cuff repairs and de-impingements in a group of 20 patients who had experienced virtually complete remission of symptoms after these procedures. Nevertheless, in 18 there was a contrast leak (full thickness) through the repaired cuff. Although "one swallow does not a summer make," yet this lone study of its kind does imply that in certain cases pain may well derive more from impingement and tendinitis than from a cuff tear. The study does not relate the size of a tear to the quantity of symptoms. In fact, there is no evidence in the literature to suggest a proportionality between cuff tear size and the particular symptom of pain (as opposed to weakness, stiffness, or instability).

Therefore, the issue that presents in treating the middle-aged, noncompetitive, recreational athlete whose chief complaint relates to pain unresponsive to conservative management is whether to consider an arthroscopic decompression without repairing the cuff. Such a consideration burns no bridges (i.e., does not preclude a subsequent cuff repair if symptoms fail to remit). Gartsman[31] has indicated that arthroscopic debridement of large cuff tears per se produces no significant benefit. Where does all of this leave the clinician? Some surgeons may elect to prescribe invasive or noninvasive treatments based upon clinical acumen and conventional roentgenography alone. However, rotator cuff tears require special diagnostics for elucidation; and of the radiographic modalities available for rotator cuff tears (partial or full thickness), efficacies ranging from variably good to consistently excellent (viz. our experience at NYU for MR) have been reported. (See Chapter 15.)

Burk et al.[10] evaluated 38 patients with suspected cuff tears using MRI and double-contrast arthrography in a double-blind manner; 23 were also evaluated by sonography, and 16 were operated upon. The authors concluded that MRI and arthrography were equivalently accurate in diagnosing full-thickness tears but sonography was considerably less accurate.

Zlatkin et al.[16] studied 8 pain-free individuals and 32 patients with clinically suspected cuff pathology by MRI. Of the patients with symptoms, 24 underwent virtually concurrent arthrography and all were operated on. The authors concluded that MRI sensitivity and specificity for partial-thickness and full-thickness tears were about 90% compared to some 70% for arthrography. Perhaps of greater interest was the correlation between the MRI prediction of cuff tear size and the actual size measured at surgery ($r = 0.95$ using a linear regression analysis in a double-blind study).

Similarly, Burk et al.[11] have indicated that MR provides an accurate assessment of cuff tear size and quality of the remaining tendon. Zlatkin et al.[16] asserted that these capacities of MRI play a significant role in surgical planning: anterior versus posterior approach, primary suture versus prosthetic material, tissue advance based on tear size and locus, edge retraction, and tissue quality. They cited Gscwend et al. (1988) as having demonstrated that the size and site of tears have prognostic import, influencing the recovery of both strength and range of motion.

With respect to tear size and tissue quality, Kilcoyne and Matsen[4] reported the efficacy of arthropneumotomography. Using this technique, they found good correlation between the predicted and actual sizes of tears and the quality of tissues observed at surgery in 33 cases. Still, the technique fails to provide as much detailed information about the elements of impingement on the capsulolabral complexes as MRI does.

Even if it is conceded that arthrography and MRI are, for the most part, equally capable of determining the presence of a full-thickness tear, Zlatkin et al.[16] cite their experience with more than a few cases in which MRI detected tears of less than 1.5 cm length that had escaped detection by arthrography. It is evident that MRI has the most to offer with respect to rotator cuff evaluation, even apart from its capacity to demonstrate elements of the glenohumeral joint and the other manifestations of impingement. It is our overwhelming choice in all instances in which special evaluation of the shoulder is indicated.

The two points to be underscored and reemphasized at this time are that

1. Each orthopedic surgeon has a philosophy of treatment and a level of expertise in utilizing advanced surgical techniques the successes of which are still anecdotal.

2. The value of recommendations to perform certain tests by radiologists and the accuracy and specificity of the reported findings are estimable only as they relate to the surgeon's philosophy and approach.

Impingement

The so-called "impingement syndrome" of the shoulder, an increasingly popular entity amongst orthopedic surgeons over the past 15 to 20 years, became a more focused issue for radiologists in the mid-1980s, since which time MRI has permitted better visualization of its constituents. Impingement and its eponyms, the "supraspinatus syndrome" and the "painful arc syndrome," have been recognized for more than 80 years.

Codman described impingement in 1906[32]; and in 1909 Meyer presented a description of impingement, as did Watson-Jones in 1943.[20] The real burgeoning of syndrome recognition, however, followed Neer's description[24] in 1972. What Neer described was largely an anterior acromial impingement of the bursa and cuff due to hypertrophic changes of the acromion (Table 16-1).

Table 16-1 Impingement

STAGE I: EDEMA AND HEMORRHAGE

Typical age	<25 yr
Differential diagnosis	Subluxation
	Acromioclavicular joint arthritis
Clinical course	Reversible
Treatment	Conservative

STAGE II: FIBROSIS AND TENDINITIS

Typical age	25 to 40 yr
Differential diagnosis	Frozen shoulder
	Calcium
Clinical course	Recurrent pain with activity
Treatment	Consider bursectomy or coracoacromial ligament division

STAGE III: BONE SPURS AND TENDON RUPTURE

Typical age	>40 yr
Differential diagnosis	Cervical radiculitis
	Neoplasm
Clinical course	Progressive disability
Treatment	Anterior acromioplasty
	Rotator cuff repair

Adapted from Neer CS: Clin Orthop 1983; 173:70-77.

In 1977 Kessel and Watson,[22] demonstrated a greater complexity of pathology under the banner of "impingement" and recognized three types distinguished primarily by location, treatment response, and the arc of abduction in which pain was manifested (Table 16-2).

The last distinguishing feature encouraged the authors to use the terminology *painful arc* in lieu of "impingement." They studied and treated nearly 100 patients with the syndrome by obtunding tender areas with local anesthetic and performing conventional roentgenography or limited arthrography. Those not responding to simple treatment (e.g., steroid injections) underwent resection of the CA ligament and/or excision of the AC joint. Results and observations are demonstrated in Table 16-2.

Kessel and Watson's classification[22] was more sophisticated in some respects than Neer's.[24] Even more sophistication and variety in examining for impingement have been developed subsequently and appear in Fig. 16-3.

During the 1970s and 1980s plain roentgenography and arthrography were of little value in determining the diagnosis of anything more than the most advanced stages of impingement in any classification. Physical signs were considered the best diagnostic tool. However, only the finding of glenohumeral instability is more definitely pathognomic of its derivative pathology than are the physical signs of impingement.

Certainly, for many orthopedic surgeons a physical examination "very positive" for impingement is sufficient grounds for surgical intervention. The clinical suspicion gained from physical examination is frequently corroborated by the "injection test" of Neer,[23,24] wherein a local anesthetic injected into the subacromial space produces a marked attenuation of pain on the impingement tests. Although this test provides additional objective evidence of a subacromial impingement, the evidence is circumstantial rather than pathognomonic; it only implies a pain source in the subacromial region. Likewise, the absence of pain relief after injection does not preclude the presence of impingement since the structures being anesthetized are only presumed to be involved. If much of the pain is derived from the acromioclavicular joint, subacromial injection may be incapable of relieving pain.

One potential advantage of injection relates to patients whose shoulder complaints include weakness as well as pain. If in these patients the injection relieves pain so that shoulder strength can be more effectively evaluated, the integrity of the rotator cuff as a participant in disability can be better surmised; then arthrography, sonography, or MRI can be considered with greater conviction. For many orthopedic surgeons the physical is so diagnostic of impingement that the only added information needed is whether the cuff is significantly torn, and this can be reasonably obtained with arthrography or sonography in most instances.

The foregoing discussion of clinical diagnosis should have pointed up two dilemmas relative to the impingement syndrome.

1. One is the difficulty in segregating sources of pain and disability by individual structure and determining the relative contributions of each to the manifested signs and symptoms.

   a. For example, how does one distinguish weakness due to pain from that due to cuff interruption . . . or lost range of motion due to pain from that due to mechanical impedance . . . or pain due to severe tendinitis from that due to AC joint hypertrophic arthritis? And which, if any, of these distinctions can be better settled by conventional or special radiography as opposed to physical examination or primary arthroscopy? Obviously the issue here may be resolved best with MRI or arthrography, but only if a cuff tear of sizable proportion is discovered.

   b. Another example, the derivation of a loss of motion in the patient with a painful shoulder, may be most easily resolved by injections of local anesthetic, which dispel pain and thereby restore motion. Otherwise, an arthrographic technique probably best serves to outline capsular dimensions and, on occasion, may even prove therapeutic by accomplishing a hydrostatic brisement.

   c. In a third example, the relative pain contributions of cuff tendinitis and AC joint arthritis may be surmised using MR, but not without clinical correlation in all cases. The injection of local anesthetic into each specific site of pathology is probably the best potential determinant of pro-

Table 16-2   Types of Impingement

Location	Age	Aggravated by	Painful arc (degrees)	ACJ, DJD	Treatment success*
1. Posterior	40s and 50s	Internal rotation	60 to 120	No	Steroids
2. Anterior	40s and 50s	External rotation	60 to 120	No	Steroids
3. Superior	40s and 50s	Neither external nor internal rotation	60 to 180	Yes	Surgery (CAL and ACJ)

CODE: ACJ, aacromioclavicular joint
    DJD, degenerative joint disease
    CAL, coracoacromial ligament
*Represents the major response in each category.
Adapted from Kessel L, Watson M: J Bone Surg [Br] 1977;59:166-172.

A   B   C

D₁   D₂

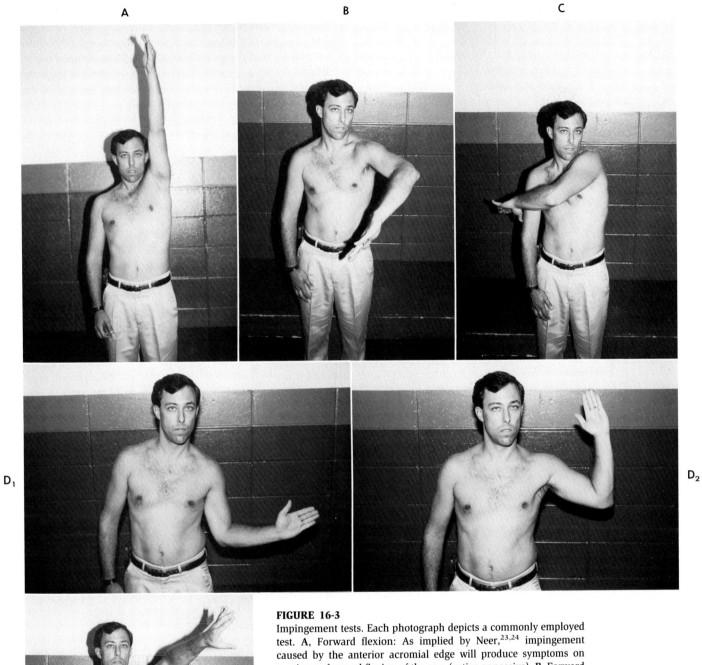

E

FIGURE 16-3

Impingement tests. Each photograph depicts a commonly employed test. **A,** Forward flexion: As implied by Neer,[23,24] impingement caused by the anterior acromial edge will produce symptoms on maximum forward flexion of the arm (active or passive). **B,** Forward flexion with internal rotation and elbow flexion: From this position the arm is further flexed forward after having been adducted to the front of the body. In this maneuver, described by Hawkins and Kennedy,[21] pain elicited implies the presence of impingement. **C,** Cross chest maneuver: The forward flexed and abducted arm is adducted across the chest. Pain implies impingement, perhaps due to AC joint disease or coracoid impingement[20] or perhaps to some other pathology. **D,** External rotation at the side or with the arm abducted (D₁ and D₂, respectively): These movements increase the leverage of the anterior capsule. The latter movement compresses the suprahumeral tissues toward the acromion. **E,** Forward flexion to about 90 degrees, internal rotation, and slight abduction: With the arm held in this position a downward force is applied to it. Pain implies rotator cuff inflammation ("the Jobe test").

portionate pain contributions. The message, if there is one thus far, seems to be that each shoulder presents a different problem and there is no place for the rote ordering of available tests.

2. The second of the two dilemmas is a natural corollary of the first: the establishment of priorities among the patient's complaints. A detailed understanding of how the patient perceives and prioritizes symptoms and complaints is important in determining the extent to which diagnostic and therapeutic pursuits are either necessary or reasonable.

   a. Is the patient disconcerted primarily by the presence of constant pain or by pain that occurs only with function? Is a loss of motion the primary complaint, even though significant pain accompanies the condition? Is loss of function the major concern (whether due to weakness, loss of motion, or instability) in a stoic patient with great pain tolerance? Does the patient wish only to eliminate the most pressing disability as he perceives it . . . or to eradicate the maximum quantity of symptoms and pathology regardless of the extent of necessary surgery . . . or to resolve the implications of pain with respect to the quantity of damage and the prognosis?

   b. The variations and many planes of priorities make it clear that except in the case of academic study there may often be a different depth of diagnostic radiographic and therapeutic pursuits even among patients with nearly identical syndromes.

The concept of impingement expressed by Neer[23,24] and by Kessel and Watson,[22] which is commonly embraced by the orthopedic and radiological communities, is that there is a *compression* occurring within the subacromial region. This concept is probably an oversimplification; compression represents but one component among many in the array of syndromes.

Most of the so-called "compressive" causes of impingement are due to tissue *excesses* within the subacromial space: cuff swelling, bursal enlargement, acromial and acromioclavicular spurs, and possibly corocoacromial and coracoid ligament hypertrophy. Impingement manifestations can occur when there is a "tissue minus" situation, as with a large cuff tear. The acromiohumeral interval is reduced. Should this circumstance be labeled compressive even though the most propitious treatment would be to restore cuff thickness while miniaturizing the anterior acromion?

There are causes of impingement that might be termed "*restrictive*"; adhesive capsules of fibroses of the bursa-cuff-arch spans are examples of disorders that restrict structure glide, create poor mechanics, and cause impingement. There are impingements that are combinations of compressive and restrictive. Glenohumeral instability may cause impingement signs but is difficult to classify. There may be no static encroachment on the subacromial space. However, the dynamic translation of the humeral head in certain arcs leads to poor mechanics and compression. Simple weakness of the shoulder girdle musculature can produce disharmony of the scapulohumeral rhythm and consequent signs and symptoms attributable to impingement. The relative multiplane rotations of the humeral head, arch, and scapula may alter the subacromial space to produce abnormal pulls and/or compression without being purely compressive or "restrictive." It is conceivable that multiplanar scapulometry (CT, MRI, or cine-MRI) performed in neutral and impingement postures may disclose alterations of the relationships of the participating bony landmarks.

For the orthopedic surgeon the importance of mechanism has been understated for two reasons. The first has been too little appreciation of the existence of mechanisms other than the "standard" compressive one. The second is that the orthopedic surgeon using the low-morbidity arthroscopic de-impingement has had a relatively high success rate without having had to relate its success to the etiological mechanism.

What, for example, creates the disability when there is a hypertrophic osteoarthritis of the AC joint with "downspurs"? Is it pain from the arthritic joint itself? . . . or the restrictive mechanics derived from reduced clavicular rotation with arm elevation? . . . or the downspurs compressing and abrading the underlying cuff? Would excising the distal end of the clavicle (while leaving the acromial side downspurs) adequately relieve symptoms by eliminating the joint pain and improving clavicular rotation? . . . or would excision of downspurs alone be more relieving? The answers to such questions could help the orthopedic surgeon minimize the surgical approach or at least make it more selective.

Of what help is special radiography in recognizing mechanistic contributions? Very little, in fact, other than to reveal the quantity of existing pathology in a static state. As stated, this is best accomplished using MRI. To this end, Stauffer et al.[15] have proposed a "staged" MRI classification of impingement that corresponds to Neer's classification[23,24] (box).

The Stauffer et al.[15] concept of staging and its correlation to clinical evidence is interesting, but two objections can be tendered:

1. Although it should not be presumed that Neer's concept is adequate to explain all clinically determined impingements, we do not wish to challenge its validity but only to point out its failure to include the entities and mechanisms discussed in the preceding paragraphs.
2. Evidence of impingement (any stage) is not necessarily quantifiably related to an expression of symptoms.

It is the latter point that is of particular import in discussing the influence of special radiography on an approach to treatment. The presence of *inflammatory* (fluid) *signs* alone might suggest that a clinical response to nonoperative management is achievable.

The study of Stauffer et al.[15] sought to determine

Stage I
A. Early AC joint hypertrophy; mild impingement on the supraspinatus tendon by the AC joint capsule or acromial spurs
B. Mildly increased signal in the supraspinatus tendon

Stage II
A. More advanced AC joint hypertrophy
B. Narrowing of the coracoacromial arch
C. Thinning of the supraspinatus tendon, with substantially increased signal intensity within the tendon; subchrondral zones of decreased signal in the posterosuperior portion of the greater tuberosity of the humerus

Stage III
A. Presence of a complete rotator cuff tear
B. Retraction; atrophy of the supraspinatus tendon and muscle
C. Advanced AC joint hypertrophy
D. Erosion of the undersurface of the acromion

From Neer CS: Clin Orthop 1983;173:70-77

whether subacromial space "congestion" could be definitively ascribed to a reversible edema or an irreversible fibrosis or bony constraint on the basis of MRI. Indeed, this is a difficult determination; reversible and irreversible components often coexist. Sequential MRI may reveal the effect of nonoperative treatment on the irreversible components; the value of sequential MRI evaluations has not yet been reported as a correlate to symptoms.

The presence of a given quantity of irreversible mechanical signs "by any radiographic technique" does not necessarily offer a prognosis for any intended surgery. The fact is that the individual mechanical contributors to impingement that can be visualized on MRI (rotator cuff, acromion, CAL, subacromial bursa) have yet to be assigned their apportioned contributions.

Therefore, the value of visualizing these structures as an aid to surgery or surgical planning is questionable. The coracoacromial ligament, for example, often implicated in the production of impingement symptoms and often excised in the hope of achieving symptomatic relief, may be visualized on MRI oblique sagittals or coronals (Fig. 16-1). Nevertheless, its visualization does not help determine whether the structure is impinging, and hence its visualization has no capacity to predict any relief that might be achieved by its resection (which results in increased bleeding from the thoracoacromial vascular arborization). The orthopedic surgeon is not certain as to which structures need be attacked and to what extent. As a result most surgeons performing de-impingements routinely attack all structures named above in a rote effort. After surgery, does the MRI still reveal evidence of impingement whether or not symptoms are present? This must still be studied (Plate 16-1).

As a rule, only patients with symptoms are submitted to MRI. The MR findings of impingement in symptomatic shoulders enforce a thrust to treat, their incidence in a symptom-free population being less well known. Flagrant mechanical impingement due to osseous projections from the acromion or the AC joint are determinable with conventional roentgenography or CT-arthrography. The primary advantage of MR for impingements is its demonstration of soft tissue abnormalities (cuff, ligaments, and bursa). As indicated, MR provides reenforcement and a measure of quantification. It is, as a rule, not a necessity for treatment.

The most critical element that may influence the extent of a treatment for impingement is the presence (and possibly the size) of an associated tear of the rotator cuff, and this information can be secured by numerous tests, as previously stated. Despite what may seem like a negative attitude about the use of MRI for impingement syndrome evaluation, we commonly implement this test. It is noninvasive, it provides the most information of all radiographic tests about impingement, it reveals the presence and gross size of existing cuff tears, it demonstrates levels of inflammatory response, and it shows other intra- as well as extracapsular pathology about the shoulder. Furthermore, it best supports any clinical suspicion of prevailing pathology.

Capsulolabral complex instability

The association between labral lesions and recurrent dislocations of the shoulder became more widely appreciated following the publication in 1938 of Bankart's study[33] on the pathology of dislocated shoulders. However, the role of isolated labral pathology was not widespread before the popularization of therapeutic shoulder arthroscopy in the early 1980s, despite the fact that shoulder arthrotomies were occasionally performed for pain, catching, and/or locking and revealed a torn labrum unrelated to instability.

Removal of the torn or bucketed portion would relieve the acute symptoms (Plate 16-2). As shoulder arthroscopy became more sophisticated, it became increasingly clear (through the reports of such workers as Andrews, Carson, and McLeod[34]) that isolated and symptom-producing tears, especially those of the superior labrum, were commonly found in the dominant shoulder of throwing athletes.

Almost concurrent with these orthopedic advances Mizuno and Hirohata[35] described the special use of arthrography to diagnose labral tears (associated with instability), thereby creating a possible diagnostic alternative to arthroscopy.

The technique, however, was too crude to serve as a reliable indicator of the need for surgery on an isolated labral lesion; actually tomography (as described in 1982 by Braunstein and O'Connor[1]) better demonstrated the superior and inferior portions of the labrum, and the double-contrast axillary slice technique of El-Khoury et al. (1979)[36] better demonstrated the anterior and posterior portions. In fact, Kleinman et al. (1984)[5] confirmed

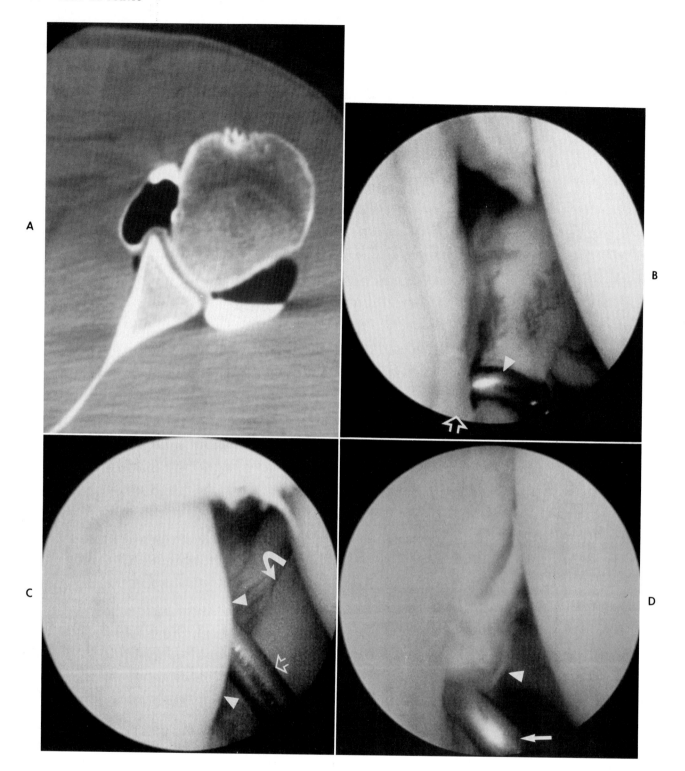

the efficacy of the latter technique, reporting 100% sensitivity and 80% specificity (based on surgical corroboration) for the detection of labrocapsular lesions.

CT arthrography proved to be even better, and a number of authors[2,3,7-9,17,18] have alluded to its merits. (For a comprehensive discussion of the subject the reader is referred to Rafii, Minkoff, and Di Stefano.[18]) These authors proclaim CT-arthrography to be "currently the most accurate radiographic means for the detection of lesions of the labrum" though not infallible [see Plate 16-2 and Fig. 16-4].) Deutsch et al. (1984)[3] claimed 100% sensitivity for anterior labral lesion discovery in a series of surgically corroborated CT-arthrographies. McNiesh and Callaghan (1987)[17] and Rafii et al. (1986 to 1989)[7-9,18] demonstrated the ability of computed arthrography to reveal not only tears and detachments but also morphological variations of the labrum.

MRI also has an excellent capacity for demonstrating

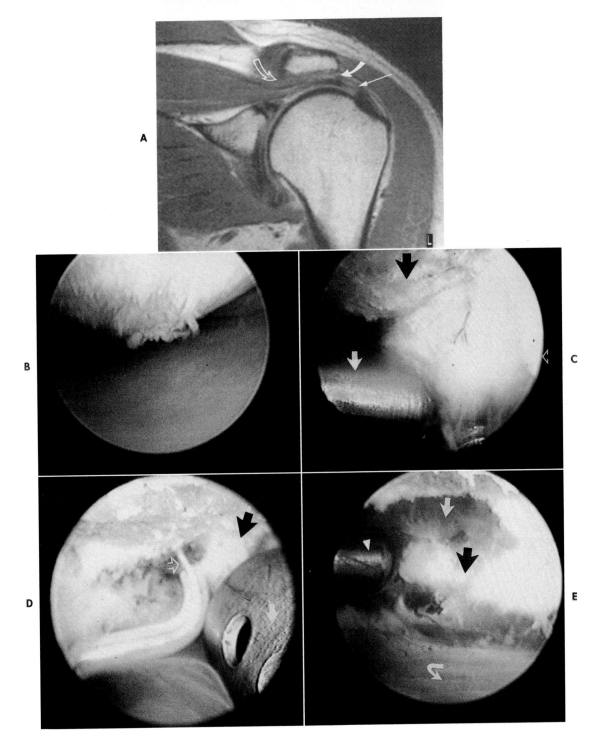

PLATE 16-1

A, Preoperative oblique coronal proton density (2100/30) MR image of the left shoulder in a middle-aged athlete with virtually all impingement tests positive on physical examination. Night pain was also exquisite. The peribursal fat signal is diminished due to a proliferative type of bursitis *(curved solid arrow)*. There is increased signal from the supraspinatus tendon, indicating tendinitis or degeneration *(straight arrow)*. Overgrowth of the acromial aspect of the AC joint may participate in the impingement *(curved hollow arrow)*. Arthroscopic photographs show the following: **B**, the degenerated undersurface of the anterolateral acromion tip prior to decompression; **C**, the undersurface of the anterior acromion denuded of its periosteal investment *(black arrow)* (with a metal shaver *[white arrow]* abutting on the white coracoacromial ligament); **D**, the transected coracoacromial ligament *(black arrow)* with a plastic insulated cautery *(open arrow)* (note the metallic inflow cannula at the lower right); and, **E**, the partially abraded undersurface of the acromion *(white arrow)* near the completion of decompression. Remnants of the coracoacromial ligament and subdeltoid bursa *(black arrow)* are being shaved out at the left *(arrowhead)*. The supraspinatus tendon demonstrates no overt pathology *(curved arrow)*.

Three months after decompression all symptoms were resolved and all impingement tests were negative. On a follow-up MRI the findings had changed minimally. One may be led to assume that the preponderance of signal in the supraspinatus tendon was due to degenerative rather than inflammatory change, since the symptoms dissipated in spite of signal persistence. The relative roles of each of the components of impingement in the production of this patient's symptoms remain undetermined.

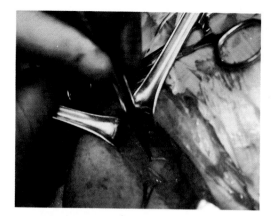

PLATE 16-2

Intraoperative photograph of the right shoulder of a middle-aged woman with a history of tolerable anterior glenohumeral instability until a few weeks prior to the operation. She suddenly began to experience pronounced and painful shifting within the joint. Arthrotomy revealed a completed bucket handle tear of the anterior labrum *(arrow)*. Of incidental note, a CT arthrogram had revealed a severely attenuated anterior labrum but failed to delineate the presence of a bucket handle tear.

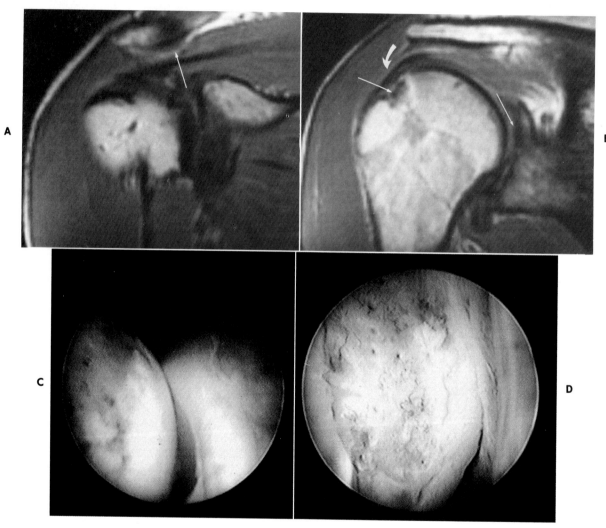

PLATE 16-3

Answers are not always easy: A 30-year-old throwing athlete presented with anterior pain about the dominant shoulder and no history of a specific traumatic episode. Clinical impingement signs were weakly positive. The opposite shoulder had undergone repair for recurrent anterior instability, but no symptoms of instability were present in the dominant shoulder. Physical therapy failed to provide relief of symptoms. **A,** Oblique coronal, proton density (2100/30) image. An acromial proliferative process *(arrow)* is visible anteriorly and may participate in the impingement. **B,** Oblique coronal, proton density (2100/30) image. More posteriorly the subdeltoid peribursal fat plane is obliterated, indicative of bursitis *(curved arrow)*. There is a degenerative irregularity of the anatomical neck of the humerus, adjacent humeral head, and glenoid *(straight arrows)*; but the implications of these are unclear (apart from arthritis). **C** and **D,** Posterior arthroscopic views of the glenohumeral joint reveal severe degenerative changes (especially in **D,** in which the posterior articular surface of the humeral head has been denuded to raw bone).

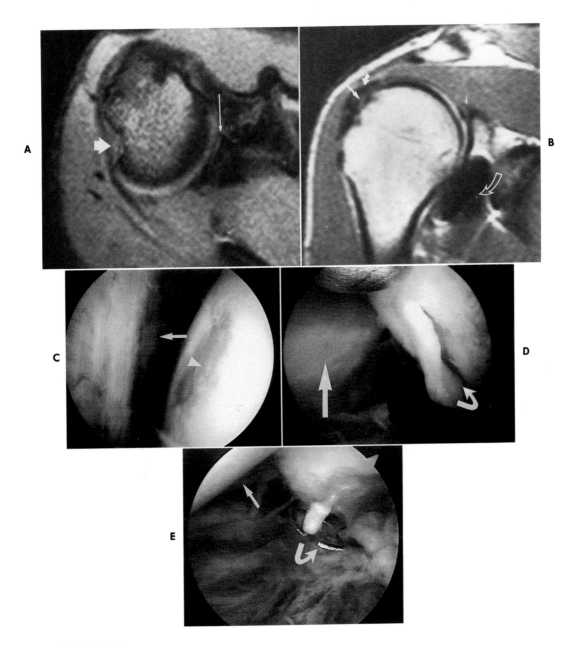

PLATE 16-4

A recreationally active man in his late 30s presented with pain and restricted range of motion in his right shoulder, which had undergone a prior Bristow operation for recurrent anterior instability. Evaluation in the office revealed no gross instability of the glenohumeral joint but a fibrotically captured joint with severe limitation of forward flexion and of abduction, extension, and external rotation (arm-cocked position). **A,** Axial gradient echo (400/18 and 70) image of the superior aspect of the glenohumeral joint. A large Hill-Sachs lesion is present *(short thick arrow),* but only a small remnant of the labrum can be seen *(long thin arrow).* Distortion of the image anteromedially is due to a metallic artifact. **B,** Oblique coronal, proton density (800/30) image. An osteochondral irregularity of the humeral head is visible *(straight arrow).* The supraspinatus tendon is intact *(curved arrow),* but only a remnant of the superior labrum is present *(small arrow).* The location of the Bristow procedure screw in the scapular neck is denoted by the signal void and slight image distortion due to a metallic artifact *(hollow arrow).* Posterior arthroscopic views of the joint demonstrate, **C,** severe erosive changes of the glenoid *(straight arrow)* on the left with erosion of the posterior humeral head on the right *(arrowhead),* **D,** the glenoid at the left *(straight arrow)* and the humeral head on the right with a large posteromedial flap of articular cartilage *(curved arrow)* (note the metallic shaving superiorly), and **E,** a pristine portion of the humeral head at the upper left *(straight arrow).* The screw from the prior Bristow operation *(curved arrow)* is seen "standing proud" from the scapular neck and retaining none of the tissue it was inserted to tether.

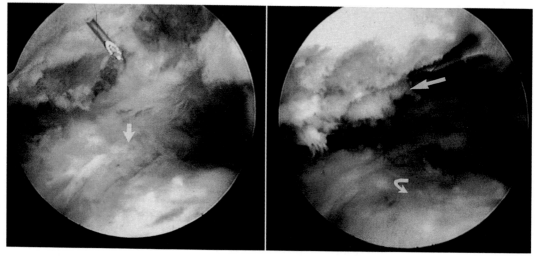

A

B

PLATE 16-5

Arthroscopic de-impingement. **A** and **B** are arthroscopic photographs of a right shoulder in the midst of a subacromial decompression. The bursa has been largely removed and the undersurface of the acromion has been stripped of its soft tissue coverings. What is apparent is that perspectives within the space are difficult to interpret with respect to what structures are producing impingement signs and to what extent debridement (e.g., partial acromionectomy) is necessary to gain relief. (In **A**, note the needle inserted through the AC joint anteriorly to help with geographic orientation. The supraspinatus tendon is seen below *[arrow]*. In **B**, a more lateral perspective, the partially denuded acromion can be seen above. The *straight arrow* resting on the metallic shaving points toward a remnant of the coracoacromial ligament. The supraspinatus tendon is seen below *[curved arrow]*.)

FIGURE 16-4

A (1985), CT arthrographic image of the left shoulder of a professional hockey player a few weeks after having sustained acute trauma. No history or symptoms of instability preexisted the injury. Other than attenuation of the anterior labrum, presumed to be degenerative in nature, the image reveals no pathology of note. Arthroscopic photographs taken within 1 week of the CT arthrogram demonstrate the glenoid on the left and humeral head on the right. **B** shows a probe surrounded by hemorrhage (*arrowhead*) at the site of disruption between the anteroinferior portion of the labrum (*hollow arrow*) and the anterior capsular structures. **C**, A more anterior and magnified view shows a probe (*hollow arrow*) lifting the detached and loosened labrum (*arrowheads*). Just behind the probe is the subscapularis tendon (*curved arrow*). **D** reveals a more inferior portion of the anterior labrum (*arrowhead*), which is torn and degenerated (as demonstrated by the probe, *straight solid arrow*).

The damaged labrum was arthroscopically debrided by shaving. The acute symptoms rapidly abated, but the patient ultimately began to have anterior instability. The accuracy and value of CT arthrography in this acute case are highly questionable, perhaps even misleading. Retrospectively, although the CT arthrogram did not show a tear of the capsulolabral complex, the characteristic location of labral attenuation and visualized expansion of the capsule were thought to have been manifestations of an occult instability. In current therapy, refixation of the complex to the glenoid by an arthroscopic technique might have been attempted to avert the progression of instability. Also a CT arthrogram or MR image might have hinted at the pathology, but only arthroscopy would have been unequivocally diagnostic as well as therapeutic.

---

lesions of the capsulolabral complex. Although we believe CT-arthrography more crisply delineates lesions of the complex, we also feel that MR coronal images reveal superior labral lesions to better advantage.

The orthopedic surgeon may deduce the possibility of an isolated labral lesion by history and physical examination. A throwing athlete, for example, with complaints of shoulder clicking, catching, or locking, and without evidence of frank instability on physical exam, would be suspected of having an isolated labral lesion.

Such evidence, though objective, is highly circumstantial. Assuming either a failure of conservative management or a special urgency, the surgeon has but two reasonable choices — to perform a diagnostic (and possibly therapeutic) arthroscopy or to attempt to prove the existence of the suspected lesion before undertaking any intervention. The choice must satisfy both patient and surgeon. If proving the existence of the lesion is the choice, any of the above-mentioned radiographic techniques may serve the purpose. If all techniques are available, the surgeon's choice should be MRI because of its ability to reveal the maximum information about other pathology that may be present, and because it is noninvasive.

The principal disadvantage of any of these techniques versus arthroscopy is the possibility, though small, that a falsely negative study will defer an appropriate treatment course (Fig. 16-4) or that a falsely positive one will encourage an unwarranted arthroscopy. In other words,

the radiographic techniques are highly accurate but arthroscopy is unerring in the evaluation of the labrum.

Of course, CT-arthrography and MRI are both excellent techniques for demonstrating the lesions of glenohumeral instability — labral abnormalities, capsular enlargements, abnormal capsular insertions.[2,7-9,17,18] However, practically speaking, the overwhelming majority of these are readily diagnosed by history and physical examination and thus there is virtually no need for computed arthrography or MRI to ascertain their existence, despite the possibility that their directions and associated pathology may require clarification. There is also little or no "downside" (other than financial) to performing a noninvasive MRI, which may confirm the suspected or reveal the unsuspected, though in other instances little will be added (Plates 16-3 and 16-4).

With respect to the case illustrated in Plate 16-3, MRI revealed no Hill-Sachs lesion of the humeral head but some evidence of ubiquitous degenerative disease of the glenohumeral joint. Examination under anesthesia revealed no glenohumeral instability, despite denudement of the posterior articular surface (which might of itself have been considered pathognomonic for anterior instability in a young man with no history of trauma or disease and a history of instability in the opposite shoulder), but the posterior lesion did not explain the anteriorly based pain and symptoms. Although some evidence of impingement based on MRI may have accounted for a few symptoms, arthroscopic decompression relieved the symptoms. A combination of MRI and arthroscopy was not adequate to explain all the ramifications of this case.

With respect to the case in Plate 16-4, upon induction of anesthesia a great amount of multidirectional instability became evident. MRI provided evidence of prior anterior instability but no insight as to why there should now be this multidirectional format (a common problem in patients who have had prior instability operations.) The MRI did suggest, however, the presence of degenerative change within the glenohumeral joint, though not with the clarity revealed by arthroscopy. In this instance it took an examination under anesthesia to reveal severe instability as a source of disability, and an arthroscopy to delineate the extent of articular damage as a possible contributor to the patient's chronic pain complaints.

There are instances in which CT-arthrography or MRI will reveal findings consistent with multidirectional instability when only a unidirectional format has been suspected.[9,18] Of course, "stress" views, especially when performed with the benefit of a general anesthetic, will usually reveal the same information, even when the physical examination is inconclusive. Oddly, though arthroscopy may disclose pathology consistent with a multidirectional (or any directional) instability, the "eye" is often almost too close in many cases to verify the magnitude and direction of displacement.

Since the middle 1980s there has been a progressive interest in and evolution of arthroscopic reconstructive techniques for the unstable shoulder[37-40] (Fig. 16-4). These procedures, which include advancement of the anterior capsule to the glenoid rim using the LCR staple system of Johnson,[38] or with sutures passed transscapularly (through its neck) from the anterior capsular to a posterior subcutaneous locus,[39] have evolved for use with arthroscopic reconstructions. One important guideline, however, is that any arthroscopic reconstructive technique be confined to unidirectional anterior instabilities. Experience with isolated posterior instabilities has not been reported.

Such an admonition might induce some surgeons to perform computed arthrography or MRI to rule out evidence of a posterior or multidirectional instability (not revealed by examination) before beginning an arthroscopic reconstruction. When the instability is multidirectional or the surgeon does not routinely perform arthroscopic reconstructions, open reconstructive techniques are recommended, often a capsular shift variety. In such cases, though cuff pathology may be associated with instability, there is little need for elaborate presurgical radiographic analysis beforehand.

The acutely injured shoulder is a potentially greater problem for both radiologist and orthopedist. The radiologist must contend with hemorrhage and swelling in discerning lesions and structural damage. MRI interpretation may be enhanced rather than compromised in this circumstance.

The orthopedist has been traditionally reluctant to intercede surgically in an acute shoulder injury, exceptions being the irreducible dislocation or a high degree of suspicion that the cuff has been ruptured. (In the latter case an arthrographic procedure would normally have preceded any exploration.) In some instances the patient is unaware of instability but has an appreciation only of pain at the time of the injury. CT-arthrography or MRI in such cases may help disclose the nature of the problem or help in planning an appropriate surgical procedure.

Injuries that initiate a progression of instability manifestations have become more and more respected in recent years. For example, in the second half of the 1980s Andrews[37] reported on a series of acute capsular disruptions that he repaired by an arthroscopic imbrication technique with screw fixation of the capsular margins to avert a progression of instability. Other authors[40] have reported similar experiences. It is easily reasoned that once such technical feats are possible there may no longer be a reason to defer reconstruction until after multiple episodes of instability have inflicted disability, time loss, and progressive damage.

Hence, in the closing years of the 1980s, a new and increasingly popular trend to arthroscope acute shoulder injuries has arisen. Workers such as Fu[41] and Baker[42] have provided evidence that acute capsulolabral repair is meritorious. Once again, MRI or CT arthrography may have presurgical value in distinguishing acute cuff lesions from those of the capsulolabral complex.

SUMMARY

Until the early 1980s orthopedic surgeons had been at a diagnostic disadvantage because of their inability to visualize soft tissue and some bony pathology of the shoulder with existing radiographic techniques. The one major exception was the ability to visualize full-thickness tears of the rotator cuff using arthrography, a technique that had come into vogue only during the 1970s. With the advent of techniques such as arthrotomography, computed arthrography, and ultimately MRI, much of the "visual" diagnostic disability was overcome. The orthopedic surgeon could then appreciate the presence and magnitude of rotator cuff tears, alterations of the bursa, tendonitides and other components of impingements, and tears and detachments of the capsulolabral complex that herald throwing and instability lesions.

While the above-cited radiographic techniques were being developed, orthopedists were becoming much more knowledgeable and their physical evaluations much more discerning with respect to cuff disease, impingement, and instability. More important, arthroscopy achieved an extremely high level of diagnostic accuracy and therapeutic ability for each of these entities during the same period.

As already indicated, the majority of glenohumeral instabilities can be discovered and treated without benefit of special radiography. Only the isolated labral tear requires a particular technique. Still, it is easily seen and treated by arthroscopy; in fact there is some concern that labral lesions may be "overtreated" simply because they can be visualized with special radiography or "undertreated" because the specificity of their definition is less reliable than the determination that "some" labral abnormality exists.

Most orthopedic surgeons consider that the physical signs of impingement are sufficient for predicating conservative or interventional treatment but a better perspective of needed therapy requires a preoperative imaging study (Plate 16-4). However, this is not true when the primary pathology resides in the rotator cuff. Physical examination is often inadequate as a basis for approaching the definitive treatment of cuff lesions. Whereas a full-thickness cuff tear may be diagnosed by arthrography alone, its size cannot be revealed by simple arthrography; nevertheless, such information is not particularly important for the majority of orthopedists.

By looking at Plate 16-4, it is possible to deduce that MRI is advantageous in these cases, providing both insight as to what structures should be keyed upon (by virtue of pathology and inflammation) and a baseline against which to compare future MRIs in the event symptoms fail to resolve or a recrudescence develops. Furthermore, the size and shape and the focus of offending tissue are less clearly appreciated by arthroscopy alone than when it is used in conjunction with MRI (which provides a truer concept of spur size, location, and magnitude and of the location of inflammatory response).

The "bottom line" is that special techniques such as CT-arthrography and MRI are valuable to orthopedic surgeons because they offer detailed information by relatively noninvasive means. Although arthroscopy has both therapeutic and diagnostic capability, it is surgically invasive (with a disability aftermath) and it does not reveal intrasubstance (cuff) pathology, extrasynovial processes (e.g., tumors), or subacromial encroachment as well as MRI does, which for these entities should be the modality of choice.

There are few times when the decision to treat and the nature of the treatment to be rendered are more significantly altered by special radiographic findings than in a setting where high sophistication and expertise (and philosophy) exist among surgeons and where special tests are expertly performed and interpreted. In our practice (devoted primarily to athletic medicine) and our community (where tests are expertly performed and evaluated) we have made frequent use of CT-arthrography (1983 to 1986) and MRI (1986 to the present) to both detail and confirm suspected diagnoses and to reveal unsuspected pathology. These modalities provide a baseline against which to compare future images of the shoulder and to help in planning surgery (arthroscopy vs. arthrotomy) and projected disability periods more accurately.

REFERENCES

1. Braunstein EM, O'Connor G: Double contrast arthrotomography of the shoulder. J Bone Joint Surg (Am) 1982;64:192-195.
2. DeHaven JP, Callaghan JJ, McNiesh LM, et al: A prospective comparison study of double contrast CT arthrography and shoulder arthroscopy. Walter Reed Army Medical Center. Presented at the AOSS San Francisco, January 1987.
3. Deutsch AL, Resnik D, Mink JH, et al: Glenohumeral joint: normal anatomy and clinical experience. Radiology 1984;153:603-609.
4. Kilcoyne RF, Matsen FA: Rotator cuff tear measurement by arthropneumotomography. AJR 1983;140:315-318.
5. Kleinman PK, Kanzaria PK, Gross TP, Pappas AM: Axillary arthrotomography of the glenoid labrum. AJR 1984;141:993-999.
6. McGlynn FJ, El-Khoury G, Albright JP: Arthrotomography of the glenoid labrum in shoulder instability. J Bone Joint Surg (Am) 1982;64:506-518.
7. Rafii M, Firooznia H, Bonamo JJ, et al: Athlete shoulder injuries: CT arthrographic findings. Radiology 1987;162:559-564.
8. Rafii M, Firooznia H, Golimbu C, et al: CT arthrography of capsular structures of the shoulder. AJR, 1986;146:361-367.
9. Rafii M, Minkoff J, Bonamo J, et al: CT arthrography of shoulder instabilities in athletes. Am J Sports Med 1988;16:352-361.
10. Burk DL Jr, Karasick D, Kurtz AB, et al: Rotator cuff tears: prospective comparison of MR imaging with arthrography, sonography, and surgery. AJR 153:87-92, 1989.
11. Burk DL Jr, Karasick D, Mitchell DG, Rifkin MD: MR imaging of the shoulder: correlation with plain radiography. AJR 1990;154:549-553.
12. Kneeland JB, Carrera GF, Middleton WD, et al: MR imaging of the shoulder: diagnosis of rotator cuff tears. AJR 1987;149:333-337.
13. Middleton WD, Kneeland JB, Carrera GF et al: High resolution MR imaging of the normal rotator cuff. AJR 1987;148:59-64.
14. Seeger LL, Gold RH, Bassett LW, Elman, H, et al: Shoulder impingement syndrome: MR findings in fifty-three shoulders. AJR 1988;150:343-347.
15. Stauffer A, Reicher M, Nottage W, et al: A comparison of MRI and conventional radiographic techniques of the shoulder with arthroscopic and surgical correlation. Presented at International Arthroscopy Association Meeting, Rome, May 1989.
16. Zlatkin MB, Iannotti JP, Roberts MC, et al: Rotator cuff tears: Diagnostic performances of MR imaging. Radiology 1989;172:223-229.
17. McNiesh LM, Callaghan, JJ: CT arthrography of the shoulder: Variations of the glenoid labrum. AJR 1987;149:963-966.
18. Rafii M, Minkoff J, Di Stefano V: Diagnostic imaging of the shoulder. In Nicholas JA, Hershman EB (eds): The upper extremity in sports medicine. St Louis, Mosby, 1990, pp 91-158.
19. Bigliani LV, Morrison DS, April EW: Morphology of acromion and its relationship to rotator cuff tears. Orthop Trans 1986;10:459-460(abstract).
20. Gerber C, Terrier F, Ganz R: The role of the coracoid process in the chronic impingement syndrome. J Bone Joint Surg [Br] 1985;67:703-708.
21. Hawkins RJ, Kennedy JC: Impingement syndrome in athletes. Am J Sports Med 1980;8:151-158.
22. Kessel L, Watson M: The painful arc syndrome. J Bone Joint Surg [Br] 1977;59:166-172.
23. Neer CS: Anterior acromioplasty for the chronic impingement syndrome in the shoulder: A preliminary report. J Bone Joint Surg [Am] 1972;54:41-50.
24. Neer CS: Impingement lesions. Clin Orthop 1983;173:70-77.
25. Ghelman B, Goldman A: The double-contrast shoulder arthrogram: evaluation of rotary cuff tears. Radiology 1977;124:251-254.
26. Goldman AB, Ghelman B: The double-contrast shoulder arthrogram. Radiology 1978;127:655-663.
27. Killoran PJ, Marcove RC, Freiberger RH: Shoulder arthrography, AJR 1968;103:658-668.
28. Middleton WD, Edelstein G, Reinus WR, et al: Sonographic detection of rotator cuff tears. AJR 1985;144:349-353.
29. Pattee GA, Snyder SJ: Sonographic evaluation of the rotator cuff: Correlation with arthroscopy. Arthroscopy 4:No. 1, 1988, 15-20.
30. Calvert PT, Packer NP, Stoker, DJ, et al: Arthrography of the shoulder after operative repair of the torn rotator cuff. J Bone Joint Surg [Br] 1986;68:147-150.
31. Gartsman GM: Arthroscopic subacromial arthroscopy for rotator cuff disease. Presented at the Fourth International Conference on Surgery of the Shoulder. New York, October 1989.
32. Ciullo JV, Koniuch MP, Teitge RA: Axillary roentgenography in clinical orthopedic practice. Orthop Trans 1982;6:451-452.
33. Bankart AS: The pathology and treatment of recurrent dislocation of the shoulder joint. Br J Surg 1938;26:23-29.
34. Andrews JR, Carson WG Jr, McLeod WD: Glenoid labrum tears related to the long head of the biceps. Am J Sports Med 1985;13:337-341.
35. Mizuno K, Hirohata K: Diagnosis of recurrent traumatic anterior subluxation of the shoulder. Clin Orthop 1983;179:160-167.
36. El-Khoury GY, Albright JP, Yousef MA, et al: Arthrotomography of the glenoid labrum. Radiology 1979;131:333-337.
37. Andrews JR: Arthroscopic evaluation of the shoulder and methods to document subluxation during arthroscopic visualization. Presented June 27, 1987, Amelia Island Plantation.
38. Johnson LC: Personal communication, 1990.
39. Morgan CD, Bodenstab AB: Arthroscopic suture repair: Technique and early results. Arthroscopy 1987;3:111-122.
40. Warren RF: Personal communication, 1987.
41. Fu F: Significance of a partial and full Bankart lesion: A biochemical comparison. Lecture presented June 17, 1989, Traverse City, Michigan.
42. Baker C: Initial anterior shoulder dislocations. Lecture presented June 17, 1989, Traverse City, Michigan.

17 Elbow

CORNELIA N. GOLIMBU

Computed tomography (CT) of the elbow has been established as a useful imaging modality for fractures, especially those that are comminuted or complicated by displacement and angulation.[1-4] Calcified intraarticular loose bodies or fragments of bone can be precisely located. Cartilaginous loose bodies, synovial pathology, and osteochondritis dissecans are best studied by CT performed immediately after double-contrast arthrography (CT-arthrography).[5]

As a result of the increasing usage of magnetic resonance imaging, however, the indications for CT of the elbow are changing. MR is preferred for its multiplanar imaging capabilities and its noninvasive nature. It can detect abnormalities in the bone marrow, capsule, ligaments, and periarticular soft tissues.[6]

MRI of the elbow is directly dependent upon the use of surface coils specialized for the imaging of extremities.[7,8] Even though it is not done as frequently as MRI of the other joints (the knee, shoulder, wrist, hip, and ankle), the demand for imaging of the elbow has been increasing.[9] This increase is mostly the result of familiarity of radiologists and referring clinicians with the large range of pathology diagnosed by MRI. A confident and prompt MR diagnosis of problem cases is the most convincing

argument in favor of MRI of the elbow. To properly treat such patients, clinicians need to know more about the layers of cartilage, the capsule and ligaments, and the tendons and other paraarticular soft tissues.

ANATOMY

The elbow is a complex joint formed by three distinct articulations: ulnohumeral, radiohumeral, and radioulnar. The first two function has as a hinge, permitting flexion and extension between the arm and forearm; the last two accomplish the pivot motion of pronation and supination and are functionally linked to the distal radioulnar joint and the wrist. These joints have a common articular cavity and share a multitude of enveloping structures — including synovium, capsule, and ligaments, which make the elbow a single anatomical unit.[10]

Bone structures

The distal end of the humerus has a characteristic shape derived from the presence of two distinct articular surfaces and the medial and lateral condyles and epicondyles.[10,11] The cross section of the diaphysis of the humerus is triangular. The metaphyseal segment widens transversely to form the lateral and medial condyles and

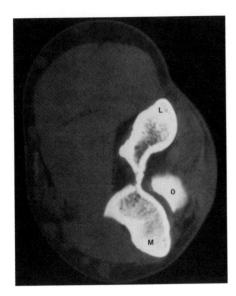

FIGURE 17-1
Normal humerus. A CT axial image through the medial *(M)* and lateral *(L)* epicondyles. *O,* Olecranon.

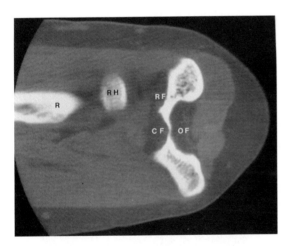

FIGURE 17-2
Olecranon and coronoid fossa of the humerus. An axial CT image shows a thin layer of bone separating the two depressions of the distal humerus: posteriorly the olecranon fossa *(OF),* anteriorly the coronoid *(CF)* and radial *(RF)* fossae. The radial head *(RH)* and diaphysis *(R)* are partially visible.

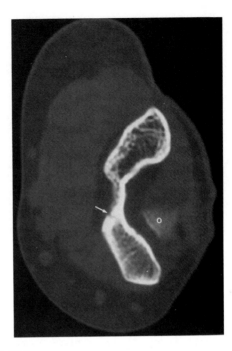

FIGURE 17-3
Normal humerus. Nutrient vessel groove. A CT axial image of the condylar segment of the humerus shows interruption of the anterior cortex *(arrow)* at the point of entry of a vessel in the coronoid fossa. The olecranon *(O)* is partially visible.

the epicondyles (Fig. 17-1). Just lateral to the medial epicondyle is a groove that contains the ulnar nerve. The central part of the humerus, between the condyles, is thin and formed mainly by cortical bone with biconcave surfaces: anterior is the shallow coronoid fossa, posteriorly the deep olecranon fossa. In flexion and extension these depressions are occupied respectively by the coronoid process and olecranon process of the ulna. Occasionally the thin cortical bone separating the olecranon from the coronoid fossa is perforated.[12] Absence of this bone wall is a normal variant and should not be confused with a zone of bony destruction (Fig. 17-2.) Nutrient vessels enter the humerus in the proximal margin of these fossae;

they are seen on CT images as low-density lines traversing the cortex on their way to the medullary cavity (Fig. 17-3).

The radial fossa is a small shallow depression on the anterolateral surface of the humerus that accommodates the radial head in flexion.

The distal humerus has two articular surfaces, the capitellum and trochlea. The capitellum has a flat posterior surface and a spherical inferior and anterior part covered by cartilage. It articulates with the concave superior surface of the radial head. A shallow groove covered by articular cartilage separates it from the trochlea; this is called the capitellotrochlear sulcus. The trochlea is an articular surface, concave in the transverse direction and convex in the anteroposterior direction, that resembles a pulley or an hourglass placed horizontally. This surfaces locks-in tightly with the proximal ulna (Fig. 17-4).

The superior end of the ulna has two components, the olecranon and the coronoid process, that together form an articular surface concave anteroposteriorly and slightly convex in the transverse dimension (the semilunar or trochlear notch). A shallow linear depression in this notch is not covered by articular cartilage, appearing like a seam of rough irregular cortical bone 2 to 3 mm long and transversely oriented across the proximal ulna. This groove is best seen on sagittal images, where the contrast between smooth articular cortex (covered by a hyaline cartilage) and the rough "seam" (devoid of cartilage) serves to distinguish the olecranon from the coronoid processes (Fig. 17-5).

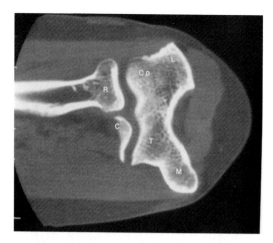

FIGURE 17-4
Distal humerus. A CT axial image shows the articulation between the head *(R)* and capitellum *(Cp)* and between the trochlea *(T)* and coronoid process *(C)*. The medial epicondyle *(M)* is large, the lateral *(L)* smaller.

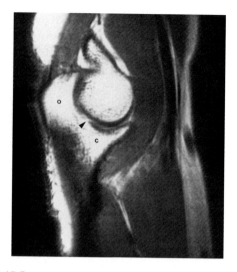

FIGURE 17-5
Normal ulna. A sagittal T1-weighted image shows the olecranon *(O)* and coronoid *(C)* separated by a line devoid of articular cartilage *(arrowhead)*.

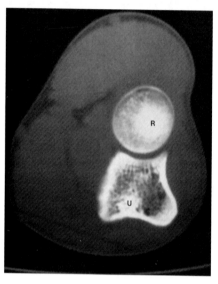

FIGURE 17-6
Normal proximal radioulnar joint. An axial CT image of the elbow shows the concave articular surface of the ulna *(U)* articulating with the round radial head *(R)*.

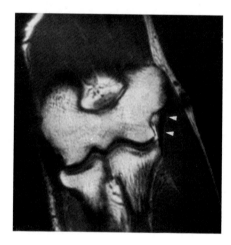

FIGURE 17-7
Ulnar collateral ligament. A coronal T1-weighted image shows the signal void of the anterior band of the ligament *(arrowheads)*.

On the lateral side of the proximal ulna is a third articular surface, the radial notch, that contacts the vertical cylindrical surface of the radial head (Fig. 17-6).

A large part of the proximal end of the radius is covered by articular cartilage. The radial head has an almost cylindrical shape with a slightly concave superior surface. Inferiorly it is mildly constricted (described as the neck).[13] More distally and toward the anteromedial side is the prominent radial tubercle, the site of insertion of the biceps brachii. The interdigitations of tendon and periosteum give a rough irregular contour to the cortical bone surface of the radial tubercle, evident on axial images, that should not be confused with periostitis (see Fig. 17-4).

Articular capsule and ligaments

As in most hinge joints, the capsule of the elbow is relatively weak and loose anteriorly and posteriorly, permitting the large range of flexion—extension. The capsule is reinforced medially and laterally by the strong collateral ligaments.

The ulnar collateral ligament has three distinct components: an anterior, a posterior, and a thick transverse band (the ligament of Cooper). The anterior and posterior bands originate on the medial epicondyle near the common origin of the superficial flexor muscles and insert on the medial surfaces of the coronoid and olecranon respectively (Fig. 17-7). The triangular space left between them is filled with a thin layer of fibrous

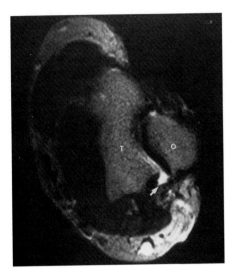

FIGURE 17-8
Ulnohumeral recess of the synovial space. A T2-weighted axial image shows a small collection of fluid *(arrow)* at the medial margin of the joint space between the olecranon *(O)* and trochlea *(T)* in a patient with no joint effusion.

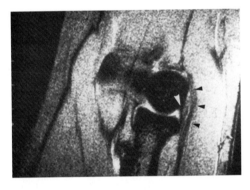

FIGURE 17-9
Radial collateral ligament. A coronal T2* shows the ligament *(white arrowhead)* originating on the humerus, beneath the common tendon of the extensor muscles *(black arrowheads).*

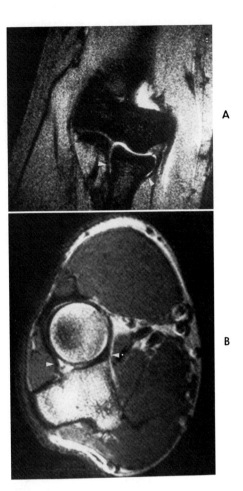

FIGURE 17-10
Annular ligament. **A,** A coronal T2*-weighted image discloses fluid within the joint outlining the inner surface of the annular ligament *(arrowhead).* **B,** An axial proton density–weighted image shows the ulnar insertion of the ligament *(arrowheads).*

tissue on which the ulnar nerve lies. Inferiorly this triangular space is marginated by the thick transverse ligament of Cooper, which stretches between the medial side of the olecranon and coronoid processes, uniting the inferior ends of the anterior and posterior bands. The inferior margin of the transverse ligament of Cooper is not attached to bone; a free space exists beneath it, through which an outpouching of synovium can be seen either with certain movements that shift the normal joint fluid to this area or in a joint overdistended by effusion (Fig. 17-8).

The radial collateral ligament is a thick band of fibrous tissue triangular in shape, with its apex attached on the lateral epicondyle, adjacent to and beneath the common origin of the extensor muscles (Fig. 17-9). From here it flares distally, forming the base of the triangle at its insertion on the anterior and posterior margins of the radial notch of the ulna and on the annular ligament itself.

The annular ligament is a thick band of fibrous tissue attached to the anterior and posterior margins of the radial notch of the ulna. It completes the four fifths of the ring in which the radial head rotates; the fifth part of this ring is provided by the articular surface forming the radial notch of the ulna (Fig. 17-10). The ligament is tighter inferiorly; this feature, as well as the slightly tilted articular surface of the ulna, provides a funnellike space for the radial head. The narrow part tightens around the radial neck, preventing the inferior displacement of the radial head.

Synovium

The synovial membrane lines the inner surface of the articular capsule of the elbow joint. It extends inferiorly under the margin of the annular ligament and reflects itself in an upward fold to insert on the neck of the radius.[12] In the olecranon and coronoid fossae, fat pads fill the loose space between the synovial membrane and articular capsule (Fig. 17-11). Joint effusions or hemarthroses displace these fat pads from their deep position in

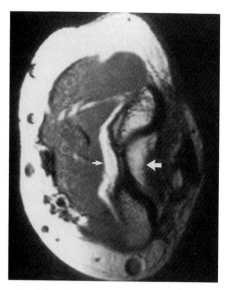

FIGURE 17-11
Normal anterior and posterior fat pads. Proton density–weighted axial image of the distal humerus (TR 2100 msec/TE 29 msec). Fat is located deep in the olecranon fossa posteriorly *(large arrow)* and the coronoid fossa anteriorly *(small arrow)*.

the two fossae, making them protrude away from the adjacent bony surface. When displaced, the olecranon fat pad becomes visible on lateral roentgenograms (positive fat pad sign).

A normal outpouching of the synovial membrane in the elbow can be seen around the radial neck, inferior to the annular ligament, as well as beneath the transverse fibers of the collateral ligament (of Cooper) and the fibers bridging horizontally the superior margin of the olecranon fossa.

Muscles and tendons

Numerous muscles and tendons originate or insert on the osseous surfaces of the elbow. Their spatial arrangement can be best described in an orderly fashion by dividing them into lateral, anterior, medial, and posterior groups.[12]

Lateral group. Three muscles are included in the lateral group: the brachioradialis, the extensor, and the supinator.

The brachioradialis is the most superficial of the lateral muscles. Its origin is on the lateral supracondylar ridge of

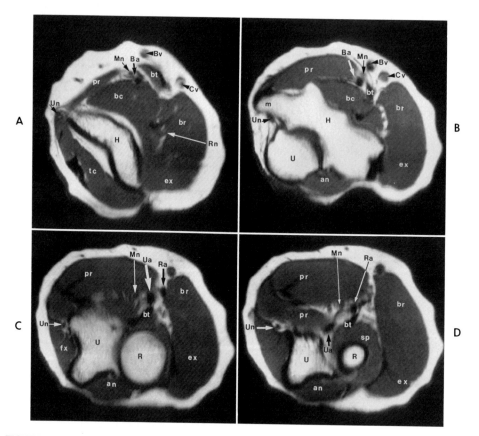

FIGURE 17-12
Cross-sectional anatomy of the elbow. MR images, **A**, through the distal humerus, **B**, through the epicondyles, **C**, through the radial head, and, **D**, through the radial neck. The following are shown: humerus *(H)*; ulna *(U)*; radius *(R)*; medial epicondyle *(m)*. Note also the *an*, anconeus muscle; *Ba*, brachial artery; *bc*, brachialis muscle; *br*, brachioradialis muscle; *bt*, biceps tendon; *Bv*, basilic vein; *Cv*, cephalic vein; *ex*, extensor muscles of the wrist; *fx*, flexor muscles of the wrist; *Mn*, median nerve; *pr*, pronator teres; *Ra*, radial artery; *Rn*, radial nerve; *sp*, supinator muscle; *tc*, triceps muscle; *Ua*, ulnar artery; and *Un*, ulnar nerve.

the distal humerus, and its fusiform flat part stretches inferiorly over the elbow joint toward the midforearm, where it becomes tendinous; further distally it inserts on the radial styloid.

Posterior and deep to the brachioradialis is the extensor carpi radialis longus. This muscle originates on the same lateral supracondylar ridge as the brachioradialis, only slightly more distally. It ends in a tendon that courses toward the dorsal part of the wrist and inserts on the posterior surface of the base of the second metacarpal. More posterior and deeper to this muscle, on the dorsal surface of the lateral epicondyle, is the common tendinous origin of the extensor carpi radialis brevis, extensor digitorum, extensor digiti minimi, and extensor carpi ulnaris. All these muscles have separate individual bellies only in the midarm; at the elbow they are united and appear in cross section as a single structure (Fig. 17-12).

The supinator is the deepest muscle in the lateral group and is completely covered by the superficial muscle layers. Its main origin is on the posterolateral surface of the ulna and the inferior surface of the lateral epicondyle, where it courses inferiorly and laterally to wrap around the proximal radius. It inserts on the anterior surface of the proximal radial diaphysis. In full pronation this muscle almost completely surrounds the proximal radius.

Anterior group. The anterior structures include the biceps and, at a deeper level, the brachialis.

The biceps originates as two separate tendons, at the coracoid (short head) and on the superior margin of the glenoid of the scapula (long head). They unite in midarm to form a common belly; further distally this tapers abruptly to a tendon that runs longitudinally in the anticubital fossa toward the dorsal part of the radial tuberosity (Fig. 17-13). A small bursa separates the volar

surface of the tuberosity from the terminal segment of the biceps tendon.

The bicipital aponeurosis, a direct continuation of the superficial surface of the musculotendinous junction of the biceps, is a band of fibrous tissues covering the brachial artery and the median nerve. It ends by joining the fascial layer that covers the origin of the pronator and flexor muscles.

The brachialis originates on a large area of the distal humerus. Its belly covers anteriorly the elbow joint and ends in a short tendon attached to the anterior surface of the proximal ulna, on a prominence called the brachialis (or ulnar) tuberosity (Fig. 17-13).

Medial group. The muscles in the medial group are arranged in three layers: Superficially and more laterally is the pronator teres. Beneath it and more medially is the common tendinous origin of the palmaris longus and the flexor muscles of the wrist and fingers (flexor carpi radialis, flexor digitorum superficialis and flexor carpi ulnaris); differentiation among these muscles is difficult at the elbow, since they do not become distinct structures until the forearm. The deep layer is formed by the flexor digitorum profundus and flexor pollicis longus. All these structures are more distinctly separated in the forearm and wrist.

Of all the medial muscles the pronator teres is the one most commonly visualized in axial images of the elbow. It has a double origin: from the distal humerus, superior to the medial epicondyle (the superficial head), and from the medial surface of the coronoid process of the ulna (the smaller deep head). The median nerve traverses the elbow beneath the deep and superficial tendons of this muscle. The pronator teres is obliquely oriented, forming the medial border of the antecubital fossa and continuing

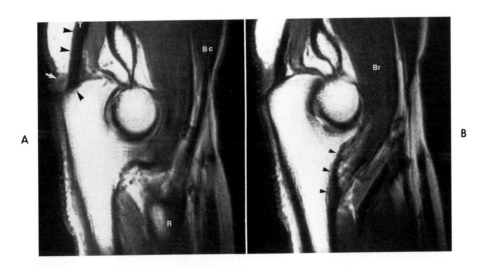

FIGURE 17-13
Three major muscles inserting at the elbow. **A,** T1-weighted sagittal image. The triceps tendon *(T)* appears as a signal void band inserting on the olecranon *(arrowheads)*. The olecranon bursa is superficial to the tendon insertion *(arrow)*. Note that the biceps *(Bc)* has its insertion *(arrowheads)* on the radial tubercle *(R)*. **B,** T1-weighted sagittal image. *Arrowheads* point to the brachialis *(Br)* insertion on the ulna.

laterally toward the midforearm to insert on the lateral surface of the middiaphysis of the radius.

Posterior group. Two muscles form the posterior group: the triceps and the anconeus.

The triceps originates near the inferior margin of the glenoid (long head) and on the mediolateral posterior surface of the humeral diaphysis (medial and lateral head). Its belly forms the fleshy contour of the posterior part of the arm. At the elbow, the triceps is represented by a broad, flat tendon inserted on the posterior surface of the olecranon process of the ulna (see Fig. 17-13).

The anconeus is a small triangular structure originating on the posterior surface of the lateral epicondyle, from where it takes an oblique direction medially toward the dorsal surface of the olecranon process.

Vessels and nerves

The brachial artery is the most important arterial vessel at the elbow. In the distal segment of the arm it descends parallel to the medial margins of the biceps muscle and tendon. In the cubital fossa it divides into the radial and ulnar arteries. Recurrent branches of these then anastomose with corresponding collateral branches of the brachial artery to form a complex network of small arteries supplying the structures of the elbow (Fig. 17-12).

The radial artery continues in the direction of the brachialis anterior to the tendon of the biceps, across the supinator and pronator teres; it is covered anteriorly by the brachioradialis muscle (Fig. 17-12).

The ulnar artery is the largest of the two terminal branches of the brachial artery. Just after its origin in the cubital fossa, it crosses obliquely and deeper under the pronator teres and flexor muscles.

The brachial, radial, and ulnar arteries are accompanied by paired veins (venae comitantes) that run parallel to the arterial channels.[14]

In addition to these deep veins, there is a network of superficial venous structures in the forearm that come together at the elbow to form two main channels: the cephalic vein (on the lateral side of the cubital fossa) and the basilic vein (on the medial side). Between these two there is an anastomotic channel, the median cubital vein, located subcutaneously. Commonly the anastomotic channels between these veins describe a letter M configuration in the subcutaneous soft tissues of the anterior elbow.

The visualization of nerves on axial images of the elbow is directly related to the amount of fat present around them. The fat provides a natural background of contrast that permits identification of the three main nerves of the elbow: median, ulnar, and radial.

The median nerve descends in the lower part of the arm alongside the brachial artery, crosses anterior to it in the cubital area, and continues inferiorly between the deep and superficial heads of the pronator teres muscle (Fig. 17-12). Further distally it is located in the middle of the anterior compartment of the forearm, between the superficial and deep flexor muscles.

The ulnar nerve crosses the elbow on the posteromedial side; only the segment that passes in the groove between the medial epicondyle and olecranon process is seen on axial images; at this point it is surrounded by an abundant fat layer (Fig. 17-14). The ulnar nerve groove is covered posteriorly by an aponeurotic layer that stretches between the epicondyle and the olecranon. Further distally, where the nerve is located between the flexors digitorum superficialis and profundus and the flexor carpi ulnaris, there is seldom enough fat for the necessary natural contrast to make this nerve identifiable on axial images.

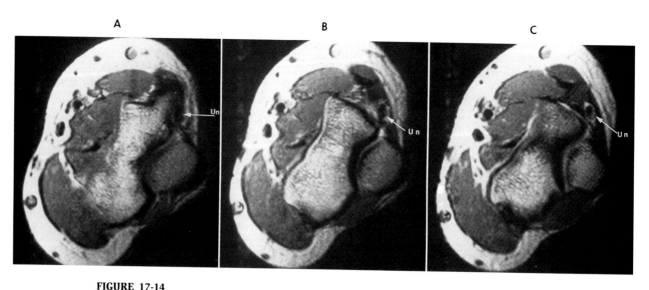

FIGURE 17-14
Normal ulnar nerve. Consecutive axial proton density–weighted images (TR 2100/TE 29). **A**, At the medial epicondyle and, **B** and **C**, more distal. The ulnar nerve *(Un)* is in the osseous groove on the posterior surface of the medial epicondyle.

The radial nerve descends in the distal segment of the arm between the brachialis and brachioradialis muscles. At the elbow it divides into thin and deep superficial branches, which are only occasionally visualized, between the supinator and brachioradialis muscles (Fig. 17-12).

COMPUTED TOMOGRAPHY
Technique

When scanning the elbow, it is most comfortable for the patient to be prone with the arm fully extended above the shoulder (Fig. 17-15). In some cases a lateral decubitus position is preferred, with the extremity to be studied in extension, abducted above the shoulder and placed on the scanner table with the volar surface up (Fig. 17-16).

Patients who have disease-related limitation of extension should be scanned with the elbow in 90 degrees of flexion and the ulnar side of the forearm on the table (Fig. 17-17). The axial images obtained through the humerus continue inferiorly with coronal representation of the structures of the forearm (Fig. 17-18).

The field of view should be limited to the minimal size necessary to encompass all the anatomical structures of the elbow, including soft tissues. Usually this is 15 to 20 cm. Targetted views facilitate visualization of the elbow placed eccentrically on the scanner table.

Slice thicknesses of 3 mm are used in most cases and represent a practical compromise between the desire to have maximum resolution of sloping bone surfaces and the need to limit the time and irradiation allowed for this examination. When small-sized loose osseous bodies are suspected, 1.5 mm thick slices limited to the zone of interest can be obtained.

Reformatted images in the sagittal or oblique plane can be made from the stack of sequential axial images.

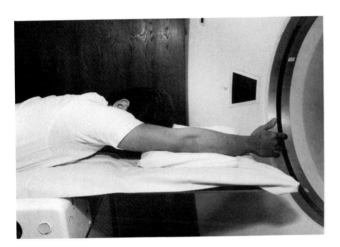

FIGURE 17-15
Technique of elbow CT. The patient is positioned prone, with arm extended above the head, medial side on the table.

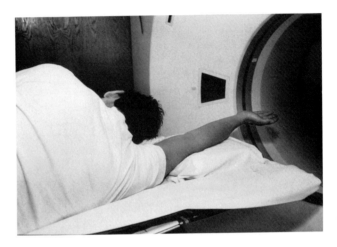

FIGURE 17-16
Technique of elbow CT. Lateral decubitus, with the arm extended, dorsal side down on the scanner table.

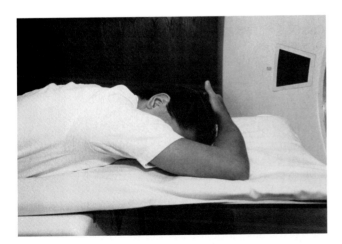

FIGURE 17-17
Technique of elbow CT. Prone, with the arm abducted above the head and the elbow flexed 90 degrees, medial side down.

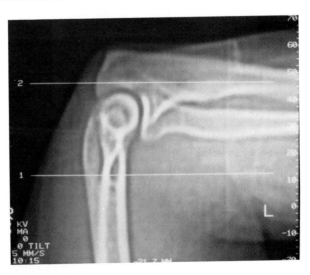

FIGURE 17-18
Technique of elbow CT. Scout view of the elbow flexed 90 degrees. The *two lines* superimposed on the image represent the most proximal and most distal slice location.

CT-arthrography

The indications for elbow CT-arthrography include detecting cartilaginous intrasynovial loose bodies and synovial abnormalities and assessing the cartilaginous surfaces and articular cortex.[15]

Double-contrast arthrography of the elbow is performed by introducing contrast through a 23-gauge needle placed lateroposteriorly and aiming at the space between the radial head and capitellum. The joint is distended by injecting 8 to 12 ml of room air; 0.5 to 1 ml of radiopaque contrast medium (Reno-M-60, diatrizoate meglumine) is usually sufficient to coat the entire joint surface. The injection is performed under fluoroscopic control, which assures correct positioning of the needle and proper distention of the synovial space, thus avoiding leakage of contrast outside the joint cavity.[16-18] After the injection routine projection roentgenograms are obtained, followed within a few minutes by the CT scan. A lapse of more than 30 minutes between injection and scanning is undesirable; the contrast coating the joint surfaces becomes diluted by newly secreted synovial fluid. When CT is performed immediately after the arthrogram, there is no need to add epinephrine to the injected contrast material.

After the injection, to avoid rupturing the fragile layer of synovium (already stretched by air distention of the joint), motion of the elbow should be kept to a minimum. The CT examination consists of 3 mm thick axial images obtained from the radial neck to the superior margin of the olecranon fossa (Fig. 17-19).

MAGNETIC RESONANCE Technique

High-resolution MR images of the elbow can be performed only with dedicated extremity coils capable of showing a small field. These may be either a flexible surface coil wrapped around the extremity or a hinged multipurpose extremity coil.[7-9] Only when extreme lateral decentering is permitted by the scanner functioning parameters is the elbow placed in the resting position, with the arm by the patient's side. Otherwise, it must be placed close to or in the scanner center by positioning the patient prone on the table with the arm extended above the head (Fig. 17-20).

When specific point tenderness or a localized small mass is the reason for the examination, it helps to mark this area with a lipid-containing marker attached to the skin (Fig. 17-21).

The first sequence consists of T1-weighted images with 7 mm thick slices at 10 mm intervals; these serve as scout views to facilitate orientation of the coronal and axial slices (Fig. 17-21).

Then spin echo T1-weighted images are obtained in the coronal or sagittal plane with a TR of 500 msec, a TE of 20 to 30 msec, two to four measurements, a 256 × 256 matrix, a field of view (FOV) of 12 to 16 cm, a slice thickness of 3 mm, and an interslice gap of 0.5 mm.

T2-weighted axial images are obtained with a TR of 1800 and 2400 msec, a TE of 80 and 100 msec, two measurements, a 256 × 256 matrix, an FOV of 12 to 16

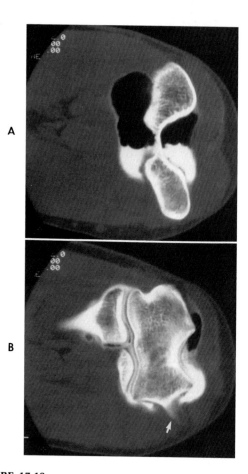

FIGURE 17-19
CT-arthrogram of the elbow. **A,** Axial image of the coronoid and olecranon fossae. The synovial spaces are distended by air and positive contrast. Bubbles of air give an irregular contour to the air/fluid level. **B,** Normal articular cartilage coated with contrast. The medial epicondyle *(arrow)* is outside the synovial space.

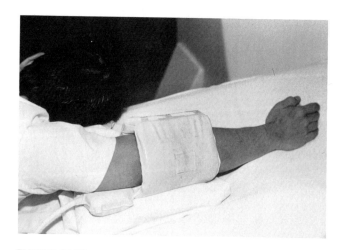

FIGURE 17-20
Technique of elbow MR using the flexible wraparound coil. The patient is positioned with elbow extended, arm above the head.

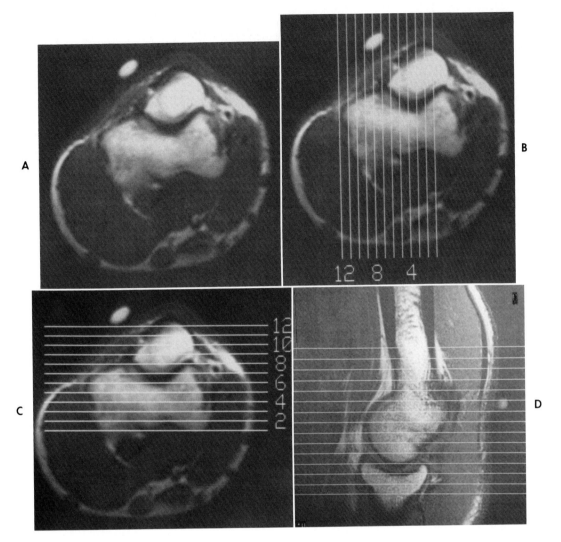

FIGURE 17-21
MRI technique. Slice orientation. **A,** Axial scout, with a marker placed on the skin at the site of point tenderness. The orientation of sagittal, **B,** and coronal, **C,** images is shown. **D,** Axial images are planned on the sagittal image.

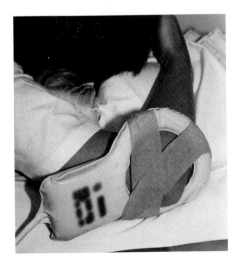

FIGURE 17-22
Technique of elbow MRI using a flat circular coil. The patient is positioned with the elbow flexed 90 degrees, and the coil is taped in place around the elbow.

cm, and slices 3 to 5 mm thick. By using a first-echo TE of 30 msec, it is possible to obtain a proton density type of image with no additional expenditure of time in each spin echo T2-weighted sequence.

Sagittal gradient-recalled or T2* images are useful in portraying the joint surfaces against a background of bright signal from the synovial fluid.[9] They are obtained with a TR of 600 and TE of 22 msec, a flip angle of 20 degrees, a matrix of 256×256 with two measurements, an FOV of 12 to 16 cm, and a slice thickness of 3 mm.

As with CT, when full extension of the elbow is not possible during an MR examination, it is preferred to scan the joint in 90 degrees of flexion rather than in an intermediary semiflexed position (Fig. 17-22). The medial side of the elbow and forearm is placed on the scanner table, which allows slices in the coronal plane of the scanner to produce sagittal views of the anatomy. Images in the sagittal plane of the scanner produce coronal views of the humerus and axial views of the radius and ulna (Fig. 17-23, *A*). Conversely, slices oriented axially in the scanner produce axial images of the humerus and coronal images of the radius and ulna (Fig. 17-23, *B*).

Intravenous administration of gadopentetate plays a role limited mostly to enhancement of the vascularized parts of mass lesions. Its usefulness as an intraarticular contrast agent is still being evaluated.[19,20]

MRI of the normal elbow

As in all other parts of the muscloskeletal system, MR images of the elbow provide exquisite differentiation between muscles, tendons, ligaments, and neurovascular and osseous structures.[21-24] In T1-weighted images the fatty marrow is seen as a homogeneous zone of bright signal in the humerus, ulna, and radius (Figs. 17-24 and 17-25). Normal low-signal horizontal striations in the distal humerus represents struts of dense compact bone traversing the spongy bone of the metaphysis (Fig. 17-26). The cortical bone is represented by a band of signal void. The hyaline articular cartilage is seen on T1-weighted images as a zone of intermediate signal (Fig. 17-27).

On T2- or T2*-weighted sequences the superficial layer of articular cartilage has a bright signal that may be summated with signal from the articular fluid to form one rather homogeneous high-signal zone (Figs. 17-28 and 17-29). The cartilage is not distinguishable from synovial fluid on T2-weighted images.

TRAUMATIC LESIONS
Tendon tears

The two most powerful muscles acting antagonistically on the elbow, the biceps and the triceps, are occasionally subjected to distracting forces that may produce an avulsion at their insertion site on the bone surface or a tear in the tendon itself. Often degenerative disease of the collagenous fibers reduces the mechanical resistance of these structures, making them prone to intratendinous tears, even after minor but repetitive trauma.

On MR images the normal triceps tendon is represented as a band of signal void (Fig. 17-30). A tear in the tendon appears as a zone of high signal intensity on T2-weighted images. In full-thickness tears this abnormal signal area can replace the signal void representing the tendon. The end of the torn tendon appears irregular and frayed. In cases of partial-thickness or intratendinous tears the high-signal zone is margined or contained by the low signal representing the remaining portion of the ligament. On proton density–type images such a tear is seen as a zone of intermediate signal intensity (Fig. 17-31).

During the acute phase of an injury, edema and hemorrhage surround the tear and are manifested as obliteration of the fat planes around the tendon by a diffuse zone of intermediate or high signal intensity. When the hematoma begins to heal, it may appear as a cystic collection of fluid with a characteristically high signal intensity in T2-weighted images and intermediate signal on T1-weighted images. The absence of normal tendon in its place of insertion and the retraction of muscle fibers are clues that the hematoma represents pathology associated with the complete tendon tear.[25]

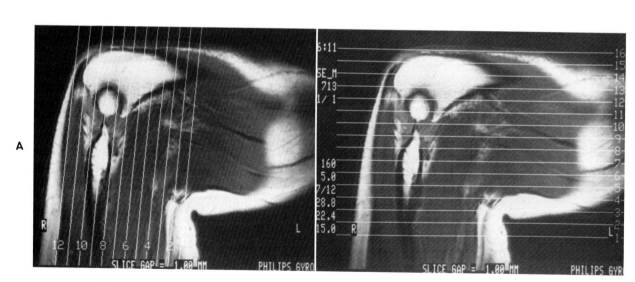

FIGURE 17-23
Technique of MRI scan planning of the elbow in flexion. The coronal plane of the scanner has produced sagittal images of the arm, elbow, and forearm. These are used to plan the next two sequences. **A,** Sagittal image of the elbow in flexion. The *lines* on the image, representing slices oriented in the sagittal plane of the scanner, portray the arm structures in a coronal plane and those of the forearm in an axial plane. **B,** Same images, this time with the lines representing slices oriented in the axial plane of the scanner. They represent axial views of the arm structures and coronal views of the forearm structures.

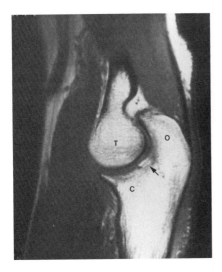

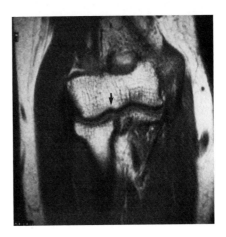

FIGURE 17-24
Normal MRI of the ulnohumeral joint. A sagittal T1-weighted image shows a central depression *(arrow)* separating the articular surfaces of the olecranon *(O)* and the coronoid *(C)*. The trochlea is denoted by *T*.

FIGURE 17-25
Normal articular surface of the trochlea and capitellum. A coronal T1-weighted image shows the cartilage-covered groove *(arrow)* separating the trochlea from the capitellum.

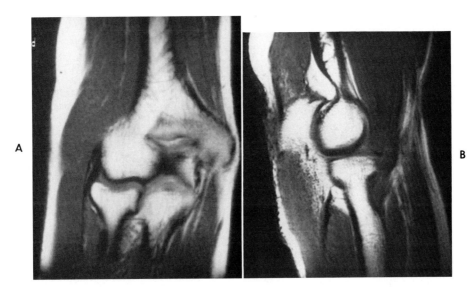

FIGURE 17-26
MRI of the normal humerus. Bone septations in the marrow space. Coronal, A, and sagittal, B, T1-weighted images show parallel signal void lines, which represents struts of compact cortical bone traversing the medullary cavity of the distal humeral metaphysis.

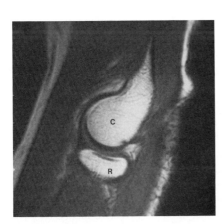

FIGURE 17-27
Normal articular cartilage of the capitellum. A sagittal T1-weighted image at the lateral site of the joint. *C* is the capitellum; *R* the radial head. The posterior surface of the capitellum is flat and not covered by articular cartilage, the anterior rounded and covered by cartilage.

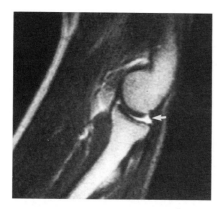

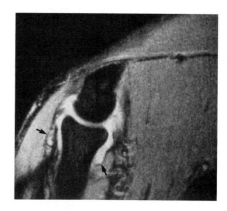

FIGURE 17-28

Normal articular fluid. A T2-weighted sagittal image of the joint between the capitellum and radius. Note the small amount of fluid, seen as a thin layer of bright signal around the capitellum *(arrow)*. The articular cartilage is not distinguishable from the fluid.

FIGURE 17-29

Synovial recess around the neck of the radius. A sagittal T2* image of the elbow joint shows the synovial space, distended by fluid, outlining the recesses around the radial neck *(arrows)*. The articular cartilage cannot be seen.

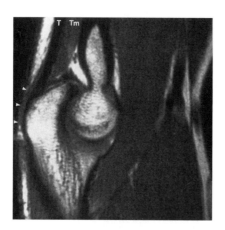

FIGURE 17-30

Normal triceps tendon. A T1-weighted sagittal image through the olecranon shows the band of signal void representing normal triceps tendon *(T)*. Anterior to it is the fleshy part of the triceps muscle *(Tm)*. Parallel to the posterior surface of the tendon is a line of intermediate signal intensity, which represents the normal olecranon bursa *(arrowheads)*.

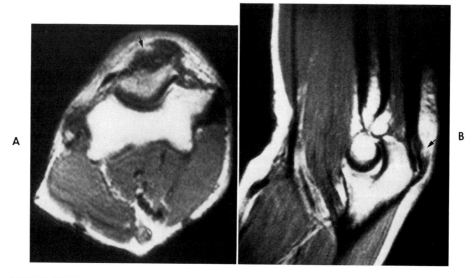

FIGURE 17-31

Partial-thickness tear, triceps tendon. **A,** Axial proton density–weighted image (TR 1900/TE 20) of the terminal segment of the triceps tendon. An incomplete tear is seen as a line of high signal obliquely intersecting the dorsal surface *(arrow)*. **B,** A sagittal T1-weighted image shows the tear of the tendon *(arrow)*.

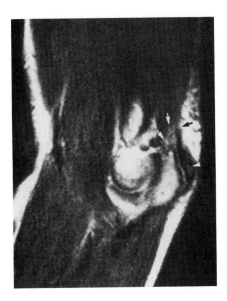

FIGURE 17-32
Chronic stage of a partial-thickness tear, triceps tendon. A sagittal proton density–weighted image (TR 1900/TE 30) shows abnormally thin tendon of the triceps muscle, just above the tip of the olecranon *(black arrow)*. Inside the terminal segment of this tendon a zone of increased signal is consistent with intratendinous tear *(arrowhead)*. Anterior to the torn segment the intermediate-signal zone represents scar *(white arrows)*.

During the chronic stage of a tear, scar tissue forms at the site of tendon injury and is perceived on MR images as a zone of intermediate signal intensity (Fig. 17-32).

A pitfall of interpretation may be encountered when imaging the triceps in older patients, who have less elastic tendons. With the elbow in 90 degrees of flexion the tendon is fully stretched, in a straight and continuous band. With the elbow extended and the extremity passive, relaxation of the muscle permits some infolding of the tendon, which develops a wavy surface. Thin coronal slices through the tendon in such a position may give the false impression of a tear, by showing interruptions of the band of signal void with interspersed zones of bright signal (fat) on T1-weighted images. The clue to solving this puzzle is forthcoming when sagittal and coronal images are compared: the waviness of the tendon is perceived only on sagittal images that are perpendicular to the surface of the band. It is therefore advisable, when the aim of the study is to evaluate the triceps tendon, to position the patient with 90 degrees of flexion in the elbow. The integrity of this structure is best seen when it is represented by a continuous straight band stretched between the muscle belly and the osseous insertion on the olecranon process.

Tennis elbow

The syndrome described in clinical practice as "tennis elbow" is characterized by chronic disabling pain in the lateral side of the elbow, with point tenderness in the epicondyle and capitellum or near the radial head. There is no localized swelling or reduction in range of motion of

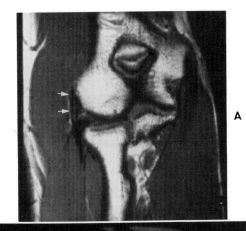
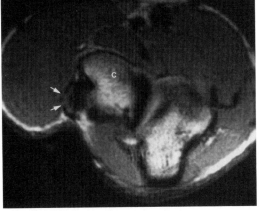

FIGURE 17-33
MRI of tennis elbow. Partial-thickness tear of the common extensor tendon. A, A coronal T1-weighted image shows nonhomogeneous signal in the common extensor tendon as it inserts on the lateral epicondyle *(arrows)*. B, Proton density axial image. The nonhomogeneous signal in the tendon plus interruption of its lateral surface indicates a partial tear *(arrows)*. C is the capitellum.

the joint, although active contraction of the extensor muscles produces pain that, in turn, limits the strength of the grasp.[26]

The etiology of this disease is unknown; it is more frequent in young and middle-aged adults who have intensive physical activities requiring frequent rotatory motion and extension of the forearm. Rarely, similar symptoms appear in the medial side of the joint when the flexor tendons are subjected to continuous stress. It is believed that the pathological process responsible is partial tearing of the tendon fibers from their attachment on the epicondyle. Continuous use of the extremity, with forceful contraction of the muscles, prevents healing. As more and more fibers of the tendon are torn, a nonspecific inflammatory reaction produces traumatic periostitis.

The MRI abnormalities seen with tennis elbow reflect these pathological features: the proximal segment of the common extensor tendon has zones of increased signal, irregular contour of its margins, and fluid collections within or beneath it (Fig. 17-33). On T2-weighted images increased signal near the bone surface indicates the zone

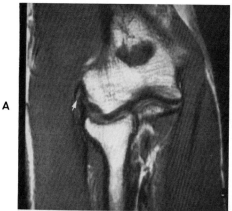

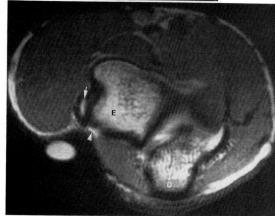

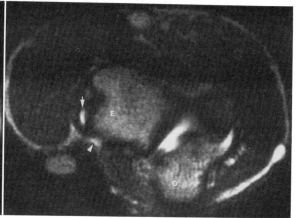

FIGURE 17-34

MRI of tennis elbow. Periostitis. **A,** A coronal T1-weighted image shows increased signal at the osseous attachment of the common extensor tendon *(arrow)*, consistent with fluid or an inflammatory reaction. **B** and **C,** Proton density–weighted and T2-weighted axial images of the lateral epicondyle *(E)* and olecranon *(O)* show fluid beneath the extensor tendon *(arrow)*. This area is extrasynovial, and the fluid from the joint space does not extend over the lateral epicondyle; therefore the explanation for it must be intrinsic abnormality of the tendon. The zone of increased signal on the posterior humeral surface signifies edema associated with periostitis *(arrowhead)*. The oval marker attached to the skin denotes the point of tenderness at clinical examination of the elbow.

of edema representing periostitis (Fig. 17-34). Conservative treatment with immobilization of the elbow in a splint and physiotherapy usually provides lasting relief. In rare cases of disabling recurrent manifestations, surgical treatment may be necessary—denervation of the lateral epicondyle by resecting the articular branch of the radial nerve or (more extensively) detachment of the tendon from the bone with periostitis, curetting the bony surface, and reinserting the tendon on the newly formed cancellous bone.[26] It is in patients who require surgical treatment that MRI has the most important role to play, as a means for presurgical evaluation. It can document abnormalities in the tendon and the extent of periostitis in the lateral epicondyle.

Dislocations

Elbow dislocations are usually diagnosed by clinical examination followed by routine roentgenograms. The most common dislocation is a posterior displacement of the ulna and radius in relation to the articular surface of the distal humerus.[27] At the time of this injury the anterior margin of the coronoid process can fracture when it is jammed against the trochlea. Attempts at reduction may further displace within the joint the fracture fragment of the coronoid or even produce a new fracture when incongruent bony surfaces are forcefully made to slide against each other. Occasionally one or more small fracture fragments will become trapped in the joint, preventing reduction of the dislocation. In such a situation any further manipulation of the joint in an attempt to reduce the dislocation not only is doomed to failure but also can injure articular cartilage and cortex hitherto intact.

The overlap of complex osseous structures in the elbow makes routine roentgenography a poor tool for detecting small entrapped fragments. When none can be seen but are suspected clinically, or when the exact position of such fragments is uncertain, CT is the most rapid and thorough radiological means of solving the problem. CT scanning should be performed immediately when intraarticular fragments are suspected as the cause of failure to reduce an elbow dislocation. Sequential 3 mm thick CT slices disclose small fracture fragments in and around the joint. However, CT images of a dislocated elbow can be confusing sometimes if one does not refer constantly to the scout view obtained at the beginning of the examination: depending upon the orientation of the slices, an abnormally large joint space or even "naked" articular cortex can be seen, the result of displacement of the radius and ulna (which are no longer in contact with the opposing surfaces of the capitellum and trochlea [Fig. 17-35]). In the abnormal gap between the dislocated articular surfaces, entrapped osseous fragments appear as dense structures. Detection and location of these fragments are most important for planning their arthroscopic or open surgical removal.

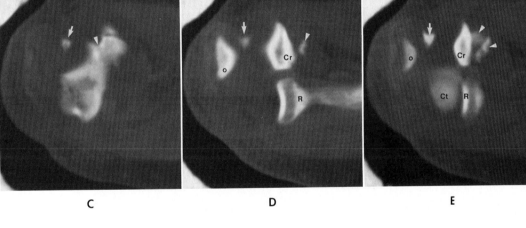

FIGURE 17-35
Irreducible elbow dislocation with a fragment of bone trapped in the ulnohumeral joint. **A,** The initial lateral roentgenogram shows posterior dislocation of the radius and ulna with a small fracture fragment near the coronoid. **B,** CT image after an attempt at reduction had failed. The lateral scout shows persistent posterior displacement of the radius and ulna. **C,** CT axial image of the trochlea. The medial margin is fractured *(arrowhead),* and there is a loose bone fragment present *(arrow).* **D,** Coronal CT image of the radial head and ulnar sigmoid notch. The normal relation with the humerus is lost: the capitellum and trochlea are not seen; instead the "naked" articular surfaces of the radius *(R),* coronoid *(Cr),* and olecranon *(o)* are visible. In the coronoid notch there is a triangular fracture fragment *(arrow).* **E,** Coronal CT image 3 mm proximal to **D** showing a loose fragment of bone *(arrow)* in the joint space near the olecranon process *(o).* Another two fracture fragments are seen inferior to the coronoid process *(Cr),* radial head *(R),* and capitellum *(Ct).*

In chronic dislocations, most often involving only the radius, conventional roentgenography is sufficient for diagnosing displacement of the radial head[28] (Fig. 17-36, *A*). However, CT is better for evaluating localized pressure erosions at points of abnormal contact between bone surfaces (Fig. 17-36, *B*) and MRI is better for the associated soft tissue abnormalities, specifically stretching or tearing of the annular ligament (Fig. 17-36, *C* to *H*). Visualization of these soft tissues is beneficial to planning of the reconstructive surgery, aimed at permanent reduction by tightening of the capsule and ligaments.

Fractures

Although most elbow fractures can be adequately diagnosed by roentenograms obtained in frontal and lateral projections,[29,30] sometimes additional views (tangential to the olecranon surface, oblique to the capitellum

and radial head) will be needed for subtle breaks.[31-33] When a simple roentgenographic evaluation fails to reveal the injury, two courses of action can be taken: (1) immobilization of the joint in a splint followed by reevaluation in 2 to 3 days or (2) immediate further study with CT and MRI for an exhaustive diagnostic work-up. Prompt diagnosis of injuries is a necessity whenever it is thought that immediate surgery will be beneficial, especially in patients for whom a rapid return to normal mobility is essential (e.g., professional athletes).

• • •

Because a full description and classification of elbow fractures is beyond the scope of this chapter, only the more common injuries will be discussed, especially those that can benefit from imaging by CT and MR.

In adults one of the most common fractures of the elbow is at the radial head or neck. Displaced fractures

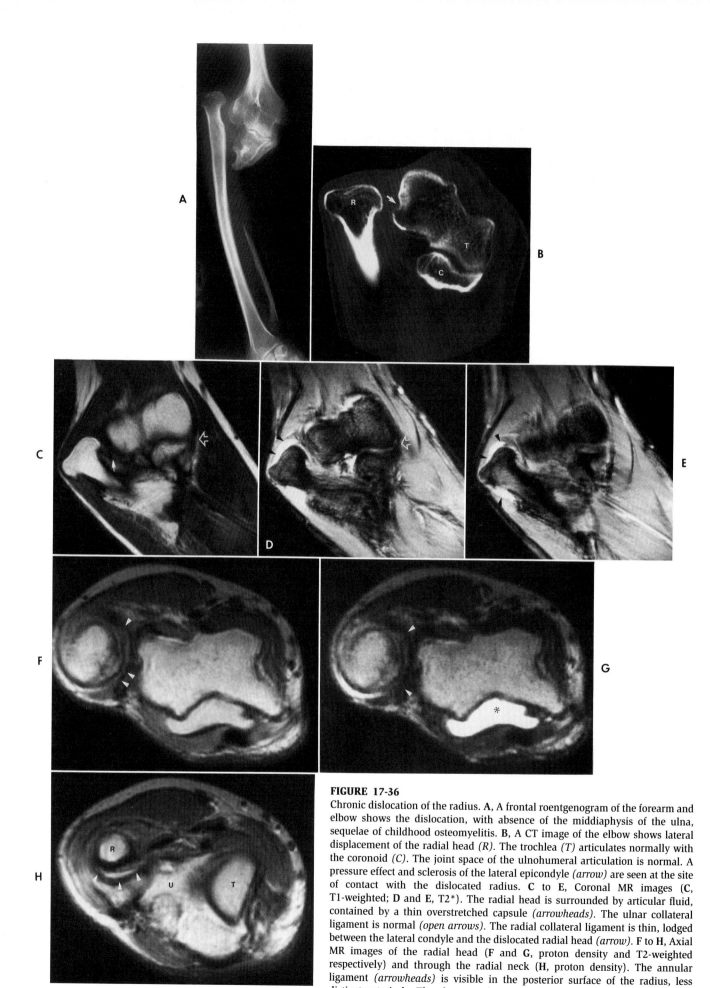

FIGURE 17-36

Chronic dislocation of the radius. **A,** A frontal roentgenogram of the forearm and elbow shows the dislocation, with absence of the middiaphysis of the ulna, sequelae of childhood osteomyelitis. **B,** A CT image of the elbow shows lateral displacement of the radial head *(R)*. The trochlea *(T)* articulates normally with the coronoid *(C)*. The joint space of the ulnohumeral articulation is normal. A pressure effect and sclerosis of the lateral epicondyle *(arrow)* are seen at the site of contact with the dislocated radius. **C** to **E,** Coronal MR images (**C,** T1-weighted; **D** and **E,** T2*). The radial head is surrounded by articular fluid, contained by a thin overstretched capsule *(arrowheads)*. The ulnar collateral ligament is normal *(open arrows)*. The radial collateral ligament is thin, lodged between the lateral condyle and the dislocated radial head *(arrow)*. **F** to **H,** Axial MR images of the radial head (**F** and **G,** proton density and T2-weighted respectively) and through the radial neck (**H,** proton density). The annular ligament *(arrowheads)* is visible in the posterior surface of the radius, less distinct anteriorly. The olecranon fossa contains synovial fluid *(asterisk)*.

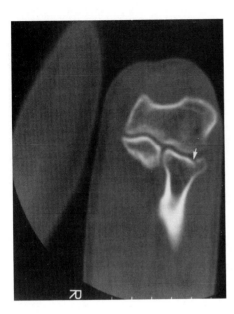

FIGURE 17-37
Fracture of the radial head. A CT image of the elbow in 90 degrees of flexion shows the fracture affecting the lateral part of the head *(arrow)*.

each of the three planes (coronal, sagittal, axial) may be seen. The cartilaginous segments of the epiphysis are also well portrayed. However, the diagnosis and reduction of elbow fractures are conducted as emergency medical procedures; rarely can MRI be performed in the first few hours after injury, when the pain is most intense and any motion of the extremity is contraindicated. The MRI examination requires some initial handling of the extremity for surface coil positioning, and subsequently immobility of the segment must be maintained for 30 to 45 minutes. This can rarely be accomplished in an acutely injured patient, especially a child, which explains why few examples of acute phase of elbow fractures are found in the recent radiological literature describing MR imaging of trauma cases. It is hoped that reduction of the scanning time and the easy availability of this examination to emergency medical care will increase the number of patients with acute injuries of the elbow who would benefit from the diagnostic power of the MRI.

CT has the practical advantages of wide availability and rapidity of study. It is indicated for a variety of cases—including complex and severe fractures, especially when associated with dislocations (Fig. 17-35), joint effusions secondary to trauma but with no identifiable fracture on conventional films, and situations in which pain and fixed contractions of muscles and capsule preclude proper radiographic positioning.[37]

CT has been of practical use in children who have a supracondylar fracture of the humerus with displacement of the distal fragment.[38] Rotation of the epiphyseal fragment around the transverse axis produces great instability: the fragment also becomes angulated in the coronal plane and tilted dorsally, and the resulting tilt produces malalignment, usually of the cubitus varus type. CT can directly detect the amount of axial rotation of the distal fragment,[38] and this should be done before therapy is planned. In children the single most preventable cause of deformity of the elbow joint resulting from trauma is malposition of a distal humeral fracture fragment.[39] If the fracture is not adequately reduced, in the healing stage a cubitus varus or valgus develops, with resulting functional and cosmetic compromise.[40]

For the CT examination the patient is positioned supine with the injured extremity in a resting position by the side of the trunk, if possible with the hand supinated (palm facing up). A frontal scout of the entire humerus including the elbow joint is obtained. A single axial image of the humeral diaphysis proximal to the fracture site portrays the humerus as a triangle in cross section. The flat posterior surface of the diaphysis (the coronal plane of the bone) is marked with a tangential line on the imaging screen. This line is transposed onto the axial image of the distal fracture segment obtained through the trochlea, and the transverse diameter of the trochlea is marked electronically. The angle formed between these two lines is measured (Fig. 17-38).

Normally there is a small degree of external rotation of

are normally quite apparent on roentgenograms. Undisplaced fractures may occasionally be difficult to detect, although they may be suspected when positive fat pad signs are seen on a lateral film of the elbow.[29,33] With a history of acute trauma and no preexisting pathology, any elbow joint effusion should be interpreted as hemarthrosis, usually caused by bleeding at the site of an intraarticular fracture. CT and MRI can detect such elusive nondisplaced fractures, by demonstrating the interruption of articular cortex in the radial head (Fig. 17-37).

In children with an elbow fracture the supracondylar segment of the humerus is the most frequent site of injury,[34] the fracture usually acquired by falling on an outstretched hand with the elbow in extension. The olecranon process of the ulna locks in the olecranon fossa, and forces transmitted axially through these two surfaces split the humerus at its weakest part (the supracondylar segment). The first to break is the anterior cortex. When the posterior cortex is also fractured, displacement of fragments can be produced. The distal humeral fragment, often still attached to intact periosteum, becomes displaced posteriorly, occasionally with a concomitant medial or lateral deviation as well. Often these are unstable fractures that can progress to further angulation and fragment displacement, which in turn may injure the brachial artery and the radial and median nerves.[35] It is most important therefore that anatomical reduction of the fragments be accomplished—first, assessing the exact position of each fragment and planning the reduction.[36]

The best information about fracture lines can be obtained with MRI, because it offers the choice of multiplanar imaging (often an advantage in complex comminuted fractures). Displacement or angulation in

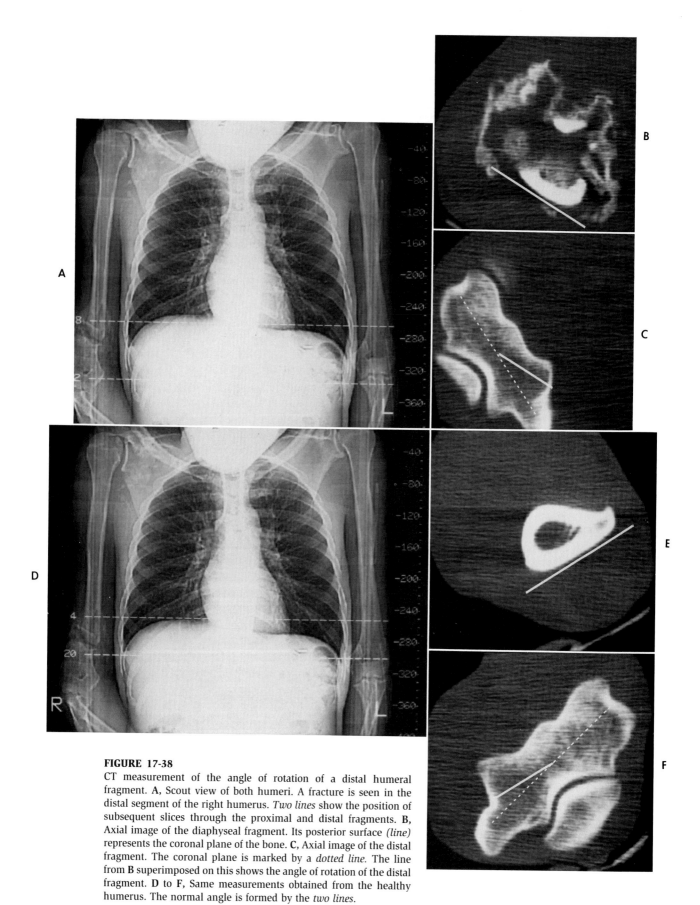

FIGURE 17-38
CT measurement of the angle of rotation of a distal humeral fragment. **A,** Scout view of both humeri. A fracture is seen in the distal segment of the right humerus. *Two lines* show the position of subsequent slices through the proximal and distal fragments. **B,** Axial image of the diaphyseal fragment. Its posterior surface *(line)* represents the coronal plane of the bone. **C,** Axial image of the distal fragment. The coronal plane is marked by a *dotted line.* The line from **B** superimposed on this shows the angle of rotation of the distal fragment. **D** to **F,** Same measurements obtained from the healthy humerus. The normal angle is formed by the *two lines.*

the distal articular surface of the humerus relative to the diaphysis and humeral head, most pronounced in adults. In children, during the normal phases of skeletal maturation this rotation of the distal humerus progressively increases. Consequently a certain degree of natural variability of the normal rotation angle exists between children of the same age and between children and adults. To compare the angle of rotation the normal elbow with that of the fractured joint requires the uninjured extremity to be included in the CT images by use of a large FOV. The normal angle of rotation is recorded as for the injured side. Only after comparison of the normal with the injured side can one be certain of the degree of abnormal rotation of the distal humeral fracture fragment (Fig. 17-38). Results of a study by Hindman et al.[38] showed that internal rotation of the distal humeral fragment more than 10 degrees resulted in a cubitus varus deformity. This could be explained by the fact that the distal humeral fragment not only is rotated but also is usually displaced or angulated in both the coronal and the

FIGURE 17-39

Osteochondral fracture of the humerus. **A,** A coronal T1-weighted image shows a defect in the articular surface of the capitellum *(arrows)* representing the fracture site. From this area, directed superiorly, a line of low signal indicates extension of the fracture in the marrow of the capitellum *(arrowheads).* Note the homogeneous intermediate signal intensity of the fluid accumulated between the radial head and the capitellum. **B** and **C,** Axial T2 and proton density images show increased signal in the marrow of the capitellum, indicating hemorrhage at the fracture site *(arrowheads).* Joint effusion has distended the synovial recess on the lateral side of the olecranon process. **D** and **E,** Sagittal T1- and T2-weighted images through the capitellum. Joint effusion is the bright-signal collection of fluid conforming to the shape of the synovial space. The concave surface of the capitellum denotes the fracture. A low-signal line adjacent to the surface of the capitellum represents a detached fracture fragment *(arrow).*

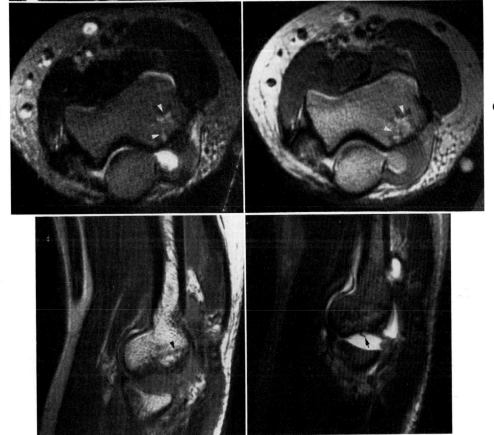

sagittal plane, which produces medial or lateral tilt (abnormality in the coronal plane) and dorsal or ventral tilt (abnormality in the sagittal plane).[41]

For reformatting images in the coronal and sagittal plane as an aid to understanding positional and alignment abnormalities, contiguous 3 mm thick CT axial slices of the entire elbow can be used. Comminuted fractures or penetrating injuries with retained foreign bodies are best seen in three-dimensional reconstruction images.[42]

OSTEOCHONDRAL FRACTURES

The most common site of osteochondral fracture in the elbow is the convex surface of the capitellum. The injury usually results from a shearing force transmitted by the radial head, which moves against the capitellum and at the same time rotates while changing from supination to pronation and from flexion to extension. This type of motion is exemplified by the pitching of a baseball; and indeed, most such injuries are seen in the dominant side of young baseball players.[43]

A splintered osteochondral fragment may be totally detached from the capitellum, in which case it moves freely in the synovial cavity. Occasionally an osteochondral fracture fragment will remain attached to the articular surface by a tag of uninterrupted cartilage. Such partially detached fragments can slide intermittently out of their bed, become entrapped between opposing surfaces of the joint, and produce locking of the elbow.

MR images of an acute osteochondral fracture show a zone of hemorrhage in the bone marrow as a band of signal abnormality surrounding the defect in the articular surface (increased signal on T2-weighted images, decreased on T1-weighted). The fragment itself is best seen on T2 or T2*-weighted images as a zone of signal void (Fig. 17-39).

AVASCULAR NECROSIS OF BONE
Osteochondritis dissecans

Avascular necrosis of bone is occasionally seen in patients predisposed to obliteration of the blood supply to the bone secondary to caisson disease, sickle cell anemia, or collagen vascular disease (e.g., lupus).

The idiopathic form in the epiphysis of the elbow (osteochondrosis) is most likely the result of trauma and usually is seen in the capitellum (Panner's disease).[44]

In traumatic osteonecrosis a pathogenic chain reaction is initiated by chronic repetitive trauma that injures the superficial layers of bone forming the convex surface of the capitellum. These injuries diminish the vascularity of the bony trabeculae in a limited zone, where the bone is most exposed to compressive forces. The covering cartilage, however, remains intact and, by virtue of its elasticity and compressibility, absorbs some of these forces without breaking. Thus, in the early stage of osteochondritis dissecans, a "button of bone" becomes necrotic but retains an intact layer of covering cartilage.

As the disease progresses, the necrotic trabeculae break under pressure and cannot renew themselves through osteoblastic activity (which requires normal blood supply). More and more such microfractures lead eventually to collapse of the bony architecture. When the articular cortex becomes fragmented, the overlapping hyaline cartilage breaks also. At this point the "button of bone" becomes detached from the surrounding normal bone. It can remain in the same location or be sloughed off as a single fragment or multiple free fragments. In these last stages avascular necrosis is manifested as the anatomopathological entity of osteochondritis dissecans.[45,46]

The role of the radiologist is not only to detect this disease but also to determine whether the necrotic piece of bone is covered by intact cartilage or is fragmented and detached, a task best accomplished by obtaining a CT-arthrogram.

Double-contrast arthrography — coating the cartilage surface with contrast and distending the synovial space with air — shows the folds of synovium and occasional bubbles of air as a confusing picture of overlapping lines on the roentgenograms obtained after injection. Small osseous fragments are difficult to visualize, and the complex articular surfaces cannot be seen tangentially in their entirety. It is precisely for this reason that CT examination after injection of contrast has been utilized: the information obtained by arthrography is enhanced,[47] and scans obtained immediately after joint injection permit a detailed study of the articular surfaces (especially when thin slices [3 mm or less] are used).[15] The integrity and thickness of the articular cartilage can be assessed (Fig. 17-40) and in the early stages will be found adequate (Fig. 17-41). Fissures in the cartilage covering the bone cortex can be used as indicators of the progression toward full-blown osteochondritis dissecans (Fig. 17-42). Fragmentation of the articular cortex and overlapping cartilage is detected in advanced stages (Fig. 17-43).

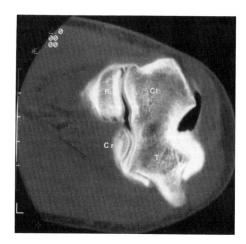

FIGURE 17-40
Normal CT-arthrogram. Positive contrast coats the articular cartilage of the capitellum *(Ct),* trochlea *(T),* coronoid *(Cr),* and radial head *(R).*

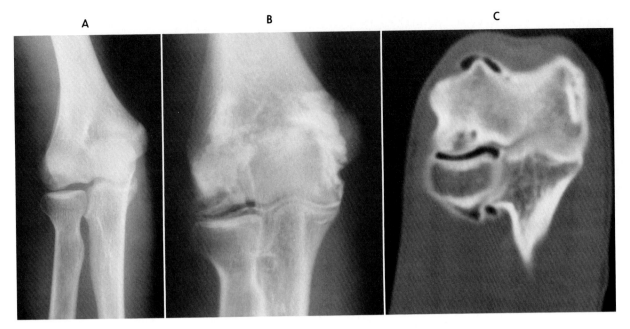

FIGURE 17-41
Osteonecrosis of the capitellum (Panner disease). **A,** A frontal roentgenogram of the elbow shows a zone of decreased density with calcifications in the capitellum. **B,** Frontal view of the arthrogram. **C,** The image through the joint between the capitellum and radial head shows normal articular surface.

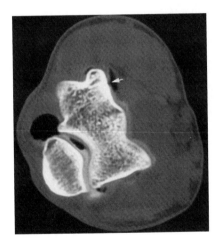

FIGURE 17-42
Osteonecrosis and cartilage fissure. CT-arthrogram. An axial image of the capitellum shows a fissure *(arrow)* in the layer of cartilage covering the dense zone of avascular necrosis.

INTRAARTICULAR OSTEOCARTILAGINOUS BODIES
Osteochondral fragments

There are three causes of loose osteochondral bodies in the joint: (1) acute trauma can splinter a fragment of the articular surface, (2) advanced osteonecrosis can slough off in the joint fragments of necrotic bone covered by cartilage, and (3) metaplasia of the synovium can produce multiple chondromatous bodies that calcify.

The osseous fragments found in the joint may be free but most often are embedded within the synovial lining. Usually they are thin splinters of bone detached from the articular surface, forced partially through and adherent to the synovium. Depending upon their location, they restrict motion by becoming entrapped between opposing articular surfaces or acting simply as a mechanical irritant to the surrounding synovial folds. The hyperemia produced in the adjacent synovium promotes invasion of blood vessels into the osseous part of the fragment, with subsequent resorption of the bone. Indeed, most of the small fragments of bone produced by acute injuries appear to become embedded within the synovium and ultimately disappear through resorption.[48] Those that remain free in the synovial space continue to grow by deposition of concentric layers of cartilage, which can calcify. A multilayered calcific rim is their characteristic feature. Often the center of these osteocartilaginous bodies (i.e., the nidus) "betrays" their osseous origin. The cartilage, receiving nourishment from the synovial fluid, continues to grow and gradually envelops the original bone fragment.

The fragment from an osteochondral fracture usually shows signs of osteonecrosis, due to interruption of its blood supply. It is therefore difficult, based on histology alone, to distinguish between an old osteochondral fracture fragment and a segment of bone that was initially necrotic and later became detached.

Regardless of their etiology, these intrasynovial bodies have common manifestations—the most characteristic being locking of the joint, produced when a body is trapped between the articular surfaces; reduced range of flexion or extension may result when numerous or voluminous osteocartilaginous bodies occupy the coronoid or olecranon fossa. The radiographic detection of

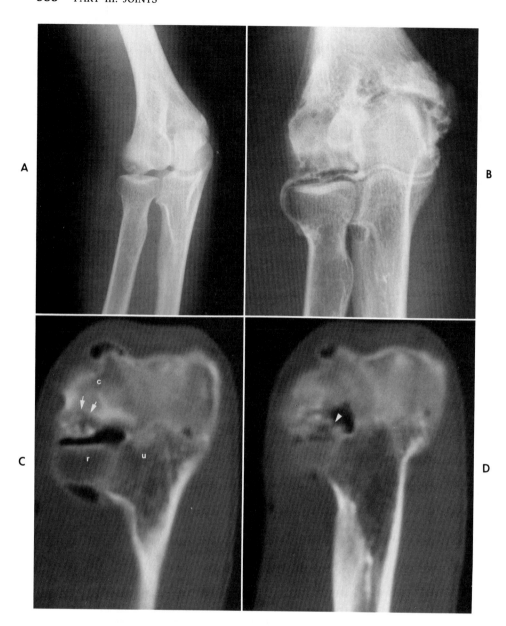

FIGURE 17-43
Osteochondritis dissecans of the capitellum. **A,** Oblique roentgenogram. Note the lucent zone with calcifications in the capitellum. **B,** Double-contrast arthrogram. The contour of the articular surface is indistinct. **C** and **D,** CT images representing adjacent slices through the posterior surface of the radius *(r),* capitellum *(C),* and ulna *(u).* The osteonecrotic part of the capitellum has nonhomogenous density *(arrows).* Fragmentation of the cortex of the posterior capitellar surface is outlined by air *(arrowhead).*

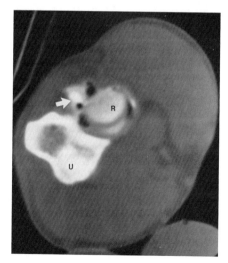

FIGURE 17-44
Loose osseous body. An axial CT-arthrogram image through the radial head shows a small osseous body *(arrow)* surrounded by contrast in the space between the radius *(R)* and ulna *(U).*

fragments trapped within the joint space following acute trauma is often difficult because of the concave and convex articular surfaces. Small osseous fragments may be obscured by the superimposed bones, and purely cartilaginous ones are not seen.

The task of detecting and precisely locating loose intrasynovial bodies (cartilaginous or osseous) is accomplished by CT-arthrography (Fig. 17-44). Purely cartilaginous bodies have a density similar to that of synovium or other soft tissue, and can be seen only when their surface is completely coated by dense positive contrast (Fig. 17-45). Pitfalls in the interpretation of CT images may be avoided by analyzing sequential slices: synovial buds or folds will appear as "loose" cartilaginous bodies when intersected by the CT slice at their free (intraarticular) edge, but adjacent slices will show continuity with the rest of the synovial surface and thus allow differentiation by the "tip of the stalactite effect" (Fig. 17-46).

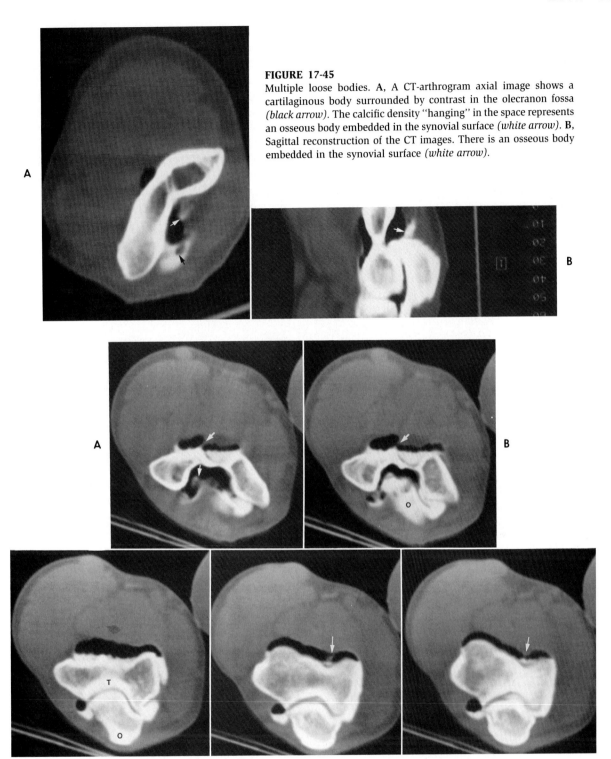

FIGURE 17-45

Multiple loose bodies. **A,** A CT-arthrogram axial image shows a cartilaginous body surrounded by contrast in the olecranon fossa *(black arrow)*. The calcific density "hanging" in the space represents an osseous body embedded in the synovial surface *(white arrow)*. **B,** Sagittal reconstruction of the CT images. There is an osseous body embedded in the synovial surface *(white arrow)*.

FIGURE 17-46

False image of loose bodies. Synovial adhesions. **A,** CT-arthrogram. Axial image of the distal humerus. Folds of synovium are silhouetted on the background of air *(arrows)*. The posterior one *(small arrow)* can be confused with a cartilaginous body. **B,** Axial image 3 mm distal to **A**. The posterior synovial fold continues directly with the tip of the olecranon *(O)*, on which it inserts. An osteophyte at the margin of the articular surface gives an irregular contour to the tip of the olecranon. The anterior fold is seen clearly as an adhesion band in the synovial cavity *(arrow)*. **C,** Axial image 6 mm distal to **B**. The olecranon *(O)*, trochlea *(T)*, and normal synovial space recesses can be seen medial and lateral to the olecranon and anterior to the trochlea. **D** and **E,** Two adjacent axial images distal to **C**. Another synovial band *(arrow)* appears in **D** as a free intrasynovial cartilaginous body. Its true nature as a synovial adhesion is revealed in **E**, which shows the tethered synovial surface. This appearance can be compared with that of a stalactite attached to the ceiling of a cave.

Osteochondral fracture fragments embedded in the synovium appear to be coated only partially by positive contrast (Fig. 17-45).

Noncontrast CT of the elbow can detect and precisely locate the bone fragments of an acute osteochondral fracture and cartilaginous bodies that are calcified (Fig. 17-47). However, it may induce underestimation of their true size and number by missing the cartilaginous parts.

MRI of the elbow can detect the loose bodies in the synovial space.[49] The parts that are calcified or consist of compact cortical bone have a typical signal void aspect

(Fig. 17-48). The cartilaginous parts have signal characteristics similar to those of synovial fluid on T2-weighted images. Only when a calcific rim exist at the periphery of such a cartilaginous body can its true size be seen and distinguished from the surrounding fluid. On T1-weighted images the layer of cartilage has intermediate signal intensity, only slightly different from that of the synovial fluid. The cartilaginous body is detected either by its shape and displacement of fat pads or by the signal characteristics of its osseous nidus containing fatty marrow and compact cortical bone (Fig. 17-49). The similarity between the signal intensity of the cartilage and that of

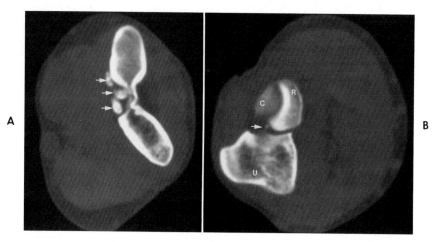

FIGURE 17-47
Calcified loose bodies. CT appearance. **A,** An axial image shows three distinct bodies in the coronoid fossa of the humerus *(arrows)*. No contrast was injected into the joint. **B,** An axial view at the joint between the capitellum *(C)*, radial head *(R)*, and ulna *(U)* shows a small calcific body trapped in the joint space *(arrow)*.

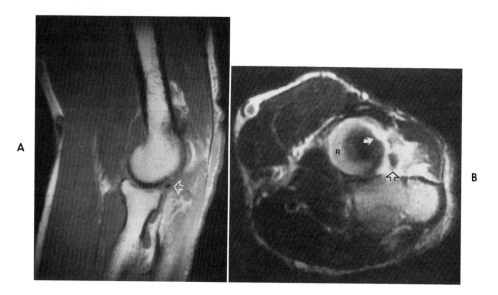

FIGURE 17-48
Osteochondral fragment loose in the joint. MRI characteristics. **A,** Sagittal T1-weighted image of the elbow. An osseous body consisting of cortical bone is seen as a dot of signal void in the posterior margin of the radiocapitellum joint *(open arrow)*. **B,** Axial T2-weighted image. The osseous body *(open arrow)* is seen against the background of synovial fluid. A defect in the radial head *(R)* indicates the site from which this fragment of bone has been detached *(curved arrow)*.

the surrounding synovial fluid makes detection of purely cartilaginous bodies often difficult on MR images.

Synovial chondromatosis

Multiple cartilaginous and osseous bodies in the articular cavity of the elbow joint can appear as a result of synovial metaplasia. Irritated synovium hypertrophies by producing abundant villous projections in the articular space. These villi can break off their connection with the synovial surface. Metaplasia from synovium to cartilage and from cartilage to bone can transform these free-floating villi into loose cartilaginous or osteocartilaginous bodies (synovial chondromatosis). The initial phase of this process produces a generalized irritation of the entire synovium; multiple villi break off from their place of origin and create a multitude of loose bodies packing the entire joint cavity.[48,49] This is in contradistinction to the few loose fragments of bone seen with advanced stages of osteochondritis dissecans. Furthermore, a single traumatic event causing an acute osteochondral fracture is likely to have one, two, or three fragments of bone rather than many as is the case with synovial chondromatosis (Fig. 17-50).

SYNOVIAL PATHOLOGY
Joint effusion

The normal elbow contains only a thin layer of fluid between the articular surfaces and in the small recesses of the synovial space (Fig. 17-51).

Fluid in the synovial cavity of the elbow joint can be due to trauma (bleeding from an intraarticular fracture), a localized inflammatory process (infectious arthritis), or a systemic inflammatory arthritis (rheumatoid, psoriatic, etc). The effusion is best seen on sagittal T2*-weighted images, which show the high signal of fluid contrasting with the low signal of the surrounding articular cortex, fat pads and capsule (Fig. 17-52). In the subacute stage of hemorrhage one can see in the elbow joint a combination of high-signal fluid distending the capsule and lower-signal blood clots (Fig. 17-53).

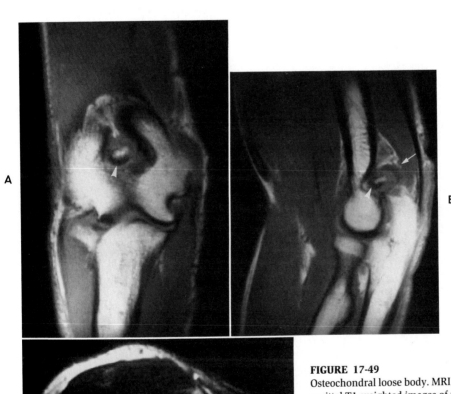

FIGURE 17-49
Osteochondral loose body. MRI characteristics. A and B, Coronal and sagittal T1-weighted images of the body in the olecranon fossa. Fatty marrow in the osseous center has bright signal, partially surrounded by a layer of cortical bone (seen as a curvilinear signal void, (arrowheads). A layer of cartilage around the bone is see as a ring of intermediate signal undistinguishable from fluid. Displacement of the posterior fat pad (arrow) and a thin low-signal rim at the periphery of the cartilage layer are clues to the actual size of the loose body. C, Axial T2-weighted image. The marrow of the loose body is low in signal, whereas the cartilage is high (white arrowhead) and could be confused with synovial fluid.

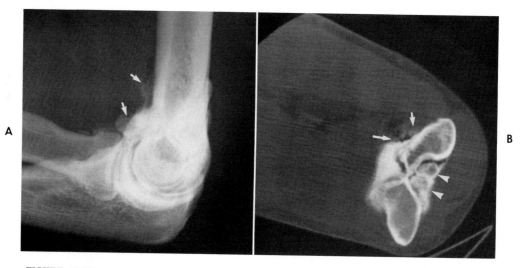

FIGURE 17-50
Synovial chondromatosis. **A,** Double-contrast arthrogram showing the granular surface of synovium anteriorly *(arrows)*. There is poor definition of cartilaginous bodies in the posterior part of the joint. **B,** CT-arthrogram. Two large cartilaginous bodies outlined by contrast are seen in the olecranon fossa *(arrowheads)*. Multiple small cartilaginous bodies *(arrows)* are seen anteriorly.

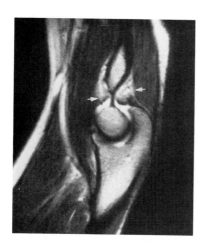

FIGURE 17-51
MRI of normal synovial fluid in the elbow joint. A sagittal T2-weighted image shows the bright signal of fluid accumulated in the coronoid and olecranon recesses of the synovial space. Fat pads in normal position *(arrows)* are located deep in the space of the olecranon and coronoid fossae.

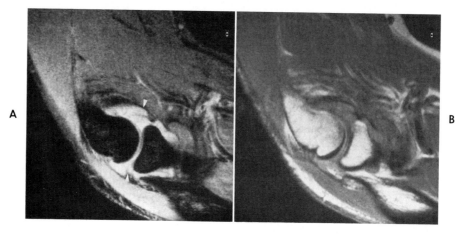

FIGURE 17-52
Joint effusion of the elbow. **A,** A sagittal T2*-weighted image shows distention of the capsule by bright-signal fluid *(arrowheads)*. **B,** Sagittal T1-weighted image at the same level. The fluid has intermediate signal and is more difficult to distinguish from the surrounding structures.

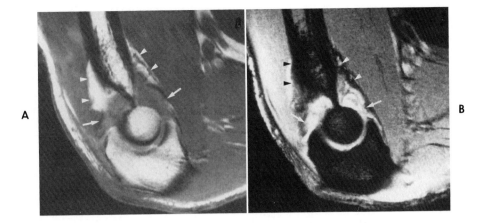

FIGURE 17-53
Acute injury causing hemarthrosis of the elbow. **A,** A sagittal T1-weighted image shows displacement of the fat pads *(arrowheads)* by fluid in the joint space *(arrows)*. **B,** A sagittal T2*-weighted image, same level, shows reversal of signal intensity: fluid in the joint appears as bright signal *(arrows)*, the fat as low signal *(arrowheads)*. Several blood clots in the fluid have intermediate signal.

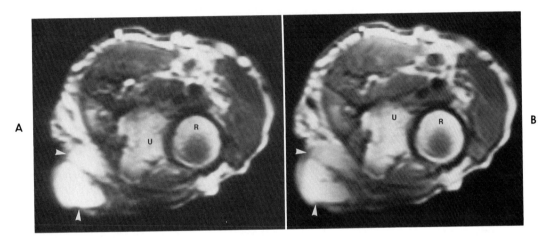

FIGURE 17-54. **A,** An axial T2-weighted shows a biloculated collection of fluid *(arrowheads)* in the subcutaneous layer, posterior to the ulna. **B,** A proton-density image (TR 1600/TE 30) at the same level shows the anatomy in better detail. However, the fluid in the olecranon bursa is not as distinct. *R,* Radial head; *U,* ulna.

Synovitis

Occasionally a chronic synovitis of any etiology will appear as granulation on the synovial surface. The small projections of hypertrophied villi give rise to elevations of the synovial surface, which then appears shaggy (Fig. 17-50). This is a nonspecific finding, common of all diseases that produce chronic inflammatory reactions in the synovial membrane. Based on the characteristic appearance of all joints affected, the only histologically specific diagnosis of synovial disease feasible by MR images is pigmented villonodular synovitis. The hemosiderin deposits with this disorder appear to be of low signal intensity on both T1- and T2-weighted images.

Olecranon bursitis

Thickening of the synovial membrane and accumulation of fluid in the olecranon bursa are the hallmarks of bursitis, appearing on MR images as increased size of the bursa and bright signal (representing the fluid and edematous synovium) (Fig. 17-54). These are nonspecific findings; they can be seen as a result of traumatic repetitive trauma and with rheumatoid arthritis or gout. MR images are not usually acquired in such cases: ultrasound is faster and less expensive.

DEGENERATIVE DISEASE OF TENDONS (CALCIFIC TENDINITIS)

Inflammation of the tendinous structures of the elbow may result from chronic trauma, producing incomplete tears (tennis elbow), or from age-related degenerative disease of the collagenous structures. Dystrophic changes of the tendons trigger an acute inflammatory reaction, with granulation tissue representing the natural repair process. Necrosis of soft tissue at the site of the inflam-

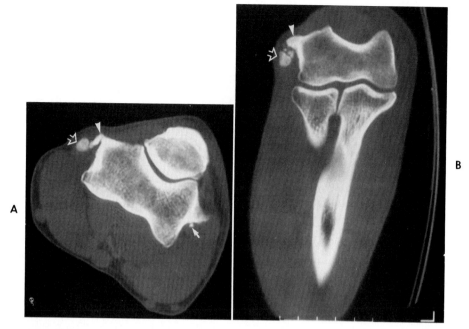

FIGURE 17-55

Calcific tendinitis. CT appearance. **A,** A axial CT image shows a spur on the lateral epicondyle *(arrowhead)* and ossification in the extensor tendon *(open arrow)*. On the medial side, calcific tendinitis appears as a single dot of density *(arrow)*. At the time of scanning the patient had symptoms only on the medial side. **B,** A coronal CT image of the elbow reveals ossification in the common tendon of the extensor muscles *(open arrow)* and stippled calcifications between spur on the lateral epicondyle *(arrowhead)* and tendon.

matory process may progress to calcification, manifested radiologically as amorphous conglomerates of calcific deposits. When present in small amounts, they are easier to detect by CT (which has better density resolution than roentgenography) (Fig. 17-55).

Calcifications are commonly seen in the bony attachments of strong ligaments of patients with diffuse idiopathic skeletal hyperostosis. When contiguous with the bone cortex, they have the characteristic appearance of osteophytes on the olecranon process and medial and lateral epicondyles. Spurs formed at the margin of the articular surfaces, the hallmark of osteoarthritis, are usually seen on routine roentgenograms; seldom is it necessary to obtain CT or MRI for their disclosure.

SUMMARY

CT and MRI are radiological examinations with great potential for solving problems in the management of bone and soft tissue pathology of the elbow.

Computerized tomography is widely available and easily performed, even in acutely traumatized patients. It represents a rapid and practical way of assessing the displacement/malalignment of fragments in comminuted fractures or those with complex multiplanar angulation. Specifically, it optimally portrays the axial rotation of a distal fragment in children with supracondylar fracture of the humerus.

CT-arthrography constitutes the most precise modality for imaging cartilaginous loose bodies in the joint.

The value of magnetic resonance is evident primarily in its ability to detect early avascular bone necrosis, tears of ligaments or tendons, and synovial pathology. It portrays osteochondral fractures quite well, although purely cartilaginous bodies may occasionally be obscured by the similarity of signal between synovial fluid and cartilage.

Technical improvements in and the wider availability of MRI will likely convince clinicians that this technique is an invaluable and practical modality for noninvasively investigating a multitude of diseases. The curve of learning and doing MRI of the elbow is expected to rise at a steep pace during the next several years and will ultimately spur new interest in the surgical repair of injuries to ligaments, capsule, and tendons that previously were undetectable by radiological investigations. By pinpointing the location of an abnormality, MRI allows the targeting of surgery with minimal trauma to healthy tissues and contributes thereby to the success of treatments for a variety of elbow disorders.

REFERENCES

1. Pitt MJ, Speer DP: Imaging of the elbow with an emphasis on trauma. Radiol Clin North Am 1990;28:293-305.
2. Newberg AH: Computed tomography of joint injuries. Radiol Clin North Am 1990:28:445-460.
3. Dalinka MK, Kricun ME, Zlatkin MB, Hibbard CA: Modern diagnostic imaging of joint disease. AJR 1989;152:229-240.
4. Kleinman PK, Spevak MR: Advanced pediatric joint imaging. Radiol Clin North Am 1990;28:1073-1109.

5. Sauser DD, Thordarson SH, Fahr LM: Imaging of the elbow. Radiol Clin North Am 1990;28:923-940.

6. Berquist TH: The elbow and wrist. Top Magn Reson Imaging 1989;1:15-27.

7. Ehrman RL: MR imaging with surface coils. Radiology 1985;157:549-550.

8. Fisher MR, Barker B, Amparo EG, et al: MR imaging using specialized coils. Radiology 1985;157;443-447.

9. Burk DL, Dalinka MK, Schiebler ML, et al: Strategies for musculoskeletal magnetic resonance imaging. Radiol Clin North Am 1988;26:653-672.

10. Warwick R , Williams PL (eds): Gray's anatomy of the human body, 36th British ed. Philadelphia, Saunders, 1980, pp 359-377, 571-583, 702-708, 1098-1103.

11. Netter FH: Atlas of human anatomy. Summit NJ, Ciba-Geigy Corp, 1989, pp 406-410, 411-425.

12. Grant JCB: An atlas of anatomy, 6th ed. Baltimore, Williams & Wilkins, 1972, pp 44-58.

13. Clemente CD: Anatomy. A regional atlas of the human body, 2nd ed. Baltimore, Urban & Schwarzenberg, 1981, pp 56-86.

14. Pernkopf E: Atlas of topographical and applied human anatomy. Philadelphia, Saunders, 1964, Vol 1, pp 74-80.

15. Singsong RD, Feldman F, Rosenberg ZS: Elbow joint: assessment with double contrast CT-arthrography. Radiology 1986;160:167-173.

16. Pavlov H, Ghelman B, Warden R: Double contrast arthrography of the elbow. Radiology 1979;130:87-95.

17. Teng M, Murphy M, Gilula Z, et al: Elbow arthrography: a reassessment of the technique. Radiology 1984;153:611-613.

18. Johansson O: Capsular and ligament injuries of the elbow joint: a clinical and arthrographic study. Acta Clin Scand (suppl) 1962;287:17-20.

19. Hajek PC, Sartoris DJ, Neumann CH, et al: Potential contrast agents for MR arthrography: in vitro evaluation and practical observations. AJR 1987;149:97-104.

20. Flannigan B, Korsunoglu-Brahme S, Snyder R, et al: MR arthrography of the shoulder: comparison with conventional MR imaging. AJR 1990;155:829-832.

21. Middleton WD, Macrander S, Kneeland JB, et al: MR imaging of the normal elbow: anatomic correlation. AJR 1987;149:543-547.

22. Bunnell DH, Fisher DA, Bassett LW, et al: Elbow joint: normal anatomy of MR images. Radiology 1987;165:527-531.

23. Bunnell DH, Bassett LW: The elbow. In MRI atlas of the musculoskeletal system. London, Martin Dunitz, 1989, pp 129-138.

24. Macrander SJ: The elbow. In Middletown WD, Lawson TL (eds): Anatomy and MRI of the joints. A multiplanar atlas. New York, Raven, 1989, pp 49-81.

25. Beltran J: The elbow. In Beltran J (ed): MRI: Musculoskeletal system, 4th ed. Philadelphia, Lippincott, 1990, pp 2-11.

26. Turek S: Orthopedics, 3rd ed. Philadelphia, Lippincott, 1977, pp 866-884.

27. Smith FM: Surgery of the elbow. Philadelphia, Saunders, 1971, pp 60-247.

28. Eklöf O, Nybonde T, Karlsson G: Luxation of the elbow complicated by proximal radio-ulnar translocation. Acta Radiol 1990;31:145-146.

29. Rogers LF: Fractures and dislocations of the elbow. Semin Roentgenol 1978;13:97-107.

30. Wilkins KE: Fractures and dislocations of the elbow region. In Rockwood CA Jr, Wilkins KE, King RE (eds): Fractures in children. Philadelphia, Lippincott, 1984, Vol 3, pp 374-501.

31. Greenspan A, Norman A: Radial head–capitellum view: an expanded imaging approach to elbow injury. Radiology 1987;164:272-274.

32. Grundy A, Murphy G, Barker A, et al: The value of the radial head–capitellum view in radial head trauma. Br J Radiol 1985;58:965-967.

33. Hall-Craggs MA, Shorvon PJ, Chapman M: Assessment of the radial head–capitellum view and the dorsal fat-pad sign in acute elbow trauma AJR 1985;145:607-609.

34. Ozonoff MB: Pediatric orthopedic radiology. Philadelphia, Saunders, 1979.

35. Culp RW, Osterman AL, Davidson RS, et al: Neural injuries associated with supracondylar fractures of the humerus in children. J Bone Joint Surg [Am] 1990;72:1211-1215.

36. Wilkins KE: The operative management of supracondylar fractures. Orthop Clin North Am 1990;21:269-289.

37. Franklin PD, Dunlop RW, Whitelaw G, et al: Computed tomography of the normal and traumatized elbow. J Comput Assist Tomogr 1988;12:817-823.

38. Hindman BW, Schreiber RR, Wiss DA, et al: Supracondylar fractures of the humerus: prediction of the cubitus varus deformity with CT. Radiology 1988;168:513-515.

39. D'Ambrosia RD: Supracondylar fractures of humerus — prevention of cubitus varus. J Bone Joint Surg [Am] 1972;54:60-66.

40. Wilkins KE: Residuals of elbow trauma in children. Orthop Clin North Am 1990;21:291-314.

41. Worlick P: Supracondylar fractures of the humerus. Assessment of cubitus varus deformity by the Baumann's angle. J Bone Joint Surg [Br] 1986;68:755-757.

42. Magid D, Fishman EK: Imaging of musculoskeletal trauma in three dimensions: an intergrated two-dimensional/three dimensional approach with computed tomography. Radiol Clin North Am 1989;27:945-956.

43. Gore RM, Rogers LF, Bowerman J, et al: Osseous manifestations of elbow stress associated with sports activities. AJR 1980;134:971-977.

44. Woodward A, Bianco A Jr: Osteochondritis dissecans of the elbow. Clin Orthop 1975;110:35-41.

45. Mitsunaga MM, Adishian DA, Bianco AJ Jr: Osteochondritis dissecans of the capitellum. J Trauma 1982;22:53-55.

46. Tivnon MC, Anzel SH, Waugh TR: Surgical management of osteochondritis dissecans of the capitellum. Am J Sports Med 1976;4:121-128.

47. Brody AS, Ball WS, Towbin RB: Computed arthrotomography as an adjunct to pediatric arthrography. Radiology 1989;1970:99-102.

48. Milgram J, Rogers L, Miller H: Osteochondral fractures: mechanism of injury and fate of fragments. AJR 1978;130:651-658.

49. Kerr R: Diagnostic imaging of upper extremity trauma. Radiol Clin North Am 1989;27:891-908.

50. Lawson JP: Symptomatic radiographic variants in extremities. Radiology 1985;157:625-631.

18 Wrist

CORNELIA N. GOLIMBU

The complexity and interdependence of the anatomical structures of the hand and wrist make possible a multitude of movements unmatched by any other segments of the human body.

Radiologists are familiar with the roentgenographic anatomy and pathology of the carpus, the metacarpals, and the phalanges. The introduction of computed tomography and magnetic resonance imaging has made possible differentiation between soft tissues such as tendons, ligaments, muscles, blood vessels, and nerves.[1-3] These structures might appear confusing at first glance; therefore, to simplify and divide them into distinct anatomical spaces, related to specific clinical entities, the first section of this chapter describes the anatomy of the wrist, with special attention to the structures of the carpal tunnel, distal radioulnar joint, and triangular fibrocartilage of the wrist. There then follows, in related order, discussion of the carpal tunnel syndrome, distal radioulnar joint dislocations, and traumatic disruptions of the triangular fibrocartilage complex. Fractures and avascular necrosis of the carpal bones are discussed separately.

ANATOMY OF THE WRIST
Carpal tunnel

The carpal tunnel is the restricted space between the rigid fibers of the flexor retinaculum and the concave arch formed by the carpal bones.[4,5] In this tunnel the flexor tendons of the digits and the median nerve course toward the hand. The bony walls of the carpal tunnel are formed medially by the pisiform and hook of the hamate, laterally by the distal pole of the navicular and trapezium. The floor of the tunnel is formed by the lunate and capitate (Plates 18-1 to 18-4 and Fig. 18-1).

The flexor retinaculum, also known as the volar carpal ligament, is a band of inelastic fibrous tissue that inserts medially on the pisiform and the hook of the hamate and laterally on the tubercle of the scaphoid and crest of the trapezium; the proximal edge of this structure is thin, the distal part thick and fibrous. The unyielding flexor retinaculum restricts the carpal tunnel to a relatively fixed volume. Increments in the thickness of the flexor retinaculum or enlargement of the tendons and their sleeves increase the pressure in the carpal tunnel and compress the median nerve, leading to carpal tunnel syndrome.

The structures traversing the carpal tunnel are arranged in a superficial and a deep layer (Fig. 18-2). A separate compartment exists for the flexor carpi radialis tendon, which is located in the lateral aspect of the wrist adjacent to the trapezium, encased between the deep and superficial layers of the flexor retinaculum. The superficial structures in the carpal tunnel are represented from lateral to medial by the tendon of the flexor pollicis longus, the median nerve, tendons of the flexor digitorum superficialis, and an inconstant vessel (the median artery).

The deep layer is formed by the four tendons of the

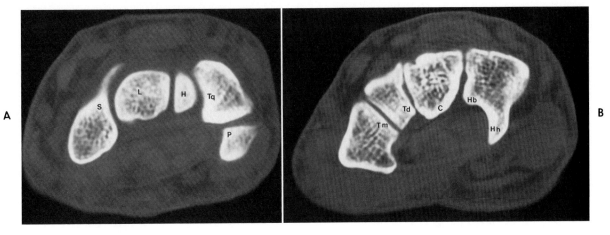

FIGURE 18-1
Bone structures forming the walls of the carpal tunnel. **A,** CT image of the proximal carpal row. The lateral wall is formed by the distal pole of the scaphoid *(S)*; the floor by the lunate *(L)* and superior part of the hamate *(H)*; the medial wall by the triquetrum *(Tq)* and pisiform *(P)*. **B,** CT axial image of the distal carpal row. The lateral wall is formed by the trapezium *(Tm)*; the floor by the trapezoid *(Td)*, capitate *(C)*, and body of the hamate *(Hb)*; and the medial wall by the hook of the hamate *(Hh)*.

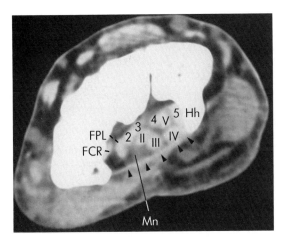

FIGURE 18-2
Soft tissue structures of the carpal tunnel. Axial CT image through the hook of the hamate *(Hh)* showing the flexor retinaculum *(arrowheads)*, flexor carpi radialis tendon *(FCR)*, flexor pollicis longus tendon *(FPL)*, median nerve *(Mn)*, flexor digitorum superficialis and flexor digitorum profundus *(2 through 5)*.

flexor digitorum profundus, from which originate the lumbrical muscles. All the flexor tendons are surrounded by a common synovial sleeve (the ulnar bursa), which assures smooth gliding motion of these structures. MRI can demonstrate these individual tendons, separated from each other by the synovial lining of their sleeves (Fig. 18-2).

Structures traversing the wrist longitudinally

The axial view is best for simultaneous identification of the individual structures traversing the wrist longitudinally.[6-13] The identity of these structures can be estab-

lished by analyzing their position, size, and shape and their relation to the adjacent structures (Fig. 18-2).

VOLAR ASPECT OF THE WRIST

Flexor carpi radialis. This muscle originates on the medial epicondyle of the humerus and inserts at the base of the second and third metacarpals (Fig. 18-3). In the distal part of the forearm it becomes tendinous, orienting itself toward the lateral and superficial aspect of the wrist, where it occupies a separate compartment formed by the groove of the trapezium and the flexor retinaculum (the latter at this level divided between a superficial and a deep layer). Thus, even though longitudinally oriented in the wrist as all other flexors, this tendon resides in a separate and distinct compartment anterior and lateral to the carpal tunnel (Fig. 18-3). The tendon of the *flexor carpi ulnaris* divides at its insertion on the pisiform, hamate, and base of the fifth metacarpal (Fig. 18-3). Another superficial structure, anterior to the flexor retinaculum, is the thin flat tendon of the *palmaris longus,* which ends by blending with the palmar aponeurosis (Fig. 18-3). These three muscles (the palmaris longus and the flexors carpi ulnaris and radialis) have a common origin on the medial epicondyle of the humerus (Fig. 18-3).

Flexor digitorum superficialis. This muscle has an arclike origin on the medial epicondyle of the humerus, the anterior aspect of the ulna, and the radius. It becomes tendinous as it approaches the wrist, where it divides into four separate tendons that pass beneath the flexor retinaculum to insert on the medial and lateral sides of the middle phalanges of digits II through V (Fig. 18-4). In the carpal tunnel the tendons of digits II and V are deeper than those of digits III and IV (Fig. 18-2).

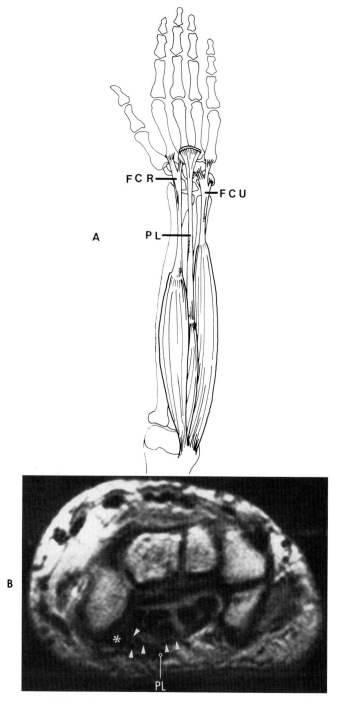

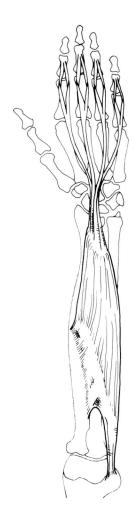

FIGURE 18-4
Flexor digitorum superficialis. Arclike origin on the medial epicondyle of the humerus, above the anterior surfaces of the radius and ulna. It divides at the wrist into four tendons, which insert on the middle phalanges of digits II through V.

FIGURE 18-3
Flexors of the carpus. **A,** Insertion of the flexor carpi radialis tendon *(FCR)* on the base of the second and third metacarpals. The flexor carpi ulnaris *(FCU)* inserts on the base of the fifth metacarpal. The palmaris longus *(PL)* inserts on the palmar aponeurosis. These three muscles have a common origin the medial epicondyle of the humerus. **B,** Axial MR image. The flexor carpi radialis tendon (*) is between the superficial and deep divisions of the flexor retinaculum *(arrowheads)* and palmaris longus *(PL),* anterior to the retinaculum.

Flexor digitorum profundus. This muscle originates on the anterior aspect of the ulna, becomes a tendon at the wrist, where its four separate divisions form the deepest layer of structures residing in the carpal tunnel, and inserts at the base of the distal phalanges of digits II through V (Fig. 18-5). The lumbrical muscles have their origin on the tendons of the deep flexor, just distal to the carpal tunnel. When the fingers are flexed the tendons slide proximally, advancing the most cranial segment of the lumbrical muscles and making them visible on axial images of the carpal tunnel.

Flexor pollicis longus. This muscle originates on the anterior aspect of the radius and inserts at the base of the terminal phalanx of the thumb (Fig. 18-6). Its tendinous segments courses obliquely along the lateral aspect of the carpal tunnel in a separate synovial sleeve (the radial bursa) next to the median nerve (Fig. 18-6).

Median nerve. The median nerve, composed of branches from the C5 through T1 nerve roots, provides innervation on the muscles of the anterior aspect of the forearm; just as it approaches the wrist, it gives off a thin

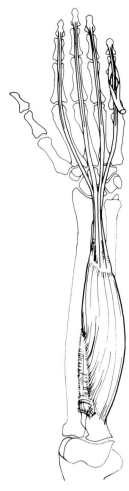

FIGURE 18-5
Flexor digitorum profundus. Origin on the anterior surface of the ulna. Its four tendons form the deepest structures of the carpal tunnel and insert on the base of the distal phalanges of digits II through V.

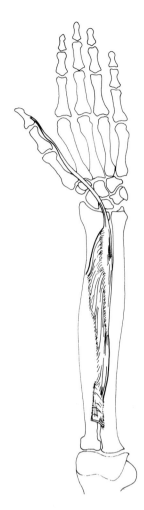

FIGURE 18-6
Flexor pollicis longus. Origin on the anterior surface of the radius; insertion on the base of the terminal phalanx of the thumb.

superficial palmar cutaneous branch. In the wrist it resides in the lateral superficial aspect of the carpal tunnel, between the flexor pollicis longus laterally, the flexor digitorum superficialis medially, and the flexor retinaculum anteriorly. It has an oval cross section measuring 2 to 4 mm. On MR images it has intermediate signal intensity, contrasting with the signal void of the tendons (Fig. 18-7). It is slightly wider at the distal end of the carpal tunnel, just before dividing into three terminal branches that supply sensory innervation to the radial half of the hand and motor innervation to the first two lumbricals and muscles of the thenar eminence (Fig. 18-8).

Muscles of the thenar eminence. These originate from the flexor retinaculum and carpal bones and are arranged in two layers. The superficial layer is formed by the *abductor pollicis brevis* and *flexor pollicis brevis,* both inserting at the base of the first phalanx. The *opponens pollicis,* in the deeper layer, inserts on the shaft of the first metacarpal (Fig. 18-9).

The *adductor pollicis* is the deepest muscle in the

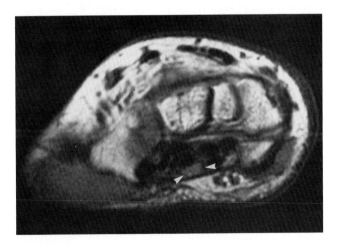

FIGURE 18-7
Median nerve. Axial MR image (SE; TR 2000 msec/TE 30 msec). The nerve *(arrowheads)* is oval on cross section and can be differentiated from the flexor tendons by its intermediate signal intensity.

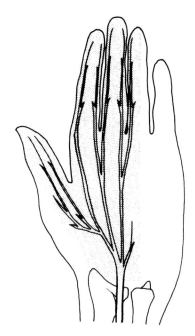

FIGURE 18-8
Median nerve branches. Sketch of the terminal branches supplying sensory innervation to the radial half of the hand and motor innervation to the muscles of the thenar eminence.

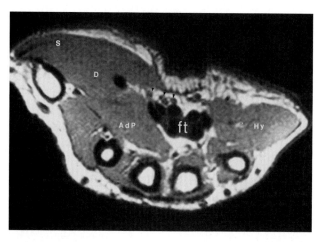

FIGURE 18-9
Anatomy of the thenar and hypothenar eminences. Axial MR image of the palm, distal to the carpal tunnel (SE; TR 1800 msec/TE 30 msec). Superficial *(S)* and deep *(D)* layers of the muscles in the thenar eminence. The adductor pollicis *(ADP)* is the deepest of the thenar eminence muscles. The hypothenar eminence muscles *(HY)* are grouped together on the medial side. The median nerve is divided into three branches *(arrowheads)* located superficially to the flexor tendon *(ft)*.

thenar eminence. It originates in the anterior aspect of the capitate and third metacarpal, inserting at the base of the first phalanx. The radial artery traverses this muscle, separating it into a proximal (oblique) and a distal (transverse) portion (Fig. 18-8).

Muscles of the hypothenar eminence. These are similar to the muscles of the thenar eminence, except that they insert on the fifth digit (Fig. 18-9). There is no adductor of

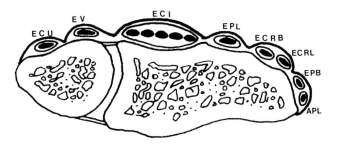

FIGURE 18-10
Extensor tendons. On the dorsal and lateral surface of the wrist, encased in six compartments separated by septations of thin extensor retinaculum. Starting with the medial side, these are the extensor carpi ulnaris *(ECU)*, extensor digiti quinti *(EV)*, extensors digitorum communis and indicis *(ECI)*, extensor pollicis longus *(EPL)*, extensors carpi radialis brevis and longus *(ECRB* and *ECRL)*, extensor pollicis brevis *(EPB)*, and abductor pollicis longus *(APL)*.

the fifth digit. The tendon of the *flexor carpi ulnaris*, superficially located in the medial side of the wrist, inserts on the pisiform.

DORSAL ASPECT OF THE WRIST

The dorsal aspect of the wrist is traversed longitudinally by the extensor tendons of the fingers and wrist and the thumb abductors. They are separated by divisions of the thin layer of fibrous tissue that forms the extensor retinaculum (Fig. 18-10).

Extensor muscles. In the center of the dorsal wrist are the four individual tendons of the *extensor digitorum communis*, which with the *extensor indicis* tendon occupy one of the compartments formed by the dorsal retinaculum. They terminate distally in the dorsal extensor tendon expansions of fingers two through five. The *extensor of the fifth finger* travels in an individual compartment medial to the extensor communis. The most medial of the extensor tendons is the *extensor carpi ulnaris*, located in a separate fibroosseous compartment formed by the extensor retinaculum and a groove between the styloid process and head of the ulna. The extensor carpi ulnaris sleeve has fibrous connections with the dorsal margin of the triangular fibrocartilage of the wrist and the meniscus homologue. Distal to these structures it ends by inserting on the base of the fifth metacarpal.

Lateral to the common extensor tendons are the structures responsible for motion of the thumb; in order, from medial to lateral, they are the extensor pollicis longus, extensor pollicis brevis, and abductor pollicis longus. Also on the dorsal side of the wrist, interposed between the extensors pollicis longus and brevis, are the tendons of the extensors carpi radialis brevis and longus. The *abductor pollicis longus* inserts at the base of the first metacarpal; the *extensor pollicis brevis*, which courses just medial to it, inserts at the base of the first proximal phalanx. Medial to this and beneath the extensor retinaculum are the tendons of the *extensors carpi radialis longus* and *brevis*, which insert respectively on the base of the second and third metacarpal.

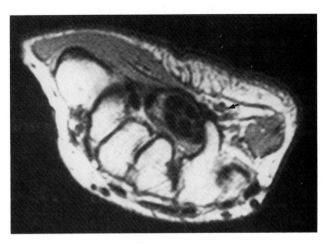

FIGURE 18-12
Guyon's canal. MRI axial view showing the ulnar nerve, artery, and vein *(arrow)* in the triangular space anterior to the hook of the hamate and anteriomedial to the palmar retinaculum.

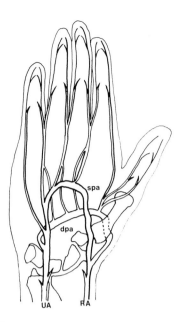

FIGURE 18-11
Arterial arches of the wrist and hand. The ulnar artery *(UA)* anastomosis with the superficial branch of the radial artery *(RA)* forms the superficial palmar arterial arch *(spa)*. The radial artery anastomosis with the deep branch of the ulnar artery forms the deep palmar arterial arch *(dpa)*. The branches of the palmar arches form the digital arteries.

Radial artery. On the lateral aspect of the radius, next to the flexor carpi radialis tendon, the *radial artery* descends from the forearm to the wrist. At the wrist it lies in the "anatomical snuff box," beneath the abductor pollicis longus and extensors pollicis brevis and longus. It perforates the first interosseous muscle and traverses the space between the thumb and index finger, entering the palm side of the hand between the lumbrical muscles and the adductor pollicis longus. Its anastomosis with the deep palmar branch of the ulnar artery forms the deep palmar arterial arch (Fig. 18-11).

Ulnar artery and nerve. The ulnar artery and nerve are located in a separate compartment on the medial side of the palmar wrist, called Guyon's canal, separated from the rest of the subcutaneous fat by two fascial layers. The medial wall of Guyon's canal is formed by the pisiform. Medial and anterior to the canal is the flexor carpi ulnaris tendon, and more lateral and deeper is the flexor retinaculum forming the anterior wall of the carpal tunnel (Fig. 18-12).

Distal radioulnar joint

The distal radius has a concave facet on its medial side, the sigmoid notch, that articulates with the ulnar head. The sigmoid notch has a sharp edge dorsally and a rounded margin anteriorly. On the dorsal surface the distal radius has a prominence called Lister's tubercle. This can be used to identify the posterior aspect in a single CT axial image of the distal radius (Fig. 18-13). The junction between the distal articular surface of the radius and the sigmoid notch is represented by a sharp ridge of

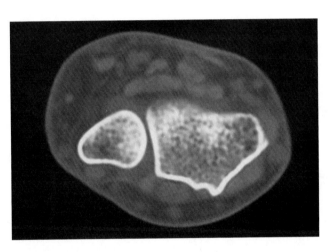

FIGURE 18-13
CT of the distal radiocarpal joint. An axial image shows the distal ulna articulating with the sigmoid notch of the radius. The prominence on the dorsal surface of the radius is Lister's tubercle.

bone that serves as the origin of the triangular fibrocartilage.

The distal radioulnar joint consists of two cylindrical opposing articular surfaces with different-sized diameters. The concave sigmoid notch is larger than the convex ulnar head, and as a result the motions permitted by this anatomical arrangement include not only rotation of the radius (with the carpus and hand) around the ulna but also posteroanterior translation of the ulnar head within the sigmoid notch.[14]

Triangular fibrocartilage of the wrist

The triangular fibrocartilage of the wrist (TFC), also known as the articular disk, is a band of fibrous tissue originating on the medial margin of the distal radius. It traverses horizontally the space between the ulna and carpal bones and inserts near the base of the ulnar

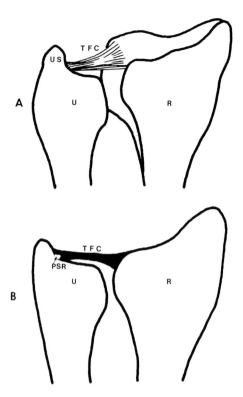

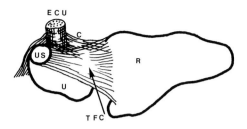

FIGURE 18-15
Connection between the triangular fibrocartilage and the sheath of the extensor carpi ulnaris tendon. The dorsal margin of the TFC has interconnecting fibers *(C)* uniting it with the sheath of the extensor carpi ulnaris tendon *(ECU)*. Ulnar styloid *(US)*, radius *(R)*, ulna *(U)*.

FIGURE 18-14
Anatomy of the triangular fibrocartilage of the wrist *(TFC)*. **A,** Anterior view. The TFC is fan shaped, with a wide origin on the margin of the sigmoid notch of the radius *(R)* and a narrow insertion near the base of the ulnar styloid *(US)*. **B,** Coronal section. The ulnar insertion is in the basistyloid fovea and at the base of the ulnar styloid. Between these two insertions is a space lined with synovium, the prestyloid recess *(PSR)*. The radial insertion on the radius is thicker than the center.

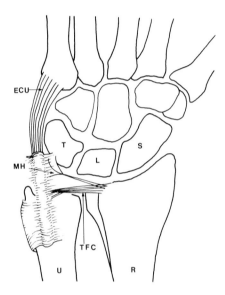

FIGURE 18-16
Dorsal view of the meniscus homologue and extensor carpi ulnaris sheath. Radius *(R)*, ulna *(U)*, triquetrum *(T)*, lunate *(L)*, scaphoid *(S)*, meniscus homologue *(MH)*, extensor carpi ulnaris tendon *(ECU)*, triangular fibrocartilage *(TFC)*. The meniscus homologue attaches to the triquetrum and radius.

styloid.[15,16] It is fan shaped, with a wide origin on the margin of the sigmoid notch of the radius and narrow converging insertion on the ulna (Fig. 18-14). Its center is formed by thin translucent chondroid fibrocartilage 1 to 3 mm thick that, as a consequence of normal aging, undergoes degeneration, often with a central perforation.[16,17] The anterior and posterior margins are thicker, bandlike, and composed of lamellar collagen fibers that blend with the dorsal and palmar radioulnar ligaments and the articular capsule of the radioulnar joint.[16] The thickest part (5 mm) of the TFC is near the ulnar insertion, where the collagenous fibers of the anterior and posterior borders converge, inserting partly on the styloid process and mostly in a shallow depression (the basistyloid fovea) between the ulnar articular surface and the base of the styloid process. These two sites are separated by a synovial space, varying in size between 1 and 5 mm, called the prestyloid recess.

The triangular fibrocartilage exchanges thin connections with the fibrous tissues of the *extensor carpi ulnaris* tendon sheath and the meniscus homologue (Fig. 18-15). The *meniscus homologue* is an inconstant anatomical structure, represented by a crescent-shaped fibrocartilage

attached to the ulnar side of the synovial lining of the medial wrist joint. It has straps attaching it to the triquetrum and, proximally, to the radius, sharing a common origin with the triangular fibrocartilage of the wrist (Fig. 18-16). It also has connections with the sheath on the extensor carpi ulnaris. Two other structures intimately connected with the margins of the triangular fibrocartilage of the wrist are the *ulnolunate* and *ulnotriquetral* ligaments. All these structures are functionally and anatomically linked in one unit, named in the surgical literature the *triangular fibrocartilage complex* (TFCC).[18]

The TFCC acts as the major stabilizing element of the distal radioulnar joint by providing a mechanism of rotation of the radiocarpal unit around the ulnar axis. It connects the ulnar side of the wrist and hand with the radius. It also cushions the impact of the forces transmitted through the ulnocarpal axis.[18]

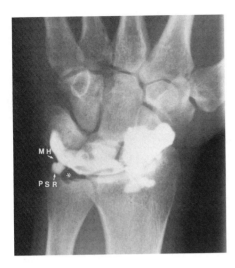

FIGURE 18-17
Normal wrist arthrogram. Contrast injected into the radiocarpal joint outlines the distal surface of the triangular fibrocartilage (*). No contrast enters the distal radioulnar joint. The thorn-shaped meniscus homologue (MH) is medial and distal to the prestyloid recess (PSR).

The TFCC separates the radioulnar joint from the radiocarpal synovial space. On arthrograms of the radiocarpal joint the flow of contrast is limited by the distal surface of the TFC. Contrast collects normally around the ulna (prestyloid recess) and outlines the "thorn" shape of the meniscus homologue, distal and medial to the ulnar styloid (Fig. 18-17).

TECHNIQUE OF WRIST CT

In our experience, when extension of the arm above the head is required for scanning, most patients prefer the prone position.

Making the patient comfortable and taping the hand with Velcro straps for immobilization of the extremity are important factors in assuring true sequential views of the anatomy when 1.5 or 3 mm slices are obtained.

The choice of slice orientation depends to some degree upon the pathology suspected: a fracture of the hook of the hamate is best detected on axial views whereas its craniocaudad displacement is better appreciated in sagittal images and can be totally missed on coronal slices. The relationship of the central carpal bones is best seen in coronal views, but sagittal views show to best advantage any tilt of the lunate or subtle perilunate-type dislocation.

The navicular bone has an oblique orientation in the wrist; thus when a fracture or complications thereof require CT scanning, it is best to obtain an oblique sagittal view through the wrist.

A dislocation of the distal radioulnar joint is best seen on axial views. By obtaining these in pronation and supination, a dynamic representation of joint alignment can be obtained, revealing a subtle unipositional subluxation.

The smallest field of view that can portray the entire

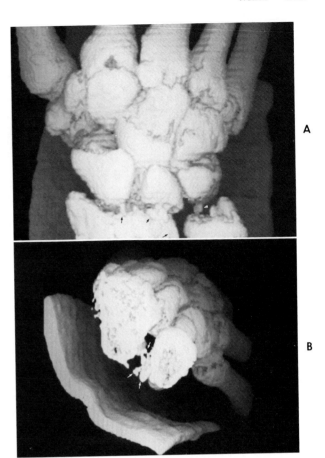

FIGURE 18-18
Three-dimensional reconstruction of CT images. **A**, Dorsal view of the wrist supported by a plaster cast placed on the palmar side. Fragment of bone interposed between ulnar head and triquetrum (arrowhead). Abnormally large space in the radioulnar joint. Comminuted fracture of the radius (arrows). **B**, View from the proximal end of the wrist. Several fragments of bone (arrows) are interposed between the distal radius and ulna, preventing reduction of the distal radioulnar joint.

anatomical site of interest is preferred (usually 10 to 15 cm). Slice thickness generally is 3 mm, though 1.5 mm may be necessary when small structures such as the navicular or hook of the hamate are being studied.[19-20]

When three-dimensional reformatting of images is planned, the 1.5 mm slice thickness gives a smoother edge to the bone structures, reducing the partial volume averaging artifacts (which give a zigzag margin to curved bone surfaces)[21,22] (Fig. 18-18).

Axial images

Position
    Arm and forearm straight, extended over the head
    Medial side on a sponge block
Scanogram: Frontal view of the wrist
Slice selection (Fig. 18-19)
    Prospective targeted images with bone algorithm
    Centered on the carpal bones
    Field of view 12 cm
    Slice thickness 3 mm

FIGURE 18-19
Technique of CT axial images. **A,** Positioning. **B,** Scanogram portraying the anatomy of the wrist in frontal view. **C,** The lines on the image mark the inferior and superior ends of the stack of contiguous axial images. **D,** CT image. Pisiform *(p)*, triquetrum *(tq)*, lunate *(l)*, scaphoid *(s)*, hamate *(h)*, and trazepium *(tm)*.

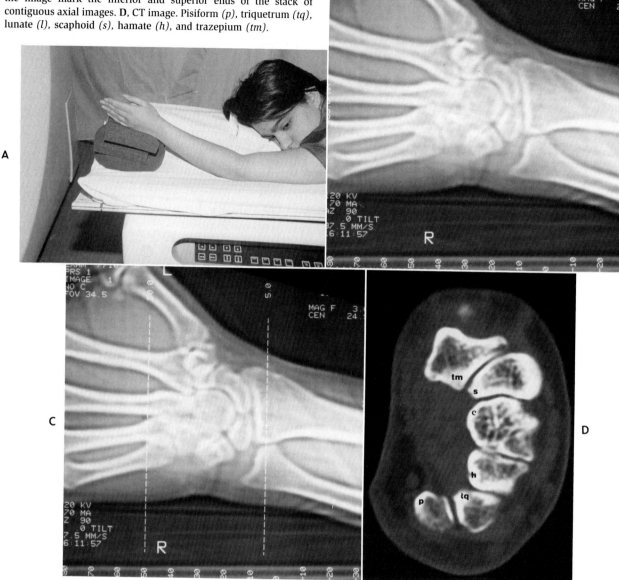

Coronal images

Position
Arm extended over the head
Elbow flexed 90 degrees
Hand resting with the ulnar side on a sponge block
Palm facing (but not touching) the crown of the head
Scanogram: Lateral view
Slice selection (Fig. 18-20)
Prospective targeted images with bone algorithm
Centered on the carpus
Field of views 12 to 15 cm
Slice thickness 3 mm

Sagittal images

Position
Arm extended over the head

Elbow flexed 90 degrees
Hand resting with the palmar surface down on a sponge block
Scanogram: Anteroposterior view
Slice selection (Fig. 18-21)
Prospective targeted images with bone algorithm
Centered on the carpus and distal radius
Field of view 15 cm
Slice thickness 3 mm

Axial images for the distal radioulnar joint

Position
Arm extended over the head
Ulnar side of the wrist down, resting on a sponge block
Scanogram: Lateral view of the wrist
Slice selection
Prospective targeted images with bone algorithm

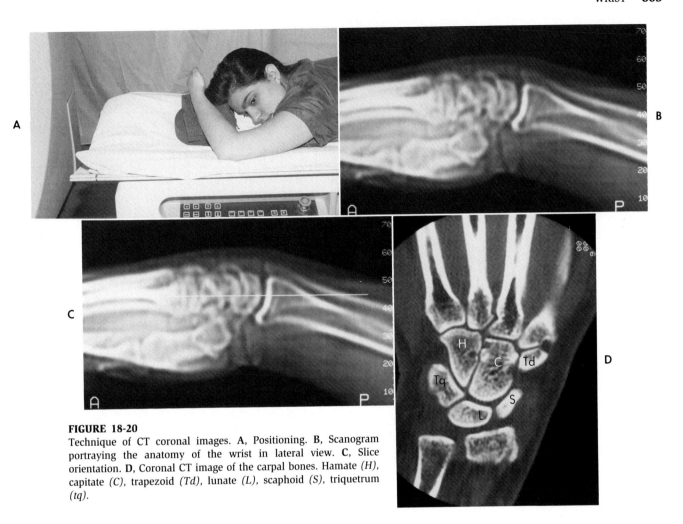

FIGURE 18-20
Technique of CT coronal images. **A,** Positioning. **B,** Scanogram portraying the anatomy of the wrist in lateral view. **C,** Slice orientation. **D,** Coronal CT image of the carpal bones. Hamate *(H),* capitate *(C),* trapezoid *(Td),* lunate *(L),* scaphoid *(S),* triquetrum *(tq).*

Centered on the distal radius
Field of view 15-20 cm
Slice thickness 3 mm
One to three slices are sufficient

Repeat scanogram and axial images after turning the hand in extreme supination (palm facing superolaterally) and pronation (palm down) (Fig. 18-22); when subtle abnormalities are suspected, both sides should be scanned (Fig. 18-23).

Oblique axial images for the navicular

Position
Arm extended over the head
Elbow flexed 60 degrees
Palm facing down on a sponge block
Hand obliquely oriented in the gantry, at 60 degrees
Slight ulnar tilt of the hand relative to the wrist
Scanogram: Frontal view
Slice selection (Fig. 18-24)
Prospective targeted images with bone algorithm
Centered on the navicular
Field of view 10 cm
Slice thickness 1.5 mm

TECHNIQUE OF WRIST MRI

Rapid progress in the development of coils dedicated to studying the extremities has led to frequent changes in the technical parameters used for scanning of the wrist.[23-28] The protocol described below applies to the 1.5 tesla Gyroscan unit.* Similar scanners might have slight variations of this technique.

Patient position (Fig. 18-25)
Prone, arm extended above the head
Hand placed on a foam block
Surface coil: Flat circular 6 or 11 cm diameter
Axial scout
Five slices, 7 mm thick
TR 500/TE 30, field of view (FOV) 250 mm
One measurement, 70% acquisition time
Scanning time 1 minute 12 seconds
T1-weighted coronal or sagittal images (Figs. 18-26 and 18-27)
Nine slices, 3 mm thick
TR 500/TE 30, FOV 100 mm
Two measurements, matrix 256/256
Scanning time 5 minutes 15 seconds

*Philips Medical Systems North America, Shelton Conn. 06484.

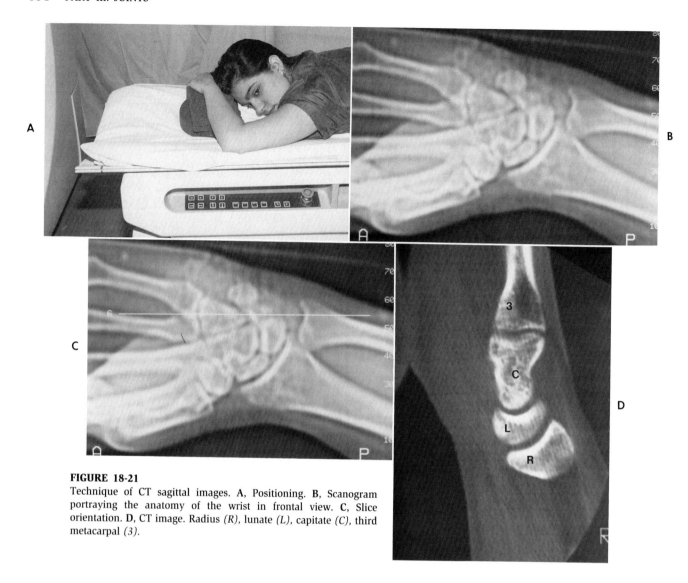

FIGURE 18-21
Technique of CT sagittal images. **A,** Positioning. **B,** Scanogram portraying the anatomy of the wrist in frontal view. **C,** Slice orientation. **D,** CT image. Radius *(R)*, lunate *(L)*, capitate *(C)*, third metacarpal *(3)*.

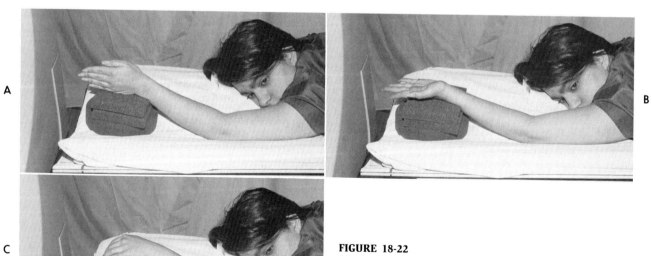

FIGURE 18-22
Positioning for study of the distal radioulnar joint. **A,** Neutral position. **B,** Supination. **C,** Pronation.

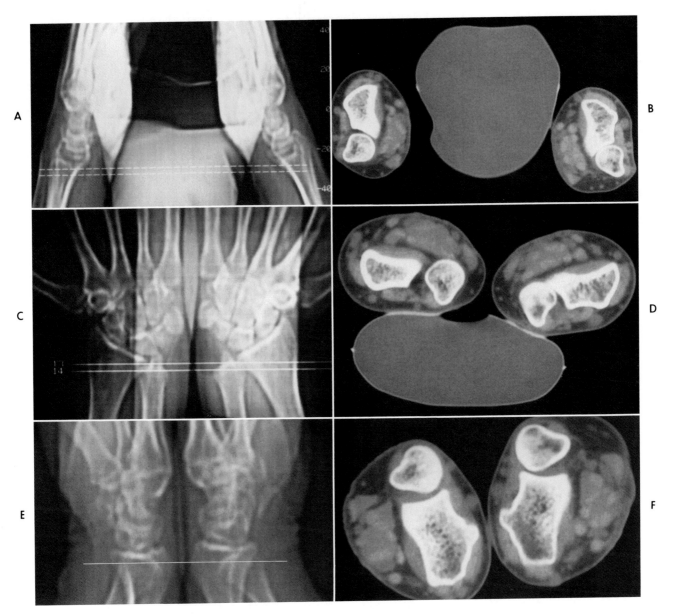

FIGURE 18-23
Technique of CT. Comparative views of both radioulnar joints. **A,** Scanogram in neutral position. **B,** Axial images of the wrists in neutral position. In the center, a water bag was used as bolus. **C,** Scanogram in supination. **D,** Axial images of both wrists in supination. **E,** Scanogram in pronation. **F,** Axial images of both wrists in pronation.

T2-weighted axial images (Fig. 18-28)
    Slice factor 1.2
    Twelve to eighteen slices, 3 mm thick
    Slice factor 1.2
    TR 2100/TE 80 FOV 100 mm
    Two measurements, 204/256 matrix
    Scanning time 14 minutes 23 seconds
Gradient-recalled echo images in coronal or sagittal orientation (T2*) (Fig. 18-29)
    Nine slices, 3 mm thick, slice factor 1.2
    TR 600/TE 20, flip angle 20 degrees, FOV 100 mm
    256/256 matrix
    Scanning time 5 minutes 13 seconds

IMAGING OF WRIST DISORDERS
Carpal tunnel syndrome

The median nerve, enclosed in the carpal tunnel with the flexor tendons, is vulnerable to compressive forces whenever the pressure increases in that compartment. The increased pressure is frequently the result of soft tissue pathology and may be caused by a multitude of factors — including traumatic tenosynovitis, arthritic processes associated with synovial hypertrophy (pannus), edema of the tendons and their synovial sleeves, calcific deposits associated with hyperparathyroidism, thickening of the palmar aponeurosis, fibrosis of the epineurium,

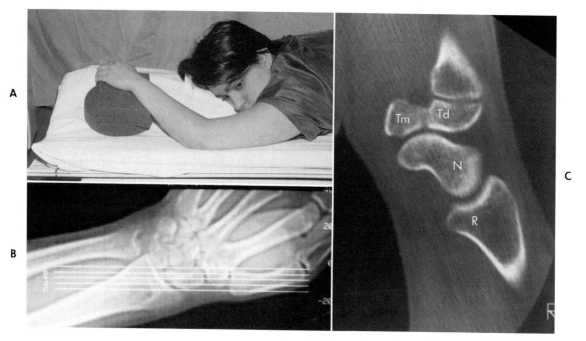

FIGURE 18-24
Technique of CT for the navicular bone. **A,** Positioning. **B,** Scanogram. **C,** CT image showing the navicular *(N)* in a longitudinal sagittal representation and its articulations with the radius *(R)*, trapezium *(Tm)*, and trapezoid *(Td)*.

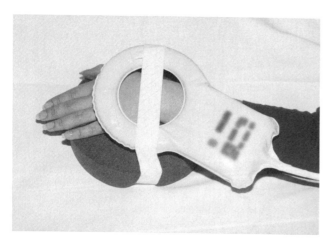

FIGURE 18-25
Technique of wrist MRI. The flat circular surface coil is positioned on the dorsal surface of the wrist.

FIGURE 18-26
Coronal MRI of the normal wrist (SE; TR 550 msec/TE 30 msec; slice thickness 3 mm; FOV 100 mm; NSA 2; 256/256 matrix). Scaphoid *(s)*, lunate *(L)*, triquetrum *(Tq)*, hamate *(H)*, capitate *(C)*, trapezoid *(Td)*, and second, third, and fourth metacarpals *(2 to 4)*.

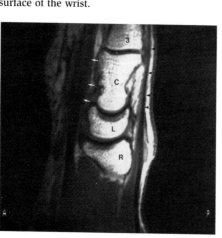

FIGURE 18-27
Sagittal MRI of the normal wrist. Radius *(R)*, lunate *(L)*, capitate *(C)*, and base of the third metacarpal *(3)*; extensor tendon *(arrowheads)* and flexor tendons *(arrows)* of the third finger.

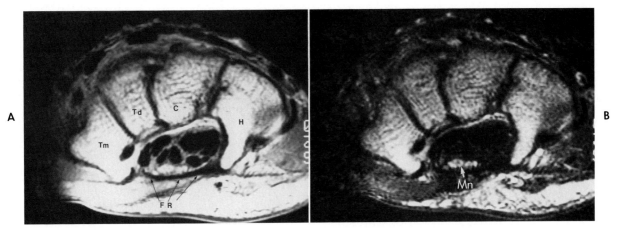

FIGURE 18-28
Axial MRI of the carpal tunnel (SE; TR 2000 msec/TE 30 and 80 msec; FOV 100 mm; slice thickness 3 mm; NSA 2; 204/256 matrix). **A,** Proton density—weighted image. **B,** T2-weighted image. Hamate *(H),* capitate *(C),* trapezoid *(Td),* and trapezium *(Tm).* The flexor retinaculum *(FR)* inserts on the trapezium and the hook of the hamate. Beneath it are the median nerve *(Mn, arrow* in **B)** and the tendons longitudinally traversing the carpal tunnel.

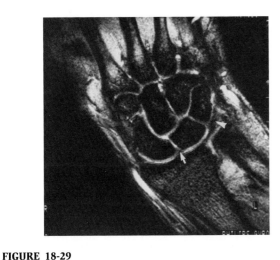

FIGURE 18-29
Gradient-recalled echo MR image; coronal view (TR 600 msec/TE 20 msec, flip angle 20 degrees; NSA 2; FOV 100 mm; slice thickness 3 mm). The fatty bone marrow, cortical bone and fibrocartilage have low signal. The articular hyaline cartilage and joint fluid are uniformly high in signal. This contrast allows for better visualization of the TFC *(arrowhead)* and the scapholunate ligament *(arrow).*

neuroma of the median nerve.[29,30] Rarely the bony walls of the canal may be abnormal, leading to constriction of the tunnel. This can be seen in fracture-dislocations of the carpal bones or in degenerative disease of the scaphotrapezial joint. Fragments of bone, dislocated carpal segments, or hypertrophic spurs oriented toward the carpal tunnel may impinge on the soft tissue structures residing within the tunnel.

Of all these tissues, the most vulnerable is the median nerve. Irritation and, later, paralysis of this nerve have been described as carpal tunnel syndrome—manifested as pain, paresthesia, and tingling in the distribution of the

nerve (muscles of the thenar eminence, first two lumbricals, and skin of the radial half of the hand).

The clinical signs of carpal tunnel syndrome are rather characteristic. Neuroconduction studies usually confirm compression of the median nerve in the carpal tunnel. Treatment consists of surgical releasing the palmar retinaculum.

Occasionally, radiological examinations are necessary to explain discrepancies between clinical and EMG findings or to detect causes of persistence of symptoms after surgery. CT and MRI have been used as imaging modalities in such situations.[31-35]

Computed tomography. CT of the carpal tunnel may reveal traumatic abnormalities of the bony walls, which are difficult to see on conventional roentgenograms. Specifically, a fracture of the hook of the hamate is well seen on axial images. Displacement of fragments and the presence of edema and hemorrhage near the fracture site may compress the structures passing through the carpal tunnel (Fig. 18-30).

Similarly spurs oriented medially from the scaphotrapezial joint may encroach on the canal and are best observed in axial CT images (Fig. 18-31). Calcific deposits in the soft tissues of the carpal tunnel are also easily seen on CT images of the wrist (Fig. 18-32).

Magnetic resonance. MR imaging is best suited for the detection of soft tissue pathology in this area—tendinitis, synovitis, ganglion cysts, neuromas, fibrous tissue masses[31,33] (Fig. 18-33). The thickness of synovium surrounding the flexor tendons must be compared with that in the normal wrist; subtle enlargement may produce carpal tunnel syndrome.

Bowing of the palmar retinaculum, which assumes a convex anterior surface, can be observed on axial images obtained at the level of the hamate and trapezium. This is

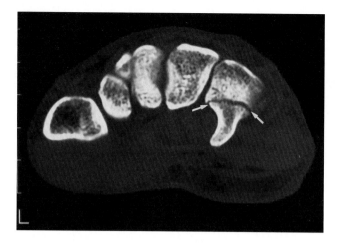

FIGURE 18-30
Bone abnormality in the wall of the carpal tunnel: fractured hook of the hamate. Axial CT image. The fracture appears as a line of separation traversing the base of the hook of the hamate *(arrows)*.

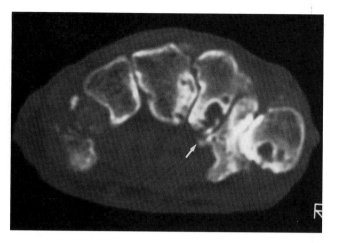

FIGURE 18-31
Impingement on the carpal tunnel secondary to osteoarthritis. Erosions of the articular surfaces are present in the trapezoid, trapezium, and first metacarpal. A spur formed at the margin of the trapeziotrapezoidal joint protrudes into the carpal tunnel *(arrow)*.

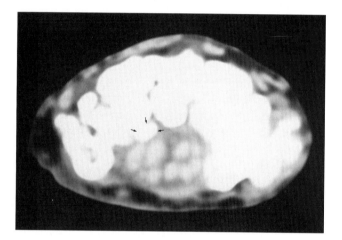

FIGURE 18-32
Carpal tunnel syndrome secondary to hyperparathyroidism. Calcific deposits are in the carpal tunnel *(arrows)*.

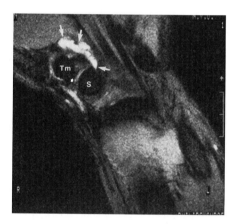

FIGURE 18-33
Carpal tunnel syndrome produced by a synovial cyst. T2* coronal MR image through the carpal tunnel. The fluid-filled cyst *(arrows)* appears as a bright-signal elongated zone adjacent to the trapezium *(Tm)* and the distal pole of the scaphoid *(S)*.

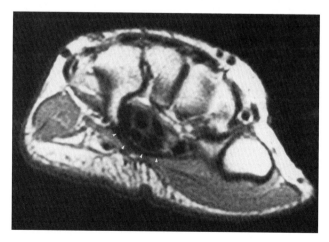

FIGURE 18-34
Carpal tunnel syndrome. MRI axial view at the level of the hook of the hamate. Bowing of the palmar retinaculum *(arrowheads)* is a nonspecific finding, reflecting increased pressure in the carpal tunnel.

a nonspecific finding and reflects increased pressure in the carpal tunnel (Fig. 18-34). The median nerve is well seen on axial MR images of the wrists, appearing as a structure with 4×2 mm ovoid cross section and intermediate signal intensity similar to that of muscle, which contrasts with the adjacent low-signal tendons and facilitates its detection on MR images.[31] In patients with carpal tunnel syndrome the median nerve may appear swollen just proximal to the "tight tunnel." To observe subtle changes in the diameter of the median nerve requires comparing the appearances of this structure on axial MR images obtained at the distal radius, pisiform, and hamate; the nerve may be enlarged just before entering the high-pressure zone of the carpal tunnel and compressed and flattened in the tunnel itself[31,33] (Fig. 18-35). The higher signal of the median nerve seen in patients with carpal tunnel syndrome may reflect perineural edema related to compression.

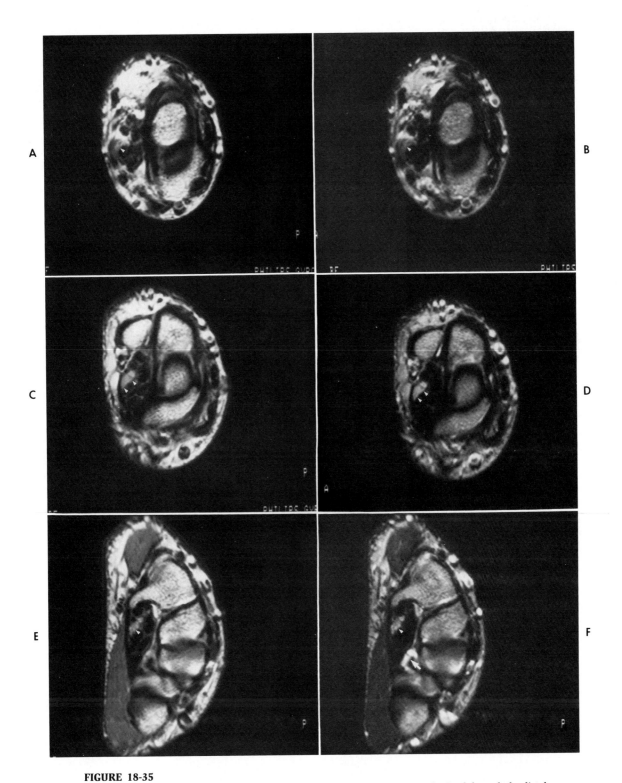

FIGURE 18-35

Median nerve compression in the carpal tunnel syndrome. Axial MR images obtained through the distal radius, **A** and **B**, pisiform, **C** and **D**, and hamate, **E** and **F** (SE; TR 1800 msec/TE 29 msec [**A, C, E**] and TE 80 msec [**B, D, F**]). The images obtained at the radius and pisiform demonstrate increased diameter and signal intensity of the nerve *(arrowheads)* at its entrance into the carpal tunnel (**C** and **D**), signifying edema just proximal to the compressed segment. The increased pressure in the canal can be explained by the presence of a synovial cyst filled with bright-signal fluid (**F**) near the trapeziotrape-zoidal joint *(arrow)*.

In successful surgical decompression the fibers of the palmar retinaculum are interrupted. Incomplete transection of this fibrous band may be seen in patients with persistent symptoms following surgery[34] (Fig. 18-36).

Pathology of the distal radioulnar joint

Axial images obtained by CT are extremely useful in studying the distal radiocarpal joint.[36-40] They can portray the sigmoid notch of the radius with its dorsal sharp border and ventral rounded margin. They can also help in assessing the integrity of the articular cortex in the radioulnar joint; this is important in fractures of the mediodistal radius (Fig. 18-37). These fractures are often associated with malposition of the fragments forming the sigmoid notch (Fig. 18-38). Reduction of the fragments is best observed on axial images.[37]

The relative position of the ulnar head in the sigmoid notch of the radius changes during normal movement of pronation/supination. The radius, carrying with it the carpal bones, rotates around the ulna in a 190-degree arc with the center next to the ulnar styloid.[40] The concavity of the sigmoid notch is larger than the convex surface of the ulnar head. This permits a translation of the ulna within the radial surface at the time of pronation and supination. In neutral position approximately 80% of the ulnar head surface has contact with the sigmoid notch of

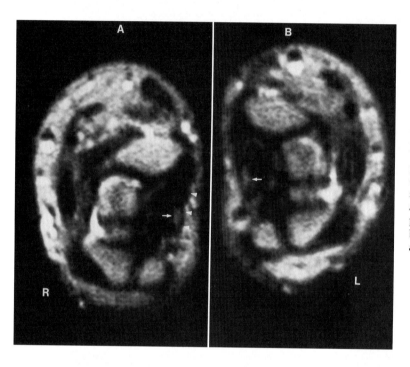

FIGURE 18-36
Incomplete transection of the palmar retinaculum. T2-weighted axial MR images of the wrists in a patient with persistent signs of right median nerve compression following surgery for carpal tunnel syndrome. The images of the normal left wrist, **B**, and the symptomatic right side, **A**, show that the palmar retinaculum *(arrowheads)* is still tightly bound to the anterior surface of the flexor tendons and median nerve *(arrow)* in the right wrist.

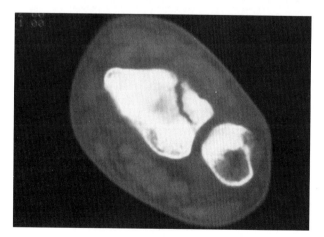

FIGURE 18-37
Fracture of the distal radius. CT of the distal radioulnar joint. A fracture line intersects the articular cortex of the sigmoid notch of the radius. The radioulnar joint space is abnormally wide.

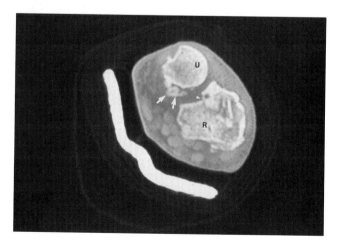

FIGURE 18-38
Incongruous surfaces of the distal radioulnar joint. An axial CT image through the sigmoid notch shows a comminuted fracture with displacement of fragments, creating a step-off deformity of the articular surface *(arrowhead)*. Fragments of bone *(arrows)* are interposed between the ulnar head *(U)* and the radius *(R)*.

the radius. In pronation the ulna slides anteriorly, which brings the palmar aspect of the sigmoid notch into contact with the ulna. In supination the ulna slides in a reverse direction and only 30% or less of the ulnar articular surface faces the dorsal aspect of the sigmoid notch. It appears that a certain degree of variability exists in the exact amount of apposition of the articular surfaces; thus it is important to compare images of the symptomatic and asymptomatic sides. Only then can one be certain that subtle subluxations are not, in fact, variants of normal capsular laxity permitting a larger range of motion in the distal radioulnar joint of individual patients (Fig. 18-39).

Instability of the distal radioulnar joint can be mani-

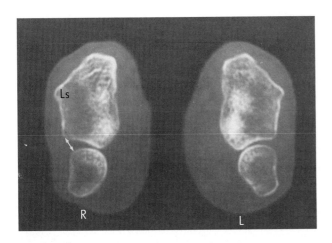

FIGURE 18-39
Subluxation of the right distal radioulnar joint. An axial CT image of both wrists obtained through the distal radius and ulna shows a subtle difference between the two sides. The right side has a larger space, mostly in the dorsal aspect of the joint *(arrow)*. The dorsal surface of the radius is recognizable by the prominent Lister tubercle *Ls*).

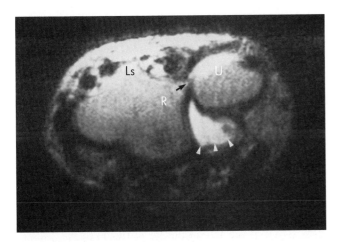

FIGURE 18-40
Dislocation of the distal radioulnar joint. Axial T2-weighted MR image. The ulna *(U)* is dislocated and impacted against the dorsal margin of the sigmoid notch of the radius *(arrow)*. The prominent Lister tubercle *(Ls)* identifies the dorsal surface of the radius *(R)*. Effusion of the radioulnar joint is manifested as a zone of bright signal *(arrowheads)*.

fested as a dorsal-volar dislocation, subluxation, or radioulnar diastasis (Fig. 18-40). Occasionally a dorsally torn triangular fibrocartilage of the wrist will slide in the sigmoid notch and prevent reduction of anterior ulnar dislocation.[41] CT and MRI can detect the cartilage fragment and establish the need for open reduction.

Computed tomography and magnetic resonance. CT has distinct advantages over MRI when study of the distal radioulnar joint alignment is necessary. It permits immediate change of position from supination to pronation; it allows study of the normal and symptomatic sides simultaneously; and it shows with great detail any interruption in the articular cortex of the radius or ulna. MRI studies require precise positioning of the surface coil on each wrist, and this precludes rapid examinations of both extremities in different positions. Consequently, at present, axial CT images remain the more practical modality for studying subtle abnormalities of the distal radioulnar joint that necessitate changes in position to become manifest.

Abnormalities of the triangular fibrocartilage

Injuries to the medial side of the wrist can produce tears of the triangular fibrocartilage. The established method for radiologically evaluating this abnormality, prior to MRI, was wrist arthrography.

Arthrography and CT-arthrography. The introduction of contrast into the radiocarpal joint outlines the distal surface of the triangular fibrocartilage (TFC). Tears are diagnosed by observing entrance of contrast in the distal radioulnar joint[42] (Fig. 18-41). Similarly, tears of the scapholunate and lunotriquetral ligaments are manifested by arthrography as extension of contrast from the radiocarpal to the midcarpal joints (Fig. 18-41). Technical refinements of arthrography (e.g., digital subtraction and video recording of flow of injected contrast) are aimed at distinguishing the exact point of communication between articular compartments, thus establishing the location of tears of ligamentous and fibrocartilaginous structures.[43,44] Furthermore, it has been shown[45] that tricompartmental injection (radiocarpal, midcarpal, and distal radioulnar joints) is necessary to visualize tears that allow only unidirectional flow of injected contrast (Fig. 18-42).

Some authors[46,57] have suggested the use of CT for studying the surface of the TFC coated with contrast: CT-arthrography of the wrist (Fig. 18-43). However, the minimal additional information obtained does not justify the radiation exposure, time, and cost incurred when performing CT following an arthrogram directed at studying the TFC.

Computed arthrotomography of the wrist has been found helpful[48] in precisely locating loose calcified intraarticular bodies. This is a rarely encountered clinical problem in the wrist joint, and it is therefore not expected that CT-arthrography will be performed frequently.

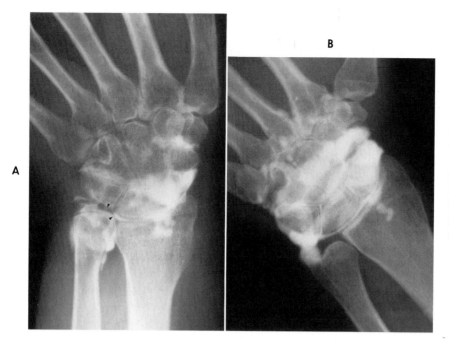

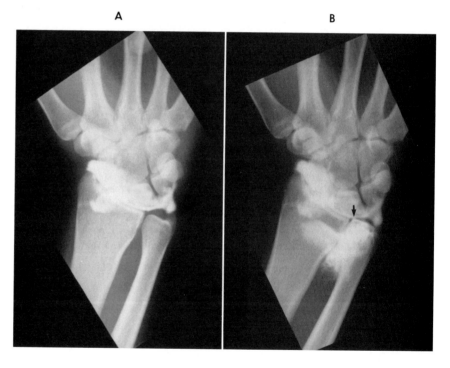

FIGURE 18-41
Abnormal arthrograms of the radiocarpal joint. **A,** Tear of the triangular fibrocartilage *(TFC).* Contrast enters the distal radioulnar joint through tears in the TFC *(arrowheads).* Contrast is also present in the midcarpal joints. **B,** Another patient, with a normal TFC but a tear in the lunotriquetral ligament permitting entrance of contrast into the middle and distal carpal joints.

FIGURE 18-42
Bicompartment wrist arthrogram. **A,** Contrast injected into the radiocarpal joint outlines the distal surface of the TFC. No tear is detected. **B,** A second injection, this time into the distal radioulnar joint, shows perforation of the TFC near the radial insertion *(arrow).*

Magnetic resonance. MRI of the wrist, obtained with dedicated surface coils and a small field of view, allows visualization of the triangular fibrocartilage,[49] which appears as a low-signal structure against the background of intermediate- or high-signal synovial fluid. The coronal images show it best, especially when thin slices (3 mm or less) are obtained to avoid partial volume averaging. The TFC appears as a band of signal void stretching from the medial margin of the radius to the base of the ulnar styloid. It is thicker near the ulnar insertion (approximately 5 mm), where it connects (posteriorly) with fibers

of the external layer of the sheath of the extensor carpi ulnaris and (medially) with the proximal aspect of the meniscus homologue (Figs. 18-14 and 18-44).

In young patients MRI images show a high or intermediate signal at the lateral border of the TFC, most likely representing the normal chondroid cartilage that extends to the margin of the radial articular surface (Fig. 18-45).

Tears in the TFC appear on MRI as high- or intermediate-signal lines interrupting the signal void of the fibrocartilage (Fig. 18-46). T2-weighted and gradient-recalled echo images produce an "arthrogram effect," which

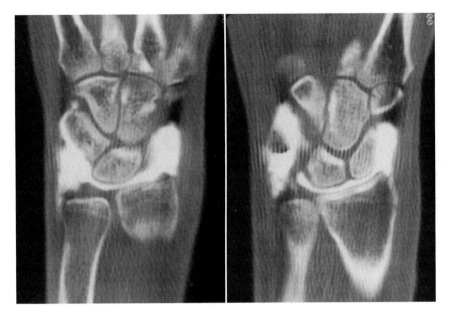

FIGURE 18-43
Normal CT arthrogram of the wrist. Direct coronal views of the wrist show contrast in the radiocarpal joint and around the medial surface of the triquetrum. The TFC is intact; the scapholunate and lunotriquetral joints do not contain contrast.

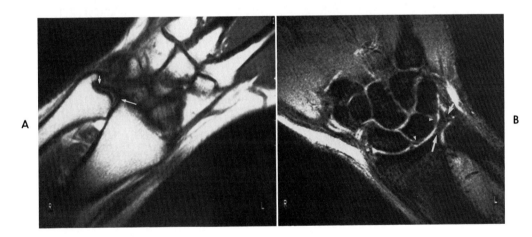

FIGURE 18-44
MRI of the normal TFC. A, Coronal T1-weighted image. The TFC appears as a thin band of signal void *(arrows)*. B, Coronal gradient-recalled image. The low-signal band of the TFC *(arrows)* contrasts with the bright signal of the articular fluid. The scapholunate and lunotriquetral ligaments are also visible *(arrowheads)*.

makes the triangular fibrocartilage stand out against the background of high-signal synovial fluid.[49] Tears appear more evident on such images (Fig. 18-47) and can be located near the radial origin, in the center, or near the ulnar insertion of the TFC (Fig. 18-48).

Occasionally an abnormal focal area of low signal will be observed in the ulnar head of a patient with a TFC tear. This is probably an area of chondromalacia resulting from pressure of the ulna on the lunate directly, or indirectly through the fragmented irregular margin of the torn TFC (Fig. 18-49).

SIGNIFICANCE OF TFC TEARS

The triangular fibrocartilage of the wrist has two histologically different parts with separate but complementary functions:

The center (consisting of chondroid cartilage) is exposed to compressive forces generated by the "corkscrew" motion that makes the ulnar head advance toward the carpus during pronation. This part of the TFC serves as a cushion to diminish the impact of the ulna on the lunate and triquetrum.

The margins (anterior and posterior) are subjected to

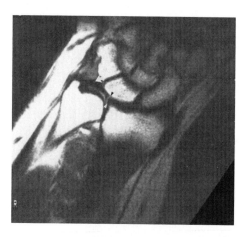

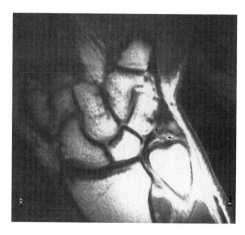

FIGURE 18-45

A T1-weighted coronal image of a 21-year-old woman shows TFC intact *(arrow)*. On its lateral margin a line of intermediate signal, parallel to the cortex of the radius, represents normal chondrocartilage of the sigmoid notch in the radius *(arrowheads)*.

FIGURE 18-46

A coronal T1-weighted image shows nonhomogeneous intermediate- and high-signal zones interrupting the TFC on its ulnar side *(arrows)*.

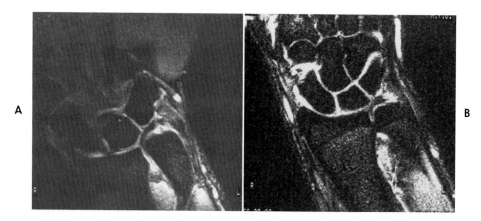

FIGURE 18-47

Tears of the TFC. Gradient-recalled echo MR images (T2*). The tear stands out as a bright-signal zone on the ulnar side. It is better seen due to the "arthrogram effect" of this type of imaging sequence.

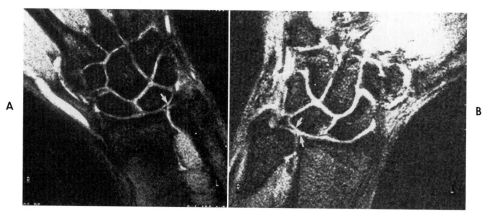

FIGURE 18-48

Tears of the central and radial part of the TFC. Coronal gradient-recalled type of MR images in two patients. **A,** Perforation in the center *(arrow)*. **B,** Tear of the radial margin *(arrows)*.

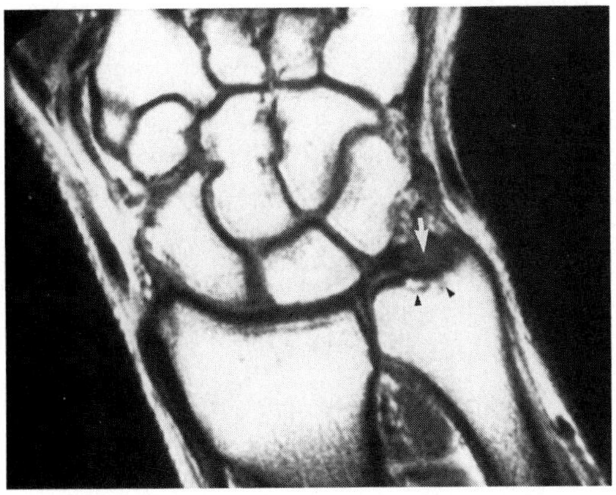

FIGURE 18-49
Tear of the TFC and chondromalacia of the ulnar head. A T1-weighted coronal image shows an area of abnormally low signal in the ulnar head (arrowheads) adjacent to a tear in the TFC (arrow).

tensile forces.[16] Fibrillar collagen is found in the thick fibrous bands of the margins (especially in their convergence at the insertion on the ulna). Together with the anterior and posterior radioulnar ligaments, these bands represent elastic stabilizers of the radioulnar joint, permitting rotation yet maintaining apposition of the radius and ulna during pronation and supination.

Tears of the ulnar TFC margin are more common in young patients with a history of trauma and are usually symptomatic.[50] On the medial side the TFC is composed mostly of collagenous fibers with multiple connections to the neighboring structures (meniscus homologue, extensor carpi ulnaris tendon sheath, and ulnotriquetral and ulnolunate ligaments). All these structures, mechanically interdependent, play an important role in the stability of the distal radioulnar joint. Tears of these connections and detachment of the ulnar insertion of the TFC likely produce joint instability and resulting pain.

In contradistinction to these traumatic peripheral lesions of the TFC, which are seen in young patients, degenerative disease of the center usually appears in asymptomatic older individuals. The center of the TFC is a 1 to 3 mm thick core of chondrocartilage, which degenerates with aging, sometimes as early as the third decade of life, leading to depressions and fissures that first develop on the ulnar surface and ultimately produce central perforations.

In anatomical dissections of normal wrists in cadavers of various ages, Mikic[17] found that 40% of those in the fifth decade had perforations of the TFC. It has therefore been concluded[51] that arthrographic demonstration of a communication between the radiocarpal and distal radioulnar joints does not necessarily imply pathology.

Reinus et al.[52] pointed out the lack of positive correlation between TFC perforations detected by arthrography and the clinical presence of pain, carpal instability, and ulnar variance in a group of 162 patients. Most individu-

als had perforations at the radial side or the center of the TFC. These data indicate that an arthrographic evaluation of the TFC is of only limited value, especially in older subjects, which factor, together with the invasive nature of the procedure, should make it less and less frequently performed for this condition.

MRI is rapidly replacing arthrography for the detection of tears in the triangular fibrocartilage.[35,49] It has the double advantage of being noninvasive and providing information regarding other associated pathological processes (tendinitis, paraarticular synovial fluid collections [ganglion cysts], edema or hemorrhage around the torn cartilage, and aseptic necrosis of bone) (Figs. 18-50 and 18-51).

At present, however, it cannot consistently distinguish all the supporting ligaments connected to the TFC. The connections between the TFC and the extensor carpi ulnaris tendon sleeve are thin bands that can be seen on T1-weighted sagittal images (Fig. 18-52). When torn, they appear on MR images to be interrupted by a high- or intermediate-signal zone representing hemorrhage, edema, or articular fluid (Fig. 18-53). Indirect signs of acute or subacute tear are localized edema in the subcutaneous tissue on the mediodorsal side of the wrist and increased signal in the tendon of the ECU (Fig. 18-54).

The intercarpal ligaments are occasionally seen in MR images, the scapholunate and lunotriquetral ligaments most frequently. They appear as signal-void bands bridging the proximal end of the corresponding intercarpal joint spaces (Figs. 18-29 and 18-55). Occasionally, tears of these ligaments are diagnosed on MR images, when absence or interruption of the signal void bands occurs (Fig. 18-56).

The future advances in MRI of the wrist are aimed at even higher spatial resolution, three-dimensional acquisition, and volumetric and surface rendering of the data, which will permit visualization of concentric layers of soft tissues and bones and allow for any particular three-dimensional representation of data to the demands of each individual case.[53]

Aseptic (avascular) necrosis of the carpal bones

The two most common sites of carpal avascular necrosis are the lunate and the proximal fragment of a fractured navicular.

LUNATE AVASCULAR NECROSIS

In 1910 Kienböck[54] described osteomalacia of the lunate, a clinicoradiological entity characterized by pain, stiffness, swelling of the wrist, and increased roentgenographic density of the lunate. It has remained in the medical literature as Kienböck's disease and is included in the list of idiopathic aseptic necroses of bone. Its cause, however, remains controversial. Attention has been focused on the precarious blood supply, explained by the

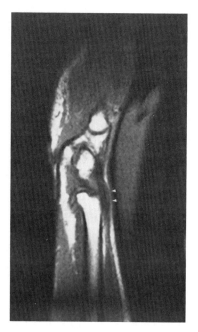

FIGURE 18-50
Tendinitis. A sagittal T1-weighted image through the ulna. Nonhomogeneous signal and fusiform swelling of the extensor carpi ulnaris tendon *(arrowheads)* near and distal to the ulnar head.

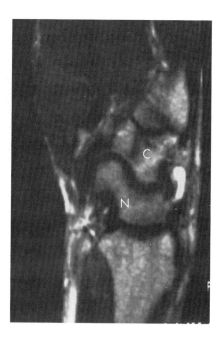

FIGURE 18-51
Ganglion cyst. A sagittal T2-weighted shows a homogeneous high-signal zone representing a fluid-filled cyst posterior to the capitate *(C)* and navicular *(N)*.

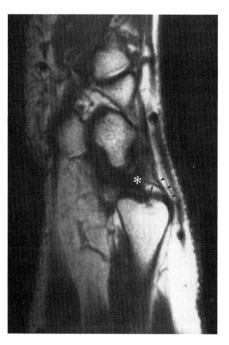

FIGURE 18-52
Fibrous connections of the TFC. A sagittal T1-weighted MR image. Low-signal bands *(arrow)* connect the dorsal margin of the TFC (*) to the sleeve of the extensor carpi ulnaris tendon *(arrowheads)*.

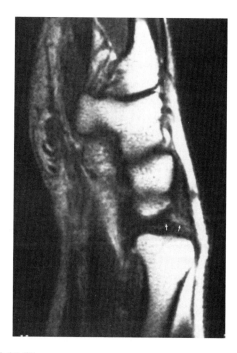

FIGURE 18-53
Torn TFC and ECU connections. A sagittal T1-weighted MR image shows irregular contour of the dorsal margin of the TFC *(arrows)* and nonhomogeneous signal replacing the bands connecting it to the extensor carpi ulnaris tendon sleeve.

fact that the lunate is covered with articular cartilage on most of its surface; the only two possible sites of entry of nutrient vessels are small areas covered with periosteum in the dorsal and ventral poles.[55] The small intraosseous arterial branches anastomose in a Y, X, or I pattern in the center of the lunate (Fig. 18-57). The subchondral zone of

the proximal part of the lunate, being less vascularized, is specifically the most frequent site of aseptic necrosis.

It has been postulated that trauma interrupts the arterial supply and leads to aseptic necrosis. It has also been observed that most of the patients with Kienböck's disease have a history of chronic repetitive stress rather

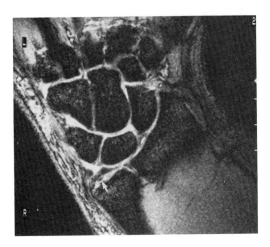

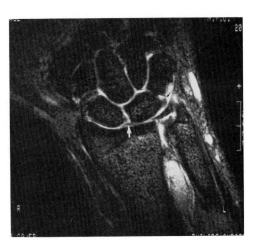

FIGURE 18-54
Acute tear of the TFC. Coronal T2* image. The tear is seen as a flap on the proximal surface of the TFC *(arrow)*. Edema of the subcutaneous soft tissue is present on the medial side of the wrist, manifested as lines of bright signal alternating with layers of low-signal fat.

FIGURE 18-55
Normal intercarpal ligaments. Coronal T2* image. Bands of low signal seen in the proximal margin of the intercarpal joints represent the scapholunate ligament *(white arrow)* and lunotriquetral ligament *(black arrow)*.

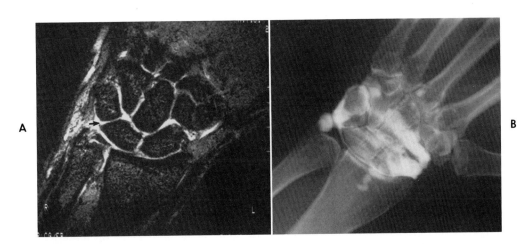

FIGURE 18-56
Torn lunotriquetral ligament. **A,** A coronal T2* image shows a gap in the proximal end of the lunotriquetral joint *(arrow).* **B,** An arthrogram reveals that contrast has entered the midcarpal joints through the gap, which was a result of the lunotriquetral ligament tear.

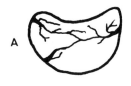

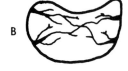

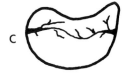

FIGURE 18-57
Vascular supply to the lunate and intraosseous anastomoses. In all these patterns of vascular distribution the proximal part of the lunate receives less abundant blood supply. **A,** Two vessels entering the ventral pole anastomose in the center of the lunate with one vessel of the dorsal pole (Y pattern). **B,** Two vessels of each pole form a central anastomosis (X pattern). **C,** Single vessels for each pole anastomose in the center (I pattern).

than a single major traumatic event. The high incidence of negative ulnar variance (ulna shorter than radius at the distal radioulnar joint) in patients with Kienböck's disease has been used as an argument in favor of chronic stress transmitted mainly through axial forces distributed along the radius-lunate-capitate, rather than shared with the ulna and triangular fibrocartilage of the wrist. The increased stress can have a "nutcracker" effect, compressing the lunate, producing microfractures, and ultimately compromising the vascularity of the bone marrow by interrupting the blood supply to the small fragments.[56] Continuation of the stress ultimately leads to fragmentation of the cortex and collapse of the lunate.

The staging of Kienböck's disease is based on its radiological aspects[57] (Fig. 18-58):

Stage I: Normal contour of the lunate; a radiolucent or radiodense line represents a compression fracture

Stage II: Resorption of bone along the fracture line

Stage III: All the changes of Stages I and II plus sclerosis of bone

Stage IV: Fragmentation or flattening of the lunate

Stage V: Arthrosis of the radiocarpal and intercarpal joints

The characterization of the process and staging are important for treatment planning. Special attention should be paid to quantitating fragmentation of the lunate, the presence of loose fragments, the integrity of the capitate-lunate joint, and proximal migration of the capitate. These abnormalities can be evaluated with

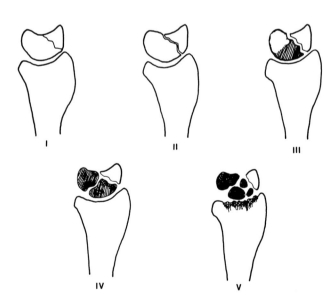

FIGURE 18-58
Staging of avascular necrosis of the lunate. Stage *I:* Normal contour of the lunate; fracture appearing as a radiolucent or radiodense line. Stage *II:* Resorption of bone at the fracture surface, widening the lucent line. Stage *III:* Sclerosis of bone in the proximal segment of the lunate. Stage *IV:* Fragmentation of the necrotic segment. Stage *V:* Arthrosis of the radiocarpal joint.

roentgenograms, radionuclide scans, conventional tomography, computed tomography, and MRI.[58] Of all these radiological modalities, MRI is the only one that can provide information about the viability of the fatty bone marrow and detect the layers of articular cartilage covering the necrotic bone. It has also the advantage of depicting the synovitis which usually accompanies the acute and subacute stages of Kienböck's disease.

Stages I and II of Kienböck's disease can be seen on T1-weighted images as a line of low signal in the marrow (representing stress fracture) (Figs. 18-59 and 18-60). In the early stage of avascular necrosis the bone marrow of a limited zone of the lunate has decreased signal intensity on T1-weighted images, but the overall contour of bone is normal (Fig. 18-61).

When collapse of the lunate has taken place, the fragmentation will appear on MR images as zigzag lines of low signal separating the segments of necrotic bone (Fig. 18-62). The shape of the lunate is altered, usually by reduction of its craniocaudal dimension and volar or dorsal displacement of fragments (Fig. 18-63). Some segments of lunate may retain their blood supply, thus showing normal fatty bone marrow, with bright signal on MR images (Fig. 18-64). Necrotic fragments show decreased signal, partially as as result of compression of the trabeculae in the dead bone. Pockets of fluid between and in the fragments may explain the patchy nonhomogeneous moderately high signal seen on T2-weighted MR images of Kienböck's disease (Fig. 18-65).

A process of synovitis is frequently present in advanced stages of Kienböck's disease. The synovial proliferation and fluid accumulation in the wrist joint are manifested as zones of intermediate signal intensity on T1-weighted and moderately high signal on T2-weighted images. The synovial pathology and dorsal-volar displacement of fragments are best observed on sagittal or axial images (Fig. 18-62). The proximal migration of the capitate can be seen in sagittal views but is more striking on coronal images, which portray the position of neighboring carpal bones (Fig. 18-66).

SCAPHOID AVASCULAR NECROSIS

Fractures of the scaphoid are frequently complicated by avascular necrosis. The main blood supply to this bone is through the distal segment; only inconstant thinner arterial branches enter through the waist of the navicular. The proximal pole derives its blood mostly from terminal branches of the arterial vessels passing through the middle segment of the scaphoid. Thus, the more cranial a fracture is located, the higher are the chances of interruption of the blood supply and aseptic necrosis of the proximal segment. It has been estimated[59] that 30% of the fractures of the waist of the navicular are complicated by avascular necrosis. It is important to determine as early as possible the viability of the fragments; long immobilization in a plaster cast can lead to healing only if the blood supply to the fragments is adequate. When there is

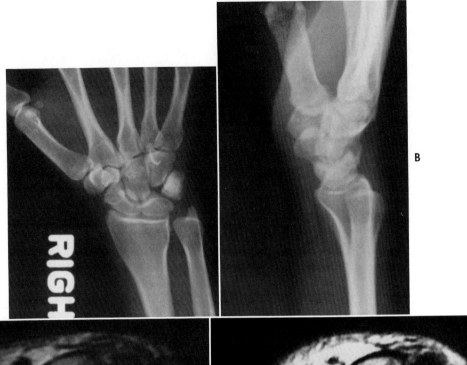

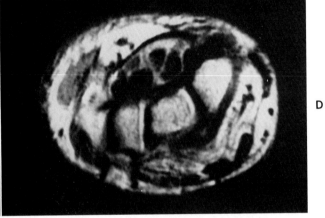

FIGURE 18-59
Stress fracture of the lunate. Stage I avascular necrosis. **A** and **B**, Frontal and lateral roentgenograms of the wrist of a 30-year-old woman with midcarpal pain. The lunate appears normal. **C**, Axial T1-weighted MR images show a line of low signal traversing the lunate *(arrows)*. This can be regarded as a Stage I avascular necrosis. **D**, Follow-up 3 months later shows return to normal signal, suggesting healing of the fracture.

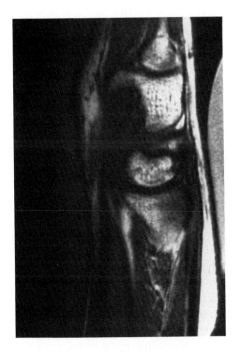

FIGURE 18-60
Stages II and III avascular necrosis of the lunate. Sagittal T1-weighted MRI. A low-signal line traverses the lunate, and the proximal segment has decreased signal in the bone marrow.

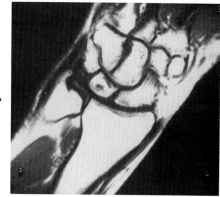

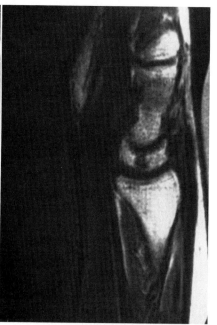

FIGURE 18-61

Stage III avascular necrosis of the lunate. A, A coronal and, B, a sagittal T1-weighted MRI. The zone of decreased signal in the bone marrow corresponds to aseptic necrosis.

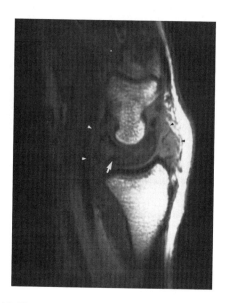

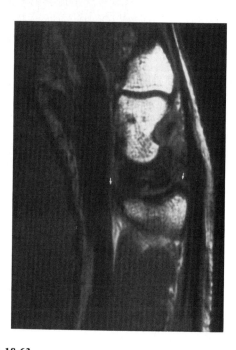

FIGURE 18-62

Stage IV avascular necrosis of the lunate. Sagittal T1-weighted images. Fragmentation of necrotic bone (arrow), loss of vertical dimension, and volar-dorsal displacement of the fragments. Synovitis is seen as intermediate-signal zones bulging in the dorsal and palmar aspects of the lunate (arrowheads).

FIGURE 18-63

Stage V avascular necrosis of the lunate and arthrosis of the radiocarpal joint. A sagittal T1-weighted MR image shows marked fragmentation and low signal in the lunate, signifying aseptic necrosis. Spurs at the margins of the articular surface of the distal radius (arrows) and narrowing of the radiocarpal joint space represent manifestations of osteoarthrosis.

avascular necrosis, early surgical intervention consisting of bone graft placement has a better chance of restoring the viability of the proximal navicular fragment. It should be performed before structural collapse of the necrotic bone has taken place.

The two most valuable studies for follow-up of navicular fractures diagnosed on conventional roentgenograms are radioisotope bone scan and MRI. The bone scan has value only when it shows a "cold" area corresponding to the segment of bone that has not received the tracer because it is devoid of vascular supply. Most often the bone scan cannot detect small zones of absent tracer activity caused by small necrotic areas. The MRI can portray changes in the bone marrow signifying necrosis before any change in contour or radiographic density of the fragments has taken place[58] (Fig. 18-67).

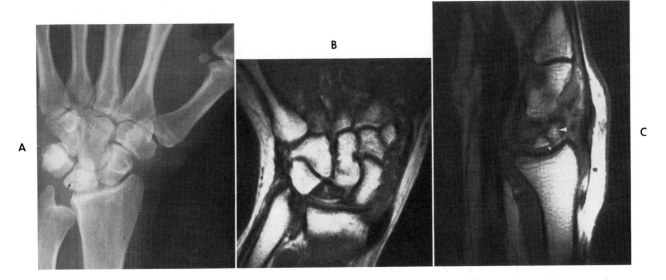

FIGURE 18-64

Avascular necrosis of the lunate; necrotic versus viable segments. **A,** Frontal projection roentgenogram of the right wrist. The lunate appears dense and is traversed by a barely visible lucent line *(arrow).* **B,** Coronal T1-weighted MRI. Low signal in the necrotic part of the lunate. **C,** Sagittal T1-weighted MRI. Several fragments of lunate can be distinguished; the palmar ones have low signal, consistent with AVN. The two dorsal fragments have bright signal in the bone marrow *(arrowheads),* indicating the high probability of a retained blood supply.

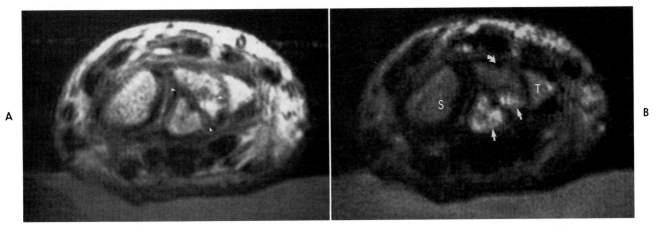

FIGURE 18-65

Avascular necrosis of the lunate. T2-weighted MRI. **A,** Axial proton density image (SE; TR 2000 msec/TE 30 msec). The lunate is separated into three individual fragments by fracture lines (best seen in a proton density image) *(arrowheads).* **B,** T2-weighted image (SE; TR 2000 msec/TE 80 msec). The nonhomogeneous bright signal in the palmar fragments can be explained by fluid accumulation between the dead bone trabeculae *(arrows).* The dorsal segment *(curved arrow)* has normal signal intensity, similar to that seen in the triquetrum *(T)* and scaphoid *(S).*

The proximal pole of the fractured navicular may have a decrease in signal intensity of the bone marrow on T1-weighted images; subsequently the contour of the cortex becomes indistinct and irregular. Changes in the shape of the bone, with significant loss of volume, represent a manifestation of advanced necrosis complicated by structural collapse. At this stage MRI has very little information to add besides the obvious pathology detected by roentgenography: increased density, fragmentation, collapse of the proximal segment of the fractured navicular.

Carpal bone fractures

Injuries to the wrist may produce fractures and dislocations of the carpal bones. Commonly these are diagnosed by means of routine roentgenography. Even special views required to study the navicular or hamate may fail to detect nondisplaced fractures. A 99mTc bone scan can be used in such cases to screen patients suspected of having carpal bone fractures. Those with abnormal focally increased uptake should be studied further, by means of CT.

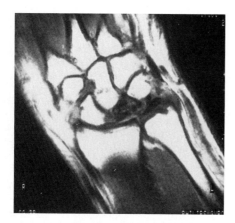

FIGURE 18-66
Advanced avascular necrosis of the lunate, proximal migration of the capitate. A coronal T1-weighted image shows abnormally low signal, fragmentation, and collapse of the lunate. The capitate has migrated cranially.

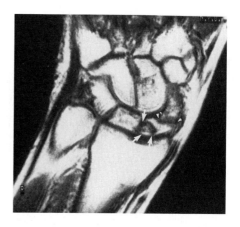

FIGURE 18-67
Aseptic necrosis secondary to a navicular fracture. A T1-weighted coronal MR image shows the fracture line in the waist of the navicular *(arrowheads)*. The proximal pole has a zone of low signal, representing aseptic necrosis *(arrows)*.

Compared with roentgenograms, CT has the advantage of eliminating overlap of the interlocking articular surfaces by portraying only narrow slices of the anatomy. In the wrist in particular, CT has one other advantage: it can obtain primary images not only in the axial plane but in the coronal, sagittal, or oblique axial plane as well. Each is suited for a specific anatomical site: the navicular is best seen on oblique axials, the hook of the hamate on axials or sagittals, the lunate on coronals and sagittals. Palmar or dorsal rotation of the lunate and rotatory subluxations of the navicular are best seen on sagittal images.

NAVICULAR FRACTURES

Fractures of the waist of the navicular are slow healing, often associated with nonunion and aseptic necrosis. These complications can be avoided by early detection and prompt immobilization. Often it is difficult to demonstrate on roentgenograms the presence of nondisplaced fractures of the navicular in their acute phase. CT can help detect such injuries by demonstrating the fracture line free of any overlap of adjacent bone structures (Fig. 18-68).

It is important to determine as early as possible whether a fracture has good potential for healing (in which case the wrist is kept in a cast for up to 3 months). When poor vascularity of the proximal segment leads to aseptic necrosis of bone or nonunion, it is futile to continue immobilization of the extremity as the only treatment applied. Surgical intervention with bone graft placement should be done. Surgery has a better chance of success when performed before structural collapse of the cortical bone has taken place in the proximal segment.

In the healing process there is transition from fibrous to calcified callus. CT can show the presence of uniform calcification obliterating the fracture gap, an indication of normal healing (Figs. 18-69 and 18-70).

CT can help early detection of complications of navic-ular fractures by demonstrating signs of nonunion: wide gap between fragments, eburnation of trabecular bone, sclerosis of the fracture surface[60,61] (Fig. 18-71).

Nonunion of the scaphoid is treated surgically with a bone graft fragment removed from the dorsal aspect of the radius and placed on the posterior surface of the fracture fragments, spanning the fracture site. Roentgenographic follow-up of the surgical results while the wrist is in a plaster cast can be difficult. The bone graft and proximal and distal fragments overlap each other. It may take several months for the calcified callus to obliterate the entire fracture gap, including the palmar side. Till then, plain roentgenograms of the wrist may show a lucent space at the fracture site, creating confusion between a partially healed fracture and a failure of healing (Fig. 18-72). In these cases further studies with conventional tomography or CT are necessary to establish the relation between the graft and the navicular fracture fragments as well as the presence of calcified callus. Conventional hypocycloidal-motion tomography has become a rarely performed examination; many radiology departments no longer have this equipment. This and the high radiation dose resulting from multiple frontal and lateral tomographic views have promoted replacement of the procedure by CT. High-resolution CT with a small field of view and thin slices (1.5 or 3 mm) provides excellent detail of the cortical and trabecular bone of the fractured navicular and can reveal progression of calcified callus from the dorsal aspect, where the graft is placed, toward the volar side of the fracture (Fig. 18-73).

Absence of callus formation and fragmentation of the bone graft itself, indicative of persistent nonunion, are best seen on sagittal CT images oriented in the long axis of the navicular. Often CT detects a gap between the grafted segment and the indigenous bone; this indicates failure of graft incorporation, most often secondary to motion (Fig. 18-74). Motion between the graft and the fragments of the navicular is directly seen on fluoroscopic

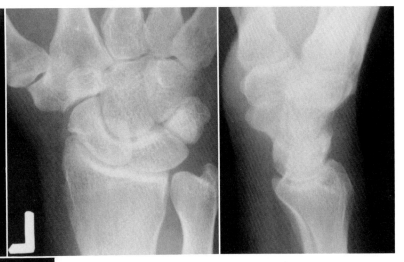

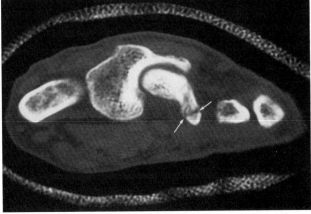

FIGURE 18-68
Occult fracture of the navicular, CT diagnosis. **A** to **C**, Roentgenograms of the wrist in a 33-year-old man with pain in the "anatomical snuff box" following a fall on the outstretched hand. No fracture was detected. Based on the clinical data, a fracture of the navicular was suspected and the wrist was casted. **D**, Sagittal CT image 3 days later showing the fracture *(arrows)* in the distal navicular.

observation of wrist motion, which is a simple, rapid, and less costly modality than CT. Conventional tomography in flexion and extension can be used to detect motion between the fragments.[62]

The other complication of navicular fractures (after nonunion), avascular necrosis of the proximal segment, is best seen in its early stage on MR images.[58] On T1-weighted images it appears as decreased signal intensity of the bone marrow in the proximal segment (Fig. 18-67). In later stages collapse of the articular cortex changes the contour of the navicular. Compressed trabecular bone will appear as low-signal zones on T1- and T2-weighted images. However, on a T2-weighted the synovial fluid interspersed between fragmented bone can give a non-homogeneous signal, with zones of high signal mixed in the pathological segment. At this late stage of aseptic necrosis plain films, CT, and MRI are equally diagnostic. The expensive and time-consuming examinations have no further information to offer once conventional roentgenograms demonstrate collapse, fragmentation, and increased density in the proximal segment of the fractured navicular (Fig. 18-75). All these signs are diagnostic for aseptic necrosis in advanced stage. For such cases all efforts should be directed to surgical treatment; MRI

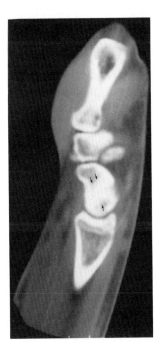

FIGURE 18-69
Healed navicular fracture. CT image showing a band of density traversing the navicular waist, indicative of fracture healing *(arrows)*.

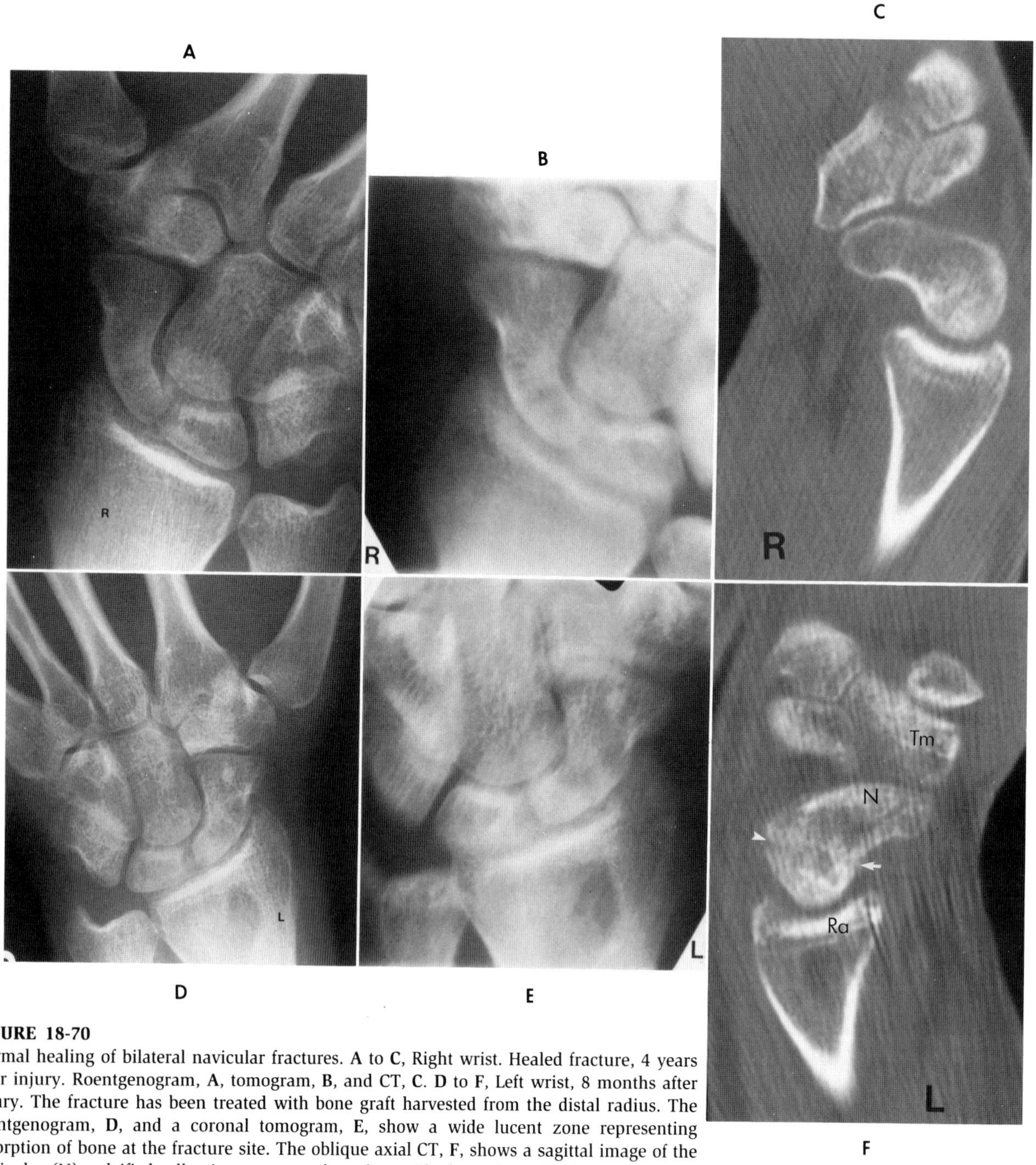

A

B

C

D

E

F

FIGURE 18-70
Normal healing of bilateral navicular fractures. **A** to **C**, Right wrist. Healed fracture, 4 years after injury. Roentgenogram, **A**, tomogram, **B**, and CT, **C**. **D** to **F**, Left wrist, 8 months after injury. The fracture has been treated with bone graft harvested from the distal radius. The roentgenogram, **D**, and a coronal tomogram, **E**, show a wide lucent zone representing resorption of bone at the fracture site. The oblique axial CT, **F**, shows a sagittal image of the navicular *(N)*; calcified callus is present on the palmar side *(arrow)*. In the dorsal margin of the fracture fibrous union is present *(arrowhead)*. Trapezium *(Tm)*, radius *(Ra)*.

should be reserved only for follow-up study, to detect the progression of healing and revascularization of the proximal fragment. Calcification of callus is best observed on CT images, which help in determining the time when removal of the cast is safe and physiotherapy programs can be initiated.

HAMATE FRACTURES

The hamate, a wedge-shaped bone in the medial border of the distal carpal row, articulates with the triquetrum, lunate, capitate, and bases of the fourth and fifth metacarpals, all of which protect it from direct trauma on most of its surface. The exception is the hamulus, also known as the hook of the hamate, which is not protected but is vulnerable to direct trauma induced either by a fall on the outstretched palm or by a sudden forceful blow from the handle of a tool or sports implement held in a tight grip (e.g., the handle of a hammer or tennis racket). The hamulus is oriented perpendicular to the palmar surface of the hamate, resembling a peg or the blade of an ax (Fig.

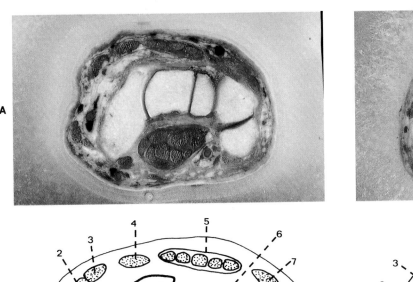

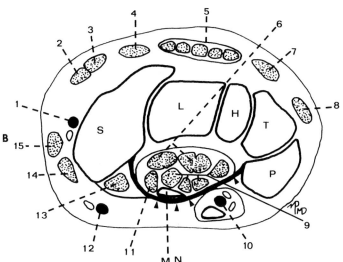

PLATE 18-1

A, Anatomical specimen. Microtome axial section through the pisiform and scaphoid. B, Schematic representation.

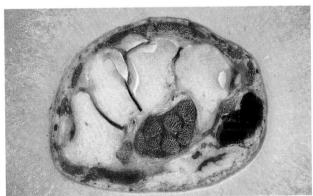

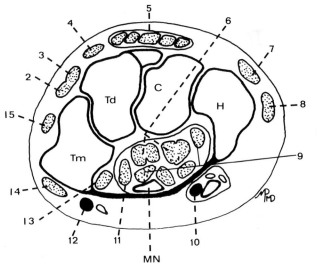

PLATE 18-2

A, Anatomical specimen. Microtome axial section through the hamate and trapezium. B, Schematic representation. Bone structures: *C*, capitate; *H*, hamate; *L*, lunate; *R*, radius; *S*, scaphoid; *T*, triquetrum; *Td*, trapezoid; *Tm*, trapezium; *U*, ulna; *Mn*, median nerve. Soft tissue structures: *1*, radial artery, dorsal branch; *2*, extensor carpi radialis longus tendon; *3*, external carpi radialis brevis tendon; *4*, extensor pollicis longus tendon; *5*, extensor digitorum communis and extensor indicis tendons; *6*, flexor digitorum profundus tendons; *7*, extensor digiti minimi tendon; *8*, extensor carpi ulnaris tendon; *9*, flexor digitorum superficialis tendons; *10*, ulnar artery (medial to it, ulnar nerve; lateral, a vein); *11*, flexor pollicis longus tendon; *12*, radial artery, superficial palmar arch; *13*, flexor carpi radialis tendon; *14*, abductor pollicis longus tendon; *15*, extensor pollicis longus tendon.

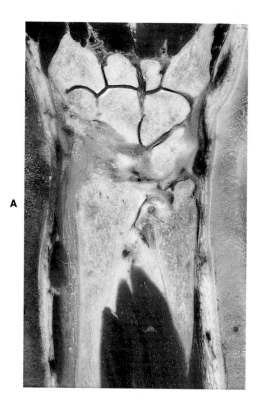

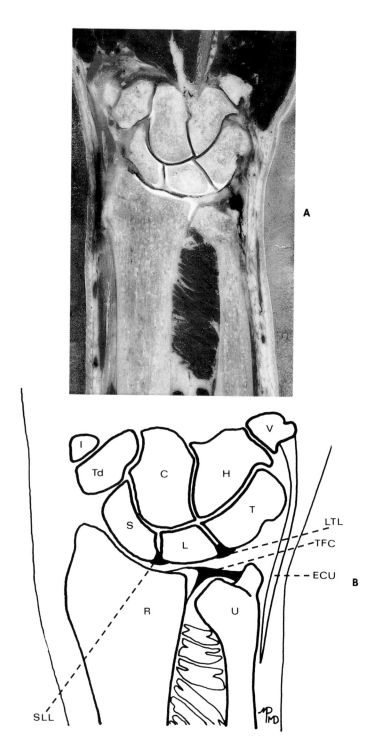

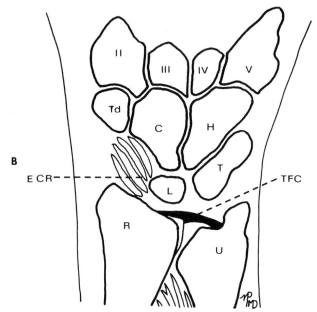

PLATE 18-3

A, Anatomical specimen. Coronal microtome section through the dorsal part of the wrist joint. **B,** Schematic representation. *II,* Second metacarpal; *III,* third metacarpal; *IV,* fourth metacarpal; *V,* fifth metacarpal; *C,* capitate; *H,* hamate; *L,* lunate; *R,* radius; *T,* triquetrum; *Td,* trapezoid; *U,* ulna; *ECR,* extensor carpi ulnaris brevis muscle; *TFC,* triangular fibrocartilage.

PLATE 18-4

A, Anatomical specimen. Coronal microtome section through the carpal bones. **B,** Schematic representation. *I,* Base of the first metacarpal; *V,* base of fifth metacarpal; *C,* capitate; *H,* hamate; *L,* lunate; *R,* radius; *S,* scaphoid; *T,* triquetrum; *Td,* trapezoid; *U,* ulna; *ECU,* extensor carpi ulnaris tendon; *LTL,* lunotriquetral ligament; *SLL,* scapholunate ligament; *TFC,* triangular fibrocartilage.

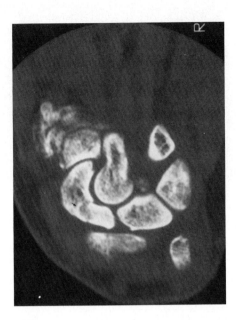

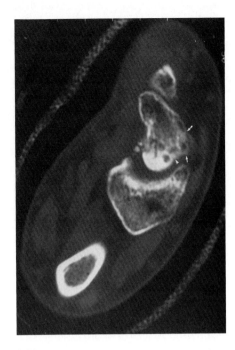

FIGURE 18-71
Nonunion of a navicular fracture. Coronal CT image showing a wide gap between the fragments, with sclerosis of the fracture surface *(arrow)*.

FIGURE 18-73
Fracture of the navicular treated with a bone graft; avascular necrosis. Sagittal CT view. The bone graft placed on the dorsal surface of the navicular *(arrows)* has been incorporated into the distal fragment. Calcified callus is bridging the dorsal margin of the fracture *(arrowhead)*. The proximal segment is dense, suggesting AVN; a pin track is visible in the proximal fragment, where impaired vascularity delays obliteration of the tunnel left after removal of the hardware.

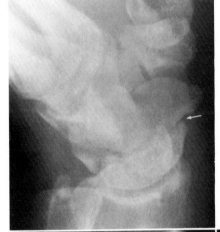

FIGURE 18-72
Healing fracture of the navicular. **A,** Roentgenogram, oblique view. The fracture line is still visible *(arrow)*. **B,** A coronal CT obtained near the palmar surface of the navicular shows part of the fracture gap *(arrowhead)*. The lateral margin is obliterated by callus. **C,** Coronal CT in the center of the navicular. Normal trabecular bone indicates healing of the fracture. No aseptic necrosis is evident.

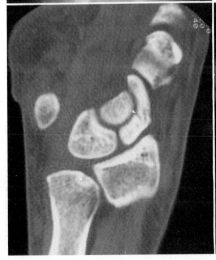

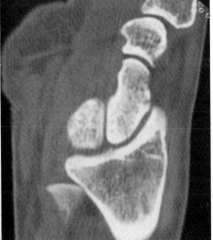

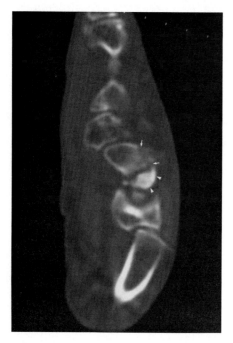

FIGURE 18-74
Navicular fracture treated with a bone graft; failure of graft incorporation. A sagittal CT image shows a gap between the grafted bone and the proximal and distal fragments of the navicular *(arrows)*. The proximal fragment has avascular necrosis, manifested as increased density *(arrowheads)*.

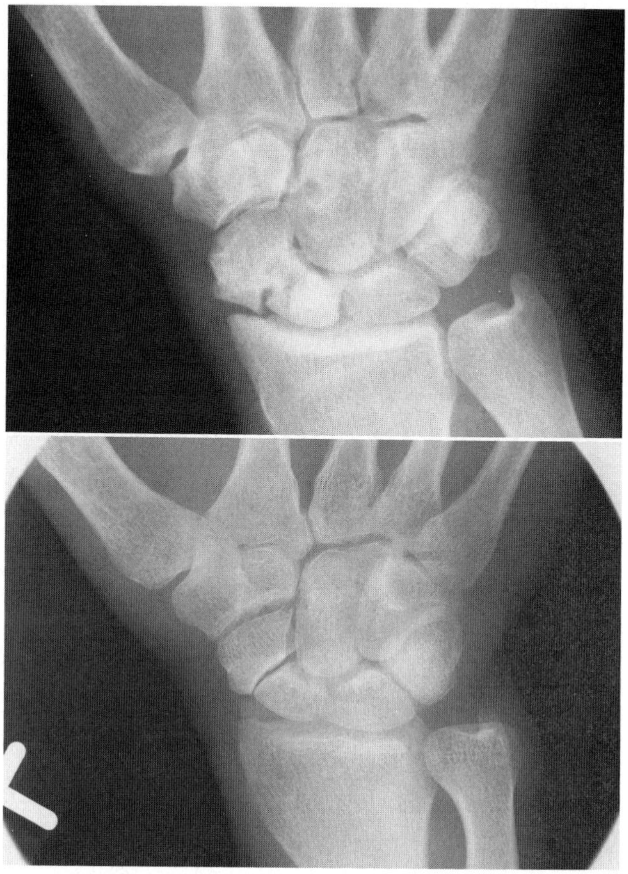

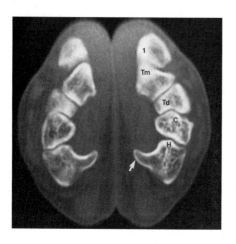

FIGURE 18-76
CT of the normal hamate. An axial view of both wrists shows the hamulus *(arrow)* as a hooklike prominence of the palmar surface of the hamate *(H)*. The capitate *(C)*, trapezoid *(Td)*, trapezium *(Tm)*, and base of the first metacarpal *(1)* are also seen in this image.

FIGURE 18-75
Complications of a navicular fracture. Roentgenographic diagnosis. **A,** Aseptic necrosis of the proximal fragment. **B,** Nonunion.

18-76). On the tip of the hook is the insertion site of the flexor retinaculum (palmar aponeurosis); lateral is the carpal tunnel; and medial and anterior is the Guyon canal, which contains the ulnar nerve and corresponding vascular structures.

Most fractures of the hook are located at its base, oriented in the coronal plane, and are difficult to see on routine roentgenograms. Special positioning (e.g., oblique and carpal tunnel views) can visualize them occasionally. A fracture of the hook of the hamate is frequently missed in the initial routine examination. This is especially important in view of the high rate of complications of untreated fractures (aseptic necrosis,

nonunion leading to persistent pain and diminished grip strength). Displaced fragments of the hook can impinge on not only the structures of the carpal tunnel but also the ulnar nerve by compressing the Guyon canal.

The best way to image the hook of the hamate and its relation with neighboring structures is the axial views of CT or MRI (Figs. 18-77 and 18-78). Fractures are easily detected by CT as interruption of the center and a linear gap traversing the base. Any mediolateral tilt or displacement can be easily seen. On sagittal images the fracture has a similar aspect, the advantage being the ability to detect craniocaudal shift or angulation.

MR images of the fractured hook are best at detecting

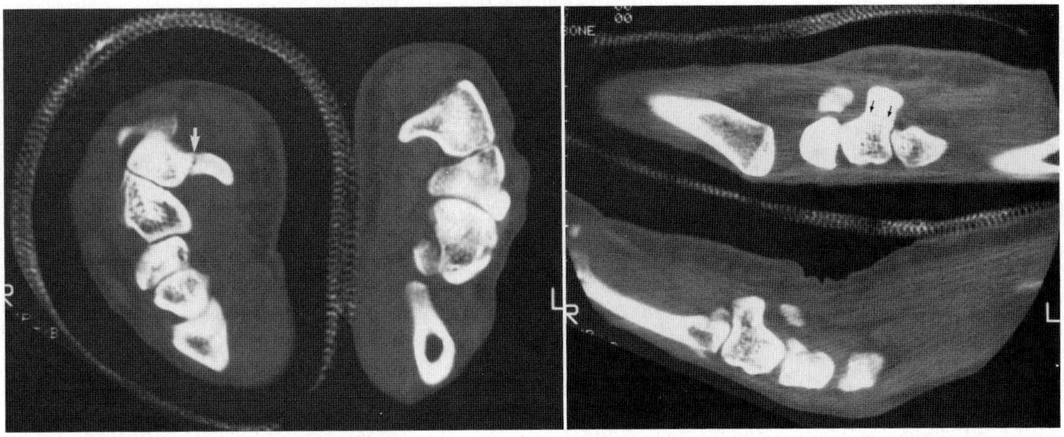

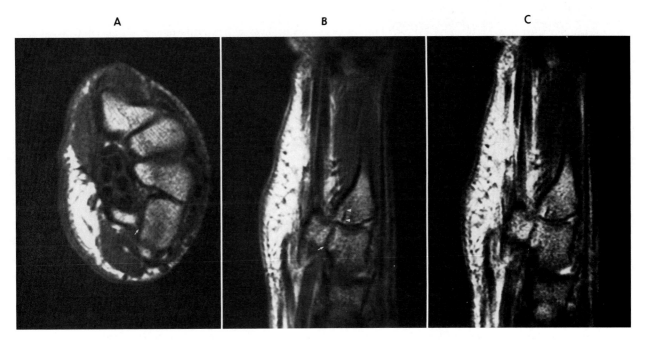

FIGURE 18-77
Fractured hook of the hamate. **A,** Axial CT image of both wrists. Fracture in the right hamate, at the base of the hook *(arrow).* **B,** Sagittal CT image of the hamate, both wrists. The right side is in a cast. Nondisplaced fracture through the base of the hook of the right hamate *(arrows).* The left side is normal.

FIGURE 18-78
MRI of a fractured hamate. **A,** Axial T1-weighted image. At the base of the hook a line of low signal represents the fracture *(arrow).* **B,** Sagittal MR (SE; TR 2100 msec/TE 80 msec). Fracture of the hook at the base *(arrow).* Note the nondisplaced fracture at the base of the fourth metacarpal *(arrowheads).* **C,** Sagittal MR (SE; TR 2100 msec/TE 30 msec). Hyperemia of the bone marrow explains the increased signal on both sides of the hamulus fracture, indicative of normal vascular supply to the hook fragment.

early stages of avascular necrosis of the hamular fragment. CT is better for demonstrating the amount of calcified callus formed at fracture site (Figs. 18-79 and 18-80). Nonunion can be diagnosed when sclerosis of the fracture surfaces and increase in the fracture gap are seen (Fig. 18-81). MR cannot distinguish between nonunion and fibrous or calcified callus, all of which have low

signal on T1-weighted images. On a T2-weighted image highly vascular granulation tissue in the early stage of normal healing may be confused with fluid filling a nonunion site. Rarely the body of the hamate bone has chip fractures that are hidden between the interlocking surfaces with the metacarpal bases and therefore silent on routine projections of standard roentgenograms. They are

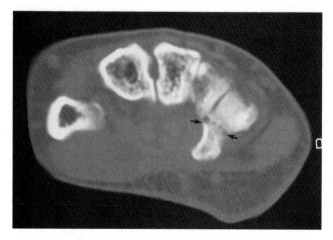

FIGURE 18-79
Healing fracture of the hamate. CT axial image. The fracture gap *(arrows)* at the base of the hamulus is partially obliterated by calcified callus.

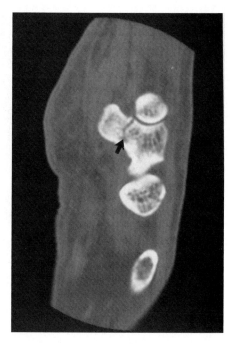

FIGURE 18-81
Nonunion of the hamate fracture. CT sagittal image. Sclerosis of the fracture surface and a large gap between the fragments suggest nonunion at the base of the hamulus *(arrow)*.

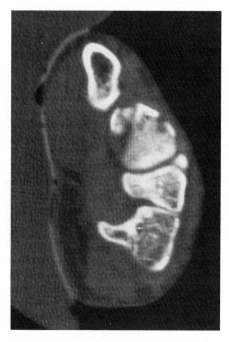

FIGURE 18-80
Healed hamate fracture. CT axial image. Calcified callus has filled in most of the fracture gap *(arrow)*.

easily seen on axial CT images (Fig. 18-82). Occasionally it will be necessary to compare axial images of the normal and injured extremity to differentiate a small displaced chip fracture from the normal bone protrusion of the interlocking surfaces of the carpometacarpal joints (Fig. 18-82).

Soft tissue masses

MRI is the most useful examination for detecting and precisely locating a mass lesion in the wrist.[63-67] However, with few exceptions, there is no specific MRI feature that can accurately and consistently distinguish a benign from a malignant tumor or the different histological types of tumors. The exception is lesions with a distinct texture and macroscopic appearance (cavernous hemangioma, lymphangioma) or a homogeneous and characteristic content (lipoma, ganglion cyst). Biopsy is necessary in most instances for a definitive histological diagnosis.

Synovial cysts. The most common soft tissue mass of the wrist is the synovial cyst, known as a "ganglion." It is a cystic cavity lined with synovial membrane surrounded by fibrous tissue and containing fluid. It may have connection to one of the synovial sleeves of the tendons crossing the dorsal aspect of the wrist, or it may be isolated. In its early stage of development it is flat and insinuates itself between the tendinous structures of its vicinity (Fig. 18-83). Progressive accumulation of fluid leads to increased volume and pressure within the cyst, which makes the mass feel firm and round. On MR images a ganglion cyst characteristically appears as a sharply defined collection of homogeneous high signal on T2-weighted images and intermediate signal on T1-weighted images.[63] It displaces the tendons in its immediate vicinity, bulging into the subcutaneous fat layer and beneath the skin.

Solid soft tissue masses. Malignant tumors of soft tissue origin are rarely seen in the wrist. In children rhabdomyosarcoma is the most common of these. In young adults a synovioma or synovial sarcoma is more common. In middle-aged or older subjects a fibrohistiosarcoma may be encountered. Most of these tumors share common MRI features — masses with high signal on T2-weighted and

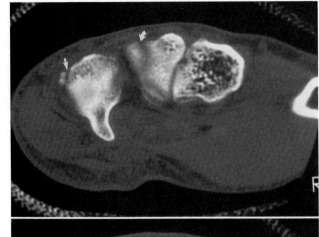

A

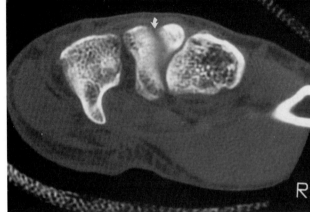

B

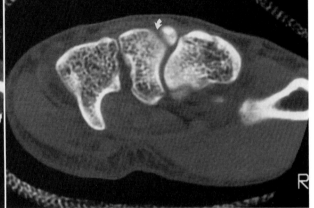

C

FIGURE 18-82

Chip fracture of the hamate; differentiation from a partial volume artifact. CT axial images of the hamate, representing adjacent 3 mm thick slices. **A,** Chip fracture of the dorsomedial margin of the hamate *(straight arrow).* **B** and **C,** The partial volume averaging of the slanted base of the third metacarpal, capitate, and their joint space represents a smoothly fading low-attenuation band, which should not be confused with a fracture *(curved arrow).*

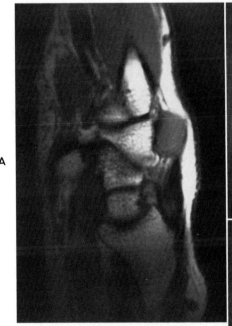

A

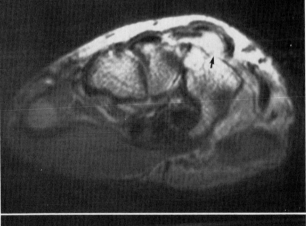

B

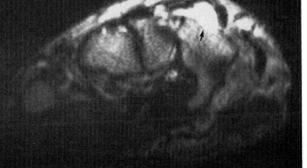

C

FIGURE 18-83

MRI of a synovial cyst. **A,** Sagittal T1-weighted image. On the dorsal surface of the hamate there is a sharply marginated mass with homogeneous signal of intermediate intensity. The bone is normal. **B** and **C,** Proton density–weighted and T2-weighted axial images. The mass has characteristic homogeneous bright signal, indicating its fluid content *(arrow).* It is located beneath the extensor tendons of the third and fourth fingers.

intermediate signal on T1-weighted images, poorly defined margins, and invasion of adjacent structures such as bone.[63] Occasionally, a malignant tumor (e.g., a synovial sarcoma) will have homogeneous signal and well-defined markings. It is therefore safe to state that certain MR features point toward an aggressive character of soft tissue masses; however, absence of such features does not exclude malignancy.

Benign soft tissue masses of the wrist include lipoma, fibroma, hemangioma, lymphangioma, and pigmented villonodular tenosynovitis.

As expected, lipomas have uniform high signal on T1-weighted images, some with a fibrous capsule appearing as a low-signal rim.[64]

Hemangiomas have ill-defined contours. Occasionally there will be dilated tortuous vessels feeding them, giving the observer a clue as to the nature of the mass. The MRI signal characteristics of hemangioma are dependent upon the amount of fat often present within these lesions and the quantity of (slow-moving) venous blood. Thus, one may see a low or high signal on T1 and a high signal on T2 and gradient echo images.

Lymphangiomas have a soft consistency that gives them the ability to engulf rather than displace neighboring structures. They have a bright signal on T2-weighted images (Fig. 18-84).

Pigmented villonodular synovitis has a fairly distinctive appearance on MR images, both T1- and T2-weighted, with low signal the result of hemosiderin deposits.[65-67]

Giant cell tumors of the tendons represent extraarticular pigmented villonodular synovitis. Depending upon the amount of hemosiderin deposited, they may have low or intermediate signal intensity in T2-weighted images (Fig. 18-85).

Occasionally localized forms of granulomatous disease such as sarcoidosis or tuberculosis will produce soft tissue masses or bone erosions that become confused with tumors (Fig. 18-86). In such instances, although the correct diagnosis can be inferred by considering the clinical history, biopsy is still necessary for confirmation.

Bone tumors

Giant cell tumors. Giant cell tumors of the distal radius have a fairly characteristic pattern — expansile, osteolytic,

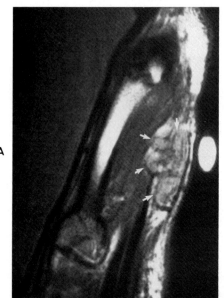
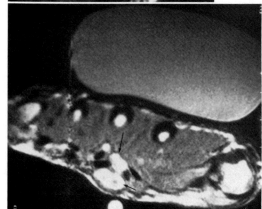
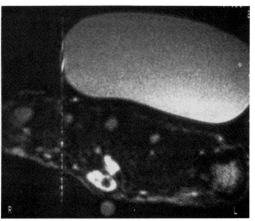

FIGURE 18-84

Lymphangioma of the hand. A pill containing oil base marks the location of a mass in the right palm. A water bag is placed on the dorsal surface of the wrist and hand. **A,** Sagittal T1-weighted image. Nonhomogeneous mass with irregular contour and subcutaneous location *(arrows)*. **B,** Axial proton density image (SE; TR 2100 msec/TE 30 msec). A bilobular mass is between the flexor tendons *(arrows)*. **C,** Axial T2-weighted image (SE; TR 2100 msec/TE 80 msec). The mass has intense but nonhomogeneous signal.

located in the epiphysis of an adult bone.[68] Some patients present first when a pathological fracture develops. MRI or CT can demonstrate extension of the lesion into soft tissues. In giant cell tumors not complicated by pathological fracture, soft tissue invasion is a strong indicator of malignant behavior.

Aneurysmal bone cysts. Aneurysmal bone cysts may be encountered in the distal metaphysis of the radius, usually in children, and is characterized on CT and MR images by the layering of fluids (blood and serum).

Enchondromas. Benign cartilaginous tumors are common in the metacarpals and phalanges, either as a single lesion or as multiple enchondromas in a patient with Ollier's disease (multiple hereditary enchondromatosis).

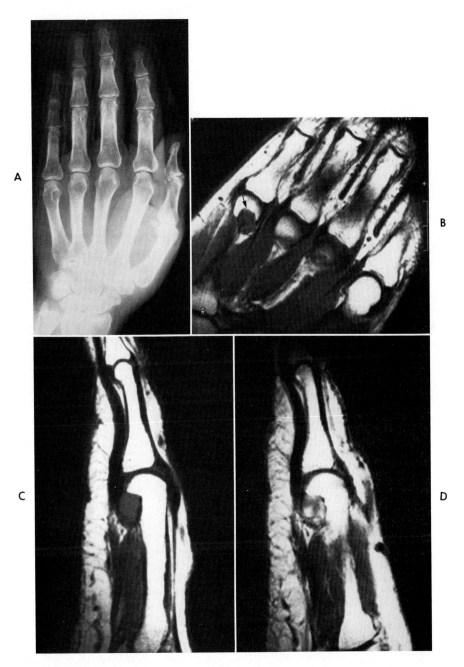

FIGURE 18-85
Giant cell tumor of the tendon sheath enhanced with gadopentetate. **A,** A frontal roentgenogram of the right hand shows the lytic lesion with a sclerotic border in the distal metaphysis of the fifth metacarpal. **B,** Coronal T1-weighted image. The tumor is sharply circumscribed and has low signal *(arrow).* **C,** Sagittal T1-weighted image. The tumor is located on the palmar surface of the fifth metacarpal head. **D,** Same as **C,** after intravenous injection of gadopentetate. Nonhomogeneous enhancement in parts of the tumor, seen as zone of bright signal. This signifies active vascularity in parts of the lesion.

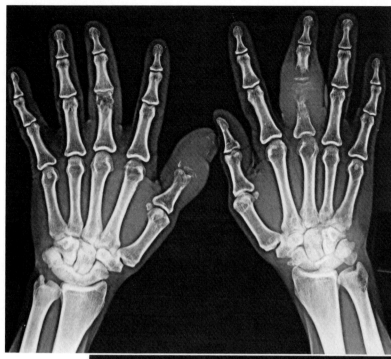

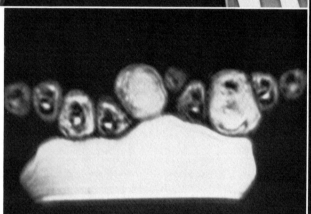

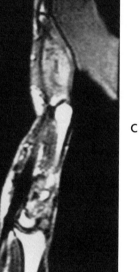

FIGURE 18-86

Sarcoidosis of bone. **A,** Frontal view of both hands. Lytic destructive lesions are present in several phalanges and the left ulna, subsequently proven by biopsy to contain noncaseating granulomas characteristic of sarcoidosis. **B,** Axial T2-weighted image through the base of the fingers. (A water bag is beneath the hand.) The high signal in the lesions is a nonspecific pattern. The signal void of cortical bone is absent in the left third finger and right thumb, a reflection of the osteolysis (better seen in plain films). **C,** Sagittal T1-weighted image through the left third finger. The bone is replaced by a nonhomogeneous mass with intermediate signal intensity.

On T2-weighted images they have a background of high signal and some dots of low signal (calcifications in the chondroid matrix).

REFERENCES

1. Dalinka MK, Kricun ME, Zlatkin MB, Hibbard CA: Modern diagnostic imaging in joint disease. AJR 1989;152:229-240.
2. Sartoris DJ, Resnick D: MR imaging of the musculoskeletal system: current and future status. AJR 1987;149:457-467.
3. Burk DL, Dalinka MK, Schiebler ML, et al: Strategies for musculoskeletal magnetic resonance imaging. Radiol Clin North Am 1988;26:653-672.
4. Clemente CD: Anatomy. A regional atlas of the human body, 2nd ed. Urban & Schwarzenberg, Baltimore, 1981, pp 87-114.
5. Pernkopf E: Atlas of topographical and applied human anatomy. Philadelphia, Saunders, 1964, Vol 2, pp 94-108.
6. Zeiss J, Skie M, Ebraheim N, Jackson WT: Anatomic relations between the median nerve and flexor tendons in the carpal tunnel: MR evaluation in normal volunteers. AJR 1989;153:533-536.
7. Jessurun W, Hillen B, Zonneveld F, et al: Anatomical relations in the carpal tunnel: a computed tomographic study. J Hand Surg [Br] 1987;12:64-67.
8. Weiss KL, Beltran J, Shamam OM, et al: High-field MR surface coil imaging of the hand and wrist. I. Normal anatomy. Radiology 1986;160:143-146.
9. Weiss KL, Beltran J, Lubbers LM: High field MR surface coil imaging of the hand and wrist. II. Pathologic correlations and clinical relevance. Radiology 1986;169:147-152.
10. Koenig H, Lucas D, Meissner R: The wrist: a preliminary report on high resolution MR imaging. Radiology 1986;160:463-467.
11. Middleton WD, Macrander S, Lawson TL, et al: High resolution surface coil magnetic resonance imaging of the joints. Anatomic correlation. Radiographics 1987;7:645-683.
12. Baker LL, Hajek PC, Björkengren A, et al: High-resolution magnetic resonance imaging of the wrist. Normal anatomy. Skeletal Radiol 1987;16:128-132.
13. Middleton WD: The wrist. In Anatomy and MRI of the joints. A multiplanar atlas New York, Raven, 1989, pp 83-120.
14. Bowers WH. The distal radioulnar joint. In Green DP (ed): Operative hand surgery, 2nd ed. New York, Churchill Livingstone, 1988, pp 939-989.
15. Palmer AK, Werner FW: The triangular fibrocartilage complex of the wrist — anatomy and function. J Hand Surg 1981;6:153-162.

16. Mikic ZD: Detailed anatomy of the articular disc of the distal radioulnar joint. Clin Orthop Rel Res 1989;245:123-132.

17. Mikic ZD: Age changes in the triangular fibrocartilage of the wrist joint. J Anat 1978;126:367-384.

18. Palmer AK: The distal radioulnar joint. Anatomy, biomechanics, and triangular fibrocartilage complex abnormalities. Hand Clin 1987;3:31-40.

19. Biondetti PR, Vannier MW, Gilula LA, Knapp P: Wrist: coronal and transaxial CT scanning. Radiology 1987;163:149-151.

20. Pennes DR, Jonsson K, Buckwalter KA: Direct coronal CT of the scaphoid bone. Radiology 1989;171:870-871.

21. Nakamura R, Horii E, Tanaka T, et al: Three-dimensional CT imaging for wrist disorders. J Hand Surg 1989;14[Br]:53-59.

22. Engel J, Salai M, Yaffe B, Tadmor R: The role of three dimension computerized imaging in hand surgery. J Hand Surg [Br] 1987: 12:349-352.

23. Hindshaw WS, Andrew ER, Bottomley PA, et al: An in vivo study of the forearm and hand by thin section NMR imaging. Br J Radiol 1979;52:36.

24. Mathaei D, Frahm J, Haase A, et al: Multipurpose NMR imaging using stimulated echoes. Magn Reson Med 1986;3:554-561.

25. Frahm J, Haase A, Matthaei D: Rapid three-dimensional MR imaging using the flash technique. J. Comput Assist Tomogr 1986;10:363-368.

26. Axel L, Constantin J, Listerol J: Intensity correction in surface-coil MR imaging. AJR 1987;148:418-420.

27. Fulmer JM, Harms SE, Flaming DP, et al: High-resolution cine MR imaging of the wrist. Radiology 1989;173(P):26.

28. Krahe T, Schindler R, Landwehr P: MRI of the hand: technical requirements. Medicamundi 1989;34:20-23.

29. Phalen GS: The carpal tunnel syndrome, clinical evaluation of 598 hands. Clin Orthop 1972;83:29-40.

30. Firooznia H, Golimbu C, Rafii M: Acute carpal tunnel syndrome as a heralding manifestation of secondary hyperparathyroidism. Arch Intern Med 1981;141:959.

31. Middleton WD, Kneeland JB, Kellman GM: MR imaging of the carpal tunnel: normal anatomy and preliminary findings in the carpal tunnel syndrome. AJR 1987;148:307-316.

32. Mesgarzadeh M, Schneck CD, Bonakdar-pour A: Carpal tunnel: MR imaging. I. Normal anatomy. Radiology 1989;171:743-748.

33. Mesgarzadeh M, Schneck CD, Bonakdar-pour A, et al: Carpal tunnel: MR imaging. II. Carpal tunnel syndrome. Radiology 1989;171:749-754.

34. Zucker-Pinchoff B, Herman G, Srinivasan R: Computed tomography of the carpal tunnel: a radioanatomic study. J Comput Assist Tomogr 1981;5:525-528.

35. Zlatkin MB, Chao P, Osterman AL, et al: Chronic wrist pain. Evaluation with high resolution MR imaging. Radiology 1989;173:723-729.

36. Sclafani SJ: Dislocation of the distal radioulnar joint. J. Comput Assist Tomogr 1981;5:450.

37. Mino DE, Palmer AK, Levensohn EM: Radiography and computerized tomography in the diagnosis of incongruity of the distal radioulnar joint. J Bone Joint Surg [Am] 1985;67:247-252.

38. Space T, Louis D, Francis I, Braunstein EM: CT findings in distal radioulnar dislocation. J Comput Assist Tomogr 1986;10: 689-670.

39. King GJ, McMurtry RY, Rubenstein JD, Ogston NG: Computerized tomography of the distal radioulnar joint: correlation with ligamentous pathology in a cadaveric model. J Hand Surg [Am] 1986;11:711-717.

40. King GJ, McMurtry RY, Rubenstein JD, Gertzbein SD: Kinematics of the distal radioulnar joint. J Hand Surg [Am] 1986;11:798-804.

41. Paley D, Rubenstein J, McMurtry RY: Irreducible dislocation of the distal radial ulnar joint. Orthop Rev 1986;15:69-72.

42. Dalinka MK, Turner ML, Osterman DL, Batra P: Wrist arthrography. Radiol Clin North Am 1981;19:217-226.

43. Resnick D, Andre M, Kerr P, et al: Digital arthrography of the wrist: a radiographic-pathologic investigation. AJR 1984;142: 1187-1190.

44. Manaster BJ: Digital wrist arthrography: precision in determining the site of radiocarpal-midcarpal communication. AJR 1986;147:563-566.

45. Levinsohn EM, Palmer AK, Coren AB, Zinberg E: Wrist arthrography: the value of three compartment injection technique. Skeletal Radiol 1987;16:539-544.

46. Brody AS, Ball WS, Towbin RB: Computed arthrotomography as an adjunct to pediatric arthrography. I. Radiology 1989;179:99-102.

47. Quinn SF, Belsole RB, Greene TL, Rayhack JM: Work in progress; Postarthrography computed tomography of the wrist: evaluation of the triangular fibrocartilage complex. Skeletal Radiol 1989;17:565-569.

48. Tehranzadeh J, Gabriele OF: Intra-articular calcified bodies: detection by computed arthrotomography. South Med J 1984;77:703-710.

49. Golimbu CN, Firooznia H, Melone CP Jr, et al: Tears of the triangular fibrocartilage of the wrist: MR imaging. Radiology 1989;173:731-733.

50. Taleisnik J: Pain on the ulnar side of the wrist. Hand Clin 1987;3:51-68.

51. Mikic ZD: Arthrography of the wrist joint: an experimental study. J Bone Joint Surg [Am] 1984;66:371-378.

52. Reinus WR, Hardy DC, Totty WG, Gilula LA: Arthrographic evaluation of the carpal triangular fibrocartilage complex. J Hand Surg [Am] 1987;12:495-503.

53. Rusineck H, Mourino MR, Firooznia H, et al: Volumetric rendering of MR images. Radiology 1987;171:269-272.

54. Kienböck R: Concerning traumatic malacia of the lunate and its consequences: degeneration and compression fractures. Clin Orthop 1980;149:4-8.

55. Gelberman RH, Bauman TD, Menon J, Akeson WH: The vascularity of the lunate bone and Kienböck's disease. J Hand Surg 1980;5:272-278.

56. Gelberman RH, Szato RM: Kienböck's disease. Orthop Clin North Am 1984;15:355-367.

57. Almquist EA: Kienböck's disease. Hand Clin 1987;3:141-148.

58. Reinus W, Conway W, Totty W, et al: Carpal avascular necrosis: MR imaging. Radiology 1986;160:689-693.

59. Taleisnick J: The wrist. New York, Churchill Livingstone, 1985, pp 239-271.

60. Hindman BW, Kulik WY, Lee G, Avolio RE: Occult fractures of the carpals and metacarpals: demonstration by CT. AJR 1989;153:529-532.

61. Bush CH, Gillespy T, Dell PC: High resolution CT of the wrist: initial experience with scaphoid disorders and surgical fusions. AJR 1987;149:757-760.

62. Tehranzadeh J, Davenport J, Pais MJ: Scaphoid fracture: evaluation with flexion-extension tomography. Radiology 1990;176:167-170.

63. Binkowitz LA, Berquist TH, McLeod RA: Masses of the hand and wrist: detection and characterization with MR imaging. AJR 1990;154:323-326.

64. Brooks ML, Mayer DP, Grannick MS, et al: Paraosteal lipoma of the finger: preoperative evaluation with computed tomography. Comput Med Imaging Graph 1989;13:481-485.

65. Patel MR, Zinberg EM: Pigmented villonodular synovitis of the wrist invading bone—report of a case. J Hand Surg [Am] 1984;9:854-858.

66. Kransdorf MJ, Jelinek JS, Moser RP, et al: Soft tissue masses: diagnosis using MR imaging. AJR 1989;153:541-547.

67. Jelinek JS, Kransdorf MJ, Utz JA, et al: Imaging of pigmented villonodular synovitis with emphasis on MR imaging. AJR 1989;152:337-342.

68. Moser RP Jr, Kransdorf MJ, Gilkey FW, Manaster BJ: Giant cell tumor of the upper extremity. Radiographics 1990;19:83-102.

19 Hip

JEFFREY C. WEINREB
NEIL M. ROFSKY

Hip pain is a common problem, and preliminary diagnostic evaluation almost always begins with radiographic studies. If conventional roentgenograms provide the information required to direct patient management, further imaging studies are not usually required. Sometimes, however, the roentgenograms are normal or equivocal and further imaging procedures, especially CT or MR, are indicated.

NORMAL ANATOMY OF THE HIP

The hip joint is a ball-and-socket (enarthroidal) joint that provides strength and stability to support the weight of the body in the erect position. It is formed by the spherical head of the femur and the cup-shaped cavity of the acetabulum.

The acetabulum is formed by the three component bones of the pelvis. It is surrounded by a fibrocartilaginous rim, called the acetabular labrum or cotyloid ligament, which acts to increase the depth of the acetabulum, enhancing the stability of the hip joint. The transverse acetabular ligament bridges the acetabular notch, a deficiency in the anteroinferior portion of the acetabular rim, thus transforming the notch into an acetabular foramen. Nerves and blood vessels pass to and from the hip joint through this foramen. The acetabulum has a centrally located pit, the acetabular fossa, which is filled with fat as well as the attachment of the ligamentum teres.

The other attachment of the ligamentum teres occurs at the fovea centralis, a small depression at the medial aspect of the femoral head. This is the only portion of the femoral head devoid of hyaline cartilage. The ligamentum teres transmits blood vessels to the femoral head. The articular surface of the femoral head is greatest at its superoanterior aspect, where the greatest weight is directed. The relationship of the femoral head and acetabulum is maintained by a fibrous capsule which encircles the joint and much of the femoral neck. This is strengthened by surrounding ligaments, including the iliofemoral, pubofemoral, and ischiofemoral.

CROSS-SECTIONAL IMAGING OF THE NORMAL HIP

Images of the normal anatomy of the hip and surrounding structures are presented in Figs. 19-1 to 19-9. The serial axial images were obtained at comparable levels with noncontrast CT and T1-weighted MR.

In the normal femoral head on CT, physiologically thickened load-transmitting trabeculae appear arranged in the form of a star, the so-called "asterisk sign" (Fig. 19-8). The raylike branches of the star usually extend to the upper surface of the femoral head. Normally there may be some clumping and thickening in the center of the star but not in the periphery.[1]

The MRI appearance of the marrow and articular cartilage of the hip joint is dependent upon age-related

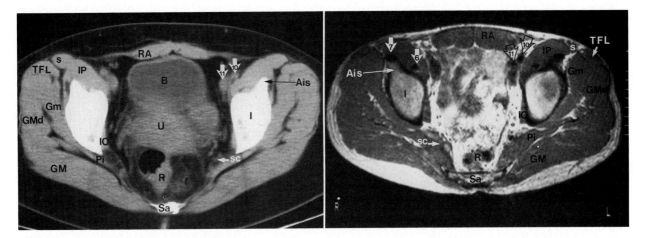

FIGURE 19-1
CT and MR images at the anterior inferior iliac spine and acetabular roof. **Muscles**—anterior group: iliopsoas *(IP)*, sartorius *(s)*; posterior group: internal obturator *(IO)*, piriformis *(Pi)*; lateral group: gluteus maximus *(GM)*, gluteus medius *(GMd)*, gluteus minimus *(Gm)*, tensor fasciae latae *(TFL)*; rectus abduminus *(RA)*. **Bone structures**—anterior inferior iliac spine *(Ais)*, ilium *(I)*, sacrum *(Sa)*. **Viscera**—bladder *(B)*, rectum *(R)*, uterus *(U)*. **Nerve**—sciatic *(sc)*. **Vessels**—external iliac artery *(10)* and vein *(11)*. Note also that MR demonstrates the **tendons** of the iliopsoas *(6)* and rectus femoris *(7)*.

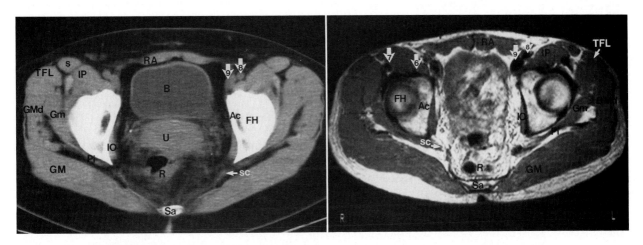

FIGURE 19-2
CT and MR images at the acetabulum. **Muscles**—anterior group: iliopsoas *(IP)*, sartorius *(s)*; posterior group: internal obturator *(IO)*, piriformis *(PI)*; lateral group: gluteus maximus *(GM)*, gluteus medius *(GMd)*, gluteus minimus *(Gm)*, tensor fasciae latae *(TFL)*; rectus abduminus *(RA)*. **Bone structures**—acetabulum *(Ac)*, femoral head *(FH)*, sacrum *(Sa)*. **Viscera**—bladder *(B)*, rectum *(R)*, uterus *(U)*. **Nerve**—sciatic *(sc)*. **Vessels**—common femoral artery *(8)* and vein *(9)*. Note that MR also demonstrates the **tendons** of the iliopsoas *(6)* and rectus femoris *(7)*.

changes. Yellow marrow, which is hematopoietically inactive, is composed predominantly of fat cells and thus demonstrates marked hyperintensity on T1-weighted images and progressively decreased signal with increasing T2 weighting. Hematopoietically active red marrow contains only approximately 40% fat and has a richer vascular network than yellow marrow. As a result, it demonstrates intermediate signal on T1-WIs and T2-WIs.[2]

In the fetus all bone marrow is hematopoietic. After birth, conversion of red to yellow marrow occurs in a predictable, but not a perfectly homogeneous or symmetrical, pattern, beginning in the distal extremities and progressing from diaphyseal to metaphyseal in the femora. By the third decade of life, the adult distribution of marrow is achieved. Differences depend upon individual variation and the body's demand for hematopoiesis. Whereas red marrow in the femur is usually restricted to the proximal metaphysis, it can occupy as much as two thirds of the femoral shaft or be restricted to just the intertrochanteric region or distinct islands. In children intermediate-signal red marrow is present throughout the

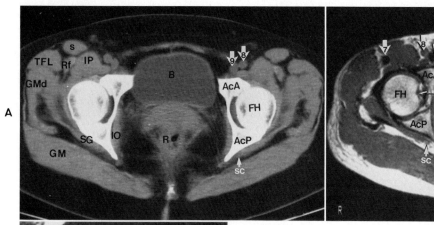
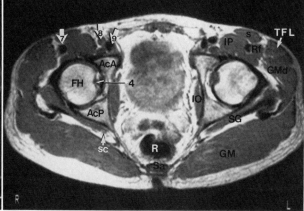
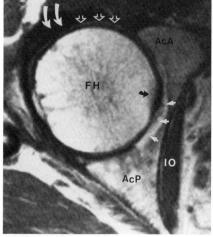

FIGURE 19-3

A and **B**, CT and MR images at the acetabulum slightly inferior to Fig. 19-2. **Muscles**— anterior group: iliopsoas *(IP)*, rectus femoris *(Rf)*, sartorius *(s)*; posterior group: internal obturator *(IO)*, superior gemellus *(SG)*; lateral group: gluteus maximus *(GM)*, gluteus medius *(GMd)*, gluteus minimus *(Gm)*, tensor fasciae latae *(TFL)*. **Bone structures**— anterior column of the acetabulum *(AcA)*, posterior column of the acetabulum *(AcP)*, femoral head *(FH)*, sacrum *(SA)*. **Viscera**— bladder *(B)*, rectum *(R)*. **Nerve**— sciatic *(sc)*. **Vessels**— common femoral artery *(8)* and vein *(9)*. Note that MR demonstrates the rectus femoris **tendon** *(7)* and the **ligamentum** teres *(4)*. **C**, A T1-weighted transaxial image at the level of the femoral head *(FH)* obtained with a surface coil and small field-of-view. The fovea centralis *(black curved arrow)* is devoid of articular hyaline cartilage *(open white arrows)*. In the central portion of the acetabulum, between the anterior column *(AcA)* and posterior column *(AcP)*, the fat-filled acetabular fossa is seen *(short white arrows)*. The internal obturator *(IO)* lies adjacent to the medial portion of the acetabulum. The low-intensity iliofemoral ligament is also visible *(curved white arrows)*.

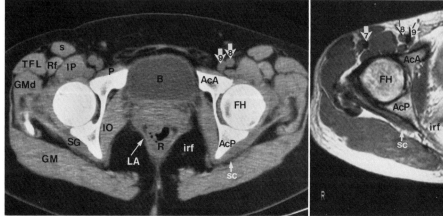
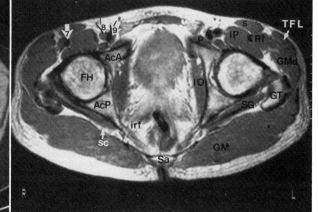

FIGURE 19-4

CT and MR images at the inferior aspect of the acetabulum. **Muscles**— anterior group: iliopsoas *(IP)*, rectus femoris *(Rf)*, sartorius *(s)*; posterior group: internal obturator *(IO)*, superior gemellus *(SG)*: lateral group: gluteus maximus *(GM)*, gluteus medius *(GMd)*, tensor fasciae latae *(TFL)*; medial group: pectineus *(P)*; levator ani *(LA)*. **Bone structures**— anterior column of the acetabulum *(AcA)*, posterior column of the acetabulum *(AcP)*, femoral head *(FH)*, greater trochanter *(GT)*, sacrum *(Sa)*. **Viscera**— bladder *(B)*, rectum *(R)*. **Nerve**— sciatic *(sc)*. **Vessels**— common femoral artery *(8)* and vein *(9)*. Note that MR also demonstrates the rectus femoris tendon *(7)* and at this level the ischiorectal fossa *(irf)* is identified.

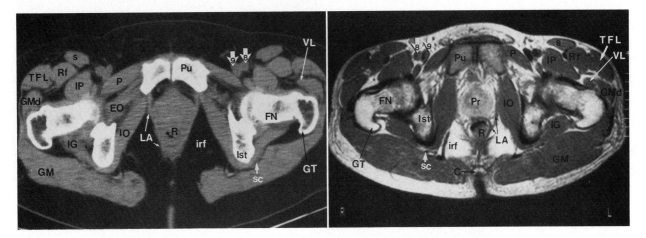

FIGURE 19-5

CT and MR images at the superior pubis and femoral neck. **Muscles**— anterior group: iliopsoas *(IP)*, rectus femoris *(Rf)*, sartorius *(s)*; posterior group: external obturator *(EO)*, internal obturator *(IO)*, inferior gemellus *(IG)*; lateral group: gluteus maximus *(GM)*, gluteus medius *(GMd)*, tensor fasciae latae *(TFL)*; medial group: pectineus *(P)*; levator ani *(LA)*; vastus lateralis *(VL)*. **Bone structures**— coccyx *(C)*, femoral neck *(FN)*, greater trochanter *(GT)*, ischial tuberosity *(IST)*, pubis *(Pu)*. **Viscera**— prostate *(Pr)*, rectum *(R)*. **Nerve**— sciatic *(sc)*. **Vessels**— common femoral artery *(8)* and vein *(9)*. The ischiorectal fossa *(irf)* is identified.

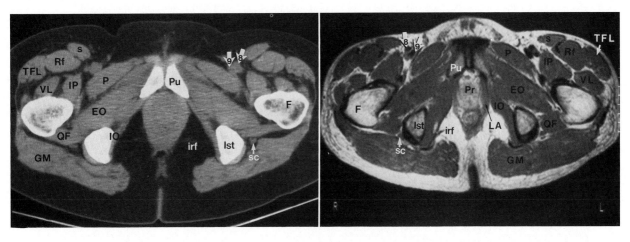

FIGURE 19-6

CT and MR images at the inferior pubis. **Muscles**— anterior group: iliopsoas *(IP)*, rectus femoris *(Rf)*, sartorius *(s)*; posterior group: external obturator *(EO)*, internal obturator *(IO)*, quadratus femoris *(QF)*; lateral group: gluteus maximus *(GM)*, tensor fasciae latae *(TFL)*; medial group: pectineus *(P)*; levator ani *(LA)*; vastus lateralis *(VL)*. **Bone structures**— femur *(F)*, ischial tuberosity *(Ist)*, pubis *(Pu)*. **Viscera**— prostate *(Pr)*. **Nerve**— sciatic *(sc)*. **Vessels**— common femoral artery *(8)* and vein *(9)*. The ischiorectal fossa *(irf)* is identified.

pelvis. Gradually it is replaced by fatty marrow, though it is common to see patchy areas of red marrow in the pelvic bones in the adult[2,3] (Fig. 19-9).

The cartilaginous capital epiphysis does not contain any marrow until it undergoes ossification early in life and is replaced by yellow marrow. Thus in the young child the femoral capital epiphysis demonstrates moderately high signal intensity, a reflection of the high water content of nonossified epiphyseal cartilage.[4] As the capital epiphysis matures, fatty marrow forms in the center of the cartilage anlage and gradually enlarges to occupy the entire epiphysis. This is seen on MR as a progressive increase in high signal volume in the epiphysis. The greater trochanter apophysis undergoes similar changes and demonstrates the high signal of fatty marrow beginning early in life.[5]

After the adult pattern of marrow distribution is attained in the mid-twenties, the fractional balance of yellow and red marrow in the femur may slowly change with advancing age. Thus, although most healthy persons

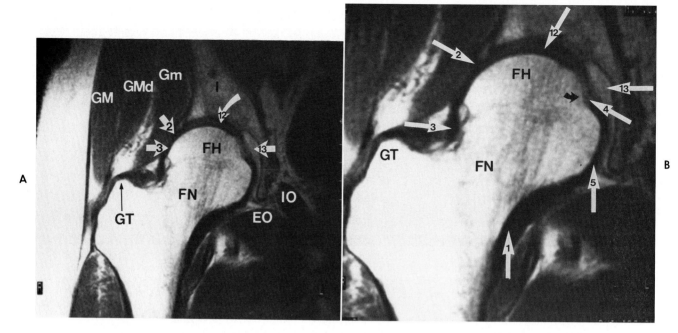

FIGURE 19-7

Normal T1-weighted coronal surface coil MR images through the femoral head *(FH)*, femoral neck *(FN)*, greater trochanter *(GT)*, and ilium *(I)*. Some of the lateral- and posterior-group muscles of the hip are indicated in **A**: gluteus maximus *(GM)*, gluteus medius *(GMd)*, gluteus minimus *(Gm)*, external obturator *(EO)*, internal obturator *(IO)*. The fibrocartilaginous and ligamentous structures exhibit very low signal intensity. Note the capsular/iliofemoral ligaments *(1)*, cotyloid ligament *(2)*, iliofemoral ligament *(3)*, and transverse ligament *(5)* in **B**. The articular hyaline cartilage *(12)* shows low to intermediate signal intensity. The fat-filled acetabular fossa *(13)* exhibits high intensity. In **B** the ligamentum teres *(4)* inserts at the fovea centralis *(curved black arrow)*.

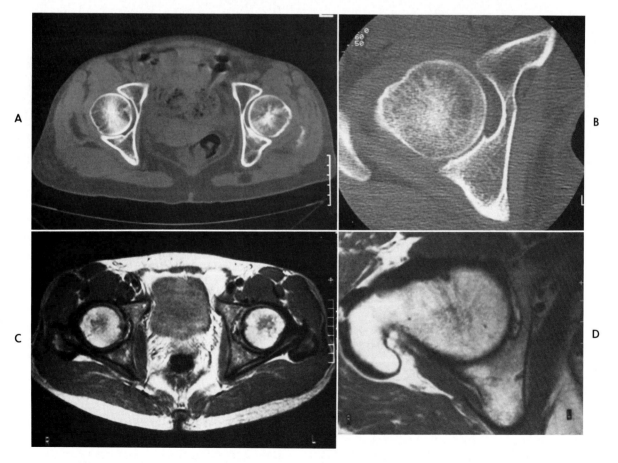

FIGURE 19-8

CT and MR of the normal femoral head. **A** and **B**, On CT the physiologically thickened load-transmitting trabeculae appear arranged in the form of a star, the so-called "asterisk sign." **C** and **D**, On MR the central low-signal area is the "asterisk sign."

FIGURE 19-9
Normal age-related patterns of cellular and fatty bone marrow distribution in the proximal femora on T1-WIs. **A,** A 10-year-old with uniform high signal in the capital femoral epiphysis and the greater and lesser trochanters (not shown). Note the low-signal epiphyseal growth plate. **B,** A 20-year-old with fatty marrow in the region inferior to the medial femoral head in addition to the areas seen in **A. C,** A 30-year-old with patchy areas of high-signal fatty marrow in the intertrochanteric region in addition to the areas seen in **B. D,** A 50-year-old with uniform high-signal fatty marrow occupying the entire proximal femur.

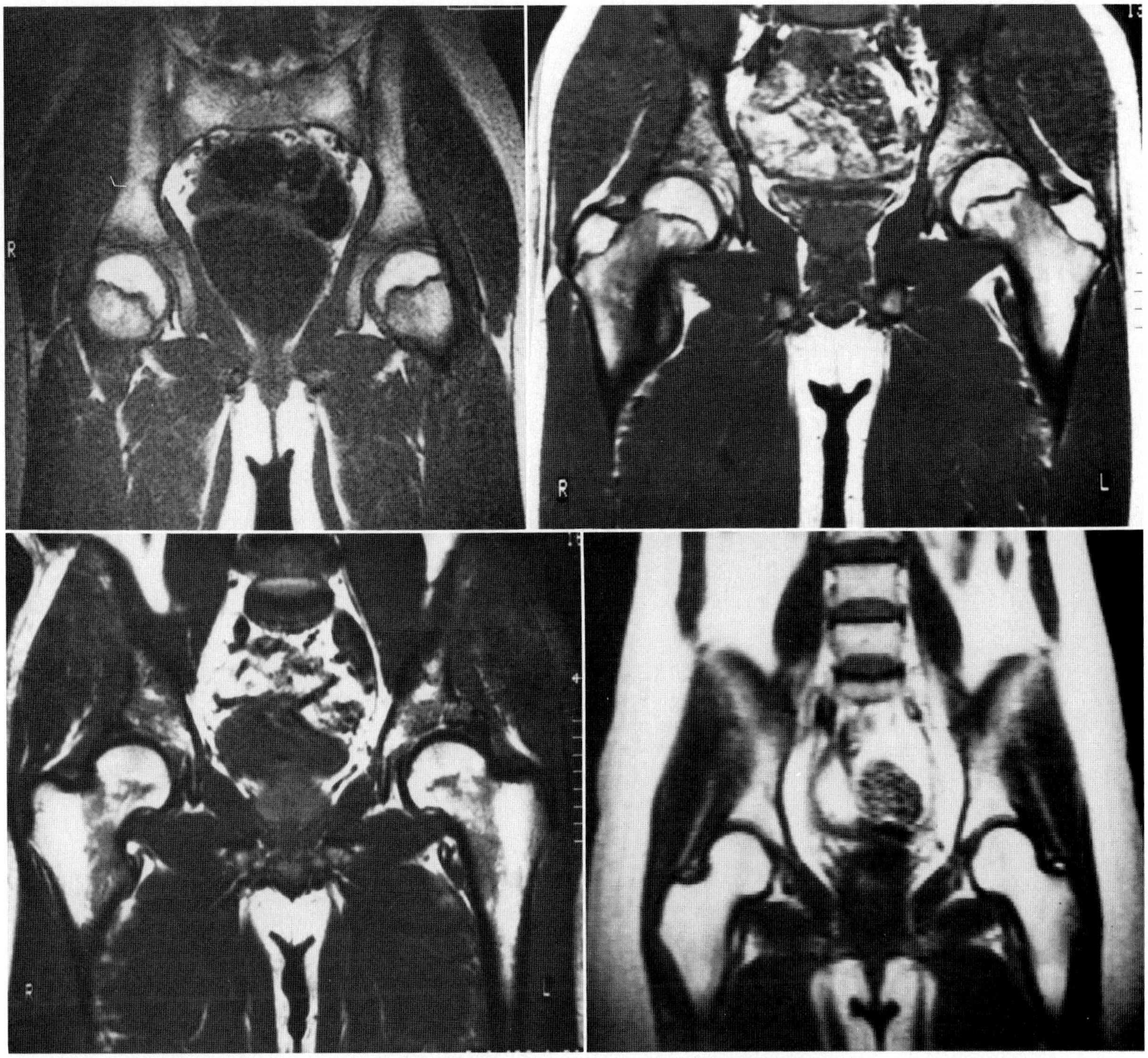

less than 50 years of age have some red marrow in the intertrochanteric region, fatty marrow predominates in almost all older individuals. These age-related changes have been attributed to a physiologic decrease in blood supply. Early fatty conversion may be a predisposing factor for AVN in the femoral head.[3] Marked deviation from the normal patterns of marrow distribution should raise the suspicion of systemic disease (Fig. 19-10).

In children a broad curvilinear low-intensity line between the capital epiphysis and metaphysis represents the physeal growth plate. With aging, the growth plate

fuses, and a thin dark line in the same location in the adult represents the dense bone of the fused physis (Fig. 19-11). The physeal scar is best appreciated on coronal or sagittal images.[5,6]

On coronal images there is frequently a vertically oriented low-intensity band extending from the inferolateral aspect of the femoral neck to the superomedial aspect of the femoral head (Fig. 19-7) that represents the central weight-bearing trabeculae, the MR equivalent of the "asterisk sign" of thickened trabeculae seen on CT. It appears dark because it contains relatively more calcium

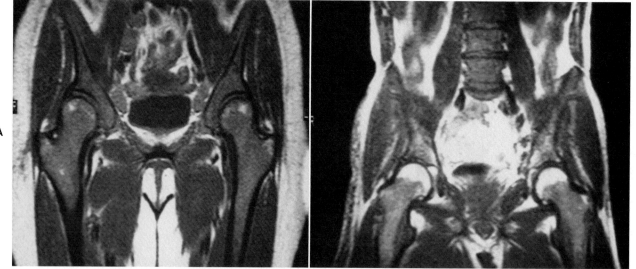

FIGURE 19-10
Abnormal bone marrow patterns in the proximal femora on T1-WIs. **A,** A 20-year-old with leukemia has almost complete replacement of high-signal fatty marrow signal. Contrast this image with that of the normal 20-year-old in Fig. 19-9, *B.* **B,** A 38-year-old with AIDs has high-signal fatty marrow apparent only in the capital femoral epiphyses. Contrast this image with that of the normal 30-year-old in Fig. 19-9, *C.*

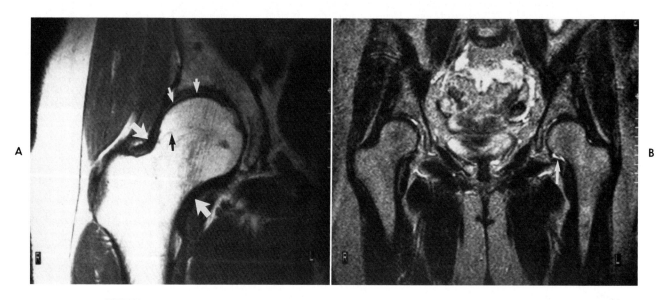

FIGURE 19-11
MR of the normal femoral head. **A,** Surface coil coronal T1-WI. The vertically oriented low intensity band represents the central weight-bearing trabeculae. The thin faint low-signal curvilinear structure *(small black arrowhead)* crossing horizontally across the femoral head is the physeal scar. Cortical bone appears as a thin, sharply defined signal void. Hyaline cartilage *(small white arrowheads)* appears as a thin rim of intermediate signal. A hypointense fibrous capsule *(large white arrowheads)* encloses the femoral neck. **B,** Coronal T2-WI. A small amount of fluid *(small arrow)* that does not extend to surround the femoral neck and distend the joint is visible in greater than 80%.

than adjacent fatty marrow. On axial sections it appears as a central area of low signal within the femoral head (Figs. 19-8, *A* and *B*, and 19-11, *A*) and should not be mistaken for an area of pathology.

The cortical bone that surrounds the marrow appears as a thin sharply defined signal void. The outline of the femoral head is smooth and round, indented medially by the fovea centralis. Articular hyaline cartilage appears as a thin intermediate-signal curvilinear band surrounding the femoral head except at the fovea centralis. The thin rim of intermediate-signal hyaline cartilage also lines the articular surface of the acetabulum. A hypointense fibrous articular capsule encloses the femoral neck and extends from an area just above the acetabular brim and labrum to the femoral neck.

A small amount of fluid may be visible in more than 80% of normal hip joints, particularly on T2-WIs, where the fluid demonstrates marked hyperintensity (Fig. 19-11, *B*). Young subjects tend to have more normal fluid than older subjects, and minor disparities between the right and left sides in the quantity of joint fluid are common. Generally fluid that does not surround the femoral neck or distend the joint should be considered normal.[7]

NONTRAUMATIC AVASCULAR NECROSIS OF THE HIP
Background

Nontraumatic avascular necrosis (AVN) or osteonecrosis of the femoral head is the result of an aseptic ischemic insult to cellular elements of the bone marrow. It is responsible for a great deal of morbidity due to unrelenting degeneration of the involved hip, leading to serious joint deformity and dysfunction. The prevalence of AVN appears to be increasing because of longer survival of the high-risk patient population. Patients with nontraumatic AVN in one hip are at greater risk for development of the disease on the contralateral side. The earliest symptoms of nontraumatic AVN of the hip include vague discomfort in the hip, knee, or groin, and often preceding radiographic evidence of AVN.

The treatment of osteonecrosis of the hip is generally determined by the course and severity of the disease at the time of presentation. Data suggest that early diagnosis is desirable because timely institution of decompression, drilling, or other relatively conservative measures may allow healing before complications occur. Once fracture, collapse, or destruction of the joint ensues, more drastic surgical intervention (e.g., varus osteotomy or total hip replacement) is mandated.[8-10]

Etiology and pathogenesis

Nontraumatic AVN is associated with a variety of conditions and is a common endpoint for a number of initiating insults. The common factor seems to be an increase in the intramedullary pressure secondary to deficient venous drainage. The fatty marrow in the adult femoral head is especially vulnerable because it is relatively hypovascular. Suggested mechanisms for venous congestion and edema include steroid effects, vasculitis, embolization, and extrinsic compression by the accumulation of marrow fat stores. Etiological factors are steroids and antimetabolic therapy, thrombosis secondary to sickle cell anemia or other hemoglobinopathies, radiation injury, alcoholism, Cushing's disease, collagen vascular diseases (e.g., systemic lupus erythematosus), Gaucher's disease, dysbaric conditions, and pancreatitis. Some cases are idiopathic.

To understand the CT and MR appearances of AVN in the femoral head, one needs an appreciation of the associated histopathological changes.

Following the ischemic insult, the initial pathological phase of AVN is characterized by the sequential death of cellular marrow components: first, the hematopoietic cells; then, osteoblastic, osteoclastic, and osteocytic elements; and, finally, the fat cells. Necrotic debris appears in the intertrabecular spaces of the devascularized area. Repair begins with a hyperemic response of the tissues surrounding the ischemic region. A reactive interface, characterized by inflammation and mesenchymal capillary proliferation, forms between the viable and necrotic tissue. Progressive bone resorption within the interface stimulates osteoblastic reinforcement of adjacent cancellous bone, with resultant trabecular thickening, leading to radiographically apparent sclerosis. Within the sclerotic margin an advancing front of fibrosis, hyperemia, inflammation, and bone marrow resorption extends into the infarcted region. Bone resorption may cause mechanical failure, producing subchondral fracture, articular collapse, and progressive joint changes.[2,11-14]

Different histological stages of the disease may be seen simultaneously in different areas of the same femoral head. There is not a good correlation between histology and clinical features.

Computed tomography

Although CT is not generally used in primary evaluation of the hip for AVN, it can be used to confirm suspected findings or detect changes not apparent on standard roentgenograms. With CT, bony architecture is visible without the overlap that may plague roentgenograms, and abnormalities are more readily detected and defined. CT is particularly valuable for the depiction of subchondral or cortical fractures for accurate staging of AVN.[1,15,16]

TECHNIQUE

The patient is positioned supine with the feet in neutral anatomic position. To prevent patient motion, the feet and knees may be taped together.

Beginning above the dome of the acetabulum, contiguous 3 to 6 mm sections are obtained to a level just below the lesser trochanter. If a multiplanar reconstruction (MPR) is anticipated, 4 mm thick sections are obtained at 3 mm intervals. Images are filmed using both bone and soft tissue window width and level settings.

FINDINGS

Staging of AVN with CT uses the same criteria developed for roentgenogram studies.[5,15] All the radiographic and CT changes of AVN occur relatively late in the course of the disease, and once these changes are detected, conservative treatment may be precluded.

Stage I disease is a histological and clinical diagnosis without CT findings. The insensitivity of roentgenograms and CT for the diagnosis of early AVN is easily understood if one considers the fact that devascularized medullary bone has the same density and architecture as live bone. The x rays used in plain roentgenograms or CT depict only the cortical and cancellous bony changes that occur long after AVN has developed in the bone marrow.

In Stage II AVN the normal arrangement of trabecular bone becomes altered. The earliest sign of AVN on CT is distortion of the "asterisk," with clumping and fusion of the peripheral rays at the interface between necrotic and viable bone (Fig. 19-12, A). There may be a halo of relative osteopenia surrounding a central core of relatively dense necrotic bone. These findings reflect the presence of hyperemic viable medullary bone surrounding the infarcted bony segment. Early findings may be subtle and difficult to appreciate. The surface and contour of the femoral head is preserved.

Stage III is characterized by a subchondral cavity or lucency due to fragmentation and collapse of the weakened necrotic segment. This is often referred to as the radiographic "crescent sign."

In Stage IV the fragmented subchondral bone leads to articular collapse and flattening of the femoral head (Fig. 19-12, B).

Finally, Stage V is characterized by acetabular involvement with joint space narrowing and secondary degenerative arthritis. Occasionally the iliopsoas bursa, which extends from the inguinal ligament to the lesser trochanter, will fill with fluid via a communication with the hip joint. This appears as a water density mass located close to the psoas muscle at the level of the hip joint.

An important shortcoming of routine transaxial CT is that it may provide only limited information about the major weight-bearing components of the hip (i.e., the superior pole of the femoral head, the upper joint space, the acetabular dome, and the anterior and posterior acetabular columns), where AVN begins.[15] This can be addressed by MPR (multiplanar reconstruction) in the coronal and sagittal planes. CT with MPR facilitates preoperative planning and supplements conventional roentgenograms and transaxial CT by providing the following information: (1) detection of subtle femoral head contour changes, (2) definition of the sclerotic cone of involvement and the remaining intact femoral head, (3) assessment of the joint space for subtle narrowings or unsuspected effusions, (4) improved assessment of the acetabular dome and weight-bearing columns.

In one study in which CT/MPR was compared with routine roentgenograms,[15] CT/MPR upgraded staging in 30% of the hips studied and made significant contributions to patient management in 54%. For instance, in some patients asymptomatic and radiographically normal contralateral hips were found to have Stage II and III disease on CT/MPR.

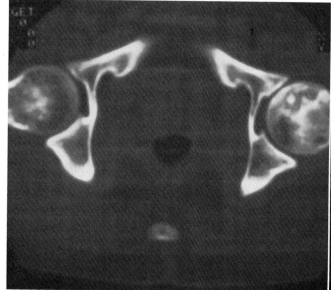 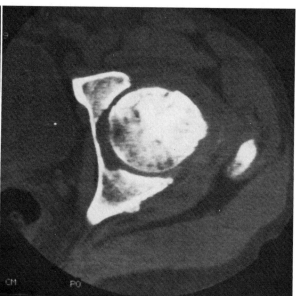

A   B

FIGURE 19-12
CT findings in AVN. **A,** Stage II; on the left there is distortion of the "asterisk," with clumping and fusion of the peripheral rays. **B,** Stage IV; fragmented subchondral bone.

Magnetic resonance imaging

MRI is now accepted as the most sensitive and specific noninvasive test for AVN.[17-23] In one study[17] it was 98% specific for the diagnosis; and it was 97% sensitive in differentiating AVN from normality, 85% sensitive in differentiating it from non-AVN disease, and 91% sensitive in differentiating it from both conditions.

TECHNIQUE

Generally both hips are imaged simultaneously with the patient supine in the body coil. At present, this may require a relatively large field of view (in the range of 32 to 40 cm) for simultaneous evaluation and comparison of both hips, an important consideration when dealing with this frequently bilateral disease. Since AVN involves primarily the anterosuperior weight-bearing surface of the femoral head, the hips should be imaged in two planes, usually coronal and axial. The diagnosis of a normal versus an abnormal hip is generally apparent on coronal T1-WIs obtained with a TR of between 400 and 900 msec and a TE in the range of 15 to 30 msec. Sections 3 to 5 mm thick are obtained with small (or no) gaps between slices. Axial or coronal T2-WIs can provide information about histopathology, the presence of fluid, and associated or alternative diagnoses. Axial images may also be useful for demonstrating the anterior and posterior acetabular margins. T2-weighted sagittal images are routinely used by some to demonstrate joint fluid and observe the signal intensity changes noted in pathological areas on the T1-WIs.

Small-FOV (16 to 20 cm) surface coil images of the femoral heads have not usually been included as part of a routine screening examination because they do not image both hips simultaneously. However, they can provide additional information about joint space narrowing, articular cartilage fracture, and other findings that might not be apparent on routine large-FOV images and they probably improve the sensitivity of the examination for AVN[24] (Figs. 19-13 and 19-17). As the capability of scanning both hips simultaneously with dual surface coils becomes available, this will probably become the routine screening technique. Sagittal small-FOV surface coil images may be particularly useful for determining the anterosuperior and superoinferior extent of the osteonecrotic segment and to facilitate lesional location for biopsy or decompression.[24]

STIR (short TI inversion recovery) and T2*-weighted gradient echo sequences can be used to supplement conventional spin echo images. T2*-weighted gradient echo images are especially useful for evaluating the articular hyaline cartilage, which will demonstrate high signal intensity, in contrast to the low−signal intensity bone marrow and even higher−signal intensity joint fluid[25] (Fig. 19-14).

Chemical-shift images reveal the distribution of water and fat in the femoral heads and can depict femoral head contour and width of the joint space better than routine spin echo sequences can. However, they do not seem to add any diagnostic sensitivity.[26,27]

Although little experience has been reported with MRI of the hip using paramagnetic intravenous contrast agents (e.g., gadopentetate), experiments in dogs suggest that

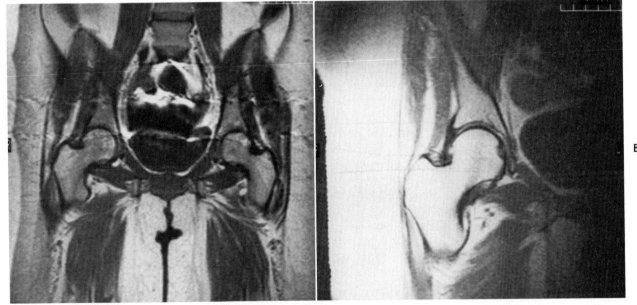

FIGURE 19-13
A 23-year-old woman with right hip pain and known AVN of the knees. **A,** The routine large FOV T1-W coronal is nondiagnostic due to relatively poor resolution and presence of artifacts. **B,** A small FOV T1-W coronal obtained with the surface coil shows improved resolution, indicating the absence of AVN findings. Note the improved visualization of articular cartilage compared to **A.**

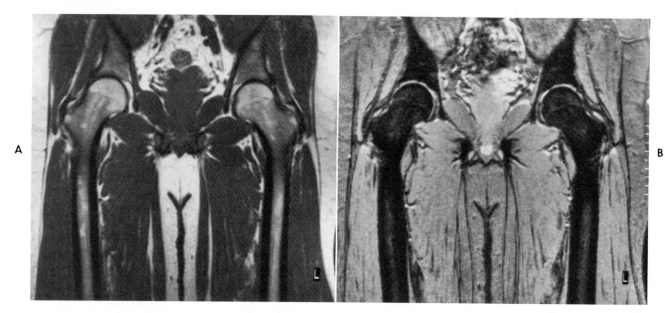

FIGURE 19-14
Normal coronal MR of the hips in a 30-year-old man. **A**, T1-WI (TR 700/TE 20). The articular cartilage is not discernible. **B**, T2* gradient-recalled echo (TR 365/TE 13 flip angle 25). Hyaline articular cartilage demonstrates high-signal intensity in contrast to the low-signal intensity of bone marrow and even higher-signal of joint fluid.

contrast-enhanced fast MRI may allow early detection of abnormal bone marrow flow. In the future this capability could be useful for evaluating patients at risk of AVN of the femoral head.

FINDINGS

Symptoms of femoral capital AVN may appear before any changes are evident on MRI[28]; and, conversely, AVN may remain asymptomatic until long after MRI abnormalities have appeared.

Three separate studies[18,21,28] have reported on small series of high-risk patients with negative MR studies who were proven to have early AVN by biopsy. Thus, routine MR may not diagnose the very earliest stages of AVN.

Bone marrow edema and congestion are an early feature of AVN and precede the appearance of a reactive interface. Not surprisingly, the earliest MR finding in AVN is probably the "edema" pattern, characterized by diffuse low signal intensity on T1-WIs without any focal abnormalities. One published report[29] described six hips with these findings. AVN was subsequently shown to be present in all six by either core biopsy or the subsequent development of characteristic focal abnormalities. A similar pattern was found in the marrow just above the acetabulum in two of the cases. This pattern is probably due to vascular congestion or edema. Thus far, it has been noted only in symptomatic hips. At present, it is not known whether it always precedes the focal findings described below or whether people with it represent a distinct subpopulation of patients with AVN. Although the diffuse "edema" pattern may be an early finding in

AVN, it is not diagnostic but has been reported in a variety of bone conditions, including transient osteoporosis,[30,31] transient edema,[32] osteomyelitis,[33] fracture,[34] and painful sickle cell crises.[35] It has also been identified with metastases, osteoarthritis, septic arthritis, and Paget's disease; and radiographic correlation and clinical history may be needed for its differentiation (Figs. 19-15 and 19-28).

The diagnosis of AVN of the femoral head with MRI has relied primarily on the presence of characteristic and highly specific focal lesions. These may be small or large, and may be irregular or appear as bands, lines, rings, or wedges (Fig. 19-16). The various patterns reflect differences in severity, chronicity, and regional variability of host response to infarction. Since MRI and radiography reflect the different parameters these modalities measure, a precise correlation between MR and radiographic staging does not exist. Mitchell et al.[19] defined an AVN classification system that correlates MRI signal patterns with histopathology. The prognostic and therapeutic implications of this classification system have not been established.

Class A (fatlike): Central region with signal characteristics of fat (i.e., high signal on T1-WIs and intermediate signal on T2-WIs) surrounded by a low-intensity reactive interface (Fig. 19-17).

The central fatlike area can represent either fat persisting within the lesion or necrotic debris with relaxation characteristics similar to those of fat. This is the most common pattern in early AVN, occurring in 43% of all affected hips[27] and in 88% of asymptomatic ones.[17] Often there is a high-signal ring within a low-signal halo on T2-WIs,

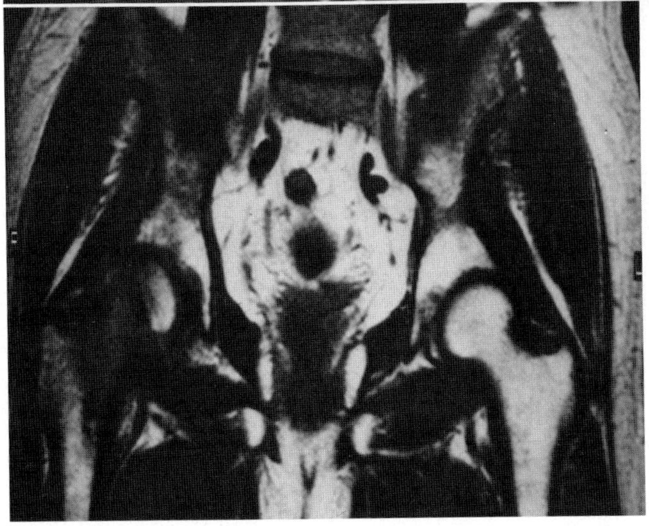

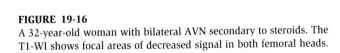

FIGURE 19-15
In addition to early AVN, there are other causes of diffuse low signal in the proximal femur on T1-WIs. **A,** Metastatic breast carcinoma (biopsy proven). **B,** Paget's disease (roentgenographically proven). **C,** Osteoarthritis (surgically proven).

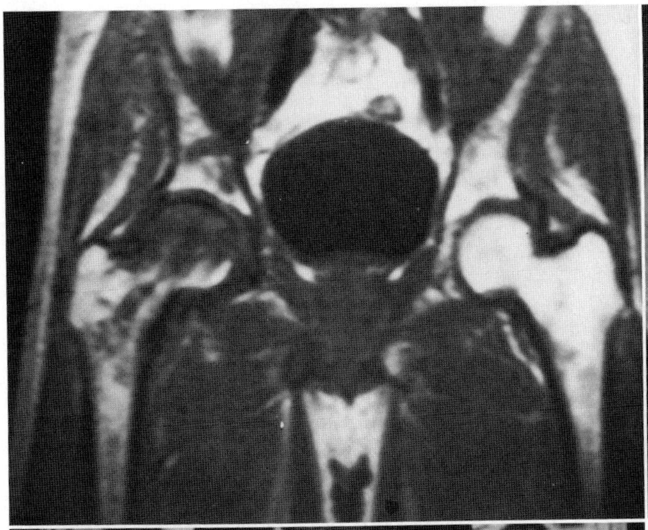

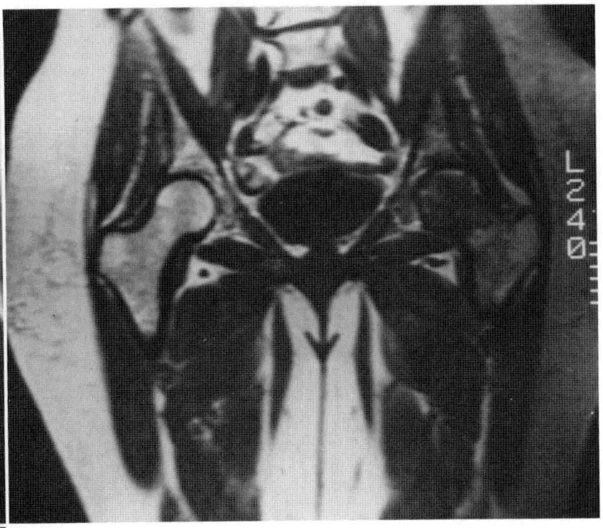

FIGURE 19-16
A 32-year-old woman with bilateral AVN secondary to steroids. The T1-WI shows focal areas of decreased signal in both femoral heads.

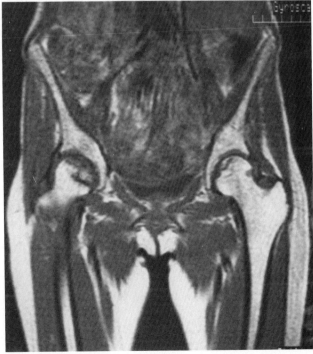

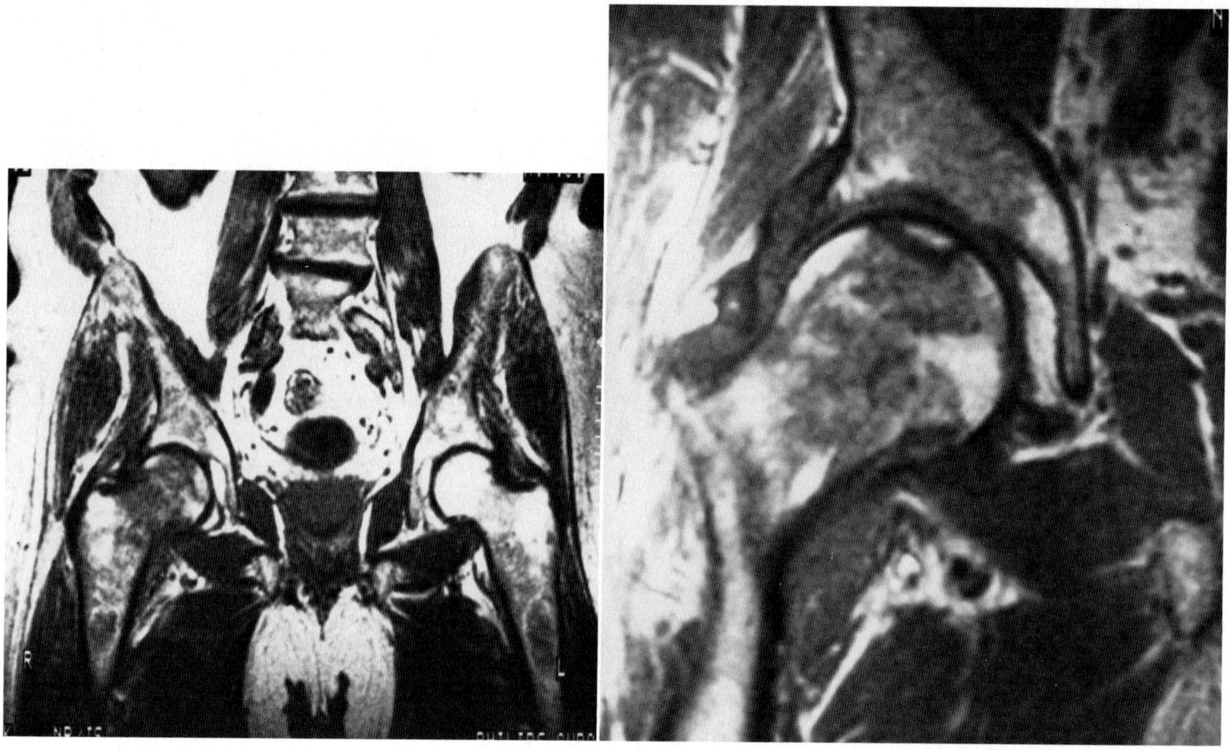

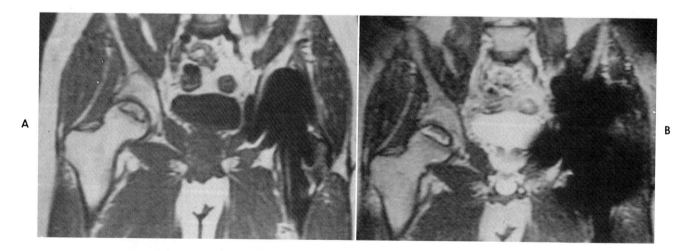

FIGURE 19-17
Class A AVN. **A,** A routine large-FOV (375 mm) coronal T1-WI shows decreased signal in the right femoral head but no focal abnormality. **B,** A small-FOV (240 mm) coronal obtained with the surface coil shows a focal abnormality in the superior femoral head, which confirms the diagnosis of AVN.

FIGURE 19-18
Class A AVN in the right hip (1.5 T). **A,** T1-WI and, **B,** T2-WI. The central region with fatlike signal on both T1-WI and T2-WI is surrounded by a low-signal reactive interface. Note the high-signal ring within the low-signal ring, the so-called "double line sign," which is thought to be a diagnostic feature of AVN. The large signal void on the left is due to the presence of a metallic hip prosthesis. (**A** and **B** courtesy Donald G. Mitchell, M.D.)

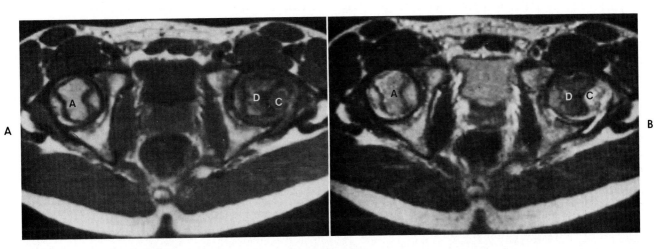

FIGURE 19-19
Class A AVN in the left hip (0.35 T). **A**, T1-WI and **B**, T2-WI. Note that the "double line sign" may be visible on images obtained with low–field strength MR units.

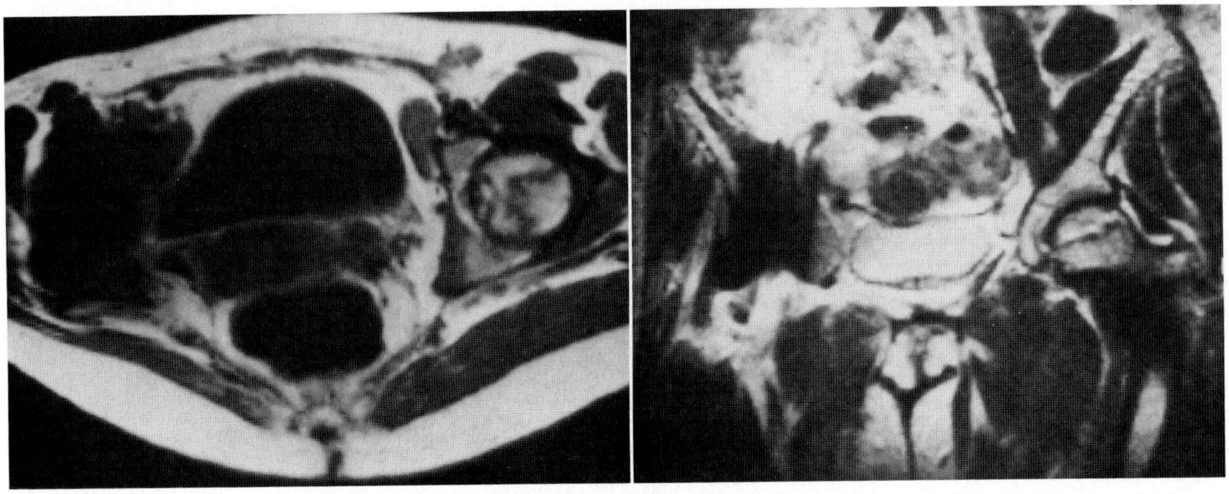

FIGURE 19-20
A 26-year-old man with left hip pain. Roentgenograms showed evidence of AVN on the left and a normal right hip. **A**, T1-WI and **B**, T2-WI. More than one class of AVN may be present in different areas of the same hip. Centrally there is a large region that demonstrates low signal fibrosis-like Class D signal on T1-WI and T2-WI. Laterally a smaller region demonstrates Class C changes in that it behaves as fluid, with low signal on T1-WI and intense signal on T2-WI. There is also obvious Class A AVN in the radiographically normal right hip.

thought to represent hyperemic granulation tissue, that has been termed the *double line sign* (Figs. 19-18 and 19-19). It is thought to be a diagnostic feature of AVN and is reported present in about 80% of lesions.[27] However, experience has shown it to be less common than this in AVN, and it has also been present in some cases of osteoarthritis.

Class B (bloodlike): High signal intensity on T1-WIs and T2-WIs, similar to subacute hemorrhage (found in 11% of hips with AVN)

Class C (fluidlike): Low signal intensity on T1-WIs and marked hyperintensity on T2-WIs, similar to fluid (Fig. 19-20) (found in 25%)

Class D (fibrouslike): Low signal intensity on both T1-WIs and T2-WIs (Fig. 19-20) (found in the later stages of AVN, when medullary sclerosis and fibrosis predominate; present in 21% of affected hips)

More than one class of AVN may be present in different areas of the same hip (Fig. 19-20).

ASSOCIATED FINDINGS

An increased amount of synovial fluid is often found in the hip joint affected with AVN, and the presence of effusion correlates with pain[7,22] (Figs. 19-21 and 19-22). However, the significance of increased joint fluid in the absence of characteristic AVN changes in the bone is not known. It could indicate a very early stage of AVN that has not yet become apparent in the bone. Another possibility is that it might predispose the patient to AVN. In any event, when abnormally increased joint fluid is present (i.e., enough to surround the femoral neck or

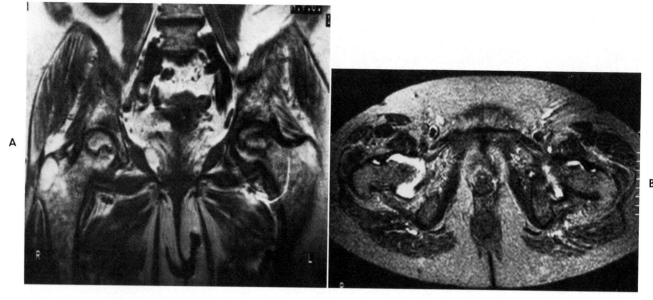

FIGURE 19-21
An 80-year-old woman with lymphoma and right hip pain. **A,** A coronal T1-WI shows evidence of bilateral AVN. **B,** An axial T2-WI shows asymmetrical joint effusions. Such effusions are commonly found with AVN.

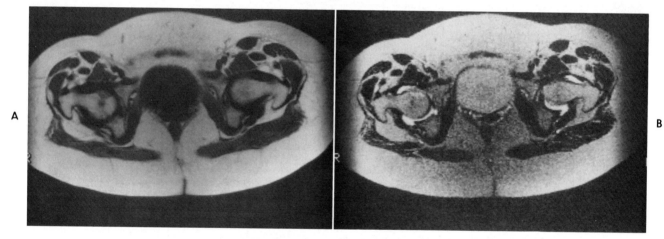

FIGURE 19-22
A 31-year-old woman receiving steroids for SLE complained of bilateral hip pain. MR demonstrated bilateral AVN (not shown). **A,** T1-WI and, **B,** T2-WI. Note the bilateral symmetric joint effusions which are distending the joint capsule and surrounding the femoral necks.

distend the joint capsule), in the absence of associated bone changes an etiology other than AVN should be sought.

The iliopsoas bursa (located between the iliopsoas muscle anteriorly and laterally and the pectineus muscle and femoral vessels medially and anteriorly) may become distended with fluid (Fig. 19-23). Although iliopsoas bursitis is not a specific finding in AVN but may be seen with a variety of inflammatory conditions, it can have important clinical implications. Patients with a distended

iliopsoas bursa may have a palpable inguinal mass, local or referred pain, paresthesias, neuropathy, urinary frequency, or lower extremity edema. Decompression of the bursa may dramatically alleviate symptoms, even in the presence of AVN.

MRI can depict areas of cartilage thinning in association with AVN as well as degenerative changes such as osteophytes, marrow changes associated with bony sclerosis, and subchondral cyst formation in secondary osteoarthritis[5,24] (Fig. 19-24).

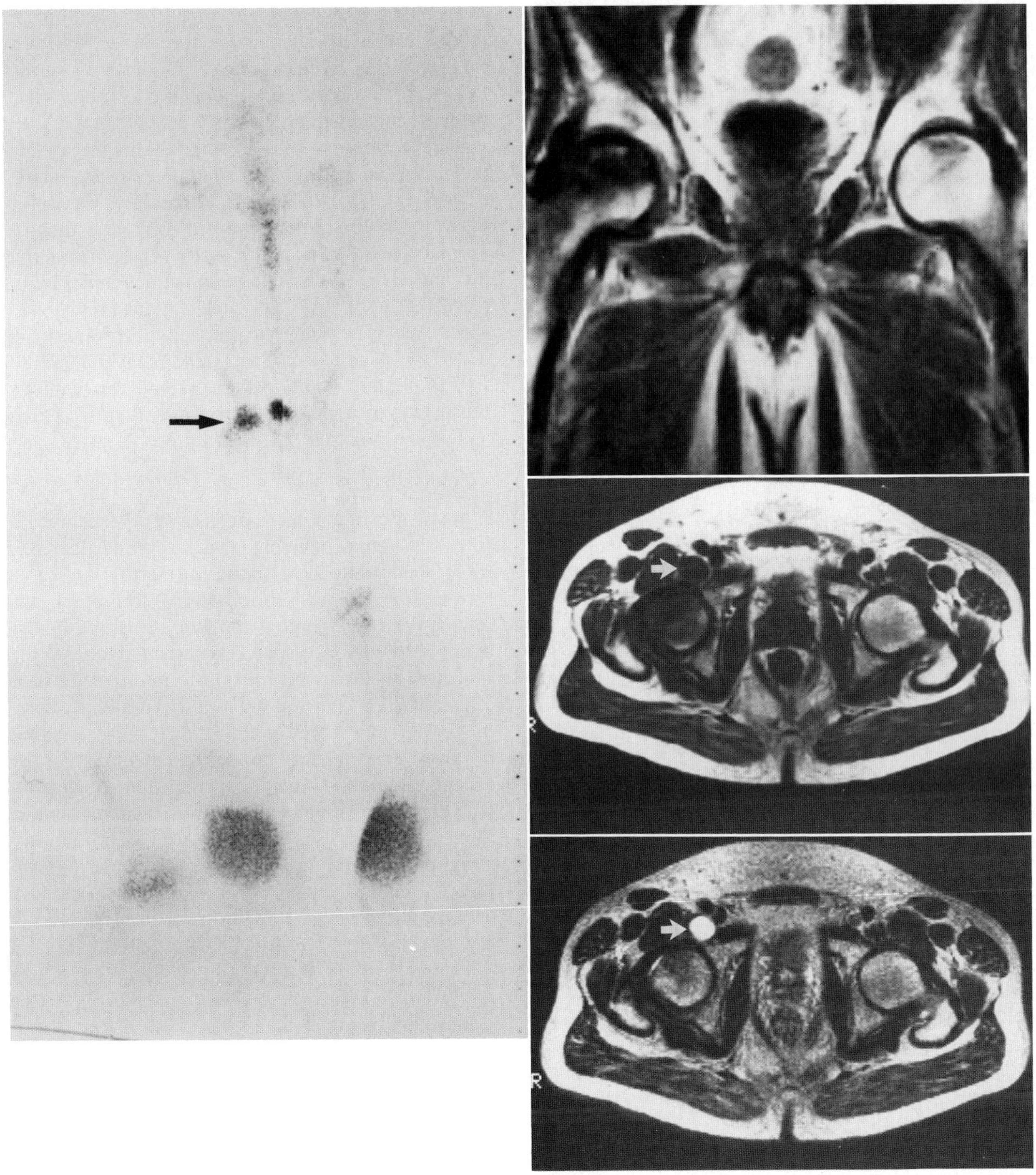

FIGURE 19-23
A 52-year-old man receiving steroids for SLE complained of right hip pain. **A,** A technetium-99m pyrophosphate bone scintigram shows increased uptake in the right hip *(arrow)* and a normal left hip. **B,** A coronal T1-WI shows obvious AVN on the right and subtle characteristic AVN changes on the left. Core biopsies confirmed bilateral AVN. **C,** Axial T1-WI. **D,** Axial T2-WI shows fluid *(arrowheads)* in the right iliopsoas bursa. Iliopsoas bursitis may accompany AVN and cause a variety of symptoms.

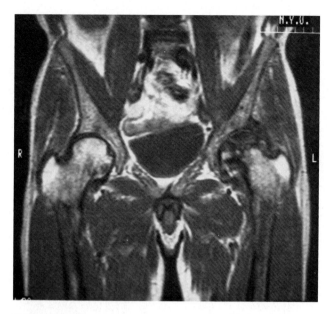

FIGURE 19-24
AVN of the left hip with severe secondary osteoarthritis. Coronal T1-WI.

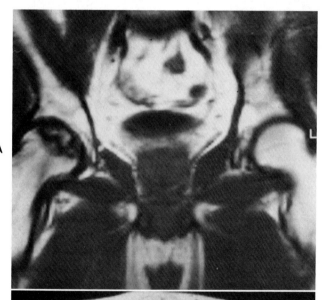

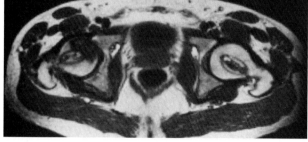

FIGURE 19-25
A 41-year-old male with an 8-month history of right hip pain. Roentgenograms and bone scan were negative. **A,** The T1-WI shows AVN on the right. The left side appeared normal. **B,** Another T1-WI following bilateral core biopsies that revealed bilateral AVN. The tracks from the large-bore needles are visible.

Other tests for avascular necrosis
NUCLEAR SCINTIGRAPHY

Technetium-99m pyrophosphate bone scintigraphy is more sensitive than conventional roentgenography or CT for detection of AVN, particularly for the early stage of the disease.[20,21] Although bone scintigraphy may detect AVN before roentgenographic and CT changes occur, the bone may appear normal in early stages of the disease, during the transition between the initial perfusion insult and subsequent hyperemic repair. Because the disease is often bilateral and interpretation is difficult in the absence of a normal contralateral hip, there is also a significant incidence of false-negative examinations (up to 18%).[21,36]

MRI is reported[20-23] to have a higher sensitivity and specificity than bone scintigraphy for Stage 0 or I AVN[20-23] (Figs. 19-23 and 19-25). Although SPECT (single photon emission tomography) can improve the sensitivity of radionuclide examination, recent studies[37,38] indicate that MRI is still probably more sensitive.

INVASIVE TESTS

Invasive tests for the diagnosis of AVN include measurement of bone marrow pressure (greater than 30 mm Hg is abnormal), the response of marrow pressure to a "stress test" (5 cc intraosseous injection of saline), intraosseous venography, and core biopsy. Although the bone marrow biopsy is usually considered the definitive test, its results may be difficult to interpret in the early stages of AVN and are subject to sampling error. The biopsy not only serves as a diagnostic tool but is thought by some investigators to be therapeutic; that is, by decompressing the medullary cavity and allowing a path for revascularization it may arrest, and in some cases reverse, the progress of the disease. A core biopsy is a surgical procedure that requires general anesthesia and a recovery time of several weeks. Significant complications occasionally develop. None of these invasive procedures can be considered a routine diagnostic test.[8,21,39]

Role of MRI

Most investigators agree that MRI is more sensitive than roentgenography, CT, or planar scintigraphy for diagnosing AVN. Does this mean that every patient with symptoms suggestive of AVN should undergo MRI?

Plain roentgenographic findings may be sufficient for diagnosis and may obviate more expensive tests. Also, the findings are used by many orthopedists for staging to determine therapy. However, bone scintigraphy or MRI is indicated when the roentgenogram is negative or equivocal on the symptomatic side. Because MRI usually costs significantly more than bone scintigraphy, the nuclear scan may be preferred for the second study. In most cases, sufficient information is obtained from the combination of clinical history, roentgenography, and scintigraphy to treat the patient. MRI should be used if other studies are negative. Even when the other studies are positive, MR may be useful. For instance, MR can be used to measure precisely the volume of diseased tissue in the femoral head. This may have important therapeutic and prognostic implications. Beltran et al.[40] have shown that MR is superior to roentgenographic staging as a predictor of collapse following therapeutic core decompression. In a series of 34 AVN hips only those with greater than 25% involvement of the weight-bearing portion of the femoral head on MR collapsed shortly after core decompression; 29 with more than 50% involvement collapsed. Decreasing volume of involved tissue after core decompression seems to correspond to clinical improvement.[5]

It should be noted that AVN of the hip may be a difficult clinical diagnosis, and the signs and symptoms can be mimicked by other problems. MR is able to provide valuable information as to other conditions that may cause hip pain and not be apparent on roentgenography or nuclear scintigraphy.

If roentgenographic findings are positive for AVN on the symptomatic side, then MRI rather than scintigraphy should be used in evaluating the asymptomatic side, which is at high risk for the development of AVN. If not prohibited by cost, MR may also be helpful in screening certain patients who are at high risk for AVN, such as those with steroid-treated systemic lupus or renal transplants.

OTHER CONDITIONS OF THE HIP
Osteoarthritis

Because osteoarthritis is so common, it is frequently encountered on MR studies for the evaluation of hip pain. The findings must be distinguished from other causes of hip complaints. With mild osteoarthritis the roentgenograms may be normal or uncertain. The MR findings are characterized by focal or generalized thinning and irregular nonhomogeneous signal in the articular cartilage. In more advanced osteoarthritis there is progressive loss of MR signal from the articular cartilage and decreased signal of the marrow as the normal fatty marrow is replaced by sclerotic bone. Both MR and roentgenograms demonstrate marginal osteophytes and synovium-filled degenerative cysts.[5,24]

Since roentgenograms adequately demonstrate the progressive sclerosis and destruction of subchondral bone in late osteoarthritis, CT and MR are not required for diagnosis of advanced stages of the disease. CT examination of the hip in patients with marked deformity secondary to arthritis may be helpful in assessment of the extent of deformity of the acetabulum and femoral head as well as preoperative surgical planning, selection of the reconstruction procedure and selection of the proper acetabulum and femoral prosthesis. However, since damage to articular cartilage can only be inferred on roentgenograms and CT, and since MR can directly image articular cartilage, MR may find a role in evaluation of early osteoarthritis. One study[41] reported that the presence of nonhomogeneity and discontinuity of high signal in articular cartilage, along with blurring of the trabecular pattern and loss of signal in the femoral head and neck, had a better correlation than roentgenographic changes with clinical symptoms in early osteoarthritis.

Rheumatoid arthritis

The MRI findings associated with synovial arthritis in the hip include cartilage thinning, joint space narrowing, joint effusion, synovial hypertrophy, and bone erosion.[42,43] Although damage to articular cartilage can only be inferred on CT, secondary changes joint space narrowing, osseous deformity, and subchondral cysts) can be appreciated (Fig. 19-26).

Trauma

Traumatic serosanguineous cysts are produced secondary to trauma and cause shearing of interfaces, usually deep to the deep fascia. This potential space then fills with serosanguineous fluid. CT and MR are useful for diagnosing traumatic serosanguineous cysts and depicting the extent of involvement (Fig. 19-27).

In the case of a femoral neck fracture the additional resolution of MR makes determination of the correct diagnosis easier than with nuclear scintigraphy. Also, since MR may show traumatic fractures earlier than scintigraphy, it should be used (if roentgenograms are negative) in the first 48 hours following trauma, when scintigraphy is usually normal. MR is particularly useful for the diagnosis of nondisplaced hip fractures, which may be difficult to recognize on roentgenograms. On T1-WIs the fracture appears as an oblique or serpiginous low-signal line surrounded by edema (which has slightly higher signal though still much lower than that of normal marrow (Fig. 19-28). On T2-WIs the fracture line retains its low signal while the surrounding edema becomes hyperintense compared to nearby normal marrow. MR is particularly useful in elderly patients because bone scans lack specificity; areas of synovitis, arthritis, and degenerative change can mimic fracture.[44]

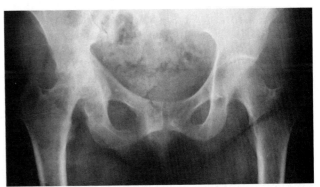

A

FIGURE 19-26
Chronic inflammatory arthritis. **A,** A frontal roentgenogram shows extensive deformity of the femoral head and acetabulum on the right side. The hip joint is markedly narrowed, and there are multiple cystic areas. *Continued.*

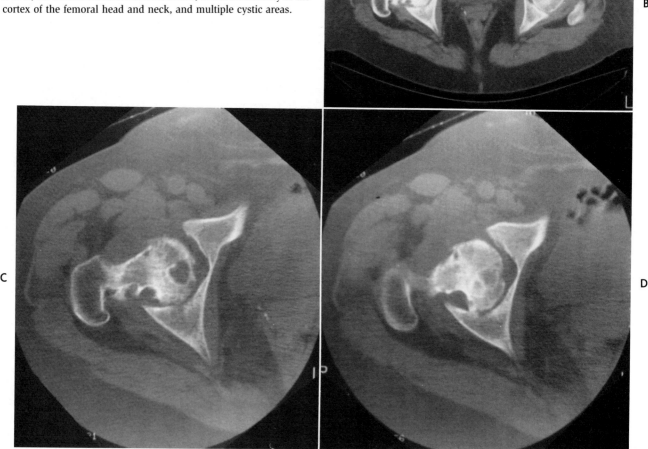

FIGURE 19-26, cont'd
B to D, CT reveals extensive osteosclerosis, marked deformity of the cortex of the femoral head and neck, and multiple cystic areas.

Stress fractures about the hip present a more difficult problem. There may be extensive marrow edema (Fig. 19-29) but no visible fracture line on MR. With no history of trauma, differentiation from a neoplastic process may be difficult. In these instances thin section high-resolution CT may display subtle cortical discontinuities not visible with MR. CT is also extremely useful in evaluating the three-dimensional nature of acetabular fractures because it provides information concerning the configuration of the fracture, the integrity of the acetabular dome, and the presence of loose bodies, factors critical for successful internal reduction and stabilization procedures.[45,46]

Fibrous dysplasia

Fibrous dysplasia is a common benign skeletal disorder that may be encountered in the proximal femur or acetabular region. Since its diagnosis is usually suggested from the roentgenographic appearance, MR plays only a limited role in its imaging work-up; but because MR is frequently used for evaluating pelvic soft tissues, this relatively common lesion may be visualized and its MR findings should be recognized.

As in other regions of the body, the fibrous dysplastic lesion causes an expanded bony contour. Sometimes it may behave as "classic" fibrous tissue and demonstrate decreased signal on both T1- and T2-WIs. Often, however, fibrous dysplasia will demonstrate marked increased signal on T2-WIs. The varying appearance of fibrous dysplasia on T2-WIs is probably related to differences in cellularity, fibrous content, cyst formation, and vascularity[47] (Fig. 19-30).

Herniation pits of the femoral neck

Herniation pits of the femoral neck are common incidental findings on roentgenograms that are sequelae of anterior hip capsule pressure on the proximal femoral neck. They represent small cortical defects with sclerotic

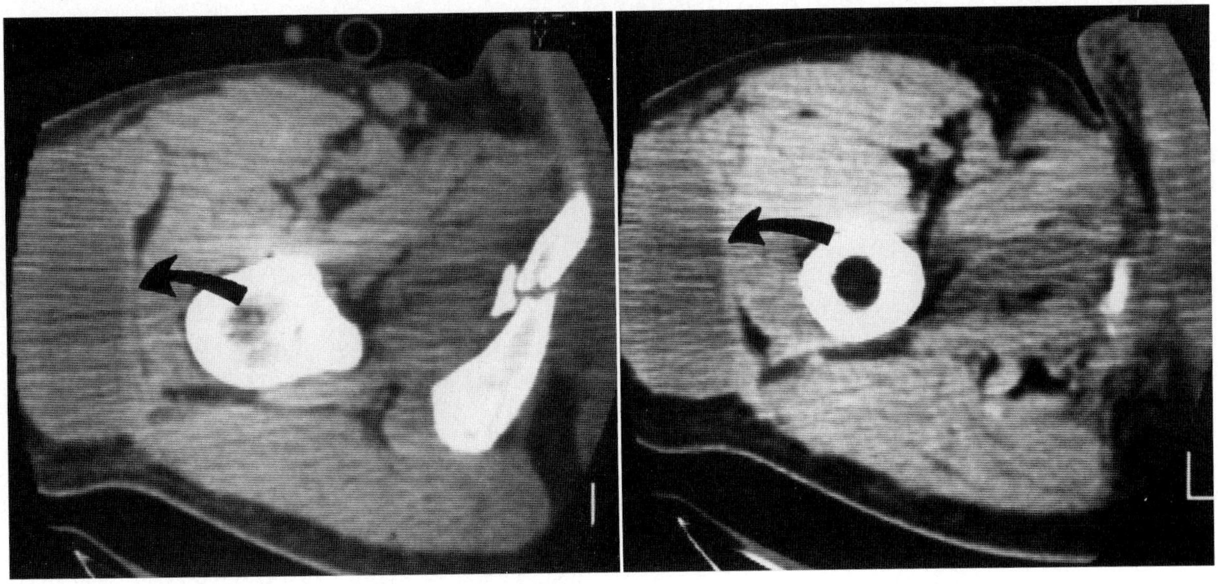

FIGURE 19-27
CT of a traumatic serosanguineous cyst presenting as painless swelling 24 hours after traumatic fracture of the pelvis. The cyst started at the level of the hip joint and extended to the middle of the thigh. There were bilateral ischiopubic fractures.

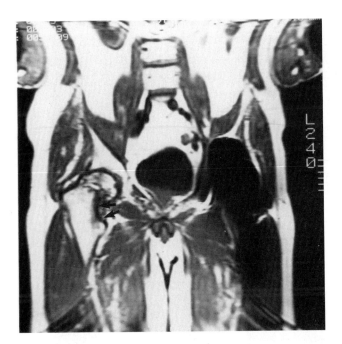

FIGURE 19-28
A 46-year-old man receiving steroids complained of pain in the right hip. He had had prior surgery on the left hip for AVN. MR showed a subcapital fracture. The T1-WI shows a broad-based low-intensity area along the medial femoral cortex *(arrowheads)*, a varus deformity, and a fracture line. There was no evidence of AVN.

borders and are filled with fibrous tissue and/or fluid. Usually they are ovoid or lobular and less than 1 cm in size. Although they are not a cause of hip pain, their characteristic MR appearance should be recognized because they are so prevalent in the adult population.

Typically herniation pits are located in the anterosuperior lateral quadrant of the femoral neck. They usually have a dark peripheral rim on T1- and T2-WIs that, presumably, corresponds to the sclerotic rim seen on roentgenograms. If they are filled with fibrous tissue, they will appear dark on T1- and T2-WIs. Of course, fluid in the pit appears dark on T1-WIs and bright on T2-WIs (Fig. 19-31). Differential considerations include osteoid osteoma, Brodie abscess, intraosseous ganglion, avascular necrosis, and metastasis. Definitive diagnosis on the basis of MR alone may be difficult, and correlation with conventional roentgenograms and clinical presentation may be helpful.[48]

Prostheses

Although patients with metallic hip prostheses may be safely studied with MR, local image distortion from the metal usually precludes the use diagnosis of prosthesis loosening or infection. Evaluation of surrounding soft tissues and the distal part of a femoral stem prosthesis is sometimes possible, depending upon the type of prosthesis as well as the pulse sequences, imaging planes, and MR magnetic field strength employed.[49]

Paget's disease and miscellaneous conditions of bone

Numerous conditions may involve the hip and are described in other chapters. Figs. 19-32 to 19-38 illustrate some of these.

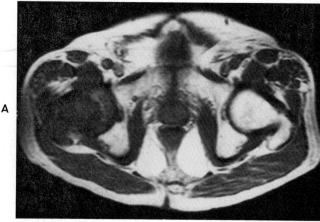

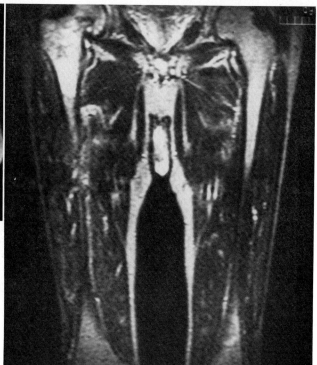

FIGURE 19-29
An 82-year-old man with lymphoma complained of right hip pain.
MR revealed a stress fracture. **A,** The T1-WI shows diffuse decreased
signal in right proximal femur. **B,** On the T2-WI there is diffusely
increased signal.

FIGURE 19-30
A 51-year-old man with right hip pain. Roentgenograms showed the
characteristic "ground glass" appearance of fibrous dysplasia. MR
was performed at 0.35 T. **A,** A coronal T1-WI clearly shows low
signal intensity involving the right femoral neck and shaft. **B,** A
coronal STIR (TR 1500/TI 100/TE 30) image reveals an area of
marked hyperintensity in comparison to the suppressed signal of
normal fatty bone marrow. **C,** Axial T1-WI. **D,** Axial T2-WI (TR
2000/TE 120).

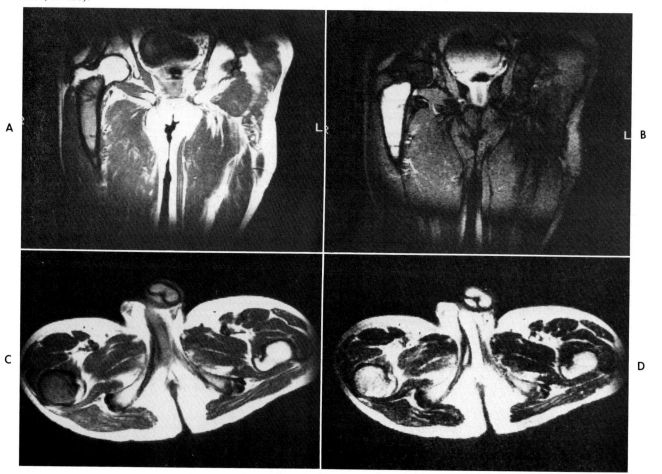

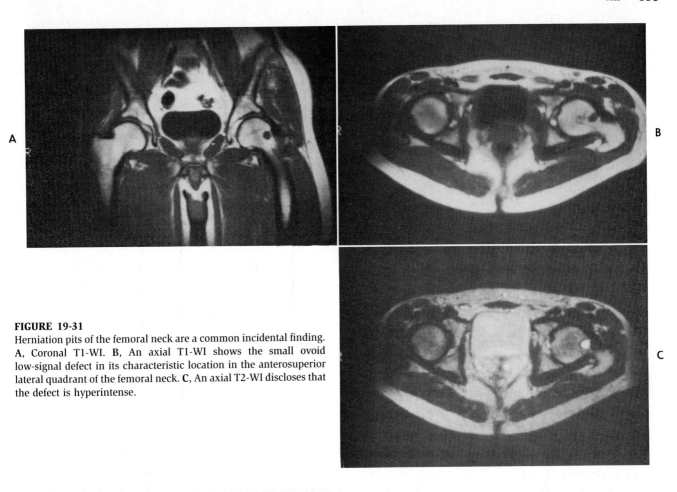

FIGURE 19-31

Herniation pits of the femoral neck are a common incidental finding. **A,** Coronal T1-WI. **B,** An axial T1-WI shows the small ovoid low-signal defect in its characteristic location in the anterosuperior lateral quadrant of the femoral neck. **C,** An axial T2-WI discloses that the defect is hyperintense.

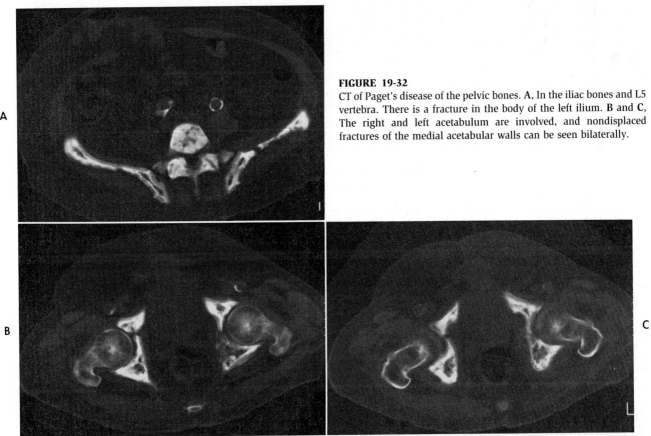

FIGURE 19-32

CT of Paget's disease of the pelvic bones. **A,** In the iliac bones and L5 vertebra. There is a fracture in the body of the left ilium. **B** and **C,** The right and left acetabulum are involved, and nondisplaced fractures of the medial acetabular walls can be seen bilaterally.

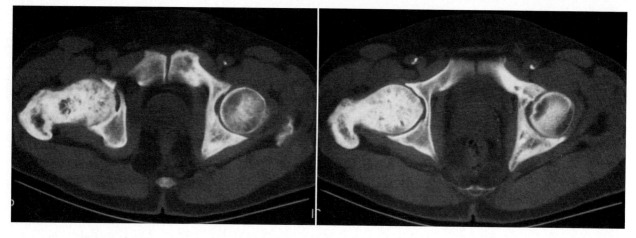

FIGURE 19-33
CT of Paget's disease. Extensive involvement of the right femoral head and left acetabulum.

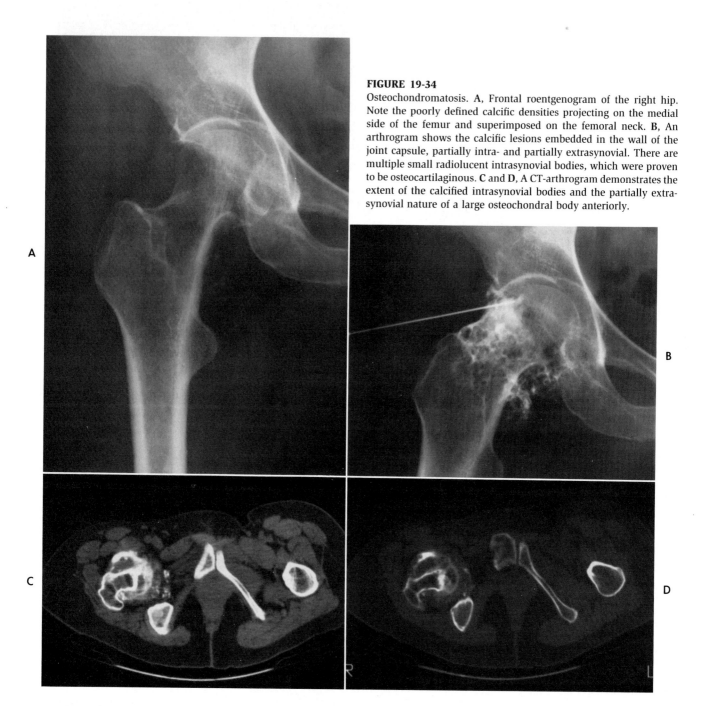

FIGURE 19-34
Osteochondromatosis. **A**, Frontal roentgenogram of the right hip. Note the poorly defined calcific densities projecting on the medial side of the femur and superimposed on the femoral neck. **B**, An arthrogram shows the calcific lesions embedded in the wall of the joint capsule, partially intra- and partially extrasynovial. There are multiple small radiolucent intrasynovial bodies, which were proven to be osteocartilaginous. **C** and **D**, A CT-arthrogram demonstrates the extent of the calcified intrasynovial bodies and the partially extrasynovial nature of a large osteochondral body anteriorly.

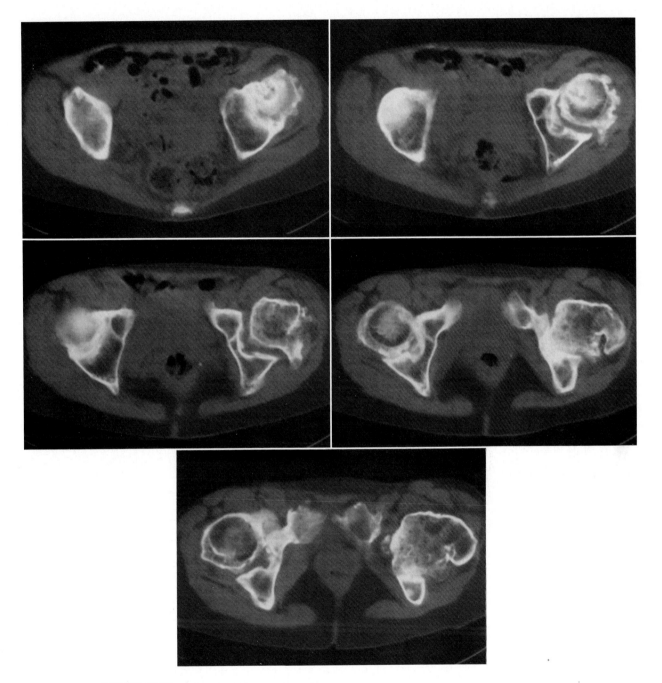

FIGURE 19-35
Multiple hereditary exostoses. Marked deformity of the femoral head, with osteocartilaginous exostoses
bilaterally. There is also osteosclerosis with deformity of the articular surface of the acetabulum in
response to the markedly deformed femoral heads.

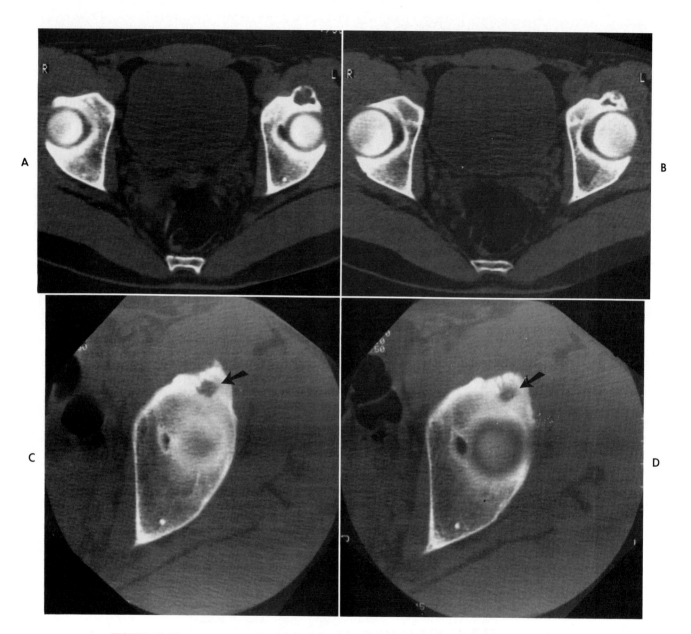

FIGURE 19-36
CT of an osteoid osteoma of the anterior acetabular wall. **A** and **B,** There is an expansile lytic lesion affecting the superoanterior wall of the left acetabulum. Soft tissue edema is directly anterior to the acetabulum. **C** and **D,** The patient returned 1 year after surgery with recurrence of pain. There was sclerosis of the anterior wall of the left acetabulum. Note the distinct area of radiolucency *(arrow)* containing a nidus of calcification. Reexploration confirmed recurrence or reactivation of the osteoma.

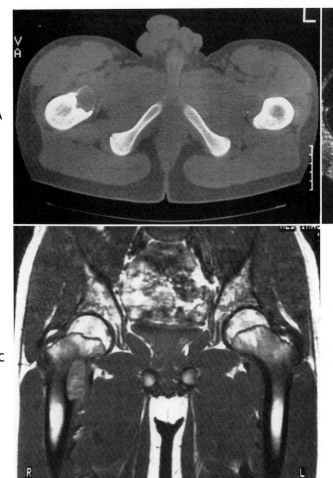

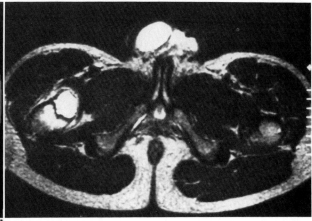

FIGURE 19-37
A 16-year-old man with chondroblastoma in the proximal femur. **A,** CT showing an eccentric expansile osteolytic lesion with a thin sclerotic rim. **B,** Axial T2-WI. The lesion has high signal with a dark rim. Note the increased signal in the adjacent bone, which appears normal on CT. This may represent edema. **C,** Coronal T1-WI. The lesion has nonhomogeneous intermediate signal. Its craniocaudal extent can be appreciated on this image.

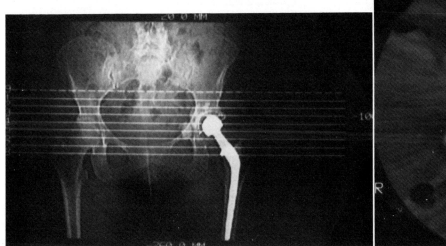

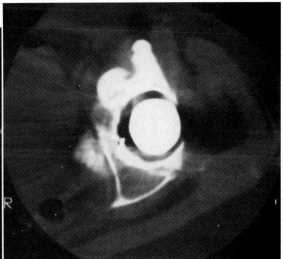

FIGURE 19-38
Femoral nerve entrapment by cement following a total hip replacement. **A,** A frontal CT scanogram shows the replacement on the left side. **B,** Note the radiopaque cement in the soft tissues anterior to the left acetabulum. The femoral nerve was found to be partially encased by cement.

REFERENCES

1. Dihlmann W: CT Analysis of the upper end of the femur: the asterisk sign ischaemic bone necrosis of the femoral head. Skeletal Radiol 1982;8:251-258.

2. Vogler JB, Murphy WA: Bone marrow imaging. Radiology 1988;168:679-693.

3. Mitchell DG, Rao VM, Dalinka M, et al: Hematopoietic and fatty bone marrow distribution in the normal and ischemic hip: new observations with 1.5-T MR imaging. Radiology 1986;161:199-202.

4. Littrup PJ, Aisen AM, Braunstein EM, Martel W: Magnetic resonance imaging of femoral head development in roentgenographically normal patients. Skeletal Radiol 1985;14:159-163.

5. Smith DK, Totty WG: Articular disorders of the hip. Top Magn Reson Imaging 1989;3:29-41.

6. Totty WG, Murphy WA, Ganz WI, et al: Magnetic resonance imaging of the normal and ischemic femoral head. AJR 1984;143:1273-1280.

7. Mitchell DG, Rao V, Dalinka M, et al: MRI of joint fluid in the normal and ischemic hip. AJR 1986;146:1215-1218.

8. Ficat RP: Idiopathic bone necrosis of the femoral head: early diagnosis and treatment. J Bone Joint Surg 1985;67B:3-9.

9. Marcus ND, Enneking WF, Massam RA: The silent hip in idiopathic aseptic necrosis: treatment by bone grafting. J Bone joint Surg [Am] 1973;55:1351-1366.

10. Hungerford DS, Zizic TM: The treatment of ischemic necrosis of bone in systemic lupus erythematosis. Medicine 1980;59:143.

11. Glimcher MJ, Kenzora JE: The biology of osteonecrosis of the human femoral head and its clinical implications. I to III. Clin Orthop 1979;138:284-309; 139:283-312; 140:273-312.

12. Sweet DE, Madwell JE: Pathogenesis of osteonecrosis. In Resnick DK, Niwayama G (eds): Diagnosis of bone and joint disorders. Philadelphia, Saunders, 1981, pp 2780-2831.

13. Lang P, Jergesen HE, Moseley ME, et al: Avascular necrosis of the femoral head: high-field-strength MR imaging with histologic correlation. Radiology 1988;169:517-524.

14. Ehman RL, Berquist TH, McLeod RA: MR imaging of the musculoskeletal system: a 5-year appraisal. Radiology 1988;166:313-320.

15. Fishman EK, Magid D, Mandelbaum BR, et al: Multiplanar (MPR) imaging of the hip. Radiographics 1986;6(1):7-54.

16. Magid D, Fishman EK, Scott WW, et al: Femoral head avascular necrosis: CT assessment with multiplanar reconstruction. Radiology 1985;157:751-756.

17. Glickstein MF, Burk DL, Scheibler ML, et al: Avascular necrosis versus other diseases of the hip: sensitivity of MR imaging. Radiology 1988;169:213-215.

18. Cohen JM, Weinreb JC, Muschler G, Erdman WA: Avascular necrosis of the femoral heads: initial screening and postoperative evaluation with MR imaging. Radiology 1986;161(P):23.

19. Mitchell DG, Rao VM, Dalinka MK, et al: Femoral head avascular necrosis: correlation of MR imaging, radiographic staging, radionuclide imaging, and clinical findings. Radiology 1987;162:702-715.

20. Mitchell DG, Kundel JL, Steinberg ME, et al: Avascular necrosis of the hip: comparison of MR, CT, and scintigraphy. AJR 1986;147:67-71.

21. Beltran J, Herman LJ, Burk JM, et al: Femoral head avascular necrosis: MR imaging with clinical-pathologic and radionuclide correlation. Radiology 1988;166:215-220.

22. Coleman BG, Kressel HY, Dalinka MK, et al: Radiographically negative avascular necrosis: detection with MR imaging. Radiology 1988;168:525-528.

23. Markisz JA, Knowles RJR, Altchek DW, et al: Segmental patterns of avascular necrosis of the femoral heads: early detection with MR imaging. Radiology 1987;162:717-720.

24. Shuman WP, Castagno AA, Baron RL, Richardson ML: MR imaging of avascular necrosis of the femoral head: value of small-field-of-view sagittal surface-coil images. AJR 1988;150:1073-1078.

25. Bongartz G, Bock E, Horbach T, Requard H: Degenerative cartilage lesions of the hip-magnetic resonance evlauation. Magnetic Resonance Imaging 1989;7:179-186.

26. Matthaei D, Frahm J, Haase A, et al: Chemical-shift-selective magnetic resonance imaging of avascular necrosis of the femoral head. Lancet 1985:370-371.

27. Mitchell DG, Joseph PM, Fallon M, et al: Chemical-shift MR imaging of the femoral head: An in vitro study of normal hips and hips with avascular necrosis. AJR 1987;148:1159-1164.

28. Genez BM, Wilson MR, Houk RW, et al: Early osteonecrosis of the femoral head: detection in high-risk patients with MR imaging. Radiology 1988;168:521-524.

29. Turner DA, Templeton AC, Selzer PM, et al: Femoral capital osteonecrosis: MR findings of diffuse marrow abnormalities without focal lesions. Radiology 1989;171:135-140.

30. Wilson AJ, Murphy WA, Hardy DC, et al: Transient osteoporosis: transient bone marrow edema? Radiology 1988;167:757-760.

31. Bloem JL: Transient osteoporosis of the hip: MR imaging. Radiology 1988;167:753-755.

32. Pay NT, Singer WS, Bartal E: Hip pain in three children accompanied by transient abnormal findings on MR images. Radiology 1989;171:147-149.

33. Unger E, et al: Diagnosis of osteomyelitis by MR imaging. AJR 1988;150:605-610.

34. Lee JK, Yao L: Stress fractures: MR imaging. Radiology 1988;169:217-220.

35. Rao VM, Fishman M, Mitchell DG, et al: Painful sickle cell crises: bone marrow patterns observed with MR imaging. Radiology 1986;161:211-215.

36. Bieber E, Hungerford D, Lennox DW: Factors in the diagnosis of avascular necrosis of the femoral head. Adv Orthop Surg 1985;147:221-226.

37. Collier BD, Carrera GF, Johnson RP, et al: Detection of femoral head avascular necrosis in adults by SPECT. J Nucl Med 1985;26:979-987.

38. Chrysikopulos H, Sartoris DJ, Resnick DL, et al: Femoral head avascular necrosis: comparison of MR imaging and SPECT. Radiology 1988;69(P):32.

39. Mitchell DG: MR of the normal and ischemic hip. In Kressel HY (ed): Magnetic resonance annual, New York, Raven Press, 1988, pp 37-69.

40. Beltran J, Knight CT, Zuelzer WA, et al: Core decompression for avascular necrosis of the femoral head: correlation between long-term results and preoperative MR staging. Radiology 1990;174:533-536.

41. Li KC, Higgs J, Sisen AM, et al: MRI in osteoarthritis of the hip; gradations of severity. Magn Reson Imaging 1988;6:229-236.

42. Beltran J, Caudill JL, Herman LA, et al: Rheumatoid arthritis: MR imaging manifestations. Radiology 1987;165:153-157.

43. Yulish BS, Lieberman JM, Newman AJ, et al: Juvenile rheumatoid arthritis: assessment with MR imaging. Radiology 1987;165:149-152.

44. Deutsch AL, Mink JH, Waxman AD: Occult fractures of the proximal femur: MR imaging. Radiology 1989;170:113-116.

45. Mack LA, Harley JD, Winquist RA: CT of acetabular fractures: analysis of fracture patterns. AJR 1982;138:407-412.

46. Saks BJ: Normal acetabular anatomy for acetabular fracture assessment: CT and plain film correlation. Radiology 1986;159:139-145.

47. Utz JA, Kransdorf MJ, Jelinek JS, et al: MR appearance of fibrous dysplasia. J Comput Assist Tomogr 1989;13(5):845-851.

48. Nokes SR, Volger JB, Spritzer CE, et al: Herniation pits of the femoral neck: appearance at MR imaging. Radiology 1989;172:231-234.

49. Lemmens JA, van Horn JR, den Boer J, et al: MR imaging of 22 Charnley-Müller total hip prostheses. ROFO 1986;145(3):311-315.

20 Knee

HOSSEIN FIROOZNIA

CT OF THE KNEE

Since the introduction of MRI the need for CT examination of the knee has steadily decreased. Nevertheless, there are disorders of the knee in which CT and CT-arthrography can be applied.

Lytic or blastic lesions

CT may be used for detecting, locating, and (at times) characterizing questionable juxtaarticular bony lesions. A large number of lesions, including neoplasms and infection, present with ill-defined foci of bone lysis. CT is often helpful in detecting and mapping the extent of these and in monitoring their response to treatment. In addition to the well-known blastic metastases and Paget's disease, several other lesions can present with a rather confusing picture of arthralgia and a poorly defined osteoblastic reaction of the intraarticular and juxtaarticular bone. These include osteoid osteoma, cortical abscess, eosinophilic granuloma, and rare instances of intracortical metastases.

Osteoid osteoma, when located in the intraarticular portion of the femur or tibia, may masquerade as an inflammatory arthritis, a situation that also applies to other joints.[1-3] Intraarticular osteoid osteoma often does not present with the usually well-recognized radiographic manifestations seen in metaphysiodiaphyseal lesions. The nidus may not be identifiable when located in a plane inaccessible to conventional roentgenography (e.g., the tibial plateau or the curvilinear and overlapping surfaces of the intercondylar notch). Thickening of the cortex due to exuberant periosteal new bone formation, a characteristic feature of metaphysiodiaphyseal lesions, is far less impressive here owing to the imperatives of anatomy. CT is helpful because of its high sensitivity in resolving osteosclerotic lesions and lesions containing calcification on a cross-sectional image (Fig. 20-1). The nidus of osteoid osteoma is usually a few millimeters wide. A tiny calcified fragment may be present in its center (Fig. 20-1, C).

A cortical abscess may have similar characteristics but be impossible to differentiate from osteoid osteoma. In some cases its "nidus" will be markedly irregular and the zone of osteosclerosis much larger.

Eosinophilic granuloma and rare solitary metastases to the cortex may present with similar characteristics. CT is generally quite helpful in the detection and location of these lesions but often not very helpful in their further characterization. A definitive diagnosis usually requires biopsy.

Meniscal injuries

We currently use knee arthrography only in individuals who cannot be examined by MRI. Based on an experience of several thousand knee MRI examinations, and an equal number of knee arthrograms prior to the MRI era, we believe MRI is superior to knee arthrography for evaluation of pathology in every one of the structures present in the knee; there is no justification for knee arthrography, unless MRI cannot be used.

COMPUTED TOMOGRAPHY

CT, without injection of contrast into the joint, has been used by some investigators for evaluating pathology in the menisci. However, it has been proven inefficacious for this purpose by many other investigators and is therefore not widely used.

CT-ARTHROGRAPHY

In our experience CT-arthrography utilizing a high-resolution state-of-the-art scanner and 1.5 mm thick slices has not proven of significant advantage over conventional arthrography in a large number of patients. Thus we believe that, when arthrography is the only alternative, conventional arthrography is sufficient in most clinical situations.

Patellofemoral disorders

Anatomy of the patellofemoral joint. The patellofemoral articulation has such an extensive range of motion that when the knee is in full extension the patella only barely articulates with the trochlear groove; also proper patellofemoral alignment is achieved only when the knee is flexed.

The characteristic shape of the articular facets of the patella (Figs. 20-2 and 20-3) and of the trochlea of the femur, which articulates with the patella, is primary and

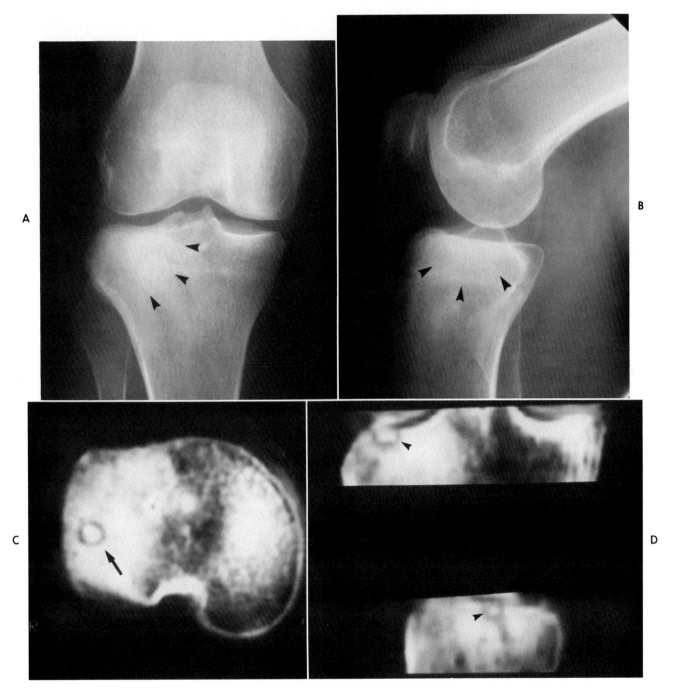

FIGURE 20-1
Osteoid osteoma. **A** and **B,** Frontal and lateral projections of the right knee reveal an area of marked osteosclerosis affecting the lateral tibial condyle extending to the level of the lateral tibial plateau *(arrowheads).* **C,** A 1.5 mm thick axial CT slice at the level of the tibial plateau shows the area of osteosclerosis surrounding a lucent nidus containing a large calcific density *(arrow).* **D,** Coronal and sagittal reformatted CT images through the osteoid osteoma show the position of the lesion just at the articular cortex of the lateral tibial plateau *(arrowhead).*

genetically determined (i.e., the facets are formed before they are ever used[4] and are not influenced by axial loading of the knee). Ficat and Hungerford[4] have stated that the only exception to this is the ridge between the medial and odd facets of the patella, which presumably develops in response to the forces and constraints applied during early life.

There are two main articular facets, a medial and a lateral (Fig. 20-3), on the posterior surface of the patella. Although significant variation exists, they have a fairly characteristic configuration on true axial views. The lateral facet is both longer and wider than the medial; and it extends further anteriorly and is situated much closer to the coronal plane than the medial facet is, which has an

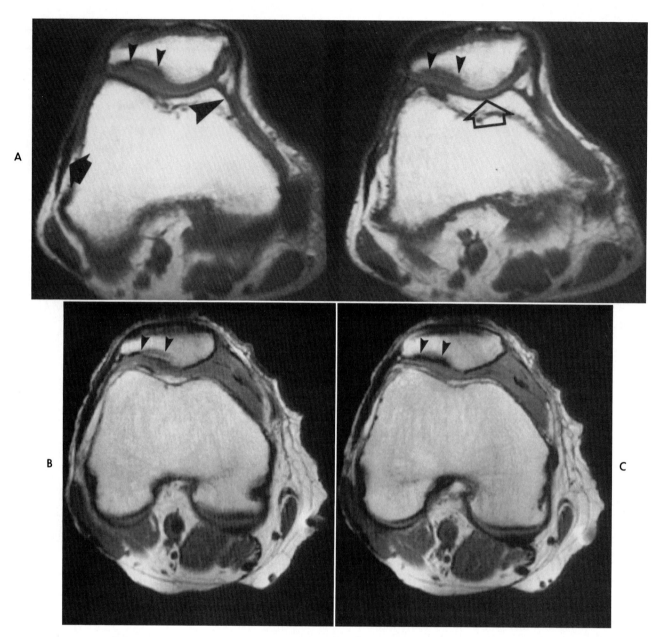

FIGURE 20-2
Normal patella. **A,** T1-WI axial view. The *hollow arrow* points to the articular cartilage of the patella. *Small arrowheads* point to the typical configuration of the lateral facet of the patella. This should not be mistaken for chondromalacia. The *large arrowhead* points to the typical bifid configuration of the medial retinaculum. The *solid arrow* points to the lateral retinaculum. **B** and **C,** T1-WI axial views in another patient. The *arrowheads* show a similar configuration in the lateral facet of a normal patella.

almost 40-degree angle to the coronal plane (Figs. 20-2 and 20-3).

As stated, a ridge separates the facets in the midportion of the patellar surface. The facets thus are roughly triangular and fit imperfectly against the trochlear surface of the femur. This median ridge runs along the longitudinal axis of the patella, and the articular facets occupy approximately 75% of the posterior surface. The lower 25% (corresponding to the posterior surface of the downward pointing apex of the triangle) is nonarticulating and has numerous orifices for a rich vascular supply, which crosses through the infrapatellar fat pad. The fat

pad itself is firmly adherent to this portion of the patella. The remaining 75% of the posterior surface of the patella (i.e., the articular facets) is covered by hyaline cartilage (Fig. 20-2). Interestingly enough, this cartilage is the thickest of any such articular covering in the body, reaching 4 to 5 mm in its central portion. It gradually becomes thinner as it approaches the margin of the patella.

The trochlear surface of the femur is immediately above the condylar articular surfaces and is separated from these by a groove that develops in adulthood. This groove corresponds to the impression of the menisci

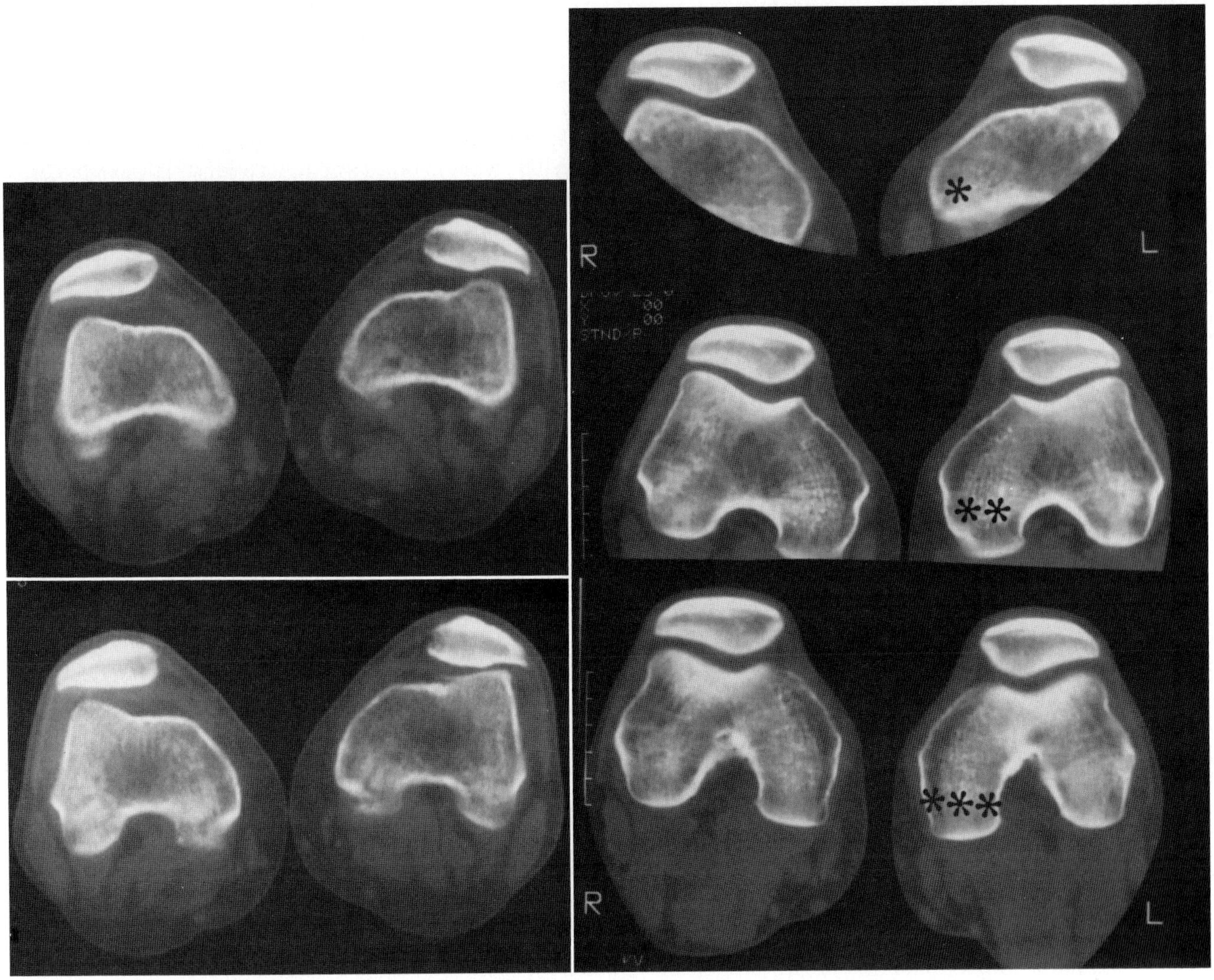

FIGURE 20-3
Normal patellofemoral joint. **A** and **B,** Axial CT images of the knee show the normally incongruent state of the patellofemoral joint in full extension. Note that the patella is deviated laterally in this position. **C,** Another patient. Axial views show the joint in full extension *(single asterisk),* 20 degrees of flexion *(double asterisks),* and 40 degrees of flexion *(triple asterisks).* Full congruity is achieved at 40 degrees in this subject.

against the femur at full extension. The trochlear surface is covered by hyaline cartilage. The medial and lateral patellar facets each form an articulation with their corresponding trochlear articular surface of the femur. The pathology of each patellofemoral compartment is frequently linked with that of the corresponding compartment of the knee joint (medial or lateral compartment). According to Ficat and Hungerford,[4] reviews of large numbers of specimens from the autopsy room suggest that pathology of the patellofemoral joint precedes that of the medial or lateral knee compartments.

Because of the extensive motion of the patella, the patellofemoral articulation (a component of the anterior aspect of the knee joint) must have a fairly wide and permissive capsule. Consequently, the capsule cannot perform its traditional stabilizing function as in other joints of the body. However, to prevent the widely moving patella from ranging too far from the functionally desirable boundaries of the joint, a number of active and passive stabilizing systems have developed.

Of the *active stabilizers,* the quadriceps tendon is the major component.

This tendon, formed from fusion of the tendons of the rectus femoris and the vasti (medialis, lateralis, and intermedius), crosses on the anterior surface of the patella, forming grooves in it, and continues as the patellar tendon.

Of the *passive stabilizers,* the patellar tendon and the medial and lateral stabilizing elements are the main components.

The patellar tendon is the continuation of the fibers of the quadriceps tendon and extends from the anterior surface and inferior pole of the patella to the tibial tubercle. It is 50 to 60 mm long, 4 to 8 mm thick, and 30 mm wide at its insertion into the apex of the patella (25 mm at its insertion into the tibial tubercle).[4] The orientation of the tendon follows roughly the long axis of the leg, though often slightly oblique laterally from proximal to distal.

The medial stabilizing elements include the medial retinaculum (Fig. 20-2, *A*) and the vastus medialis. The capsule of the knee has a tough fibrous layer that inserts into the superior two thirds of the posteromedial border of the patella. This forms the patellofemoral ligament, which extends from the patella to the medial femoral epicondyle. Another condensation of of the capsule connects the patella anteriorly and inferiorly to the anterior horn of the medial meniscus (patellomeniscal ligament).

The lateral stabilizing elements are the lateral retinaculum (Fig. 20-2, *A*), the vastus lateralis, and the iliotibial tract. On the lateral side there is a condensation of the capsule that forms the lateral patellofemoral ligament, connecting the patella to the lateral epicondyle. Similarly, the lateral meniscopatellar ligament, which is more developed than its medial counterpart, connects the patella to the anterior horn of the lateral meniscus. There is also a band of soft tissue extending from the fascia lata to the lateral border of the patella. The lateral stabilizers of the patella are significantly stronger than their medial counterpart, which accounts for the tendency of the patella to be deviated laterally when the knee is extended and other stabilizers are lax.

Physiological motion of the patellofemoral joint. In the fully extended knee the patella only minimally contacts the trochlear articular surface (Fig. 20-3, *A* and *B*). The medial compartment of the joint is wide open, and the patella is situated in a lateral position. On axial CT views the patella appears dislocated (Fig. 20-3, *A* and *B*). This is normal and due to the stronger pull of the lateral stabilizing elements than of the medial. When the knee is gradually flexed, both the medial and the lateral facets of the patella come into proper contact with the trochlear articular surfaces and stay in this position until full flexion[5] (Fig. 20-3, *C*).

Although it is not clearly established, the general impression is that two thirds of normal knees attain the congruent state at about 40 to 50 degrees of flexion. In this state there is an almost perfect match between the articular surfaces of the patella and femur. If abnormalities of patellar tracking develop, optimal congruence is not achieved until the knee is flexed further. In patients with a hypoplastic patella, dysplastic and deformed trochlear articular surfaces, or other abnormalities, the optimal congruence may not be achieved regardless of the degree of flexion. This is an uncommon occurrence.

COMPUTED TOMOGRAPHY

Abnormalities of the patellofemoral joint are not limited to bone; deformities of the articular cartilage are at least as important as, if not more important than, bony abnormalities. The articular cartilage cannot be evaluated on CT without intraarticular contrast (although CT is suitable for demonstrating bony congruence of the patellofemoral joint). Evaluation of patellofemoral congruence by conventional roentgenography is unsatisfactory because a true axial view of the knee joint in less than 30 degrees of flexion is practically impossible to obtain with the design of x-ray tubes currently available in the United States. A large number of conventional roentgenography techniques have been described,[6-12] including one with an extension at the end of the x-ray table[8] designed to position the knee in multiple degrees of flexion, but none can deliver an axial view in full extension or in 0 to 30 degrees of flexion. The best that can be achieved is an axial view at about 35 degrees of flexion. Conventional roentgenography can provide satisfactory axial views when the knee is flexed more than 35 degrees. At the present time it is unnecessary to use conventional roentgenography and settle only for axial views with the knee flexed more than 40 degrees, because it is critical to assess the patellofemoral joint during 0 to 40 degrees of flexion, when maltracking is likely to occur. Another important consideration is the amount of radiation that may reach the patient's pelvic region and gonads when conventional roentgenography semiaxial views are obtained. This problem is eliminated by computed tomography.

Technique. The technique for patellofemoral joint evaluation by CT is as follows:

With the patient supine, the knees are placed absolutely symmetrically in the midplane of the gantry.

A lateral scout view is obtained with a large body calibration.

Three to four consecutive slices, 3 to 5 mm thick, are obtained with the equator of the patella at the center of the slices and the knee in full extension.

Then the procedure, including the lateral scout, is repeated with the knee in 15, 30, 45, and 60 degrees of flexion (Fig. 20-3, *C*).

Assessment of joint alignment. The patellofemoral joint has traditionally been studied on axial, though also on AP and lateral, views utilizing conventional roentgenography.[6,13-15] However, it is virtually impossible to obtain axial views in less than 30 degrees of flexion with the x-ray tubes available in the United States. Because of the size of the tube housing, the apparatus cannot be lowered enough to obtain satisfactory views in less than 30 degrees of flexion. Evidently, in Europe, this is possible because the tubes do not have such a large housing unit.

The lack of ability to obtain axial images of the knee in full extension, prior to CT and MRI, led to the interesting (and erroneous) concepts that (1) a normal patellofemoral joint is in a congruent state at all times and (2) the patella rests in the trochlear groove with the knee in full extension. Experience with CT and MRI has shown both these statements to be incorrect. The patella does not rest in the trochlear groove, and the patellofemoral joint is not in a congruent state at full extension. At full extension the medial facet of the joint is open and the patella is displaced laterally. It is possible to obtain conventional roentgenography axial views of the patellofemoral joint with the knee in flexion of 35 degrees or more. Thus no information from 0 degrees to 35 degrees of flexion can be obtained on conventional roentgenography. However, this information may be important, particularly when dislocation or dislocatability of the patella is being investigated with the knee in extension or flexion of less than 35 degrees. It is obvious therefore that a meaningful evaluation of the patellofemoral articulation during its full arc of motion is not possible on conventional roentgenography.

As the knee is flexed, the medial and lateral retinacula begin to tighten and the patella descends and returns to the midline from its lateralized position in full extension. Also, the medial facet begins to close until the articular facets of the patella and trochlea coincide. Eventually an almost congruent state is reached, with matching of the patellar and trochlear articular facets. Exactly at what degree of flexion this normal state of congruent alignment is reached we do not know; what we do know is that the state of optimal congruence occurs in a normal knee at a lesser degree of flexion than in an abnormal knee. Almost all normal individuals have a satisfactory congruence and midline position of the patella at 90 degrees of knee flexion. (Obviously, there will be no congruence of the articular surfaces in the presence of marked deformity or dysplasia of the trochlear surface or patellar facets [Fig. 20-4].) At about 60 degrees of flexion the patella is

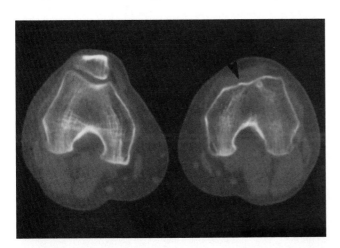

FIGURE 20-4
The *arrowhead* points to a markedly deformed trochlear articular surface of the left femur in a patient with recurrent dislocation of the patella who had had the patella surgically removed. The right patellofemoral joint is normal.

centered and there is optimal congruence in 84% of all asymptomatic individuals. At 30 degrees of flexion a centrally located patella and optimal congruence of the facets are noted in only 26% of individuals. At full extension, almost all persons show a lateral position of the patella and the patellar facets are in only partial contact with the trochlear surfaces.

The position of the patella relative to the midline axis of the knee is dependent upon the stabilizing apparatus of the patella. According to Imai et al.,[5] when the patellofemoral joint is in the incongruent state (i.e., full extension) the medial retinaculum is more lax than the lateral. In the congruent state both are equally tense. Nevertheless, in full extension or small degrees of flexion the patellofemoral joint may appear congruent; but this may be deceptive. The clue is the laxity of the medial retinaculum and patellar tendon. If the congruence is real, both retinacula will be tense. Therefore it seems that a proper evaluation of the patellofemoral joint requires stressing of the joint, which is not surprising since the necessity of stress roentgenography in other joints of the body is well understood and accepted. If clinically indicated, one may apply pressure to the medial and lateral borders of the patella and obtain axial CT views to investigate the possibility of false congruence and dislocatability of the patella in a moderately flexed knee.

One can also evaluate deformities of the subchondral surface of the patella and trochlea on CT. It must be emphasized, however, that lesions of the articular cartilage of the patella cannot be evaluated on CT without intraarticular contrast.

CT-ARTHROGRAPHY

Computed tomography of the patellofemoral joint may be obtained following injection of intraarticular contrast. The technique is similar to what has already been described for CT of this joint. CT-arthrography is helpful for evaluating the articular cartilage of the patella, although this information can also be obtained by MRI (Fig. 20-2). In our experience double-contrast arthrography is superior to single positive contrast arthrography for this purpose.

CT-arthrography is able to show various abnormalities of the patellar articular cartilage—including erosion, attenuation, and disruption. Erosion and deformity of the subchondral bone are also visualized.

Assessment of joint dynamics. The ideal method for assessing the dynamics of patellofemoral joint motion would be a technique that provided images during the act of walking. So far, this has not been possible. A modification of the supine stationary axial views of the patellofemoral joint attempts to obtain several axial views with incremental flexion using either CT or MRI[16-18]; these are then looped together and a semikinetic study is created. Although this is not actually a kinematic study, it may be helpful for a rapid demonstration of the changing relationships of the patella and trochlea, indicators of patellar maltracking, during various degrees of flexion.

Chondromalacia patellae

Chondromalacia patellae is present when there is softening of the articular cartilage of the patella (Fig. 20-5). It may be primary or secondary in origin[19] and may present idiopathically in teenagers and young adults, with chronic knee pain as its major manifestation. The condition usually subsides with no significant complication. A secondary form, also occurring in teenagers, has been described as a consequence of direct trauma to the patella or secondary to trauma of repeated episodes of patellar subluxations. This form may lead to degenerative arthritis of the patellofemoral joint (and the knee joint proper) with advancing age. Another secondary form with manifestations in adult life may begin during the teens. Asymptomatic degenerative changes of the patellofemoral articulation and the knee joint proper may develop and eventually become symptomatic in middle age or beyond (Figs. 20-6 and 20-7).[19]

In chondromalacia the articular cartilage of the patella may show a blister, presenting as a smooth hemispherical swelling of the patella. The cartilage may be significantly thicker, most likely due to edema. In later stages it shows fibrillation, fraying, fissuring, and splitting. Eventually complete disintegration of all or part of the articular cartilage is noted. There may be marked attenuation of the cartilage with almost complete loss of it in the later stages. Osteochondritis dissecans of the patella may also be present. Eventually, hypertrophic changes of the articular surface and margins of the patella are noted.[19,20]

MRI OF THE KNEE
Technical considerations

Position of the patient. The patient is placed supine, with the knee in the most comfortable position. If possible, full extension is desirable; if not, the knee should be in the least degree of flexion. If the knee is flexed more than a few degrees, the anterior cruciate ligament may not be optimally visualized. After the knee is in the surface coil, the legs are placed in supporting

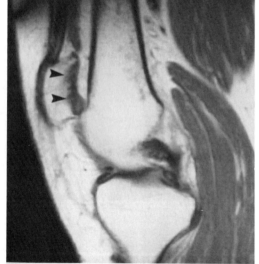

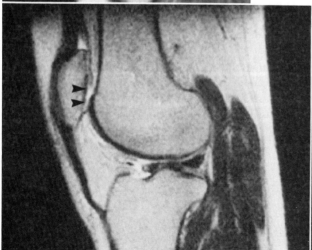

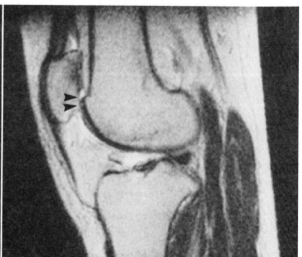

FIGURE 20-5
Chondromalacia patellae. **A,** T1-WI sagittal. Note the erosion of subchondral bone *(arrowheads).* **B** and **C,** T2-WI sagittals showing erosion of the patellar articular cartilage *(arrowheads).*

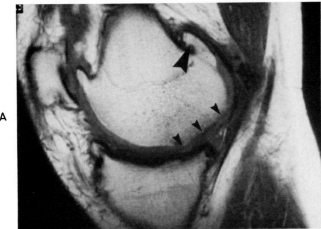

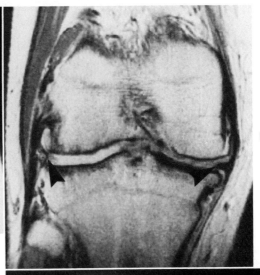

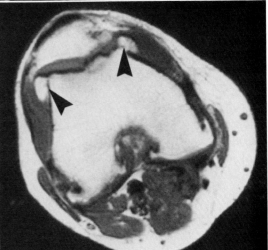

FIGURE 20-6
Severe primary degenerative arthritis of the knee in a 40-year-old man. **A**, T1-WI anatomical sagittal view. The *large arrowhead* points to an osteophyte. The *small arrowheads* mark irregularities in the subchondral cortex of the medial femoral condyle. There is also attenuation of the femoral articular cartilage. The posterior and anterior horns of the medial meniscus are missing. **B**, SD coronal view. The *arrowhead* points to a capsular remnant of the lateral and medial menisci. Almost all of the lateral meniscus has been eroded and torn. On the medial side only a small segment of capsular margin of the medial meniscal body remains. The rest has been eroded and torn. The joint is markedly narrowed. On the lateral side there is nearly complete destruction of the articular cartilages of the femur and tibia. The ACL is torn. **C**, T1-WI axial view. Note the severe degenerative patellofemoral arthritis, with large hypertrophic osteophytes *(arrowheads)* arising from the margins of the trochlear articular surface of the femur.

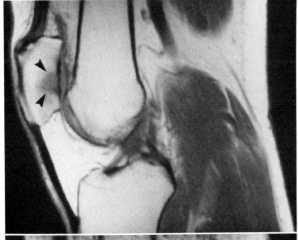

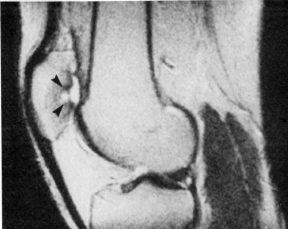

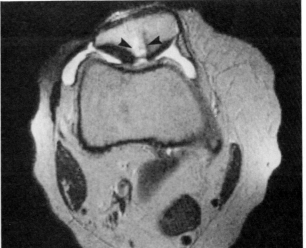

FIGURE 20-7
Degenerative disease. **A**, A sagittal T1-WI and, **B** and **C**, sagittal and axial T2-WI images. There is severe degenerative disease affecting the articular cartilage of the patella. Note the erosion of patellar subchondral bone. The *arrowheads* in all these views point to the erosion, which is filled with fluid (exhibiting high SI on T2-WI).

molded foam rubber to assure comfort and immobilization.

Surface coil. There is unanimous agreement that a dedicated surface coil is necessary for optimal imaging of the knee. We have used a flexible wrap-around coil as well as a rigid cylindrical one. The former, a receive-only antenna, is designed to cover the entire circumference of the knee and provide uniform signal intensity throughout the examined volume. The latter, a transmit-receive device, has all the attributes of the flexible surface coil, with the additional benefits of a longer life, higher signal-to-noise, and lower incidence of artifacts. Other surface coils (e.g., loop-gap resonators) are also satisfactory. A flat surface coil, similar to the spine coil, usually placed beneath the knee, is not sufficient for an optimal examination because there is a significant dropoff of signal intensity in the more anterior portions of the knee, which interferes with proper visualization of the anterior knee structures.

The success of the MRI examination is dependent, to a significant degree, upon the ability of the patient to stay motionless during the procedure. Thus, it is essential to design an examination that can be completed in a reasonably short time (25 minutes or less) and make every effort to allay patient anxiety. Accumulated experience with a large number of patients indicates that a thorough explanation of the MRI procedure and reassurance are very helpful. Some patients do remarkably well if they are taught relaxation exercises a few days prior to the examination. If necessary a mild short-acting sedative may be given prior to the procedure.

Imaging protocols

MRI of the knee is performed for a variety of disorders. The most common by far is internal derangement, which includes disorders of the menisci, articular cartilages, cruciate ligaments, collateral ligaments, and capsule. Disorders of the patellofemoral joint are next. Other indications for MRI of the knee are to investigate suspected bone and soft tissue neoplasms, infection, popliteal artery aneurysm, and deep venous thrombosis (DVT).

INTERNAL DERANGEMENT
1. Scout: Axial T1-weighted images (T1-WI)
2. Anatomical sagittals, T1-WI and T2-WI, 4 to 5 mm thick
3. Oblique sagittals, T2-WI, 4 mm thick, angled 12 to 15 degrees to the anatomical midsagittal plane
4. Coronals, spin density (SD) and T2-WI, 3 mm thick, at a 90-degree angle to the T1-weighted sagittals (anatomical sagittals)

Additional sequences and alternatives are
1. Sagittal and coronal gradient echo images
2. Axial T1-WI and T2-WI
3. Radial images

Scout. With an FOV of 20 × 20 cm and a reduced matrix, the scout axial T1-weighted images are obtained in about 1 minute. To derive coordinates for the sagittal and coronal views, an axial slice that shows the middle or lower portion of the femoral condyles is selected.

The most comfortable position for the patient is usually with the knee in minimal flexion and 10 to 15 degrees of external rotation (i.e., the axial scouts show external rotation). We program the sagittal T1-WI and T2-WI and the coronal SD and T2-WI parallel to the true anatomical sagittal and coronal planes of the knee. Thus, the anatomical sagittals are parallel to the true midline sagittal plane and the coronals are at 90 degrees to them. We obtain true anatomical sagittals for evaluation of the menisci, because there is no distortion of the critically important posterior horns on these images. Anatomical sagittals are also better suited for imaging the posterior cruciate ligament (PCL). Oblique sagittal views are useful for evaluating the anterior cruciate ligament (ACL). They also may be programmed on the axial scouts, or the coronal images. The desired oblique sagittal plane on the axial scout is at about 15 degrees to the anatomical midsagittal plane, extending anteriorly to posteriorly and medially to laterally, and should result in a radially oblique view that corrects for the medial-to-lateral and anterior-to-posterior tilt of the ACL. The prescription for the desired oblique sagittal on coronal images has a coronal view showing the midportion of the menisci with the oblique sagittal plane parallel to the anatomical course of the ACL: cephalad to caudad, lateral to medial, about 15 degrees to the anatomical sagittal plane.

The body of the ACL is seen satisfactorily on either oblique technique. The tibial insertion of the ACL is visualized equally well on the anatomical or oblique sagittals. The attachment to the femur is displayed optimally on both the axial and the oblique sagittal views.

The PCL is better delineated on anatomical sagittals than on oblique sagittals. In almost all patients the combination of anatomical sagittals and coronals is sufficient for its evaluation. Occasionally, however, it may become necessary to obtain T2-WI axial views for evaluation of the femoral insertion of the PCL. The body of the ligament and the attachment of the PCL to the tibia are well seen on anatomical sagittals and coronals. The attachment of the ligament to the medial femoral condyle is often well visualized on the axials and anatomical coronals.

Technical parameters. In most patients we utilize the following technical parameters: An FOV of 16 × 16 cm is optimal for the average adult. This permits visualization of the distal portion of the quadriceps tendon as well as the proximal metaphysis of the tibia. In children an FOV of 12 × 12 cm is sufficient. The acquisition matrix is 256 × 256. We obtain 4 to 5 mm thick anatomical sagittal and oblique sagittal cross sections. Thinner slices may be obtained, although we have not found them advantageous in our everyday practice. For coronal cross sections we prefer 3 mm thick slices and SD to T1-WI (Fig. 20-8) because the menisci are significantly better delineated on SD than on T1-WI coronals. On SD the articular cartilage is of intermediate signal intensity (SI) (Fig. 20-8, *A, B,* and *E* to *H*). This is helpful in delineating the superior and inferior articular surfaces of the menisci on the coronal views. The T1-WI coronal views (Fig. 20-9), on the other hand, do not usually provide a satisfactory SI difference between the articular cartilage and the menisci on routine window settings, consequently, the superior and inferior articular surfaces of the menisci are not well delineated. On the sagittal cross sections, the hemispherical configuration of the femoral condyles, and probably other factors, permit a satisfactory delineation of the menisci on T1-WI (Fig. 20-10). Thus, strictly for this purpose, it is not

necessary to obtain SD sagittal views.

The sagittal views are helpful for assessing the anterior and posterior horns of the menisci, the cruciate ligaments, articular cartilage of the femoral condyles, the subarticular cortex of the femur and tibia, and the bone marrow. The soft tissues of the popliteal fossa are also better visualized on these views.

The coronal views are essential for evaluating the capsule, tibial collateral ligament, body of the menisci, femoral articular cartilages, subchondral cortex of the tibia and femur, and bone marrow. They are also helpful in assessing the cruciate ligaments. An assessment of abnormalities in the capsule and tibial collateral ligament, capsulomeniscal junction, and cruciate ligaments usually requires a T2-WI sequence.

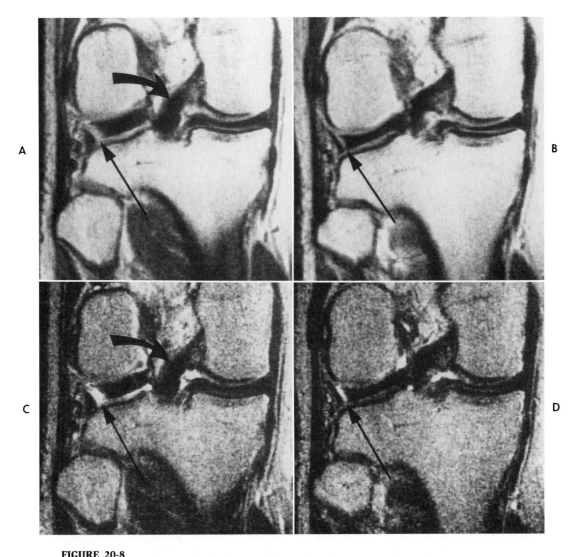

FIGURE 20-8
Anatomy of the normal menisci. **A** and **B**, Spin density and, **C** and **D**, T2-weighted coronal views of the posterior horns of the menisci. The *straight arrow* points to the zone of increased signal due to synovial tissue and is minimal fluid within the synovial bursa surrounding the popliteus tendon as it obliquely crosses the posterolateral aspect of the posterior horn of the lateral meniscus. The *curved arrow* points to the posterior cruciate ligament.
Continued.

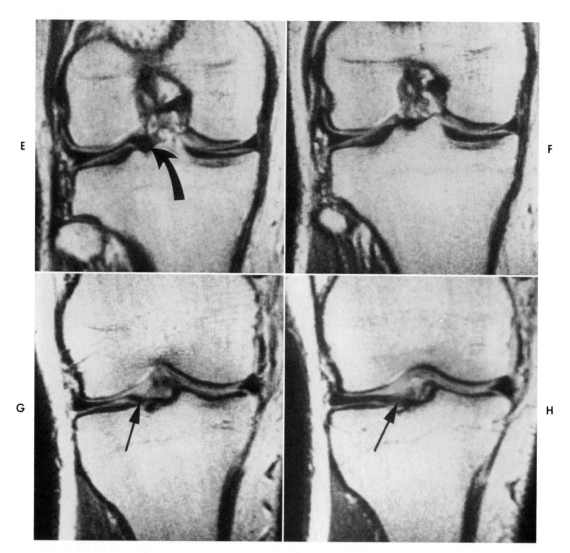

FIGURE 20-8, cont'd
E to H, Coronal spin density views showing the body and anterior horn of the menisci. The *curved arrow* in E points to the central attachment of the posterior horn of the lateral meniscus. The midportions of the bodies of the menisci are well seen in **F**. **G**, Slice 20 mm anterior to E. The anterior horn of the lateral meniscus is visible. The *arrow* points to the central attachment of the anterior horn. **H**, Anterior horns of both menisci. The *arrow* points to the central attachment of the anterior horn of the lateral meniscus. Slice **G** is close to the free margin of the anterior horn. Thus the anterior horn appears thin. Slice **H**, 4 mm anterior to **G**, is closer to the capsular margin of the anterior horn. The anterior horn is thicker in this region.

The gradient echo (T2*) sequence may be obtained as a substitute for T2-WI. However, it should be noted that it may exaggerate the signal abnormalities of the menisci, particularly at the capsulomeniscal junction (Fig. 20-10, B and D), and lead to false-positive diagnoses of a meniscal separation or peripheral tear. It may also exaggerate the signal abnormalities of the cruciate ligaments, quadriceps tendon, and patellar tendon. Thus, if this is the sole imaging sequence available, a definitive diagnosis of abnormalities of the capsule and ligaments should be made with caution.

Axial views are helpful for evaluating the patellofemo-ral articulation, femoral attachments of the cruciates, intraarticular bodies, and subtle instances of bone trauma and for locating tumors and cysts.

Radial images may become necessary for revealing pathology at the junction of the anterior and posterior horns with the bodies of the menisci, because this segment of the menisci may not be optimally imaged on either sagittal or coronal views. The anatomical sagittals are most useful where the plane of the image is at right angles to the capsular margin of the meniscus (i.e., the anterior and posterior horns). The coronals are best suited for visualization of the bodies of the menisci. The

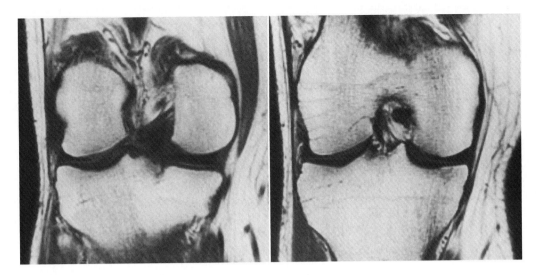

FIGURE 20-9
Coronal T1 weighted images of the knee. With routine window settings the menisci are not clearly differentiated from the adjacent articular cartilage on these images.

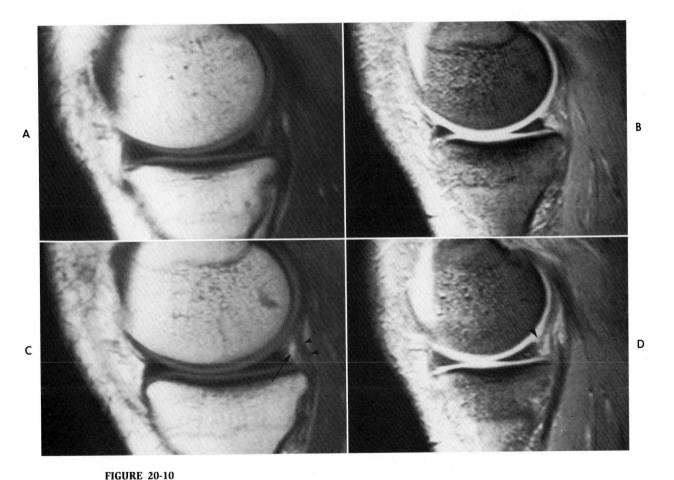

FIGURE 20-10
Normal medial meniscus. **A** and **C**, Sagittal T1-WI and, **B** and **D**, sagittal T2*. (**A** and **D** show approximately the same region of the medial meniscus.) There is a minimal amount of increased SI in the posterior horn, better seen in the T2*. Note also that the peripheral margin of the meniscus (*arrowhead* in **D**) has significantly higher SI in T2* than in T1-WI. In **C** the *arrow* points to fat, which may normally be present between the posterior horn of medial meniscus and the capsule at the apex of the posterior horn. The *two small arrowheads* designate the capsule, which is bowed toward the middle of the knee. Note the configuration of the capsulomeniscal junction and the capsule in **B**.

radial images have the advantage of being perpendicular to the capsular margin along the entire circumference of the meniscus. At present they are practical only with a gradient echo pulse sequence. They are not, however, necessary in the great majority of the patients. Although it is desirable to have an MR imager with radial capability, this is not essential. One can simply obtain an additional set of 45-degree views.

PATELLOFEMORAL JOINT

Our MRI protocol for internal derangement does not include an evaluation of the patellofemoral joint. We believe this joint requires a separate study consisting of 3 to 4 mm thick axial slices, utilizing T1-WI and T2-WI or T2* sequences, preferably with the knee flexed.

NEOPLASMS AND CYSTS

The protocol for detecting, locating, and if possible characterizing neoplasms, infection, DVT, popliteal fossa cysts, and cystic lesions must be individually decided on but usually includes axials in T1-WI and T2-WI sequences encompassing the area of suspected pathology and T1-WI or spin density (SD) in another appropriate plane (sagittal or coronal).

The protocol for routine MRI of the knee must be selected by each institution based on the type of patients referred to it and the experience and beliefs of its imaging and referring physicians. Many investigators do not obtain, and do quite well without, anatomic sagittals but get only oblique sagittals with the knee positioned purposefully in external rotation. Others obtain axial images in all patients and include an assessment of the patellofemoral joint as a routine component of knee MRI. Still others include axial and sagittal gradient echo images along with the sagittal and coronal spin echo views as a routine part of their knee MRI protocol. All these protocols are acceptable, as long as they contain both sagittal (anatomical and/or oblique) and coronal views, at least one T1-WI and one T2-WI, preferably two T2-WI (one in the sagittal and one in the coronal plane), with slice thicknesses of no more than 5 mm (3 to 4 mm in the coronal plane) and the least possible interslice gap.

NORMAL ANATOMY
Menisci

The menisci (semilunar cartilages) are two fibrocartilaginous crescentic lamellae situated on the peripheral portion of the tibial articular surfaces that create a concave surface to accommodate the convex femoral condyles[21,22] (Plate 20-1). Their peripheral borders (capsular margins) are convex and 4 to 7 mm thick, their free margins a millimeter or less thick. They are composed of a fairly firm, dense, and avascular fibrocartilaginous tissue, except for the peripheral zone (about 20% to 30% of the width of the posterior horn, 2 to 3 mm of the body and less of the anterior horn), which is softer, vascularized, and innervated.

Lateral meniscus. The lateral meniscus[23-25] is shaped about like a three-quarter circle (Fig. 20-11). When viewed from above, it is of almost the same width (7 to 10 mm), except for the extreme anterior and posterior horns, the regions just proximal to the site of attachment of the meniscus to bone (central attachments), which are significantly narrower. The central attachments are relatively irregular in outline. The posterior horn is attached to bone just posterior to the intercondylar eminence of the tibia and just anterior to the attachment of the posterior horn of the medial meniscus. The anterior horn is attached to the tibia in front of the intercondylar eminence. This region is some 3 to 4 mm posterior, and slightly lateral, to the site of attachment of the ACL to the tibia. The fibers attaching the anterior horn to bone may actually blend with the ACL.

The *meniscofemoral ligaments*[26-30] are inconstant 3 to 4 mm thick fibrous bands that arise from the posterior horn of the lateral meniscus (Figs. 20-11 to 20-15). The meniscofemoral ligament of Wrisberg (Figs. 20-13 and 20-14) (also referred to as the ligament of Robert) arises from the posterosuperior margin of the posterior horn (Fig. 20-15, *A* to *C*), usually just lateral and 7 to 10 mm proximal to the innermost segment of the horn (Fig. 20-16), extends superiorly and medially on the posterior surface of the PCL (Fig. 20-15, *D* and *G*), and attaches to the lateral surface of the medial femoral condyle. The ligament of Humphrey usually shares a common origin with the ligament of Wrisberg and extends superiorly, anteriorly, and medially on the anterior surface of the PCL. It often blends with the PCL,[29] although it may continue as a separate bundle of fibers just anterior to the PCL until it reaches the medial femoral condyle.[22]

The peripheral margin of the lateral meniscus is attached to the capsule, except posterolaterally, where the popliteus tendon crosses it obliquely, laterally, and upward (Fig. 20-12, *A* and *B*). The inner portion of the posterior horn, just prior to its central attachment, is not attached to the capsule. The capsule does not extend this far anteriorly into the joint. The attachment of the peripheral margin of the lateral meniscus to the capsule is less firm than that of its medial counterpart. There is a thin layer of loose connective tissue and fat between the anterior portion of the body and anterior horn of the lateral meniscus and the capsule.

The *popliteus* itself[21,22,25,31] (Figs. 20-12 and 20-17) covers the floor of the lower half of the popliteal fossa (Fig. 20-18). It is a flat and triangular muscle originating on the medial side of the posterior surface of the tibia above the soleal line. In this region it also merges into the tendinous expansion that covers it. It extends laterally and upward, in roughly a 45-degree angle. It has a lateral and a medial component. The lateral component is the popliteus tendon, which extends superiorly and laterally (Figs. 20-8, *A* and *B*, and 20-19 to 20-21) and is attached to the anterior portion of the popliteus groove on the lateral surface of the lateral femoral condyle. The tendon

Text continued on p. 680.

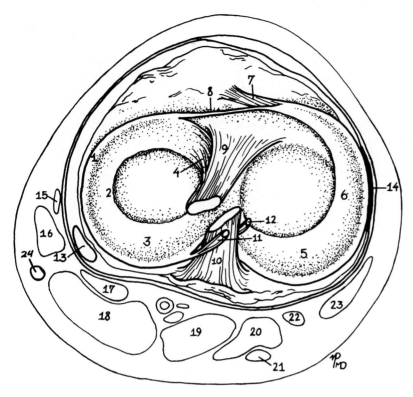

FIGURE 20-11
Normal axial anatomy of the knee joint. *1,* Capsular margin of the lateral meniscus; *2,* free margin of the body of lateral meniscus; *3,* posterior horn of lateral meniscus; *4,* central attachment of the anterior horn of lateral meniscus; *5,* posterior horn of medial meniscus; *6,* body of medial meniscus; *7,* central attachment of the anterior horn of medial meniscus; *8,* transverse ligament; *9,* ACL; *10,* PCL; *11,* ligament of Wrisberg; *12,* ligament of Humphrey; *13,* popliteus tendon; *14,* tibial collateral ligament; *15,* fibular collateral ligament; *16,* biceps; *17,* plantaris; *18,* gastrocnemius (lateral head); *19,* gastrocnemius (medial head); *20,* semimembranosus; *21,* semitendinosus; *22,* gracilis; *23,* sartorius; *24,* common peroneal nerve.

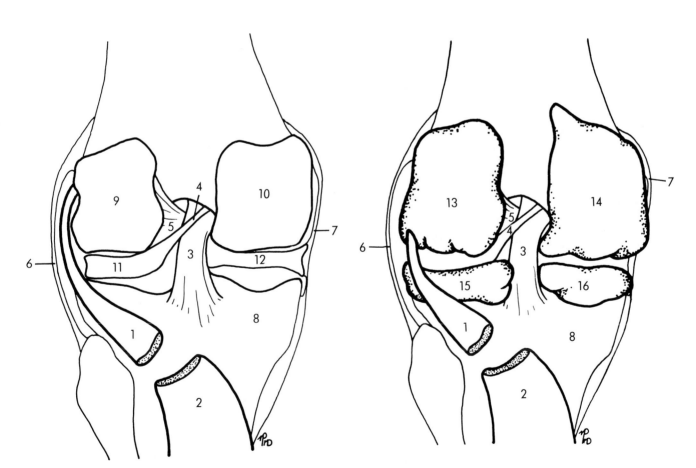

FIGURE 20-12
Normal anatomy of the knee. *1* and *2,* Popliteus muscle and tendon; *3,* PCL; *4,* ligament of Wrisberg; *5,* ACL; *6,* fibular collateral ligament; *7,* tibial collateral ligament; *8,* medial tibial condyle; *9,* lateral femoral condyle; *10,* medial femoral condyle; *11,* posterior horn of lateral meniscus; *12,* posterior horn of medial meniscus; *13, 14, 15,* and *16,* synovial coverings of the posterior compartment of the knee joint.

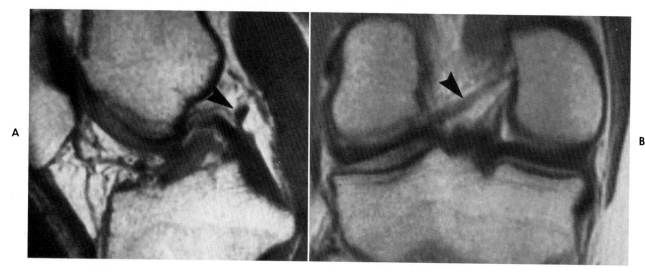

FIGURE 20-13
Meniscofemoral ligament of Wrisberg. **A,** A T1-WI sagittal and, **B,** a spin density coronal. The *arrowhead* points to the ligament.

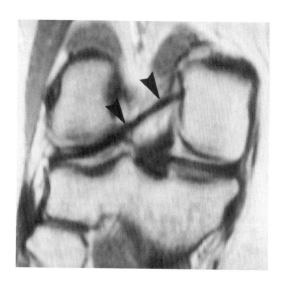

FIGURE 20-14
Coronal SD. The *arrowheads* point to the ligament of Wrisberg.

FIGURE 20-15
Normal meniscofemoral ligament of Wrisberg mimicking a tear of the inner portion of the posterior horn of lateral meniscus. **A** and **B,** T2* sagittal and, **C** to **G,** T1-WI sagittal views. The small *arrowhead* in **A** points to the Wrisberg ligament at its point of takeoff from the inner portion of the posterior horn of the lateral meniscus *(large arrowhead)*. The *small arrowhead* in **B** signifies that the Wrisberg ligament is now completely separate from the inner portion of the posterior horn of the lateral meniscus *(large arrowhead)*. The *curved arrow* points to joint effusion. **C** and **D** are from another patient. In **C** the *small arrowhead* points to the Wrisberg ligament at its origin. The *large arrowhead* points to the inner portion of the posterior horn of the lateral meniscus. In **D** the *small arrowhead* points to the Wrisberg ligament. The *large arrowhead* points to the PCL. The *arrow* designates the ACL. In **E** to **G,** from another patient, the *small arrowhead* points to the Wrisberg ligament at its takeoff (**E**) and just medial to its takeoff (**F**) while the *large arrowhead* points to the inner portion of the posterior horn of the lateral meniscus. In **G** the *arrowhead* points to the Wrisberg ligament, the *arrow* points to the PCL, and the *curved arrow* points to joint effusion.

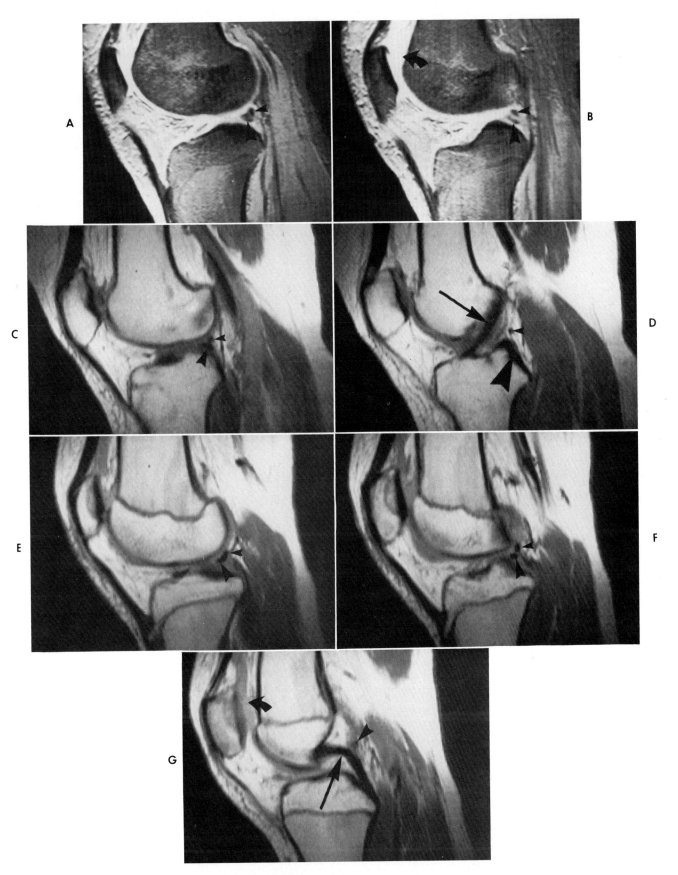

FIGURE 20-15
For legend see opposite page.

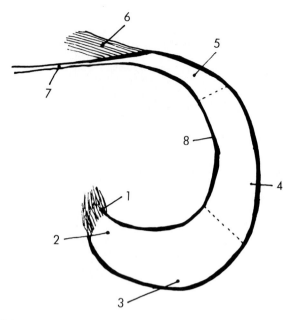

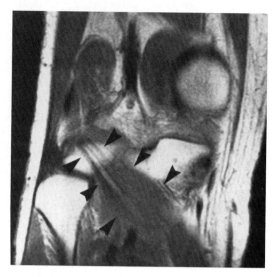

FIGURE 20-16

The medial meniscus. *1,* Central attachment of the posterior horn; *2,* the most inner portion of the posterior horn, just proximal to the central attachment; *3,* apex of the posterior horn; *4,* body of the medial meniscus; *5,* anterior horn; *6,* central attachment of the anterior horn; *7,* transverse ligament; *8,* free margin of the body of the meniscus. The designations of various segments of the medial meniscus are identical for the lateral meniscus.

FIGURE 20-17

Normal popliteus muscle *(arrowheads).* Coronal SD.

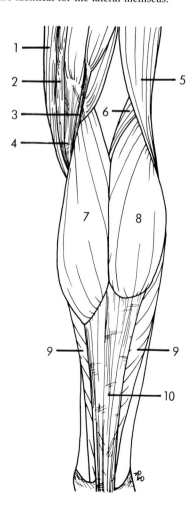

FIGURE 20-18

Muscles of the popliteal fossa and calf. *1,* Gracilis; *2* and *3,* semimembranosus; *4,* semitendinosus; *5,* biceps femoris; *6,* plantaris; *7* and *8,* medial and lateral heads of gastrocnemius; *9,* soleus; *10,* Achilles tendon.

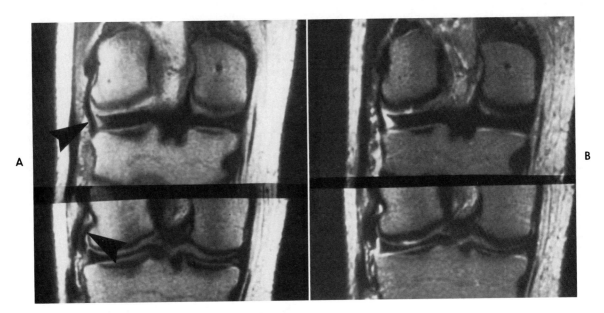

FIGURE 20-19
A, Spin density and, B, T2-WI. The *arrowheads* in A point to the popliteus tendon. In B the synovial tissue and fluid are shown with increased SI.

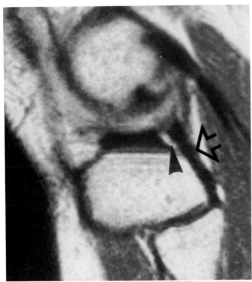

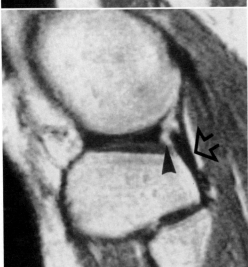

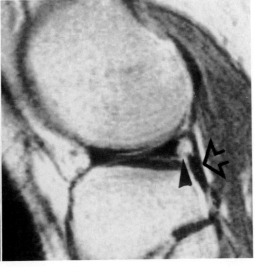

FIGURE 20-20
Normal lateral meniscus and the popliteus tendon. Spin density sagittal views 3 mm thick. In A the peripheral segment of the midportion of the body is shown. B and C, Extending further inside the lateral compartment, show the posterior and anterior horns of the lateral meniscus. The *arrowhead* points to the line of increased signal due to synovial tissue surrounding the popliteus tendon, which is seen crossing the posterolateral aspect of the posterior horn obliquely *(hollow arrow)*.

is approximately 25 mm long and 3 to 6 mm wide. The medial component of the muscle is attached to the posterior surface of the posterior horn of the lateral meniscus; it also blends with the portion of the fibrous capsule that is adjacent to the lateral meniscus.

There is a depression on the posterior surface of the

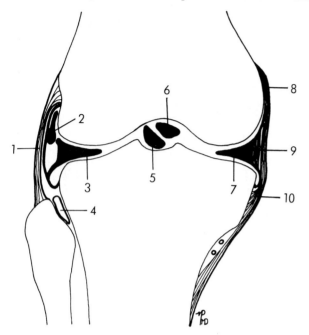

FIGURE 20-21
Normal anatomy of the midcoronal plane of the knee joint. *1*, Fibular collateral ligament; *2*, popliteus tendon; *3*, lateral meniscus; *4*, proximal tibiofibular joint; *5*, ACL; *6*, PCL; *7*, medial meniscus; *8*, femoral attachment of the tibial collateral ligament; *9*, intraligamentous bursa between the superficial and deep fibers of the TCL adjacent to the peripheral margin of the medial meniscus; *10*, proximal tibial attachment of the TCL.

lateral tibial plateau, along with a similar groove on the posterior border of the posterior horn of the lateral meniscus, for the popliteus tendon. At the joint line the tendon penetrates the capsule and becomes intracapsular. At the level of the meniscus, its outer surface is usually adherent to the inner surface of the capsule (Fig. 20-21). More superiorly, this attachment becomes less extensive and is absent where the tendon curves inward to attach to its groove on the lateral femoral condyle (Figs. 20-8, *A* and *B* and 20-19). The fibular collateral ligament (Figs. 20-21 and 20-22) is situated distinctly separate from the capsule and is obviously lateral to the popliteus tendon, which is intracapsular. There is a synovial bursa (Fig. 20-12), usually an extension of the synovial lining of the knee joint proper, that is situated deep to the popliteus tendon and extends between it and the posterior surface of the lateral meniscus and the lateral femoral condyle (subpopliteal bursa). The attachment of the posterolateral border of the lateral meniscus to the capsule is interrupted opposite the popliteus tendon.[23,24,32] In this region the meniscus is attached to the capsule via a superior and inferior fascicle (Figs. 20-19 and 20-21).[32]

The *transverse ligament* (Figs. 20-23 and 20-24) is an inconstant fibrous band that extends from the superoanterior margin of the anterior horn of the lateral meniscus to the medial side. Its course is from lateral to medial and slightly posterior to anterior (Fig. 20-11). It passes in front of the ACL (Fig. 20-24, *C*), just above the ligament's insertion on the tibia, and then merges with the superior margin of the posterior segment of the anterior horn of the medial meniscus. In some individuals the ligament may originate from a point slightly below the superior margin of the anterior horn of the lateral meniscus, rather than from the superior margin itself. This ligament is

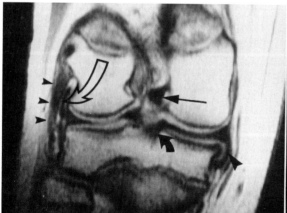
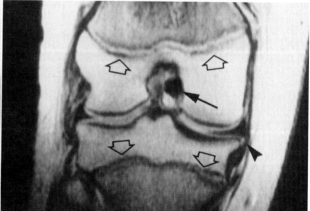

FIGURE 20-22
Spin density coronal views. The *short hollow arrows* designate the normal physeal line separating the epiphysis (containing fatty marrow) from the metaphysis (containing mostly red marrow) in a 14-year-old boy. The *straight arrow* points to the PCL. The *large arrowhead* points to the coronary ligament, exceptionally well seen in this case, with a prominent inferior synovial recess on the medial side. The *solid curved arrow* points to the central attachment of the posterior horn of the medial meniscus, the *hollow curved arrow* to the popliteus tendon, and the *small arrowheads* to the FCL.

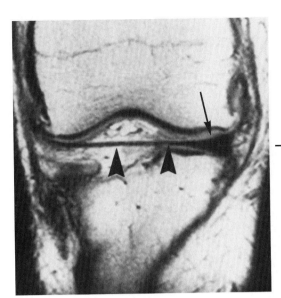

FIGURE 20-23
Normal transverse ligament. Spin density coronal image. The transverse ligament *(arrrowheads)* can be seen extending to the superior margin of the anterior horn of the medial meniscus *(arrow)*.

FIGURE 20-24
Normal lateral meniscus and transverse ligament. **A** to **D**, Spin density oblique sagittal views from the lateral to the medial side. The *straight arrow* in all images points to the transverse ligament. The *arrowheads* in **A** and **B** point to the anterior horn of the lateral meniscus. The transverse ligament can be seen arising from the superior margin of the anterior horn of the lateral meniscus. The *curved arrow* in **C** points to the ACL. The transverse ligament crosses in front of the ACL. The *large arrowhead* in **D** points to the anterior horn of the medial meniscus, with the transverse ligament *(arrow)* joining its superior margin. The *small arrowhead* points to the normal markedly slanting capsular margin of the inner portion of the posterior horn of the medial meniscus.

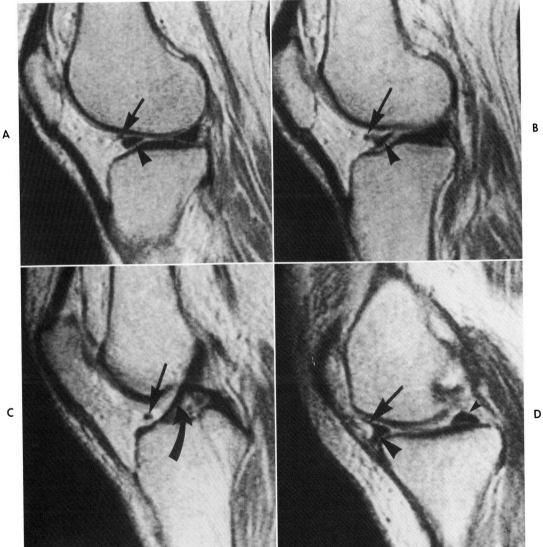

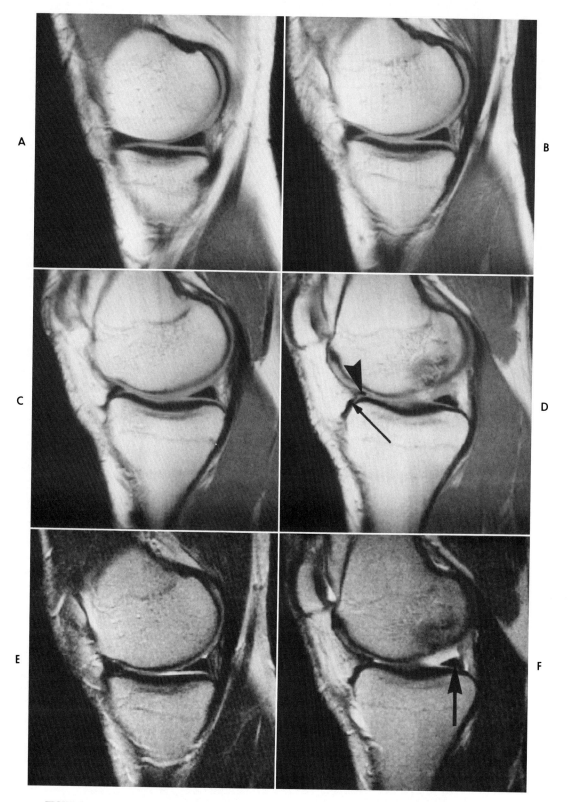

FIGURE 20-25
Normal medial meniscus. **A** to **D**, Sagittal SD and, **E** and **F**, sagittal T2-WI. The posterior and anterior horns of the medial meniscus are shown as triangles of signal void. The *arrowhead* in **D** points to a very thin transverse ligament. The *arrow* points to the innermost portion of the anterior horn of the medial meniscus. In **F** the *arrow* points to the innermost portion of the posterior horn of the medial meniscus. Note that this segment may be surrounded by synovial tissue and fluid and not attached to the capsule.

variable in thickness, ranging from just a millimeter to 3 or 4 mm.

Medial meniscus. The medial meniscus is shaped more like the letter C, or a half circle, whose radius is about twice that of its lateral counterpart (Fig. 20-11). Its posterior horn may be slightly larger than the posterior horn of the lateral meniscus. Unlike the lateral meniscus, the medial meniscus is not of uniform width throughout but is wider in the posterior horn. It then tapers gradually and continuously to the tip of the anterior horn. The posterior horn is attached to the posterior intercondylar area of the tibia (central attachment) (Figs. 20-8, *A* and *B*,

and 20-11), just posterior to the attachment of the lateral meniscus, and approximately 3 to 5 mm anterior to the anterior border of the PCL. The anterior horn of the medial meniscus essentially has two parts. One, the most anterior and inferior portion (anteroinferior segment), is attached to the anterior intercondylar area of the tibia (Figs. 20-11 and 20-16), some 5 to 8 mm anterior to the tibial attachment of the ACL. The other part is the superior margin of the anterior horn, which is more posteriorly situated; it gives rise to the transverse ligament (Figs. 20-23 and 20-25). The anteroinferior portion of the anterior horn is 10 to 14 mm anterior to the anterior

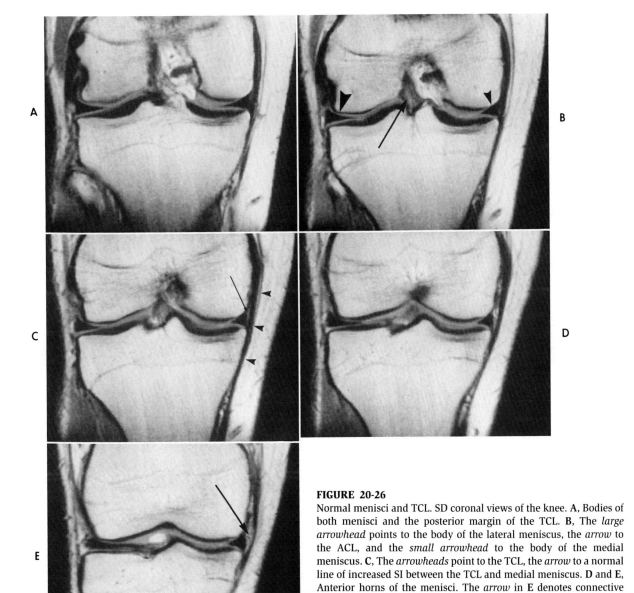

FIGURE 20-26
Normal menisci and TCL. SD coronal views of the knee. **A,** Bodies of both menisci and the posterior margin of the TCL. **B,** The *large arrowhead* points to the body of the lateral meniscus, the *arrow* to the ACL, and the *small arrowhead* to the body of the medial meniscus. **C,** The *arrowheads* point to the TCL, the *arrow* to a normal line of increased SI between the TCL and medial meniscus. **D** and **E,** Anterior horns of the menisci. The *arrow* in **E** denotes connective tissue and fat between the capsule and the anterior horn of the medial meniscus.

horn of the lateral meniscus and lies in the floor of a small valley just medial to the middle anterior margin of the tibia (Fig. 20-11). The periphery of the medial meniscus is firmly attached to the inner surface of the capsule (Fig. 20-8) and, via the coronary ligament (Fig. 20-22), to the margin of the medial tibial plateau. The attachment of the anterior horn of medial meniscus to the capsule is more substantial than that of its lateral counterpart; nevertheless, a layer of rather loose connective tissue and fat may be present between the anterior horn and the capsule (Figs. 20-8, G and H, 20-11, 20-26, and 20-27). A small amount of fat may be present normally between the apex of the posterior horn and the capsule (Fig. 20-10, C). The

innermost portion of the posterior horn is not attached to the capsule (Fig. 20-11).

Joint capsule

The knee is the largest and most complex joint in the body. It is better thought of as a compound joint formed by the merging of three separate joints[21-33,34]: a sellar joint (patellofemoral) and two condylar hinge joints (medial and lateral femorotibial compartments). This explains some of the complexities and peculiarities of its anatomy. For example, the cruciate ligaments may be thought of as collateral ligaments, hence their extrasynovial position. The peculiar synovial investments of these

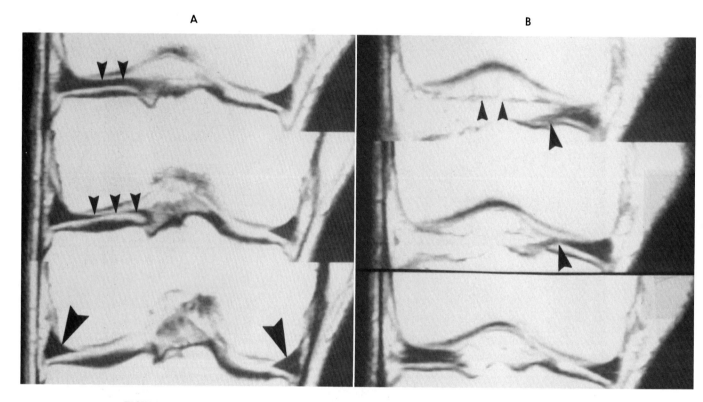

A   **B**

FIGURE 20-27
Normal anterior horns of both menisci, coronal spin density, meniscal windows. **A,** Anterior portion of the bodies of the medial and lateral menisci *(large arrowheads)* and the anterior horns of both menisci. The *three small arrowheads* point to the inner margin of the anterior horn of the lateral meniscus as it curves inward to attach to the tibia. The *two small arrowheads* identify the anterior horn, slightly more anterior to the free margin of the meniscus. **B,** Anterior horns of both menisci. The *large arrowheads* point to the most anterior portion of the medial meniscus as it turns to attach to the tibia. The *two small arrowheads* point to the transverse ligament as it extends to attach to the superior margin of the anterior horn of the medial meniscus.

FIGURE 20-28
Normal capsule and TCL. **A** and **B,** Sagittal and, **C** to **H,** coronal spin density views of the knee. Note the normally concave margin of the posteromedial joint capsule *(large arrowhead in A to D).* The *arrowhead* in **E** identifies the posterior margin of the TCL. The TCL is best seen in **F** and **G,** posterior and anterior to the midcoronal plane of the knee. The *arrow* in **G** points to a normal line of increased SI between the TCL and body of the medial meniscus due to the presence of fat or a small bursa in this region. **H,** Anterior portion of the body of the medial meniscus. The *arrowhead* points to the capsule. Note the increased SI between the margin of the meniscus and the capsule (due to loose connective tissue and fat). The *small arrowheads* in **A** and **B** point to the pes anserinus tendons.

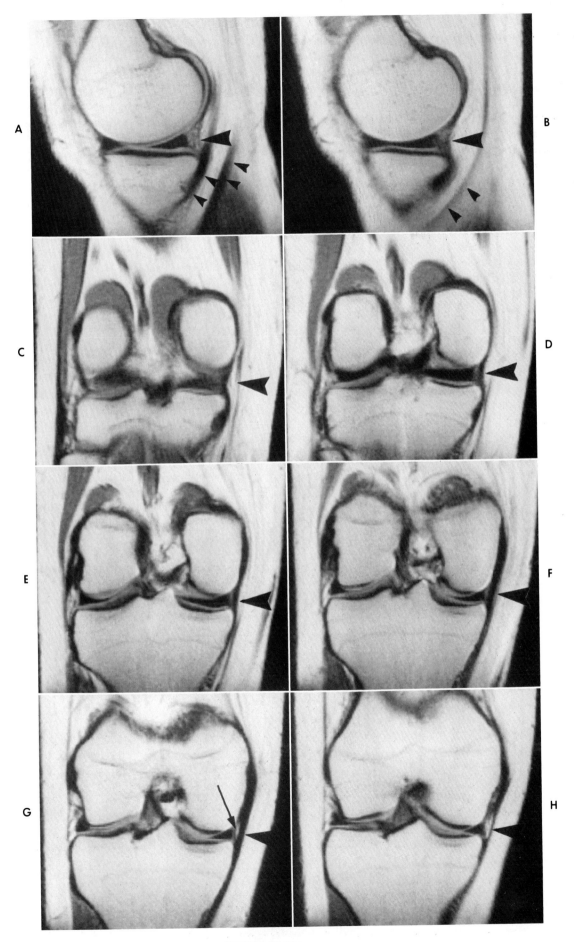

FIGURE 20-28
For legend see opposite page.

ligaments do not resemble those of truly intraarticular ligaments; thus they are more faithfully described as communicating synovial bursae interposed between the collateral ligaments and the synovial cavity of the joint proper.

The fibrous capsule of the knee is a complex structure, entirely absent anteriorly and consisting elsewhere essentially of expansions, extensions, and reinforcements by various tendons, muscle aponeuroses, and ligaments.[4,21,22] Anteriorly the aponeuroses of the vasti extend from the lateral margins of the quadriceps tendon, the patella, and the patellar tendon posteriorly on each side as far back as the corresponding collateral ligament and inferiorly to the condyles of the tibia. This passive stabilizing apparatus is also referred to as the medial and lateral patellar retinacula. On the medial side the fibrous capsule is attached to the medial surface of the femoral condyle (Fig. 20-28), just above the margin of the articular cartilage, and to the tibia just below the medial margin of the tibial plateau. The medial meniscus is attached to the inner surface of the capsule/tibial collateral ligament complex (Fig. 20-11), although there may be a small bursa (Fig. 20-21) interposed between them. That portion of the capsule that attaches the inferior margin of the capsular border of the menisci to the tibia is called the coronary ligament (Fig. 20-22).

Tibial collateral ligament

The joint capsule on the medial side is reinforced by the tibial collateral ligament (TCL) (Fig. 20-11), a broad and flat band (2 to 3 mm thick and 20 mm wide at the joint line) attached to the medial epicondyle of the femur immediately below the adductor tubercle. It may be thought of as a downward extension of the adductor magnus tendon.[21,22,35-38] Extending from the femur inferiorly, the TCL attaches to four places (Fig. 20-29). The deep fibers, which are considered part of the fibrous capsule (Figs. 20-12, 20-21, and 20-26, *A* to *C*), attach loosely to the peripheral margin of the body of the medial meniscus (a small bursa or a minimal amount of fat may be interposed here) and then firmly to the tibia just below the joint line, in the process forming the coronary ligament (Fig. 20-22). The superficial fibers continue the attachment to the cortex of the medial tibial condyle inferiorly for about 2 cm, and then extend 3 to 4 cm more inferiorly (as a bowstring stretched across the hollow between the condyle and the shaft) to attach to the shaft of the proximal tibia (Fig. 20-29). In this region, some fat and fairly constant anteroposteriorly coursing vessels are interposed between the ligament and the tibial cortex.

Laterally the capsule originates on the lateral femoral condyle, just above the popliteus tendon groove (Fig. 20-21), and extends inferiorly, covering the popliteus tendon and then the lateral meniscus; further inferiorly it attaches to the lateral surface of the tibia just below the joint line.[21,22,35,39,40] The popliteus tendon is attached to the inner surface of the capsule along most of its course (Figs. 20-19, 20-21, 20-22). The capsule also sends expansions externally to the head of the fibula. The lateral meniscus is joined to the inner surface of the capsule along its entire border, except posteriorly, where the popliteus muscle is attached to the meniscus, and imme-

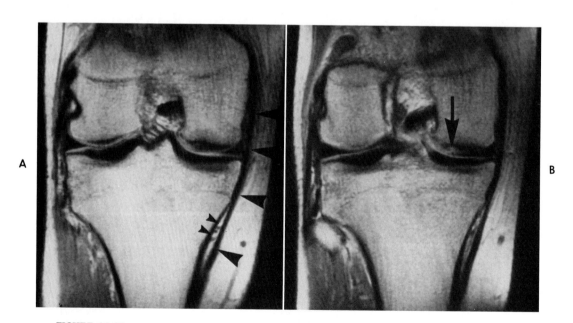

A

B

FIGURE 20-29
Normal TCL. A and B, Spin density coronal views. *Large arrowheads* point to the ligament. A thin line of increased signal is usually present between the peripheral margin of the body of the meniscus and the TCL. It may be due to fat or a small bursa. The *small arrowheads* point to venous channels, with fat surrounding them, normally present between the distal portion of the TCL and the tibia. The *arrow* in **B** points to a small area of osteochondral defect due to previous trauma.

diately adjacent to it, where the popliteus tendon is interposed between the meniscus and the capsule.

Fibular collateral ligament

The fibular collateral ligament (FCL) (Figs. 20-11, 20-12, and 20-20 to 20-22) is a round cord attached to the lateral epicondyle of the femur superiorly just above the popliteus groove, in which region it merges with the outer surface of the capsule. From this point the FCL extends inferiorly and posteriorly to attach to the anterior portion of the apex of the fibular head. It stands clear of the capsule. There is a small amount of fat between it and the capsule, through which the lateral inferior genicular vessels and nerve pass. The FCL is partly attached to the tendon of the biceps femoris, which itself adheres to the apex of the fibula.

Posteriorly the fibrous capsule is attached to the margins of the femoral condyles and the intercondylar region, and it extends inferiorly to attach to the posterior margin of the tibial condyles, just below the articular margin, and to the posterior border of the intercondylar area, blending with the posterior fibers of the posterior cruciate ligament.

Synovial membrane

The synovial membrane (Fig. 20-12) of the knee, like the capsule, is the most extensive and complex of all the joints in the body. The inner surface of the joint capsule medially and laterally is covered by the synovial membrane, which extends up to the level of the attachment of the menisci to the capsule. The synovial membrane does not cover the surfaces of the menisci, but covers the inner surface of the coronary ligaments, which attach the inferior margin of the capsular borders of the menisci to the tibia.

Laterally the synovial membrane sends an extension, through the opening in the capsule posterolaterally, to be interposed between the popliteus tendon and the posterolateral surface of the lateral meniscus and, further inferiorly, between the tendon and the posterior surface of the tibia. This bursal extension is called the subpopliteal recess. It may communicate with the superior tibiofibular joint. The synovial membrane also sends an extension that partially covers the popliteus tendon in the popliteal groove on the lateral surface of the lateral femoral condyle.

Anteriorly the synovial membrane extends as a distinct bursa superiorly between the quadriceps tendon and the femur. This is called the suprapatellar bursa (Fig. 20-30). The suprapatellar bursa is formed as an independent synovial cavity of the originally separate patellofemoral joint, but shortly later it communicates with the synovial cavity of the femorotibial articulations. Anteriorly the suprapatellar bursa is attached to the patella along the

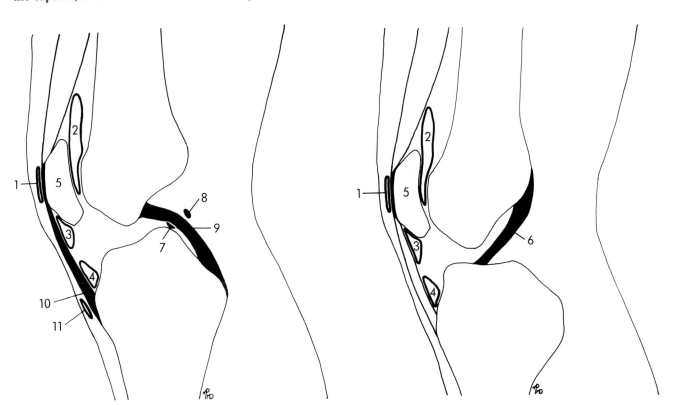

FIGURE 20-30
Normal anatomy of the midsagittal plane of the knee. The following are shown: *1,* Prepatellar bursa; *2,* suprapatellar bursa; *3* and *4,* infrapatellar bursae deep to the patellar tendon (also called the deep infrapatellar bursa); *5,* patella; *6,* ACL; *7,* ligament of Humphrey; *8,* ligament of Wrisberg; *9,* PCL; *10,* patellar tendon; and *11,* superficial intrapatellar bursa.

margins of the patellar articular cartilage. From each side of the patella it extends to the sides of the femur, merging with the synovial lining of the medial and lateral compartments. From the inferior margin of the patella it extends posteriorly and downward. The fat pad of Hoffa is interposed between the patellar tendon and the synovial membrane in this region. Further posteriorly the synovial membrane joins the anterior part of the synovial cavity of each femorotibial compartment. The synovial membrane extending inferiorly from the patella has a central fold called the ligamentum mucosum, on each side of which are accessary alar folds. The posterior wall of the suprapatellar bursa is attached to the femur along the margin of the articular cartilage, and it then merges with the lining of the inner surface of the fibrous capsule medially and laterally.

Cruciate ligaments

ACL. The anterior cruciate ligament attaches just on the medial side of midline in the anterior intercondylar area, well posterior to the anterior margin of the tibia (Figs.

20-11, 20-30, *A,* and 20-31). The attachment is posterior to the transverse ligament (Fig. 20-24, *C*). The tibial origin of the ACL is not in the coronal plane; it is slightly oblique, with the medial end more anterior than the lateral. Thus, it may be thought of as being anteromedial and posterolateral.[41-44] In some subjects, the ligament seems to have two, sometimes more, distinct bundles, separated by thin bands of looser connective tissue, or a minimal amount of fat (Fig. 20-31, *A, B,* and *E*). This arrangement is evident at its origin and along a quarter to a half (rarely all) of its length. The ligament extends superiorly, laterally, and posteriorly, twisting on itself in its middle and upper portion, and fans out to become attached on the posterior part of the medial surface of the lateral femoral condyle.

PCL. The posterior cruciate ligament originates on the posterior surface of the posterior intercondylar region of the tibia (Figs. 20-11, 20-31, *A,* and 20-32 to 20-34), well below the level of the tibial articular margin, and extends superiorly, at first in the anatomical sagittal close to the vertical plane, and then almost abruptly, anteriorly and

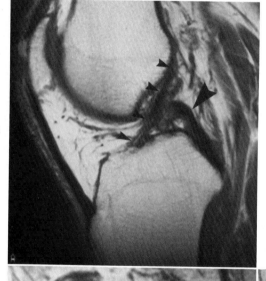

A

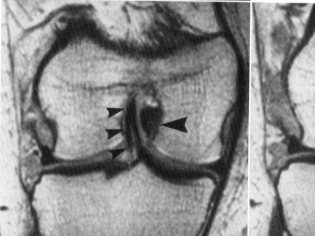

B

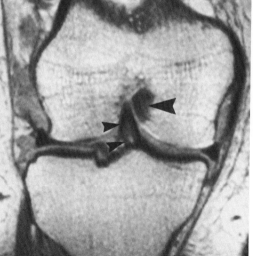

C

FIGURE 20-31
Normal ACL and PCL. **A,** A T1-WI anatomical view, **B** and **C,** SD coronal views.

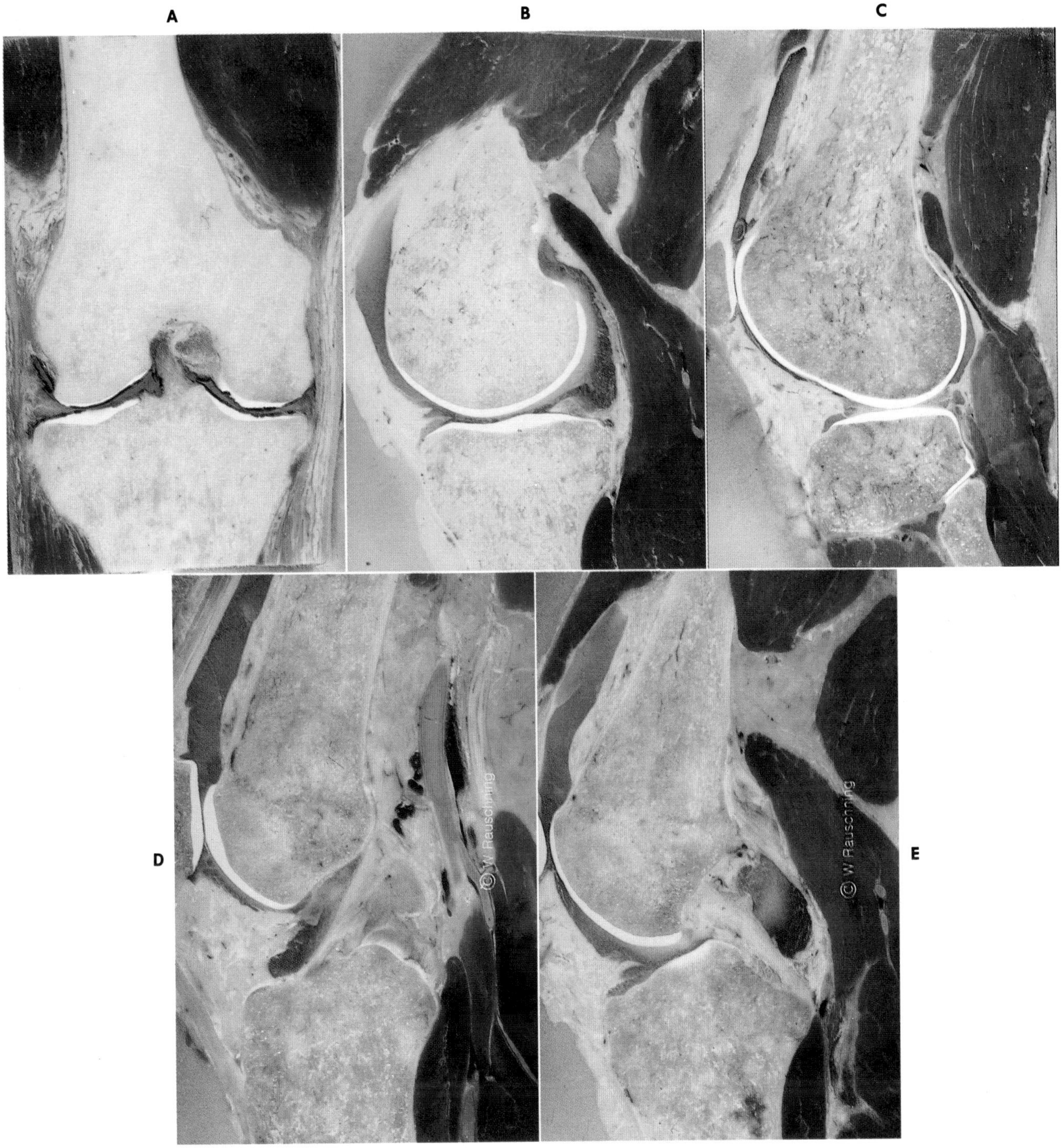

PLATE 20-1
Cryomicrosections of the knee. **A,** A midcoronal section shows the bodies of the medial and lateral menisci and the ACL. **B,** A parasagittal section through the medial compartment showing the anterior and posterior horns of the medial meniscus. **C,** Another parasagittal section, this time through the lateral compartment, shows the anterior and posterior horns of the lateral meniscus. **D,** An immediately lateral paramedian section displays the ACL and, **E,** an immediately medial paramedian shows the PCL.

medially and nearly horizontally, to attach to the middle and anterior portion of the lateral surface of the medial femoral condyle[45,46] (Figs. 20-30, *B*, and 20-31, *A*). This ligament is significantly wider, and moderately thicker, than the ACL.

Synovial covering. The cruciate ligaments are partially intracapsular, but totally extrasynovial. Nevertheless, they are partially invested with synovial membrane.

These ligaments are usually classified as intracapsular, but such a view is open to serious challenge. The PCL may be considered to be *on the anterior side* of that portion of the capsule covering the posterior aspect of the knee. The designation of the position of the ACL as either intra- or extracapsular is not easy, with the ligament being some distance away from the capsule posteriorly and there being no distinct capsule anteriorly.

The synovial investment of the cruciate ligaments deserves careful scrutiny if one is to identify injuries to the ligaments or the synovial membrane within the intercondylar notch. The synovial membrane forms a narrow tentlike structure with a perforated roof in the intercondylar fossa. The ACL acts as an inside pole holding up the anterior and inferior extremities of the tent. The femoral attachment of the PCL, with the synovial membrane in front of it, forms the anterosuperior corner of the tent. Thus the anterior surface of the femoral attachment of the PCL, and almost all of the anterior surface of the ACL are covered by the synovial membrane.[21,22,47] The synovial membrane then extends posteriorly, in the process covering the medial and lateral sides of the ACL and PCL. From this point it reflects on the inner surface of the posterior capsule, reaching the capsular surface sides of midline and leaving the midportion (opposite the PCL) uncovered. In some individuals the synovial membrane sends a small diverticulum-like extension, from the lateral side to the medial, interposed

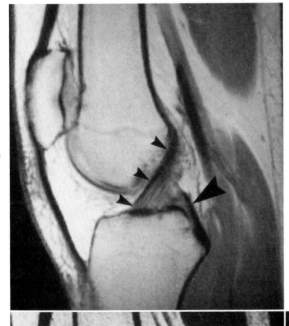

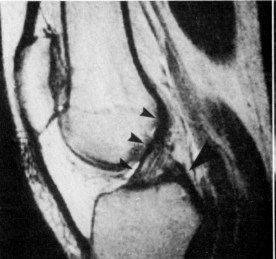

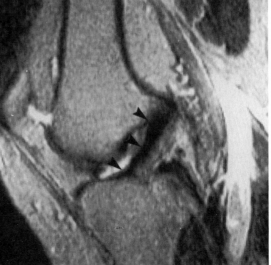

FIGURE 20-31, cont'd
D, Anatomical sagittal SD. *E,* Anatomical sagittal T2-WI and, *F,* oblique sagittal T2-WI. In all these images the *small arrowheads* point to the ACL and the *large arrowhead* to the PCL. Note the normally high-SI synovial tissue and fluid in front of the ACL. In *F* the minimal redundancy and laxity of the ACL and about 10 degrees of knee flexion can be appreciated.

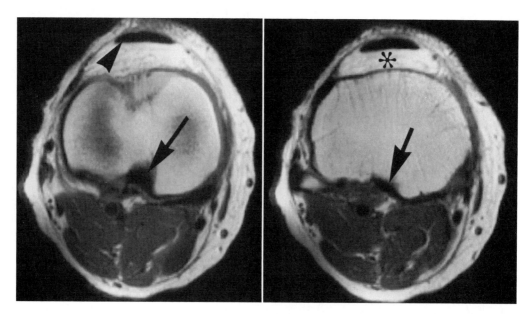

FIGURE 20-32
Normal axial anatomy. T1 weighted images just below the tibial plateau. The *arrow* points to the origin of the PCL, the *asterisk* is on the infrapatellar fat pad, and the *arrowhead* points to the patellar tendon.

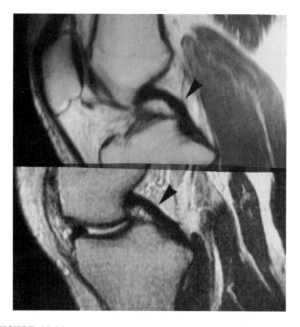

FIGURE 20-33
Normal PCL. Anatomical sagittal T1 weighted *(upper image)* and oblique sagittal T2 weighted *(lower image)*. The *arrowheads* point to the PCL. Note its flattened curve, which is occasionally seen on oblique sagittals, even with the knee in full extension.

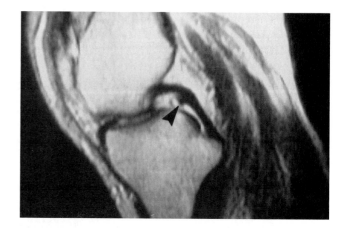

FIGURE 20-34
Normal PCL and the anterior meniscofemoral ligament of Humphrey *(arrowhead)*. T2-WI sagittal view.

between the ACL and PCL. Thus a small segment of the posterior surface of the ACL and anterior surface of the PCL may also appear to be covered by the synovial membrane.

SYNOVIAL BURSAE, CYSTS, AND GANGLION CYSTS

A bursa is a flat, synovium-lined, closed cavity usually containing a small amount of fluid. When distended, it is called a cyst; when inflamed, bursitis.

The synovial lining of the bursae has a fairly high signal intensity (SI) on T1-WI, more so on SD, T2-WI, and T2* sequences. A cyst is usually well delineated on MRI as an egg-shaped or spherical cavity with smooth walls containing fluid.[37,48,49] The cyst contents, if synovial fluid, are of low SI on T1-WI and high SI on T2-WI and T2*. When the cyst contains a fluid with a thick proteinaceous debris, it is usually of low or medium SI on all pulse sequences. The cyst may contain calcification, osteochondral bodies, or organized hematoma, which will have signal characteristics peculiar to them. If there are hemosiderin deposits (e.g., in a giant cell tumor of the tendon sheaths) or repeated bleeding into a cyst (rheumatoid calf cysts, hemophilia), there will be zones of signal void, more prominently on T2-WI. This is secondary to the well-known lowering of T2 of nearby water molecules by the ferric (Fe^{3+}) iron of hemosiderin.[50]

Most cystic lesions around the knee are adequately seen and located on the MRI protocol designed for internal derangement. However, for cysts extending away from the knee region, calf cysts, and giant dissecting or ruptured popliteal cysts, additional sets of images may have to be obtained.

There are numerous bursae interposed between the ligaments, tendons, and muscles associated with the knee joint. The most important and frequently encountered are discussed next.

Bursae and cysts in the popliteal fossa

The medial and lateral gastrocnemius bursae are situated between the corresponding heads of the muscle and the capsule covering the femoral condyles (Figs. 20-11 and 20-18). The medial gastrocnemius (G) bursa is present in all individuals and almost always communicates with the semimembranosus (SM) bursae. In children the G-SM bursa seldom communicates with the knee joint.[51,52] We have noted that in adults the communication is seen in at least 50% of patients with internal derangement referred for arthrography. The percentage of the communication increases significantly with increased severity and duration of knee pathology. The most important causes of this communication, or opening of a preexisting channel, are persistent and chronic joint effusion and increased intraarticular pressure. Thus all knee disorders that cause persistent joint effusion may also cause a popliteal cyst. The most common are internal

derangement, osteoarthritis, and chronic inflammatory arthritis of the knee (e.g., rheumatoid arthritis).

The combined G-SM bursa is usually the one that fills with synovial fluid consequent to long-standing joint effusion and increased intraarticular pressure, and it presents as a cyst in the popliteal fossa, referred to as the popliteal cyst or Baker cyst (Figs. 20-35 and 20-36). A popliteal cyst may be produced also by extension of a cyst into the popliteal fossa or enlargement of other bursae. These are uncommon and, in descending order of frequency, include the lateral gastrocnemius bursa, a posteriorly extending medial parameniscal cyst, and the subpopliteal bursa.

A popliteal cyst may rupture into the posteromedial compartment of the calf and produce a clinical picture indistinguishable from deep venous thrombosis (DVT). A large popliteal cyst may markedly displace and compress the popliteal vein and contribute to or cause DVT.[53-55] A clinical presentation similar to DVT may also be noted in patients with bleeding into a calf cyst. Calf cysts are usually walled-off ruptured popliteal cysts, rarely a consequence of a dissecting but not ruptured popliteal cyst. They are seen in patients with long-standing inflammatory arthritis (e.g., rheumatoid or psoriatic). The patient with rheumatoid arthritis has a tendency to bleed into the calf cyst also.

Bursae on the medial side of the knee

Numerous bursae may be interposed between the TCL and medial femoral or tibial condyles, and between the superficial and deep layers of the TCL. A thin layer of fat may also be present between the deep and superficial layers.

The tendons of the sartorius, gracilis, and semitendinosus (pes anserinus) (Fig. 20-37) cross obliquely, superiorly to inferiorly and posteroanteriorly over the surface of the lower portion of the TCL. A bursa is usually interposed between these tendons and the TCL (pes anserinus bursa). The TCL bursae and pes anserinus bursa may be injured by direct trauma, sprain, or tear of their respective tendons, or severe twisting injuries (see pp. 707 to 711).

Bursae on the lateral side of the knee

On the lateral side there usually is a bursa between the FCL and the biceps femoris tendon, and another between the FCL and the capsule. The latter bursa is often a prolongation of the subpopliteal recess (subpopliteal bursa), itself an extension of the synovial cavity of the lateral compartment. The subpopliteal bursa may enlarge and present as a cyst in the popliteal region.

Bursae on the anterior side of the knee

Anteriorly there are several bursae associated with the patella and the patellar tendon[21,25,56] (Fig. 20-30). The suprapatellar bursa, at this stage of human evolution, is better regarded as an extension of the synovial cavity of

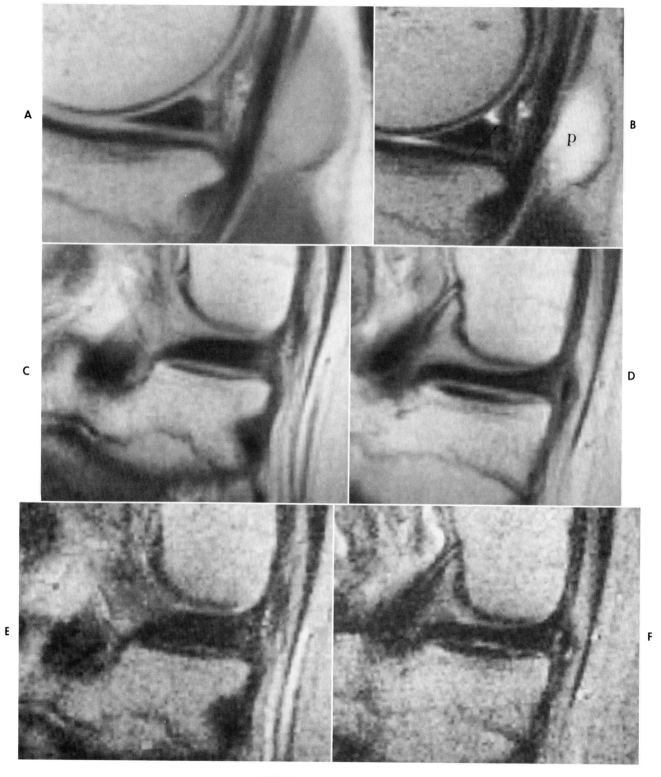

FIGURE 20-35
For legend see opposite page.

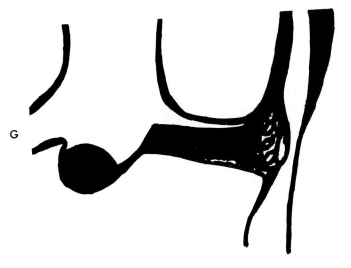

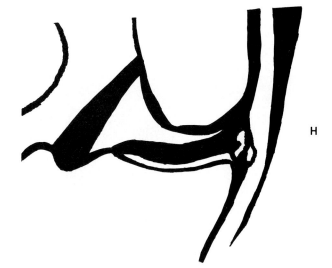

FIGURE 20-35

Capsulomeniscal injury, joint effusion, and a popliteal cyst. **A** and **B**, SD and T2-WI sagittal views through the midportion of the posterior horn of the medial meniscus. There is minimal disruption of the capsulomeniscal junction superiorly. Note the irregular outline of the area containing bright fluid in **B**. The superior recess is disrupted at its base *(arrow)*. There is thickening of the capsulomeniscal junction, with a microtear of the capsule evidenced by the presence of fluid in it. *P* is a small popliteal cyst. **C** and **D**, Spin density and, **E** and **F**, T2-WI coronal cross sections show the posterior horn of the medial meniscus. **G** and **H** are schematics of **E** and **F**. There are multiple small areas of increased signal on T2-WI in the substance of the joint capsule and in the capsulomeniscal junction, indicating the presence of microtears. Note that the capsule is bulging out in **F** and contains tiny bubbles of fluid. **I**, Midsagittal T2-WI. A popliteal cyst can be seen extending in front of *(p)* and behind *(P)* the medial gastrocnemius muscle.

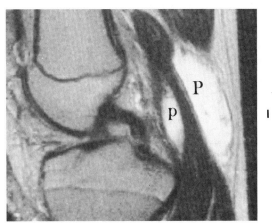

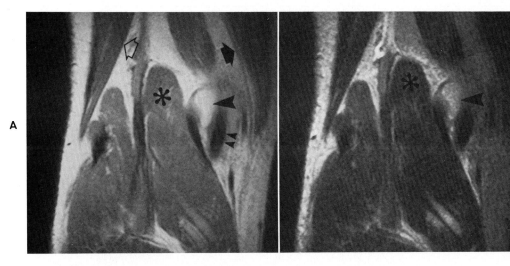

FIGURE 20-36

Popliteal cyst extending superiorly, medially, and anteriorly. **A** and **B**, Spin density and T2-WI coronal views of the popliteal fossa. The *hollow arrow* in **A** identifies the biceps femoris. The *solid wide arrow* points to the displaced sartorius and gracilis, the *two small arrowheads* to the semimembranosus. The *asterisk* is on the medial head of the gastrocnemius.

Continued.

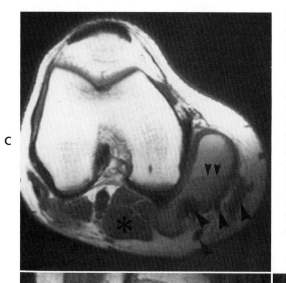

C

FIGURE 20-36, cont'd

C, A T1-WI axial through the midportion of the femoral condyle. The *asterisk* is on the medial head of the gastrocnemius. The cyst is dissecting between that muscle and the semitendinosus, semimembranosus, gracilis, and sartorius (designated by *arrowheads* in **C,** respectively, medially to laterally). The cyst contains hemorrhagic fluid. The fluid level between the more cellular fraction, accumulating in the dependent portion of the cyst, and the serous fluid is shown by *two arrowheads* in **C. D** and **E,** Spin density and T2-WI coronal views at the level of the posterior surface of the femoral condyles. The *asterisk* is on the cyst. The *hollow arrow* points to the displaced sartorius and gastrocnemius. Note the significantly lower signal intensity of the cellular elements of blood precipitating to the bottom of the cyst on T1-WI, **C,** and T2-WI, **B** and **E.** There is markedly increased signal of these same regions on the spin density, **A** and **D.** The serous fluid is of moderately high signal intensity on spin density, **F,** and is of high signal intensity on T2-WI, **G.** The *small arrowheads* in **F** point to the normal anterior portion of the bodies of the medial and lateral menisci, the *large arrowhead* to the anterior margin of the TCL.

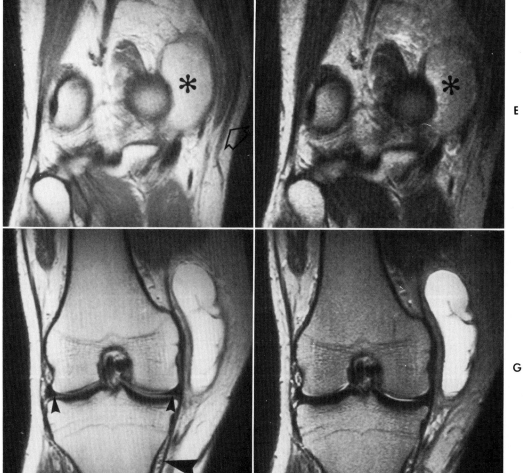

D

E

F

G

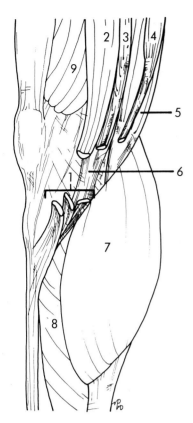

FIGURE 20-37
Muscles and tendons on the medial side of the knee. *1,* Pes anserinus; *2,* sartorius, *3,* gracilis; *4,* semitendinosus; *5,* semimem-branosus; *6,* tibial collateral ligament; *7,* gastrocnemius (medial head); *8,* soleus.

the femorotibial articulations and thus part of the synovial cavity of the joint rather than a periarticular bursa. However, a plica may cause the suprapatellar bursa in adults to become separated from the femorotibial compartments.

Anterior to the patella one often finds a rather large bursa, the prepatellar bursa (Fig. 20-30, *A*), interposed between the inferior half of the anterior surface of the patella and the skin. There are other similar bursae occasionally encountered interposed between the patellar tendon and the skin.[22] There is often a small bursa between the distal portion of the patellar tendon, just proximal to its insertion on the tibial tubercle, and the anterior surface of the tibia. This is called the deep infrapatellar bursa (Fig. 20-30, *A*). Occasionally, other smaller bursae are found between the anterior surface of the distal portion of the patellar tendon and the tuberosity of the tibia or the overlying skin. These bursae when inflamed, or injured (e.g., by direct trauma or kneeling) present as distended cysts, easily identified on T2-WI.

Ganglion cysts around the knee

A ganglion is a cyst that develops along the tendon sheaths. It is thought to form consequent to herniation of

the synovial lining of a joint, a tendon sheath, or even a nerve covering. The communication with the donor site is usually lost and the cyst migrates toward the subcutaneous tissue, in the process insinuating itself between the tendons in its path. A ganglion often contains clear fluid, which is of high SI on T2-WI and T2*, but it may contain hemorrhagic fluid or a proteinaceous jelly-like substance[37] with debris that are of low SI on T2-WI and T2*.

Although most ganglions are felt to be of synovial origin, the histology of the lining of an old ganglion is difficult to characterize. A ganglion may be situated close to bone and cause pressure erosion.

In the knee region (Fig. 20-38) a ganglion can occur in various locations, although the most frequent site is in the vicinity of the tibiofibular joint, where it is called a peroneal nerve ganglion cyst.

Peroneal nerve ganglion cyst. This small cyst develops lateral to the head of the fibula. Its exact pathogenesis is not known. According to Parkes[57] ganglia of the common peroneal nerve arise from the proximal tibiofibular joint and extend along the sheath of the small recurrent superior tibiofibular articular branch of the common peroneal nerve to the main nerve. Once the ganglion has arrived at the main sheath and become situated within it, marked enlargement and cystic degeneration can take place. Some authors[58-60] have suggested that these ganglia may merely represent cystic degeneration of the nerve sheath.

Compression of the peripheral nerves by ganglion cysts can strongly mimic central nerve root compression.[61] The diagnosis is not suspected unless one is aware of the entity. There are reports[62] of laminectomies having been performed in patients with a peroneal nerve ganglion cyst on the basis of clinical findings and equivocal myelography results. The initial complaint is usually pain, which is first localized to the upper lateral aspect of the leg and then may be referred downward and over the dorsum of the foot and toes. The pain can occur anywhere along the distribution of the cutaneous supply of the peroneal nerve. Varying degrees of paresis of the muscles supplied by the common peroneal nerve is also usually present. A small mass, posterolaterally adjacent to the neck of the fibula, may be the presenting symptom; it may be asymptomatic for a number of months or years, and in approximately 20% of patients a palpable mass may not be present.

Although ganglion cysts are common, they rarely involve the peripheral nerves. According to Stack et al.,[62] Hartwell[63] in 1901 was the first to describe peripheral nerve involvement by a ganglion cyst. In his patient the median nerve was affected. Sultan[64] in 1921 reported a patient with paralysis of the common peroneal nerve caused by a cystic tumor. Since then a relatively large number of cases have been reported,[58-62,65,66] most of which include involvement of the common peroneal nerve. In 1961 Parks[57] reported on a series of nine ganglia involving the common peroneal nerve. He treated eight patients within a period of approximately 6 years and concluded that this problem was not rare.

MRI OF THE NORMAL MENISCI

The configuration of a cross section of the menisci depends upon the angle of the image plane with the capsular margin and the thickness of the section. When the plane of the section is at 90 degrees to the capsular margin, the cross section of the menisci is more or less triangular. Otherwise, the menisci appear as a band of varying thickness depending on the segment imaged.

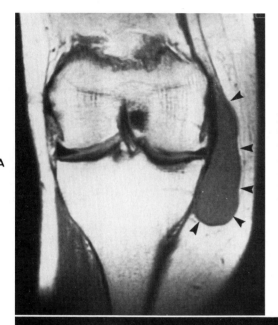

A

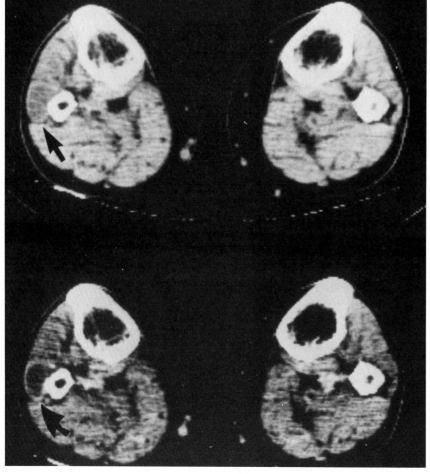

B

FIGURE 20-38
Ganglion cyst. **A,** SD midcoronal view of the knee. There is no communication between this large cyst and the knee joint. The medial meniscus was relatively small, but otherwise normal, at surgical exploration. **B,** Axial CT images obtained through the neck of the fibula in another patient. Note the distinct cystic structure with enhancing margins lateral to the neck of the right fibula *(arrow).*

SAGITTAL VIEWS

On anatomical sagittal cross sections the midportion of the posterior horns of the menisci (Figs. 20-39 to 20-42), usually the largest parts on both sides, is triangular. The vascular peripheral segment of the posterior horn of the medial meniscus is broadest in width, possibly 4 to 6 mm. The central attachment of the posterior horns to the tibia, not well seen on sagittal cross sections, is often better appreciated on coronal images (Fig. 20-22, *A*). The menisci just prior to their central attachments may appear irregular with nonhomogeneously increased SI. This is due to the presence of vascularity and synovial tissue and should not be confused with a tear.

The posterior horn of the medial meniscus (Fig. 20-25, *A* to *C*) is normally triangular in cross section. The sides of the triangle (the superior and inferior articular surfaces of the meniscus) are approximately twice as long as the base (capsular margin). The anterior horn (Fig. 20-25, *A* to *C*) is about a half to a third the size of the posterior horn. The junction between the vascular and nonvascular portions is a coronal plane that is tilted a few degrees anteriorly and superiorly to inferiorly (Fig. 20-28, *A* and *B*). In the innermost portion of the posterior horn, just prior to the central attachment, this boundary plane is more rounded and tilted a few degrees more anteriorly (Fig. 20-39).

The apices (midportions) of the posterior and anterior horns of the lateral meniscus appear almost of equal size on anatomical sagittal views (Fig. 20-40). Cross sections through the midportion of the posterior horn of the lateral meniscus show it to be of almost the same size as the corresponding segment of the medial meniscus (Fig. 20-29, *A* and *B*). Some texts of anatomy and surgery state that the lateral meniscus is slightly broader than the medial meniscus. This statement is certainly correct for the body and anterior horn; but the posterior horn, as seen on anatomical sagittal views, does not appear to be broader than its medial counterpart. In some patients it actually appears slightly narrower. The posterior horn of the lateral meniscus is not continuously attached to the capsule, because of the interposition of the popliteus tendon between the two (Figs. 20-19 to 20-22). Instead, the meniscus is attached to the capsule via a superior and an inferior fasicle. These are occasionally visualized on sagittal and coronal views. The popliteus tendon is often well delineated on the oblique sagittal views (Fig. 20-20) as it crosses on the posterior aspect of the posterior horn of the lateral meniscus. A linear area of increased SI, due to the synovial tissue partially surrounding the popliteus tendon, is seen on sagittal (Fig. 20-20) and coronal views (Figs. 20-8 and 20-19) crossing the posterior horn of the lateral meniscus. This should not be mistaken for a tear. The capsular margin of the posterior horn of the lateral meniscus describes a vertical coronal plane (Figs. 20-40 and 20-42). The origin of the ligament of Wrisberg, from the superior margin of the posterior horn of the lateral meniscus, is usually well seen on sagittal views (Fig. 20-15, *A* to *C, E,* and *F*). The cross section of the ligament appears as a black circle attached, or just next, to the superior margin of the posterior horn. This should not be mistaken for a tear. The ligament then can be followed, on subsequent slices extending medially across the intercondylar notch, to its insertion on the femur.

The anterior horn of the lateral meniscus (Figs. 20-40 and 20-42) is similar in configuration to the posterior horn, although usually somewhat smaller. The inner portion of the anterior horn is significantly narrower and

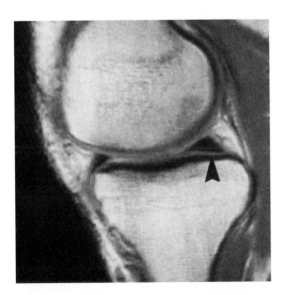

FIGURE 20-39
Normal medial meniscus. The *arrowhead* designates the posterior horn just prior to its central attachment on bone. Note the steeply inclined surface of the capsular border.

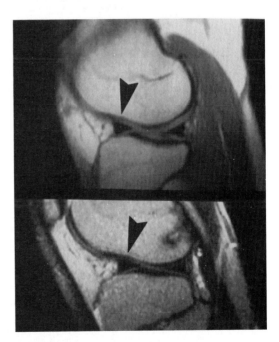

FIGURE 20-40
Sagittal T1-WI *(upper image)* and T2-WI *(lower image)* of the knee. Note the normal depression of the lateral femoral condyle *(arrowheads)*.

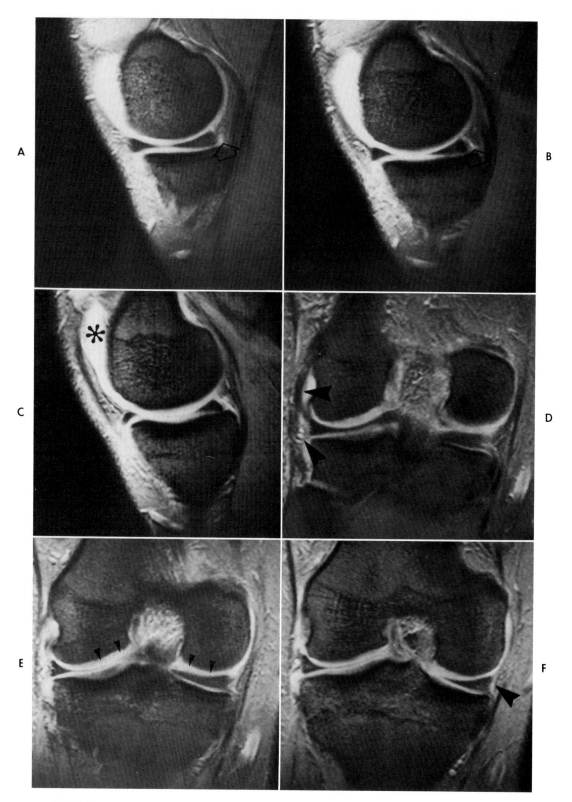

FIGURE 20-41

Normal anatomy on gradient echo (T2*) imaging (TR 720/TE 13, RF angle 30 degrees). **A** to **C**, Sagittal and, **D** to **F**, coronal views. The *hollow arrowhead* in **A** and **B** points to an area of markedly increased SI within the vascular segment of the posterior horn of the medial meniscus. This is normal and should not be mistaken for a tear. The *asterisk* in **C** identifies effusion within the suprapatellar bursa. **D**, The *upper arrowhead* designates the popliteus tendon, the *lower arrowhead* the inferior genicular veins running along the peripheral margin of the lateral meniscus. **E** and **F** show the meniscal anatomy in the midcoronal plane of the knee. The *arrowheads* in **E** mark the articular cartilage of the femoral condyle, which is of high SI, The *arrowhead* in **F** points to a line of increased SI between the peripheral margin of the medial meniscus and the TCL. Note that this normal line of increased signal, due to a small bursa or a minimal amount of fat, is exaggerated on T2*.

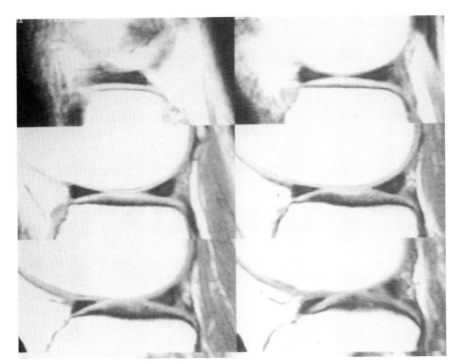

FIGURE 20-42
Normal lateral meniscus, sagittal T1-WI, meniscal windows.

thinner and may appear as a band (Fig. 20-27, *A*). It is notably more posteriorly positioned than its medial counterpart, which is on the very edge of the anterior margin of the tibia (Fig. 20-11).

On sagittal views the anterior horn of the medial meniscus is sitting on an inclined facet in the extreme anterior edge of the articular margin of the tibia (Fig. 20-25, *C* and *D*). The transverse ligament (TL) joins the anterior horn superiorly and may cause the anterior horn/transverse ligament complex to appear V shaped. The V is horizontally placed, with its apex pointing posteriorly. On the lateral side, sagittal views show the TL as a dark circle directly in front of the upper margin (Fig. 20-24, *A* and *B*) of the anterior horn of the lateral meniscus (less frequently somewhat lower). This should not be mistaken for a tear of the anterior horn.

Sagittal views are useful mainly for assessing the integrity of the posterior and anterior horns of the menisci. The bodies of the menisci, the capsule adjacent to them, and the TCL are not optimally seen on these views. Sagittal slices on the peripheral surface of the medial and lateral compartments cross through the bodies of the menisci. On the medial side the body is long, has a relatively gradual curve, and appears flat. The next sagittal slices go through the midportion of the body and then the free margin. These slices (on both the medial and the lateral side) must be interpreted with caution because the curvatures of the menisci and their thin free margins may produce an image that suggests a tear. A tear of the free margin of the body suspected on sagittal images should always be confirmed on coronal views. On the lateral side, because the lateral meniscus is part of a significantly smaller circle, the sagittal cross sections going through the body will show a flat band and, immediately thereafter, a bow tie configuration.

CORONAL VIEWS

These images are useful mainly for evaluating the bodies of the menisci, the capsule, the TCL, and the FCL. The posterior and anterior horns are also seen. The first coronal images touching the posterior horns show the menisci as flat bands (Fig. 20-13). On the lateral side the popliteus muscle is visualized as it extends upward and laterally at an approximate angle of 45 degrees (Fig. 20-8, *A* and *B*). The popliteus tendon crosses the posterior horn of the lateral meniscus posterolaterally, also at an approximate angle of 45 degrees, to reach its attachment on the lateral femoral condyle. The medial portion of the popliteus muscle attaches to the posterior surface of the lateral meniscus. The lateral portion, which forms the popliteus tendon, penetrates the joint capsule and interposes itself between the capsule and the posterolateral aspect of the lateral meniscus. There is often a groove on the posterior surface of the meniscus for the popliteus tendon. A synovial prolongation extends inferiorly through the opening in the joint capsule and lies between the tendon and the joint capsule. It also extends superiorly and lies between the tendon and the lateral surface of the lateral femoral condyle. The synovial membrane surrounding the popliteus tendon causes an oblique linear area of medium signal intensity on spin density images, and high signal on T2-WI views (Fig. 20-8, *A* to *D*). This line crosses on the posterolateral aspect of the posterior horn of the lateral meniscus with an approximate angle of 45 degrees inferiorly to superiorly and medially to laterally. There is often a small amount of fluid present in the synovial prolongation surrounding the popliteus tendon (subpopliteal bursa), which is clearly identified on T2-WI. In some patients there is a communication between this synovial prolongation and the superior tibiofibular articulation.[21,22]

The attachments of the posterior horns of both menisci to the tibia (central attachments) (Figs. 20-8, *E,* 20-11, and 20-22, *A*) are often well seen on coronal views. The medial meniscus is attached to the tibia just anterior to the PCL. The attachment of the lateral meniscus is anterior to that of the medial meniscus (Fig. 20-11). The PCL, likewise, is well visualized on the coronal views. The meniscofemoral ligament of Wrisberg (Figs. 20-13, *B,* and 20-14) and, occasionally, the ligament of Humphrey are also well seen.

Coronal views in the midportion of the knee joint best show the bodies of both menisci (Figs. 20-21 and 20-26, *B* and *C*), each with a triangular configuration. The body of the lateral meniscus often is a little larger than that of the medial (Fig. 20-26, *B* and *C*). On the lateral side the capsule is a millimeter or so thick. On the medial side, because of reinforcement of the capsule by the TCL, the capsuloligamentous complex is about 2 to 4 mm thick at the midcoronal plane of the knee, for approximately 20 mm anteroposteriorly. The medial meniscus is seen to be attached to the inner surface of the capsuloligamentous complex. A very thin bursa or, more commonly, a minimal amount of fat may be seen interposed between the medial meniscus and the capsule (Figs. 20-21 and 20-26, *C*). More anteriorly the anterior horn of the lateral meniscus is seen to curve inward toward its insertion on bone (Figs. 20-8, *G* and *H,* and 20-27, *A*). The anterior portion of the body of the medial meniscus is seen on these coronal images. It is quite small (Figs. 20-26, *E,* and 20-27, *A*), in some patients no more than 3 to 4 mm wide and thick. Coronal slices that go through the free margin of the anterior horn of the lateral meniscus, the portion that is almost in the coronal plane, show a thin band of meniscal tissue (Fig. 20-27, *A*). One or two slices more anteriorly the central attachment and the true size (thickness) of the anterior horn of the lateral meniscus are shown. Further anteriorly the plane of the image is anterior to the anterior horn of the lateral meniscus but still shows the anterior horn of the medial meniscus (Fig. 20-27, *B*), because of its significantly more anterior extension. Still further anteriorly the transverse ligament is visualized (Fig. 20-23), and even further the attach-

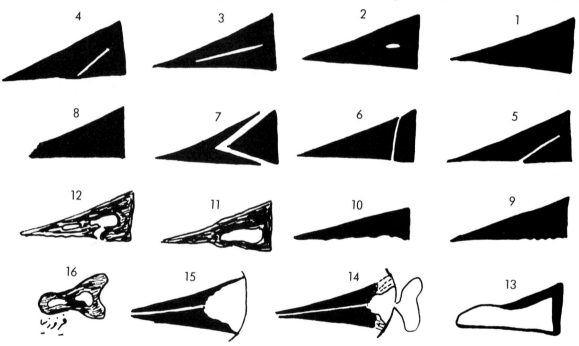

FIGURE 20-43

Meniscal tears. *1,* Normal; *2,* focal zone of increased SI, commonly seen in adults; *3,* intrasubstance, closed tear (the line of increased signal does not communicate with the articular surfaces of the meniscus); *4,* intrasubstance tear reaching just beneath the inferior articular surface of the meniscus, but not quite penetrating through it (there is a focal area of irregularity on the inferior articular surface at the point where the intrasubstance tear approaches the articular surface); *5,* partial thickness oblique/horizontal tear communicating with the inferior articular surface; *6,* full-thickness peripheral vertical tear (when this type runs along a significant portion of the meniscus, it will produce a bucket handle tear); *7,* in this form of bucket handle tear, when the handle of the bucket is displaced into the intercondylar fossa, the capsular remnant may be mistaken for a normal meniscus; *8,* amputation of the free margin; *9,* degenerative disease causing erosion of the inferior articular surface of the meniscus (note that the meniscus is slightly thinner than normal); *10,* far advanced degenerative erosion of the inferior articular surface (a horizontal tear with displacement of the undersurface of the meniscus will produce a similar configuration); *11,* advanced degenerative disease, with diffuse nonhomogeneity of signal and irregularity of the articular surfaces of the menisci; *12,* advanced degenerative disease with a tear extending to the inferior articular surface; *13,* most of the substance of the meniscus is replaced by degenerative tissue, causing cystic expansion and deformity; only a thin shell of meniscal tissue remains; *14,* horizontal cleavage tear of the medial meniscus with intra- and parameniscal cysts; *15,* horizontal tear of the lateral meniscus with an intrameniscal/parameniscal cyst; *16,* far advanced degenerative disease, causing marked deformity of the meniscus (there are two microcysts in the substance of the meniscus).

ment of the anterior horn of the medial meniscus to the tibia may be noted.

Signal characteristics of normal knee structures

The signal characteristics of various components of the knee are dependent upon their composition. The menisci, joint capsule, collateral ligaments, quadriceps tendon, patellar tendon, and cortical bone all appear essentially as zones of signal void (i.e., black on all pulse sequences) (Fig. 20-8). The hyaline articular cartilage has low to intermediate signal on T1-WI (Fig. 20-10, *C*) and intermediate to high signal on SD, T2-WI, and T2* (Fig. 20-10, *B* and *D*). The synovial fluid is of low signal on T1-WI (Fig. 20-10, *C*) but high signal on T2-WI and T2* (Figs. 20-10, *C*, and 20-41). As elsewhere in the body, the signal intensity of the bone marrow is dependent upon the age of the individual. In children the epiphyses have relatively high signal on T1-WI and intermediate to high signal on T2-WI, because of the high fat content of the marrow. The metaphyses, on the other hand, may have significantly lower signal intensity because of the larger fraction of red marrow and nonfatty elements in this age group. In older individuals the marrow of the epiphyses and metaphyses may be identical in signal intensity, exhibiting high signal intensity on T1-WI and intermediate to high signal on T2-WI. In many individuals multiple zones of low signal on T1-WI are noted in the marrow of the distal femur and proximal tibia. These presumably represent remnants of red marrow or reconversion of the yellow marrow to red marrow.

Signal characteristics of normal menisci

The avascular portions of the menisci appear as an area of signal void on all pulse sequences. The peripheral vascular zones are of low to medium SI on T1-WI (Figs. 20-10, *A*, and 20-25, *B*) and SD, and of medium to fairly high SI on T2* images (Figs. 20-10, *B*, and 20-41). A normal meniscus in a child often is homogeneously black. However, with increasing age, and particularly when imaging is done on a high-field magnet, multiple focal but indistinct areas of medium to high SI may normally be visualized in the vascular and avascular segments of the menisci on T1-WI and SD. In a significant number of asymptomatic adults, indistinct focal areas of increased SI (on T1-WI and SD) are seen in the avascular portions of the posterior horns of the menisci, particularly on the medial side (Fig. 20-43). These probably represent minute zones of degeneration, although definitive proof is not yet available. In children, and less commonly in adults, one may see distinct focal zones of brightness in the peripheral portion of the body of the medial meniscus. These most likely represent venous and arterial channels visualized end-on. On the lateral side the inferior geniculate veins run in the peripheral margin of the anterior horn and anterior portion of the body of the meniscus (Fig. 20-44) and are fairly constantly visualized on MRI.

MRI OF ABNORMAL MENISCI
SIGNAL CHARACTERISTICS

With increasing age there is a definite increase in the prevalence of zones of increased SI in the menisci. In our experience the zones of increased SI have been present in the posterior horn and posterior aspect of the body of the medial meniscus (in absence of other signs of degenerative disease or a traumatic tear) in some 32% of individuals 30 years of age or older. Some of these zones of increased SI in the posterior horn of the medial meniscus may be due to an intrameniscal area of condensation or ligamentlike modification of the substance of the menis-

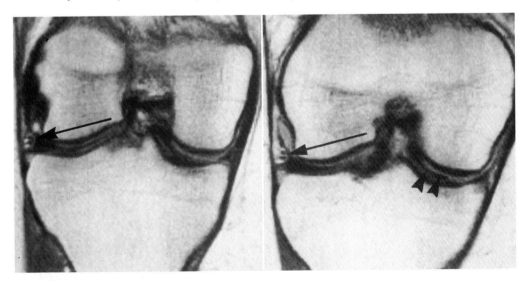

FIGURE 20-44
Normal lateral meniscus. Coronal spin density views. The *arrow* points to venous channels in the peripheral segment of the meniscus. This patient has a bucket handle tear of the medial meniscus that extends into the anterior horn. The anterior horn is detached from the remainder of the medial meniscus and displaced *(arrowheads).*

cus. The great majority of them, however, are produced by focal areas of degeneration.

• • •

Meniscal tears have traditionally been divided into two categories: traumatic and degenerative.

TRAUMATIC MENISCAL TEARS

Traumatic tears typically occur in children and young adults and are characteristically longitudinal (i.e., they extend anteroposteriorly along the length of the meniscus). They may be localized to one segment of the meniscus, usually the posterior horn, less commonly the body, or the anterior horn. The plane of a tear is generally oblique superiorly to inferiorly, posteriorly to anteriorly, and from without inward. This results in the typical oblique/vertical tear so commonly seen extending from the superior to the inferior surface of the meniscus and pointing in the direction of the midportion of the joint (Fig. 20-45). A longitudinal tear is produced when the femoral condyle compresses the meniscus superiorly to inferiorly, posteriorly to anteriorly, and from without inward (Fig. 20-46).

In children the articular cartilage and menisci are thick, soft, and elastic and can absorb sideways strain. Consequently, this common strain does not readily cause a tear of the menisci. However, in maturity and several years thereafter the liability to longitudinal tears becomes maximal, because the cartilage and meniscus have lost their relative increased thickness and elasticity. Conse-

quently, a longitudinal tear is produced precisely along the direction of the force exerted on the meniscus (i.e., superior to inferior, posterior to anterior, and from without inward) (Fig. 20-46). The advance of the aging process in both articular cartilage and meniscus causes a progressively increasing liability to horizontal cleavage tears.[67]

Capsulomeniscal injuries

Because the meniscus is attached to the capsule, the capsulomeniscal junction comes under remarkable stresses when the meniscus is forced forward and inward (Fig. 20-46). The capsulomeniscal junction is pulled inward, stretched, and elongated by microtears or a full-thickness tear.[56,57] Under these circumstances the meniscus can be more easily pushed forward and inward and thus is more easily and frequently torn. The important point to realize is that capsulomeniscal injury is a common problem, in fact more so than tears of the meniscus. Capsulomeniscal injury often precedes the meniscal tear and, for a time, may be the only abnormality present.

Classification of traumatic tears

Longitudinal tears can be classified as extraperipheral (capsulomeniscal) and peripheral[68] (Fig. 20-45). A longitudinal tear may be segmental (usually limited to the posterior horn) or may extend into the body and the anterior horn. Most are said to be closer to the peripheral margin than to the free margin of the

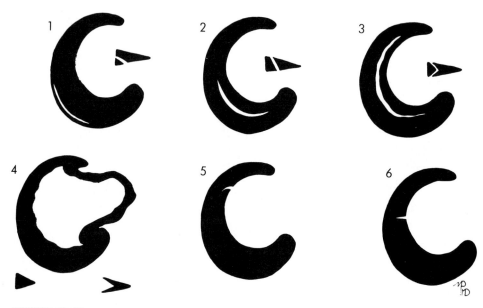

FIGURE 20-45
Meniscal tears. *1,* Extreme peripheral tear separating the inferior segment of the capsular margin of the meniscus; *2,* longitudinal tear within the midportion of the meniscus; *3,* extensive longitudinal tear, bucket handle type (the handle of the bucket is not displaced). (The term "bucket handle" is usually applied to a displaced longitudinal tear.) *4* is a bucket handle tear with displacement of the handle to the middle and anterior portion of the knee joint (in this particular kind of tear the remaining capsular margin, although short and with steeply sloping articular surfaces, may mimic a normal meniscus); *5* is a parrot beak tear, and *6,* a small radial tear of the free margin.

meniscus; hence the designation peripheral tear. However, a significant number are almost in the midportion of the substance of the menisci.

A *bucket handle tear* (Fig. 20-45) extends longitudinally from the posterior to the anterior horn. The peripheral (capsular) segment of the meniscus is the "bucket," and the "handle" the torn inner portion of the meniscus, which is displaced into the intercondylar notch.

An *incomplete (partial-thickness)* tear (Fig. 20-43) is one that has affected only a portion of the superior to inferior thickness of the meniscus. It is commonly seen in the posterior horns of both menisci extending obliquely from a point within the substance of the posterior horn into the inferior articular surface in an anteroposterior direction and from without inward. Eventually such tears are converted to complete tears by repetitive injury.

Isolated longitudinal tears of the anterior horn are uncommon and, when encountered, are usually on the lateral side (and in women).

Longitudinal meniscal tears are traumatic lesions seen in the healthy menisci of youngsters and young adults, although they may also be encountered in older individuals with healthy menisci. They should be differentiated from horizontal tears, which are seen almost exclusively in degenerated menisci and in older individuals, and represent disease of the aging meniscus.[68]

Twisting injuries and locking of the knee. Longitudinal tears of the menisci are preceded by a distinct twisting trauma to the knee. This is followed usually by sudden pain, moderate swelling and locking of the knee.[69] The clinical picture is particularly prominent in the classic cases of bucket handle tears of the menisci. Locking of the knee (i.e., inability to place the knee in full extension) has been shown[69] to be due to the interposition of a segment of the meniscus between the femur and the tibia at a point anterior to the midcoronal plane of the joint. It occurs when a longitudinal tear extends into the anterior meniscal segment.

Locking of the knee in association with a twisting injury is an important diagnostic sign of a torn meniscus. However, it is not always due to a torn meniscus, nor is it universally present in all individuals with a longitudinal tear. Locking occurs in about 24% of patients proven to have a longitudinal tear. Acute locking of the knee may be produced, or simulated by a number of conditions, including intraarticular bodies, tear of the ACL, and hematoma in the anterior peripheral attachment of the menisci.[69]

In young individuals, particularly during the first injury, the displaced handle of a bucket handle tear may immediately return to its normal position. In subsequent injuries it may not return to its normal position immediately. When the displaced fragment stays in the intercondylar notch for an extended time, it may compress and distort the anterior cruciate ligament or lead to its rupture.[67]

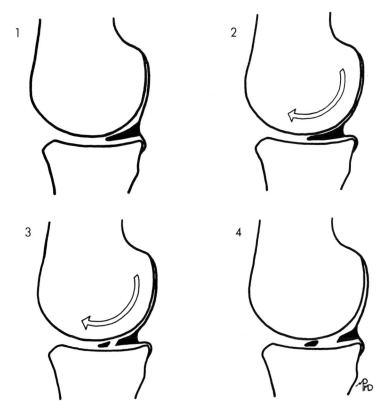

FIGURE 20-46
Biomechanics of meniscal injury. *1*, Normal; *2*, the meniscus and capsule are pulled toward the center of the joint; *3*, an oblique vertical tear extends superiorly to inferiorly and from without inward; *4*, the torn fragment is displaced into the center of the joint, with return of the capsular segment and capsule to normal position. (From Smillie IS. In Smillie IS [ed]: Injuries of the knee joint, 5th ed. New York, 1978, Churchill Livingstone, p 79.)

MR findings in traumatic tears of the menisci
EXTRAPERIPHERAL MENISCAL, CAPSULOMENISCAL, AND CAPSULAR INJURIES

Injury to the most peripheral portion of the meniscus and the capsulomeniscal junction is a common occurrence, its incidence depending upon the type of patients examined at each MRI facility. In a practice dealing with acute as well as chronic knee problems, it may constitute as much as 20% to 25% of all lesions of the knee. It occurs more frequently along the border of the posterior horn and body of the meniscus.

Unless relatively large tears are present, the clinical and imaging diagnosis of capsular and capsulomeniscal injury is difficult. The diagnosis is rarely made on arthrography, except when detachment of the meniscus from the capsule is present or when a complete tear of the capsule permits extravasation of contrast beyond it. MRI has improved our ability significantly in the diagnosis of capsulomeniscal injuries. However, it is likely that a sizable proportion of these injuries still escape detection, given the capabilities of the state-of-the-art MRI imagers in 1991.

A careful histological examination of the peripheral margin of the medial meniscus (on knee specimens) shows this region to be composed of uninterrupted, vascular, and innervated connective tissue contiguous with the capsule. There may be some fat normally between the apex of the posterior horn and the capsule. This ideal state is seen only in children and young adults without any evidence of degeneration or trauma. With advancing age scarring, tissue gaps, and small irregular islands of fat appear in the region. These findings are indicative of multiple episodes of trauma causing small tears of the capsule and capsulomeniscal junction, with

subsequent scarring or persistence of the tear, with or without accumulation of fat. We have no histological experience with knee specimens with an acute tear of this region. However, it is probably safe to assume that an acute tear may show zones of tissue disruption, bleeding, and granulation tissue formation.

The anatomical arrangement of the lateral side is similar to that of the medial side, except in the posterior horn of the lateral meniscus, where there is interposition of the popliteus tendon between the meniscus and the joint capsule. Our preliminary impression, based on histological examination, is that the incidence of injury to the peripheral portion of the lateral meniscus and capsule is significantly less common than to the medial meniscus and capsule.

CAPSULOMENISCAL INJURIES

The MR diagnosis of microtears in the peripheral portion of the menisci, capsulomeniscal junction, and capsule is difficult. Findings include ill-defined dots or lines of increased SI, irregularities of the border between the vascular and avascular portions of the menisci, and evidence of edema and thickening or irregularity of the capsular outline. These abnormalities, barely visible on T1-WI, are moderately conspicuous on SD. On T2-WI edema/hemorrhage within and in the vicinity of the capsule and the peripheral vascular segment of the menisci is seen as zones of increased SI.

Medial capsulomeniscal injuries. The capsule is about a millimeter or so thick and forms a concave or vertical supporting wall for the posterior horn and the posteromedial segment of the body of the medial meniscus (Fig. 20-28, *A* to *C*). Injuries to this region may cause an incomplete or complete (full-thickness) tear of the cap-

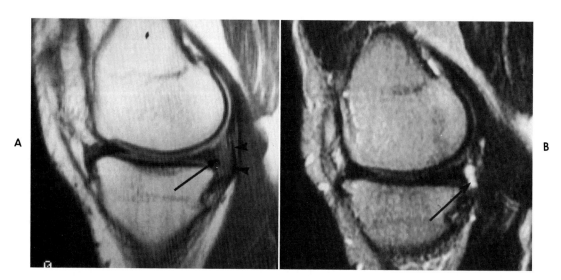

FIGURE 20-47
Detached but not displaced posterior horn of the medial meniscus. **A,** T1-WI and **B,** T2-WI sagittal views. In **A** the capsule is swollen and bulges outward *(arrowheads)*. The *arrow* points to a markedly irregular capsular margin of the posterior horn. In **B,** note the effusion between the meniscus and capsule *(arrow)*, indicating detachment of the meniscus from the capsule. The meniscus is not displaced inward.

sule (Figs. 20-35, *A* and *B* and *F* to *H,* and 20-47 to 20-52), partial or complete detachment of the meniscus from the capsule (Figs. 20-47, *B,* 20-50, and 20-51), or a tear of the meniscus itself (Fig. 20-53).

Incomplete (intrasubstance) tears of the capsule lead to bleeding and edema within it, which cause it to become thickened and to protrude outward (Figs. 20-35, *F* to *H,* 20-47, *A,* and 20-49, *B*). The tears of the meniscocapsular junction also lead to bleeding and edema and, unlike tears of the nonvascular segment of the meniscus, may not be visualized as linear areas of increased SI (Figs. 20-35, *B* and *E* to *H,* and 20-52) on T1-WI and SD. Thus these lesions may go undetected if no other pulse sequence is used. On T2-WI and gradient echo T2* images most of the lesions are visualized as regions of markedly increased SI due to accumulation of fluid within them. When there is a complete tear of the capsule, T2-WI images usually show extension of fluid through the substance of the capsule to a point beyond it.

One must be cautious, however, in making a diagnosis of capsular and capsulomeniscal injury on gradient echo images (Fig. 20-41), without confirmation of the findings on T2-WI. Gradient echo images may exaggerate the apparent abnormalities of this region and lead to false-positive diagnoses.

Detachment of the posterior horn of the medial meniscus. The posterior horn and body of the medial meniscus are more fixed in position than the corresponding parts of the lateral meniscus and have a fairly constant relationship to the articular margin of the tibia. Thus, on anatomical sagittal views the boundary between the avascular and vascular segments of the posterior horn normally is within 2 to 4 mm of the posterior edge of the tibial plateau (Fig. 20-25, *A* to *C* and *E*).

When there is stretching, a microtear, or a full-thickness tear (including separation of the meniscus from the capsule), the meniscus may be forced to sit further from the posterior margin of the tibial plateau, and closer to the midportion of the joint. This is an indirect sign of capsulomeniscal injury. In the presence of stretching but no definite tear, there may be no other abnormality. In these cases a definitive diagnosis is difficult. With more extensive injuries (focal tears or partial separation of the meniscus from the capsule) it is often possible to identify

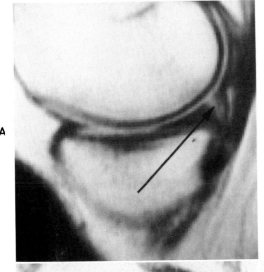

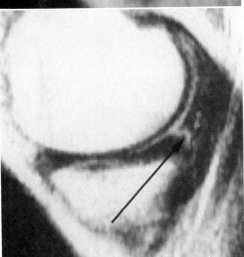

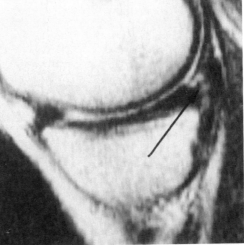

FIGURE 20-48
Capsulomeniscal junction tear, posterior horn of the medial meniscus. **A,** A T1-WI anatomical sagittal and, **B** and **C,** T2-WI oblique sagittal views. The *arrow* in all images points to the disruption of the capsulomeniscal junction.

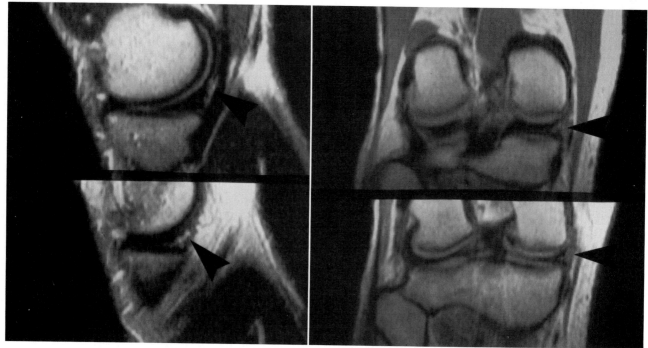

FIGURE 20-49

Tear of the capsulomeniscal junction and peripheral margin of the medial meniscus. A, T2-WI sagittal, and B, spin density coronal. In A the *arrowheads* point to an irregular area of increased SI due to tearing of the capsulomeniscal junction. B, The *arrowheads* show the swollen outwardly convex capsule of the posteromedial region. A normal capsule here would be straight or concave toward the central portion of the knee. Note the increased SI and tearing of the peripheral margin of the posterior horn.

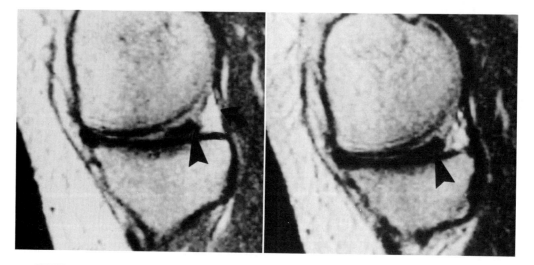

FIGURE 20-50

Tear at the capsulomeniscal junction. T2-WI sagittals. The posterior horn of the medial meniscus *(arrowhead)* is displaced away from the capsule *(curved arrow)*. High–signal intensity fluid occupies the space between the capsule and the meniscus. Note the increased distance between the capsule and posterior margin of the tibial plateau and the meniscus.

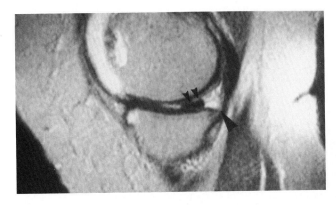

FIGURE 20-51

Detachment of the posterior horn of the medial meniscus from the capsule. T2-WI anatomical sagittal view. The *small arrowheads* point to the posterior horn, which is displaced anteriorly. The meniscus has markedly irregular outline due to degenerative disease. The *large arrowhead* points to the capsule and posterior edge of the medial tibial plateau. The space between the meniscus and the capsule is filled with effusion.

irregularity, nonhomogeneity, and abnormal zones of increased SI, particularly on SD, along with an accumulation of focal zones of fluid on T2-WI at the peripheral margin of the meniscus. With complete separation of the meniscus from the capsule a gap between the two (Figs. 20-50, *A*, and 20-51), containing fluid, is clearly identified on T2-WI or T2*.

Trauma to the tibial collateral ligament. Sprain of the TCL is quite common. On MRI, the ligament is thicker and has slightly increased internal signal due to intraligamentous edema. Fluid may be noted on both sides of it (Figs. 20-54 and 20-55). These findings are particularly evident on SD and T2-WI. Instrasubstance tears are seen as fairly irregular zones of fluid accumulation within the ligament (Fig. 20-54, *C* and *D*). Partial tears are diagnosed when a definite plane of abnormal increased SI is identified in the substance of the ligament, extending to the superficial or deep surface. With complete tears the ligament is discontinuous and fluid extends beyond the margin of it.[35,36,38]

A Grade I sprain consists of minimal intrasubstance tears and edema surrounding the ligament. A Grade II sprain shows moderate intrasubstance tears or an incom-

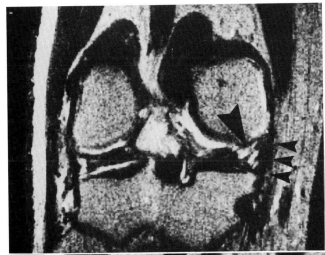

A

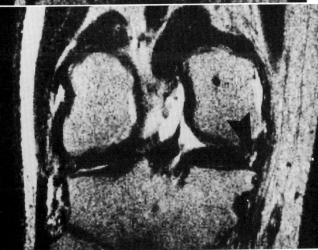

B

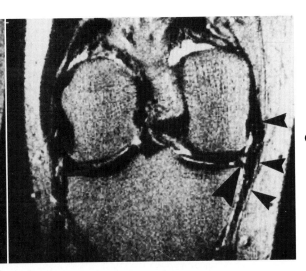

C

FIGURE 20-52

A thickened and torn capsule with a tear of the capsulomeniscal junction of the posterior horn and body of the medial meniscus. Coronal T2-WI. **A,** The *large arrowhead* points to the capsule and capsulomeniscal junction. The *small arrowheads* point to the thickened capsule, which is bulging outward. In this region the capsule normally is only a millimeter or so thick and often concave toward the middle of the joint. **B,** The *arrowhead* points to the tear at the capsulomeniscal junction and capsular margin of the meniscus. The capsule is thick. **C,** The *large arrowhead* points to the tear. Note also a small tear of the inferior articular surface. The *small arrowheads* point to the thickened and outwardly displaced capsule-TCL complex.

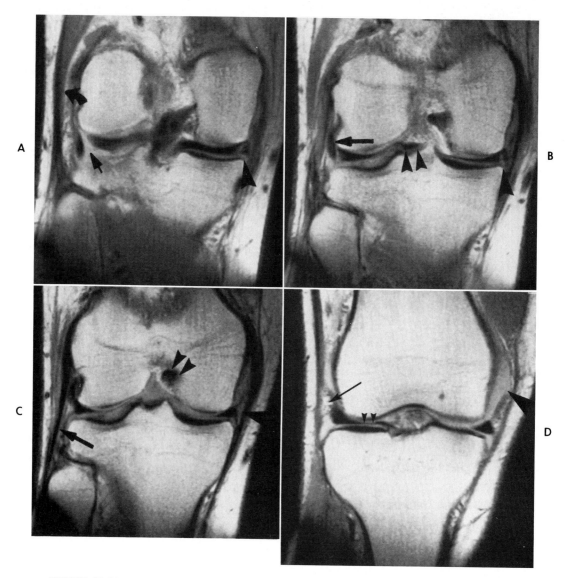

FIGURE 20-53

Peripheral tear of the medial meniscus. Spin density coronal views. **A,** The *arrowhead* points to a vertical tear in the posterior horn of the meniscus. Note the capsular thickening. The *curved arrow* points to the biceps femoris, the *arrow* to increased SI because of synovial tissue surrounding the popliteus tendon. **B,** The *large arrowhead* points to the vertical peripheral tear. The capsule is displaced away from the medial compartment. *Two arrowheads* point to the central attachment of the posterior horn of the lateral meniscus, the *arrow* to the popliteus tendon. **C,** The *large arrowhead* marks detachment of the medial meniscus from the TCL-capsule complex. The *two smaller arrowheads* point to the attachment of the PCL to the medial femoral condyle. The *arrow* points to the FCL. **D,** The *large arrowhead* shows distention of the medial aspect of the suprapatellar bursa by effusion. The *arrow* points to the inferior genicular vessels, the *two small arrowheads* to the inner margin of the anterior horn of the lateral meniscus just proximal to its central attachment.

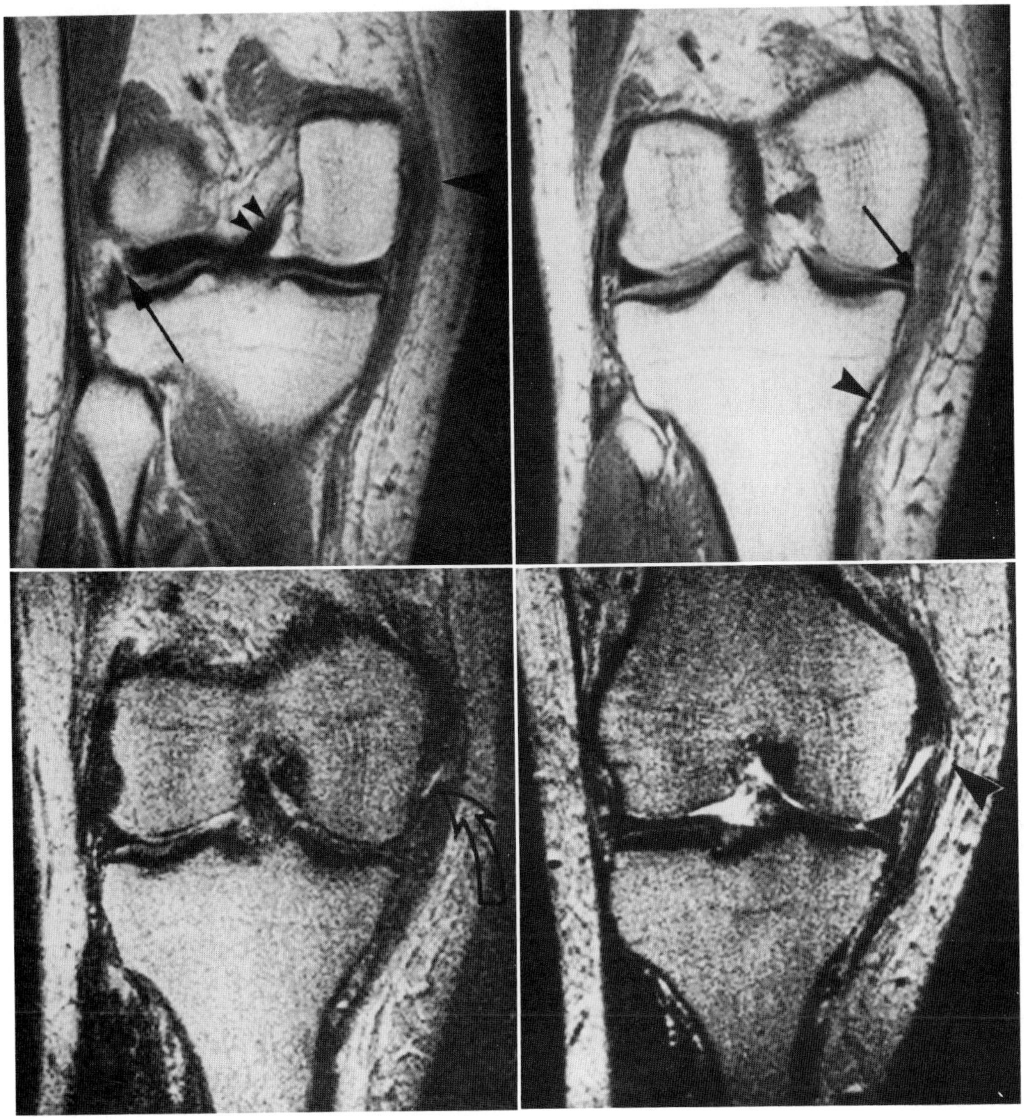

FIGURE 20-54

Thickening and tear of the TCL. **A** and **B**, Proton density and, **C** and **D**, T2-WI coronal images of the knee. There is severe thickening of the capsule-TCL complex. **A**, Marked thickening of the complex *(large arrowhead)*. *Two small arrowheads* point to the normal PCL, the *arrow* to the normal line of lucency produced by the synovial investment of the popliteus tendon as it crosses on the posterolateral surface of the lateral meniscus. **B**, The *arrow* points to the normal area of increased SI in the midcoronal plane of the knee between the body of the medial meniscus and the capsule-TCL complex *(arrowhead)*. It is slightly exaggerated in this patient. An area of high SI is due to the presence of a small bursa or minimal fat in this region. Note the distal attachment of the TCL to the tibia. Normally there is a small amount of fat here (through which small venous channels extend) between the cortex of the tibia and the TCL. This should not be mistaken for stripping of the TCL from bone. **C**, Further anteriorly. The *curved arrow* points to a line of increased SI due to accumulation of fluid in an incomplete intrasubstance tear of the TCL. **D**, Still further anteriorly. Note the more extensive tears of the TCL *(arrowhead)*. In patients with distention of the suprapatellar bursa, the posterior aspect of the distended bursa may cause a line of increased SI in this region that could be mistaken for a tear. In this patient there was no effusion in the bursa.

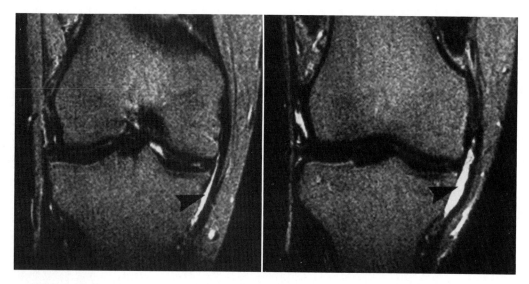

FIGURE 20-55
Tear and stripping of the capsuloligamentous complex from the medial meniscus and tibia. T2-WI coronal views show effusion dissecting between the TCL and bone *(arrowhead)*. The medial meniscus and ACL were also torn in this patient.

plete tear and extensive edema. A Grade III sprain is diagnosed when a complete tear is present.

Injury to the medial compartment and TCL may be accompanied by rupture of the coronary ligament, separation of the meniscus from the capsuloligamentous complex, peripheral tear of the meniscus, and stripping of the ligament from its attachment to the femur or the medial surface of the tibial condyle (Fig. 20-55). The last abnormality is diagnosed when fluid can be seen dissecting between the TCL and tibia on T2-WI. With severe injuries the ligament may be completely separated from its femoral or tibial attachments. A large amount of hemorrhagic fluid may dissect on the medial side between the bone and the displaced and torn capsuloligamentous complex. Hemorrhagic edema may also be noted in the subcutaneous tissues.

Long-standing and repetitive injury to the ligament can occur secondary to athletic overuse and abuse of the knee. In these individuals there is marked thickening of the ligament, which is seen as a band of soft tissue with low SI on all pulse sequences. A normal TCL is about 2 to 4 mm thick in the midcoronal plane of the knee (Fig. 20-28). In the absence of acute trauma, there should be no increased diffuse internal SI or distinct zones of increased SI on T2-WI to signify the presence of edema or microtears. There may be a thin layer of fat between the superficial and deep layers of the ligament (Fig. 20-28, *G*), evident as a fine line of increased SI on T1-WI but losing some of its SI on T2-WI, as is expected for fat. Intraligamentous hemorrhage/edema, on the other hand, becomes of higher SI on T2-WI (Fig. 20-54).

In many patients there may be calcification of the ligament, particularly at its attachment on the femoral condyle. Hypertrophic changes of the cortex of the medial femoral condyle may also be present.

Thickening of the TCL also occurs consequent to degenerative disease of the medial compartment and may be associated with marginal joint osteophytes and partial or complete extrusion of the body and anterior horn of the medial meniscus beyond the margins of the medial compartment. There may be associated bursitis of the TCL in these patients.

Tibial collateral ligament bursitis. Several bursae are associated with the medial capsuloligamentous complex,[35,37,38,70,71] and any one can be affected by injury to the medial aspect of the knee.

Distention of the TCL bursae may occur in the following conditions:

1. Bursitis (i.e., isolated inflammatory bursitis [uncommon])
2. Trauma to the medial aspect of the joint with, or without, associated tear or swelling of the TCL
3. Capsulomeniscal injury with microtears or a complete tear of the capsuloligamentous complex, usually with detachment of the meniscus from the capsule and injury to the medial compartment, with or without medial meniscal tears
4. Degenerative arthritis of the medial compartment with articular margin osteophytes and partial or complete extrusion of the medial meniscus

Isolated TCL bursitis should be diagnosed when there is accumulation of fluid in the bursa, best identified on T2-WI or T2* images. The fluid in the bursa should be isointense with joint effusion. The outline of the fluid collection should be smooth, typically only a few millimeters in width, but possibly 1 or 2 cm long (superiorly to inferiorly) (Fig. 20-56). The TCL should be visualized as a black band, 2 to 3 mm thick, extending from the femur to the tibia on the outer surface of the cyst. Isolated TCL bursitis is unrelated to meniscal and meniscocapsu-

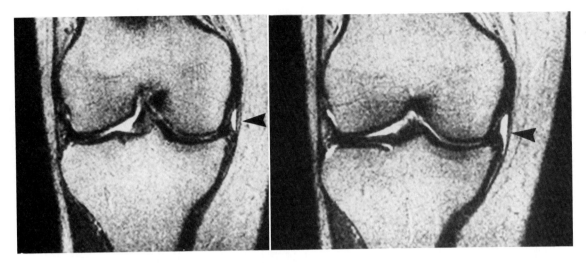

FIGURE 20-56
TCL bursitis. Coronal T2-WI views. The *arrowhead* points to the distended bursa.

lar injury. Its diagnosis therefore can and should be made in the absence of these lesions. However, because the abnormalities of the medial compartment and medial meniscus are common in adults, it may be impossible to tell whether the pathology of the medial compartment is, or is not, the cause of the TCL bursitis.

In some individuals a bursa is interposed between the TCL and its proximal tibial insertion. Following injury to the medial compartment and rupture of the coronary ligament, the medial compartment ruptures into this bursa and fills it with hemorrhagic effusion. The presence of the bursa is strongly suspected when a distinct, smooth, slender, elliptical cavity containing fluid, straddling the joint line and beneath the TCL, is identified.

Injury to the medial side of the knee is more frequently accompanied by tearing and stripping of the TCL from the tibia than by traumatic bursitis. The former cause dissection of hemorrhagic fluid between the medial surface of the tibia and the torn displaced TCL (Fig. 20-55). The irregular outline of the fluid collection should be contrasted with the less common TCL bursal distention, in which the outline of the fluid-filled cavity is smooth and distinct.

Pes anserinus bursitis. Pes anserinus bursitis (Fig. 20-36) is diagnosed when a fluid-containing distended bursa is seen at or anterior to the midcoronal plane of the knee, usually well below the joint line but superficial to the distal portion of the TCL. In most instances it is readily identified because of its characteristic location. Only rarely does the bursa become sufficiently large to extend superiorly and posteriorly and be confused with TCL bursitis.

Injuries to the anterior segment of the anterior horn of the medial meniscus and the joint capsule are less common. When encountered, however, they have MRI findings similar to those of the posterior horn region.

Lateral capsulomeniscal injuries. Injuries to the capsulomeniscal junction of the posterior horn of the lateral

meniscus are also common. However, a definitive diagnosis is difficult because the visualization of the meniscal fasicles is not routinely achieved (in 1991) even on high-resolution thin section (3 mm) images generated on state-of-the-art MR imagers. These tears are usually better seen on T2-WI, or T2*, than on other pulse sequences. Traumatic injuries of the peripheral margin of the body and anterior horn of the lateral meniscus are less common. The vascular capsular margin of the lateral meniscus is not as broad as the corresponding segment of the medial meniscus, and consequently its traumatic lesions are not usually isolated (being accompanied often by tears of the body and anterior horn).

Tears of the FCL and lateral joint capsule are usually secondary to serious injuries, such as a high-velocity varus force. They may involve the fasciculi of the posterior horn of the lateral meniscus, FCL, biceps femoris, popliteus tendon, and iliotibial band. The peroneal nerve may also be injured, resulting in long-term disability.[72] Serious injuries of the lateral capsuloligamentous complex are often associated with tears of the ACL and PCL.[40,73] Avulsion fractures of the fibula, Gerdy's tubercle, or a Segond fracture (lateral capsular sign)[40,71-76] may also be present.

The MRI findings depend upon the extent and nature of the injury. There is usually considerable bleeding into the soft tissues with edema (Fig. 20-57) and disruption of various ligamentous structures, which exhibit zones of increased SI on T2-WI and T2* at the sites of disruption and tearing.

Traumatic tears of the avascular portion of the meniscus

Tears of the menisci usually present as linear areas of increased SI communicating with one or both articular surfaces. Lotysch et al., Crues et al., and Mink et al.[77-81] have proposed a grading system for evaluating signal abnormalities of the menisci. The system is based on the

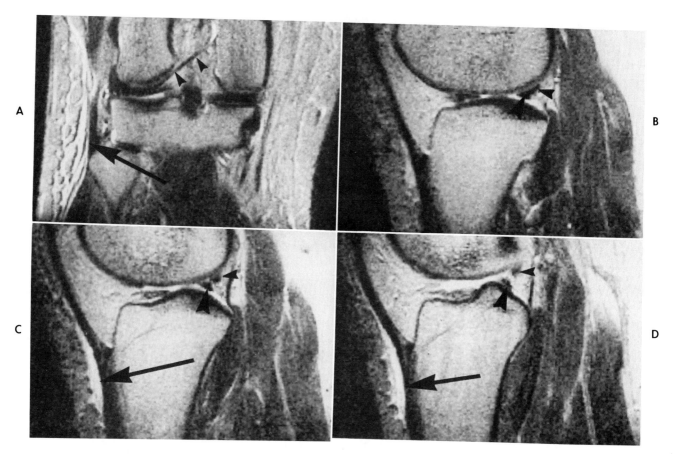

FIGURE 20-57

A, Coronal and, B to D, sagittal T2-WI. In A the *arrow* points to the hemorrhage/edema in the subcutaneous tissues outside the biceps femoris and FCL. The *arrowheads* point to the ligament of Wrisberg. In B to D the *large arrowhead* points to the inner portion of the posterior horn of lateral meniscus. The *small arrowhead* points to the ligament of Wrisberg. The takeoff of the ligament, visible in B, moves superiorly and medially. The *arrow* in C and D points to hemorrhage/edema anterior to the patellar tendon at its insertion on the tibial tuberosity. The tendon itself is normal.

morphology of the intrameniscal signal and its relationship to the articular meniscal surfaces. The articular surfaces are the superior and inferior meniscal surfaces. The capsular margin is not an articular surface. The free margin has an importance identical to that of the articular surfaces. Stoller et al.[82] compared this grading system to pathological findings in 12 menisci obtained from fresh cadavers and above-the-knee amputations. The classification of the intrameniscal signal, originally described by Mink, Reicher, and Crues,[77] is as follows:

Grade 1: a focal zone of increased SI that is not adjacent to either the superior or the inferior articular meniscal surfaces: a grade 1 signal abnormality corresponds to a stage 1 histological classification of degeneration, in which the menisci show foci of mucinous, hyaline, or myxoid degeneration in areas of hypocellularity[77]

Grade 2: primarily a linear area of increased SI that does not extend to an articular surface; typically, however, it does abut the capsular margin; this abnormality corresponds to a stage 2 histological classification, in which more extensive bands of mucinous degeneration border

hypocellular regions of the meniscus; although no distinct fibrocartilaginous separation is observed in this stage, microscopic areas of collagen fragmentation are present[77]

The middle perforating collagen bundles are fibers that horizontally divide the meniscus into superior and inferior portions and are said not to be visualized by MRI in normal menisci.[77] This statement is most likely correct in the great majority of the cases; however, we have seen two histologically documented cases in which a linear area of increased SI was present in normal menisci in this region (in the absence of degeneration or a tear). This region is a preferred location for increased accumulation of mucopolysaccharide ground substance.[77]

Grade 3: zones of increased SI that reach one or both meniscal articular surfaces; a grade 3 signal abnormality has been further subdivided into grade 3A (which consists of a smooth linear intrameniscal signal communicating with an articular surface) and grade 3B (in which the signal abnormality has an irregular outline);

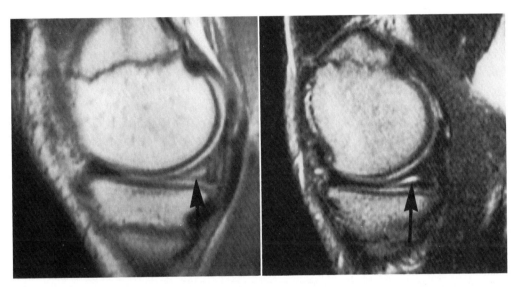

FIGURE 20-58
Horizontal tear running into the inferior articular surface, posterior horn, medial meniscus. **A,** T1-WI and, **B,** T2-WI sagittal views. The *arrow* points to the tear. Note the increased SI fluid within the tear (in **B**). The *arrowhead* marks joint effusion.

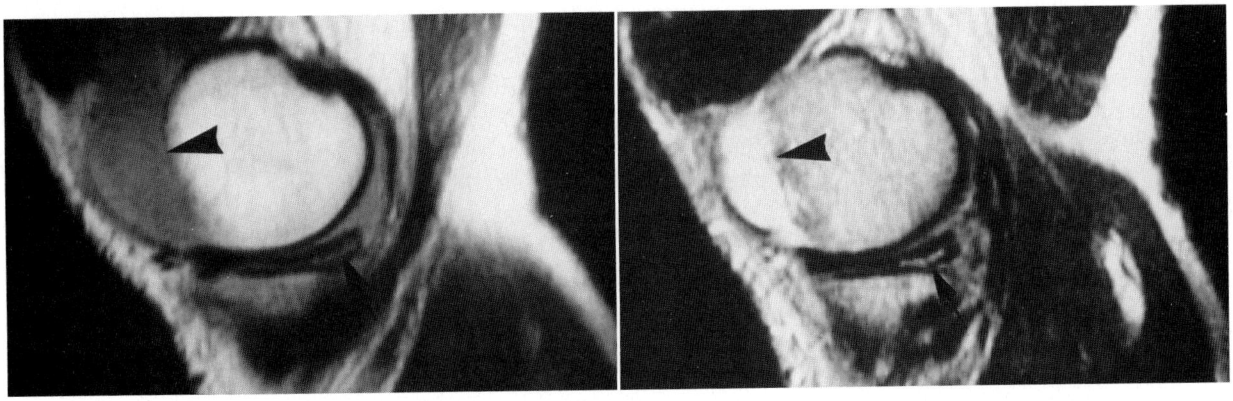

FIGURE 20-59
Tear, medial meniscus. Sagittal T1-WI and T2-WI. When there is fluid within a tear, it is often better delineated on T2-WI, as in this surgically documented tear of the posterior horn *(arrow).*

both grade 3A and grade 3B are associated with stage 3 degeneration of the menisci, showing a tear within the fibrocartilaginous meniscus, with or without grossly visible surface extension; grade 3B lesions are associated with more extensive degenerative change in the surrounding meniscus[77]

Accumulated experience with a large number of MRI examinations, correlated with findings at arthroscopy, has shown the usefulness of this system and its high negative predictive value.

This grading system and the contributions of other investigators[83,84] have helped to elucidate the MRI manifestations of various meniscal pathologies. Nevertheless, considerable confusion still exists regarding the significance and relationship of various MRI signal abnormalities to meniscal pathologies. To overcome this problem,

we have chosen not to elaborate on or classify the observed MRI signs in our reports but rather to state directly the probable pathologies they represent (tear, degenerative disease, degenerative tear, effusion).

TEARS

A tear of the meniscus is diagnosed when a linear area of increased SI is noted extending to its articular surfaces or free margin. A tear usually presents as a line of increased SI on T1-WI (Figs. 20-43 and 20-45), often more so on SD and T2* images. It may actually be obscured on T2-WI, owing to its lower SI. However, when there is synovial fluid within the tear (with or without separation of the fragments), the fluid-filled space is revealed as an area of high SI on T2-WI (Figs. 20-58 and 20-59). The T2-weighted images are also helpful in identification of an amputated free margin, a displaced torn meniscal fragment, or an intrameniscal/parameniscal cyst.

A true traumatic tear, at least in its early phases, usually has well-defined margins (i.e., the line of increased SI is distinct and sharp, often obliquely extending superiorly to inferiorly and from without inward [Fig. 20-45]). As the tear gets older, its margins become indistinct and irregular. The tear becomes wider and more extensive. The process of meniscal degeneration (Fig. 20-60) is accelerated, sometimes very significantly. Degenerative microcysts may appear, and the tear becomes more complex and extensive.

A linear area of increased SI that communicates with the free margin of the meniscus is also a complete and true tear of the meniscus.

Closed tear. An intrasubstance tear (closed tear)[68] (Fig. 20-43) is diagnosed when a plane of increased SI is noted within the meniscus but without actually reaching the articular surfaces or the free margin of it. To qualify as a plane, the zone of increased SI must be visualized on at least two (preferably more) sagittal or coronal views. Often a plane of increased SI extends to a point just beneath the articular surface, but does not actually penetrate it. There may be a focal area of deformity (e.g., a small bump, at the intersection of the plane of SI and the meniscal articular surface). Sometimes there is a step-off configuration in this region. These findings indicate that the meniscal substance has been divided in two segments, one above and one below the plane of the tear, albeit still confined within the most superficial layer of the substance of the meniscus (which acts as a capsule or retaining shell).

Bucket handle tear. In patients with a bucket handle tear (Figs. 20-61 to 20-66) the inner portion of the meniscus (the handle of the bucket) is displaced into the

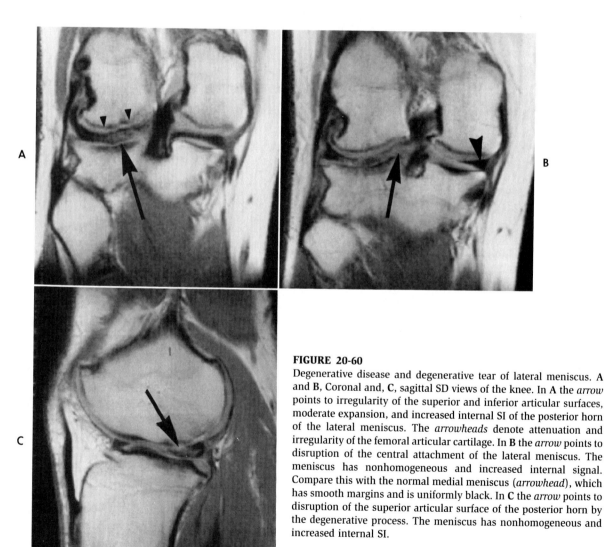

FIGURE 20-60
Degenerative disease and degenerative tear of lateral meniscus. A and B, Coronal and, C, sagittal SD views of the knee. In A the *arrow* points to irregularity of the superior and inferior articular surfaces, moderate expansion, and increased internal SI of the posterior horn of the lateral meniscus. The *arrowheads* denote attenuation and irregularity of the femoral articular cartilage. In B the *arrow* points to disruption of the central attachment of the lateral meniscus. The meniscus has nonhomogeneous and increased internal signal. Compare this with the normal medial meniscus (*arrowhead*), which has smooth margins and is uniformly black. In C the *arrow* points to disruption of the superior articular surface of the posterior horn by the degenerative process. The meniscus has nonhomogeneous and increased internal SI.

intercondylar notch (Figs. 20-43 and 20-45). The remaining peripheral margin appears irregular and significantly narrower than normal. In some patients the tear is so close to the capsular margin that most of the substance of the meniscus is torn and displaced into the intercondylar notch and only a narrow rim of tissue is left along the capsular margin (Figs. 20-62, *B*, and 20-63, *F*). Occasionally this may mimic a postmeniscectomy status. In some patients the remaining capsular margin is substantial in size and may superficially resemble a normal meniscus (Figs. 20-43 and 20-45). This happens when the planes of the tear are more or less parallel to the articular surfaces of the meniscus. In such situations the inner margin (the site of tearing) of the remaining capsular segment resembles the free margin of a normal meniscus. In some patients remodeling of the remaining capsular segment occurs, causing it to appear somewhat like a normal meniscus. However, a careful examination shows that the

remaining capsular segment is quite fat and significantly narrower from without inward. The articular surfaces have a steep grade in contradistinction to the gently sloping surfaces of a normal meniscus.

The displaced fragment inside the intercondylar fossa is usually jammed against the ACL. A significant portion of it, however, may be forced anteriorly beneath the intercondylar region of the femur. On the sagittal cross sections the displaced fragment may be visualized as a linear band of low signal, more or less in a horizontal or semicircular plane, extending anteroposteriorly, anterior and inferior to the PCL (Figs. 20-62, *E*, 20-63, *D*, 20-64, *B*, and 20-67, *C*). The ACL may be distorted or torn and impossible to identify. There may be multiple irregular low-signal regions in the intercondylar fossa (Figs. 20-61, *C* and *D*, 20-63, *F*, 20-64, *G* and *I*, and 20-67, *B*) and anteriorly along the midsagittal plane on the surface of the tibia beneath (and often continuous) with the ACL

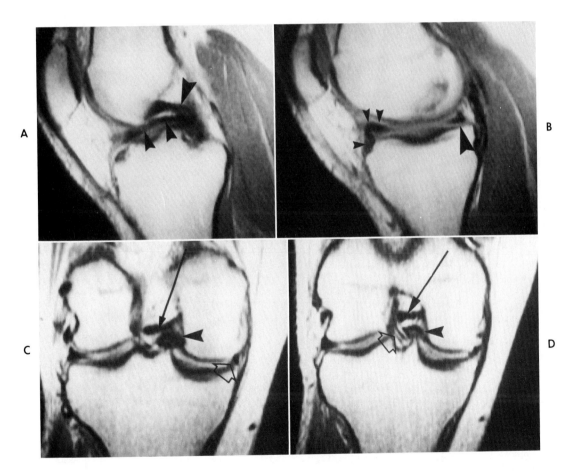

FIGURE 20-61
Extreme peripheral tear of the body of the medial meniscus (bucket handle type) and tear of the posterior horn (displaced into the notch). **A** and **B**, T1-WI anatomical sagittals. The *large arrowhead* in **A** points to the PCL. The *two smaller arrowheads* identify the displaced meniscus in the notch. The *large arrowhead* in **B** denotes a small portion of the posterior horn that remains at the capsular margin. The *single small arrowhead* designates the anterior horn. The *two small arrowheads* point to the displaced torn meniscus superior to the anterior horn. **C** and **D**, SD coronal views. The *arrowhead* points to the torn displaced meniscus in the notch. The *arrow* points to the PCL. The *hollow arrow* in **C** marks the small capsular remnant of the medial meniscus, the *hollow arrow* in **D** to the ACL.

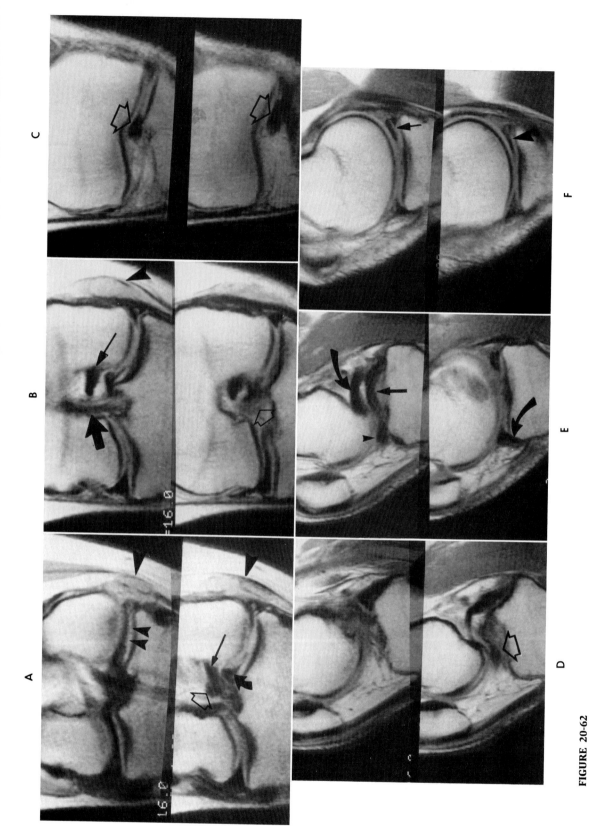

FIGURE 20-62

Bucket handle tear of the medial meniscus and a parameniscal cyst. A to C, Coronal spin density and, D to F, sagittal T1-WI. The *large arrowhead* in A points to the parameniscal cyst, the *two smaller arrowheads* to the tear in the posterior horn. Almost all the inferior aspect of the posterior horn and most of its capsular margin have been displaced. The *curved arrow* points to the posterior horn of the medial meniscus proximal to its central attachment. The *arrow* identifies the PCL. The *hollow arrow* indicates a torn fragment of meniscus displaced into the intercondylar notch. In **B** the *arrowhead* identifies the parameniscal cyst. The *thin arrow* points to the femoral attachment of the PCL, the *big arrow* to the ACL. The *hollow arrow* points out the displaced fragment of torn meniscus. Note that only a small amount of the capsular margin remains in place. In **C** the *hollow arrow* points to the large fragment of bucket handle that has been displaced anteriorly. The *hollow arrow* in **D** indicates a fragment of tear displaced into the intercondylar notch. **E**, The *curved arrow* in the upper image points to the PCL, the *straight arrow* to the handle (displaced into the intercondylar notch). The *arrowhead* identifies a large fragment displaced anteriorly, directly above the anterior horn of the medial meniscus. The *curved arrow* in the lower image points to the superimposition of torn fragment on the anterior horn. **F**, The *arrow* in the *upper image* shows a tear of the posterior horn of the medial meniscus extending into its inferior articular surface, the *arrowhead* in the *lower image* an irregular area of increased SI within the substance of the meniscus and erosion of the inferior articular surface of the posterior horn.

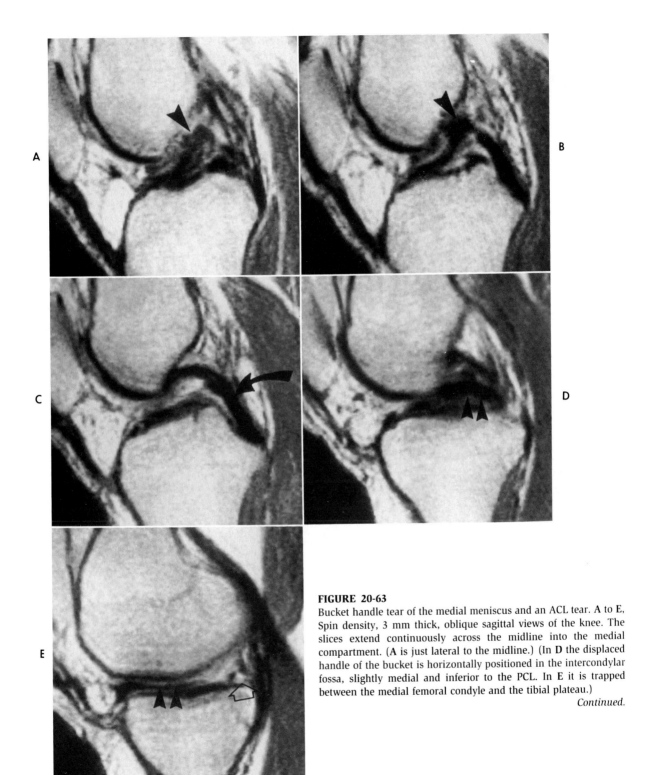

FIGURE 20-63
Bucket handle tear of the medial meniscus and an ACL tear. A to E, Spin density, 3 mm thick, oblique sagittal views of the knee. The slices extend continuously across the midline into the medial compartment. (A is just lateral to the midline.) (In **D** the displaced handle of the bucket is horizontally positioned in the intercondylar fossa, slightly medial and inferior to the PCL. In **E** it is trapped between the medial femoral condyle and the tibial plateau.)

Continued.

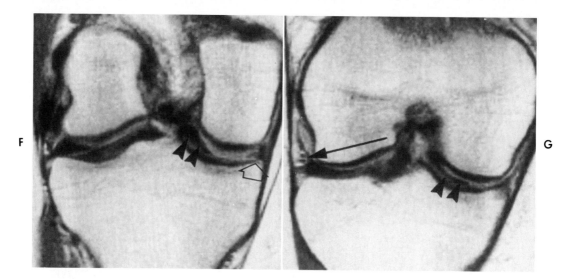

FIGURE 20-63, cont'd

F and G, Spin density coronal cross sections (F just posterior to the midcoronal plane of the knee, G through the anterior horns of the menisci). The *single arrowheads* point to almost complete avulsion of the ACL from the femur. The *curved arrow* denotes the PCL, which is normal. The *two arrowheads* designate the medial meniscus. The *two arrowheads* in F and G point to the displaced torn anterior portion of the body and anterior horn of the medial meniscus. The *hollow arrow* in E and F points to the torn peripheral segment of the medial meniscus. The *arrow* in G indicates the venous channels in the peripheral segment of the lateral meniscus.

FIGURE 20-64

Complete tear of the posterior horn and body of the lateral meniscus at the capsulomeniscal junction. The posterior horn and body are displaced into the intercondylar notch anteriorly. **A** to **C**, T1-WI anatomical sagittals. In **A** the *arrowhead* points to empty space belonging to the posterior horn of the lateral meniscus. The anterior horn appears markedly enlarged and deformed, because the body of the meniscus has been displaced into the anterior compartment (better seen in **D**). The large *arrowhead* in **D** indicates the body of the meniscus, the *small arrowhead* the anterior horn of the lateral meniscus. In **B** the *large arrowhead* points to the PCL, the *small arrowheads* to the lateral meniscus (displaced into the intercondylar notch). The *large arrowhead* in **C** points to a partial volume effect with the torn meniscus in the intercondylar notch, the *small arrowheads* to the PCL.

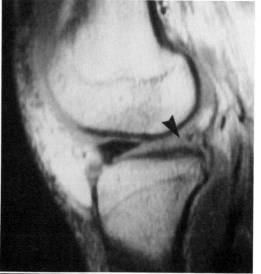

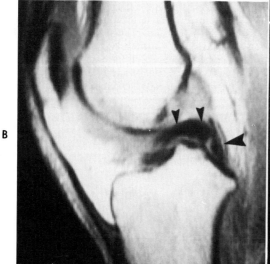

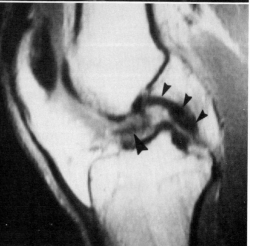

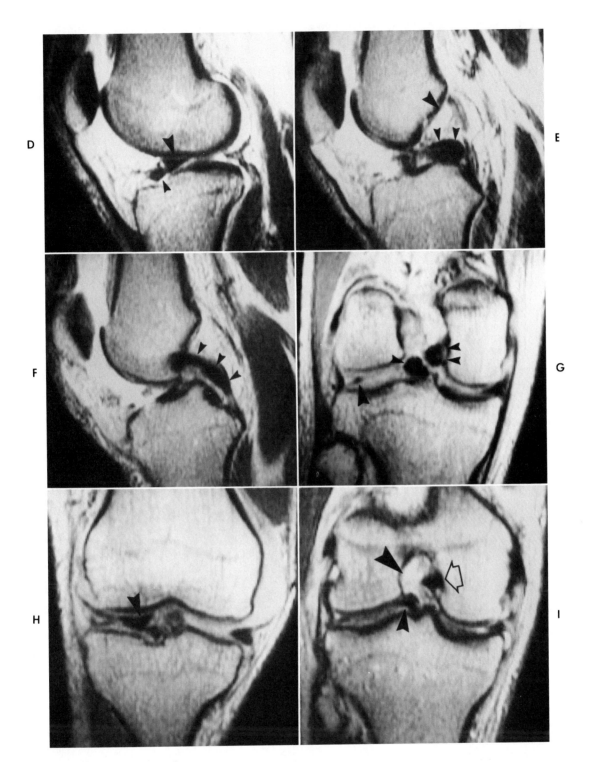

FIGURE 20-64, cont'd
D to F, T2-WI oblique sagittals. G and H, Coronal SD, and I coronal T2-WI. In **E** the *large arrowhead* indicates bright edema/hemorrhage at the femoral insertion of the ACL, which is completely torn in this patient. The *small arrowheads* signify displaced lateral meniscus in the notch. The *arrowheads* in F point to the PCL, which is normal. In **G** the *large arrowhead* identifies a small fragment of the body of the lateral meniscus remaining in the lateral compartment. *One small arrowhead* points to the displaced lateral meniscus in the intercondylar notch. *Two small arrowheads* show the PCL. In **H** the *arrowhead* points to the displaced body of the lateral meniscus into the anterior compartment. Note also the multiple small fragments of torn meniscus and ACL medial to the displaced medial meniscus. **I**, The *hollow arrow* points to the femoral insertion of the PCL. The *large arrowhead* points to the site of insertion of the ACL, which now is occupied by edema/hemorrhage. The *small arrowhead* identifies the displaced torn body of the lateral meniscus.

due to torn displaced meniscal fragments. Occasionally a fragment of the torn free margin will be pushed to a point right above the anterior horn of the meniscus (Figs. 20-65, *A* and *B*, and 20-67, *C*). This causes the anterior horn to appear quite large, thick, and irregular.

Coronal views are often very helpful in identifying the displaced central portion of a bucket handle tear. The displaced portion is seen end-on as an irregular area of low SI in the intercondylar notch. One must be careful not to confuse the normal central attachments (Figs. 20-8, *E*, 20-11, 20-16, and 20-22, *A*) of the posterior horns with the displaced central portion of a bucket handle tear. The central attachments of the posterior horns are near the midsagittal plane of the tibia and may appear as torn fragments on thin coronal images. However, careful scrutiny will show the central attachments to be contiguous with the cortex of the tibia and connected to the posterior horns, medially and laterally. The posterior

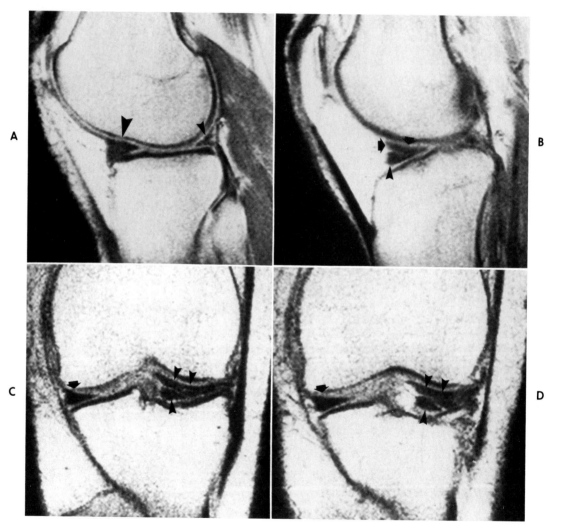

FIGURE 20-65
Bucket handle tear affecting the entire length of the lateral meniscus, with displacement of the torn handle of the bucket anteriorly, superior to the anterior horn. **A** and **B**, Sagittal T1-WI. In **A** the *small arrowhead* points to the remaining portion of the posterior horn. The remnant, although triangular in cross section, is significantly smaller than normal. The *large arrowhead* points to the anterior horn, which is very large and deformed. The torn displaced fragment is riding on top of the anterior horn. In **B**, A sagittal section closer to the midline, the *arrowhead* designates the anterior horn of the lateral meniscus and the *arrows* the displaced torn handle of the bucket. **C** and **D**, Coronal SD. The arrow points to the normal anterior horn of the medial meniscus. The *upper arrowheads* identify the displaced handle of the bucket. (It is not possible to identify the anterior horn of the lateral meniscus.) The *lower arrowhead* points to another torn fragment of the meniscus.

horns just proximal to the central attachments are separated from the tibial cortex by the line of increased SI of the articular cartilage. A displaced torn fragment may be jammed against the tibial cortex (but more frequently will be several millimeters above it) and may extend anteroposteriorly, its posterior extremity often anterior to the meniscal central attachments.

Complete tear along the capsular margin. Occasionally trauma to the knee strips the entire posterior horn and body of the meniscus from the capsule (Figs. 20-66 to 20-68). The meniscus is then usually flipped over anteriorly and forced to a point above the anterior horn. These tears can affect either meniscus. MRI shows an empty space, where one would expect to find the posterior horn and body of the meniscus. The anterior horn appears deformed and very large.

Parrot-beak tear. This is a small radial tear (Fig. 20-69) affecting the free margin of the body of the lateral meniscus, less commonly the medial meniscus. It is often better visualized on coronal cross sections. When high-resolution 3 mm thick coronal cross sections are used, it

is seen as a linear area of increased SI affecting the free margin. It may be missed on thicker cross sections.

The parrot-beak tear is considered a form of horizontal cleavage tear (which are usually thought to be of degenerative origin[68]) but it may occur in an otherwise normal meniscus.

Free margin tear. As a rule tears of the free margin of the posterior and anterior horns are optimally seen on sagittal views, and those of the body on coronal views. They appear as zones of unsharpness, irregularity, fraying, or amputation of the free margin. Occasionally, distinct small radial tears of the free margin may also be visualized. Diagnosis of a tear of the free margin often is not reliably made on sagittal views because the semicircular configurations and sloping articular surfaces of the menisci interfere with proper visualization of the free margin. This is also true for the free margin of the posterior and anterior horns on coronal views.

Erosion, fraying, fibrillation, and minor tears of the free margin of the menisci are usually considered due to degenerative disease.

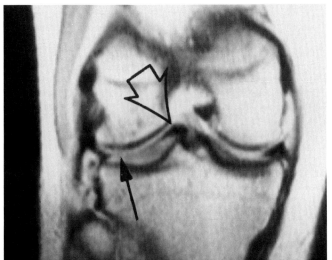

A

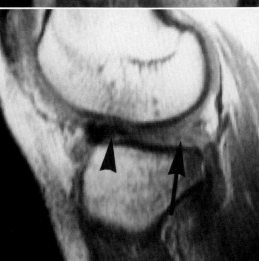

B

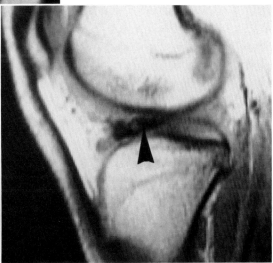

C

FIGURE 20-66
The posterior horn and body of the lateral meniscus are completely separated from the capsule and displaced anteriorly. **A**, SD coronal and, **B** and **C**, T1-WI sagittal views. In **A** the *solid arrow* points to the empty space belonging to the posterior segment of the body of the lateral meniscus. The *hollow arrow* points to the central attachment of the posterior horn, which is also torn and displaced superiorly and medially. In **B** and **C**, the *arrowhead* in these images points to the anteriorly displaced and torn lateral meniscus. The *arrow* in **B** shows the empty space belonging to the posterior horn of the lateral meniscus.

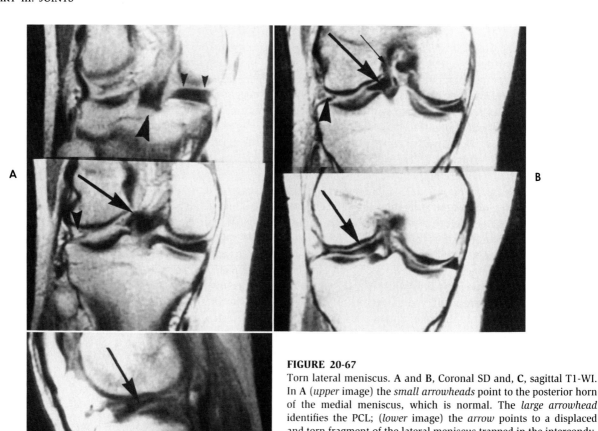

FIGURE 20-67

Torn lateral meniscus. **A** and **B**, Coronal SD and, **C**, sagittal T1-WI. In **A** (*upper* image) the *small arrowheads* point to the posterior horn of the medial meniscus, which is normal. The *large arrowhead* identifies the PCL; (*lower* image) the *arrow* points to a displaced and torn fragment of the lateral meniscus trapped in the intercondylar notch lateral to midline just in front of the PCL, the *arrowhead* to the missing posterior horn of the lateral meniscus. The posterior horn and body were detached from the capsule and displaced into the intercondylar notch. In **B** (*upper* image) the *large arrow* points to the displaced torn fragment of the lateral meniscus, just lateral to the ACL, the *small arrow* to the ACL, and the *arrowhead* to the missing body of the lateral meniscus; (*lower* image) the *arrow* points to the displaced torn fragment of the lateral meniscus, mimicking a discoid meniscus. In **C** (*upper* image) the *arrow* points to the horizontally lying torn and displaced lateral meniscus; (*lower* image) the *arrow* points to the torn meniscal fragment, the *arrowhead* to the anterior horn of the lateral meniscus. There is also moderately increased SI of the anterior horn due to a degenerative microcyst.

DEGENERATIVE DISEASE AND DEGENERATIVE TEARS OF THE MENISCI

Degenerative disease. The menisci are prone to accelerated degeneration because of their lack of vascularity (excluding the peripheral margin) and the incredible amount of stress to which they are subjected during axial loading of the knee. The degenerative process is manifested histologically as death of the chondrocytes and accumulation of acellular mucopolysaccharide ground substance in the meniscal fibrocartilage. The accumulation, or increased production, of mucopolysaccharide ground substance within the meniscal fibrocartilage has been variously termed mucoid, myxoid, or hyaline degeneration.[82,85]

The degenerive process occurs, in descending order of frequency, in the posterior horn and body of the medial meniscus; in the anterior horn, body, and posterior horn of the lateral meniscus; and in the anterior horn of the medial meniscus. The posterior horn of the medial meniscus is more prone to degenerative disease and to degenerative tear and traumatic tears than are the body and anterior horn of the medial meniscus or all of the lateral meniscus. These abnormalities of the posterior horn of the medial meniscus account for (conservatively) about 70% of similar pathologies that affect both menisci.

The MR manifestations of degenerative disease are abnormalities of signal and deformity of the meniscus.

The *signal abnormalities* commence with small globular zones of medium-increased SI (Figs. 20-70 and 20-71), usually in the posterior horn of the medial meniscus.

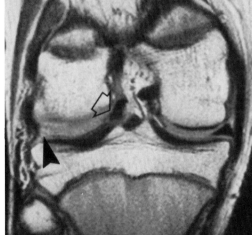

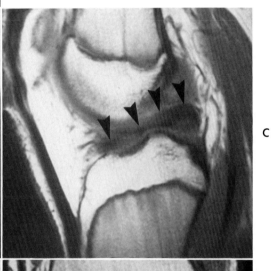

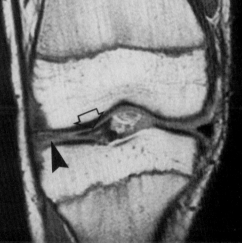

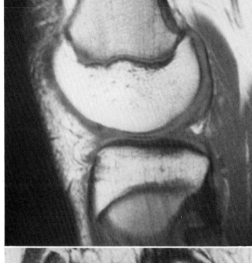

FIGURE 20-68
Complete tear of the entire lateral meniscus with displacement into the notch. **A** to **C,** T1-WI sagittal views. In **A** the *arrowheads* point to the empty spaces belonging to the posterior and anterior horns of the lateral meniscus. In **B** the lateral meniscus is absent. In **C** the torn and displaced lateral meniscus *(arrowheads)* is just lateral to the midsagittal plane of the tibia. **D** and **E,** Coronal SD. In **D** the *arrowhead* points to the empty space belonging to the posterior aspect of the body of the lateral meniscus, the *hollow arrow* to the displaced meniscus on the lateral side of the intercondylar notch. In **E** the *arrowhead* points to the empty space belonging to the anterior horn of the lateral meniscus, the *hollow arrow* to the displaced torn meniscus in the intercondylar notch.

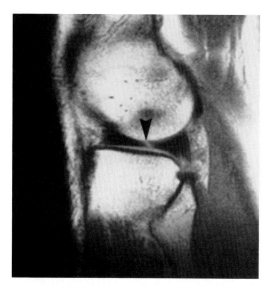

FIGURE 20-69
Radial tear of the free margin of the lateral meniscal body. Sagittal SD. The *arrowhead* marks the tear.

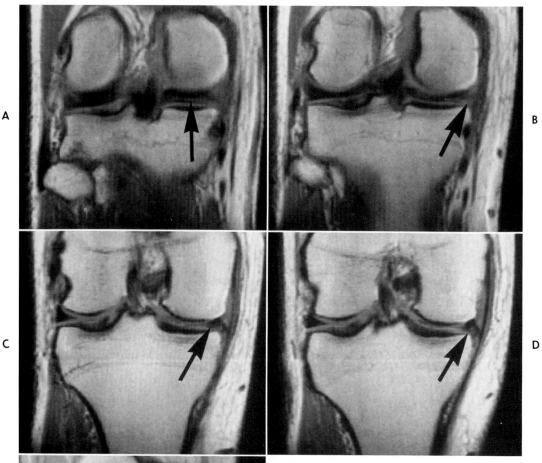

A

B

C

D

E

FIGURE 20-70
Degenerative disease of the medial meniscus. SD coronal views. The *arrow* in **A** points to a horizontal line of increased SI just above the inferior articular surface of the posterior horn of medial meniscus. This is a horizontal tear that has reached the inferior articular surface in the more anterior portion of the posterior horn (*arrow* in **B**) and has caused erosion of the inferior articular surface. Note the nonhomogeneity and increased SI of the posterior horn due to degenerative disease. The *arrow* in **C** shows an amputated free margin of the body, with erosion of the inferior articular surface. There is also marked irregularity of the body, with degenerative erosion and a tear affecting the inferior articular surface and free margin (*arrow* in **C** and **D**). **E**, SD sagittal view. The *arrowhead* points to joint effusion, the *arrow* to signal nonhomogeneity and moderately increased SI of the posterior horn. The inferior articular surface is quite eroded and irregular.

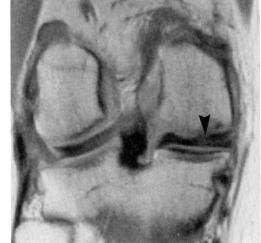
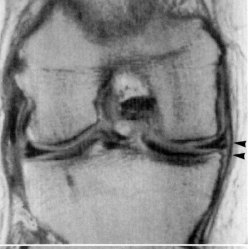
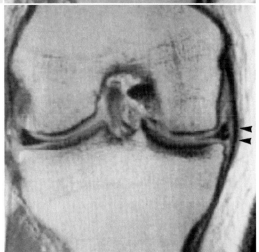

FIGURE 20-71
Degenerative disease, medial meniscus. Spin density coronal views.
A, The *arrowhead* points to moderate irregularity of the superior articular surface and the diffuse internal signal nonhomogeneity of the posterior horn of medial meniscus. **B,** The *arrowheads* point to the moderately outward-bowing joint capsule. The meniscus is minimally extruded beyond the margins of the medial compartment. **C,** The *arrowheads* point to a more prominent bowing out of the capsule, and the meniscus is slightly more extruded beyond the margins of the medial compartment. There was partial detachment of the meniscus from the capsule, confirmed on T2-WI (not shown).

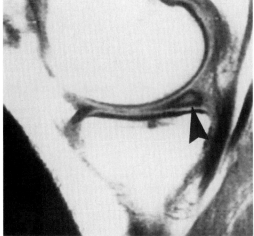

FIGURE 20-72
Degenerative disease of the medial meniscus. T1-WI sagittal and spin density coronal views, meniscal windows. The substance of the meniscus is almost completely replaced by a medium- to high-signal degenerative tissue. Only a thin shell of normal meniscal tissue remains. The meniscus, however, has maintained its normal configuration.

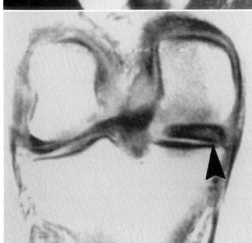
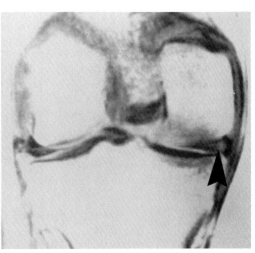

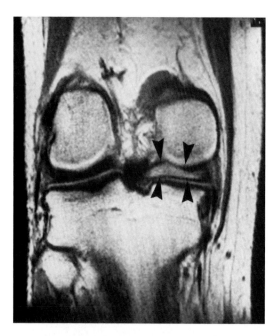

FIGURE 20-73
Coronal SD. The *arrowheads* point to cystic expansion of the posterior horn of the medial meniscus. The degenerative process has replaced almost all the substance of the meniscus except for its peripheral shell.

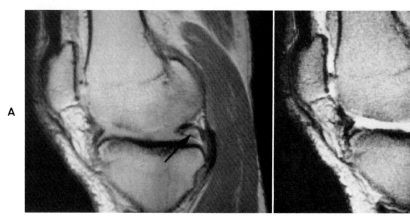

FIGURE 20-74
Degenerative disease, medial meniscus. **A**, SD and, **B**, T2-WI sagittal views. The *arrow* points to a degenerative microcyst within the substance of the posterior horn, which is moderately deformed. There is increased SI of the microcyst on SD, even more on T2-WI.

With more advanced disease the zones of increased SI get larger, until in far-advanced stages the entire substance of the meniscus, except for a thin peripheral shell, is occupied by the degenerative tissue (Figs. 20-72 to 20-74). In some patients the degenerative process may produce a localized microcyst, causing expansion of that segment of the meniscus. This is seen commonly in the midportion of the body and anterior horn of the lateral meniscus, but also in the body and the posterior and anterior horns of the medial meniscus (Fig. 20-75).

Some investigators[67] believe that a closed tear of the posterior horn of the medial meniscus is essentially a manifestation of degenerative disease. This is probably correct in most instances, although we have seen definite instances of this lesion in otherwise normal menisci following trauma in children and young adults.

The small and moderate-sized zones of increased SI within the substance of the menisci, due to degeneration

FIGURE 20-75
Degenerative disease, horizontal tear, and degenerative cystic deformity of the medial meniscus. **A** and **B**, T1-WI sagittal views. The *arrow* denotes a horizontal tear of the posterior horn. The *arrowhead* in A identifies the cystic degenerative expansion of the anterior horn, the *arrowhead* in **B** a fairly well-defined cyst directly anterior to the tibial origin of the ACL. The cystic expansion of the anterior horn has extended across the midline to the lateral side. **C** to **F**, Spin density coronal views. The *arrowhead* in **C** shows the horizontal tear of the posterior horn, the *arrowhead* in **D** the body of the medial meniscus (which is more than 50% thinner in the superior to inferior dimension because of erosion due to degenerative disease and a degenerative horizontal tear). The torn inferior segment has been displaced. No definite large fragments were identified in the intercondylar notch on MRI. At arthroscopy multiple small fibrocartilaginous fragments were found. The *arrowhead* in **E** points to degenerative cystic expansion of the peripheral portion of the anterior horn. The *small arrowheads* in **F** show the horizontal tear of the anterior horn. The *large arrowheads* point to the cystic expansion of the anterior horn. Note that the cyst arising from the anterior horn near its central attachment has extended across the midline to the lateral side.

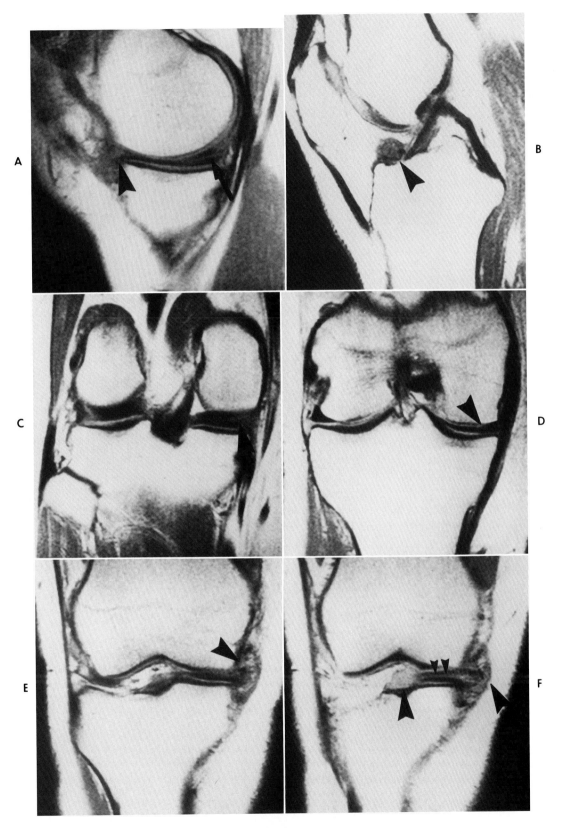

FIGURE 20-75
For legend see opposite page.

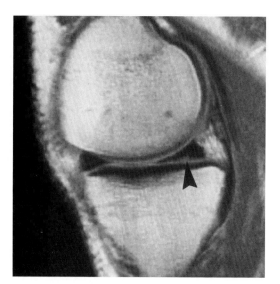

FIGURE 20-76
Degenerative erosion *(arrowhead)* of the inferior articular surface of the medial meniscus. SD sagittal view.

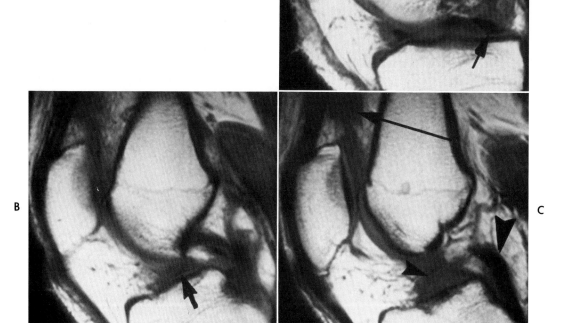

FIGURE 20-77
Tear of the ACL and degenerative disease with degenerative tear of the medial meniscus. **A** to **C**, Oblique sagittal views. In **A** (4 mm medial to midline) the *arrow* points to a torn displaced fragment of the ACL. In **B** (midline) the *arrow* points to a thin portion of the ACL lying almost horizontally. In **C** (4 mm lateral to midline) the *large arrowhead* denotes the PCL. The *small arrowhead* points to fluid accumulation in the expected position of the ACL, the *arrow* to effusion in the suprapatellar bursa. **D** and **E**, Spin density coronal views. (In **D** the *curved arrow* points to the PCL, the *straight arrow* to the body of the lateral meniscus, the *arrowhead* to the inner portion of the posterior horn of the medial meniscus adjacent to its insertion on the tibia. In **E** the *straight arrow* indicates a defect of the inferior articular surface of the body of the medial meniscus, representing an incomplete tear secondary to degenerative disease. Note that the body of the medial meniscus is at least 30% to 40% thinner in the superior to inferior direction than expected. The *curved hollow arrow* points to the displaced fragment of the ACL, which is lying in an oblique horizontal position.) **F** and **H**, Spin density and, **G** and **I**, corresponding T2-WI coronal views. The *curved hollow arrow* points to a loose fragment. The *straight arrow* shows the remaining 15% or so of fibers of the ACL. The *curved solid arrow* points to the PCL. The tear of the inferior articular surface of the body of the medial meniscus is also seen in **F**, extending into the anterior horn in **H**. At surgery extensive degenerative disease and a degenerative tear affecting the inferior articular surface of the medial meniscus were found. The anterior cruciate ligament was split longitudinally, with most of the medial fibers torn and displaced in a horizontal direction *(curved hollow arrow* in **E**). The origin of the loose fragment could not be determined.

or a closed tear, do not cause any apparent deformity of the menisci. Thus they are not detected on arthrography or arthroscopy. Some intrasubstance (closed) tears, when they come close to an articular surface, cause a focal deformity, but not discontinuity, of the articular surface. An experienced arthroscopist is usually able to find the intrasubstance tear by careful probing at the precise spot pinpointed by the MRI.

With advancing degeneration there is *deformity of the meniscus,* minimal at first but ending in gross distortion of its morphology. The deformity is due to erosion of the articular surfaces (Fig. 20-76) and free margin, degener-

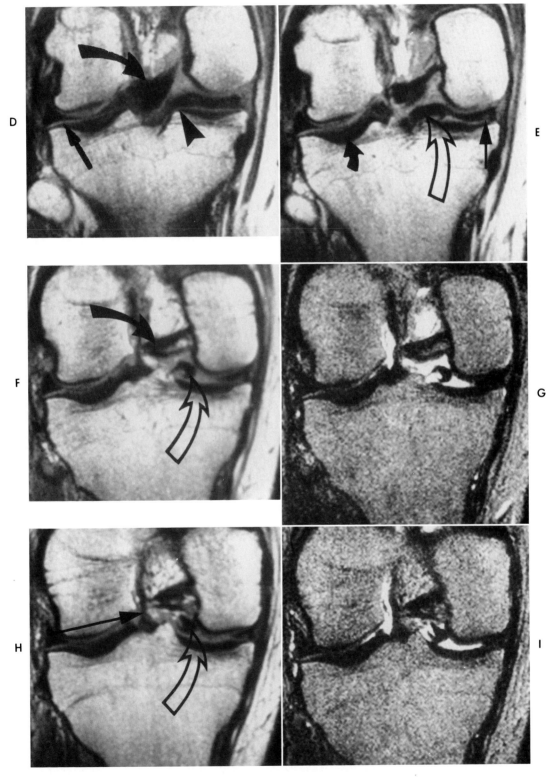

FIGURE 20-77
For legend see opposite page.

ative tearing, expansion and distortion by the degenerative microcysts, and secondary deformities by articular margin osteophytes biting into the menisci (Figs. 20-77 and 20-78).

The degenerative process starts in the subsurface of the inferior articular surface of the meniscus[67] and is usually encountered in the posterior horn of the medial meniscus. It may lead to a horizontal intrasubstance tear, subsequently extending to the inferior articular surface and separating and displacing that surface away from the rest of the meniscus. The meniscus becomes thinner, with a deformed and frayed inferior articular surface. However, the thinning may be due not to a horizontal tear but to gradual erosion of the inferior articular surface. The resulting meniscal deformity often has the same appearance on MRI, regardless of etiology.

Degenerative tears. The degenerative process causes internal disruption of the substance of the meniscus, eventually leading to tears communicating with the articular surfaces (Fig. 20-79). These tears are irregular and usually accompanied by various-sized irregular zones of degeneration manifesting as regions of increased SI. The tears are usually wider than traumatic tears, have irregular and indistinct margins, and often are horizontal or horizontal/oblique terminating in the inferior articular surface (most often) or the free margin. They also may extend into the capsular margin, causing the degenerative microcysts to rupture into this region and leading to a partial or complete separation of the meniscus from the capsule or disruption and microtears of the capsule.

Characteristic degenerative tears of the menisci are the horizontal cleavage tears, intrasubstance tears, horizontal tears affecting the inferior articular surface, tears in the menisci containing obvious globular zones of increased SI, and erosion of the free margin.

Horizontal cleavage tear of the lateral meniscus. The classical cleavage tear of the lateral meniscus is a horizontal tear that affects the body of the meniscus and is often associated with an intrameniscal/parameniscal cyst (Figs. 20-80 to 20-85). In Smillie's[68] operative material cystic degeneration of the lateral meniscus was 7.8 times that of the medial. We have found the incidence of a horizontal tear with an intrameniscal/parameniscal cyst to be almost the same for both menisci on MR studies. Occasionally the tear is very fine and difficult to visualize. Most cleavage tears communicate with the free margin or one of the articular surfaces of the meniscus. However, in some patients no definite communication can be found either to the articular surfaces or to the free margin. We have seen several such examples on pathological examination.

Intrameniscal/parameniscal cyst of the lateral meniscus. The degenerative process first forms small microcysts near the peripheral margin of the body of the meniscus,[67,86] which are seen as fairly well-delineated areas of slightly to moderately increased SI on T1-WI and SD.[37,48,87] As long as the cyst is within the confines of the meniscus, it should be called an intrameniscal cyst (Fig. 20-80). However, with progression of the disease the intrameniscal cyst enlarges, expands the peripheral margin of the meniscus, and extends into the capsulomeniscal junction, expanding it and displacing the capsule outward (Figs. 20-81 and 20-82). At this stage a parameniscal cyst is born. Because there is room on the lateral

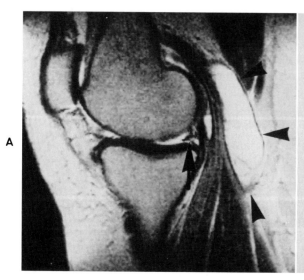
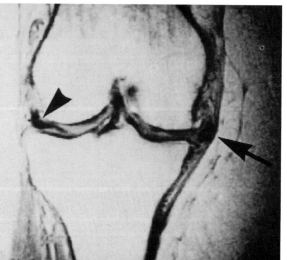

FIGURE 20-78
Degenerative disease of the menisci and a popliteal cyst. **A,** T2-WI sagittal and, **B,** spin density coronal views. This is an example of long-standing degenerative disease of the medial compartment with complete degenerative fragmentation of the posterior horn (*arrow* in **A**) and extrusion of the body and anterior horn of the medial meniscus (*arrow* in **B**). There is also degenerative disease of the lateral compartment with a degenerative tear of the lateral meniscus. The *arrowhead* in **B** points to an osteophyte causing erosion of the superior articular surface of the lateral meniscus. The *arrowheads* in **A** point to a popliteal cyst.

side of the capsule for expansion, with the only retaining structure the cordlike FCL (which is situated several millimeters away from it), the lateral capsule is able to bulge out with relative ease.[68] Thus, for a long time, unlike the situation on the medial side, the lateral capsule is not violated and the parameniscal cyst does not

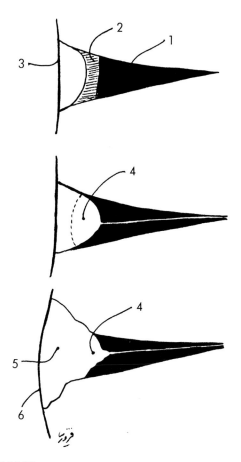

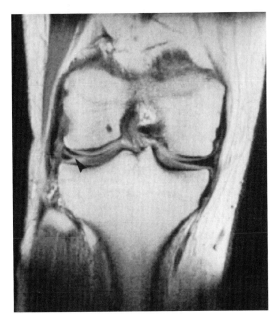

FIGURE 20-79
Coronal SD. The *arrowhead* point to a tear of the lateral meniscus that extends into the inferior articular surface and free margin of the meniscus.

FIGURE 20-80
Posterior horn of the lateral meniscus, a horizontal cleavage tear, and an intrameniscal/parameniscal cyst. *1*, Avascular zone of the meniscus; *2*, peripheral zone; *3*, fibrous capsule; *4*, intrameniscal cyst; *5*, parameniscal cyst; *6*, fibrous capsule bowed out by the large parameniscal cyst.

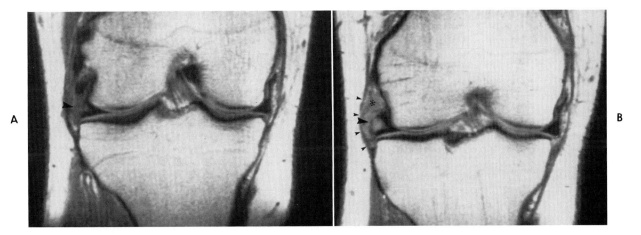

FIGURE 20-81
SD coronal views showing a horizontal tear of the body of lateral meniscus with an intrameniscal/parameniscal cyst. **A,** The *arrowhead* identifies the cyst. Note the configuration of the capsular margin of the lateral meniscus in this patient, characteristic of such tears. In some patients prior to the formation of an obvious parameniscal cyst, this is the only abnormality noted. **B,** The *large arrowhead* points to the intrameniscal cyst, which is expanding the peripheral margin of a more anterior portion of the body. The *asterisk* is on the cyst. The *small arrowheads* point to the laterally bulging capsule of the lateral compartment.

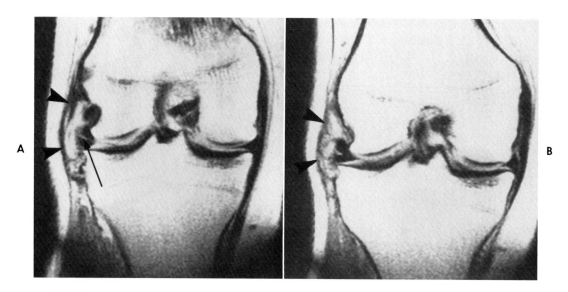

FIGURE 20-82
Horizontal tear of the lateral meniscus and a parameniscal cyst. Coronal SD. **A,** The *arrow* identifies the tear. The *arrowheads* point to the cyst. Note the externally bulging capsule and FCL. **B,** The *arrowheads* point to the cyst. The tear is evident as a line of increased SI in the midportion of the meniscus.

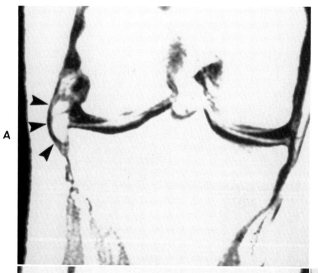

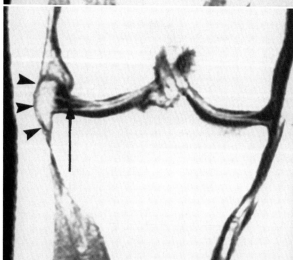

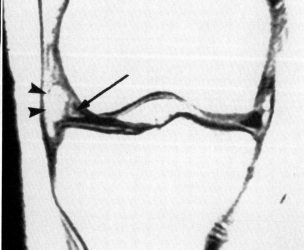

FIGURE 20-83
Horizontal tear of the lateral meniscus and a parameniscal cyst. SD coronal views, meniscal windows. The *arrowheads* in all images point to the cyst, which has high SI. The *arrow* in **B** points to the tear, the *arrow* in **C** an intrameniscal cyst adjacent to the parameniscal one.

penetrate it. Parameniscal cysts of the lateral meniscus do not usually become very large and do not extend away from their place of origin for any appreciable distance.

Within these cysts is thought to be synovial fluid of the joint, gaining access via the tear. Thus the contents of the cyst are of moderately increased SI on T1-WI and SD, and markedly increased SI (isotense with the synovial fluid) on T2-WI. However, in some patients the content of the cyst differs from synovial fluid. These cysts contain a viscous, jelly-like, proteinaceous substance, occasionally with synovial debris and evidence of old hemorrhage.[68] The cysts may be of medium or low SI on most pulse sequences (Fig. 20-84). In these patients the meniscal tear may not communicate with the articular surfaces or the free margin of the meniscus.

The intrameniscal/parameniscal cysts are formed as a direct consequence of the degenerative disease of the

luc FLuio vs cyst

meniscus. The cyst contents are a mixture of the products of degenerative disease and, in those who have a tear communicating with the articular cavity of the knee, synovial fluid.

Parameniscal cysts rarely cause erosion of bone. However, we have encountered several such cases, all surgically documented parameniscal cysts secondary to a meniscal tear, and all on the lateral side (Fig. 20-85).

Cleavage tear and intrameniscal/parameniscal cyst of the medial meniscus. Cleavage tears of the medial meniscus (Figs. 20-86 to 20-89) frequently rupture into the capsular margin of the posterior horn (Fig. 20-87), posterior to the TCL, rather than the midportion of the body. The fibrous capsule on the medial side is tight and (unlike the lateral side) cannot be forced outward to any great extent. Thus an intrameniscal/parameniscal cyst of the medial meniscus, prior to violation of the capsule, is

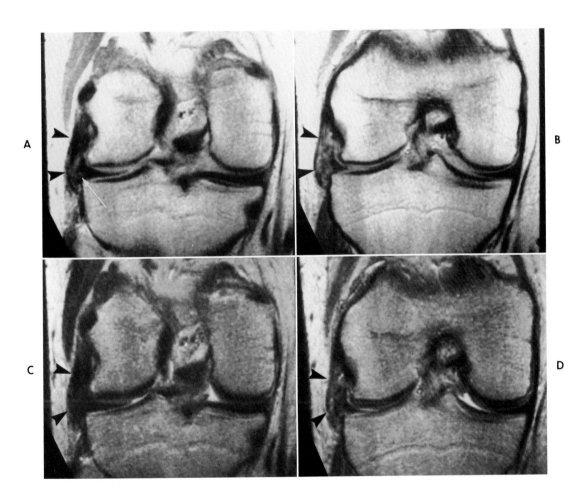

FIGURE 20-84
Incomplete horizontal tear of the lateral meniscus, not communicating with the joint, and a parameniscal cyst. **A** and **B,** SD and, **C** and **D,** T2-WI coronal views. The *arrowheads* in all images show the outwardly bulging capsule of the lateral compartment due to the cyst. The cyst contained a highly viscous proteinaceous fluid with debris, which accounts for its low SI. Note the marked irregularity of the outline and amputation of the free margin of the meniscus (best seen in **B**). There is also irregularity of the capsular margin of the meniscus in **A** and **B.** A small intrameniscal cyst *(white arrow)* is present in **A.** At exploration an incomplete horizontal tear, not communicating with the articular surfaces or the free margin of the meniscus, was found. One reason for a tear's being poorly visualized is the low SI of the fluid within the tear in patients with this type of parameniscal cyst.

usually smaller than its lateral counterpart. The degenerative process and the small intrameniscal/parameniscal cyst erode through the capsule (rather than pushing it out as on the lateral side) and permit the intrameniscal cyst to extend to the outer side of the capsule[68] (Fig. 20-86). These cysts may also develop in other segments of the meniscus, although this is less common. However, their behavior is similar to that of a posterior horn intrameniscal cyst in that they are small when confined to the meniscus and, with enlargement, they dissect through the capsuloligamentous complex and form parameniscal cysts that are on the outside of the capsule. The medial parameniscal cysts have a tendency to become very large and to extend posteriorly, medially, and superiorly for a significant distance away from their site of origin.[68] They may present as a popliteal cyst. In some patients the communication with the meniscus may be blocked by adhesions and fibrosis and the cyst may be completely

Text continued on p 740.

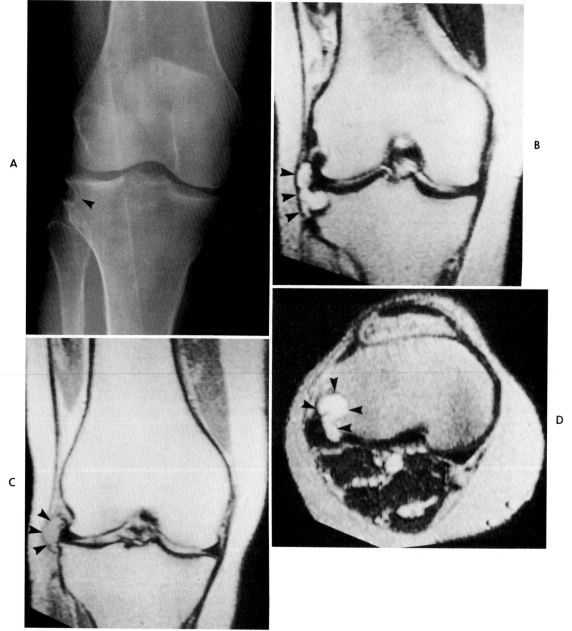

FIGURE 20-85
Parameniscal cyst with erosion of the tibia. **A,** An AP projection of the knee shows a well-marginated area of erosion of the tibia just below the joint line *(arrowhead).* **B,** T2-WI coronal view. The *arrowheads* point to the fluid-filled cyst corresponding to the image seen on the conventional film. **C,** SD coronal view 5 mm anterior to **B.** The typical parameniscal configuration of the cyst *(arrowheads)* can be appreciated. **D,** Axial T2-WI just below the joint line. *Arrowheads* point to the fluid-filled cyst within the tibial erosion. At surgical exploration a horizontal tear of the lateral meniscus associated with the parameniscal cyst was found. Erosion of bone secondary to a parameniscal cyst is unusual, being more common secondary to a ganglion cyst.

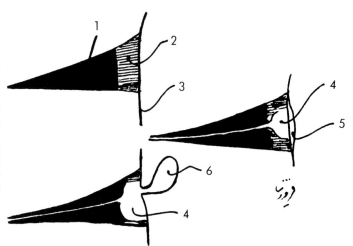

FIGURE 20-86
Cleavage tear of the medial meniscus with an intrameniscal cyst and a parameniscal cyst. The posterior horn of the medial meniscus is shown. *1,* Avascular zone of the meniscus; *2,* peripheral zone; *3,* fibrous capsule (normally the capsulomeniscal junction is straight or slightly concave inward); *4,* the intrameniscal cyst and a cleavage tear; *5,* edema and bulging of the fibrous capsule; *6,* the parameniscal cyst. The capsule has been disrupted. Parameniscal cysts on the medial side may become quite large and dissect both posteriorly and superiorly. Occasionally the connection to the meniscus and the joint will become obliterated and the cyst will migrate away from the joint region.

FIGURE 20-87
Tear, medial meniscus, and a parameniscal cyst. **A**, SD sagittal, **B** and **C**, SD and T2-WI coronal, and, **D** and **E**, SD and T2-WI axial views. In **A** the *arrow* points to a horizontal oblique tear of the posterior horn. In **B** and **C** the *small arrowheads* identify the parameniscal cyst. The *large arrowhead* in **B** points to a horizontal tear that has completely destroyed the inferior articular surface of the posterior horn. In **D** the *large arrowhead* points to the TCL. Note that disruption of the capsule has occurred posterior to the TCL. In **E** *arrowheads* show the parameniscal cyst.

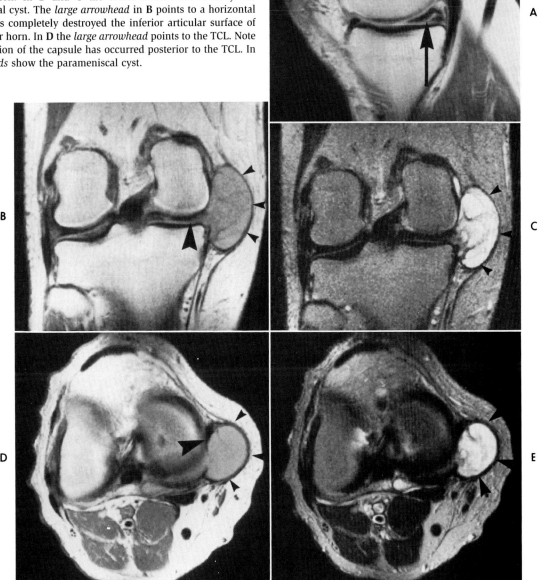

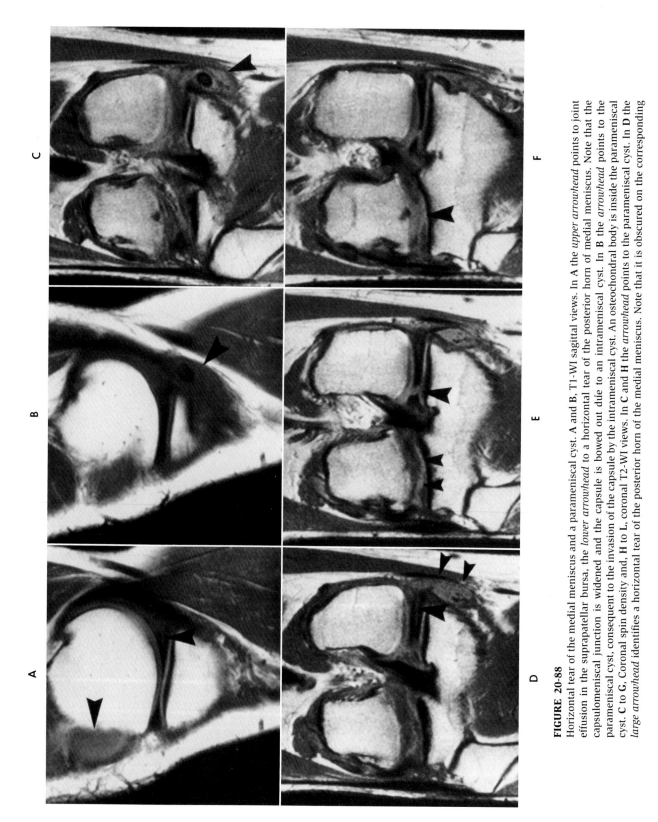

FIGURE 20-88

Horizontal tear of the medial meniscus and a parameniscal cyst. **A** and **B**, T1-WI sagittal views. In **A** the *upper arrowhead* points to joint effusion in the suprapatellar bursa, the *lower arrowhead* to a horizontal tear of the posterior horn of medial meniscus. Note that the capsulomeniscal junction is widened and the capsule is bowed out due to an intrameniscal cyst. In **B** the *arrowhead* points to the parameniscal cyst, consequent to the invasion of the capsule by the intrameniscal cyst. An osteochondral body is inside the parameniscal cyst. **C** to **G**, Coronal spin density and, **H** to **L**, coronal T2-WI views. In **C** and **H** the *arrowhead* points to the parameniscal cyst. In **D** the *large arrowhead* identifies a horizontal tear of the posterior horn of the medial meniscus. Note that it is obscured on the corresponding

T2-WI view (**I**). The *small arrowheads* in **D** point to the parameniscal cyst, which has moderately increased SI on spin density and markedly increased SI on T2-WI. The *large arrowhead* in **E** points to a tear of the posterior horn of the medial meniscus just proximal to its central insertion. Note the degenerative fragmentation of the lateral meniscus (*arrowheads*). A minimal amount of fluid is visible within the substance of the meniscus in **J** (*arrowhead*). In **F** and **K** the *arrowhead* points to marked degenerative fragmentation of the lateral meniscus. Fluid occupies the space previously taken by the meniscus. There is also severe degenerative disease of the articular cartilage of the lateral femoral condyle. In **G** and **L** note further evidence of degenerative fragmentation of the lateral meniscus (*arrowheads*).

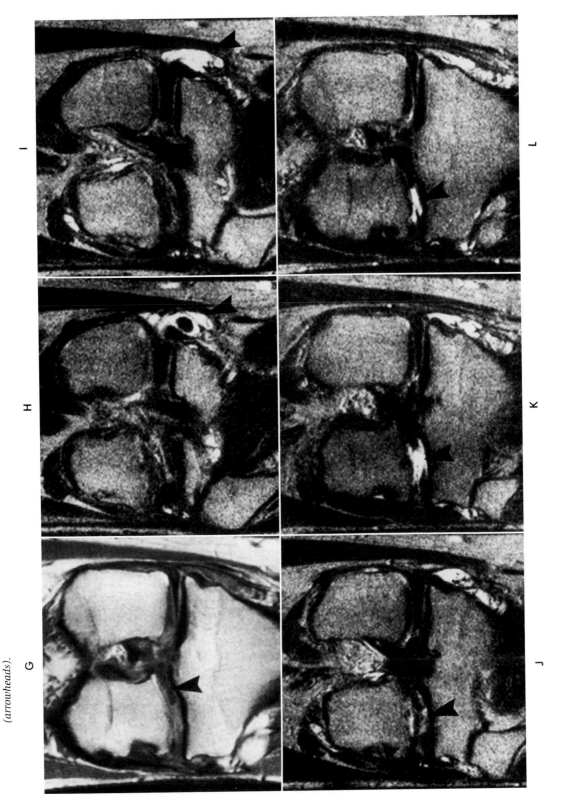

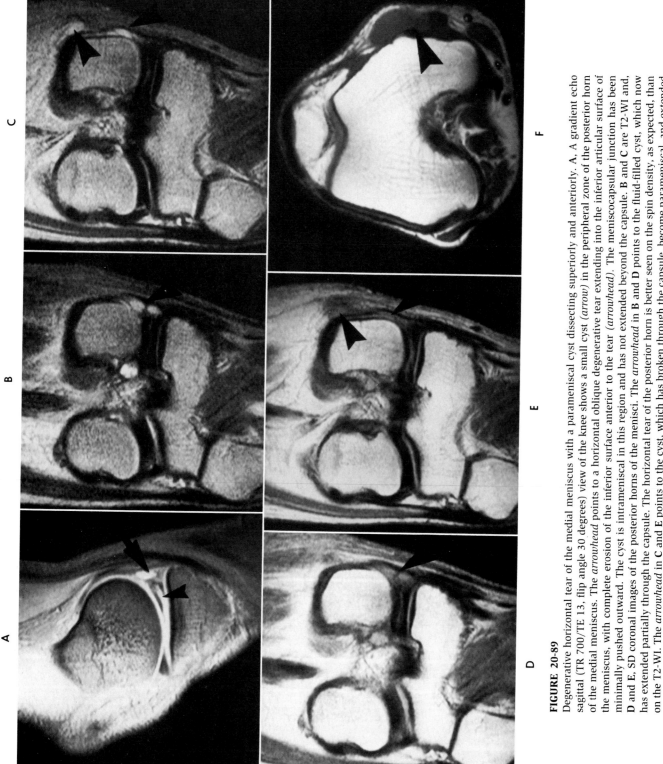

FIGURE 20-89

Degenerative horizontal tear of the medial meniscus with a parameniscal cyst dissecting superiorly and anteriorly. A, A gradient echo sagittal (TR 700/TE 13, flip angle 30 degrees) view of the knee shows a small cyst (*arrow*) in the peripheral zone of the posterior horn of the medial meniscus. The *arrowhead* points to a horizontal oblique degenerative tear extending into the inferior articular surface of the meniscus, with complete erosion of the inferior surface anterior to the tear (*arrowhead*). The meniscocapsular junction has been minimally pushed outward. The cyst is intrameniscal in this region and has not extended beyond the capsule. B and C are T2-WI and, D and E, SD coronal images of the posterior horns of the menisci. The *arrowhead* in B and D points to the fluid-filled cyst, which now has extended partially through the capsule. The horizontal tear of the posterior horn is better seen on the spin density, as expected, than on the T2-WI. The *arrowhead* in C and E points to the cyst, which has broken through the capsule, become parameniscal, and extended

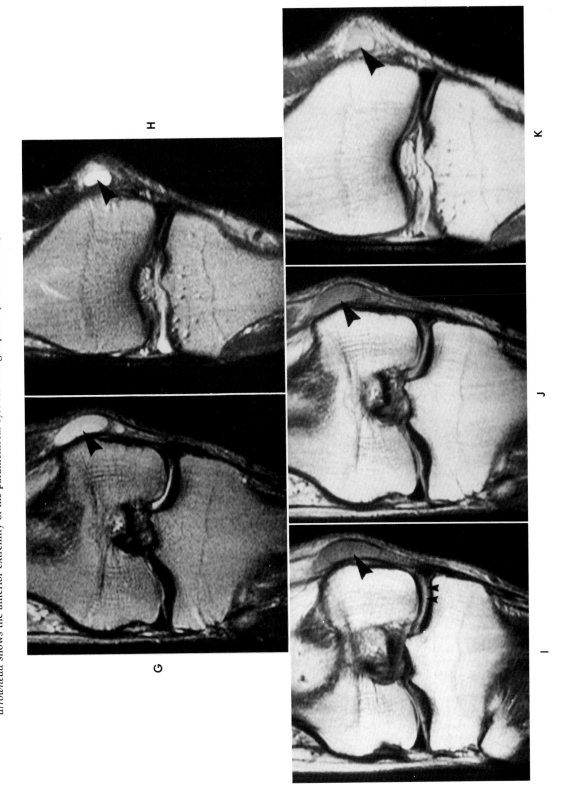

superiorly. **F,** T1-WI axial view. The *arrowhead* shows the fluid-filled cyst adjacent to the medial femoral condyle. **G** and **H,** T2-WI and, **I** to **K,** spin density cross sections of the midportion of the body and anterior horn. The *large arrowhead* in **G** to **K** points to the fluid-filled cyst, clearly outside the capsule of the joint. **I** and **J** show the midportion of the bodies of the menisci. The *large arrowhead* points to the fluid-filled cyst, clearly outside the joint capsule and extending superiorly. The *small arrowheads* in **I** point to the large horizontal tear of the body of the medial meniscus, which has almost completely eroded most of the substance of the meniscus. Only a small portion of the capsular margin and the superior articular margin of the meniscus remain in place. The body of the lateral meniscus is normal. **H** and **K,** Coronal images through the anterior horn of the medial meniscus but anterior to the anterior horn of the lateral meniscus. The *arrowhead* shows the anterior extremity of the parameniscal cyst dissecting superiorly and anteriorly.

detached from the joint. Then the parameniscal cyst masquerades as a ganglion cyst.

Intrameniscal/parameniscal cyst of the anterior horn of the meniscus. The anterior horn of the lateral (Figs. 20-90 and 20-91) and, less commonly, the medial (Figs. 20-75 and 20-92) meniscus may also be affected by a degenerative tear and a degenerative meniscal cyst. The anterior horn is expanded by a microcyst, which commonly is connected to a small cyst adjacent to it. The parameniscal cyst seems to form in response to the extrusion of fluid and other degenerative products from the anterior horn microcyst. Surgical exploration shows a small walled-off cyst formed by connective tissue that is communicating with the microcyst of the anterior horn.

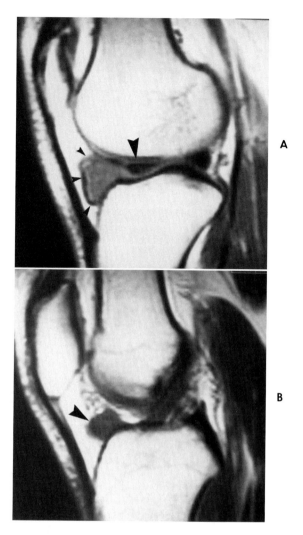

A

B

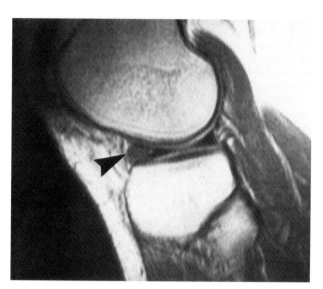

FIGURE 20-90
Degenerative disease of the lateral meniscus. T1-WI anatomical sagittal of the lateral compartment. The *arrowhead* points to a degenerative cyst affecting the anterior horn of the lateral meniscus.

FIGURE 20-91
Anterolateral synovial cyst. Sagittal T1-WI. **A,** The *large arrowhead* points to the anterior horn of the lateral meniscus. The *small arrowheads* point to the synovial cyst. In **B** the *arrowhead* denotes the synovial cyst. The anterior horn of the lateral meniscus was normal in this patient at surgical exploration. Small synovial cysts are fairly common in patients with degenerative disease and tear of the anterior horn of the lateral meniscus. However, occasionally in patients with a normal meniscus a synovial cyst will be encountered that completely surrounds the anterior horn.

FIGURE 20-92
Torn medial meniscus and a parameniscal cyst extending anteriorly. A and B, Coronal SD, C to E, coronal T2-WI, and, F, sagittal T2-WI views. In A and C (coronal views through the midportion of the body of the menisci) the *arrow* points to a minimal capsular remnant of the body of the medial meniscus. Most of the substance of the meniscus has been torn and displaced. *Arrowheads* denote the thickened and outwardly displaced TCL, which has been stripped away from the bone. There is marked fibrosis between the TCL and the medial surfaces of the femur and tibia. The medial compartment is slightly widened. In **B** (7 mm anterior to A) and **D** (11 mm anterior) the *arrow* points to the parameniscal cyst. The *hollow arrow* in **D** identifies the torn anterior horn of the medial meniscus. In **E** (18 mm anterior to A) the *arrrowheads* point to the anteromedial parameniscal cyst, the *hollow arrow* to the torn anterior horn of medial meniscus. In **F** the *arrow* points to the horizontal tear of the anterior horn of medial meniscus, and the *hollow arrow* points to a small capsular remnant of the posterior horn. The *arrowheads* show the parameniscal cyst extending anteriorly.

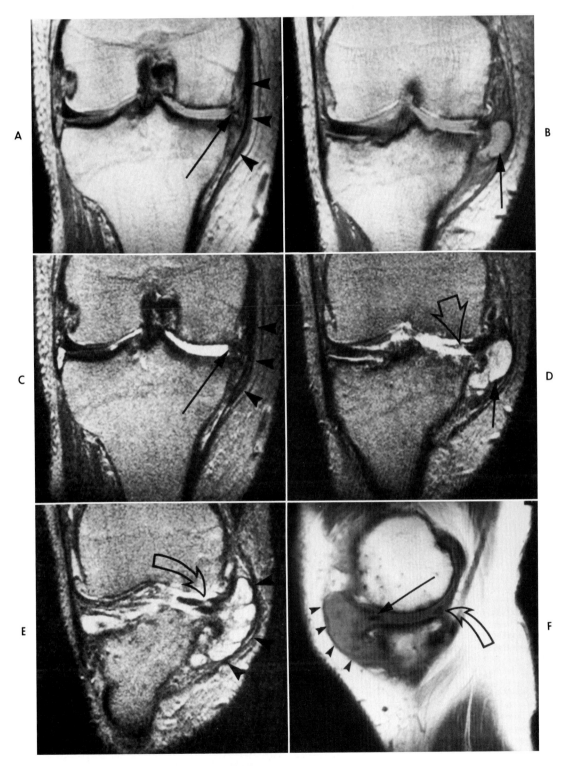

FIGURE 20-92
For legend see opposite page.

DEGENERATIVE DISEASE OF THE FEMOROTIBIAL JOINT AND OF THE MENISCI

Degenerative disease of the menisci is independent of degenerative disease of the femorotibial compartments. It usually precedes the latter. However, it is likely that meniscal degeneration accelerates the process of femorotibial arthrosis (Fig. 20-93).

In patients with femorotibial degenerative arthritis the peripheral margin of the meniscus may become adherent to the marginal osteophytes. As the femorotibial compartment narrows consequent to the degenerative attenuation of the articular cartilages, and articular margin osteophytes progressively enlarge, the meniscus (mostly the body and anterior horn) is pulled out of the joint (Figs. 20-94 and 20-95). In advanced cases the meniscus is completely extruded beyond the margins of the joint (Fig.

20-95) and is forced between the capsule and bone, often to a point above or below the joint level.

DISCOID LATERAL MENISCUS

The discoid lateral meniscus is a congenital anomaly that represents persistence of the fetal configuration of the menisci. In fetuses the menisci are flat oval cartilaginous disks the size of their respective tibial articular surfaces. After birth the central portion is resorbed, resulting in the normal crescentic configuration of the adult meniscus. If the resorption does not occur or is incomplete, the meniscus retains its fetal discoid configuration.[88] A discoid meniscus may be a flat disk or a disk with various degrees of depression of its midportion. The condition is usually encountered on the lateral side, rarely on the medial.

A discoid meniscus is prone to degeneration and

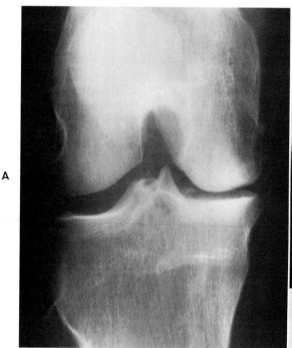

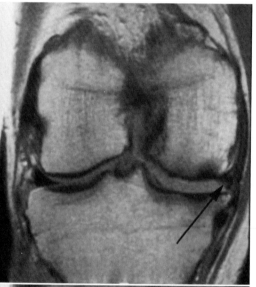

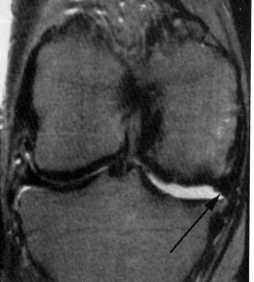

FIGURE 20-93

Degenerative disease of the medial compartment following an old tear of the medial meniscus. **A,** Tunnel view of the knee. There is osteosclerosis of the articular surfaces of the medial compartment. Note also the small hypertrophic osteophytes at the joint margins. **B,** SD and, **C,** T2-WI coronal views of the knee. The *arrow* in **B** and **C** shows the irregular remnant of the medial meniscus body. The remainder of the meniscus has been torn and displaced. The meniscal remnant resembles a postoperative meniscus. However, there was no history or evidence of previous surgery. The capsular remnant adheres to the articular margins of the femoral condyle and tibial plateau, the capsule-TCL complex is moderately thickened, and the articular cortices of the femur and tibia are irregular, with osteosclerosis of the subchondral bone secondary to degenerative disease of the medial compartment. A focal zone of osteonecrosis also may be present.

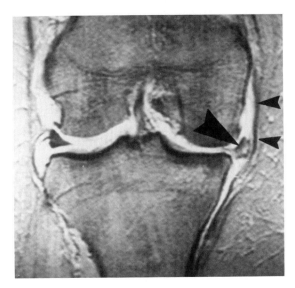

FIGURE 20-94
Degenerative disease of the medial compartment and medial meniscus. Coronal gradient echo (TR 700/TE 13, flip angle 30°) through the bodies of the menisci. There is marked deformity, with signal nonhomogeneity, of the medial meniscus (*large arrowhead*). The free margin of the meniscus has been completely eroded, the capsular margin is deformed, and there is marked narrowing of the medial compartment with attenuation of the articular cartilage of the medial femoral condyle. The meniscus is about 90% extraarticular, being extruded from the medial compartment. The joint capsule is displaced away (*small arrowheads*).

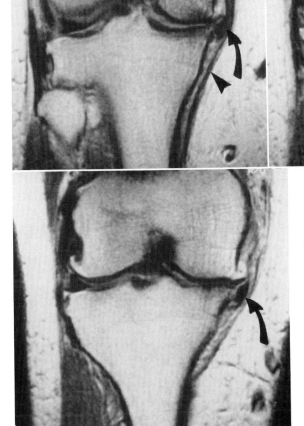

FIGURE 20-95
Degenerative disease of the medial compartment with extrusion of the meniscus. Spin density coronal views showing severe degenerative disease of the medial compartment, with almost complete obliteration of the joint. There are hypertrophic osteophytes arising from the joint margin. The body of the medial meniscus has been completely extruded from the joint (*curved arrow*). The capsule-TCL complex is stripped away from the bone and displaced outward (*arrowhead*).

tearing. It often contains multiple degenerative cysts, or a large cyst, sometimes with marked expansion of the meniscus. The expanded meniscus may protrude beyond the margins of the lateral compartment. The cyst may rupture into the capsulomeniscal zone and create a parameniscal cyst.

MRI of the discoid meniscus

On MRI the diagnosis of a discoid meniscus is made when the meniscus is significantly wider than normal. All imaging planes show the entire meniscus, including its body, to be very wide, extending from the peripheral margin of the lateral compartment to the midsagittal plane of the tibia[89] (Figs. 20-96 to 20-98). Prior to cystic degeneration a discoid meniscus is often triangular in cross section (i.e., the free margin is significantly thinner than the capsular margin) and wider than normal. The MRI appearance of intrameniscal degenerative cysts and tears of the discoid meniscus are similar to those of nondiscoid menisci.

POSTMENISCECTOMY MENISCUS

Persistence or reccurence of symptomatology in patients with previous meniscectomy is usually the reason for reexamination of the knee. The clinical symptomatology may be due to a tear of the meniscal remnant, its detachment from the capsule, loose bodies, a parameniscal cyst, or pathology or structures other than the ones previously operated on. The modern techniques of arthroscopic surgery do not cause distortion of the knee anatomy and do not interfere with the diagnosis of pathologies of structures not operated upon. The important issue is clarification of the status of the previously operated meniscus.

The MRI findings of postmeniscectomy menisci are dependent upon the extent and type of surgical resection employed. If only a minimal to moderate shaving was done, there may be no significant alteration of the meniscal configuration (Fig. 20-99). Otherwise, the meniscus is short with an irregular contour and diffuse increased internal SI (Fig. 20-100). The contour irregularity may be very marked.

The MRI diagnosis of a tear of the meniscal remnant is difficult because of the irregularity of meniscal contour (Fig. 20-100, *B* and *C*) and diffusely increased SI (Fig. 20-100, *A*); however, this is not true with full-thickness tears that have separation of fragments. Incomplete tears are impossible to identify, except on identically performed comparison studies.

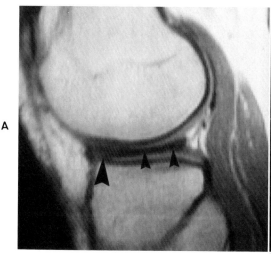

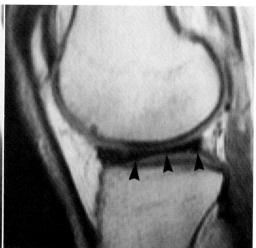

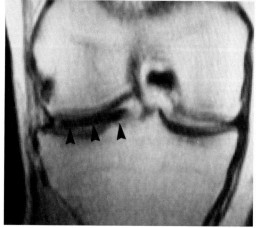

FIGURE 20-96

Discoid lateral meniscus. **A** and **B**, Sagittal T1-WI and, **C**, coronal SD. In **A** the large *arrowhead* points to the degenerative expansion and tear of the anterior horn of the discoid meniscus, and the *small arrowheads* to the intact portion of the meniscus. In **B** and **C** the *arrowheads* point to the discoid meniscus. In this patient the meniscus was actually thinner than expected but quite wide, extending from the peripheral margin to the midsagittal plane of the tibia on all sagittal and coronal views.

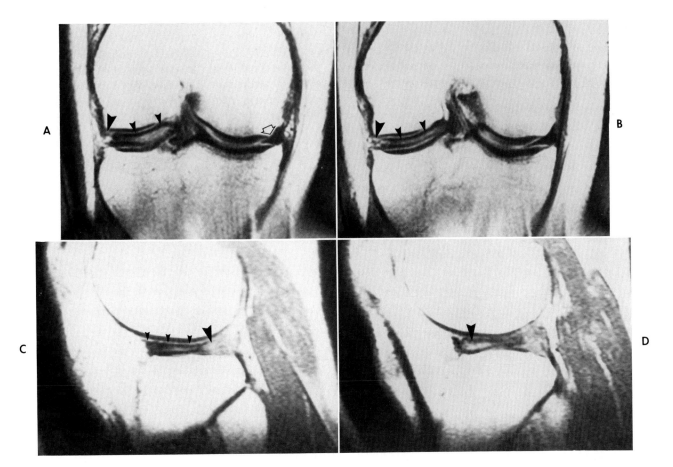

FIGURE 20-97

Discoid lateral meniscus with cystic degenerative expansion and tear. A and B, Coronal SD. The *hollow arrow in* A identifies the body of the medial meniscus, which is normal. The *large arrowhead* in A and B points to the capsular margin of the body, which is torn. The *small arrowheads* point to cystic expansion of the body. Note that the body extends all the way into the midportion of the knee joint. **C** and **D**, Sagittal T1-WI, meniscal windows. In **C** the *large arrowhead* points to severe degenerative cystic expansion and tear of the posterior horn of the lateral meniscus, the *small arrowheads* to the anterior horn of the meniscus (which shows evidence of high SI due to degenerative disease). In **D** the *arrowhead* points to cystic clublike expansion of the anterior horn due to degenerative cyst formation.

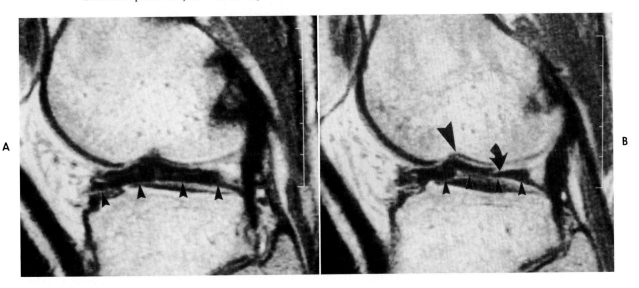

FIGURE 20-98

Torn discoid lateral meniscus. SD oblique sagittal views. The *small arrowheads* in B point to the discoid nature of the meniscus. The *large arrowhead* points to an exaggeration of the normal focal depression of the lateral femoral condyle, which is abnormally deep because of the long-standing cystic degeneration and expansion of the meniscus. The meniscus is both expanded in its center and torn. The *curved arrow* points to another tear.

The reported experience with MRI findings of menisci after surgery is limited.[77,90,91] Smith and Totty[90] reported their experience with 55 menisci treated by means of partial meniscectomy and subsequent arthroscopy. They found a spectrum of MR findings in the meniscal remnants. Menisci with minimal shaving were almost of normal length and similar configuration to menisci not operated on, although signal nonhomogeneity (56%) and a blunted meniscal tip were present in most segments. Menisci with more extensive surgical resection had a varied appearance, ranging from a shortened but otherwise normal configuration and SI to marked irregularity

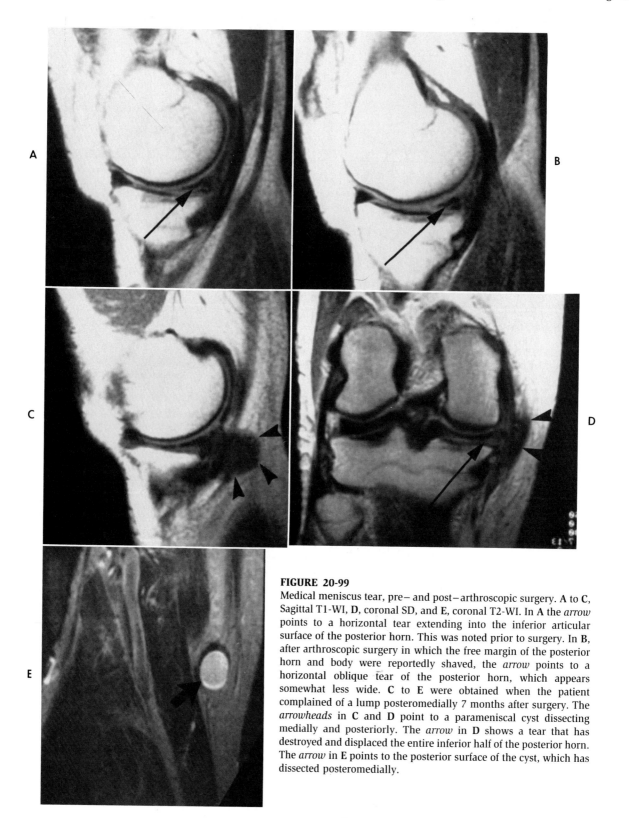

FIGURE 20-99

Medical meniscus tear, pre– and post–arthroscopic surgery. A to C, Sagittal T1-WI, D, coronal SD, and E, coronal T2-WI. In A the *arrow* points to a horizontal tear extending into the inferior articular surface of the posterior horn. This was noted prior to surgery. In B, after arthroscopic surgery in which the free margin of the posterior horn and body were reportedly shaved, the *arrow* points to a horizontal oblique tear of the posterior horn, which appears somewhat less wide. C to E were obtained when the patient complained of a lump posteromedially 7 months after surgery. The *arrowheads* in C and D point to a parameniscal cyst dissecting medially and posteriorly. The *arrow* in D shows a tear that has destroyed and displaced the entire inferior half of the posterior horn. The *arrow* in E points to the posterior surface of the cyst, which has dissected posteromedially.

of contour and nonhomogeneity of signal. There were three meniscal remnant tears missed on MRI but discovered at arthroscopy in this series. All these tears occurred in menisci with marked contour irregularity.

Moderate to marked contour irregularity and internal signal nonhomogeneity are normal findings in postoperative menisci. These characteristics of the meniscal remnant interfere with identification of partial tears. However, when a full-thickness tear is present, or the torn fragments are separated, a positive diagnosis of a tear should be made. The criteria for diagnosing traumatic lesions of the capsule, detachment of the meniscal remnant, and pathologies of other structures in a postmeniscectomy knee are the same as in nonoperated knees.

When a significant portion of meniscus is removed surgically, the chances of developing a degenerative disease of the femorotibial compartments are greatly increased (Figs. 20-100, *G,* and 20-101). For this reason the current tendency is to preserve as much of the menisci as possible.

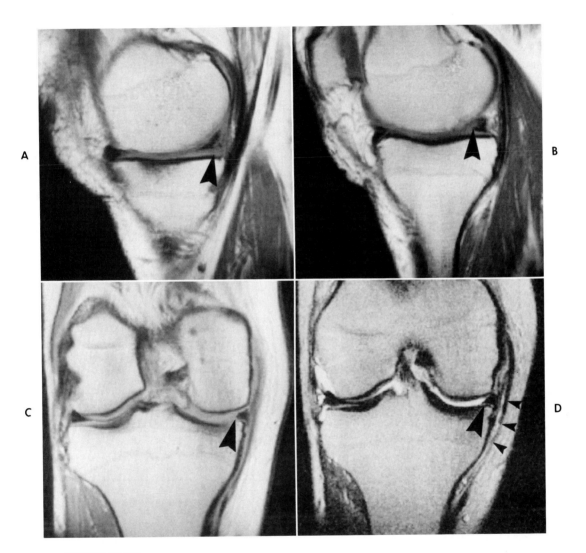

FIGURE 20-100
Postoperative meniscus in four patients. **A** and **B,** T1-WI sagittal views, normal postoperative status. In **A** the *arrowhead* points to the posterior horn of the medial meniscus. There is diffuse and nonuniformly increased SI of the posterior horn. In **B** the free margin and approximately two thirds of the width of the posterior horn have been surgically resected *(arrowhead).* The margin of the capsular remnant is irregular. **C,** Coronal SD and, **D,** coronal T2-WI from another patient. In **C** the *arrowhead* points to the free margin (site of surgical resection) of the remaining capsular segment of medial meniscus. There is thickening of the TCL-capsule complex. In **D** the *large arrowhead* points to the capsular remnant of medial meniscus, the *small arrowheads* to an intrasubstance tear of the TCL-capsule complex. Although the meniscus shows a normal postoperative configuration in this patient, there is an intrasubstance tear of the TCL-capsule complex accounting for the recurrent postoperative symptomatology.
Continued.

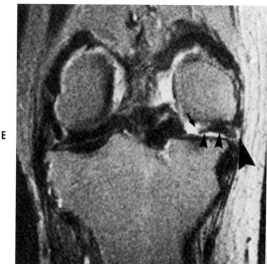

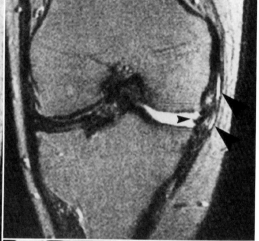

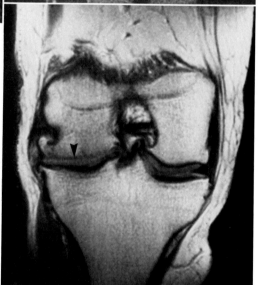

FIGURE 20-100, cont'd
E and F, Coronal T2-WI from another patient. In E the *large arrowhead* points to a zone of high SI at the capsulomeniscal junction on the posteromedial aspect of the posterior horn, indicating partial separation. The *two small arrowheads* point to a large portion of the posterior horn that was not resected, the *arrow* to the portion that was, just medial to its apex. In F the *large arrowheads* point to a linear area of increased SI due to an intrasubstance tear of the capsuloligamentous complex. The *small arrowhead* denotes a markedly irregular remnant of the anterior portion of the meniscal body. Despite their irregularity, the meniscal remnants have a normal postoperative configuration. However, there is thickening with an intrasubstance tear of the medial capsuloligamentous complex. G, Coronal SD in another patient. Note the moderately advanced degenerative disease of the lateral compartment *(arrowhead)*. This patient underwent lateral meniscectomy 6 years prior to this MR study.

FIGURE 20-101
Coronal T2-WI. The *large arrowheads* show marked irregularity and attenuation of the articular cartilage of the medial femoral condyle in this patient following medial meniscectomy. A similar process on the tibial articular cartilage is present. The *small arrowheads* point to a focal zone of aseptic necrosis of the medial tibial plateau.

INJURIES TO THE ANTERIOR CRUCIATE LIGAMENT

The ACL is usually best visualized on oblique sagittal views. However, in a significant number of patients it is satisfactorily visualized on anatomical sagittal views as well (Figs. 20-102 and 20-103). We also rely on coronal and axial views to assess the integrity of this ligament. An optimal visualization of tears in the ACL usually requires a T2-weighted sequence.

Isolated injuries of the ACL occur in about 30% of patients. The remaining 70% usually have other intraarticular injuries as well, particularly tears of the posteromedial capsule and capsulomeniscal junction, medial

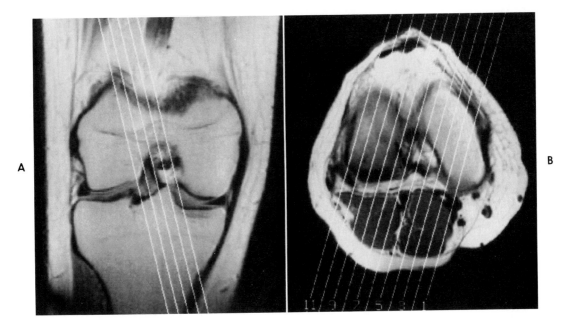

FIGURE 20-102
Oblique sagittal views for the ACL prescribed on coronal, **A**, and axial, **B**, images.

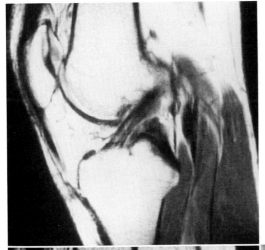

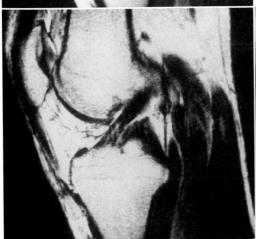

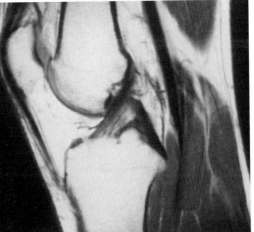

FIGURE 20-103
Normal ACL. A spin density oblique sagittal, **A**, and a T2-WI oblique sagittal, **B**, show the ligament's femoral insertion quite well. **C**, A T2-WI anatomical sagittal shows the ACL and PCL. Although the tibial insertion of the ACL is equally well seen on anatomical and oblique sagittals, assessment of its integrity of femoral insertion often requires oblique sagittals.

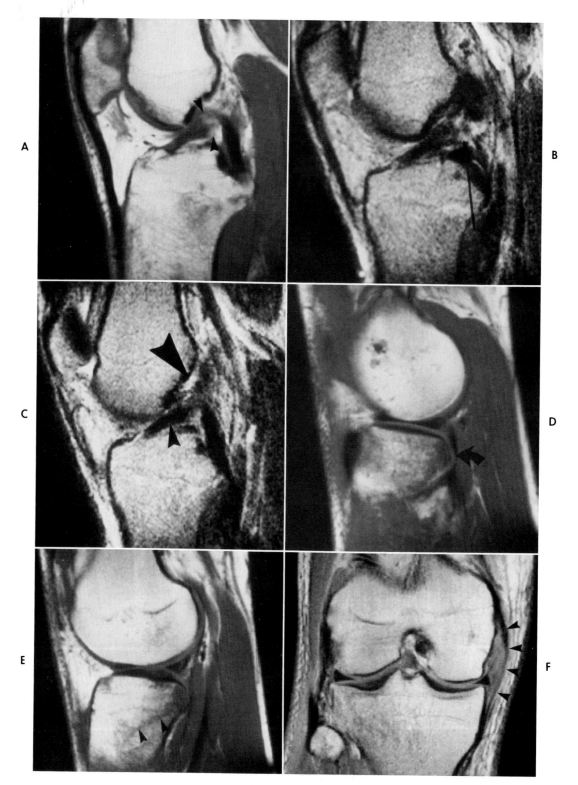

FIGURE 20-104

Tear of the ACL and TCL with fracture of the lateral tibial condyle. A is a T1-WI anatomical sagittal. The midportion of the ACL is widened and interrupted, with irregular margins *(arrowheads)*. **B** and **C** are T2-WI oblique sagittal views. In **B** there is high-SI hemorrhage/edema in the disrupted ligament *(arrow)*. In **C** the *large arrowhead* points to the high-SI hemorrhage/edema at the femoral insertion of the ACL. The *small arrowhead* points to the inferiorly displaced lower half of the ligament. **D** and **E,** T1-WI sagittal views. In **D** the *arrow* shows an area of low SI on the posterior aspect of the lateral tibial condyle due to hemorrhage/edema secondary to bone contusion. In **E** the *arrowheads* point to fracture of the proximal tibia. **F,** SD coronal view. The *arrowheads* show a grade 1 to 2 disruption of the TCL, with almost complete detachment of the body of the meniscus from the capsuloligamentous complex.

meniscus, or TCL (Fig. 20-104). Tears of the ACL frequently occur in its proximal portion, less commonly in its midportion. Complete or partial avulsions occur more frequently at the femoral than at the tibial insertion. However, avulsion fractures are more common at the tibial insertion.

An acute complete tear is typically accompanied by a large hemarthrosis, which develops immediately.[92] Incomplete and intrasubstance tears are usually accompanied by a less dramatic clinical picture and are difficult to identify clinically.[93,94]

The MRI findings of ACL injury[91,95-99] depend upon the extent and age of the lesion and consist of alterations in SI and deformity of the contour of the ligament. Generally, acute tears cause various degrees of hemorrhage and edema. Although these are strongly suspected on T1-WI

and SD (as zones of low and medium SI, and usually more SI than in the intact ligament), they are definitely more conspicuous and easier to identify on T2-WI (as zones of markedly increased SI).

Intrasubstance microtears of the ACL may cause no noticeable contour deformity. However, because hemorrhage and edema are usually present within the ligament, there often is unsharpness of the margins with blurring of the boundaries between the fasciculi within the ligament on T1-WI and SD. On T2-WI multiple small intraligamentous zones of increased SI are noted (Fig. 20-105). The larger intrasubstance tears may cause a small mass of edema and hemorrhage within and surrounding the zone of tear that is of low SI on T1-WI and high SI on T2-WI.

Incomplete and complete tears can produce a 2 to 4 cm mass of edema and hemorrhage, usually surrounding the

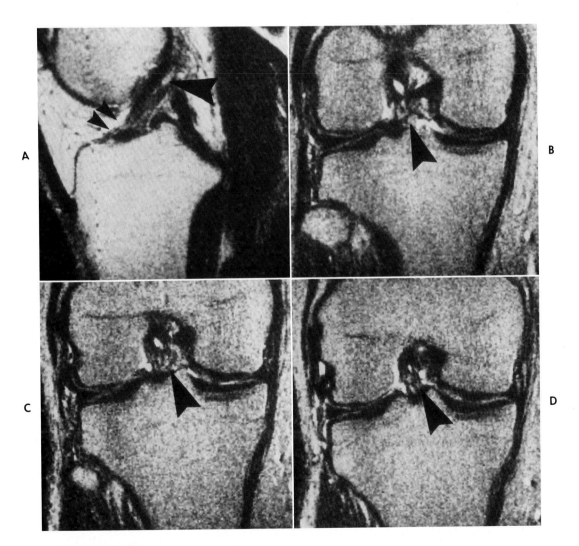

FIGURE 20-105
Intrasubstance and superficial tears of the ACL. **A** is a T2-weighted oblique sagittal, and **B** to **D** are T2-weighted coronals. In **A** the *two small arrowheads* point to the normal synovial fold containing fluid anterior to the anterior cruciate ligament. The *large arrowhead* points to one of the focal regions containing fluid within the substance of the ligament. The *arrowheads* in the coronal views show the ACL, with a number of high-signal areas due to microtears containing fluid in the substance of the ligament. At arthroscopy multiple superficial tears, bleeding, and edema were observed.

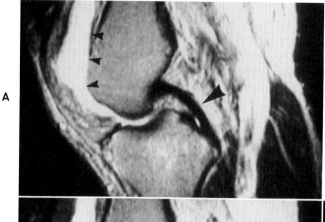

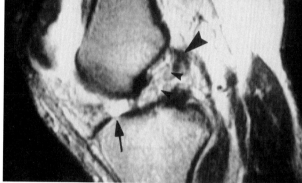

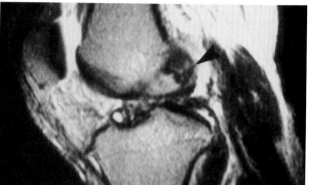

FIGURE 20-106

Tear of the ACL. Oblique sagittal T2-WI views. In **A** the PCL is normal *(arrowhead)*. The *small arrowheads* point to effusion in the suprapatellar bursa. In **B** the *small arrowheads* point to increased SI in the ACL due to edema and bleeding. The *large arrowhead* points to a minimal partial volume effect with the medial cortex of the lateral femoral condyle. The *arrow* points to a defect in the cortex of the tibia just anterior to the insertion of the ACL. Note the increased-SI effusion/blood directly above this region. In **C** the *arrowhead* points to the medial cortex of the lateral femoral condyle. At exploration an extensive tear of the ACL, avulsion fracture of the tibial insertion (with the fracture extending anteriorly), and profuse bleeding and effusion were found.

proximal part of the ACL and in the vicinity of its femoral attachment,[100] less commonly elsewhere along the course of the ligament (Figs. 20-106 to 20-108). On T1-WI this mass of edema/hemorrhage may be mistaken for a partial volume effect with the inner surface of the lateral femoral condyle (Fig. 20-108). However, on T2-WI the hemorrhagic mass shows increased SI whereas none is evident if the apparent mass is due to a partial volume effect.

With both complete and incomplete tears the ligament may have a normal course or may exhibit sagging and bowing posteriorly (Figs. 20-109 to 20-114). It is important to realize that although a complete tear may be present the ligament can have a normal course. Thus differentiation of a complete from an incomplete tear based solely on the presence or absence of contour abnormality cannot be made. An acute complete tear is positively identified when a full interruption of the fibers is seen. High-SI hemorrhage and edema are usually seen in the interrupted area on T2-WI. A complete avulsion of the ligament also causes disruption at the site of attachment on bone and may be accompanied by an avulsion fracture, usually of the tibia (Figs. 20-115 and 20-116). The tibial insertion of the ACL is usually well delineated on sagittal and coronal images and most pulse sequences. The displacement of the tibial cortex, or a larger piece of bone, with bleeding and edema at the fracture site, is usually well seen on T1-WI and T2-WI. However, visualization of the femoral insertion may require additional T2-weighted axial and oblique sagittal views.

The deformities of contour of the ACL are important

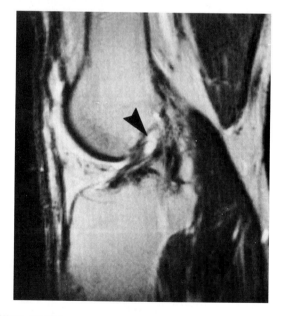

FIGURE 20-107

T2-WI oblique sagittal. The *arrowhead* points to a focal zone of increased SI at the femoral insertion of the ACL. At surgery a partial detachment of the ACL from the femur was found.

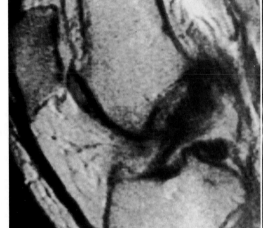

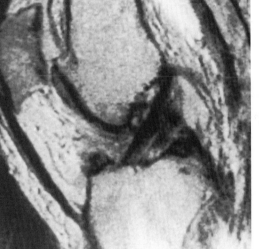

FIGURE 20-108
Partial volume effect with the lateral femoral condyle. **A** is a T2-WI oblique sagittal from one patient, and **B** and **C** are SD oblique sagittals from another. The partial volume effect with the cortex of the lateral femoral condyle is seen in **A** and **B**. The ACL is normal in **C**.

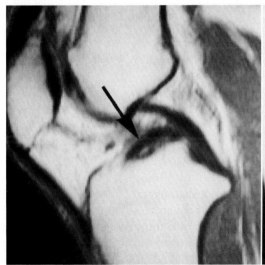

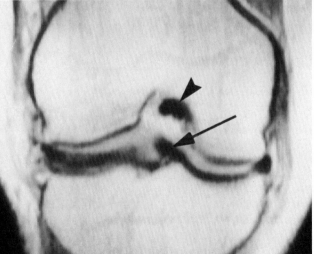

FIGURE 20-109
Tear of the ACL. **A** is a T1-WI sagittal and, **B**, a spin density coronal. In **A** the *arrow* points to the torn ACL, which is in an almost horizontal position. In **B** the *arrow* points to the lower portion of the ACL, just above its tibial insertion, which is intact. The *arrowhead* points to the attachment of the PCL to the medial femoral condyle. A partially discoid lateral meniscus is also present.

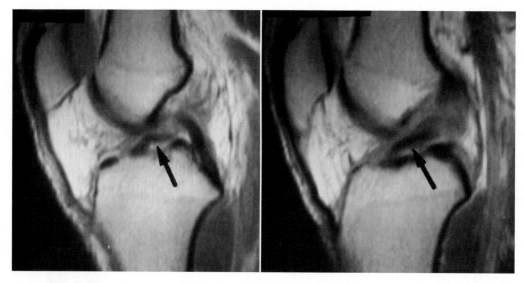

FIGURE 20-110
ACL tear. T1-WI sagittal views show the ligament, which is detached from its femoral insertion and partially buckled *(arrow)*.

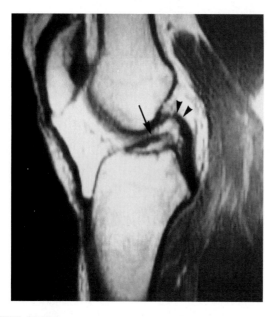

FIGURE 20-111
ACL tear. The ligament is detached from its femoral insertion and lies almost horizontal *(arrow)*. The *arrowheads* point to buckling of the PCL, a secondary sign of the ACL tear.

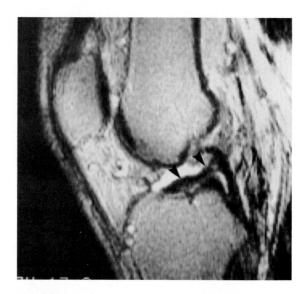

FIGURE 20-112
ACL tear. Sagittal T2-WI. The *arrowheads* point to the detached and inferiorly displaced ligament.

signs of ligament injury. When the knee is in full extension, the ACL is taut with smooth and straight margins at about 60 to 65 degrees to the horizontal plane. It is important to realize that the ligament may appear lax if the knee is flexed more than 5 degrees. A true laxity of the ACL, on the other hand, without evidence of abnormality, may be due to old, incomplete, small tears. In addition to hemorrhage and edema, incomplete avulsions cause laxity and bowing of the ligament. When there is detachment of the ligament from the femur, a longitudinal splitting of ligamentous fibers may also occasionally

be present. With a complete tear of the proximal segment or avulsion of the femoral attachment, the ligament can have a course ranging from normal to horizontal, as if it has fallen free into the joint. In other cases it may be bowed or folded upon itself.

An indirect sign of ACL laxity or tear is buckling of the PCL (Fig. 20-111), which occurs secondary to the anterior movement of the tibia relative to the femur. However, one must be careful in assessment of PCL buckling. Occasionally the PCL will appear buckled in a person with a perfectly normal ACL and PCL. This is more likely to be

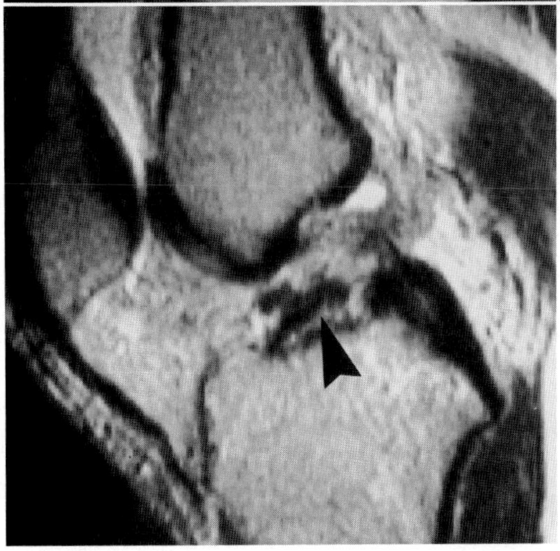

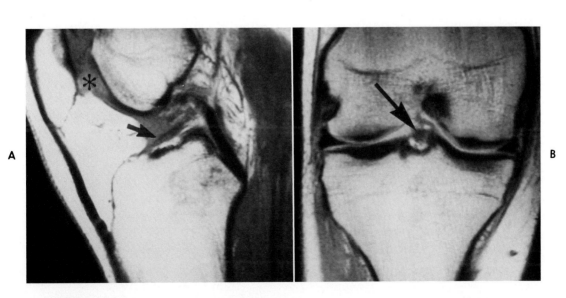

FIGURE 20-113
Tear of the ACL in three patients. **A**, T1-WI anatomical sagittal view. The *curved arrow* points to the PCL. The *arrow* points to the proximal portion of the ACL, which is displaced posteriorly. The *arrowheads* point to hemorrhage/edema surrounding the torn lower half of the ACL. **B**, T1-WI anatomical sagittal view. The *arrowhead* indicates hemorrhage/edema in the expected position of the ACL. **C**, T2-WI oblique sagittal view. The *arrowhead* points to the torn distal half of the ACL, which is displaced inferiorly.

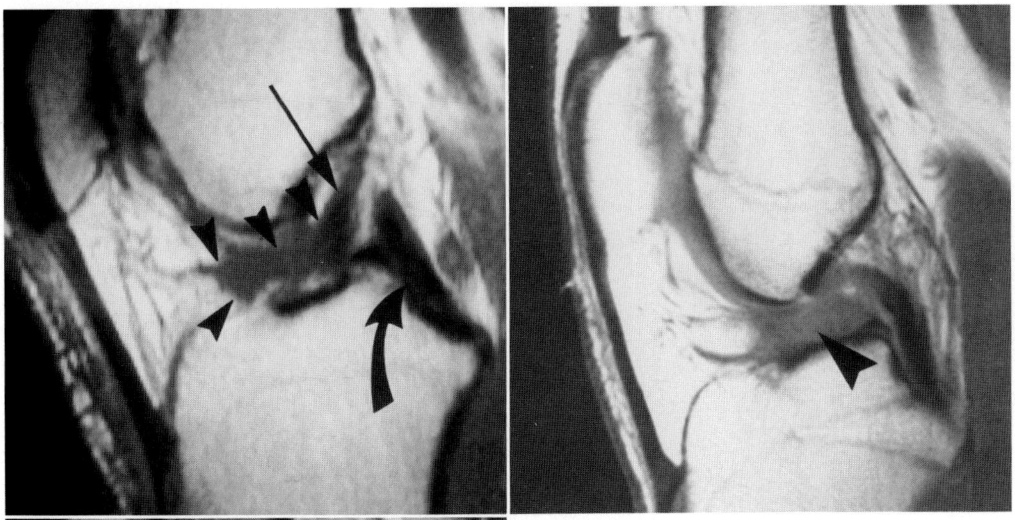

FIGURE 20-114
ACL tear. **A**, Sagittal T1-WI and, **B**, coronal spin density views. The *arrows* point to the torn and inferiorly displaced ligament. The *asterisk* is on joint effusion.

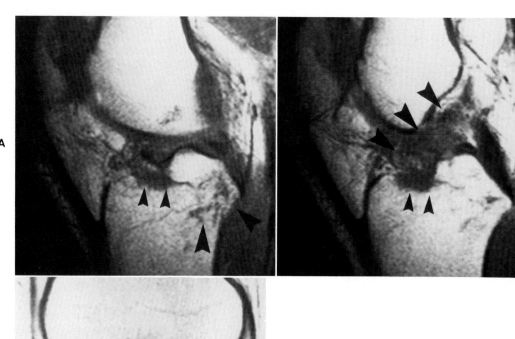

FIGURE 20-115

Avulsion fracture at the tibial insertion of the ACL. **A** and **B**, Sagittal T1-WI and, **C**, coronal SD. The *small arrowheads* in all images point to the fracture at the site of insertion of the ACL. The *large arrowheads* in **A** point to a fracture of the posterior portion of the tibia, the *large arrowheads* in **B** to edema/hemorrhage surrounding the torn ACL. This patient also had a tear of the TCL and medial joint capsule.

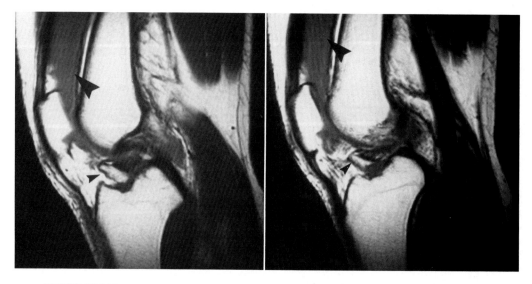

FIGURE 20-116

Tear of the ACL and an avulsion fracture of the tibia. T1-WI sagittal views. The *large arrowhead* points to joint effusion, the *small arrowhead* to the fracture, which is displaced superiorly.

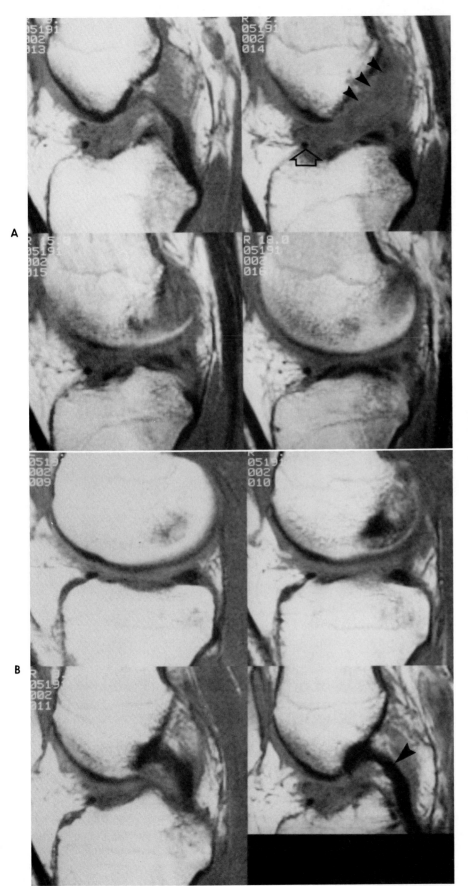

FIGURE 20-117
Old ACL tear. Sagittal T1-WI. **A,** The *hollow arrow* points to the transverse ligament, the *arrowheads* to the position of the ACL (which is missing). **B,** The *arrowhead* points to the normal PCL.

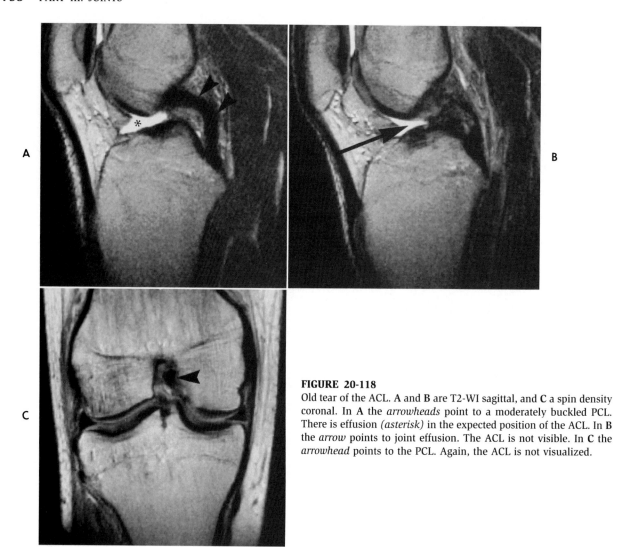

FIGURE 20-118
Old tear of the ACL. **A** and **B** are T2-WI sagittal, and **C** a spin density coronal. In **A** the *arrowheads* point to a moderately buckled PCL. There is effusion *(asterisk)* in the expected position of the ACL. In **B** the *arrow* points to joint effusion. The ACL is not visible. In **C** the *arrowhead* points to the PCL. Again, the ACL is not visualized.

seen on oblique than on anatomical sagittal views and occurs in individuals in whom the proximal part of the PCL makes an abrupt turn medially.

Chronic incomplete tears lead to laxity, sparsity of the fibers, and diffuse or nonhomogeneous moderately increased SI on T1-WI and SD.

In patients with a bucket handle tear and displacement of the handle of the bucket into the intercondylar notch, an initially intact ACL may become markedly distorted and torn.[67] The torn meniscal fragment and the ACL are jammed together in the intercondylar notch and indistinguishable from each other on MRI.

In many older patients with advanced degenerative disease of the knee there are multiple zones of moderately increased SI on T1-WI in the substance of the ligament. The ligament may be irregular of outline, very thin with few visible moderately increased SI fibers, or the fibers may be altogether absent (Figs. 20-117 and 20-118). In these patients the combination of advanced degenerative disease and multiple episodes of ligamentous tear are most likely responsible for the abnormalities observed.

MRI of the ACL after surgical reconstruction

Reconstruction of the ACL may be performed utilizing patellar, semitendinosus, gracilis, or other tendons.[101,102] In recent years, because of favorable long-term results,[103] synthetic materials (Dacron and Gortex) have become increasingly acceptable.

There are several surgical techniques for reconstruction of the ACL.[104-108] They involve the creation of tunnels in the femur and tibia, positioning the ACL substitute, and fixing it at the ends of the tunnels. When highly ferromagnetic screws and staples are used near the joint line, there may be so much interference with the magnetic field that essentially no image can be obtained. On the other hand, when the metallic objects are at least 3 cm (or more) away from the joint line, it is usually possible to obtain a reasonably good MR study.

A normal reconstructed ACL is usually visualized (on sagittal and coronal views) as a homogeneously dark band on all pulse sequences within the femoral and tibial tunnels and as it crosses the joint (Fig. 20-119). The reconstructed ligament often appears significantly thicker

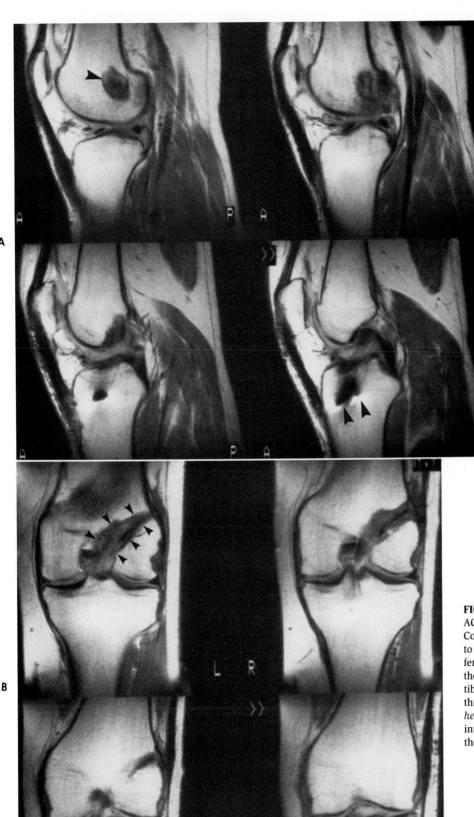

FIGURE 20-119
ACL reconstruction. **A,** Sagittal T1-WI. **B,** Coronal SD. A *single arrowhead* in **A** points to the end of the femoral tunnel in the lateral femoral condyle. *Two arrowheads* indicate the end of the tunnel in the anteromedial tibia. An artifact due to the metallic screw in this region is also present. In **B** the *arrowheads* identify the tunnel extending from the intercondylar notch to the lateral border of the femur.

Continued.

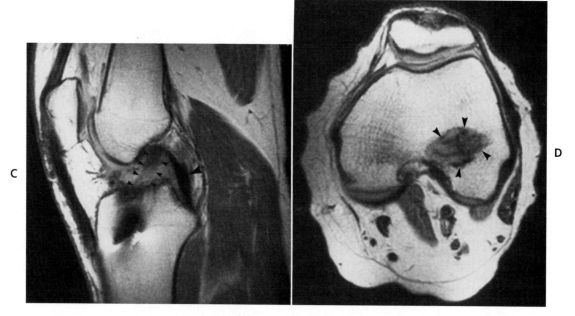

FIGURE 20-119, cont'd
C, Sagittal T1-WI, magnified view. D, Axial T1-WI. In C the *large arrowhead* points to the normal PCL, the *small arrowheads* to the reconstructed ACL. In D the *arrowheads* denote the tunnel in the lateral femoral condyle.

than a normal ACL. In our experience, when marked adhesions are present, and in patients with persistent or recurrent postoperative inflammation, the margins of the reconstructed ligament may be poorly seen or not visualized at all. Then the tibial and femoral tunnels, and the joint itself, appear to be full of irregular low-SI tissues (adhesions and fibrosis), with interspersed focal areas of high SI on T2-WI, and a definite reconstructed ligament often is not identifiable (Fig. 20-120). Furthermore, it may be impossible to detect a partial or even a complete tear of a reconstructed ACL in these patients. On the other hand, when there is a tear of a reconstructed ACL (biological tissue or synthetic fibers) in an otherwise reasonably normal knee, focal zones of high SI (on T2-WI and T2*) are seen in the torn ligament and its vicinity.[103]

The bony femoral and tibial tunnels are usually well seen on the coronal and sagittal views. However, if there is any question regarding their integrity, it is advisable to obtain axial views also. Computed tomography of the

knee is also helpful in evaluation of these patients (Fig. 20-121), particularly with stenosis of the intercondylar notch[109,110] or calcification of the reconstructed ligament.

Stenosis of the intercondylar notch, usually secondary to osteophytes, is thought to contribute to susceptibility of the ACL to tearing and is often well delineated on T1-WI coronal views when there is bone marrow within the osteophytes. However, when the notch is not well seen on MRI and appears to be full of low-SI tissues, the possible presence of calcification (Fig. 20-122) or dense osteosclerotic osteophytes within it should be considered. Computed tomography is indicated in these patients for delineation of the abnormalities.

INJURIES TO THE POSTERIOR CRUCIATE LIGAMENT

Tears of the PCL are infrequent and occur usually as a consequence of a severe sports-related injury or motor vehicle accident.[111-113] They are often accompanied by

FIGURE 20-120
Status—post ACL reconstruction. A and B, Coronal SD and, C and D, coronal T2-WI. In A the *large arrow* points to a metallic artifact at the proximal end of the femoral tunnel, the *small arrows* to the tunnel in the lateral femoral condyle. There is extensive fibrosis in this patient, making visualization of the reconstructed ACL almost impossible. In B the *arrow* points to the tunnel in the proximal tibia. In C the *solid arrow* points to the tunnel in the lateral femoral condyle, and the *hollow arrow* to a focal cystic lesion containing fluid. Note the markedly low-signal fibrosis filling the femoral tunnel. In D the *solid arrow* points to the tibial tunnel, the *hollow arrow* to a localized cystic area containing fluid. E and F are sagittal T1-WI. The *solid arrow* in both points to the metallic artifact at the distal end of the tibial tunnel. Because the metallic screws and staples were away from the joint region, there was no degradation of the image in this patient. The *hollow arrow* in E points to extensive fibrosis within the joint, the *arrowhead* in F to the tibial tunnel.

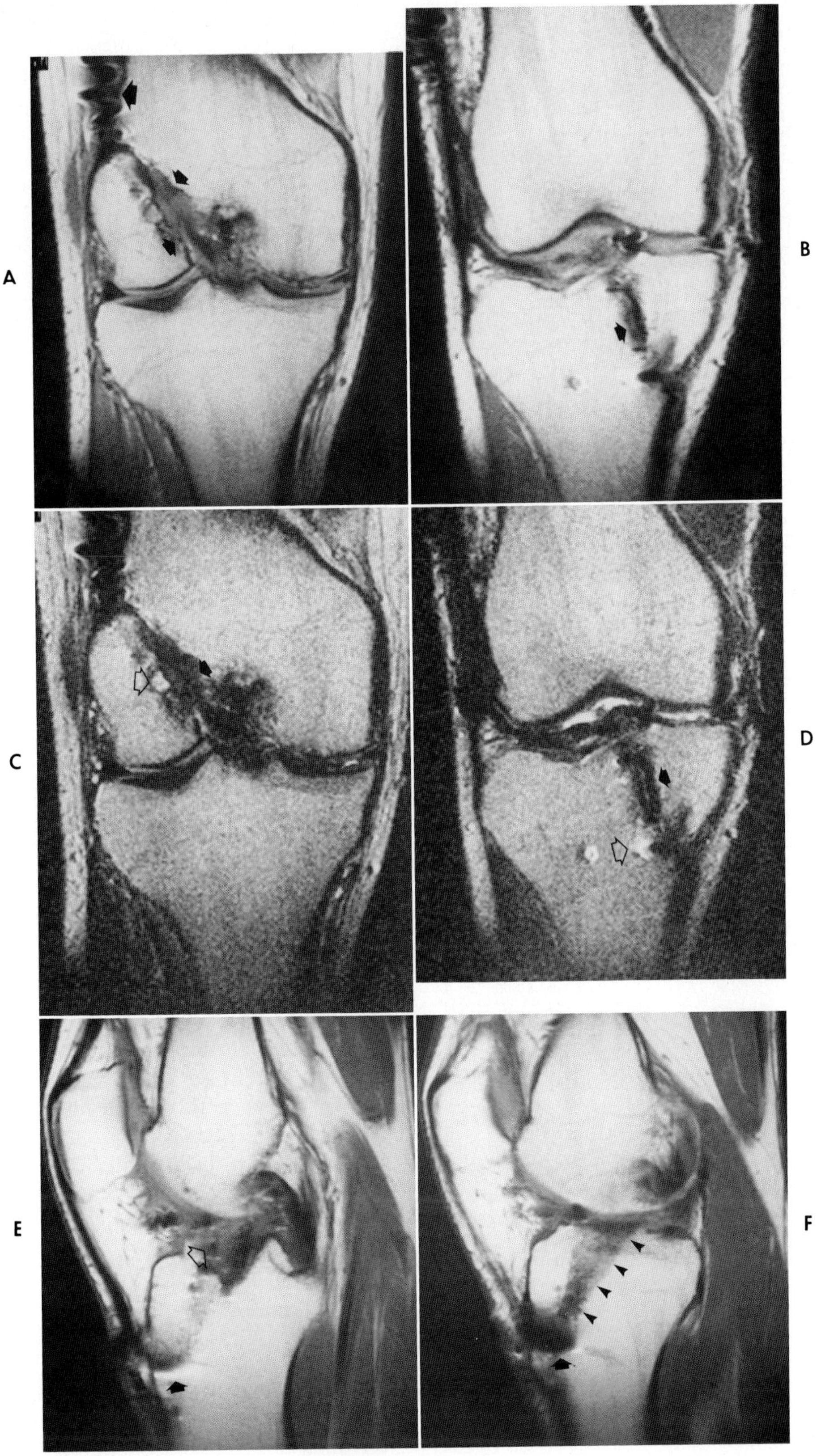

FIGURE 20-120
For legend see opposite page.

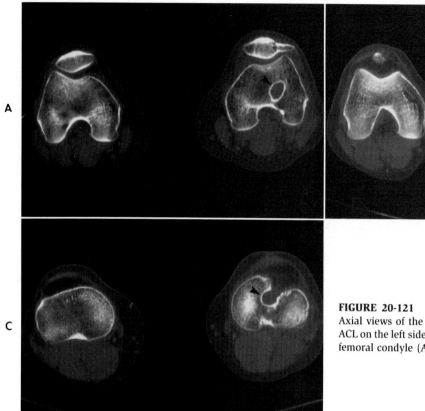

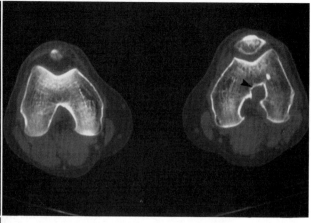

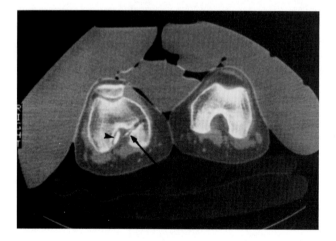

FIGURE 20-121
Axial views of the knee, status–post surgical reconstruction of the ACL on the left side. The *arrowhead* points to the tunnel in the lateral femoral condyle (**A** and **B**) and the tibia (**C**).

FIGURE 20-122
Axial CT. The *arrow* points to a calcified reconstructed PCL as it enters the femoral tunnel. The *arrowhead* points to a calcified ACL in the intercondylar notch.

tears of the ACL, medial meniscus, and TCL. Most PCL tears are incomplete and occur in its midportion. The next most common injury is tear of the tibial insertion of the ligament, which may be accompanied by an avulsion fracture of the tibia.

Acute incomplete intrasubstance tears produce irregular zones of increased SI on T2-WI secondary to hemor-

rhage and edema. Complete tears show discontinuity of the ligamentous fibers[111] (Fig. 20-123). Avulsion of the tibial insertion, often with a bony fragment displaced superoanteriorly, is usually well delineated on most pulse sequences.

Chronic tears (Figs. 20-124 to 20-131) are associated with fibrosis, enlargement, irregularity of ligamentous outline, occasionally calcification, deposits of fat, and degenerative replacement of the tendon fibers. These abnormalities cause the PCL to lose its usually normal dense homogeneously black and smooth characteristic and become less black with minimally to moderately increased SI on T1-WI and SD. On T2-WI there is no increased SI. In many individuals the milder form of this condition is asymptomatic.

SYSTEMIC AND LOCAL DISORDERS AFFECTING THE KNEE

The knee, more than any other joint, is involved in a large number of systemic and local disorders. For example, approximately 50% of all primary benign and malignant neoplasms of bone involve the distal femur and proximal tibia. The knee joint and its constituent bones are also a frequent site of involvement in rheumatoid arthritis (RA), hemophilia, infection, and fracture.

Neoplasms of bone usually do not masquerade as internal derangement and are better diagnosed on con-

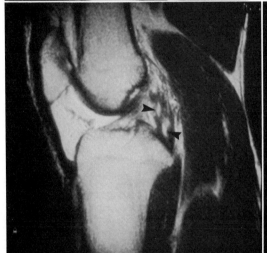

A

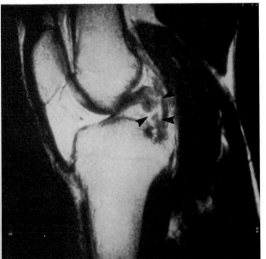

B

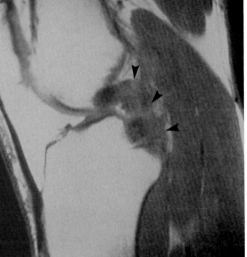

C

FIGURE 20-123
PCL tear. **A** is a sagittal anatomical T1-WI. Note the markedly irregular, thickened, and buckled PCL *(arrowheads),* with its nonhomogeneously increased internal SI. The ACL was also torn in this patient. **B** and **C** are T2-weighted anatomical sagittals. The multiple zones of increased SI in the substance of the PCL indicate tears of the ligament *(arrowheads).*

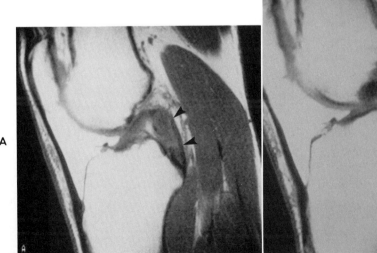

A

B

FIGURE 20-124
Tear of the PCL (old). **A** and **B**, Anatomical sagittal T1-weighted images. The PCL is markedly irregular, thickened, buckled and has increased nonhomogeneous internal signal *(arrowheads).*

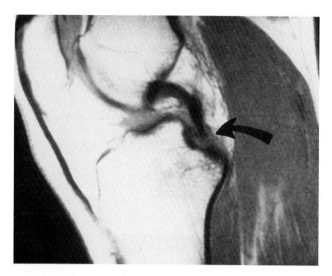

FIGURE 20-125
PCL tear. Sagittal T1-WI. There is avulsion of PCL from its tibial insertion *(arrow)*. Joint effusion and bone bruise of the posterior tibia are also present.

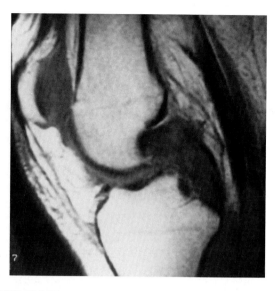

FIGURE 20-127
Old tear and degenerative disease of the PCL. A sagittal T1-WI shows marked enlargement, deformity, and moderately increased SI of the PCL, which was functionally deficient.

FIGURE 20-126
Old PCL tear. **A,** T1-WI coronal and, **B,** T1-WI sagittal views of the knee. The *arrowhead* in all images points to the PCL. Note that it is buckled and significantly thicker than expected, with moderately increased internal SI and markedly irregular borders. This patient had a history of previous injury to the PCL. In addition, the TCL and medial meniscus were torn. A partial tear of the ACL is also present.

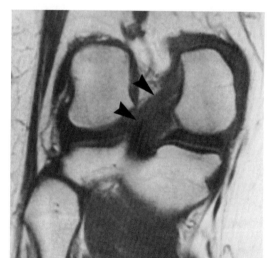

A

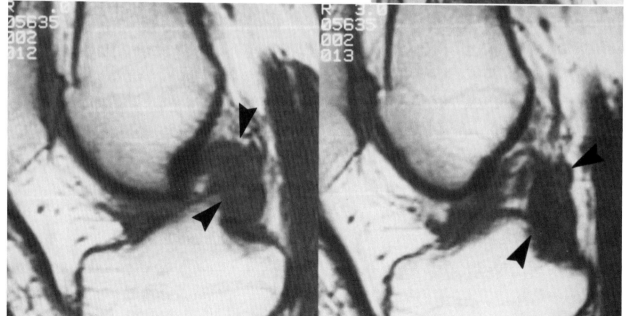

B

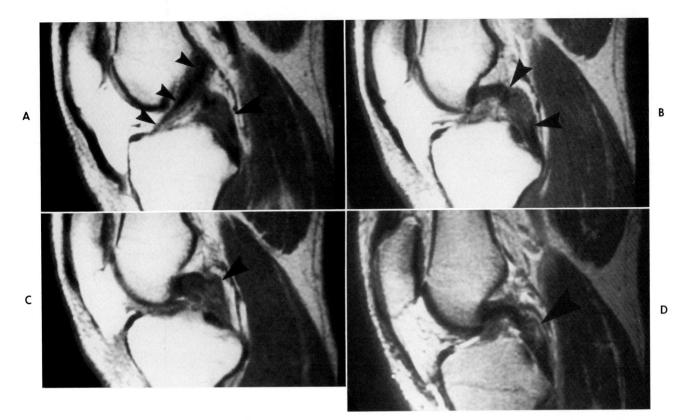

FIGURE 20-128
Old PCL tear. **A** to **C** are T1-WI, and **D** a T2-WI anatomical sagittal views. The *small arrowheads* in **A** point to the normal ACL, the *large arrowhead* to the PCL (which has moderately increased SI and is thick and deformed). In **B** and **C** the *arrowheads* show marked deformity and enlargement with moderately increased intraligamentous SI of the PCL. In **D** the *arrowhead* points to the same region as in **B**. There is minimally increased intraligamentous SI. This patient had a history of previous midsubstance tear of the PCL, treated conservatively.

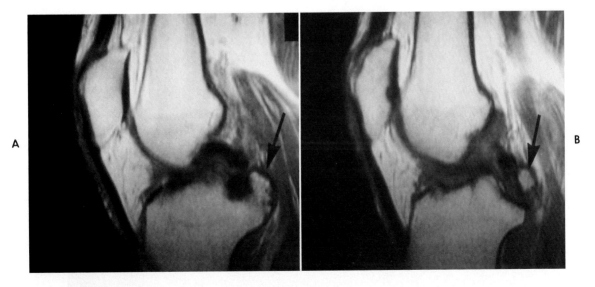

FIGURE 20-129
Old tear of the PCL with an avulsion fracture of the tibia. T1-WI sagittal views reveal marked deformity of the posterior aspect of the tibia due to an old fracture. The *arrow* points to hypertrophic deformities extending from the medial to the lateral side secondary to an avulsion fracture at the tibial insertion of the PCL.

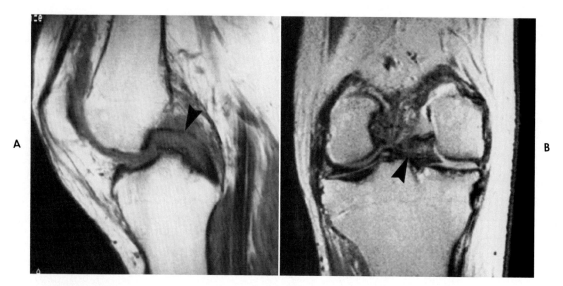

FIGURE 20-130
Long-standing degenerative disease and tear of the PCL and ACL. **A,** T1-WI sagittal. **B,** Coronal SD. There is marked distortion of the PCL. A *thin black line* (*arrowhead* in **A**) identifies the superior margin of the PCL. The remainder of the PCL has moderately increased SI. No definite PCL can be identified on the coronal view. Instead, low SI and nonhomogeneous SI tissues are seen to occupy the expected position of the PCL (*arrowhead* in **B**). The medial meniscus has been surgical resected.

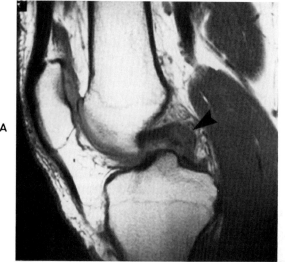

FIGURE 20-131
Chronic PCL tear. **A** is a T1-WI anatomical sagittal, **B** a coronal SD, and **C** a coronal T2-WI. In **A** the *arrowhead* points to marked buckling of the PCL, which has an abnormal contour and high internal SI. Note the moderate anterior displacement of the femur relative to the tibia. In **B** and **C** no distinct PCL is identified.

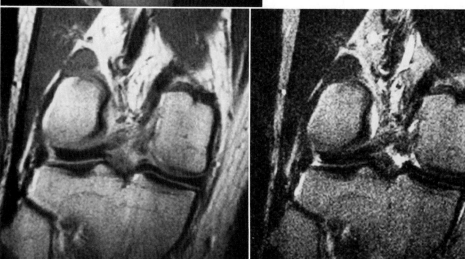

ventional roentgenography. However, CT and MRI may become necessary in these patients for a more definitive location and assessment of the extent of marrow involvement. Nevertheless, bone marrow neoplasms may present with ill-defined pain and a normal roentgenogram (Fig. 20-132), and the patient may be referred to rule out internal derangement prior to the establishment of a definitive diagnosis. The patient with a known diagnosis of storage disorder (e.g., Gaucher's disease [Fig. 20-133]) may also develop a clinical picture suggestive of a meniscal or ligamentous tear.

Infectious disease and neoplasms have been discussed in Chapters 9 and 11. The important clinical aspects and other features of many disorders of the knee have been dealt with in Chapter 21, which should be reviewed in conjunction with the present chapter. Discussion of these lesions will not be repeated here. The MRI features of some of the other conditions mentioned above, particularly those peculiar to the knee, common, or masquerading as internal derangement, and not covered in Chapter 21, will be discussed in this section.

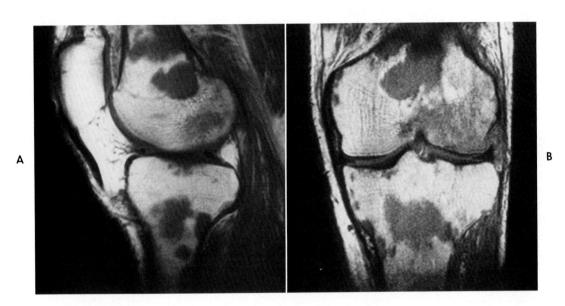

FIGURE 20-132
Leukemia. **A,** T1-WI sagittal and, **B,** spin density coronal views of the knee. There are multiple areas of low SI in the marrow in this patient.

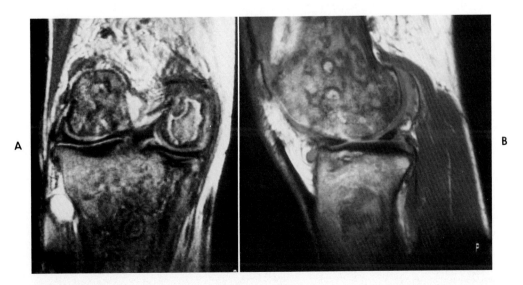

FIGURE 20-133
Gaucher's disease. **A,** Coronal SD, and **B,** sagittal T1-weighted images. The bone marrow is infiltrated by low-SI storage tissue in this patient. Note the large area of bone necrosis affecting the medial femoral condyle. The menisci are normal.

Rheumatoid arthritis

RA is a good model of chronic inflammatory arthritis for demonstrating the various joint abnormalities on MRI (Fig. 20-134). The uniform thinning of cartilage, an early manifestation, is fairly well seen.[112] In our experience the articular cartilage is optimally seen on SD and T2* images with medium and high SI respectively. The T2-WI sequence is particularly helpful when joint effusion is also present, because it renders the articular cartilage of medium SI while joint effusion is of high SI; thus the zones of cartilaginous irregularity, erosion, or destruction are well outlined at the cartilage/effusion interface. It

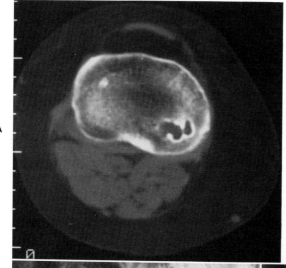

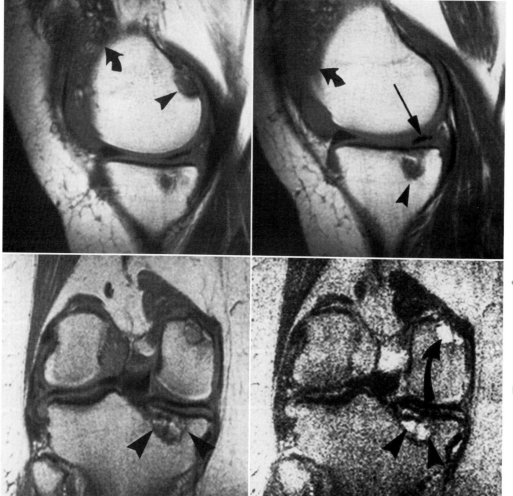

FIGURE 20-134
Subchondral synovial cyst in a patient with rheumatoid arthritis. **A** is an axial CT, **B** and **C** are sagittal T1-weighted, and **D** and **E** are coronal SD and T2-weighted images. Note the well-delineated cystic lesion of the medial tibial plateau in **A**. Subchondral cysts with rheumatoid arthritis may not have such sharply defined sclerotic margins as in this patient. In **B** the *arrowhead* denotes a synovial cyst of the medial femoral condyle. The *curved arrow* points to joint effusion and proliferative changes of the synovium, which present as high-SI nodular lesions. In **C** the *straight arrow* points to a remnant of the torn and eroded posterior horn of the medial meniscus. The *curved arrow* points to joint effusion, the *arrowhead* to the subchondral synovial cyst. The *arrowheads* in **D** and **E** show the synovial cyst of the tibia. The *curved arrow* in **E** points to the synovial cyst of the medial femoral condyle.

should be pointed out that arthroscopy is often superior to MRI in detecting the early stages of cartilage erosion — be it secondary to inflammatory arthritis, degenerative arthritis, or trauma. Subchondral sclerosis often appears as a 2 to 3 mm thick band of low SI on all pulse sequences. Subchondral cysts, of inflammatory or degenerative origin, exhibit low SI on T1-WI and high SI on T2-WI. In many patients with chronic arthritis, inflammatory or degenerative, fairly large focal zones of low SI on T1-WI are noted that often prove due to aseptic necrosis.

Joint effusion and synovitis

Joint effusion is usually seen as a homogeneous area of high SI on T2-WI and T2*. Acutely inflamed synovial tissue and pannus often are of low SI on T1-WI and exhibit a subtle nonhomogeneity of the signal due to small zones of slightly higher SI. On T2-WI they are of medium to high SI, often not as homogeneous and high in SI as effusion. Nevertheless, in some cases it may not be possible to distinguish an acutely inflamed pannus from joint effusion.[112-114] After intravenous injection of gadopentetate, effusion remains of low SI on T1-WI while acutely inflamed pannus shows increased SI.[112]

Rheumatoid arthritis is characterized by a recurrent inflammation of the synovial tissues of the joints, tendons, and bursae.[115,116] As the disease progresses, hypertrophy and villous transformation of the synovium occur. Eventually the hypertrophied synovium (pannus), in the form of granulation tissue, causes erosions of the cartilage and bone.[112,117] Although acutely inflamed pannus may

be of moderate to high SI on T2-WI, old quiescent pannus, essentially a mass of scar tissue, is low in SI, often with scattered small zones of moderately high SI.

In patients with long-standing RA, one may encounter a soft tissue mass within the synovial cavity. This mass, which may contain zones of low SI or signal void, usually proves to be old fibrotic granulation tissue/pannus with focal areas of hemosiderin deposit. It is most likely due to the well-known tendency of RA patients to bleed into the joints, bursae, and calf cysts.

Hemophilia

In hemophiliacs severe erosion and almost complete destruction of the articular cartilages develop fairly rapidly. Eventually, the joint space may become almost completely obliterated (Fig. 20-135). The femoral and tibial articular cortex and menisci become markedly deformed, irregular, and fragmented. MRI shows moderately to markedly low SI throughout the joint, at the articular surfaces, and within the frequently occurring irregular subchondral cysts. These abnormalities are secondary to repeated episodes of hemorrhage, leading to scarring, fibrosis, and the deposition of hemosiderin.[118,119] Depending upon the stage of evolution of the lesions and the amount of hemosiderin present, one may encounter low-SI intrasynovial irregular masses, small loose bodies, high- or low-SI effusions, and old subchondral cysts with low SI (fibrosis and hemosiderin deposits) or medium-high SI (serosanguineous cysts).

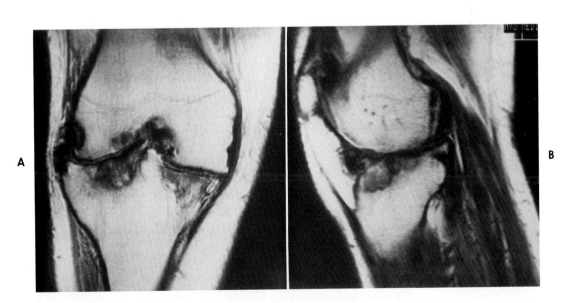

FIGURE 20-135
Hemophilia. **A**, Coronal SD and, **B**, sagittal T1-WI. There is almost complete obliteration of the joint space, with marked irregularity of the articular surfaces, complete distortion of the menisci and articular cartilages, and moderate hypertrophic changes. A fairly large subchondral cyst of the tibia is visible, along with multiple small intraarticular mass lesions. The low SI of these lesions is a consequence of repeated bleeding episodes.

Fractures

One bonus of knee MRI is the detection of various forms of fracture. This, we now know, with the benefit of hindsight, should have been anticipated from the outset. It has turned out that many fractures around the knee, masquerading as internal derangement or arthritis, were never diagnosed prior to the MRI era. Furthermore, the concept of contusional fracture — bone bruise or subchondral trabecular microfracture — has become crystallized on MRI. A variety of fractures with more or less specific MRI features have been identified.[91,120-122]

We have seen subtle, and not so subtle, fractures masquerading as internal derangement (Figs. 20-136 to 20-138) in 10% to 15% of the patients referred for routine knee MRI. The protocol suggested for internal derangement is also designed to detect the various forms of fracture encountered around the knee, so no modification is necessary for this purpose.

BONE BRUISE

This lesion is thought to be due to microfractures of bony trabeculae with hemorrhage and edema.[122] It

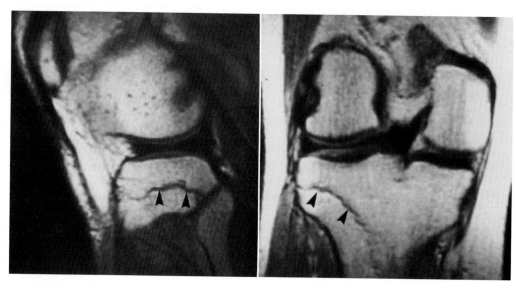

FIGURE 20-136
Fracture of the tibia. Sagittal and coronal T1-weighted images. The *arrowheads* point to the lateral condylar fracture.

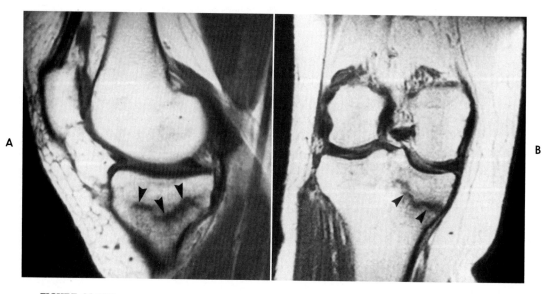

FIGURE 20-137
Fracture of the tibia. **A** is a T1-WI anatomical sagittal, and **B** a spin density coronal. *Arrowheads* denote the fracture. This 73-year-old man had gradual onset of pain without definite preceding trauma. He had been treated for arthritis during the preceding 7 weeks. This MR examination was requested to rule out internal derangement.

essentially involves the subchondral bone (Figs. 20-139 to 20-141) and presents as zones of low SI on T1-WI and moderate to high SI on T2-WI or T2*. It may be missed on SD (Fig. 20-141, *E*). The cortex is normal, with no definite fracture line evident. The lesion is localized and geographic or stellate in configuration[123] (Fig. 20-141, *B*) and may occur in either the medial or the lateral distal femur or proximal tibia (epiphysis), more commonly on the lateral side. A bone bruise is often simultaneously created by acute injuries that cause a tear of the ACL, TCL, or medial meniscus.[124,125] There is usually no significant abnormality on conventional roentgenography or arthroscopy, provided no articular cartilage injury has occurred. The bone scan shows increased tracer uptake. A bone bruise often resolves in 6 to 8 weeks. At the present time, (1991) there are no long-term studies available; nevertheless, it is interesting to speculate about the possible consequences of a bone bruise (i.e., subchondral cyst or increased susceptibility to degenerative arthritis).

A bone bruise, by definition, should not involve the articular cartilage or cortex. However, fractures of bone *may* be looked upon as a continuum, with bone bruise at one end representing closed trabecular microfractures and comminuted displaced fractures at the other. Thus,

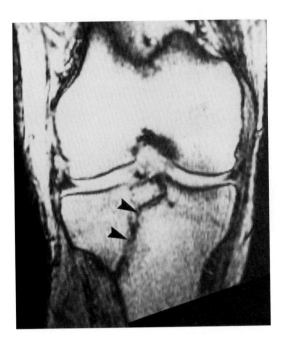

FIGURE 20-138
Tibial fracture. Coronal T2*. Note the fracture extending from the medial tibial plateau to the cortex of the proximal tibia on the lateral side *(arrowheads).*

FIGURE 20-139
Bone bruise. Trabecular fracture and hemorrhage/edema of the subchondral bone following an injury to the lateral compartment. **A** is a sagittal T2-WI, **B** a coronal SD, and **C** a coronal T2-WI. The *arrowheads* point to a zone of hemorrhage/edema accompanying the trabecular bone fracture.

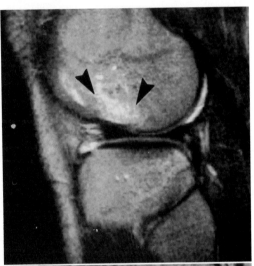

A

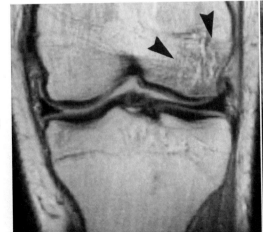

B

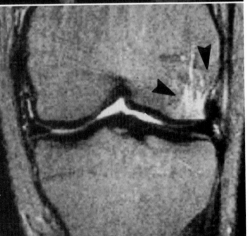

C

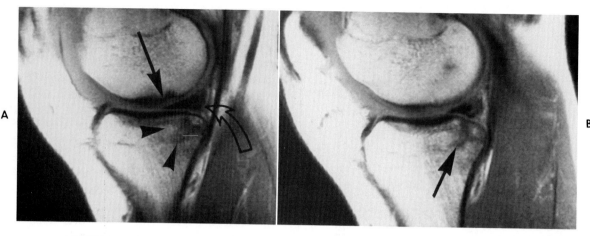

FIGURE 20-140

Peripheral tear of the medial meniscus with a bone bruise and cortical and osteochondral fractures. Sagittal T1-WI images. In **A** the *curved hollow arrow* points to the peripheral tear of the posterior horn, which extends from the midsubstance of the capsular margin into the inferior articular surface. The *arrowheads* point to the bone bruise in the posterior aspect of the tibia, the *arrow* an area of osteochondral defect due to a previous injury. In **B** the *arrow* points to a small impacted fracture. A slightly depressed fracture of the cortex is also present.

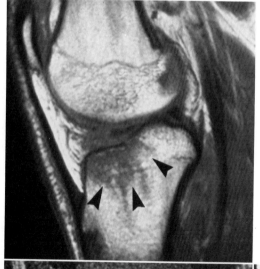

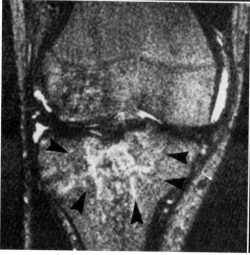

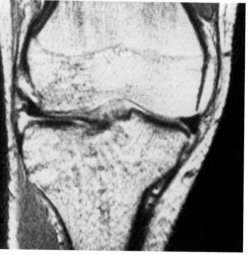

FIGURE 20-141

Skiing accident. **A**, T1-WI sagittal, **B**, T2-WI, and, **C**, SD coronal views. In **A** the *arrowheads* point to a zone of decreased SI due to edema/hemorrhage within the marrow of the anterior proximal tibia. A minimally depressed cortical fracture may also be present. In **B** the *arrowheads* point to the same region of the tibia. Note the high SI of edema/hemorrhage secondary to fracture of the trabeculae (bone bruise). In **C** these abnormalities may not be apparent.

various fractures may coexist simultaneously (Fig. 20-140) and a bone bruise may be present at the periphery of a more serious fracture.

OSTEOCHONDRAL FRACTURE

An osteochondral fracture is a closely related (Figs. 20-140 and 20-142) but more serious injury than a bone bruise that almost always is accompanied by a bone bruise, and, in about 40% of the cases, a torn medial meniscus, TCL, or ACL. It is more common on the lateral side and is identified as zones of cartilaginous and cortical bone disruption. Both T1-WI and T2-WI views can display the coexisting bone bruise. The osteochondral fracture itself is also well seen on T1-WI and T2-WI sagittals. On the coronal views, SD and T2-WI are more helpful for delineation of these fractures. If necessary, T2* images should be obtained to verify the presence of subtle cartilage disruption. The articular cartilage is displayed with high SI on T2* views.

TIBIAL PLATEAU FRACTURE

This fracture is more common on the lateral side (Figs. 20-143 and 20-144), and may be accompanied by injuries of the ACL and TCL. On MRI the fracture is evident as lines of decreased SI (on T1-WI) extending to the tibial plateau. There is usually increased SI due to edema/hemorrhage on T2-WI. When the injury is old, the fracture line is of low SI on all pulse sequences. The magnitude of depression of the tibial plateau and associated intra-articular abnormalities are also well seen on MRI.

Open reduction and internal fixation of a depressed tibial plateau fracture may become necessary not only because of the magnitude of the plateau depression (more than 5 to 7 millimeters), but also presence of ACL and TCL instability. MRI is unique amongst all imaging modalities used for evaluation of this fracture, including CT, arthrography and tomography, by the virtue that it can establish the diagnosis of a fracture, provide an accurate estimation of the magnitude of tibial plateau depression and simultaneously display injuries of the ACL, TCL and menisci, all noninvasively and not hampered by lipohemarthrosis.

It is well known that conventional roentgenography is conducive to gross underestimates of the magnitude of comminution and plateau depression.[126] For this reason planar tomography[127] and CT[126] were advocated. CT is capable of revealing the extent of comminution and plateau depression better and with less demand on the patient than planar tomography. However, CT cannot help rule in or rule out possible accompanying intraarticular injuries of the menisci, TCL, and ACL. An accurate assessment of the extent of injury of these ligaments is essential, because if ligamentous instability is present open reduction and internal fixation become necessary.[127-129]

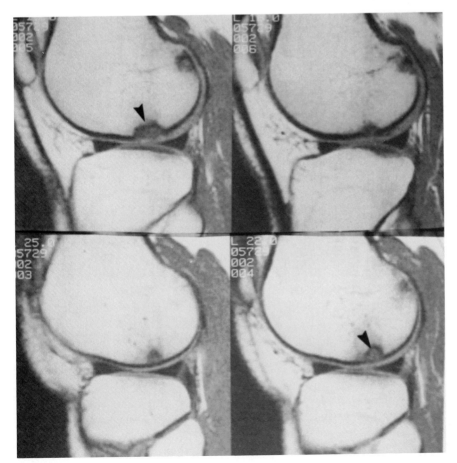

FIGURE 20-142
A 3-month-old osteochondral fracture of the lateral femoral condyle in a 22-year-old woman. The *arrowhead* points to the defect. There was a focal area of articular cartilage injury at arthroscopy, but the cartilage appears almost intact on this examination.

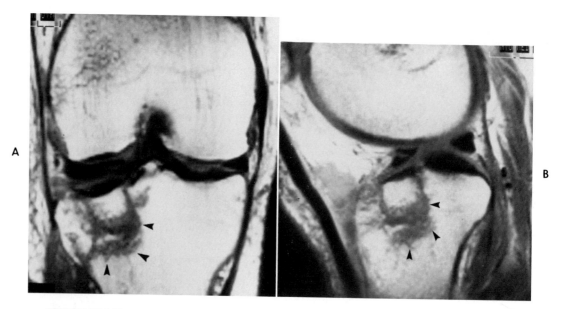

FIGURE 20-143
Fracture of the tibia. **A,** Coronal SD and, **B,** sagittal T1-WI. The *arrowheads* point to hemorrhage/edema at the base of a comminuted depressed fracture of the lateral tibial plateau.

STRESS FRACTURE

At least two kinds of fracture are recognized in this category. The first occurs in a normal bone secondary to excessive usage. This injury is what is generally understood as a stress fracture. Examples are a fatigue fracture (Fig. 20-145) and a march fracture, which may occur in the metatarsals, calcaneus, proximal tibia, and middle and proximal femur (among other places). In the second kind, fracture occurs in a weakened bone (osteoporosis, osteomalacia, Paget's, fibrous dysplasia[130]) secondary to normal usage. An example of this would be insufficiency fracture of the sacrum or other bones (Fig. 20-146).

A stress fracture is often difficult to recognize in its initial phase on conventional roentgenography (Fig. 20-145, *A*). Consequently the diagnosis is delayed for several weeks. The radiographic findings, often appreciated retrospectively, depend upon the location of the fracture. In the knee region fatigue fractures involve the cortical bone of the proximal tibial shaft, often in athletic teenagers and young adults following excessive physical exertion (jogging, running, dancing), whereas insufficiency fractures occur in the predominantly trabecular bone of the tibial metaphysis, mostly in osteopenic sedentary older women.

The roentgenographic findings in fatigue fractures of the tibia consist of a fracture line (usually at 90 degrees to the long axis of the tibia), endosteal thickening, and periosteal reaction. This triad becomes evident about 4 to 6 weeks after the onset of fracture. Depending upon its age and whether the subject continues walking and running on the injured member despite pain, the fracture may be a barely visible straight lucent line, a dense line, or a mixture of these (signifying disruption, resorption, and impaction of cortical bone, occurring simulta-

neously). The periosteal new bone formation does not become obvious for at least 10 to 14 days after the onset of fracture. It is often indistinct and subtle at first.

An insufficiency fracture usually exhibits, on conventional roentgenography, barely visible wavy lines of increased density in the metaphysis (Fig. 20-146, *A*) due to impaction of the trabeculae and cortex. There is seldom a definite lucency, endosteal thickening, or periosteal reaction.

Both a fatigue and an insufficiency fracture of the tibia may present with pain perceived by the patient as emanating from the knee, and thus referral is made to exclude internal derangement.

In our experience MRI has played a major role in bringing the magnitude of this problem to attention, by establishing the diagnosis in a proportionately large group of patients, in most of whom the correct diagnosis would not have been made. In our practice the number of patients referred for MRI to rule out internal derangement who eventually are found to have a stress fracture is at least 10 times greater than the number referred for knee arthrography prior to the MRI era. In other words, at least 90% of all stress fractures in these patients were missed in the past, at least initially.

A fatigue fracture often exhibits spectacular findings on MRI,[121,130,131] rendering this diagnosis almost impossible to miss (Fig. 20-145, *B, E,* and *F*). The bony elements in the periosteal reaction are of low SI on all pulse sequences. On T2-WI and T2* there is often an obvious wide band of increased SI surrounding the bone secondary to granulation tissue formation, congestion, and edema of the periosteal reaction. Usually also a large area of edema involves the bone marrow.

Tibial metaphyseal insufficiency fractures (Fig. 20-146,

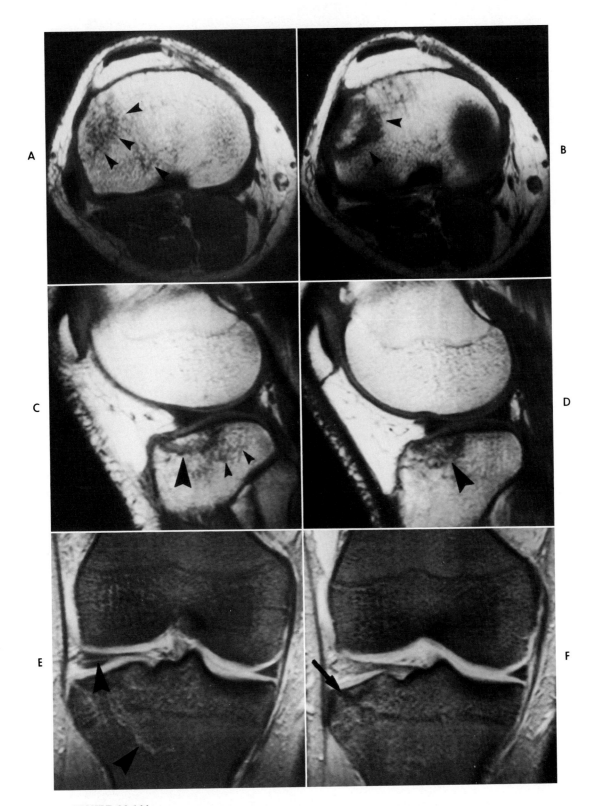

FIGURE 20-144

Tibial fracture and tear of the lateral meniscus. **A** and **B**, T1-WI axial views. *Three arrowheads* point to an area of decreased SI due to the fractured lateral tibial plateau. A single *arrowhead* posteriorly points to the area of bone bruise. **B**, *Arrowheads* point to a depressed fracture of the lateral tibia plateau. **C** and **D**, Sagittal T1-WI. The *large arrowheads* point to a slightly depressed fracture of the lateral tibial plateau. The small *arrowheads* in **C** point to the bone bruise. **E** and **F**, T2* coronal views. In **E** the *upper arrow* indicates a horizontal tear of the body of the lateral meniscus, confirmed at arthroscopy. The *lower arrow* shows the fracture extending into the metaphysis of the tibia. In **F** the *arrow* points to the depressed lateral tibial plateau fracture.

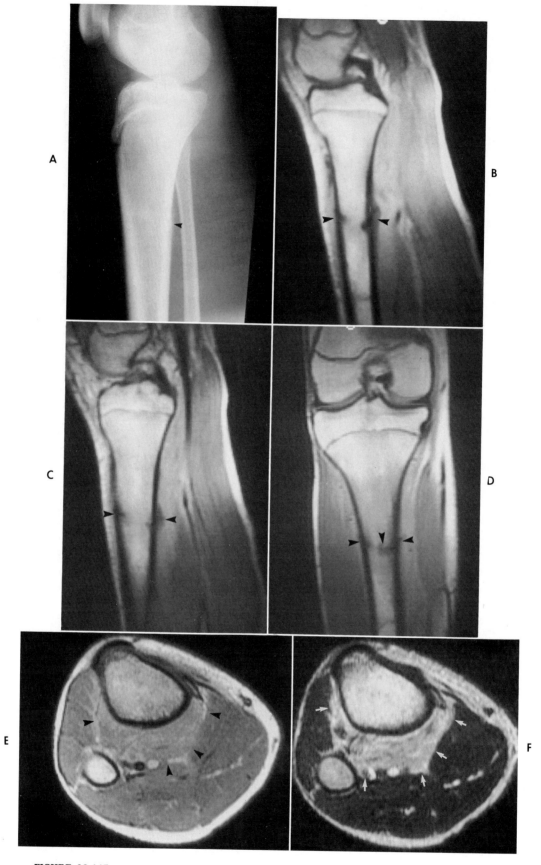

FIGURE 20-145
Fatigue fracture of the proximal tibia. **A,** A lateral roentgenogram of the proximal tibia shows minimal periosteal reaction *(arrowhead).* There is a questionable area of increased density directly anterior to this region. **B** to **D,** Sagittal and coronal T1-W images. The *arrowheads* point to the fracture in the proximal tibia. **E,** Axial SD and, **F,** axial T2-WI. The *arrowheads* show a large amount of edema surrounding the proximal shaft of the tibia. There is also extensive edema within the medullary cavity of the tibia.

B and *C*) exhibit a fairly large area of low SI on T1-WI (due to edema of the marrow) that becomes of higher SI on T2-WI. In the right clinical setting, and with the typical serpentine dense metaphyseal lines on conventional roentgenography, the diagnosis is easily reached. However, other marrow processes, such as neoplasia, must be excluded. This is facilitated by the lack of a soft tissue mass, by cortical destruction, and by the characteristic marrow extension.[131,132]

Osteochondritis dissecans

In OCD there is partial or complete separation of the articular cartilage and subchondral bone from the host bone (usually the nonweightbearing lateral surface of the medial femoral condyle, less commonly other areas of the medial femoral condyle). The lateral femoral condyle is involved in about 15% to 20% of patients. The least common sites of involvement are the middle and inferior portions of the medial facet of the patella.[133-136] In 25% of patients with a symptomatic OCD of one knee, the other knee (though symptom free) is found to be involved.[136-139] Asymptomatic bilateral involvement is also occasionally encountered. OCD is usually discovered in youngsters, between the ages of 11 and 18, less commonly in other age groups.

The clinical findings are nonspecific and consist of intermittent pain and swelling of the knee. When a detached fragment is present, locking of the knee also occurs.

The pathogenesis of OCD is not known, although most investigators believe that chronic repetitive trauma plays a major role. Whatever the cause, OCD may involve the articular cartilage alone or both the articular cartilage and the subchondral bone. The bone fragment may become completely detached from its bed and "fall" into the joint, creating an intraarticular body, which may remain loose, or become embedded in the synovial membrane. If the fragment is only partially separated from its bed, it often heals and merges with the bed, leaving no scar or only minimal deformity.

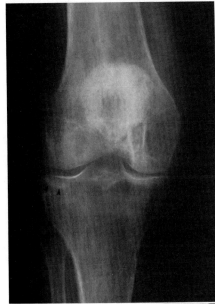

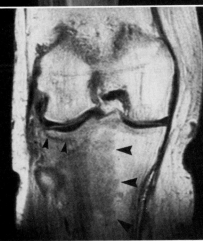

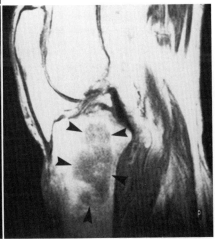

FIGURE 20-146
Insufficiency fracture of the tibia. **A,** An AP projection of the knee shows a serpentine line of increased density secondary to the fracture. There is also disuse osteopenia in this 72-year-old woman complaining of knee pain of five weeks' duration. **B,** Coronal SD. The *small arrowheads* identify the fracture, the *large arrowheads* an extensive area of edema within the marrow of the proximal tibia. **C,** Sagittal T1-WI, meniscal windows. The *arrowheads* point to edematous marrow.

Conventional roentgenography shows the characteristic lesions of OCD when the subchondral bone is involved. If the lesion is limited to the articular cartilage, roentgenograms are normal.

MRI can show lesions of the articular cartilage, the extent of detachment of an OCD fragment from its bed, and any loose bodies (calcified or not, but usually 5 mm or larger in diameter), and for this reason it is superior to all other imaging modalities. The disruption of articular cartilage is usually best seen on T2-WI or T2* (Figs. 20-147 and 20-148), appearing as lower SI than the neighboring normal cartilage, with possibly a zone of signal void due to calcification. The OCD fragment is also of low SI relative to the neighboring normal bone. When a ring of high SI is noted at the base of an OCD fragment (on T2-WI or T2*), it signifies the presence of granulation tissue or fluid at the interface between the OCD fragment and its bed. With complete detachment, the OCD fragment is completely surrounded by a ring of high SI; otherwise, the detachment is partial.[136,138]

Primary aseptic necrosis of the medial femoral condyle

This condition is seen in middle-aged and elderly adults and affects the weightbearing surface of the medial femoral condyle, less commonly and in descending order of frequency, the medial tibial plateau, lateral femoral condyle and lateral tibial plateau.[140,141]

The pathological basis of this lesion is necrosis and disintegration of the subchondral bone and overlying articular cartilage. The condition is indistinguishable histologically from secondary bone necrosis (e.g., following corticosteroid therapy). Bone necrosis leads to microfractures, which progress to larger fractures and cause collapse of the subchondral bone with fragmentation of the articular cartilage. These abnormalities, in turn, lead to narrowing of the joint space and secondary osteoarthritis. The condition is three times more frequent in women than in men and presents rather acutely. The patient usually complains of fairly constant pain that, unlike the pain of arthritis, is not relieved by rest and may actually get worse at night.[142] In our experience patients also complain of a peculiar sense of heaviness of the knee. The pain usually subsides in 6 to 8 weeks, although a vague sense of discomfort and soreness of the knee may persist. A moderate amount of joint effusion is almost always present. The pre-MRI clinical diagnosis has generally been incorrect in most patients.[143,144]

Conventional roentgenography is usually noncontributory initially, although in some patients a small increased density and blurring of the margins of the bony trabeculae of subchondral bone are demonstrated on high-

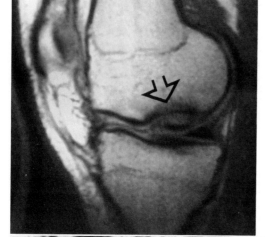

A

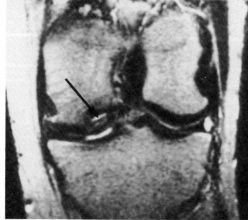

B

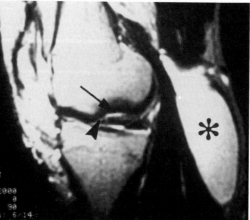

C

FIGURE 20-147
Osteochondritis dissecans. **A** is a T1-WI sagittal, and **B** and **C** are coronal and sagittal T2-WI. In **A** the *hollow arrow* designates an area of low SI (representing osteosclerosis) at the base of the osteochondral lesion in the lateral femoral condyle. In **B** the *arrow* points to an area of high SI at the base of the lesion. In **C** the *arrow* points to a zone of high SI at the base of the lesion, and the *arrowhead* to a disruption of the femoral cortex and articular cartilage in the anterior portion of the lesion. This osteochondral fragment is not attached to bone. The zone of high SI is due to granulation tissue or effusion surrounding the fragment. At exploration the fragment was found to be unstable and detached from its bed. The *asterisk* is on a popliteal cyst.

resolution fine-grain films. Minimal flattening followed by a minute step-off, signifying the boundary between normal and necrotic bone and affecting the subchondral cortex of the medial femoral condyle, usually slightly on the medial side of its midportion, is noted. Further progression of the disease leads to an obvious collapse and a depressed fracture. The subchondral bone becomes poorly defined and dense. A poorly defined zone of lucency develops in the region and, with further progression of the disease, evolves into a small cystic lesion surrounded by osteosclerosis.

MRI usually (Fig. 20-149) demonstrates a poorly defined zone of decreased SI on T1-WI, affecting the subchondral bone, as early as 6 or more months prior to establishment of the diagnosis on conventional roentgenography.[143-146] On T2-WI, a poorly defined ring of moderately high SI may be noted surrounding the lesion. MRI is also useful for excluding other conditions that may be confused clinically with spontaneous osteonecrosis. These include a tear of the medial meniscus, a stress fracture, and osteoarthritis. In our experience a degenerative tear of the medial meniscus coexists with spontaneous medial femoral osteonecrosis in about 28% of the patients. Stress fractures of the insufficiency type usually

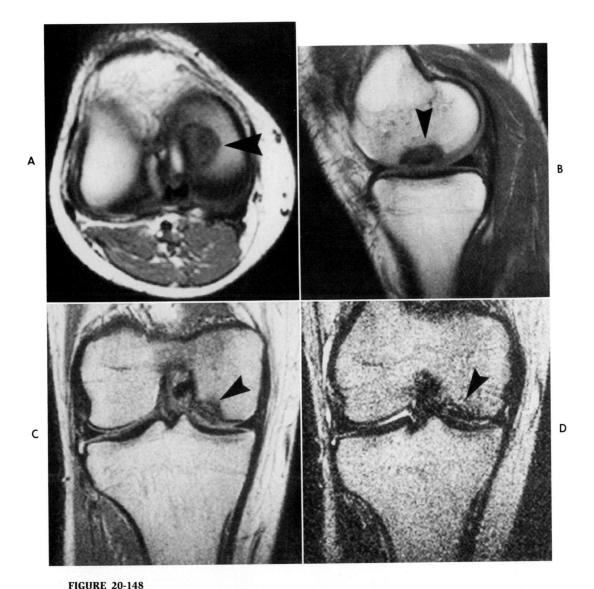

FIGURE 20-148
Osteochondritis dissecans. **A** and **B** are axial and sagittal T1-weighted images. **C** is a spin density coronal and, **D**, a T2-WI coronal view. In **A** and **B** the *arrowhead* points to the defect of the medial femoral condyle. In **C**, the *arrowhead* points to the base of the osteochondral defect; the articular cartilage of the medial femoral condyle is markedly irregular. In **D** the *arrowhead* points to a 2 to 3 mm area of increased SI, representing granulation tissue, or fluid; at the base of the lesion. Therefore, except for this region, the lesion is everywhere attached to the surrounding bone. When a ring of high SI completely surrounds an osteochondral fragment, it implies that the fragment is unstable or loose.

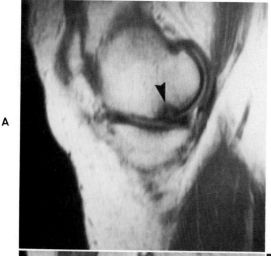

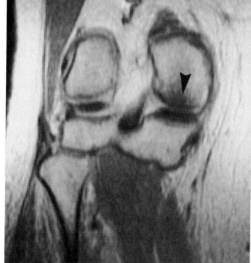

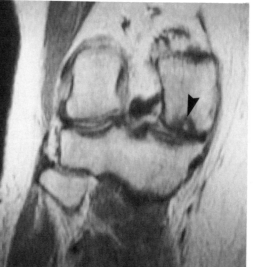

FIGURE 20-149
Primary aseptic necrosis of the medial femoral condyle. **A** is an anatomical sagittal T1-WI. The *arrowhead* points to an area of low SI surrounding a cystic lesion of the subchondral bone and a defect in the cortex of the medial femoral condyle. **B** and **C**, SD coronal views, show the area of low SI *(arrowhead)*. In **C** a cystic lesion is also present. In addition, there is narrowing of the medial compartment with marked attentuation of the articular cartilage of the condyle. The moderate to severe erosion of the free margin of the body of the medial meniscus is due to degenerative disease.

affect the metaphysis of the tibia and do not involve the articular cortex. Primary osteonecrosis, on the other hand, is typically seen in the femur and affects the articular cortex and subchondral bone. Degenerative arthritis may be present in a patient with primary osteonecrosis, particularly an elderly person. In addition, in patients without preexisting osteoarthritis, primary osteonecrosis may lead to a rapidly evolving degenerative arthritis of the medial tibiofemoral joint. In some patients a rapidly evolving destructive process affecting the medial femoral condyle (Fig. 20-150) develops, causing marked deformity before degenerative arthritis has a chance to occur.

Secondary osteonecrosis

The knee region is the second most common site (after the hip) of involvement by secondary osteonecrosis. The etiology and pathological bony changes are identical. Secondary osteonecrosis affects multiple locations, a situation that is most unlikely in the primary form. Another significant difference is the age of the patient. Primary osteonecrosis of the medial femoral condyle

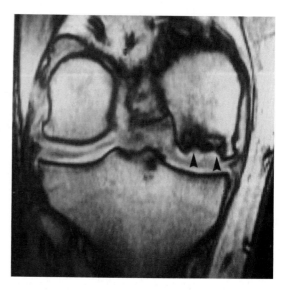

FIGURE 20-150
Spontaneous osteonecrosis of the medial femoral condyle. Gradient echo coronal view (TR 286/TE 12, FA 60) purposely obtained to show the bone necrosis better. *Arrowheads* point to the deformed medial femoral condyle. There is also a marked decrease in SI of the condyle.

occurs in patients 50 years and older whereas the secondary form can occur in practically any age group.

The clinical and roentgenographic findings of secondary osteonecrosis are similar to those of the primary form, except that the lesion may be seen in multiple locations simultaneously — for example, both femoral condyles and the tibial plateaus of both knees (Fig. 20-151). The lesion of secondary is usually much larger than the lesion of primary osteonecrosis, and it may involve a large segment of the metaphysis and extend into the diaphysis. Calcification of the marrow may also be present.[140,147-149]

Intraarticular bodies

A wide variety of knee disorders can produce an intraarticular body. These include osteochondritis dissecans, tears of the menisci and cruciate ligaments, synovial osteochondromatosis, and osteochondral fractures. An intraarticular body may be loose, or adherent to or embedded in the synovial lining of the knee.

Meniscal and ligamentous fragments are often trapped in the intercondylar fossa, although they may be forced beyond the margins of the joint to a point above or below the joint line between the capsule and bone. In osteoarthritis the menisci may be extruded beyond the joint margin in a similar fashion. Intraarticular bodies can be found not only in the intercondylar fossa but also in the suprapatellar pouch, medial and lateral parapatellar gutters, and medial and lateral posterior synovial compartments as well as in a popliteal cyst. They may be cartilaginous, fibrous, or osteocartilaginous in origin. Secondary calcification, ossification, and enlargement may occur. The clinical findings consist of intermittent joint effusion, restricted range of motion, and locking. The diagnosis may be suggested on conventional roentgenography if there is calcification or ossification of the intraarticular bodies. However, it is not possible to visualize the noncalcified component of these lesions, which may be quite large, on roentgenograms.

MRI reveals the cartilaginous bodies and torn fragments of the menisci and articular cartilages usually as zones of decreased SI on T1-WI. Calcified bodies show zones of markedly decreased SI on all pulse sequences. Osteocartilaginous bodies may contain bone marrow exhibiting high SI on T1-WI that moderately decreases on T2-WI (Figs. 20-152 to 20-155).

The MRI protocol for routine screening of internal derangement is also useful for detecting loose bodies. We obtain an additional set of axial T1-WI and T2-WI, or T1-WI and gradient echo T2*, images also in these patients. Axial images are useful for the detection and location of intraarticular bodies (Fig. 20-152, *J* and *K*). The T2-WI or T2* images are useful because joint effusion is rendered of markedly high SI and forms a suitable contrast for detection of loose bodies, particularly those with low SI. It should be pointed out that a significant number of loose bodies may be missed on MRI, particularly in the case of small (less than 5 mm) fibrocartilaginous or calcified lesions.

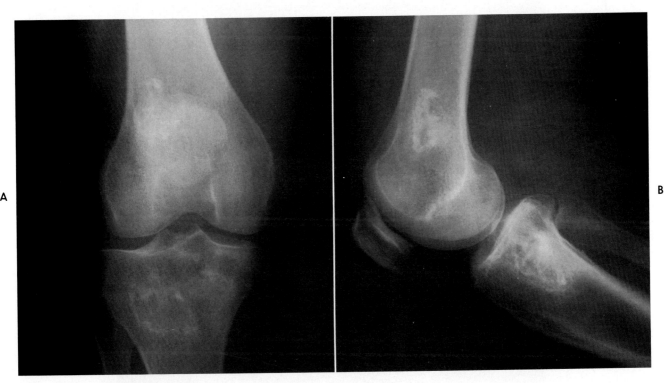

A   B

FIGURE 20-151
Sickle cell disease. **A** and **B**, AP and lateral views of the knee in a patient with moderately severe involvement.

Continued.

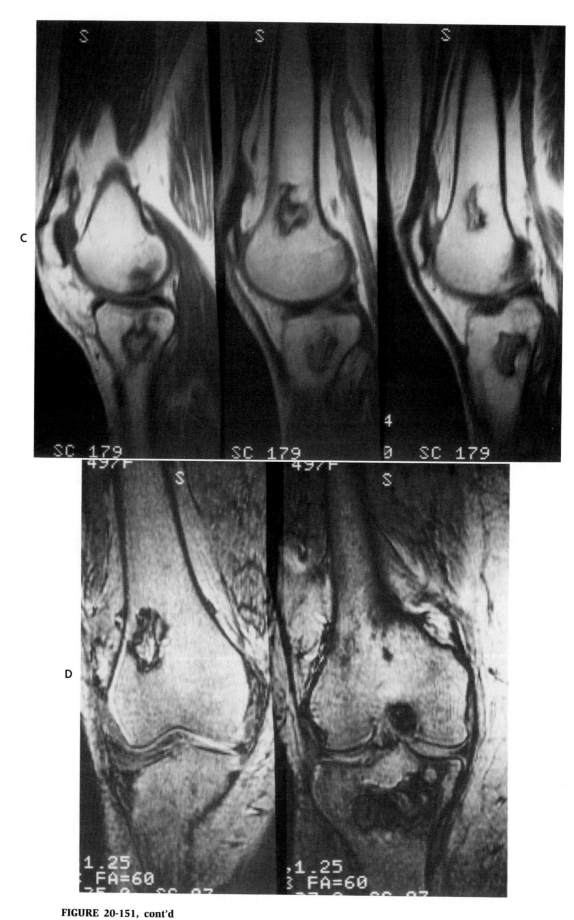

FIGURE 20-151, cont'd
C is a T1-WI sagittal, and D a gradient echo coronal. The extensive bone and medullary infarctions noted on conventional roentgenography are well demonstrated on MR image.

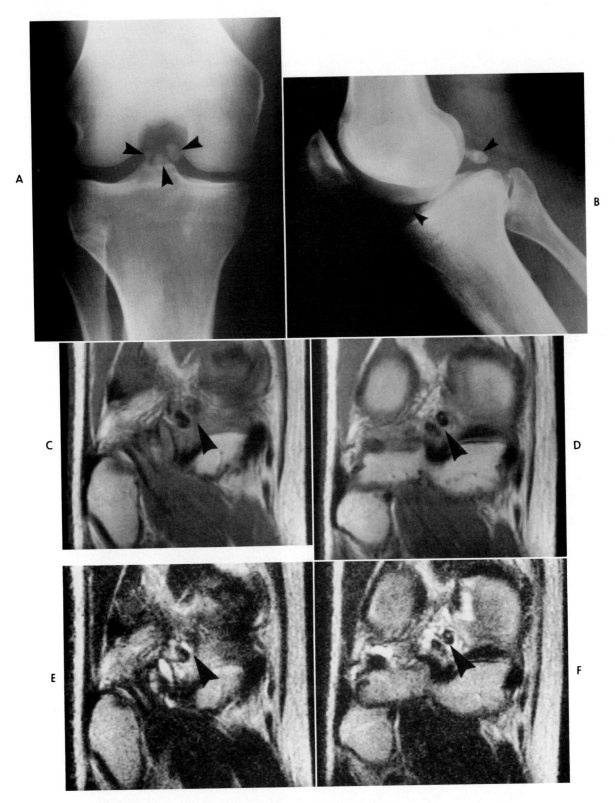

FIGURE 20-152
Intraarticular osteochondral bodies. **A** and **B**, AP and lateral roentgenograms of the right knee. The *arrowheads* point to two such bodies. **C** and **D**, Spin density and, **E** and **F**, T2-WI coronal views show osteochondral bodies in the posterior aspect of the knee *(arrowhead).*   *Continued.*

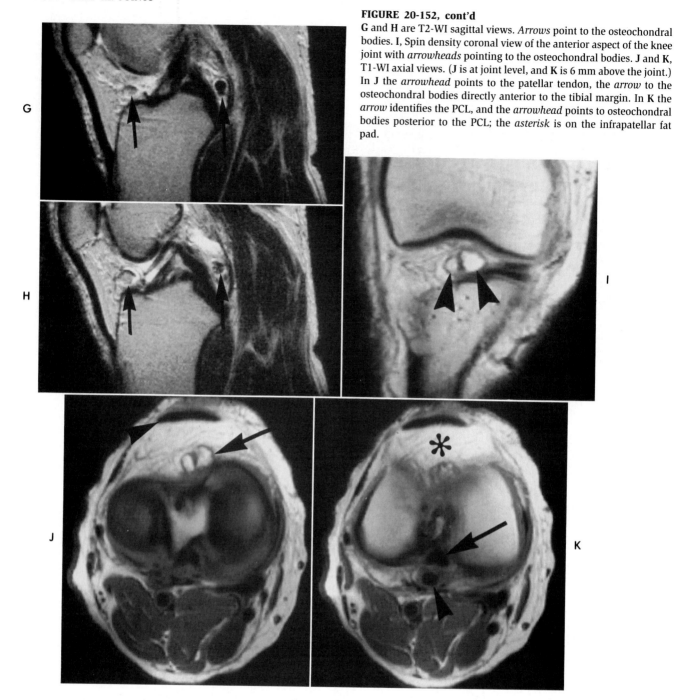

FIGURE 20-152, cont'd
G and **H** are T2-WI sagittal views. *Arrows* point to the osteochondral bodies. **I,** Spin density coronal view of the anterior aspect of the knee joint with *arrowheads* pointing to the osteochondral bodies. **J** and **K,** T1-WI axial views. (**J** is at joint level, and **K** is 6 mm above the joint.) In **J** the *arrowhead* points to the patellar tendon, the *arrow* to the osteochondral bodies directly anterior to the tibial margin. In **K** the *arrow* identifies the PCL, and the *arrowhead* points to osteochondral bodies posterior to the PCL; the *asterisk* is on the infrapatellar fat pad.

Injuries to the quadriceps tendon

A tear of the quadriceps tendon may occur spontaneously, although this is rare.[150,151] Spontaneous tears are due to degeneration of the tendon with disruption of its fibers, occasionally with calcification. A tear of the tendon may also occur, either spontaneously[152] or following a minor exertional trauma, in patients with gout and tophaceous involvement of the tendon, and in hyperparathyroidism.[153]

Traumatic tears of the tendon usually occur at, or just proximal to, its insertion on the patella and are occasionally associated with an avulsion fracture. Thy usually occur insidiously, but may be secondary to a major traumatic incident, in which case a tear of the quadriceps muscle also is sometimes present (Fig. 20-156).

MRI is ideally suited for detecting tears of the quadriceps muscle and tendon. These tears cause disruption of muscle and tendon fibers, which appear of low SI on T1-WI and high SI on T2-WI. Although complete tears of the tendon are clinically obvious, MRI is indispensable in following them after surgical repair and in detecting incomplete intratendinous tears, which are difficult or impossible to assess accurately clinically.

To ensure proper visualization of the quadriceps

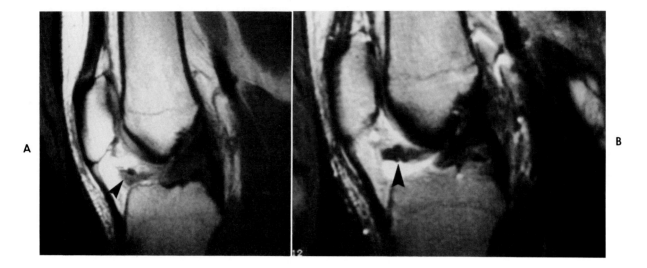

FIGURE 20-153
Intraarticular bodies. **A**, T1-WI and, **B**, T2-WI sagittal views of the knee. The *arrowheads* point to an osteocartilaginous body in the anterior aspect of the knee joint, extending into the intrapatellar fat pad. The patient had osteochondritis dissecans. At arthroscopy, multiple other small fibrocartilaginous bodies, some of which were calcified, were found.

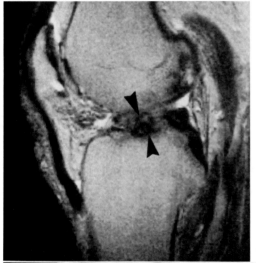

FIGURE 20-154
Intraarticular fibrocartilaginous bodies. These lesions contain multiple areas of calcification. *Arrowheads* in the T2-weighted sagittal views show, **A**, one irregular body in the joint, and **B** and **C**, another in the same joint. The patient had degenerative disease of the medial compartment, with an old tear of the medial meniscus; only the capsular margin of the meniscus remained in place at the time of MR examination. There was also an old tear of the ACL.

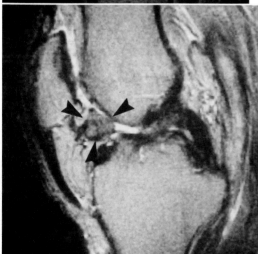

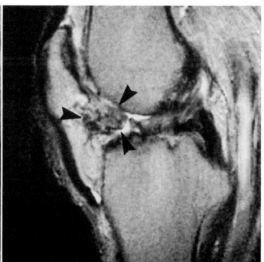

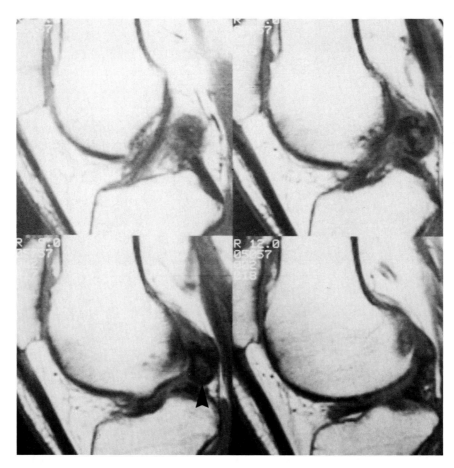

FIGURE 20-155
Intraarticular osteocartilaginous body *(arrowhead)*. T1-WI sagittal view, meniscal windows.

muscle and tendon, a larger field of view (of about 20 × 20 cm) should be utilized. Sagittal and axial T2-WI views are usually necessary for a satisfactory assessment of injuries.

Patellar tendon abnormalities

The pathogenesis of injuries to the patellar tendon is similar to that of quadriceps tendon injuries. Tears of this tendon occur near the lower pole of the patella (Fig. 20-157) or the tibial tubercle (Fig. 20-158). The tendon becomes redundant, with the torn region showing disruption of the normally solid low-SI tendon fibers and replacement with high SI (on T2-WI) due to hemorrhage/edema.

Insidious and repetitive injury to the patellar tendon can lead to formation of a moderately painful cyst of the tendon (Fig. 20-159). This condition may also be seen without any apparent cause. The cyst of the tendon usually has somewhat higher internal SI than the tendon itself does on T1-WI but is of high SI on T2-WI.

Trauma to the anterior aspect of the knee, particularly repetitive subtle trauma such as frequent kneeling, may lead to prepatellar bursitis (Figs. 20-160 and 20-161). Direct trauma can cause prepatellar hemorrhage and edema (Fig. 20-57, *C* and *D*).

Pigmented villonodular synovitis

PVNS is a rare, usually monoarticular, proliferative disorder of the synovial membrane. The pigmentation is due to deposits of hemosiderin. The synovial membrane in PVNS exhibits numerous villi. On macroscopic inspection the lesion may have a rusty or chocolate-brown color. The villi are often matted together and appear as nodules and masses of variable size. On microscopic examination there are numerous multinucleated giant cells and lipid-laden macrophages (foam macrophages) with a characteristic pigmentation due to both intra- and extracellular hemosiderin.[154-157] PVNS has both a local and a diffuse form. The local form is usually seen in the wrist and hand region, where it forms a small tumor arising from the tendon sheaths (giant cell tumor of the tendon sheath). The diffuse form affects practically the entire surface of the synovial lining of a joint, usually a major joint.

PVNS occurs most commonly in the knee (almost 70% to 80% of all the cases[155,156,158]), followed by the hip and ankle and the elbow and shoulder. The clinical findings are nonspecific, and consist of intermittent pain, a sense of tightness with decreased range of motion, or a mass in the knee. The definitive diagnosis is usually delayed, sometimes for several years, after the onset of clinical findings.[155-157,159-161]

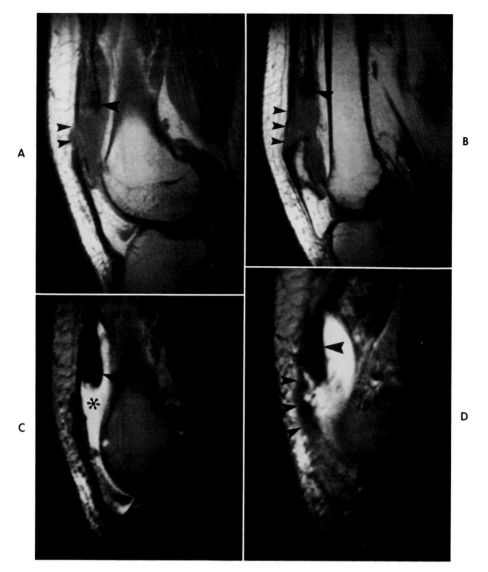

FIGURE 20-156
Torn quadriceps tendon and muscle. **A** and **B** are anatomical sagittal T1-WI views. The *large arrowhead* shows the torn and retracted muscle, the *small arrowheads* a tear in the quadriceps tendon. **C** and **D**, T2-WI anatomical sagittal views. The *large arrowhead* in these images points to the torn and retracted muscle, the *small arrowheads* in **D** to the torn distal portion of the vastus lateralis. The *asterisk* is on effusion.

The roentgenographic manifestations of PVNS consist of effusion and cystic erosions of bone, which occur in up to 50% of patients.[154,156,160] The lesions of bone usually occur in the immediate vicinity of the articular surfaces, have fairly distinct margins, and are less common in the knee than in the hip. The soft tissue lesions of PVNS do not contain calcification, and there is usually no proliferative reactive bone formation or juxtaarticular osteopenia.

The MRI findings in the local form consist of a mass lesion with low SI in the T1-WI and T2-WI that has been reported to affect the infrapatellar fat pad. In the diffuse form (Fig. 20-162), the proliferative masses of the synovium are seen as zones of low SI or signal void on all pulse sequences. The cystic lesions of bone may contain a mixture of inflamed synovium and villi of PVNS, with signal characteristics reflecting the same (i.e., high SI for inflamed synovium, low SI or no SI for hemosiderin-containing synovial masses on T2-WI. Joint effusion is usually present and is seen as high SI on T2-WI, although it may have low SI, probably due to the presence of hemosiderin.

The low SI of PVNS on T2-WI is due to the ferric iron of the hemosiderin, which lowers the T2 of the adjacent water molecules.[50] Therefore the differential diagnosis must include other disorders that are secondary to or accompanied by hemorrhage and lesions that contain zones of markedly low SI. The former would be, for example, an organizing hematoma, hemophilia, synovial

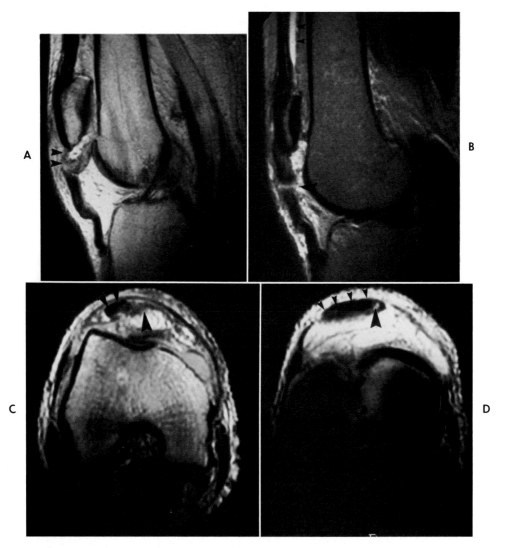

FIGURE 20-157
Patellar tendon tear. **A,** SD anatomical sagittal. The *arrowheads* point to a tear at the tendon's insertion on the inferior pole of the patella. A portion of the tendon and fat have been displaced superiorly. **B,** T2-WI anatomical sagittal. The *large arrowhead* points to a tear of the tendon approximately 2 cm below the inferior pole of the patella. *Small arrowheads* indicate effusion in the suprapatellar bursa. Note the rippling and redundancy of the tendon. **C** and **D,** SD axial views. (In **C,** just below the patella, the *two small arrowheads* mark a minor portion of the lateral patellar tendon that is not torn; the *large arrowhead* points to the torn region of the tendon. In **D,** at about the joint level, approximately 2 cm below the tear, the *large arrowhead* marks an area of increased SI within the substance of the tendon, probably representing a small intrasubstance tear; the *small arrowheads* point to an intact portion of the tendon.) The MRI examination in this patient was deliberately performed with a flat surface coil on the anterior surface of the knee; hence the marked drop-off of signal in the posterior aspect of the knee.

hemangioma, and RA. The latter would be calcified lesions and osteochondromatosis. The synovial masses of PVNS do not contain calcification. This fact is helpful in excluding calcified lesions. Rheumatoid arthritis and hemophilia are diagnosed on clinical and laboratory grounds. However, it must be emphasized that RA patients have a tendency to bleed and may have hemosiderin deposits in the synovial membrane, even in a popliteal or calf cyst. Furthermore, RA and PVNS may coexist.[156,159] A definitive diagnosis of synovial hemangioma is usually not possible without a biopsy. Furthermore, according to Spitzer et al.[156] five cases of coexistng synovial hemangioma and PVNS have been reported in the literature.

Blount's disease

Blount's disease (or tibia vara, osteochondrosis deformans tibiae, and ischemic necrosis of the medial tibial

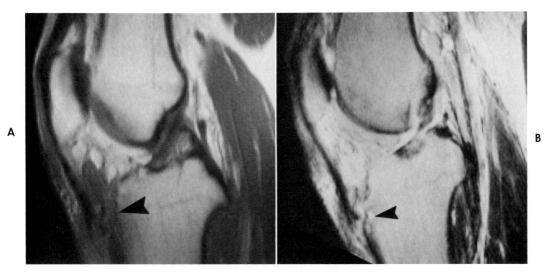

FIGURE 20-158
Traumatic tear and avulsion of the patellar tendon at its tibial insertion. **A,** T1-WI and, **B,** T2-WI sagittal views. The *arrowhead* points to an area of hemorrhage/edema at the tibial insertion of the tendon. There is avulsion of the tendon, with a tear in its distal portion.

FIGURE 20-159
Cyst of the patellar tendon. **A,** T1-WI sagittal and, **B,** SD axial views. An *arrowhead* points to the cyst. **C,** SD and, **D,** T2-WI axial views in another patient. Again, an *arrowhead* points to the cyst.

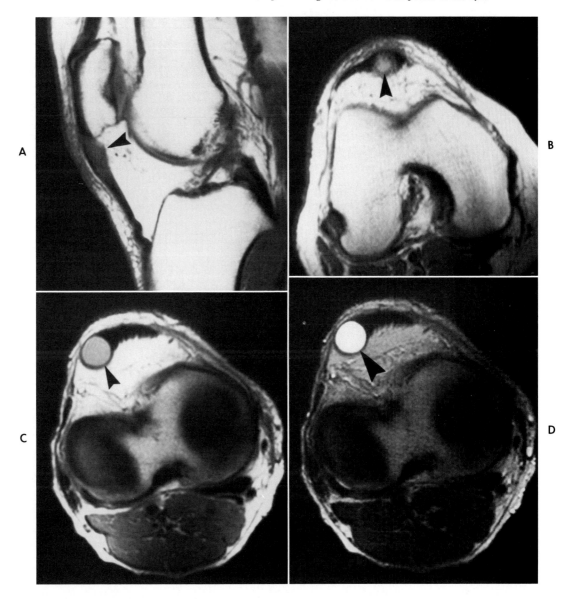

metaphysis[162]), has an infantile form, which is almost always bilateral, and a unilateral adolescent form. The clinical presentation and pathological anatomy of the two forms are similar. The most important clinical finding is lateral bowing of the leg, which is always present prior to the development of necrosis. Caffey[162] believed that Blount's lesion is a forerunner and complication of bowing rather than a cause.

The roentgenographic findings include enlargement and a beaklike deformity of the medial tibial metaphysis.

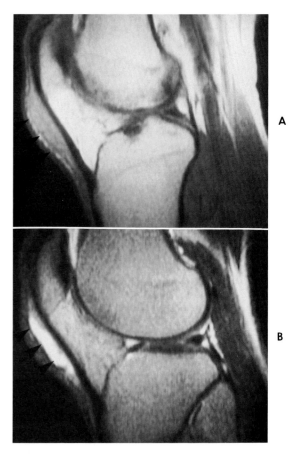

FIGURE 20-161
Prepatellar bursitis. **A**, A T1-WI anatomical sagittal and, **B**, a T2-WI oblique sagittal. *Arrowheads* point to the fluid-distended bursa.

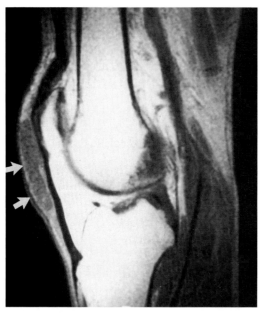

FIGURE 20-160
Sagittal T1-WI. The *arrows* point to a distended prepatellar bursa. The fluid within the bursa is of low SI, as expected on T1-WI.

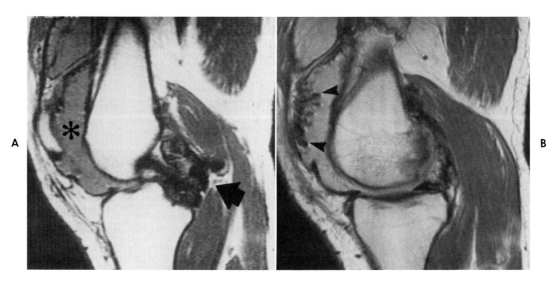

FIGURE 20-162
For legend see opposite page.

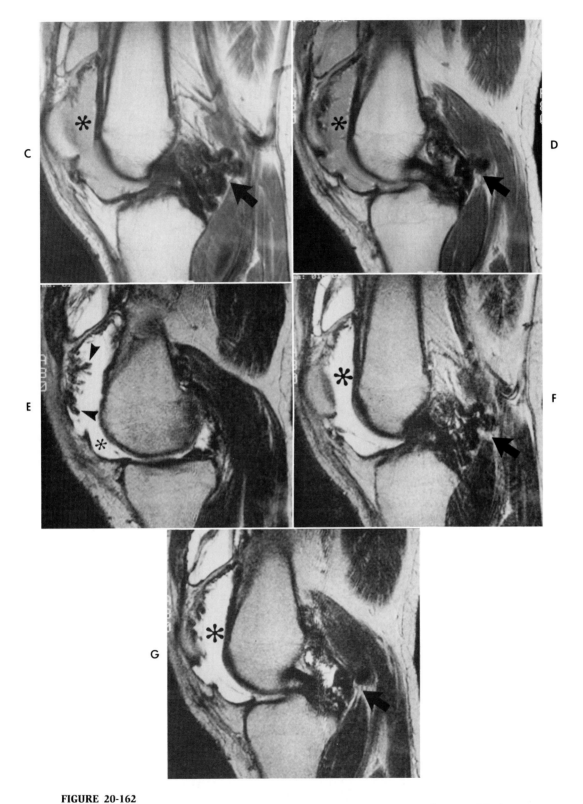

FIGURE 20-162

Pigmented villonodular synovitis. **A**, T1-WI, **B** to **D**, SD, and **E** to **G**, T2-WI sagittal images of the knee. The *asterisk* is on the distended suprapatellar bursa (which contains a large amount of effusion). *Arrowheads* point to the hypertrophic villi within the bursa, *arrows* to the hypertrophic villi in the posterior compartment.

Similar deformities may be present in the distal femur. The growth plate is inclined medially and inferiorly, causing a similar deformity of the epiphysis.[162,163] MRI has no definite advantage over conventional roentgenography in demonstrating the deformity of the metaphysis (Fig. 20-163). However, it may be of value in the presurgical assessment of these patients because it can display not only the bony defects but also defects in the articular cartilage.

Synovial plicae

In the embryo of about 9 weeks the knee joint has three compartments — the patellofemoral and the medial and lateral tibiofemoral — separated by the embryonic synovial membrane. By the twelfth week the fibrous membrane partitioning these compartments has involuted and a joint consisting of a single cavity is formed.[164-166] The involution often is not complete; up to 80%[167] of adult knees may contain remnants of these embryonic synovial

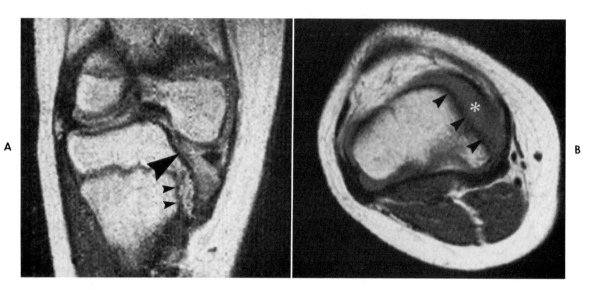

FIGURE 20-163
Blount's disease. **A,** Coronal SD. There is marked deformity of the medial side of the epiphysis and metaphysis of the tibia. The *large arrowhead* points to the medially and inferiorly inclined cortex of the tibial epiphysis. *Small arrowheads* point to a similarly inclined provisional zone of calcification. **B,** Axial T1-WI. *Arrowheads* point to the inferiorly inclined margin of the epiphysis. The *asterisk* is on the thickened cartilage.

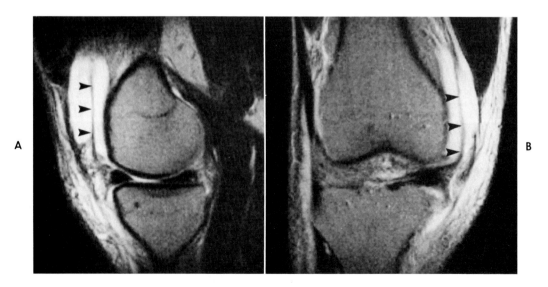

FIGURE 20-164
Plica. Sagittal and coronal T2-WI. There is a mediopatellar plica (shown as a membrane of low SI, *arrowheads*) within the high-SI joint effusion in the median parapatellar synovial gutter.

membranes, which are called synovial plicae.[168] The synovial plicae of the knee are classified according to their location into suprapatellar, mediopatellar, and infrapatellar.[169] Although this classification is convenient, one often finds incomplete fibrous septa and folds that are difficult to put into any specific category. Furthermore, different plicae may coexist.

The suprapatellar plica is an oblique horizontal fibrous membrane or fold extending anteroposteriorly in the suprapatellar pouch. It may form a complete septum separating the suprapatellar pouch from the femorotibial compartments. More commonly the septum is not intact but has an opening in its center (the porta). The mediopatellar plica originates on the medial wall of the knee joint, near the upper pole of the patella, and extends inferiorly to insert on the synovial covering of the infrapatellar fat pad.[166] The infrapatellar plica (ligamentum mucosum) is a fan-shaped, delicate, frondlike, fibrous structure that originates with a narrow base in the intercondylar notch and attaches to the inferior and medial aspect of the patella. It is directly anterior to the ACL.[169]

The plica syndrome[165,169,170] refers to the constellation of clinical findings believed to be generated by a thickened and relatively rigid plica, usually the mediopatellar plica.[166] Its pathogenesis is not known, although repetitive trauma and intraarticular bodies probably play a role.[165,169] Pathological plicae are thick and rigid, with clinical findings that include joint effusion, clicking, and a palpable or audible snap during walking. The patient may also complain of pain localized to the medial aspect of the patella and suprapatellar region. There is usually no locking or giving way of the knee, unless a torn meniscus and intraarticular bodies are also present.

Synovial plicae are visualized on MRI (Fig. 20-164) as membranes or folds of low SI on all pulse sequences, usually more conspicuous on T2-WI or T2* as a low-SI septum against the high-SI synovial effusion.

PITFALLS IN THE INTERPRETATION OF KNEE MRI

Errors in the interpretation of MRI are due to a lack of familiarity with the normal anatomy and anatomical variants, misinterpretation of the observed pathological changes, and failure to recognize the limitations of MRI in demonstration of certain lesions. Some of the most common pitfalls are as follows:

1. On sagittal views the transverse ligament, visualized just after its takeoff from the anterior horn of the lateral meniscus, may mimic a tear of the anterior horn (Figs. 20-11, 20-23, and 20-24, *A* and *B*).

2. On sagittal views the transverse ligament, as it joins the anterior horn of the medial meniscus, may cause the superior margin of the meniscus to appear elongated and deformed (Fig. 20-24, *D*). Note the normal configuration of the extreme anterior segment of the anterior horn and transverse ligament (Fig. 20-25, *C* and *D*).

3. On sagittal views the ligament of Wrisberg, as it takes off from the superior margin of the posterior horn of the lateral meniscus, may cause the posterior horn to appear torn (Figs. 20-13, *B*, 20-14, 20-15, *A* to *C*, *E*, and *F*, and 20-57, *C* to *E*). Note that the ligament of Wrisberg takes off from the posterior horn of the lateral meniscus in its posteromedial, not its posterolateral, segment, where the popliteus tendon is situated.

4. The ligament of Wrisberg, seen end-on, may mimic an intracapsular body on midsagittal and medial parasagittal views just proximal to its attachment on the medial femoral condyle (Figs. 20-13, *A*, and 20-15, *D* and *G*).

5. A fairly thick and low-lying ligament of Humphrey may resemble a torn fragment of the meniscus displaced into the intercondylar fossa on midsagittal and medial parasagittal views.

6. The superior aspect of the posterior horn of both menisci, just proximal to their central attachment (Fig. 20-16), may appear irregular and have nonhomogeneous SI. This is normal. This portion of the menisci is not attached to the capsule. The synovial membrane and a small amount of effusion, exhibiting high SI on T2-WI, may normally partially surround this region of the meniscus. This is normal and does not indicate a tear or pathological separation of the meniscus from the capsule.

7. The popliteus tendon, accompanied by its synovial covering, crosses on the posterolateral aspect of the posterior horn of the lateral meniscus. The synovial tissue causes an oblique line of moderately high SI on SD and high SI on T2-WI of coronal and oblique sagittal views. This should not be mistaken for a tear (Figs. 20-8, *A* and *C*, 20-19, *A* and *B*, 20-20, *A* to *C*, 20-53, *A*, and 20-165).

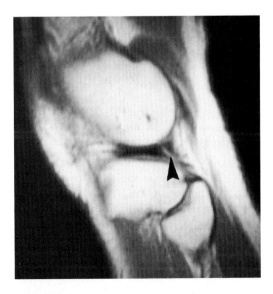

FIGURE 20-165
Oblique sagittal T1-WI. The *arrowhead* points to a line of increased SI produced by synovial tissue accompanying the popliteus tendon. It should not be mistaken for a tear.

8. A normal popliteus tendon may resemble a meniscal remnant on coronal and oblique sagittal views in patients with prior meniscectomy or patients with a complete meniscocapsular separation and displacement of the entire posterior horn and body of the lateral meniscus into the intercondylar notch or anteriorly (Figs. 20-66, *A,* 20-67, *A,* and 20-68, *D*).

9. In patients with a bucket handle tear of the menisci the plane of the tear may be V shaped, with the V horizontally oriented and pointing toward the free margin of the meniscus. When the handle of the bucket is displaced into the intercondylar notch, the capsular remnant may resemble a normal meniscus. However, careful examination shows the capsular remnant to be fat and short, with articular surfaces that are sloping downward quite steeply, unlike the gently sloping articular surfaces of a normal meniscus (Figs. 20-43 and 20-45).

10. The ACL is normally lax when the knee is flexed. This may occur even with minimal flexion. Therefore, it is important to check the position of the knee whenever the diagnosis of ACL laxity is entertained.

11. The ACL may be only a few millimeters thick. It often has more internal SI than the PCL and (unlike the PCL, which is homogeneously black) may be gray-black. In some individuals the ACL normally shows two or more distinct fasciculi.

12. In our experience using a state-of-the-art high-field magnet, a normal ACL must be visualized on at least one view, either sagittal or coronal. A lack of visualization may be due to marked obliquity of the sagittal views or poor technical capability of the MRI system. Otherwise, lack of visualization of the ACL has proven to be due to a tear.

13. A normal PCL will occasionally appear buckled on sagittal views. This is due to its making a particularly abrupt turn medially as it extends toward its attachment on the medial femoral condyle. Often a repeat sagittal view, positioned a few millimeters laterally, shows the ligament to be normal.

14. Although obvious, it nevertheless deserves repeating: A focal area of increased SI within the substance of the menisci not reaching the articular surfaces is a zone of degeneration, *not* a tear. A plane of increased SI, seen on at least two consecutive views, within the substance of the menisci, but not reaching the articular surfaces, may be a closed (intrasubstance) tear. When the articular surfaces are normal, a closed tear cannot be seen at arthroscopy.

15. Intraarticular bodies, particularly those adherent to or embedded in the synovial membrane, fibrous or cartilaginous, not calcified, and usually smaller than 5 mm, may be completely missed on MRI. Occasionally, small calcified intraarticular bodies are also missed.

16. The difficulty of differentiating PVNS from RA and other lesions should be kept in mind.

17. Early and moderate erosions of the articular cartilage, particularly the tibial articular cartilage, may be missed on MRI.

18. A satisfactory MR examination of the knee requires both sagittal and coronal views, both T1-WI and T2-WI or T2*. A knee MRI consisting of only sagittal views is not acceptable because it is virtually impossible to evaluate the bodies of the menisci and the TCL, fibular collateral ligament, and meniscocapsular junction in the midcoronal plane of the knee on sagittal views.

19. An optimal assessment of injuries to the cruciate ligaments requires a T2-WI set of images, preferably in both the coronal and the sagittal planes.

20. The gradient echo T2* sequence is useful for making tears and degenerative changes of the menisci more conspicuous. However, it may exaggerate meniscocapsular signal abnormalities and, on some MRI imagers, lead to the erroneous diagnosis of meniscocapsular separation. Similarly, it may exaggerate minor zones of increased SI within the ligaments of the knee, particularly the ACL and patellar tendon, and lead to an erroneous diagnosis of degeneration or tear of these structures.

REFERENCES

1. Kattapuram SV, Kushner DC, Phillips WC, Rosenthal DI: Osteoid osteoma: an unusual cause of articular pain. Radiology 1983;147:383-387.
2. Mahboubi S: CT appearance of nidus in osteoid osteoma versus sequestration in osteomyelitis. J Comput Assist Tomogr 1986; 10:457-459.
3. Firooznia H, Rafii M, Golimbu C: Computed tomography of osteoid osteoma. J Comput Tomogr 1985;9(3):265-268.
4. Ficat RP, Hungerford DS: Disorders of the patellofemoral joint. In Ficat RP, Hungerford DS (eds): Disorders of the patellofemoral joint. Baltimore, Williams & Wilkins, 1979, p 4.
5. Imai N, Tomatsu T, Takeuchi H, Noguchi T: Clinical and roentgenological studies on malalignment disorders of the patello-femoral joint. I. Classification of patello-femoral alignments using dynamic skyline-view arthrography with special consideration of the mechanism of the malalignment disorders. J Japan Orthop Assoc 1987;61:1-15.
6. Carson WG, James SL, Larson RL, et al: Patello-femoral disorders: physical and radiographic evaluation. II. Radiographic examination. Clin Orthop 1984;185:178-186.
7. Laurin CA, Dussault R, Levesque HP: The tangenital x-ray investigation of the patello-femoral joint: x-ray techniques, diagnostic criteria and their interpretation. Clin Orthop 1979; 144:16-26.
8. Merchant AC, Mercer RL, Jacobsen RH, Coal CR: Roentgenographic analysis of patello-femoral congruence. J Bone Joint Surg [Am] 1974;56:1391-1396.
9. Hughston JC: Subluxation of the patella. J Bone Joint Surg [Am] 1968;50:1003-1026.
10. Wiberg G: Roentgenographic and anatomic studies of the patello-femoral joint. Acta Orthop Scand 1941;12:319-326.
11. Cross MJ, Waldrop J: The patella index as a guide to the understanding and diagnosis of patello-femoral instability. Clin Orthop 1975;110:174-176.
12. Laurin CA, Lévesque HP, Dussault R, et al: The abnormal lateral patellofemoral angle: a diagnostic roentgenographic sign of recurrent patellar subluxation. J Bone Joint Surg [Am] 1978;60:55-60.

13. Insall J, Goldberg V, Salvatti E: Recurrent dislocation and the high riding patella. Clin Orthop 1972;88:67-69.

14. Insall J, Salvatti E: Patella position in the normal knee joint. Radiology 1971;101:101-104.

15. Labelle H, Lauren CA: Radiological investigation of normal and abnormal patellae. J Bone Joint Surg [Br] 1976;57B:530.

16. Schutzer SF, Ramsby GR, Fulkerson JB: The evaluation of patello-femoral pain using computerized tomography: A preliminary study. Clin Orthop 1976;204:286-293.

17. Schutzer SF, Ramsby GR, Fulkerson JB: Computerized tomographic classification of patello-femoral joint pain patients. Orthop Clin North Am 1986;17:235-248.

18. Shellock FG, Mink JH, Fox JM: Patello-femoral joint: Kinematic MR imaging to assess tracking abnormalities. Radiology 1988;168:551-553.

19. Turek SL: Chondromalacia patellae. In Turek SL (ed): Orthopedics; principles and their application, 4th ed. Philadelphia, Lippincott, 1984, pp 1339-1345.

20. Cave ET, Rowe CR: The patella in derangement of the knee. J Bone Joint Surg [Am] 1950;32:542-549.

21. Clemente CD: Anatomy: a regional atlas of the human body, 3rd ed. Baltimore, Urban & Schwarzenberg, 1987.

22. Warwick R, Williams PL: Gray's anatomy, 35th British ed. Philadelphia, Saunders, 1973.

23. Harley JD: An anatomic arthrographic study of the relationships of the lateral meniscus and the popliteus tendon. AJR 1977;128:181-187.

24. Wickstrom KT, Spitzer RM, Olsson HE: Roentgen anatomy of the posterior horn of the lateral meniscus. Radiology 1975;116:617-619.

25. Last RJ: The popliteus muscle and the lateral meniscus. J Bone Joint Surg [Br] 1950;32:93-99.

26. Watanabe AT, Carter BC, Teitelbaum GP, et al: Normal variations in MR imaging of the knee: appearance and frequency. AJR 1989;153:342-344.

27. Heller L, Langman J: The meniscofemoral ligaments of the human knee: J Bone Joint Surg [Br] 1964;46:307-313.

28. Kaplan EB: The embryology of the menisci of the knee joint. Bull Hosp Joint Dis 1955;16:111-124.

29. Kaplan EB: Discoid lateral meniscus of the knee joint. J Bone Joint Surg [Am] 1957;39:77-87.

30. Kaplan EB: The lateral menisco-femoral ligament of the knee joint. Bull Hosp Joint Dis 1956;17:176-182.

31. Last RJ: Some anatomical details of the knee joint. J Bone Joint Surg [Br] 1948;30:683-688.

32. Jelaso DV: The fascicles of the lateral meniscus: an anatomic arthrographic correlation. Radiology 1975;114:335-339.

33. Pipkin G: Lesions of the suprapatellar plica. J Bone Joint Surg [Am] 1950;32:363-369.

34. Gray DJ, Gardner E: Prenatal development of the human knee and superior tibofibular joints. Am J Anat 1950;86:235-287.

35. Lee JK, Yao L: Tibial collateral ligament bursa: MR imaging. Radiology 1991;178:855-857.

36. Warren LF, Marshall JL: The supporting structures and layers on the medial side of the knee. J Bone Joint Surg [Am] 1979;61:56-62.

37. Burk DL Jr, Dalinka MK, Kanal E, et al: Meniscal and ganglion cysts of the knee: MR evaluation. AJR 1988;150:331-336.

38. Brantigan OC, Voshell AF: The tibial collateral ligament: its function, its bursae, and its relation to the medial meniscus. J Bone Joint Surg [Am] 1943;25:121-131.

39. Seebacher JR, Inglis AE, Marshall JL, Warren RF: The structures of the posterolateral aspect of the knee. J Bone Joint Surg [Am] 1982;64:536-541.

40. Hughston JC, Andrews JR, Cross MJ, et al: Classification of knee ligament instabilities. II. The lateral compartment. J Bone Joint Surg [Am] 1976;58:173-179.

41. Kennedy JC, Weinberg HW, Wilson AS: The anatomy and function of the anterior cruciate ligament. J Bone Joint Surg [Am] 1974;56:223-235.

42. Stoller DW: The knee. In Stoller DW (ed): Magnetic resonance imaging in orthopedics and rheumatology, Philadelphia, Lippincott, 1989, p 128.

43. Kneeland JB, Jesmanowicz A, Hyde JS: Enhancement of parallel MR image acquisition by rotation of the plane of section. Radiology 1988;166:886-887.

44. Clemente CD: Gray's anatomy, 13th ed. Philadelphia, Lea & Febiger, 1985.

45. Grover JS, Bassett LW, Gross ML: Posterior cruciate ligament: MR imaging. Radiology 1990;174:527-530.

46. Van Dommelen BA, Fowler PJ: Anatomy of the PCL: a review. Am J Sports Med 1989;17:24-29.

47. Hollinshead WH: Anatomy for surgeons, 3rd ed. New York, Harper & Row, 1982. Vol 3, pp 563-583.

48. Sundaram M, McGuire MH, Fletcher J, et al: Magnetic resonance imaging of lesions of synovial origin. Skeletal Radiol 1986;15:110-116.

49. Coral A, van Holsbeeck M, Adler RS: Imaging of meniscal cyst of the knee in three cases. Skeletal Radiol 1989;18:451-455.

50. Gomori JM, Grossman RI, Goldberg HI. Intracranial hematomas: imaging by high field MR. Radiology 1985;157:87-93.

51. Mink JH, Reicher MA, Crues JV III: A spectrum of knee joint disorders. In Mink JH, Reicher MA, Crues JV III(eds): Magnetic resonance imaging of the knee. New York, Raven, 1987, p 130.

52. Lindgreen PG, Willen R: Gastrocnemius-semimembranosus bursa and its relation to the knee joint. Anatomy and histology. Acta Radiol [Diagn] 1977;18:497-512.

53. Swett HA, Jaffe RB, McIff EB: Popliteal cysts: presentation as thrombophlebitis. Radiology 1975;115:613-615.

54. Choyke PL, Kressel HY, Axel L, et al: Vascular occlusions detected by magnetic resonance imaging. Magn Reson Med 1985;2:540-554.

55. Erdman WA, Weinreb JC, Cohen JM, et al: Venous thrombosis: clinical and experimental MR imaging. Radiology 1986;161:233-238.

56. Smillie IS: Biomechanics of rotation: mechanism of injuries of the menisci and sequelae. In Smillie IS (ed): Injuries of the knee joint, 5th ed. New York, Churchill Livingstone, 1987, p 79.

57. Parkes A: Intraneural ganglion of the lateral popliteal nerve. J Bone Joint Surg [Br] 1961;43:784-790.

58. Clark K: Ganglion of the lateral popliteal nerve. J Bone Joint Surg [Br] 1971;43:778-783.

59. Ferguson LK: Ganglion of the peroneal nerve. Ann Surg 1937;106:313-316.

60. Wadstein T: Two cases of ganglia in the sheath of the peroneal nerve. Acta Orthop Scand 1931;2:221-231.

61. Firooznia H, Golimbu C, Rafii M, Chapnick J: Computed tomography in diagnosis of compression of the common peroneal nerve by ganglion cysts. Comput Radiol 1983;7:343-345.

62. Stack RE, Younku AJ, McCarthy CS: Compression of the common peroneal nerve by ganglion cysts. Report of nine cases. J Bone Joint Surg [Am] 1965;47:773-778.

63. Hartwell AS: Cystic tumor of median nerve; operation: restoration of function. Boston Med Surg J 1901;144:582-583.

64. Sultan C: Ganglion der Nervenscheide des nervus peroneus. Zentralbl Chir 1921;48:963-965.

65. Brooks DM: Nerve compression by simple ganglia. A review of thirteen collected cases. J Bone Joint Surg [Br] 1952;34:391-400.

66. Jenkins SA: Solitary tumors of peripheral nerve trunks. J Bone Joint Surg [Br] 1952;34:401-411.

67. Smillie IS: Biomechanics of rotation. Ref 56, pp 77-82.

68. Smillie IS: Surgical pathology of the menisci. In Ref 56, pp 83-111.

69. Smillie IS: Clinical features of internal derangements relative to the menisci. In Ref 56, pp 112-126.

70. Stuttle FL: The no-name and no-fame bursa. Clin Orthop 1959;15:197-199.

71. Kerlan RK, Glousman RE: Tibial collateral ligament bursitis. Am J Sports Med 1988;16:344-346.

72. Towne LC, Balzina ME, Marmor L, et al: Lateral compartment syndrome of the knee. Clin Orthop 1971;76:160-168.

73. DeLee JC, Riley MB, Rochwood CA: Acute straight lateral instability of the knee. Am J Sports Med 1983;11(6):404-410.

74. Woods GW, Stanley RF, Tullos HS: Lateral capsular sign: X-ray clue to a sign of knee instability. Am J Sports Med 1979;7: 27-34.

75. Grana WA, Janssen T: Lateral ligament injury of the knee. Orthopedics 1987;10(7):1039-1044.

76. DeLee JC, Riley MB, Rockwood CA: Acute postero-lateral rotatory instability of the knee. Am J Sports Med 1983; 11(4):199-206.

77. Mink JH, Reicher MA, Crues JV III. The menisci. In Ref 51, pp. 60-88.

78. Crues JV, Mink J, Levy TL, et al: Meniscal tears of the knee: accuracy of MR imaging. Radiology 1987;164:445:448.

79. Lotysch M, Mink J, Crues JV, et al: Magnetic resonance imaging in the detection of meniscal injuries. Magn Reson Imaging 1986;4:94.

80. Lotysch M, Crues JV, Mink J, et al: Scrutinizing knee joints: MRI offers new insight. Diagnostic Imaging 1986;7:90-94.

81. Lotysch M, Mink J, Levy T, et al: Detection of meniscal injuries using magnetic resonance imaging. Radiology 1986;161(P): 238.

82. Stoller DW, Martin C, Crues JV, et al: MR imaging — pathologic correlation of meniscal tears. Radiology 1987;163:731-735.

83. Quinn SF, Muus C, Sara A, et al: Meniscal tears: pathologic correlation with MR imaging. Radiology 1988;166:580-586.

84. Hajek PC, Gylys-Morin VM, Baker LL, et al: High signal intensity meniscus of the knee: magnetic resonance evaluation and in vivo correlation. Invest Radiol 1987;22:883-889.

85. Stoller DW: The knee In Stoller DW (ed): Magnetic resonance imaging in orthopedics and rheumatology. Philadelphia, Lippincott, 1990, p. 108.

86. Coral A, van Holsbeeck M, Adler RS: Imaging of meniscal cyst of the knee in three cases. Skeletal Radiol 1989;18:451-455.

87. Ferrer-Roca O, Vilalta C: Lesions of the meniscus. II. Horizontal cleavages and lateral cysts. Clin Orthop 1980;146:301-307.

88. Turek SL: Congenital discoid menisci. In Turek SL (ed): Orthopedics, principles and their application, 4th ed. Philadelphia, Lippincott, 1984, pp 1285-1287.

89. Silverman JM, Mink JH, Deutch AL. Discoid menisci of the knee: MR imaging appearance. Radiology 1989;173:351-358.

90. Smith DK, Totty WG: The knee after partial meniscectomy: MR imaging features. Radiology 1990;176:141-144.

91. Reicher MA, Hartzman S, Bassett LW, et al: MR imaging of the knee. I. Traumatic disorders. Radiology 1987;162:547-551.

92. DeHaven KE: Diagnosis of acute knee injuries with hemarthrosis. Am J Sports Med 1980;8:9-14.

93. Jonsson T, Althoff B, Peterson L, Renström P: Clinical diagnosis of ruptures of the anterior cruciate ligament: a comparative study of the lachman test and the anterior drawer sign. Am J Sports Med 1982;10:100-102.

94. Katz JW, Fingeroth RJ. The diagnostic accuracy of ruptures of the ACL comparing the Lachman test, the anterior drawer sign and the pivot shift test in acute and chronic knee injuries. Am J Sports Med 1986;14(1):88-91.

95. Lee JK, Yao L, Phelps CT, et al: Anterior cruciate ligament tears: MR imaging compared with arthroscopy and clinical tests. Radiology 1988;166:861-864.

96. Mandelbaum BR, Finerman GA, Reicher MA, et al: Magnetic resonance imaging as a tool for evaluation of traumatic knee injuries. Am J Sports Med 1986;14;5:361-370.

97. Mink JH, Reicher MA, Crues JV III: The ligaments of the knee. In Ref 51, pp 93-112.

98. Mink JH, Levy T, Crues JV III: Tears of the anterior cruciate ligament and menisci of the knee: MR imaging evaluation. Radiology 1988;167:769-774.

99. Stoller DW: The knee. In Stoller DW (ed): Magnetic resonance imaging in orthopedics and rheumatology, Philadelphia, Lippincott, 1990, p 128.

100. Mink JH, Reicher MA, Crues JV III: Ref 97, p 95.

101. Cho KO: Reconstruction of the anterior cruciate ligament by semitendinosus tenodesis. J Bone Joint Surg [Am] 1975; 57:608-612.

102. McMaster JM, Weinert CR, Scranton P: Diagnosis and management of isolated anterior cruciate ligament tears: preliminary report on reconstruction with gracilis tendon. J Trauma 1974;14:230-235.

103. Stoller DW: Ref 99, p 133.

104. Jackson DW, Jennings LD: Arthroscopically assisted reconstruction of the anterior cruciate ligament using a patellar tendon bone autograft. Clin Sports Med 1988;7(4):785-800.

105. Wilcox PG, Jackson DW: Arthroscopic anterior cruciate ligament reconstruction. Clin Sports Med 1987;6(3):513-524.

106. Clancy WG: Arthroscopic anterior cruciate ligament reconstruction with patellar tendon. Techn Orthop 1988;2:13-22.

107. Arnoczky SP, Warren RF, Ashlock MA: Replacement of the anterior cruciate ligament using a patellar tendon allograft. J Bone Joint Surg [Am] 1986;68:376-385.

108. Zarins B, Rowe CR: Combined anterior cruciate ligament—reconstruction using semitendinosus tendon and iliotibial tract. J Bone Joint Surg [Am] 1986;68:160-177.

109. Kieffer DA, Curnow RJ, Southwell RB, et al: Anterior cruciate ligament arthroplasty. Am J Sports Med 1987;12(4):301-311.

110. Houseworth SW, Mauro VJ, Mellon BA, et al: The intercondylar notch in acute tears of the anterior cruciate ligament; A computer graphics study. Am J Sports Med 1987;15:221-224.

111. Grover JS, Bassett LW, Gross ML, et al: Posterior cruciate ligament: MR imaging. Radiology 1990;174:527-530.

112. Loos WC, Fox JM, Blazina ME, et al: Acute PCL injuries. Am J Sports Med 1981;9:86-92.

113. Bianchi M: Acute tears of the PCL: clinical study and results of operative treatment in 27 cases. Am J Sports Med 1983;11:308-314.

114. Beltran J, Noto AM, Herman LJ, et al: Joint effusions: MR imaging. Radiology 1986;158:133-137.

115. Goldie I: Pathomorphologic features in original and regenerated synovial tissues after synovectomy in rheumatoid arthritis. Clin Orthop 1971;77:295-304.

116. Resnick D, Niwayama G: Diagnosis of bone and joint disorders, 2nd ed. Philadelphia, Saunders, 1988, pp 894-1067.

117. Gilkeson G, Polisson R, Sinclair H, et al: Early detection of carpal erosions in patients with rheumatoid arthritis: a pilot study of magnetic resonance imaging. J Rheumatol 1988;15: 1361-1366.

118. Yulish BS, Lieberman JM, Strandjord SE, et al: Hemophilic arthropathy: assessment with MR imaging. Radiology 1987; 164:759-762.

119. Kulkarni MV, Drolshagen LF, Kaye JJ, et al: MR imaging of hemophiliac arthropathy. J Comput Assist Tomogr 1986; 10:445-449.

120. Yao L, Lee JK: Occult intraosseous fracture: detection with MR imaging. Radiology 1988;167:749-751.

121. Lynch TCP, Crues JV, Morgan FW, et al: Bone abnormalities of the knee: prevalence and significance at MR imaging. Radiology 1989;171:761-766.

122. Mink JH, Deutsch AL: Occult cartilage and bone injuries of the knee: detection, classification, and assessment with MR imaging. Radiology 1989;170:823-829.

123. Berquist TH, Ehman RL: The knee. In Berquist TH (ed): MRI of the musculoskeletal system, 2nd ed. New York, Raven, 1990, p 240.

124. Berquist TH, Morin RL: General technical considerations in musculoskeletal MRI. In Ref 123, p 57.

125. Berquist TH, Morin RL: Ref 124, p 64.

126. Rafii M, Firooznia, H, Golimbu C, Bonamo J: Computed tomography of tibial plateau fractures. AJR 1984;142:1181-1186.

127. Anderson PW, Harley JD, Maslin PU: Arthrography evaluation of problems with united tibial plateau fractures. Radiology 1976;119:75-78.

128. Burri C, Bartzke G, Coldewey J, Muggler E: Fractures of the tibial plateau. Clin Orthop 1979;138:84-93.

129. Perry CR, Evans LG, Rice S, et al: A new surgical approach to fractures of the lateral tibial plateau. J Bone Joint Surg [Am] 1984;66:1236-1240.

130. Mink JH, Reicher MA, Crues JV III: Ref 51, p 134.

131. Stafford SA, Rosenthal DI, Gebhardt MC, et al: MRI in stress fracture. AJR 1986;147:533-556.

132. Stoller DW: Ref 42, p 183.

133. Mink JH, Reicher MA, Crues JV III. Osteonecrosis, osteochondrosis, and osteochondritis. In Ref 51, p 118.

134. Hughston JC, Hergenroeder PT, Courtenay BG: Osteochondritis dissecans of the femoral condyles. J Bone Joint Surg 1984;66:1340-1348.

135. Linden B: The incidence of osteochondritis dissecans in the condyles of the femur. Acta Orthop Scand 1976;47:664-667.

136. Mesgarzadeh M, Sapega AA, Bonakdarpour A: Osteochondritis dissecans: analysis of mechanical stability with radiography, scintigraphy, and MR imaging. Radiology 1987;165:775-780.

137. Berquist TH, Ehman RI: The knee. In Ref 123, pp 240-242.

138. Aichroth P: Osteochondritis dissecans of the knee: a clinical survey. J Bone Joint Surg 1971;53:440-447.

139. Mink JH, Reicher MA, Crues JV III: Ref 51, pp 120-121.

140. Ahlback S, Bauer GCH, Bohne WH: Spontaneous osteonecrosis of the knee. Arthritis Rheum 1968;11:705-733.

141. Williams JL, et al: Spontaneous osteonecrosis of the knee. Radiology 1973;107:15-19.

142. Berquist TH, Ehman RL: Ref 123, p 243.

143. Pollack MS, Dalinka MK, Kressel HY, et al: Magnetic resonance imaging in the evaluation of suspected osteonecrosis of the knee. Skeletal Radiol 1987;16:121-127.

144. Lotke PA, Ecker ML: Current concepts review. Osteonecrosis of the knee. J Bone Joint Surg 1988;70:470-473.

145. Mink JH, Reicher MA, Crues JV III: Ref 133, p 116.

146. Mink JH, Deutsch AL: Occult cartilage and bone injuries of the knee: detection, classification, and assessment with MR imaging. Radiol 1989;170:823-829.

147. Crues RL: Osteonecrosis of bone, current concepts as to etiology and pathogenesis. Clin Orthop Rel Res 1986;208:30-39.

148. Citron ND, Patterson FW, Jackson AM: Neuropathic osteonecrosis of the lateral femoral condyle in childhood. J Bone Joint Surg [Br] 1986;68:96-99.

149. Aglietti P, Insall JN, Buzzi R, et al: Idiopathic osteonecrosis of the knee — etiology, prognosis, and treatment. J Bone Joint Surg [Br] 1983;65:588-597.

150. Firooznia HF, Seliger G, Abrams R, et al: Bilateral spontaneous and simultaneous rupture of the quadriceps tendon. Bull Hosp Joint Dis 1973;34:65.

151. Scuderi C: Rupture of the quadriceps tendon, study of twenty tendon ruptures. Am J Surg 1958;95:626-635.

152. Levy M, Seelenfreund M, Maor P, et al: Bilateral spontaneous and simultaneous rupture of the quadriceps tendons in gout. J Bone Joint Surg [Br] 1971;53:510-513.

153. Preston FS, Adicoff A: Hyperparathyroidism with avulsion of three major tendons. N Engl J Med 1962;266:968-971.

154. Jelinek JS, Kransdorf MJ, Utz JA, et al: Imaging of pigmented villonodular synovitis with emphasis on MR imaging. AJR 1989;152:337-342.

155. Dowart RH, Genant HK, Johnston WH, et al: Pigmented villonodular synovitis of synovial joints: clinical, pathologic, and radiologic features. AJR 1984;143:877-885.

156. Spitzer CE, Dalinka MS, Kressel HY: Magnetic resonance imaging of pigmented villonodular synovitis: report of two cases. Skeletal Radiol 1987;16:316-319.

157. Kottal RA, Vogler JB, Matamoras A, et al: Pigmented villonodular synovitis: a report of magnetic resonance imaging in two cases. Radiology 1987;163:551-553.

158. Docken WP: Pigmented villonodular synovitis: a review with illustrative case reports. Semin Arthritis Rheum 1979;9:1-22.

159. Myers BW, Masi AT: Pigmented villonodular synovitis and tenosynovitis: a clinical epidemiologic study of 166 cases and literature review. Medicine 1980;59:223-238.

160. Smith JH, Pugh DG: Roentgenographic aspects of articular pigmented villonodular synovitis. AJR 1962;87:1146-1156.

161. Jaffe HL, Lichtenstein L, Sutro C: Pigmented villonodular synovitis, bursitis, and tenosynovitis. Arch Pathol 1941;31:731-765.

162. Caffey J: Blount's disease. In Caffey J (ed): Pediatric diagnosis, 5th ed. Chicago, Year Book, 1967, pp 924-927.

163. Blount P: Tibia vara: osteochondrosis deformans tibiae. J Bone Joint Surg 1937;19:1-29.

164. Gray DJ, Gardner E: Prenatal development of the human knee and superior tibiofibular joints. Am J Anat 1950;86:235-287.

165. Pipkin G: Lesions of the suprapatellar plica. J Bone Joint Surg [Am] 1950;32:363-369.

166. Deutsch AL, Resnick D, Dalinka MK, et al: Synovial plicae of the knee. Radiology 1981;141:627-634.

167. Mink JH, Reicher MA, Crues JV III: Ref 51, p 135.

168. Apple JS, Martinez S, Hardaker WT, et al: Synovial plicae of the knee. Skeletal Radiol 1982;7:251-254.

169. Hardaker WT, Whipple TL, Bassett FH III. Diagnosis and treatment of the plica syndrome of the knee. J Bone Joint Surg [Am] 1980;62:221-225.

170. Pipkin G: Knee injuries: the role of the suprapatellar plica and suprapatellar bursa in simulating internal derangements. Clin Orthop 1971;74:161-176.

21 MRI of the Knee: Orthopedic Applications and Expectations

JOHN J. BONAMO

Recent years have witnessed a major evolution in the treatment of the injured or painful knee. Subspecialization, rehabilitative and surgical advances, and the advent of arthroscopy have raised the expectations of both patient and surgeon for optimal functional results. These subjective expectations, however, inevitably reflect an objective pretreatment diagnosis toward which a multiplicity of radiological tests are available to supplement the orthopedic surgeon's clinical impression.

With the development of arthroscopy a surgical diagnostic tool became available for directly assessing intraarticular knee pathology. Regardless of the preoperative diagnosis, prearthrotomy arthroscopy allowed the surgeon to proceed more confidently to surgical treatment, to desist if the diagnosis was not confirmed, or to alter treatment if unexpected findings were revealed. Indeed, Dandy and Jackson[1] noted that diagnostic arthroscopy changed their therapeutic management in 51% of cases. Earlier controversies concerning the diagnostic accuracy of arthroscopy related mainly to its dependence on operator experience and its adequacy for consistent and correct evaluation of the posterior horn of the medial meniscus. However, as a result of improved technology, increased experience, and subspecialty training, the current diagnostic accuracy of knee arthroscopy exceeds 95%[2-4] (Plate 21-1, *A*) and it has rapidly evolved into the primary surgical tool for most intraarticular knee problems. With increasing confidence in its diagnostic and therapeutic effectiveness, the orthopedic surgeon is now more likely to proceed to arthroscopy on clinical judgment alone.

Arthroscopy is, however, an invasive procedure, requiring some form of anesthesia; and regardless of its intraarticular accuracy, it does not allow direct visualization of extrasynovial structures. Despite its relatively low morbidity rate, arthroscopy is not a completely benign procedure. In their series of 2640 cases Sherman et al.[5] reported an 8.2% complication rate, of which more than half were considered significant. Complications included infection, hemarthrosis, adhesions, peripheral nerve injury, reflex sympathetic dystrophy, broken instruments, and anesthetic difficulties. Despite these limitations, arthroscopy has remained the standard against which all other diagnostic modalities must be compared.

Early reports of the capability of MRI to delineate normal anatomical structures clearly[6-13] and promising preliminary studies with surgical confirmation in pathological states[12-21] led to justified enthusiasm. The fact that MRI is noninvasive and painless, that it requires no anesthesia or manipulation, and that it avoids exposure to ionizing radiation resulted in general patient acceptance. Growing evidence of the accuracy of MRI — together with its applicability to acute injury (despite the presence of pain, limited motion, or effusion), its effectiveness in allowing simultaneous assessment of intraarticular and extraarticular elements, and its capacity to permit evaluation of both the interstitial and the surface anatomy of all structures — has led to its common usage.

THE MENISCI

Because many intraarticular and extraarticular abnormalities may masquerade as a torn meniscus, the accurate clinical diagnosis of a meniscal tear can be difficult. The overall diagnostic accuracy of clinical evaluation alone for meniscal tears is disappointingly low[2,22,23] and is even less reliable for the lateral meniscus.[4,22] Moreover, even if the existence of a tear of either meniscus is correctly diagnosed, the type, site, and extent of the lesion are unlikely to be positively determined.[22]

Until recently, double-contrast arthrography was the most common means for radiological confirmation of a meniscal tear. Despite some reports describing a high degree of arthrographic accuracy,[4,24-26] others[2,22,27,28] have noted a much poorer correlation with arthrotomy or arthroscopic findings and have questioned its value compared to careful clinical evaluation. Arthrography is also less accurate for the lateral meniscus.[2,4,22,25,27] Single-contrast arthrography, computed tomography, arthrotomography, sonography, vibration arthrography, and radionuclide imaging have been advocated for meniscal evaluation, with accuracy rates generally comparable or inferior to those of double-contrast arthrography.[29-37]

Arthrographic false-negative findings most commonly involve nondisplaced horizontal or degenerative tears of the lateral meniscus[27,38] or bucket handle tears of the medial meniscus.[39,40] Most false-positive diagnoses are due to misinterpretations caused by overlapping contrast-filled structures such as the popliteal tendon sheath or communicating popliteal cysts.[22,38,41] The debatable reliability of arthrography, combined with the increased use of arthroscopy as a diagnostic tool, led to a significant reduction in the number of knee arthrograms even before the recent development of MRI.[42] If the patient's history and physical examination were clearly consistent with a meniscal tear, the orthopedic surgeon was likely to proceed to arthroscopy without the benefit of preoperative arthrography or, indeed, despite arthrographic findings at variance with a strong clinical impression.

MRI of the menisci

Although promising, early reports of magnetic resonance imaging for meniscal tears were often anecdotal, unconfirmed by surgical findings, or limited in significance by the relatively small number of cases analyzed.[12-15,17-20] Burgeoning interest in the potential of MRI has produced a second generation of studies involving significant numbers of patients who have undergone confirmatory arthroscopy.[3,43-49] These studies have uniformly demonstrated MRI's high reliability in evaluating the menisci and its superiority to clinical diagnosis, arthrography, and other radiological modalities.

The reliability of MRI as expressed by the parameters of sensitivity, specificity, accuracy, negative predictive value (NPV), and positive predictive value (PPV), is obvious (Tables 21-1 and 21-2). Of particular note is its relative equality in correctly evaluating the medial and lateral menisci. The one exception relates to its sensitivity for lateral meniscal tears. The data clearly indicate MRI's

Table 21-1 Medial meniscus and MRI

	Percentages				
	Sensitivity	Specificity	Accuracy	NPV	PPV
Polly et al.[43]	96	100	98	96	100
Mandelbaum et al.[47]	96	82	90	93	88
Jackson et al.[44]	98	89	93	98	89
Mink et al.[3]	97	89	94		
Schlesinger et al.[45]	94	82	89	90	88
Bonamo[46]	99	85	94	97	93
MEAN	97	88	93	95	92

NPV, Negative predictive value; *PPV,* positive predictive value.

Table 21-2 Lateral meniscus and MRI

	Percentages				
	Sensitivity	Specificity	Accuracy	NPV	PPV
Polly et al.[43]	67	95	90	94	80
Mandelbaum et al.[47]	75	95	91	94	80
Jackson et al.[44]	85	99	97	97	92
Mink et al.[3]	92	91	92		
Schlesinger et al.[45]	71	94	86	85	87
Bonamo[46]	76	97	90	89	93
MEAN	78	95	91	92	86

superiority to clinical diagnosis and arthrography for both menisci. This advantage is also illustrated by my own comparative diagnostic studies[22,46] (Tables 21-3 and 21-4). In addition, comparison of the analyses by Schlesinger et al.[45] and Bonamo[46] (Tables 21-1 and 21-2) suggests the probability of future improvements in reliability. These studies were performed at a 2-year interval, and the same radiologists and arthroscopists were employed. Because there was no change in the arthroscopic technique or criteria for meniscectomy, the uniform increase of all reliability parameters in the more recent study would indicate improvements in technical acquisition and greater experience in interpretation.

Of perhaps greatest significance to the treating surgeon is MRI's high NPV for both the medial and the lateral meniscus. Although claims of 100% NPV[18,49] have not been reproduced, the chance of failing to detect a clinically significant meniscal tear is certainly low.[3,43-48,51] Therefore, in treating a symptomatic patient with the clinical suspicion of a meniscal tear but a negative MRI, the orthopedic surgeon is more likely to recommend a conservative approach or reevaluate the patient for a possible nonmeniscal source of symptoms rather than suggest arthroscopy. Although clinical judgment must still be employed, the high NPV of MRI will undoubtedly continue to diminish the numbers of purely diagnostic and nontherapeutic arthroscopies. Conversely, MRI's extraordinary sensitivity and high PPV for medial meniscal tears complement arthroscopic evaluation by stimulating the arthroscopist to a more persistent examination when evaluating the posterior horn in a "tight" knee.

Pitfalls of meniscal MRI

Despite the evidence for MRI's reliability in diagnosing meniscal tears, some erroneous diagnoses are still made. False-negative reports have consistently related to either displaced bucket handle tears[50,52,53] or nondisplaced radial or oblique tears involving the free edge of the meniscus.[3,48,50-52] With a bucket handle tear the centrally displaced fragment may be overlooked on sagittal views alone and, if the remnant rim is devoid of degenerative change and presents without abnormal signal, the diagnosis may be missed (Plate 21-1, *B* and *C*). In cases of nondisplaced radial or oblique tears, findings on MRI can be subtle and the lesion may often be seen on only one image or not at all. The fact that these nondisplaced radial or oblique tears most commonly involve the lateral meniscus would explain the higher incidence of false-negative interpretations and the lower sensitivity of MRI for lateral meniscal tears. Unfortunately, this deficiency coincides with similar noted difficulties in the clinical or arthrographic evaluation of the lateral meniscus. The true incidence of false-negative MRI results for significant meniscal tears is difficult to establish because of increasing confidence in its NPV; thus patients with negative findings are less likely to proceed to surgery. Ongoing studies in which persistently symptomatic patients whose MRI findings are negative or equivocal (for a gross tear) undergo arthroscopy will help determine the true incidence of and reasons for false-negative MRI interpretations.

Normal anatomical structures are common and predictable sources of false-positive MRI diagnoses of meniscal tears. The fat plane within its tibial attachments or the fatty separation between the anterior horn of the lateral meniscus and the transverse ligament may lead to a false-positive interpretation of a tear.[50,52-55] The popliteal tendon may be misinterpreted as a vertical tear of the posterior horn of the lateral meniscus or, in the case of a previous total lateral meniscectomy, be mistaken for a retained horn.[50,54,55] The ligaments of Humphry and Wrisberg may be erroneously interpreted as meniscal fragments.[54] With increased recognition of these well-documented normal variations, false-positive diagnoses of meniscal tears have become less frequent.

Of greater controversy are false-positive MRI diagnoses

Table 21-3 Medial meniscus — comparison of clinical diagnosis, arthrography, and MRI

	Percentages				
Method	**Sensitivity**	**Specificity**	**Accuracy**	**NPV**	**PPV**
Clinical	99	62	88	95	86
Arthrography	96	53	78	77	78
MRI	99	85	94	97	93

Adapted from Bonamo JJ, Schulman G: Orthopedics 1988;11:1041-1046, and Bonamo JJ: Unpublished data, 1990.

Table 21-4 Lateral meniscus — comparison of clinical diagnosis, arthrography, and MRI

	Percentages				
Method	**Sensitivity**	**Specificity**	**Accuracy**	**NPV**	**PPV**
Clinical	59	94	81	80	85
Arthrography	57	83	73	76	66
MRI	76	97	90	89	93

Adapted from Bonamo JJ, Shulman G: Orthopedics 1988;11:1041-1046, and Bonamo JJ: Unpublished data, 1990.

of tears in the posterior horn of the medial meniscus. Some* have suggested that the majority of these apparently erroneous diagnoses are attributable to false-negative arthroscopic evaluations because of a tight knee or surgical inexperience. However, a more likely explanation relates to histologically significant but "closed" intrasubstance tears, which most commonly occur in the posterior horn of the medial meniscus.[3,48-50] The arthroscopist, limited to evaluation of the surface architecture, is unable to see such a tear directly inasmuch as no extension to an articular margin is present. Therefore, despite maximum relaxation of the patient and the use of tourniquets and thigh holders, angled scopes, multiple portals, and thorough probing, an undetermined percentage of significant intrasubstance "closed" tears may not be confirmed by arthroscopic evaluation. As will be discussed, the clinical significance and appropriate treatment of these "closed" lesions remain in doubt.

Despite the frequency with which arthroscopic partial meniscectomy is performed, little data have been accumulated concerning the value of MRI in assessing the knee after partial meniscectomy. Conflicting statements without statistical analysis have been made concerning this problem area. Some[53] have suggested that the menisci of asymptomatic patients who have undergone partial meniscectomy are distinguishable on MRI from those with incomplete removal of the tear or those with a subsequent secondary tear following surgery. Others[49] have stated that normal postoperative changes within the menisci may be indistinguishable on MRI from findings in patients with recurrent or retained tears. Because appropriate arthroscopic technique calls for removal of only mobile fragments and the retention of as much of the peripheral rim as possible, signal abnormalities on MRI, after partial meniscectomy, may be due either to the irregular edge at the site of resection or to insignificant horizontal degenerative changes extending toward the perimeter of the meniscus from the site of resection (Plate 21-1, *D*). Several of my patients after partial meniscectomy, who at significant intervals following their surgery suffered an injury to the unoperated meniscus of the same knee, have had MRI findings consistent with a retained or recurrent tear despite the absence of symptoms or subsequent arthroscopic findings localized to the site of the previous partial meniscectomy. Such inconsistent MRI information can confuse the surgeon and diminish the reinjured patient's confidence in proposed treatment.

Open or arthroscopic repair of tears in the peripheral vascular zone of the meniscus has become a common alternative to partial or total meniscectomy[57-60] (Plate 21-2). These peripheral tears are especially common with anterior cruciate ligament injury.[61] Little information is available at present concerning the appearance of the repaired meniscus in its various stages of healing. Some[51] suggest that following meniscal repair the abnormal signal within the meniscus disappears and the meniscus again takes on a normal appearance. However, others[14] believe that the repaired meniscus may never return to a completely normal appearance on MRI. In view of the increasing frequency of meniscal repair, the incidence of failed repairs in the unstable knee[57,59] and the growing interest in meniscal transplantation,[62] further data concerning the MRI appearance of healing or healed meniscal repairs are needed to determine the results of treatment and to time appropriately the patient's safe return to stressful physical activity.

Degenerative meniscal tears

Degenerative tears of the menisci are part of the normal aging process.[63-66] In Smillie's large series of 6500 arthrotomies for meniscal pathology[63] 54.5% were for horizontal cleavage tears. Noble and Hamblen,[64] in their study of cadavers with an average age of over 65 years, described a 60% incidence of degenerative tears. Noble[66] reported a 19% incidence of degenerative tears in cadavers under the age of 55 years and noted that microscopic signs of degeneration were seen in 76% of the grossly normal medial menisci examined.

Stoller et al.[50] were the first to correlate experimentally progressive pathological changes in the meniscus with grades of MRI signal intensity. They showed a 100% correlation between histological stages of meniscal degeneration and grades of MRI signal abnormality and concluded that MRI signal abnormalities represent a continuum of pathological change in the meniscus that can be used to predict gross and histological appearance. In this cadaver study all Grade III MRI signal abnormalities correlated with histologically documented fibrocartilaginous separation (degenerative Stage III). Of the eight MRI Grade III lesions, six were gross tears extending to the articular surface of the meniscus and two were intrasubstance horizontal cleavage tears without extension to an articular margin. The investigators postulated that these latter "closed" but significant lesions, all of which involved the posterior horn of the medial meniscus, were potentially symptomatic. Because these closed lesions are not directly visible on arthroscopic evaluation, they are, as previously noted, a presumed explanation for the fact that the majority of false-positive MRIs involve the posterior horn of the medial meniscus.

The extraordinary ability of MRI to reveal accurately both the surface characteristics and the intrasubstance architecture of the meniscus, plus the fact that very few patients over the age of 40 years have absolutely no meniscal signal abnormality on MRI,[48] has renewed interest in the natural history, clinical relevance, and appropriate treatment of degenerative meniscal tears. This previously unavailable information concerning interstitial meniscal pathology raises certain yet-unresolved questions. What is the true incidence of nontraumatic abnormal meniscal findings on MRI relative to age, and what percentage of these "abnormal" menisci are or will

---

*References 3, 18, 47, 48, 51, 56.

become symptomatic? Do all Grade II MRI signal abnormalities eventually progress to Grade III? Do all "closed" Grade III lesions inevitably become structurally significant tears with extension to an articular margin? Are all menisci with Grade III signal abnormalities including "closed" lesions, clinically symptomatic? Inasmuch as recently documented neurological structures within the meniscus are limited to the peripheral 20%,[67] and "closed" tears have no grossly mobile fragments, do weight-bearing forces cause sufficient mechanical distortion in the meniscus with an interstitial tear to create tension on sensible peripheral structures (the accepted final common pathway of pain production)?

The functional importance of the meniscus in load bearing, shock absorption, stabilization, and lubrication has been clearly established,[68-74] and the relationship of total meniscectomy to the development of degenerative arthritis and long-term poor results is well documented.[68,75-78] Preservation of a meniscal rim allows significant continued load-bearing effect and permits a more normal pattern of pressure distribution to the articular surfaces.[72,79] Even menisci with horizontal cleavage tears have been shown to maintain some load-bearing function.[80-82] It has been experimentally shown that the amount of secondary articular cartilage degeneration after partial meniscectomy is directly related to the amount of meniscus removed.[73] The current concept of partial meniscectomy, therefore, although clearly preferable to total meniscectomy, maintains a relationship to subsequent degenerative arthritis.

Moreover, noncausally related degenerative meniscal tears and degenerative arthritis commonly coexist.[64,81,83] Poorer results after open or arthroscopic partial meniscectomy, particularly in older patients, have been shown to be directly related both to the type of tear and to the condition of the articular cartilage at the time of surgery.[83-87] McBride et al.,[85] for example, reported 98% patient satisfaction following arthroscopic partial medial meniscectomy for nondegenerative tears and only 65% satisfactory results with degenerative tears in patients over the age of 40.

Current evaluation is based on an understanding of the functional importance of the meniscus, the frequency of nonsymptomatic degenerative meniscal tears, the common coexistence of degenerative tears and degenerative arthritis in older patients, the uncertain pathomechanics of pain production with "closed" lesions, the poorer results of partial or total meniscectomy for degenerative tears with or without coexisting arthritic changes, and the well-founded current emphasis on meniscal preservation. Thus the MRI diagnosis of a closed degenerative tear is not sufficient evidence that the lesion is the source of the symptoms or that partial meniscectomy will resolve the patient's complaints. The arthroscopist, in evaluating a degenerative meniscus with intact articular margins, is rightfully reluctant to proceed to piecemeal resection in the expectation of finding a significant interstitial structural lesion as determined by MRI evaluation. Despite the logical assumption that closed Grade III meniscal lesions will eventually progress to more significant tears, we have not yet extended our concepts of care to include prophylactic meniscectomy. Even with MRI demonstration of extension of a degenerative tear to an articular surface or, indeed, even with evidence of meniscal fragmentation, the percentage of symptoms caused by the meniscal tear as opposed to possible coexisting degenerative arthritis cannot always be precisely determined before surgery (Plate 21-3). Unless symptoms are of relatively acute onset or truly mechanical in nature, partial meniscectomy in patients with significant coexisting degenerative arthritis may have no immediate therapeutic effect and can lead to more rapid breakdown of the articular cartilage. This is not to imply that significant degenerative tears in older patients are unworthy of surgical treatment, particularly if conservative care has failed, but rather to emphasize that since the well-being of the knee is ultimately dependent upon the integrity of the articular cartilage, and the meniscus is its primary protector, caution must be employed and the patient's expectations tempered when arthroscopic surgery is based primarily on MRI demonstration of any variety of degenerative meniscal tear.

ANTERIOR CRUCIATE LIGAMENT

Conservative treatment of the ACL-deficient knee — incorporating arthroscopy for associated meniscal tears or osteochondral fractures, appropriate rehabilitation, the use of functional braces, and activity modification — has been reported to give acceptably good results.[88-92] However, when considering this conservative approach, the physician and patient must face the disconcerting facts of permanent instability, a high incidence of secondary reinjury, the time-related development of degenerative arthritis, and progressive disability.[93-99] Despite the current trend — earlier surgical repair or reconstruction, the advantages of arthroscopically assisted reconstructive procedures,[100-102] and rehabilitative advances[103-105] — controversies persist concerning the technical aspects, results, morbidity, and specific indications for reparative or reconstructive surgery in acute or chronic ACL deficiencies.

Therefore the diagnosis in itself of an ACL tear is insufficient to determine the best treatment for each patient. Individual factors such as age, occupation, type and level of sports participation, presence and degree of associated injuries, attitude concerning future activity modification, and willingness to accept a major operative procedure with long-term rehabilitation are involved in the decision-making process. Indeed, the patient's nonmedical, practical, social, and economic considerations are often the deciding factors regardless of the physician's recommendation. Clearly, the process of choosing the best alternative for each individual begins with an accurate comprehensive diagnosis, not only of the type and degree of anterior cruciate injury but also of its context (whether it is isolated or associated with other ligamentous, meniscal, chondral, or bone pathology).

The acute tear of the ACL is usually secondary to an external valgus force or to a noncontact injury related to sudden deceleration or a change of direction. An audible "pop" is described by the patient in approximately 80% of the cases.[106] Although not pathognomonic, a rapidly developing hemarthrosis after an acute injury is strongly suggestive of an ACL tear.[107] The clinical diagnosis is primarily dependent upon the assessment of stability utilizing the Lachman test[108,109] and various modifications of the pivot shift test.[110-112] The unreliability of the anterior draw test has been well documented.[108,113] However, after an acute injury physical examination without anesthesia may be inconclusive because of pain, a tense hemarthrosis, hamstring spasm, or the presence of a displaced meniscal tear.[61] Caution must be used in examining children with open physes since an undetected epiphyseal plate injury may be misinterpreted as a ligament tear on stability testing.

Instrumented testing for anterior laxity has recently become a useful aid to physical diagnosis.[106,114,115] Daniel et al.[106,114] demonstrated that, although a wide range of anterior laxity exists in normal patients, there is a small right-left difference in each individual. They showed that 92% of normal subjects demonstrated a right-left difference in anterior laxity of less than 2 mm, whereas 96% of patients with an ACL tear had an injured knee–normal knee difference in anterior displacement of greater than 2 mm. A recent report[116] has also indicated the applicability of the Genucom system in the objective measurement of knee joint laxity with a high correlation to clinical evaluation.

Since avulsions represent less than 5% of all ACL tears[117] and not all of these are associated with a detached bone fragment, routine x-ray examination is usually of little value. Woods et al.[118] have described the lateral capsular sign — an avulsion of bone from the proximal lateral tibia with tears of the lateral capsular ligament — as an indirect sign of ACL injury.[118] Double-contrast arthrography may accurately demonstrate the integrity of the ACL,[4,119,120] but its reliability in this regard has been questioned.[2,22,24,25] Although single-contrast arthrography has been advocated as more accurate for the ACL it would be less dependable in determin-

ing the presence of associated meniscal tears.[29,121,122] It is generally agreed, in view of the extrasynovial location of the ACL and the arthrogram's ability to assess only its surface architecture, that the reliability of arthrography is limited in determining the existence of a partial ACL tear.[22,29,119]

The diagnostic benefit of arthroscopically examining the acutely injured knee with a hemarthrosis and equivocal physical findings is well appreciated.[107,123-125] In cases of uncertain diagnosis, a stability examination under anesthesia, combined with diagnostic arthroscopy, will establish the status of the ACL. In candidates for reconstructive surgery, immediate open repair, arthroscopically assisted repair, or reconstruction can be performed. In patients in whom a more conservative approach has been chosen, immediate attention can be given to probable coexisting meniscal tears or articular surface damage. However, if the acute ACL tear is combined with significant damage to collateral or capsular ligaments, there is a danger of fluid extravasation during arthroscopy. Moreover, if the prearthroscopic diagnosis is uncertain, the patient has no definite foreknowledge of the injury's extent and must rely, in this instance, on the preoperative discussion of contingencies relative to the possibility of more extensive immediate surgery.

MRI of the anterior cruciate ligament

Preliminary reports[12-16,21,47,49] suggested the value of MRI in evaluating the anterior cruciate ligament. Recent larger studies[3,43-46] have confirmed MRI's reliability in the diagnosis of ACL tears. The data obviously indicate MRI's superiority to arthrography and other radiological tests in helping determine the ACL's integrity (Table 21-5). Comparison again of the data of Schlesinger et al.[45] and Bonamo[46] suggests that improved technique and greater experience in interpretation have led to increased reliability.

However, MRI's advantage over clinical evaluation for the ACL alone remains unclear. Lee et al.,[126] in a comparison of physical examination and MRI, showed that the sensitivities of the Lachman test and MRI were 89% and 94% respectively and the specificity for both was 100%. My own comparison of arthrographic diagnosis, clinical evaluation without anesthesia, and MRI indicates

Table 21-5 Anterior cruciate ligament and MRI

	Percentages				
	Sensitivity	Specificity	Accuracy	NPV	PPV
Polly et al.[43]	100	97	97	100	86
Jackson et al.[44]	100	96	97	100	70
Mink et al.[3]	92	95	95		
Schlesinger et al.[45]	78	81	80	90	64
Bonamo[46]	83	90	88	93	78
MEAN	91	92	91	96	75

that physical diagnosis of the ACL using MRI is superior to that using arthrography in all respects and that MRI is better than arthrography in all parameters except specificity[22,46] (Table 21-6). The comparison of MRI and clinical evaluation shows similar consistency in determining the status of the ACL. However, despite MRI's equality to clinical diagnosis for the ACL, its excellent overall reliability and particularly its high negative predictive value (NPV) make it a valuable complement to physical examination. More important, because the appropriate treatment of acute and chronic ACL deficiencies rests not only on the correct diagnosis of injury to the ligament itself but also on the nature of the injury — partial or complete, midsubstance or avulsion, isolated or associated with other ligamentous damage, chondral or osteochondral fractures, occult fractures or meniscal tears — it is MRI's ability to evaluate simultaneously all intraarticular and extraarticular structures and their interstitial architecture that defines its advantage in ACL injuries.

Associated meniscal tears

Coexisting meniscal tears reportedly are present in as many as 75% of all acute ACL injuries and up to 90% of untreated chronic deficiencies.* Since the importance of preserving the meniscus in the unstable knee has been established and resection of significant portions of the menisci in an ACL-deficient knee results in increased instability and progression to significant degenerative arthritis,[129-135] the extent and type of associated meniscal tears are major factors in choosing appropriate treatment. The presence of coexisting, extensive, nonreparable meniscal tears will often lead to a recommendation for reconstructive ligament surgery concurrent with significant partial or subtotal meniscectomy. Tears in the reparable peripheral vascular zone of the meniscus are particularly common with ACL injury,[57,61,127,128] and the high failure rate for repair of these peripheral tears in nonstabilized anterior cruciate deficiencies is well known.[57,59] Therefore the preoperative MRI diagnosis of a peripheral meniscal tear in an equivocal reconstructive case might indicate simultaneous ACL reconstruction and meniscal repair to improve the chances for meniscal preservation.

*References 57, 94, 107, 127, 128.

Location and extent of the ACL tear

MRI currently cannot reliably distinguish midsubstance tears from avulsions.[16,49,126] It also cannot consistently differentiate between partial and complete tears.[16,45,49] This creates a diagnostic gap. Partial tears represent a significant proportion of all ACL injuries.[61,123,136] Arthrography is notoriously unreliable in the diagnosis of partial ACL tears.[22,29,119] In one series[22] 40% (10/25) of all arthrographic false negative results were documented at arthroscopy to be partial ACL tears. The clinical determination of a partial tear of the ACL may also be difficult. In the same comparative study[22] 60% (6/10) of false-negative clinical evaluations without anesthesia, and 90% (9/10) of false-negative clinical impressions under anesthesia, were found to be partial tears at the time of arthroscopy. The relatively low PPV of MRI for complete ACL tears is presumably due to its confusing of abnormal signals from relatively insignificant interstitial damage (Grade I) or partial gross injury (Grade II) and complete tears (Grade III) (Plate 21-4). Inasmuch as the conservative treatment of partial ACL tears produces uniformly good results,* the reliable MRI diagnosis of partial tears would eliminate the need for arthroscopy except in patients with other intraarticular pathology.

Most ACL tears are localized to the proximal portion of the ligament,[117,138] and recent reports[138,139] have described their relationship to underlying stenosis of the intercondylar notch. Routine x-ray examination will usually identify avulsions associated with a bone fragment. The current inability of MRI to distinguish clearly between a complete substance tear and an avulsion can be clinically relevant. In the patient who is unequivocally a candidate for reconstructive surgery, preliminary arthroscopy will reveal whether unaugmented primary repair, repair with augmentation, or primary reconstruction is indicated. However, in the equivocal case or in an adolescent with open physes the decision relative to reparative or reconstructive surgery often is affected by the site of the tear, and this determination, if unclear on MRI, would require direct observation by diagnostic arthroscopy.

*References 93, 100, 136, 137.

Table 21-6 Anterior cruciate ligament — comparison of clinical diagnosis without anesthesia, arthrography, and MRI

Method	Percentages				
	Sensitivity	Specificity	Accuracy	NPV	PPV
Arthrography	26	86	66	69	50
Clinical	71	97	88	87	92
MRI	83	88	88	93	78

Adapted from Bonamo JJ, Shulman G: Orthopedics 1988;11:1041-1046, and Bonamo JJ: Unpublished data, 1990.

Associated chondral and bone injury

DeHaven[107] noted that x-ray negative osteochondral fractures were the source of acute posttraumatic knee hemarthrosis in 6% of cases. Arthroscopically documented chondral or osteochondral fractures have been reported in approximately 20% of all acute ACL injuries.[61,123,128] Mink and Deutsch[140] were able to identify, by MRI, displaced chondral and osteochondral fractures of the femoral condyles or patella following acute trauma. They also noted nondisplaced impacted osteochondral fractures of the anterior portion of the lateral femoral condyle in 20% of acute ACL tears. Others,[15,44,141] however, have suggested that MRI is not effective in the diagnosis of purely chondral or osteochondral loose bodies less than 5 to 10 mm in diameter. In my own series all arthroscopically identified loose fragments less than 1 cm in diameter were missed on preoperative MRI. In nonreconstructive candidates with an acute ligament injury and no associated meniscal tear the ability of MRI to identify occult chondral or osteochondral fractures would allow otherwise unlikely immediate arthroscopic attention.

In evaluating patients with acute ligament tears, several authors* have commented on MRI findings consistent with occult fractures of the metaphysis and/or epiphysis of the proximal tibia or distal femur. The common coexistence of such occult subchondral injuries with acute ligament damage introduces a new dimension to the diagnosis and treatment of acute ligament tears. Mink and Deutsch[140] recently reported on a series of 30 such occult lesions and termed them *bone bruises*. Some (7) were secondary to direct trauma, but most (23) were related to acute tears of the collateral ligament or ACL. Those associated with collateral ligament injury (5/5) were all on the contralateral side of the joint, and those related to ACL tears (18/25) all involved the lateral compartment. These bone changes were not noted on routine x-ray examination or seen at arthroscopy. Although histological confirmation was not possible, the clear historical relationship to acute injury, confirmation by positive bone scan, and subsequent spontaneous resolution on MRI are strong evidence supporting the concept of acute occult trabecular fractures secondary to compressive force. Their relevance to potential permanent sequelae with early postinjury weight bearing is still to be determined. The high reported incidence of these occult bone injuries therefore represents another indication for MRI as an extension of the physical examination of an acutely injured knee.

POSTERIOR CRUCIATE AND COLLATERAL LIGAMENTS

Injury to the posterior cruciate ligament is relatively uncommon. The usual mechanism is sudden forced hyperflexion or direct pretibial trauma to the flexed knee.

The diagnosis of a PCL tear is made on the basis of the history of injury, the development of a mild bloody effusion (less than in ACL injuries), the presence of a posterior sag, a positive posterior draw test, and a negative Lachman test. Routine x-rays are of little value unless the injury is associated with a bone avulsion, usually from the tibia. Arthrography has been notoriously unreliable in evaluating the status of the PCL. Arthroscopy, although helpful in assessing the PCL via the intercondylar notch with angled scopes or by means of posteromedial portals, is limited in its ability to reveal the entire course of the ligament.

Repair or reconstruction for midsubstance PCL tears has produced varied outcomes.[144-148] Although some[149] still recommend operative repair in acute cases, most[147,150,151] reserve surgical intervention only for those PCL tears associated with a bone avulsion (usually from the tibia) or those combined with injury to other ligaments. Conservative treatment of isolated, complete PCL tears has yielded uniformly good subjective and functional results.[150-155] Parolie and Bergfeld[152] reported 80% patient satisfaction and 84% return to previous sports in patients treated nonoperatively. In Fowler and Messieh's series of conservatively treated PCL tears,[150] all patients returned to previous activity without limitation and had good subjective and functional ratings. Both groups concluded that isolated complete tears of the PCL are essentially nondisabling, and acceptable functional results can be achieved by nonoperative treatment, provided appropriate muscular rehabilitation is completed.

The common injury to the medial collateral ligament is usually the result of a valgus force applied to the lateral aspect of the knee. Physical examination with attention to external ecchymosis and swelling, tenderness along the course of the ligament, and stability testing is essentially 100% accurate in the diagnosis of complete tears.

Traditionally, conservative treatment has been recommended for partial injuries and operative repair for complete MCL tears.[156,157] However, comparative studies of operative and nonoperative care for isolated complete MCL tears[157-160] have shown that conservative treatment, including initial immobilization, controlled early motion, and progressive muscular rehabilitation, produces equal or superior objective and functional results with less recovery time and minimal morbidity.

Injuries to the lateral ligament complex of the knee are less frequent but more disabling. They usually are the result of a violent high-velocity varus force rather than an athletic injury.[161,162] The structures involved may include the lateral capsular ligament, lateral collateral ligament, arcuate ligament, popliteus tendon, iliotibial band, and biceps tendon. There are also frequently simultaneous tears of the PCL and/or ACL[161-163]; and in severe combined injuries the peroneal nerve may be damaged.[164] The history and physical examination will usually indicate the magnitude of the more serious combined injury. Routine x-rays may demonstrate a

---

*References 48, 51, 53, 140, 142, 143.

lateral capsular sign[118] or avulsion fractures of the fibular head or Gerdy's tubercle. Operative repair is the treatment of choice.[161-165]

Direct evaluation of the collateral ligaments cannot be accomplished by the use of arthrography unless the injury is associated with a capsular ligament tear. Nor can arthroscopy directly visualize these extrasynovial structures; it is used primarily for the diagnosis and treatment of associated intraarticular pathology.

On MRI the PCL is clearly identified because of its thickness and the enhancement effect of the posterior capsule. Limited reports of MRI's ability to allow correct evaluation of the PCL[12,13,16,49] have been confirmed by larger studies clearly establishing its high reliability[3,43,45,46,51] (Table 21-7). MRI's excellent accuracy and particularly its high NPV for the PCL can be of great assistance to the treating surgeon in establishing a correct diagnosis, especially when faced with equivocal physical findings. However, the true sensitivity and PPV of MRI for PCL injury are still unclear since all reported series contain relatively few surgically documented tears.

MRI is also highly reliable in evaluating the integrity of the collateral ligaments.[13,16,21,49,51] However, in view of the accuracy and well-established criteria of physical examination, the practical value of MRI in corroborating the presence of a complete collateral ligament tear is questionable.

Because the current trend is toward nonoperative treatment for isolated complete tears of the PCL or collateral ligaments, open repair or reconstruction usually is indicated only for more serious combined ligament injuries, and arthroscopy is used primarily for associated intraarticular pathology. However, confidence in the nonoperative treatment for PCL or collateral ligament tears depends upon confirmation that the injury is truly isolated. Although MRI may aid in confirming an equivocal diagnosis and help differentiate between partial and complete tears of the PCL or collateral ligaments, its main value in these cases lies in its capabilities in terms of simultaneous evaluation of other intraarticular structures and determination of the presence of associated injuries that may alter treatment and prognosis.

ARTICULAR CARTILAGE

The common development of degenerative arthritis with increasing age is well known.[64,81,83] Noble and Hamblen[64] reported an 85% incidence in cadavers over

the age of 65, and Dandy and Jackson[83] found the incidence at arthroscopy to be three times more common in patients over the age of 40 years. The relationship to partial or total meniscectomy and ligamentous instability also has been shown.* Although the patient's history, physical examination, and routine x-rays may constitute presumptive evidence of articular surface damage, they do not allow direct assessment. The reliability of arthrography in evaluating the articular cartilage has been variable.[4,25,166,167] Computed tomography and arthrotomography have been recommended as more accurate[168-171]; and some have advocated evaluation by sensitive but nonspecific scintigraphy,[37,172] SPECT,[173] vibration arthrography,[35,174] or thermography.[175] At present, arthroscopy, with its ability to disclose the articular surfaces directly, remains the ultimate diagnostic method for documenting articular cartilage pathology[176-178] (Plate 21-5).

Initial comments concerning MRI's capabilities in evaluating the articular cartilage and defining gross defects were mostly undocumented by arthroscopy or arthrotomy.† These reports were also in conflict concerning MRI's relative value in the patellofemoral and femorotibial compartments. More recently Wojtys et al.[180] evaluated, by MRI, experimentally created lesions of the femoral condyles and patellas in cadavers. Although they were unable reliably to determine surface and texture changes without cartilage substance loss, they did document partial- or full-thickness loss in 81% of cases. They also defined focal defects at least 1 mm in depth (18/21) or greater than 3 mm in diameter (15/16), and they noted that the presence of intraarticular air or fluid helped delineate these lesions. Crues and Ryu[143] also indicated that MRI was not accurate in the determination of superficial lesions of the articular cartilage but reported 80% sensitivity for lesions that extended to bone. Yulish et al.[181] correlated MRI findings with arthroscopically confirmed articular surface changes of the patella. Although they also were unable accurately to determine the presence of softening (Grade I), they defined Grade II, Grade III, and Grade IV stages of articular surface damage with 89% accuracy. Gylys-Morin et al.,[182] in a cadaver study, were able consistently to identify on MRI 3 to 4 mm focal defects in the articular cartilage with intraarticular

---

*References 68, 73, 75-78, 83, 95-97.
†References 6, 10, 12, 14, 15, 43, 48, 179.

Table 21-7 Posterior cruciate ligament and MRI

	Percentages				
	Sensitivity	**Specificity**	**Accuracy**	**NPV**	**PPV**
Polly et al.[43]		100	100	100	100
Mink et al.[3]	92	95	95	—	—
Schlesinger et al.[45]	50	97	95	97	50
Bonamo[46]	73	100	99	99	100

saline, and in lesions as small as 2 mm with gadopentetate as a contrast agent. The impression of others[183] regarding MRI's ability to assess articular surface changes correctly is more pessimistic. In my own patients the sensitivity of prearthroscopy MRI for clinically significant chronic articular surface lesions of Grade III (gross fragmentation) or Grade IV (exposure of subchondral bone) has been less than 50% on early MRI studies. However, there has been significant improvement in accuracy on recent MRI examinations.

If MRI could be used to evaluate accurately the extent and depth of articular lesions, with or without paramagnetic contrast agents,[56,182-184] it would establish, without the need for diagnostic arthroscopy, specific criteria for conservative treatment versus palliative arthroscopic debridement, tibial or femoral osteotomy, or total knee replacement. It would also allow the establishment of more reasonable expectations in patients undergoing surgery for the combination of meniscal tear and degenerative arthritis. In patellofemoral disorders MRI's potential capacity to document accurately the degree of chondromalacia would permit the orthopedic surgeon to determine more appropriately, before diagnostic arthroscopy, the specific indications for ongoing conservative treatment, patellar debridement, realignment, decompression, or patellectomy.

OSTEOCHONDRITIS DISSECANS

Osteochondritis dissecans is readily diagnosed on the basis of routine x-ray results. More relevant and of greater difficulty in determining are the stability of the lesion and the condition of the overlying articular cartilage. Even at arthroscopy the stability of the lesion cannot always be assessed if the overlying articular cartilage is intact. Mesgarzadeh et al.[185] have evaluated the stability of osteochondritic lesions by x-ray, bone scan, and MRI. They showed that x-ray and bone scan were reasonably accurate in assessing lesional stability but that MRI allowed direct differentiation of in situ loosening and grossly unstable fragments. MRI also disclosed fluid at the fragment−underlying bone interface (92% sensitivity) and distinguished loose from stable lesions (90% specificity). If these data are reproducible, the ability of MRI to reveal the stability of osteochondritic lesions and simultaneously to help assess the condition of the overlying articular cartilage will assist orthopedic surgeons in determining the relative indications for conservative treatment, in situ drilling, bone grafting with internal fixation, fragment removal with curettage, and/or subchondral drilling or replacement with allograft; and, just as important, it will aid in following the effect of each form of treatment.

STRESS FRACTURES

Although relatively uncommon, stress fractures can occur in the region of the knee, typically involving the posteromedial aspect of the proximal tibia.[186,187] Results of routine x-rays often are insensitive on initial evaluation.[188] Although highly sensitive, bone scan is nonspecific because of the possibility of coexisting arthritis, osteonecrosis, or meniscal tears.[140,187] Several authors* have reported on the MRI diagnosis of stress fractures. Although stress fractures may be confused with acute occult fractures on MRI, the patient's history of insidious onset of symptoms and the fact that stress fractures are usually limited to the metaphysis and/or diaphysis, rather than the epiphysis, serve to differentiate the two. MRI therefore appears to be the most sensitive and specific single test available for the early diagnosis and follow-up of stress fractures.

OSTEONECROSIS

Spontaneous osteonecrosis is characterized by the sudden onset of monoarticular pain, persistent symptoms at rest, and involvement of the weight-bearing area of the medial femoral condyle. X-ray evidence of subchondral cysts is usually long delayed after the onset of symptoms. The differentiation of osteonecrosis from degenerative arthritis and degenerative meniscal tears is difficult before specific x-ray changes develop. Even a bone scan may not confirm the diagnosis or cause plans for treatment to be altered. Coexisting degenerative medial meniscal tears and/or degenerative arthritis often lead to arthroscopic meniscectomy or articular surface debridement. Unless arthroscopy unexpectedly uncovers subchondral cystic lesions, the diagnosis of osteonecrosis is still obscured. Despite preoperative expectations, symptoms worsen postoperatively as secondary articular cartilage collapse occurs. The efficacy of MRI in the early diagnosis of osteonecrosis has been reported by many,† and Schlesinger et al.[45] noted that the diagnosis of osteonecrosis by means of MRI is possible at least 6 months before determination by routine x-ray. The early diagnosis by MRI of otherwise unsuspected osteonecrosis in patients with coexisting but relatively nonsymptomatic meniscal tears and/or degenerative arthritis may, therefore, eliminate ineffective arthroscopic meniscectomy and debridement and lead to earlier appropriate treatment.

PARAMENISCAL CYSTS

Arthrography can demonstrate only parameniscal or popliteal cysts that have intraarticular communication. Noncommunicating and atypically located cysts or bursae are reliably documented by CT or sonography.[193-196] At present, the indications for cyst removal are limited and surgical treatment is usually directed only to associated intraarticular lesions. Burk et al.[197] have shown the efficacy of MRI in the diagnosis of parameniscal and popliteal cysts of all types. Inasmuch as 90% of popliteal cysts are secondary to meniscal pathology[198] and essentially all nonganglionic parameniscal cysts (usually lat-

---

*References 140, 186, 188, 189.
†References 14, 45, 48, 51, 53, 140, 141, 143, 190-192.

eral) are related to horizontal meniscal tears,[197] the major advantage of MRI over other diagnostic tests is its ability to display simultaneously both the cyst and the meniscus.

Reports of the MRI diagnosis of synovial lesions have been limited to pigmented villonodular synovitis and pseudotumors.[199-206] MRI's potential in differentiating synovial lesions from other forms of intraarticular pathology can prevent preoperative confusion and help determine in advance the type and extent of surgery required.

EXTENSOR TENDONS

Injury to the quadriceps or patellar tendon is usually of insidious onset and secondary to overuse; but it can also be the result of a single traumatic episode. The damage almost invariably occurs at the site of tendinous attachment to bone, at the superior or inferior pole of the patella, or at the tibial tubercle. The most pertinent physical finding is localized tenderness at the site of injury or, in the case of a complete tear, inability to extend the knee against gravity or resistance. A few acute tears may have x-ray evidence of avulsed bone fragments at the point of tendinous attachment. The treatment of microscopic interstitial tears (tendonitis) or gross partial tears is usually conservative. For complete tears surgical repair is required. At times surgery is appropriate for repair of partial injuries, depending upon the degree of tear. In chronic unremitting tendonitis, debridement of necrotic and fibrotic tissue may sometimes be necessary. Because the diagnosis of a complete tear is usually obvious, the need to confirm the diagnosis by MRI may be superfluous. However, MRI's capacity for evaluation of the interstitial architecture of the tendon, determination of the extent of a partial tear, and differentiation of partial from gross tears are clearly relevant to treatment planning. The accuracy of MRI in this regard has been well documented.[15,49,51,53]

PATELLOFEMORAL JOINT

Peripatellar or retropatellar symptoms are perhaps the most common reason for orthopedic knee consultation. Patellofemoral symptoms are often due to malalignment of the extensor mechanism and/or interrelated or independently explained abnormal patellar tracking. Instability or asymmetrical compression of the patella in the trochlear groove of the femur produces symptoms and possible secondary chondromalacia. The symptoms must be differentiated from those of quadriceps or patellar tendonitis and from the less common medial plica syndrome.[207,208] In addition to the patient's history and a thorough physical examination, routine x-rays are obtained to show the relationship of the patella to the trochlear groove. The lateral view will help establish the presence and extent of related patella alta or infra.[209-212] Tangential patellar views by different techniques[212-215] permit assessment of the patellar configuration[216] and allow computation of a variety of quantitative parameters such as the sulcus angle,[214,215] patellar index,[215,217]

congruence angle,[214] lateral patellofemoral angle,[213,218] and patellofemoral index.[213,218] However, these determinations are indirect attempts by static x-ray to evaluate the dynamics of the patella within the trochlear groove and therefore are of limited value. Studies utilizing cine-CT,[219-222] with imaging of the patellofemoral joint during the first 30 degrees of flexion and extension, have shown that in this range of motion patellar tracking abnormalities are most apparent.

Shellock et al.[223] were the first to report on kinematic MRI studies of the patellofemoral joint. Multiple sequential axial images obtained within the early (0 to 32 degrees) phases of flexion were viewed in a cine loop format. The authors concluded that these studies clearly demonstrated the relationship of the patella to the trochlear groove and were potentially useful in the evaluation of abnormal patellar tracking. Although more information is obtained by such techniques than by routine x-ray, with the additional benefit of articular cartilage evaluation these "kinematic" studies are still adynamic inasmuch as the knee is sequentially and statically positioned at various degrees of flexion. The effects of weight bearing and muscular activity therefore cannot be appreciated. Truly dynamic studies are needed for the clinician to make specific and quantitative assessment of patellofemoral abnormalities, choose the appropriate conservative or operative treatment, and determine the posttreatment or surgical results. A recent report of "MRI fluoroscopy"[224] suggests the potential for development of a technique adapting MRI to the study of dynamic musculoskeletal phenomena.

CONCLUSIONS

The major advantage of MRI lies in its ability to reliably and simultaneously facilitate evaluation of all intraarticular and extraarticular structures, affording both the physician and the patient a more confident and comprehensive pretreatment diagnosis and prognosis without multiple and overlapping diagnostic testing. Patient acceptance of MRI is high because of its minimal morbidity, uncommon contraindications, noninvasive and painless nature, lack of exposure to ionizing radiation, and absence of need for anesthesia or manipulation.

From the perspective of the orthopedic surgeon further improvements are needed. MRI's ability to facilitate direct evaluation of the interstitial architecture of all structures should allow better differentiation of partial injuries of the cruciate ligaments, more accurate evaluation of the status of ligament repairs or reconstructions, and a clearer understanding of the natural history of meniscal degeneration. Improvements in technical acquisition and greater experience with interpretation should diminish the already low incidence of erroneous diagnoses, improve criteria for evaluation of the post–partial meniscectomy or repaired meniscus, and more accurately document the status of articular cartilage lesions. The development of techniques for dynamic studies has the potential to ensure true kinematic analysis of unstable or reconstructed knees and understanding of the pathomechanics of the patellofemoral joint. Although MRI should not supplant careful physical examination and the application of clinical judgment, it has, despite its relative infancy and current limitations, already become an indispensible tool in the evaluation of injured or painful knees.

• • •

TERMINOLOGY

sensitivity, True-positives / true-positives + false-negatives; the percentage of positive MRI findings in patients who have a tear

specificity, True-negatives/true-negatives + false-positives; the percentage of negative MRI findings in patients who do not have a tear

accuracy, True-positives + true-negatives / number of patients; the percentage of correctly classified structures

negative predictive value (NPV), True-negatives / true-negatives + false-negatives; the confidence that can be attached to a negative MRI diagnosis

positive predictive value (PPV), True-positives / true-positives + false-positives; the confidence that can be attached to a positive MRI diagnosis

REFERENCES

1. Dandy DJ, Jackson RW: The impact of arthroscopy on the management of disorders of the knee. J Bone Joint Surg [Br] 1975;57:346-348.
2. Selesnick FH, Noble HB, Bachman DC, Steinberg FL: Internal derangement of the knee: diagnosis by arthrography, arthroscopy, and arthrotomy. Clin Orthop 1985;198:26-30.
3. Mink JH, Levy T, Crues JV III: Tears of the anterior cruciate ligament and menisci of the knee: MR imaging evaluation. Radiology 1988;167:769-774.
4. Levinsohn EM, Baker BE: Pre-arthrotomy diagnostic evaluation of the knee: review of 100 cases diagnosed by arthrography and arthroscopy. AJR 1980;134:107-111.
5. Sherman OH, Fox JM, Snyder SJ, et al: Arthroscopy — "no problem surgery": an analysis of 2640 cases. J Bone Joint Surg [Am] 1986;68:256-265.
6. Soudry M, Lanir A, Angel D, et al: Anatomy of the normal knee as seen by magnetic resonance imaging. J Bone Joint Surg [Br] 1986;68:117-210.
7. Kean DM, Worthington BS, Preston B, et al: Role of NMR in the evaluation of musculoskeletal disease. Appl Radiol 1984;4:102-108.
8. Moon KL Jr, Genant HK, Helms CA, et al: Musculoskeletal applications of nuclear magnetic resonance. Radiology 1983;147:161-171.
9. Li KC, Henkelman RM, Poon PY, Rubenstein J: MR imaging of the normal knee. J Comput Asst Tomogr 1984;8:1147-1154.
10. Reicher MA, Rauschning W, Gold RH, et al: High resolution magnetic resonance imaging of the knee joint: normal anatomy. AJR 1985;145:895-902.
11. Kean DM, Worthington BS, Preston BJ, et al: Nuclear magnetic resonance imaging of the knee: examples of normal anatomy and pathology. Br J Radiol 1983;56:355-364.
12. Beltran J, Noto AM, Mosure JC, et al: The knee: surface coil MR imaging at 1.5 T. Radiology 1986;159:747-751.
13. Gallimore GW Jr., Harms SF: Knee injuries: high resolution MR imaging. Radiology 1986;160:457-461.
14. Burk DL, Kanal E, Brunberg JA, et al: 1.5-T surface coil MRI of the knee. AJR 1986;147:293-300.
15. Reicher MA, Bassett LW, Gold RH: High-resolution magnetic resonance imaging of the knee joint: pathologic correlations. AJR 1985;145:903-909.
16. Turner DA, Prodromos CC, Petasnick JP, Clark JW: Acute injury of the ligaments of the knee: magnetic resonance imaging. Radiology 1985;154:717-722.
17. Lotysch M, Mink J, Crues JV III, Schwartz A: Magnetic resonance imaging in the detection of meniscal injuries. Magn Reson Imaging 1986;4:94.
18. Reicher MA, Hartzman S, Duckwiler GR, et al: Meniscal injuries: detection using MR imaging. Radiology 1986;159:753-757.
19. Beltran J, Noto AM, Mosure JC, et al: Meniscal tears: MR demonstration of experimentally produced injuries. Radiology 1986;158:691-693.
20. Ehman RL, Berquist TH: Magnetic resonance imaging of musculoskeletal trauma. Radiol Clin North Am 1986;24:291-319.
21. Li DK, Adams ME, McConkey JP: Magnetic resonance imaging of the ligaments and menisci of the knee. Radiol Clin North Am 1986;24:209-227.
22. Bonamo JJ, Shulman G: Double contrast arthrography of the knee: a comparison to clinical diagnosis and arthroscopic findings. Orthopedics 1988;11:1041-1046.
23. DeHaven KE, Collins HR: Diagnosis of internal derangements of the knee: the role of arthroscopy. J Bone Joint Surg [Am] 1975;57:802-810.
24. Nicholas JA, Freiberger RH, Killoran PJ: Double-contrast arthrography of the knee. J Bone Joint Surg [Am] 1970;52:203-220.
25. Brown DW, Allman FL Jr, Eaton SB: Knee arthrography: a comparison of radiographic and surgical findings in 295 cases. Am J Sports Med 1978;6:165-172.
26. Dumas JM, Eddé D: Meniscal abnormalities: prospective correlation of double-contrast arthrography and arthroscopy. Radiology 1986;160:453-456.
27. Roper BA, Levack B: The arthrogram in diagnosis of meniscal lesions in the fourth decade of life. Clin Orthop 1986;210:213-215.
28. Rao S, Tregonning RJA: Arthroscopy and arthrography of the knee menisci. J Bone Joint Surg [Br] 1986;68:678 (abstract).
29. Reider B, Clancy W, Langer LO: Diagnosis of cruciate ligament injury using single contrast arthrography. Am J Sports Med 1984;12:451-454.
30. Tegtmeyer CJ, McCue FC III, Higgins SM, Ball DW: Arthrography of the knee: a comparative study of the accuracy of single and double contrast techniques. Radiology 1979;132:137-141.
31. Passariello R, Trecco F, DePaulis F, et al: Meniscal lesions of the knee joint: CT diagnosis. Radiology 1985;157:29-34.
32. Manco LG, Kavanaugh JH, Lozman J, et al: Diagnosis of meniscal tears using high-resolution computed tomography: correlation with arthroscopy. J Bone Joint Surg [Am] 1987;69:498-502.
33. Ghelman B: Meniscal tears of the knee: evaluation by high resolution CT compared with arthrography. Radiology 1988;157:23-27.
34. Selby B, Richardson ML, Nelson B: Sonography in the detection of meniscal injuries of the knee: evaluation in cadavers. AJR 1987;149:549-553.
35. McCoy GF, McCrea JD, Beverland DE, et al: Vibration arthrography as a diagnostic aid in diseases of the knee: a preliminary report. J Bone Joint Surg [Br] 1987;69:288-293.
36. Marymount JV, Lynch MA, Henning CE: Evaluation of meniscus tears of the knee by radionuclide imaging. Am J Sports Med 1983;11:432-435.
37. Mooar P, Gregg J, Jacobstein J: Radionuclide imaging in internal derangement of the knee. Am J Sports Med 1987;15:132-137.
38. Hall FF: Pitfalls in the assessment of the menisci by knee arthrography. Radiol Clin North Am 1981;19:305-328.

39. Kaye JJ, Frieberger RH: Arthrography of the knee. Clin Orthop 1975;107:73-80.

40. Shakespeare DJ, Rigby HS: The bucket handle tear of the meniscus. J Bone Joint Surg [Br] 1983;65:383-387.

41. Kaye JJ, Nance EP Jr: Pain in the athlete's knee. Clin Sports Med 1987;6:873-883.

42. Hall FM: Arthrography: past, present and future. AJR 1987;149:561-562.

43. Polly DW, Callaghan JJ, Sikes RA, et al: The accuracy of selective magnetic resonance imaging as compared with the findings of arthroscopy of the knee. J Bone Joint Surg [Am] 1988;70:192-198.

44. Jackson DW, Jennings LD, Maywood RM, Berger PE: Magnetic resonance imaging of the knee. Am J Sports Med 1988;16:29-38.

45. Schlesinger I, Bonamo JJ, Firooznia H, et al: Correlation of arthroscopy and magnetic resonance imaging of the knee. Orthop Trans 1988;12:544-545

46. Bonamo JJ: Unpublished data, 1990.

47. Mandelbaum BR, Finerman GAM, Reicher MA, et al: Magnetic resonance imaging as a tool for evaluation of traumatic knee injuries. Am J Sports Med 1986;14:361-370.

48. Crues JV III, Mink J, Levy TL, et al : Meniscal tears of the knee: accuracy of MR imaging. Radiology 1987;164:445-448.

49. Reicher MA, Hartzman S, Bassett LW, et al: MR imaging of the knee. I. Traumatic disorders. Radiology 1987;162:547-551.

50. Stoller DW, Martin C, Crues JV, et al: Meniscal tears: pathologic correlation with MR imaging. Radiology 1987;163:731-735.

51. Mink JH, Deutsch AL: Magnetic resonance imaging of the knee. Clin Orthop 1989;244:29-47.

52. Crues JV III, Ryu R: MRI of the knee. I. Surg Rounds Orthop 1989;3:17-25.

53. Mink JH, Reicher MA, Crues JV: Magnetic resonance imaging of the knee. New York, Raven Press, 1987.

54. Watanabe AT, Carter BC, Teitelbaum GP, Bradley WG Jr: Common pitfalls in magnetic resonance imaging of the knee. J Bone Joint Surg [Am] 1989;71:857-862.

55. Herman LJ, Beltran J: Pitfalls of MR imaging of the knee. Radiology 1988;167:775-781.

56. Sartoris DJ, Resnick D: MR imaging of the musculoskeletal system: current and future states. AJR 1987;149:457-467.

57. DeHaven KE: Meniscus repair in the athlete. Clin Orthop 1985;198:31-35.

58. Graf B, Docter T, Clancy W: Arthroscopic meniscal repair. Clin Sports Med 1987;6:525-536.

59. Rosenberg TD, Scott SM, Coward DB, et al: Arthroscopic meniscal repair evaluated with repeat arthroscopy. Arthroscopy 1986;2:14-20.

60. DeHaven KE: Rationale for meniscus repair or excision. Clin Sports Med 1985;4:267-273.

61. DeHaven KE: Decision making in acute anterior cruciate ligament injury. Instructional course lectures. St. Louis, Mosby, 1987. Vol 36, pp. 201-203.

62. Arnoczky SP, McDevitt CA, Cuzzell JZ, et al: Meniscal replacement using a cryopreserved allograft — an experimental study in the dog. Orthop Trans 1984;8:293.

63. Smillie IS: Injuries of the knee joint, ed 5, Edinburgh, Churchill Livingstone, 1978.

64. Noble J, Hamblen AL: The pathology of the degenerative meniscus lesion. J Bone Joint Surg [Br] 1975;57:180-186.

65. Ferrer-Roca O, Vilalta C: Lesions of the mensicus. I. Macroscopic and histological findings. Clin Orthop 1980;146:289-300.

66. Noble J: Lesions of the meniscus. J Bone Joint Surg [Am] 1977;59:480-485.

67. Day B, Mackenzie WG, Shim SS, Leung G: The vascular and nerve supply of the human meniscus. Arthroscopy 1985;1:58-62.

68. Krause WR, Pope MH, Johnson RJ, Wilder DG: Mechanical changes in the knee after meniscectomy. J Bone Joint Surg [Am] 1976;58:599-604.

69. Seedhom BB, Dowson D, Wright V: Proceedings: Functions of the menisci. A preliminary study. Ann Rheum Dis 33:111, 1974.

70. Walker PS, Erkman PJ: The role of the meniscus in force transmission across the knee. Clin Orthop 1975;109:184-192.

71. Kettelcamp DB, Jacobs AW: Tibiofemoral contact area — determination and implications. J Bone Join Surg [Am] 1972;54:349-356.

72. Kurosawa H, Fukubayashi T, Nakajima H: Load bearing-mode of the knee joint: physical behavior of the knee joint with or without menisci. Clin Orthop 1980;149:283-290.

73. Cox JS, Nye CE, Schaeffer WW, Woodstein IJ: The degenerative effects of partial and total resection of the medial meniscus in dogs' knees. Clin Orthop 1975;109:178-183.

74. Grood ES: Meniscal function. Adv Orthop Surg 1984;7:193-197.

75. Fairbank TJ: Knee joint changes after meniscectomy. J Bone Joint Surg [Br] 1948;30:664-670.

76. Johnson RJ, Kettelcamp DB, Clark W, et al: Factors affecting late results after meniscectomy. J Bone Joint Surg [Am] 1974;56:719-729.

77. Jackson JP: Degenerative changes in the knee after meniscectomy. Br Med J 1968;2:525-527.

78. Tapper EM, Hoover NW: Late results after meniscectomy. J Bone Joint Surg [Am] 1969;51:517-526.

79. McGinty JB, Geuss LF, Marvin RA: Partial or total meniscectomy. J Bone Joint Surg [Am] 1977;59:763-766.

80. Noble J, Turner PG: The function, pathology and surgery of the meniscus. Clin Orthop 1986;210:62-68.

81. Fahmy NR, Williams EA, Noble J: Meniscal pathology and osteo-arthritis of the knee. J Bone Joint Surg [Br] 1983;65:24-28.

82. Casscells SW: The torn or degenerated meniscus and its relationship to degeneration of the weight-bearing area of the femur and tibia. Clin Orthop Rel Res 1978;132:196-200.

83. Dandy DJ, Jackson RW: Meniscectomy and chondromalacia of the femoral condyle. J Bone Joint Surg [Am] 1975;57:1116-1119.

84. Jones RE, Smith EC, Reisch JS: Effects of medial meniscectomy in patients older than 40 years. J Bone Joint Surg [Am] 1978;60:783-786.

85. McBride GG, Constine RM, Hofman AA, Carson RW: Arthroscopic partial medial meniscectomy in the older patient. J Bone Joint Surg [Am] 1984;66:547-551.

86. Jackson RT, Rouse DW: The results of partial arthroscopic meniscectomy in patients over 40 years of age. J Bone Joint Surg [Br] 1982;64:481-485.

87. Ferkel RD, Davis JR, Friedman MJ, et al: Arthroscopic partial medial meniscectomy: an analysis of unsatisfactory results. Arthroscopy 1985;1:44-52.

88. Walla DJ, Albright JJ, McAuley E, et al: Hamstring control and the unstable anterior cruciate ligament–deficient knee. Am J Sports Med 1985;13(1):34-39.

89. Jokl P, Kaplan N, Stovell P, Keggi K: Non-operative treatment of severe injuries to the medial and anterior cruciate ligaments of the knee. J Bone Joint Surg [Am] 1984;66:741-744.

90. McDaniel WJ, Dameron JB: Untreated ruptures of the anterior cruciate ligament: a follow up study. J Bone Joint Surg [Am] 1980;62:696-705.

91. Giove TP, Miller SJ III, Kent BE, et al: Non-operative treatment of the torn anterior cruciate ligament. J Bone Joint Surg [Am] 1983;65:184-192.

92. Odensten M, Hamberg P, Nordin M, et al: Surgical or conservative treatment of the acutely torn anterior cruciate ligament: a randomized study with short-term follow-up observation. Clin Orthop 1985;198:87-93.

93. Noyes FR, Matthews DS, Mooar PA, et al: The symptomatic

anterior cruciate deficient knee. II. The results of rehabilitation, activity modification and counseling on functional disability. J Bone Joint Surg [Am] 1983;65:163-174.

94. Bonamo JJ, Fay C, Firestone T: The conservative treatment of the anterior cruciate deficient knee. Paper presented at the annual meeting of the American Orthopedic Society for Sports Medicine, Palm Springs Calif, June 1988.

95. Arnold JA, Cohen TP, Heaton LM, et al: Natural history of anterior cruciate tears. Am J Sports Med 1979;7(6):305-313.

96. Fetto JF, Marshall JL: The natural history and diagnosis of anterior cruciate ligament insufficiency. Clin Orthop 1980;147:29-38.

97. Sherman MF, Warren RF, Marshall JL, Savatsky GL: A clinical and radiographical analysis of 127 anterior cruciate insufficient knees. Clin Orthop 1987;227:229-237.

98. Hawkins RJ: Follow up of the acute non-operated isolated anterior cruciate ligament tear. Am J Sports Med 1986;14(3):205-210.

99. Kannus P, Järvinen M: Conservatively treated tears of the anterior cruciate ligament. J Bone Joint Surg [Am] 1987;69:1007-1012.

100. Jackson DW, Jennings LD: Arthroscopically assisted reconstruction of the anterior cruciate ligament using a patella tendon bone autograft. Clin Sports Med 1988;7:785-800.

101. Wilcox PG, Jackson DW: Arthroscopic anterior cruciate ligament reconstruction. Clin Sports Med 1987;6:513-524.

102. Clancy WG: Arthroscopic anterior cruciate ligament reconstruction with patellar tendon. Techniques Orthop 1988;2:13-22.

103. Huegel PT, Indelicato PA: Trends in rehabilitation following anterior cruciate ligament reconstruction. Clin Sports Med 1988;7:801-811.

104. Bilko TE, Paulos LE, Feagin JA Jr, et al: Current trends in repair and rehabilitation of complete (acute) anterior cruciate ligament injuries: analysis of 1984 questionnaire completed by ACL study group. Am J Sports Med 1986;14(2):143-147.

105. Noyes FR, Mangine RE, Barber S: Early knee motion after open and arthroscopic anterior cruciate ligament reconstruction. Am J Sports Med 1987;15(2):149-160.

106. Daniel DM, Stone ML, Sachs R, Malcolm L: Instrumented measurement of anterior laxity in patients with acute cruciate ligament disruption. Am J Sports Med 1985;13(6):401-407.

107. DeHaven KE: Diagnosis of acute knee injuries with hemarthrosis. Am J Sports Med 1980;8(1):9-14.

108. Torg JS, Conrad W, Kalen V: Clinical diagnosis of anterior cruciate ligament instability in the athlete. Am J Sports Med 1976;4(2):84-93.

109. Jonsson T, Althoff B, Peterson L, et al: Clinical diagnosis of ruptures of the anterior cruciate ligament: a comparative study of the Lachman test and the anterior drawer sign. Am J Sports Med 1982;10:100-102.

110. Galway HR, MacIntosh DL: The lateral pivot shift: a symptom and sign of anterior cruciate ligament insufficiency. Clin Orthop 1980;147:45-50.

111. Losee RE: Concepts of the pivot shift. Clin Orthop 1983;172:45-51.

112. Noyes FR, Grood ES, Butler DL, Malek M: Clinical tests and functional stability of the knee: biomechanical concepts. Clin Orthop 1980;146:84-89.

113. Katz JW, Fingeroth RJ: The diagnostic accuracy of ruptures of the ACL comparing the Lachman test, the anterior drawer sign, and the pivot shift test in acute and chronic knee injuries. Am J Sports Med 1986;14(1):88-91.

114. Daniel DM, Malcolm LL, Losse G, et al: Instrumented measurement of anterior laxity of the knee. J Bone Joint Surg [Am] 1985;67:720-726.

115. Markoff KL, Amstutz HA: The clinical relevance of instrumented testing for ACL insufficiency: experience with UCLA clinical knee testing apparatus. Clin Orthop 1987;223:198-207.

116. Oliver JH, Coughlin LP: Objective knee evaluation using the Genucom knee analysis system: clinical implications. Am J Sports Med 1987;15:571-578.

117. Sherman MF, Bonamo JR: Primary repair of the anterior cruciate ligament. Clin Sports Med 1988;7:739-750.

118. Woods GW, Stanley RF, Tullos HS: Lateral capsular sign: x-ray clue to a significant knee instability. Am J Sports Med 1979;7:27-33.

119. Pavlov H, Warren RF, Sherman MF, Cayea PD: The accuracy of double contrast arthrographic evaluation of the anterior cruciate ligament. J Bone Joint Surg [Am] 1983;165:175-183.

120. Pavlov H: The radiographic diagnosis of the anterior cruciate ligament deficient knee. Clin Orthop 1983;172:57-64.

121. Wang JB, Marshall JL: Acute ligamentous injuries of the knee: single contrast arthrography — a diagnostic aid. J Trauma 1975;15:40-43.

122. Tongue JR, Larson RL: Limited arthrography in acute knee injuries. Am J Sports Med 1980;8:19-23.

123. Noyes FR, Bassett RW, Grood ES, Butler DL: Arthroscopy in acute traumatic hemarthrosis of the knee. J Bone Joint Surg [Am] 1980;62:687-695.

124. DeHaven KE: Arthroscopy in the diagnosis and management of the anterior cruciate ligament deficient knee. Clin Orthop 1983;172:52-56.

125. Gillquist J, Hagberg G, Oretorp N: Arthroscopy in acute injuries of the knee joint. Acta Orthop Scand 1977;48:190-196.

126. Lee JK, Yao L, Phelps CT, et al: Anterior cruciate ligament tears: MR imaging compared with arthroscopy and clinical tests. Radiology 1988;166:861-864.

127. Cerabona F, Sherman MF, Bonamo JR, Sklar J: Patterns of meniscal injury with acute anterior cruciate ligament tears. Am J Sports Med 1988;16:603-609.

128. Indelicato PA, Bittar ES: A perspective of lesions associated with ACL insufficiency of the knee. Clin Orthop 1985;198:77-80.

129. Levy M, Torzilli PA, Warren RF: The effect of medial menisectomy on anterior-posterior motion of the knee. J Bone Joint Surg [Am] 1982;64:883-888.

130. Patterson FW, Trickey EL: Menisectomy for tears of the meniscus combined with rupture of the anterior cruciate ligament. J Bone Joint Surg [Br] 1983;65:388-390.

131. Shoemaker SC, Markolf KL: The role of the meniscus in the anterior-posterior stability of the loaded anterior cruciate deficient knee. J Bone Joint Surg [Am] 1986;68:71-79.

132. Ferkel RD, Markolf K, Goodfellow D, et al: Treatment of the anterior cruciate ligament — absent knee with associated meniscal tears. Instrumented testing and clinical evaluation of two patient groups. Clin Orthop 1987;222:239-248.

133. Losse CM, Daniel DM, Malcolm LL, Burkes RT: The effect of meniscus surgery on anterior laxity of the knee. Orthop Trans 1983;7:280 (abstract).

134. Warren RF, Levy M: Meniscal lesions associated with anterior cruciate ligament injury. Clin Orthop 1988;172:32-37.

135. Satku K, Kumar VP, Ngoi SS: Anterior cruciate ligament injuries: to counsel or to operate? J Bone Joint Surg [Br] 1986;68:458-461.

136. Sandberg R, Balkfors B: Partial rupture of the anterior cruciate ligament. Clin Orthop 1987;220:176-178.

137. McDaniel WJ: Isolated partial tear of the anterior cruciate ligament. Clin Orthop 1976;115:209-212.

138. Kieffer DA, Curnow RJ, Southwell RB, et al: Anterior cruciate ligament arthroplasty. Am J Sports Med 1987;12:301-311.

139. Houseworth SW, Mauro VJ, Mellon BA, Kieffer DA: The intercondylar notch in acute tears of the anterior cruciate ligament: a computer graphics study. Am J Sports Med 1987;15(3):221-224.

140. Mink JH, Deutsch AL: Occult cartilage and bone injuries of the knee: detection, classification and assessment with MR imaging. Radiology 1989;170:823-829.

141. Hartzman S, Reicher MA, Bassett LW, et al: MR imaging of the knee. II. Chronic disorders. Radiology 1987;162:553-557.

142. Yao L, Lee JK: Occult interosseous fractures: detection with MR imaging. Radiology 1988;167:749-751.

143. Crues JV III, Ryu R: MRI of the knee. II. Surg Rounds Orthop 1989;3:27-33.

144. Hughston JC, Dagenhardt TC: Reconstruction of the posterior cruciate ligament. Clin Orthop 1982;164:59-77.

145. Hughston JC, Bowden JA, Andrews JR, et al: Acute tears of the posterior cruciate ligament: results of operative treatment. J Bone Joint Surg [Am] 1980;62:438-450.

146. Loos WC, Fox JM, Blazina ME, et al: Acute posterior cruciate ligament injuries. Am J Sports Med 1981;9(2):86-92.

147. Torisu T: Isolated avulsion fractures of the tibial attachment of the posterior cruciate ligament. J Bone Joint Surg [Am] 1977;59:68-72.

148. Clancy WG Jr, Shelbourne KD, Zoellner GB, et al: Treatment of knee joint instability secondary to rupture of the posterior cruciate ligament. J Bone Joint Surg [Am] 1983;65:310-322.

149. Barton TM, Torg JS, Das M: Posterior cruciate insufficiency: a review of the literature. Sports Med 1984;1:419-430.

150. Fowler PJ, Messieh SS: Isolated posterior cruciate ligament injuries in athletes. Am J Sports Med 1987;15(6):553-557.

151. Torg JS, Barton TM, Pavlov H, Stine R: Natural history of the posterior cruciate ligament–deficient knee. Clin Orthop 1989;246:208-216.

152. Parolie JM, Bergfeld JA: Long-term results of nonoperative treatment of isolated posterior cruciate ligament injuries in the athlete. Am J Sports Med 1986;14(1):35-38.

153. Cross MJ, Powell JF: Long-term follow-up of posterior cruciate ligament rupture: a study of 116 cases. Am J Sports Med 1984;12(4):292-297.

154. Cain TE, Schwab GH: Performance of an athlete with straight posterior knee instability. Am J Sports Med 1981;9(4):203-208.

155. Dandy DJ, Pusey RJ: The long-term results of unrepaired tears of the posterior cruciate ligament. J Bone Joint Surg [Br] 1982;64:92-94.

156. Ellsasser JC, Reynolds FC, Omohundro JR: The non-operative treatment of collateral ligament injuries of the knee in professional football players: an analysis of 74 injuries treated non-operatively and 24 injuries treated surgically. J Bone Joint Surg [Am] 1974;56:1185-1190.

157. Fetto JF, Marshall JL: Medial collateral ligament injuries of the knee: a rationale for treatment. Clin Orthop 1978;132:206-218.

158. Indelicato PA: Non-operative treatment of complete tears of the medial collateral ligament of the knee. J Bone Joint Surg [Am] 1983;65:323-329.

159. Jones RE, Henley MB, Francis P: Non-operative management of isolated grade III collateral ligament injuries in high school football players. Clin Orthop 1986;213:137-140.

160. Sandberg R, Balkfors, Nilsson B, Westlin N: Operative vs. non-operative treatment of recent injuries to the ligaments of the knee. J Bone Joint Surg [Am] 1987;69:1120-1126.

161. DeLee JC, Riley MB, Rockwood CA Jr: Acute straight lateral instability of the knee. Am J Sports Med 1983;11(6):404-410.

162. Grana WA, Janssen T: Lateral ligament injury of the knee. Orthopedics 1987;110:1039-1044.

163. Hughston JC, Andrews JR, Cross MJ, Moschi A: Classification of knee ligament instabilities. II. The lateral compartment. J Bone Joint Surg [Am] 1976;58:173-179.

164. Towne LC, Balzina ME, Marmor L, Lawrence JF: Lateral compartment syndrome of the knee. Clin Orthop 1971;76:160-168.

165. DeLee JC, Riley MB, Rockwood CA Jr: Acute posterolateral rotatory instability of the knee. Am J Sports Med 1983;11(4):199-207.

166. Horns JW: The diagnosis of chondromalacia by double contrast arthrography of the knee. J Bone Joint Surg [Am] 1977;59:119-120.

167. Ficat RP, Phillippe J: Contrast arthrography of the synovial joints. New York, Masson, 1981.

168. Ihara H: Double-contrast CT arthrography of the cartilage of the patellofemoral joint. Clin Orthop 1985;198:50-55.

169. Boven F, Bellemans MA, Geurts J, et al: The value of computed tomography scanning in chondromalacia patellae. Skeletal Radiol 1982;8:183-185.

170. Boven F, Bellemans MA, Geurts J, Potvliege R: A comparative study of the patello-femoral joint on axial roentgenogram, axial arthrogram, and computed tomography following arthrography. Skeletal Radiol 1982;8:179-181.

171. Sartoris DJ, Kursunoghi S, Pineda C, et al: Detection of intra-articular osteochondral bodies in the knee using computed arthrotomography. Radiology 1985;154:175-177.

172. Dye SF, Boll DA: Radionuclide imaging of the patellofemoral joint in young adults with anterior knee pain. Orthop Clin North Am 1986;17:249-262.

173. Collier DB, Johnson RO, Carrera GF: Chronic knee pain assessed by SPECT: comparison with other modalities. Radiology 1985;157:795-802.

174. Kerohan WG, Beverland DE, McCoy GF, et al: The diagnostic potential of vibration arthrography. Clin Orthop 1986;210:106-112.

175. Devereaux MD: Thermographic diagnosis in athletes with patello-femoral arthralgia. J Bone Joint Surg [Br] 1986;68:42-44.

176. Jackson RW: The role of arthroscopy in the management of the arthritic knee. Clin Orthop 1974;101:28-35.

177. Leslie IJ, Bentley G: Arthroscopy in the diagnosis of chondromalacia patellae. Ann Rheum Dis 1978;37:540-547.

178. Dandy DJ: Arthroscopy in the treatment of young patients with anterior knee pain. Orthop Clin North Am 1986;17:221-229.

179. Buckwalter K, Braunstein EM, Wilson MR, et al: Evaluation of hyaline cartilage of the knee with MR imaging. Radiology 1986;161(P):239.

180. Wojtys E, Wilson M, Buckwalter K, et al: MRI of knee hyaline cartilage and intraarticular pathology. Am J Sports Med 1987;15:455-463.

181. Yulish BS, Montanez J, Goodfellow DB, et al: Chondromalacia patellae: assessment with MRI imaging. Radiology 1987;164:763-766.

182. Gylys-Morin VM, Hajek PC, Sartoris DJ, Resnick D: Articular cartilage defects: detectability in cadaver knees with MR. AJR 1987;148:1153-1157.

183. Barronian AD, Zoltan JD, Bucon KA: Magnetic resonance imaging of the knee: correlation with arthroscopy. Arthroscopy 1989;5(3):187-191.

184. Hajek PC, Baker LL, Sartoris DJ, et al: MR arthrography: anatomic pathology investigation. Radiology 1987;163:141-147.

185. Mesgarzadeh M, Sapega AA, Bonakdarpour C, et al: Osteochondritis dissecans: analysis of mechanical stability with radiography, scintigraphy, and MR imaging. Radiology 1987;165:775-780.

186. Stafford SA, Rosenthal DI, Gebhardt MC, et al: MRI in stress fracture. AJR 1986;147:553-556.

187. Engber WD: Stress fractures of the medial tibial plateau. J Bone Joint Surg [Am] 1977;59:767-769.

188. Lee JK, Yao L: Stress fractures: MR imaging. Radiology 1988;169:217-220.

189. Lynch TC, Crues JV III, Sheehan W, et al: Stress fractures of the knee: MRI evaluation. Magn Reson Imaging (abstract). 1988;6:10.

190. Pollack MS, Dalinka MK, Kressel HY, et al: Magnetic resonance imaging in the evaluation of suspected osteonecrosis of the knee. Skeletal Radiol 1987;16:121-127.

191. Dalinka MK, Kricun ME, Zlatkin MB, Hubbard CA: Modern diagnostic imaging in joint disease. AJR 1989;152:229-240.

192. Burk DL Jr, Dalinka MK, Schiebler ML, et al: Strategies for

musculoskeletal magnetic resonance imaging. Radiol Clin North Am 1988;26:653-672.

193. Schwimmer M, Edelstein G, Heiken JC, Gilula LA: Synovial cysts of the knee: CT evaluation. Radiology 1985;154:175-177.

194. Lee KR, Cox GG, Neff JR, et al: Cystic masses of the knee: arthrographic and CT evaluation. AJR 1987;148:329-334.

195. Hall FM, Jaffe N: CT imaging of the anserine bursa. AJR 1988;150:1107-1108.

196. Lee KR, Tines SC, Price HI, et al: The computed tomographic findings of popliteal cysts. Skeletal Radiol 1983;10:26-29.

197. Burk DL Jr, Dalinka MK, Kanal E, et al: Meniscal and ganglion cysts of the knee: MR evaluation. AJR 1988;160:331-336.

198. Wolfe RD, Colloff B: Popliteal cysts: an arthrographic study and review of the literature. J Bone Joint Surg [Am] 1972;54:1057-1063.

199. Mandelbaum BR, Grant TT, Hartzman S, et al: The use of MRI to assist in diagnosis of pigmented villonodular synovitis of the knee joint. Clin Orthop 1988;231:135-139.

200. Weisz GM, Gal A, Kitchener PN: Magnetic resonance imaging in the diagnosis of aggressive villonodular synovitis. Clin Orthop 1988;236:303-306.

201. Wilson DA, Prince JR: MR imaging of hemophilic pseudotumors: case report. AJR 1988;150:349-350.

202. Spitzer CE, Dalinka MK, Kressel HY: Magnetic resonance imaging of pigmented villonodular synovitis: report of two cases. Skeletal Radiol 1987;16:316-319.

203. Kottal RA, Vogler JB, Malamorer A: Pigmented villonodular synovitis: a report of magnetic resonance imaging in two cases. Radiology 1987;163:551-553.

204. Jelinek JS, Kransdorf MJ, Utz JA, et al: Imaging of pigmented villonodular synovitis with emphasis on MR imaging. AJR 1989;152:337-342.

205. Yulish BS, Lieberman JM, Strandjord SE, et al: Hemophilic arthropathy: assessment with MR imaging. Radiology 1987;164:759-762.

206. Sundaram M, McGuire MH, Fletcher J, et al: Magnetic resonance imaging of lesions of synovial origin. Skeletal Radiol 1986;15:110-116.

207. Patel D: Arthroscopy of the replica synovial folds and their significance. Am J Sports Med 1978;6:217-225.

208. Patel D: Plica as a cause of anterior knee pain. Orthop Clin North Am 1986;17:273-277.

209. Insall J, Goldberg V, Salvati E: Recurrent dislocation and the high-riding patella. Clin Orthop 1972;88:67-69.

210. Insall J, Salvati E: Patella position in the normal knee joint. Radiology 1971;101:101-104.

211. Labelle H, Laurin CA: Radiological investigation of normal and abnormal patellae. J Bone Joint Surg [Br] 1976;57:530 (abstract).

212. Carson WG, James SL, Larson RL, et al: Patello-femoral disorders: physical and radiographic evaluation. II. Radiographic examination. Clin Orthop 1981;185:178-186.

213. Laurin CA, Dussault R, Lévesque HP: The tangential x-ray investigation of the patellofemoral joint: x-ray technique, diagnostic criteria and their interpretation. Clin Orthop 1979;144:16-26.

214. Merchant AC, Mercer RL, Jacobsen RH, Coal CR: Roentgenographic analysis of patellofemoral congruence. J Bone Joint Surg [Am] 1974;56:1391-1396.

215. Hughston JC: Subluxation of the patella. J Bone Joint Surg [Am] 1968;50:1003-1026.

216. Wiberg G: Roentgenographic and anatomic studies on femorapatellar joint, with special reference to chondromalacia patellae. Acta Orthop Scand 1941;12:319-410.

217. Cross MJ, Waldrop J: The patella index as a guide to the understanding and diagnosis of patellofemoral instability. Clin Orthop 1975;110:174-176.

218. Laurin CA, Lévesque HP, Dussault R, et al: The abnormal lateral patellofemoral angle: a diagnostic roentgenographic sign of recurrent patellar subluxation. J Bone Joint Surg [Am] 1978;60:55-60.

219. Martinez S, Korobkin M, Fondren FB, et al: Diagnosis of patellofemoral malalignment by computed tomography. J Comput Assist Tomogr 1983;7:1050-1053.

220. Delgado-Martins H: A study of the position of the patella using computerized tomography. J Bone Joint Surg [Br] 1979;61:443-444.

221. Schutzer SF, Ramsby GR, Fulkerson JP: The evaluation of patellofemoral pain using computerized tomography: a preliminary study. Clin Orthop 1986;204:286-293.

222. Schutzer SF, Ramsby GR, Fulkerson JP: Computerized tomographic classification of patellofemoral joint pain patients. Orthop Clin North Am 1986;17:235-248.

223. Shellock FG, Mink JH, Fox JM: Patellofemoral joint: kinematic MR imaging to assess tracking abnormalities. Radiology 1988;168:551-553.

224. Farzaneh F, Riederer SJ, Lee JN, et al: MR fluoroscopy; initial clinical studies. Radiology 1989;171:545-549.

ABBREVIATIONS (PLATES 21-1 TO 21-5)

Muscle	**Abbreviation**
External obturator	EO
Gluteus maximus	GM
Gluteus medius	GMd
Gluteus minimus	Gm
Iliopsoas	IP
Inferior gemellus	IG
Internal obturator	IO
Levator ani	LA
Pectineus	P
Piriformis	Pi
Quadratus femoris	QF
Rectus abdominus	RA
Rectus femoris	Rf
Sartorius	S
Superior gemellus	SG
Tensor fasciae latae	TFL
Vastus lateralis	VL
Bone	
Acetabulum	Ac
Acetabulum, anterior	AcA
Acetabulum, posterior	AcP
Anterior inferior iliac spine	Ais
Coccyx	C
Femur	F
Femoral head	FH
Femoral neck	FN
Greater trochanter	GT
Ilium	I
Ischial tuberosity	IT
Pubis	P
Viscera	
Bladder	B
Prostate	Pr
Rectum	R
Uterus	U
Nerve	
Sciatic	Sc

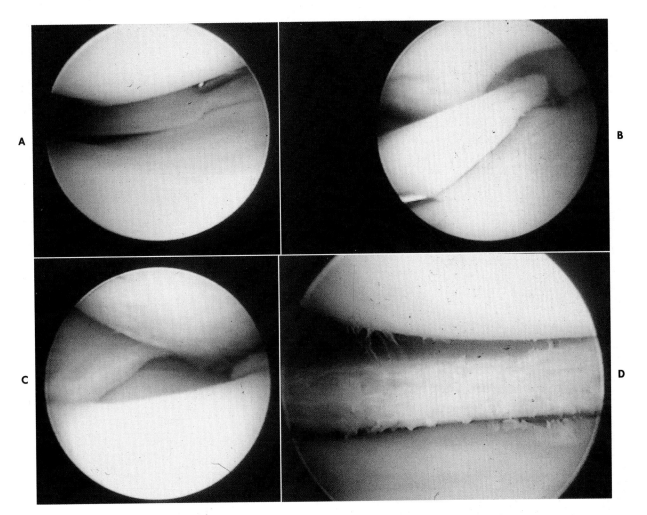

PLATE 21-1

A, Routine view of the posterior horn of the medial meniscus in a stable knee utilizing 30-degree arthroscope, thigh holder, and valgus stress in approximately 20 degrees of flexion. **B,** Centrally displaced fragment of a chronic bucket handle tear of the medial meniscus. On MRI the fragment may be missed with sagittal views alone. **C,** Centrally displaced fragment in the foreground with a peripheral intact rim of the bucket handle tear behind it. If the rim is also devoid of abnormal signal on MRI, the diagnosis may be missed. **D,** Remnant meniscal rim following partial medial meniscectomy. Irregular edges at the site of resection or degenerative changes (as indicated by *pink areas*) extending toward the perimeter could be misinterpreted on MRI as a persistent or secondary tear.

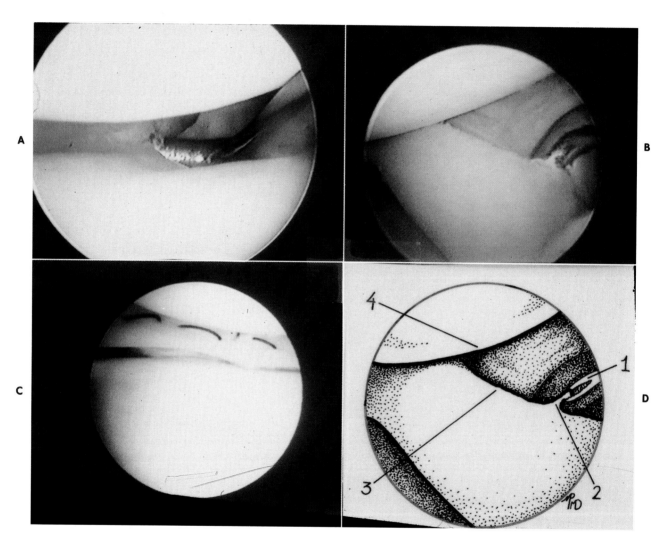

PLATE 21-2

A, Relatively small peripheral detachment of the medial meniscus at the meniscosynovial junction. The probe points to the locally disrupted capsular attachment, with the tear extending posteriorly from that site. B, Larger peripheral tear of the medial meniscus. The probe tip lies between the meniscus and the synovium, just anterior to the tear. C, Arthroscopically placed sutures, before fixation, during repair of the peripherally detached medial meniscus. D, Drawing of B. *1* is the probe; *2,* the crux of the tear; *3,* the meniscosynovial (meniscocapsular) junction; *4,* the oral condyle.

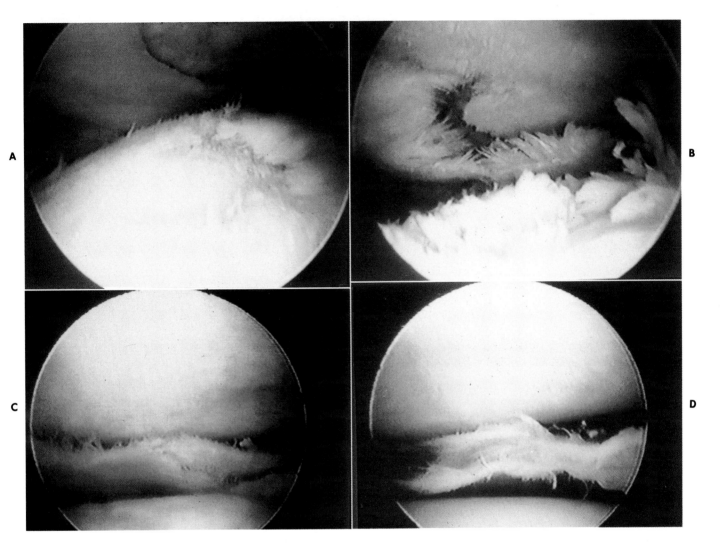

PLATE 21-3
A, Degenerative tear of the free edge of the posterior horn of the medial meniscus without associated degenerative articular cartilaginous changes. Good prognosis following partial meniscectomy.
B, Degenerative tear of the posterior horn of the medial meniscus with early Grade II articular cartilaginous changes involving particularly the femur. The short-term prognosis remains good.
C, Extensive degenerative tear of the medial meniscus with diffuse Grade III degenerative changes involving the femur and extensive Grade III and IV (bone exposed) changes of the tibial articular surface. Poor prognosis, despite partial meniscectomy and debridement. **D,** Significant Grade III and IV changes of the medial femoral and tibial articular surfaces with minimal visible changes in the meniscus.

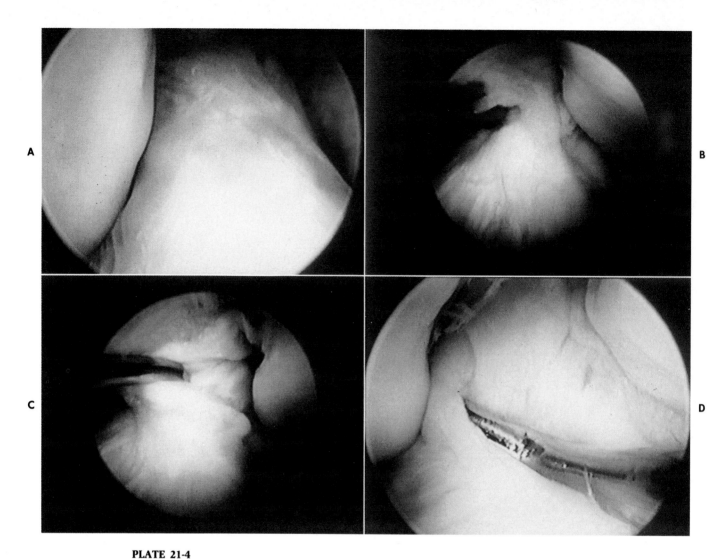

PLATE 21-4
A, ACL in continuity but with chronic induration, lack of a normal-appearing synovial sheath, and mild laxity on probing. Indicative of a chronic partial-thickness (Grade I) injury, which on MRI could be interpreted as normal. B, ACL in apparent gross continuity, interpreted as normal on MRI. However C, the probe indicates complete loss of functional integrity of the anteromedial band, with the posterolateral band remaining functionally intact. The nature and degree of injury (particularly in the chronic state) are often difficult to determine in such cases by MRI alone. D, ACL with gross continuity and an intact sheath. However, the probe indicates complete loss of functional integrity consistent with a Grade III interstitial tear, which may not be distinguishable on MRI from a partial-thickness injury.

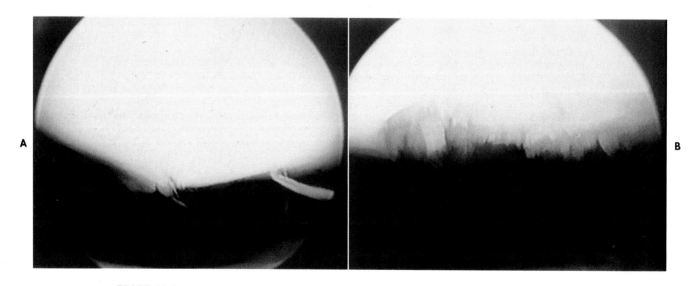

PLATE 21-5
A, Small focal area of chondromalacia patellae, difficult to identify on MRI even with special technique.
B, Diffuse Grade III (fragmentation) chondromalacia patellae, which may be undiagnosed by MRI unless axial views and special techniques are applied.

22 Ankle and Foot

CORNELIA N. GOLIMBU

ANATOMY OF THE ANKLE AND FOOT

The development of CT and MRI, radiological modalities that make possible multiplanar visualization of bones, ligaments, muscle, tendons, and fascial compartments, has rekindled the interest in the complex anatomy of the ankle and foot.[1-14] These structures are all interdependent in forming a spring mechanism that provides the weight-bearing support and mobility required for standing, walking, running, and jumping.

A review of pertinent anatomy as it applies to newer imaging modalities will be presented.

Bone structures

The ankle joint is formed by the tibia, fibula, and talus, arranged in a hingelike structure that permits dorsiflexion and plantarflexion but assures stability by restricting motion in the coronal and axial planes. The ankle mortise is represented by the horizontal surface of the tibia (tibial plafond), articulating with the convex surface of the dome of the talus, continued medially by the articulation of the talus with the medial malleolus. On the lateral side the talus articulates with the fibular malleolus. The tight fit of this joint is assured by the strong fibrous union between the distal tibia and fibula, the ankle syndesmosis, the interosseous membrane, and the anterior and posterior tibiofibular ligaments.[15,16] The mechanics of this joint are so perfect that the articular cartilage is well protected from the "wear and tear" seen in other joints that undergo degenerative change as the person ages. Indeed, primary osteoarthritis is rarely encountered in the ankle joint.

The subtalar joint separates the talus from the calcaneus. It is composed of three articulations formed by the posterior, middle, and anterior facets.

The posterior facet, the largest, supports most of the body of the talus on the convex surface of the calcaneus (Fig. 22-1). Anterior to this surface and separating it from the middle and anterior facets is the tarsal canal, which contains the strong interosseous ligament, blood vessels, and fat. This canal widens laterally to form the sinus tarsi.[14] The middle facet is formed by the sustentaculum tali, a shelflike projection on the medial side of the calcaneus, articulating with the medioinferior surface of the talus. The long axis of the talus is oriented 15 degrees medially to the long axis of the calcaneus. Consequently the sustentaculum tali and the entire middle subtalar joint have important functions in providing weight-bearing support to the medial side of the ankle. The anterior facet is the smallest; it may be independent of or contiguous with the middle facet, constituting with that facet a single articular surface in the shape of a racket, concave on the calcaneal side.

The anterior and middle facets of the subtalar joint form a functional and anatomical unit with the joint between the head of the talus and the navicular, with which they share a common synovial space, sometimes called the talocalcaneal navicular joint. Functionally these complex articulations create a type of ball-and-socket joint: the round head of the talus is surrounded by the concave surfaces of the navicular, the plantar calcaneonavicular (spring) ligament, the anterior fibers of the deltoid ligament, and the anterior and middle facets of the calcaneus — all forming an acetabulum-like surface.

Lateral and anterior to the os calcis is the cuboid, which in turn articulates with the base of metatarsals IV and V. The navicular articulates with the three cuneiforms, and these join metatarsals I through III. The metatarsal bases are thus interlocked in irregular zigzag-shaped joints with the tarsal bones. The metatarsal heads articulate with the proximal phalanges and continue further with the distal phalanx of the hallux or middle and distal phalanges of the other toes.

Ligaments

A complex system of ligaments provides support and stability to the ankle.

Deltoid ligament. One of the most important structures is the deltoid ligament (Fig. 22-2). It provides stability to the medial side of the ankle, completing the support offered by the short medial malleolus. The origin of the deltoid ligament is on the medial malleolus, and from here the deep fibers of the deltoid ligament fan out to their insertion on the medial surface of the talus. The superficial fibers form three distinct bundles — a vertical band inserts directly inferiorly on the sustentaculum tali (tibiocalcaneal ligament); and fibers obliquely oriented form the anterior and posterior parts, which take their name from their insertion (anterior is the *tibionavicular ligament;* posterior is the *tibiotalar ligament*). The inferior margin of the tibionavicular ligament blends with the fibers of the plantar calcaneonavicular ligament (spring ligament) (Fig. 22-2).

Spring ligament. The plantar calcaneonavicular ligament (also known as the spring ligament) is a strong fibrocartilaginous band providing support for the head of the talus (Fig. 22-2). It originates on the anterior and medial surface of the sustentaculum tali and inserts on the medial and plantar surfaces of the navicular. Its fibers are reinforced by the anterior division of the deltoid ligament.

Lateral ankle ligaments. The lateral aspect of the ankle is crossed by the ligaments originating on the fibular malleolus and inserting on the adjacent bone structures. They are, in order from anterior to posterior, the anterior talofibular ligament, the calcaneofibular ligament, and the posterior talofibular ligament (Fig. 22-3).

Syndesmosis ligaments. The tibia and fibula are connected by the anterior and posterior tibiofibular ligaments (Fig. 22-4). These horizontally oriented bands of fibrous tissue at the inferior margin of the syndesmosis provide

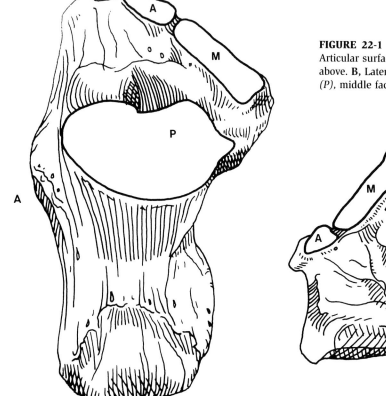

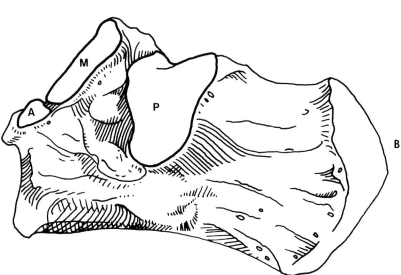

FIGURE 22-1
Articular surfaces of the calcaneus. **A,** Right calcaneus viewed from above. **B,** Lateral view. Posterior articular facet of the subtalar joint *(P),* middle facet *(M),* and anterior facet *(A).*

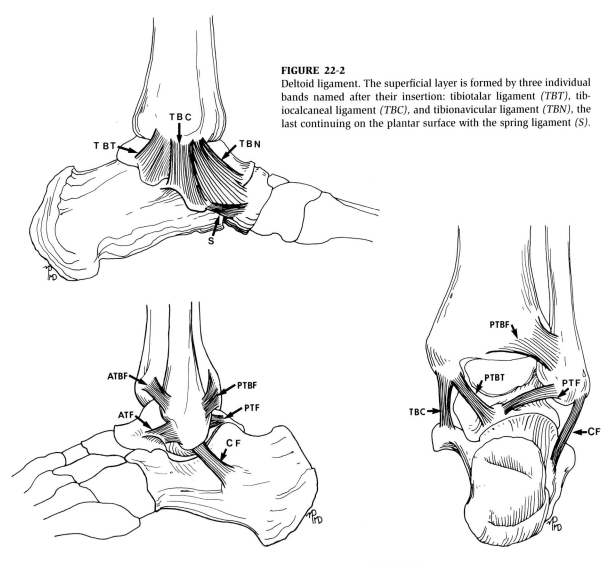

FIGURE 22-2
Deltoid ligament. The superficial layer is formed by three individual bands named after their insertion: tibiotalar ligament *(TBT)*, tibiocalcaneal ligament *(TBC)*, and tibionavicular ligament *(TBN)*, the last continuing on the plantar surface with the spring ligament *(S)*.

FIGURE 22-3
Ligaments on the lateral side of the ankle: anterior talofibular *(ATF)*, calcaneofibular *(CF)*, posterior talofibular *(PTF)*, anterior tibiofibular *(ATBF)*, and posterior tibiofibular *(PTBF)*.

FIGURE 22-4
Posterior view of the ankle ligaments: posterior tibiofibular *(PTBF)*, posterior talofibular *(PTF)*, calcaneofibular *(CF)*, posterior tibiotalar *(PTT)*, and tibiocalcaneal *(TBC)*.

stability to that joint. Another structure that binds the tibia and fibula together is the interosseous membrane.

Interosseous ligament. The interosseous ligament (also known as the talocalcaneal ligament) is the strongest band of fibrous tissue binding the talus to the calcaneus. It is obliquely oriented in the tarsal sinus, the funnellike space formed by the concave grooves that separate the posterior from the middle articular surfaces of the talus and calcaneus.

Tendons

Achilles tendon. In the superficial layer of the posterior ankle resides the most powerful tendon of the body, the tendo Achillis (calcaneus tendon). It has a vertical orientation from the fleshy part of the gastrocnemius and soleus down to the middle part of the posterior calcaneus. A small bursa is interposed between the anterior surface of the tendon and the superior margin of the calcaneus.

Another bursa is located between the skin and the posterior surface of the tendon near its calcaneal insertion.

Medial tendons. Crossing from the posterior to the medial side of the ankle are three tendons—posterior tibialis, flexor digitorum longus, and flexor hallucis longus (Fig. 22-5). In a shallow groove on the posterior surface of the medial malleous is the posterior tibialis tendon, and posterior to it is the flexor digitorum longus tendon (on which the posterior tibial artery and the tibial nerve lie). Lateral to the artery and nerve is the flexor hallucis longus tendon. As these structures bend around the tip of the medial malleolus, they course anteriorly superficial to the deltoid ligament. The posterior tibialis tendon fans out in multiple fascicles that insert on the plantar lateral aspect of the sustentaculum tali, the tubercle of the navicular, and the plantar surfaces of the first cuneiform and second, third, fourth, and occasionally fifth metatarsals.

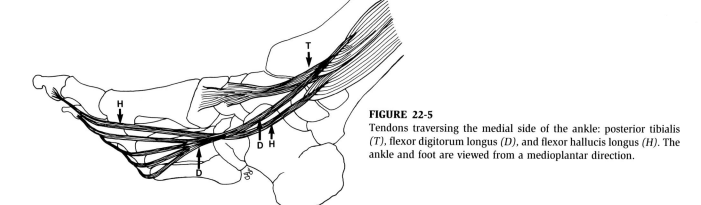

FIGURE 22-5
Tendons traversing the medial side of the ankle: posterior tibialis *(T)*, flexor digitorum longus *(D)*, and flexor hallucis longus *(H)*. The ankle and foot are viewed from a medioplantar direction.

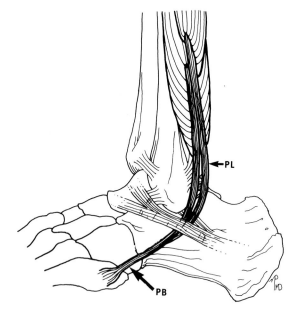

FIGURE 22-6
Tendons traversing the lateral side of the ankle: posterior to the lateral malleolus, the peroneus brevis *(PB)* and the peroneus longus *(PL)*, covered by a thin fibrous layer of retinaculum.

Lateral tendons. A similar configuration of tendons is encountered on the lateral side of the ankle — exactly behind the lateral malleolus is the peroneus brevis tendon, posterior to it is the peroneus longus tendon, and medial to these is the peroneal artery (Fig. 22-6). These structures cover the lateral collateral ligaments and course anteriorly to insert on the base of the fifth metatarsal (peroneus brevis) and plantar surface of the first tarsometatarsal joint (peroneus longus).

Anterior tendons. On the anterior surface of the ankle, beneath the thin layer of fibrous tissue forming the extensor retinaculum (ligamentum transversum cruris), from medial to lateral are the following tendons: tibialis anterior, extensor hallucis longus, and extensor digitorum longus. The anterior tibial artery and the deep peroneal nerve are located between the extensor hallucis longus and the most medial division of the extensor digitorum longus. The anterior tibial artery continues distally alongside the peroneal nerve as the dorsalis pedis artery, superficially located above the dorsal surfaces of the talus and navicular and the ligaments uniting the first and second cuneiforms.

Plantar structures. The plantar surface of the foot is arranged in successive layers — fasciae, muscles and tendons, ligaments, and the concave arch of the tarsal and metatarsals.[16,17]

The *plantar aponeurosis* is a flat band of fibrous tissue originating on the tubercle of the calcaneus; and from here thick central bundles stretch anteriorly and divide in the distal segment of the foot into five fascicles, one for each toe. At the base of the toes it inserts on the deep transverse metatarsal ligament and the base of the proximal phalanges. A function of the plantar aponeurosis is to preserve the arch of the foot by acting as a tie between the two pillars: the calcaneus and the metatarsophalangeal joints. The medial and lateral sides of the plantar aponeurosis are thinner and continue with the fascia in the dorsum of the foot. On the lateral side a reinforcement of the plantar aponeurosis forms the calcaneometatarsal ligament, which connects the lateral tubercle of the calcaneus with the base of the fifth metatarsal.

Deeper to the aponeurosis are intrinsic muscles of the foot, arranged in several layers — first and most superficial is the layer made up of the *abductor digiti quinti, flexor digitorum brevis,* and *abductor hallucis;* second is the layer containing the *quadratus plantae* and the *lumbricals* interspaced with divisions of the flexor digitorum longus tendon; third is the layer of the *flexor hallucis brevis, abductor hallucis,* and *flexor digiti quinti brevis;* fourth and deepest is the layer of the interossei.

Compartments. The anatomical structures of the foot are divided into three separate compartments; most often each is involved as a unit in infections or infiltrative neoplastic processes. The great toe and its metatarsal form the medial compartment; similarly the fifth toe and fifth metatarsal are the lateral compartment. The second through fourth toes and their corresponding metatarsals form the intermediate compartment, which continues through the flexor tendons and their sleeves toward the calf. This anatomical communication explains how an infection in the intermediate compartment of the foot can spread proximally toward the posterior leg muscles.

CT AND MRI TECHNIQUE OF THE ANKLE AND FOOT

The new imaging modalities, CT and MRI, are particularly useful in evaluating abnormalities of the ankle and foot. The most important advantage, offered especially by MRI, is the ability to image soft tissues as well as bones. When these structures are portrayed in multiplanar sections, great detail of the interlocking bone surfaces and complex ligaments, tendons, and other soft tissues is obtained.

CT is best at evaluating cortical bone and the calcification in soft tissue masses. MR has the added advantage of further discrimination between soft tissue structures such as muscle, tendon, cartilage, synovium, fat, blood vessels; and it can produce images in any plane.

Computed tomography

Both extremities are scanned at the same time, first, for ease of patient positioning and, second, for the added advantage of comparison with the normal side. To facilitate the comparison between normal and abnormal findings in each image, it is beneficial for both sides to be positioned exactly symmetrical.

Axial CT images are obtained when the lower extremities are extended supine and the foot is in anatomical position. The scanogram obtained at the beginning of the study in an anteroposterior or lateral direction helps to establish the correct positioning (Fig. 22-7).

Modified coronal CT images require tilt of the gantry and placement of the foot with the plantar surface down on the scanner table. The knees are bent in 90 degrees of flexion (Fig. 22-8). A lateral scanogram helps to establish the degree of tilt necessary for images perpendicular to the tibial plafond.

In young children undergoing CT scans, immobilization with wood boards and foot rests attached to canvas tennis shoes has been proposed.[18] However, similar results can be accomplished by taping the feet to a firm rectangular sponge; this arrangement is preferred because it permits direct inspection of the feet as the scanning proceeds and it alerts the technician to motion of the extremities, in which case collection of CT data should be temporarily interrupted.

A tilting extension attached to the scanner table has been used to facilitate positioning of the feet for coronal images.[19] In our experience such positioning devices are rarely needed; they only prolong unnecessarily the time required for setting up the scanner.

The best results are obtained when the scanning technique is tailored according to the pathology suspected: the distal tibiofibular syndesmosis, talar dome, and navicular and calcaneocuboidal joints are best seen on axial images (Figs. 22-9 to 22-14). The distal tibial articular surface, ankle mortise, subtalar joint, and plantar compartments of the foot are particularly well seen on coronal images (Figs. 22-15 to 22-18).

Most CT examinations of the ankle and foot consist of 5 mm thick contiguous sections. The choice of slice thickness depends again upon the pathology suspected: small cortical avulsion fractures or subtle erosions of bone may require 1.5 or 3 mm slices of a limited region.

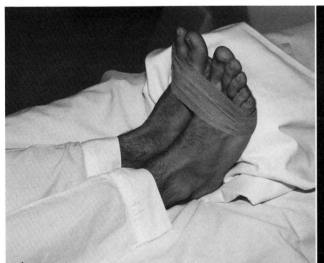
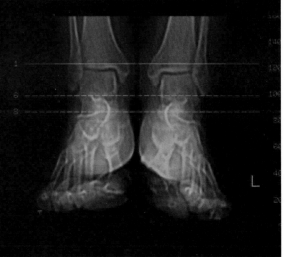

A   B

FIGURE 22-7
CT technique, axial views of the ankle. **A,** Position of the patient. **B,** Scanogram and orientation of the slices.

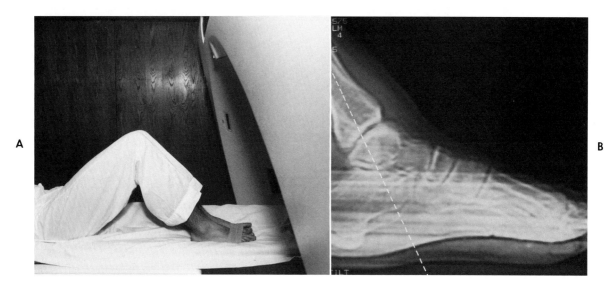

FIGURE 22-8
CT technique. Modified (tilted) coronal views. **A,** Position of the patient. **B,** Scanogram and orientation of the slices.

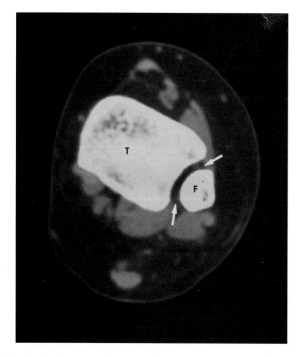

FIGURE 22-9
CT of tibiofibular syndesmosis. An axial CT image of the left ankle shows the tibia *(T)* and fibula *(F)* separated by the concave surface of the tibiofibular syndesmosis *(arrows)*.

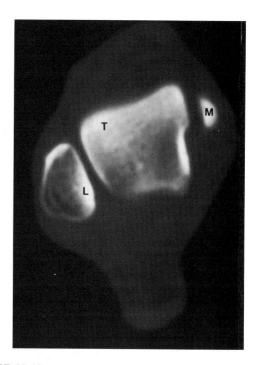

FIGURE 22-10
CT of the talar dome. Axial view of the talus. The surface of the dome is seen as a rectangular structure *(T)* between the medial malleolus *(M)* and the lateral malleolus *(L)*.

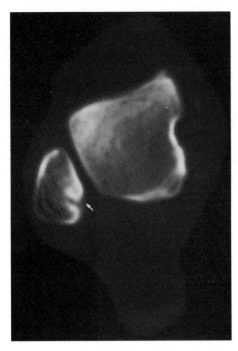

FIGURE 22-11
CT of the talus and lateral malleolus. The concave posterior surface of the fibula *(arrow)* is of normal appearance (peroneal groove). It provides stability to the peroneal tendons.

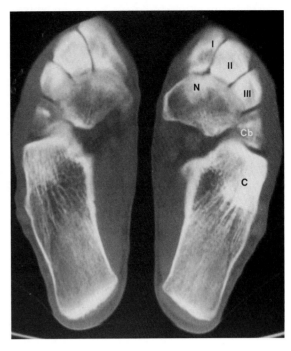

FIGURE 22-12
CT of the tarsal bones. An axial image of both feet shows the calcaneus *(C)*, cuboid *(Cb)*, navicular *(N)*, and the medial *(I)*, intermediate *(II)* and lateral *(III)* cuneiforms.

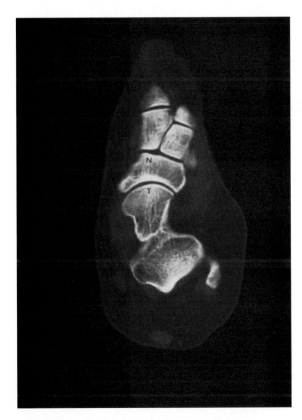

FIGURE 22-13
CT of the talonavicular joint. An axial CT image of the left foot shows the articulation between the talus *(T)* and navicular *(N)*.

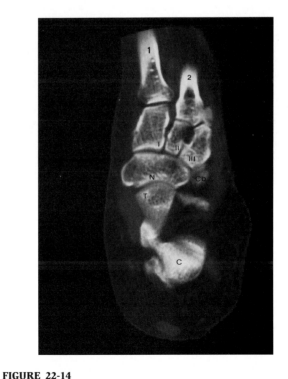

FIGURE 22-14
CT of the tarsometatarsal joints. An axial CT image of the foot shows the base of the first and second metatarsals *(1 and 2)* and their articulation with the medial *(I)*, intermediate *(II)*, and lateral *(III)* cuneiforms. The navicular *(N)* articulates with the cuneiforms and talus *(T)*. Only partial views of the calcaneus *(C)* and cuboid *(Cb)* are provided by this section.

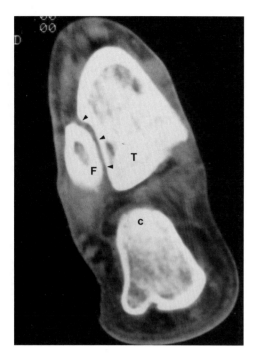

FIGURE 22-15
Coronal CT of the tibiofibular syndesmosis. Oblique coronal section through the syndesmosis *(arrowheads)*. Calcaneus *(C)*, tibia *(T)*, and fibula *(F)*.

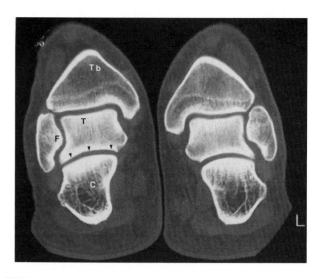

FIGURE 22-16
Coronal CT of the ankle mortise and posterior subtalar joint. The subtalar joint has a horizontal orientation *(arrowheads)*. Calcaneus *(C)*, talus *(T)*, fibula *(F)*, and tibia *(Tb)*.

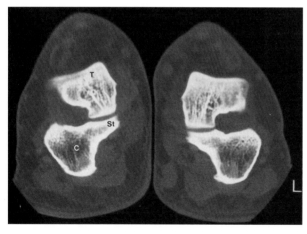

FIGURE 22-17
Coronal CT of the middle subtalar joint. The talus *(T)* articulates with the sustentaculum tali *(St)*, the medial articular process of the calcaneus *(C)*.

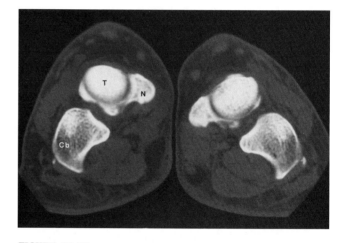

FIGURE 22-18
Coronal CT of the tarsal bones. The head of the talus *(T)* is seen as a round structure articulating with the navicular *(N)*. There is a normal space between the navicular and the cuboid *(Cb)*, which should not be misinterpreted as a dislocation. Only in occasional cases does one find a joint between the cuboid and navicular (normal variant).

When reformatted images or three-dimensional representations are needed for better understanding of the spatial orientation of structures, it is necessary to obtain contiguous 1.5 or 2 mm slices or 3 mm slices spaced at 2 mm intervals.

The radiation dose to the skin delivered by a CT examination of the foot consisting 5 mm thick slices (coronal and axial) is on the order of 3.4 rads (0.34 Gy); this is significantly less than with conventional tomography consisting of 20 slices, which delivers a dose of 18 rads (0.18 Gy).[20] This consideration, together with better density resolution (which permits simultaneous visualization of bone and soft tissues), represents a strong reason for replacing conventional tomography with CT.

Axial CT images can be easily obtained in patients who have a plaster cast on the lower extremities. For coronal images of the ankle and foot, flexion of the knee and tilt of the scanner gantry are necessary. Therefore coronal images are feasible only in patients whose cast begins below the knee.

Artifacts from metallic orthopedic fixation devices interfere to a certain degree with the resolution of adjacent soft tissue; however, in most of such cases the bone structures of the ankle and foot can be seen in sufficient detail.

Sagittal CT of the foot can be performed by positioning the patient in lateral decubitus, with the extremity to be studied at the end of the scanner table (Fig. 22-19). Inversion of the ankle and tilt of the plantar surface inferiorly make possible acquisition of primary CT images of the foot in the sagittal plane.[21] However, the difficulty of positioning limits the number of patients who can be scanned in this fashion. Thus this type of scanning is reserved for cases in which reformatted sagittal images, based on primary axially collected data, provide insufficient detail.

The most expeditious way to measure discrepancies of leg length is accomplished by using the anteroposterior CT scanogram (scout view). This is, in fact, a digital recording of a roentgenogram. Cursors are placed at the ends of each bone and its length is calculated by the computer and printed on the image (Fig. 22-20).

THREE-DIMENSIONAL RECONSTRUCTION

Three-dimensional representation of the bony structures of the ankle and foot helps in understanding the complex anatomy of the tarsals and metatarsals.[22-24] The data base is acquired by obtaining CT images that represent contiguous slices 1.5 or 3 mm thick. These are processed for either surface- or volume-rendering algorithms. Viewing the structures from different angles (lateral, medial, plantar, etc.) facilitates understanding their spatial orientation (Fig. 22-21). Thus displacement or angulation of fragments in complex comminuted fractures can be immediately perceived[25] (Fig. 22-22).

Two important scanning factors have major impact on the quality of the reconstructed images — slice thickness and immobilization of the patient. Although these might appear to be contradictory goals, the following should

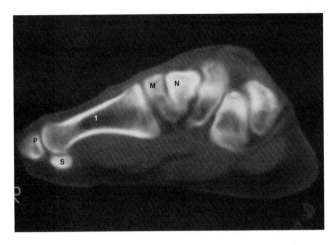

FIGURE 22-19
Direct sagittal CT image of the foot. The image obtained through the medial side portrays the longitudinal alignment of the proximal phalanx *(P)*, first metatarsal *(1)*, medial sesamoid *(S)*, medial cuneiform *(M)*, and navicular *(N)*.

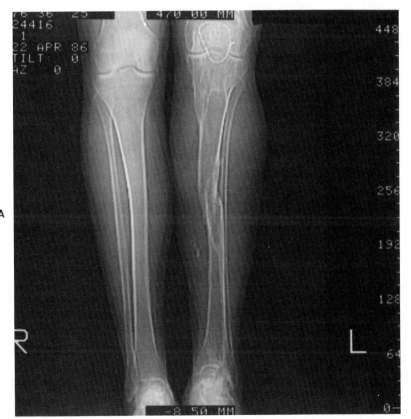

FIGURE 22-20
CT evaluation of length discrepancy in the lower extremities. **A,** An AP scanogram of both legs shows deformity of the left tibia secondary to an old displaced fracture. There is marked shortening of the left lower extremity.

Continued.

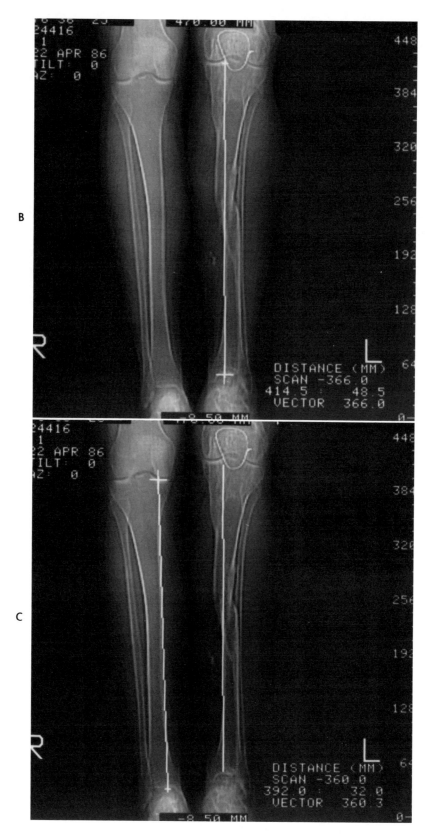

FIGURE 22-20 cont'd
B, Measurement of the length of the left tibia from the tibial plateau to the plafond, registered on the image as 366 mm. **C,** Measurement of the normal right side, registered as 360 mm. It becomes apparent that the shortening of the left leg is produced not only by the tibial deformity but also by a more proximal abnormality that has shortened the left femur.

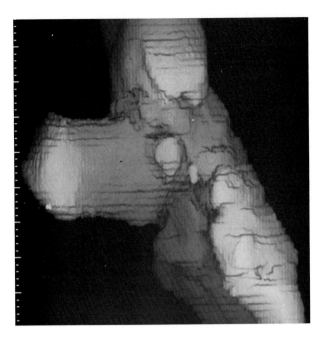

FIGURE 22-21
Tridimensional reconstruction of a normal ankle viewed from the medial side.

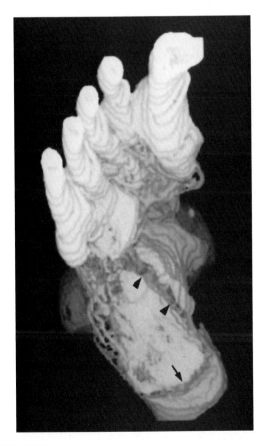

FIGURE 22-22
Tridimensional reconstruction of a fractured calcaneus viewed from the plantar surface. A sagittal fracture gap *(arrowheads)* is seen; the sustentaculum tali is medially displaced. Another fracture line is transversely oriented in the posterior part of the calcaneus *(arrow).* The lateral surface is comminuted and small displaced fragments give it the appearance of a sieve.

serve to explain: (1) the best rendering of structures is obtained with a slice thickness of 1.5 mm, (2) imaging a whole foot and ankle necessitates many thin slices, requiring a long scanning time, and (3) whenever the scanning time is long there is an increased probability that the patient will move during the examination (which obviously would distort reconstructed images). A practical compromise between the need to shorten the study and the need for informative images must be reached. In most cases this represents a sequence of adjacent 3 mm thick slices. Immobilization of the extremity is very important; any change in position from one slice to the next will distort the representation of spatial interrelationships.

Magnetic resonance

MR images of the ankle are usually obtained with the circular coil used for examinations of the head. This provides the advantage of comparison between the two sides. The feet can also be scanned in the head coil; however, occasionally a small field of view is necessary for detecting minimal abnormalities of the toes or metatarsals, in which case surface coils can be used. In such instances the most comfortable position for the patient is supine, with moderate flexion of the knees and plantar surfaces on the surface coil placed on the scanner table. If anatomical (neutral) position is preferred, a foot rest or other motion-restricting device can be used.

MRI examinations of both ankles and feet require a 20 cm field of view and a 256 × 256 matrix; this produces a pixel size of 0.78 × 0.78 mm. Reduction of matrix to 128 × 256 decreases the time of examination but diminishes the spatial resolution. Slice thickness may be 3 or 5 mm.

When the zone of pathology is small, the study is performed with extremity surface coils, which permit imaging of small fields of view (10 to 12 cm). The slice thickness is 3 or 5 mm; 1 mm thick slices are preferred for visualization of small ligaments.[26]

Most examinations of the ankle or foot can be completed in 30 minutes. They usually consist of coronal or sagittal T1-weighted images (TR 5 to 700 msec/ TE 2 to 30 msec) and axial T2-weighted and proton density images (TR 1800 to 2200 msec/ TE 30 and 80 msec) (Figs. 22-23 to 22-27). The proton density images provide a better definition of the anatomy and are used as a guide when interpreting the noisier T2-weighted images of the same slice (Fig. 22-28).

Gradient-recalled images (T2* weighted) are obtained with a TR 600 msec/ TE 20 msec and flip angle of 20 degrees (Fig. 22-29).

As everywhere else in the body, the general principle of portraying structures in orthogonal planes applies to the ankle and foot. Occasionally all three planes (coronal, sagittal, and axial) are used, for better definition of complex abnormalities.

To facilitate understanding MR images of the foot, we

refer to slice orientation as *perpendicular* to the plantar surface (coronal views) or *parallel* to the plantar surface (axial views). Such terminology simplifies the planning of scans and eliminates the need to specify the position of the foot (neutral, plantarflexed, or intermediary) (Fig. 22-30).

Three-dimensional representation of the data acquired by MR images helps in understanding the spatial arrangement of the complex anatomy of the ankle and foot.[27,28]

CONGENITAL ABNORMALITIES

With the advent of CT and MRI there has been a great increase in clinical and radiological interest in the diagnosis and treatment of congenital osseous abnormalities that affect the feet.

Tarsal coalition

Tarsal coalition represents fusion of one or more intertarsal joints; it results from failure of mesenchymal

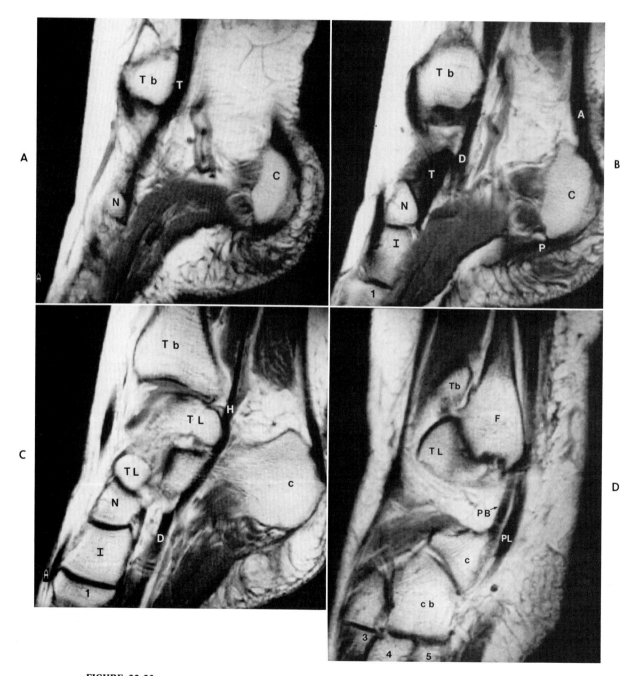

FIGURE 22-23
Sagittal T1-weighted MR images of the ankle. **A** to **C,** Adjacent sections in the medial side of the ankle. **D,** Section in the lateral side of the ankle. Osseous structures are the tibia *(Tb),* talus *(TL),* calcaneus *(C),* cuboid *(Cb),* navicular *(N),* medial cuneiform *(I),* metatarsals *(1 to 5).* Tendons are the extensor digitorum longus *(E),* tibialis posterior *(T),* flexor digitorum longus *(D),* flexor hallucis longus *(H),* peroneus brevis *(PB),* peroneus longus *(PL),* Achilles *(A),* and the plantar aponeurosis *(P).*

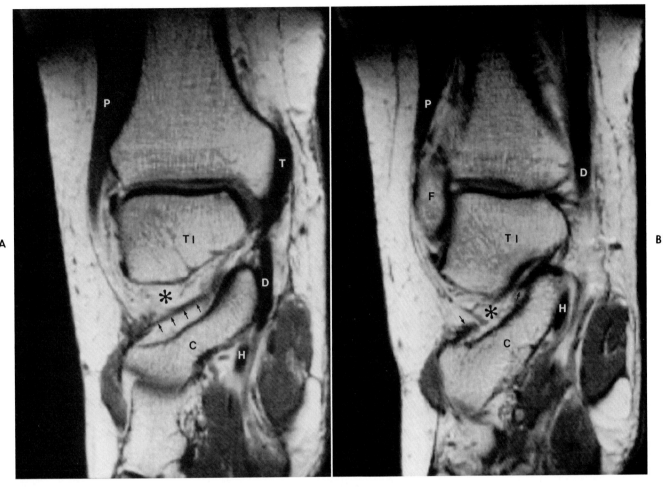

FIGURE 22-24
Coronal T1-weighted image of the ankle and foot. **A.** Tibiotalar joint and, **B,** tarsal sinus. Osseous structures are the talus *((Tl),* calcaneus *(C),* and fibula *(F).* The sinus tarsi *(asterisk)* is a triangular space open laterally between the talus and the calcaneus. It contains the interosseous ligament *(arrows)* and fat. Tendons are the tibialis posterior *(T),* flexor digitorum longus *(D),* and flexor hallucis longus *(H),* seen as they cross obliquely on the medial side. The peroneal muscles *(P)* are seen on the lateral side.

segmentation during embryonic development of the foot. Even though it is present since birth, tarsal coalition usually does not become symptomatic until age 10 to 12 years, when a combination of chondromalacia and traumatic arthritis and synovitis appears as a result of abnormal motion in the subtalar joint.[29]

Some congenital tarsal coalitions seem to be inherited as an autosomal dominant trait.[30] In the families of patients with a painful hindfoot secondary to tarsal coalition a number of asymptomatic persons can be found to have this abnormality.[31] It is therefore difficult to determine what its true frequency is in the general population, but the incidence has been estimated[32] at less than 1%.

Many types of tarsal coalition have been described[33,34]: talocalcaneal, calcaneonavicular, talonavicular, cuboidonavicular, and calcaneocuboidal (Figs. 22-31 and 22-32). Another form is massive intertarsal fusion present since birth, but this is rarely seen.

Routine roentgenograms disclose most tarsal coalitions; however, talocalcaneal fusions are seldom seen unless special views (posterior axial projection, also known as Harris view) or tomography are employed. The difficulty in diagnosing talocalcaneal fusion derives from the complexity of the normal anatomy of these two bones. The interlocking of convex-concave surfaces prevents tangential visualization of more than a limited part of the joint spaces in any given position. CT has the advantage of portraying these structures in detail, overcoming the problem of superimposed bone surfaces. It has been found to be superior to conventional roentgenography and tomography.[35,36]

In the past calcaneonavicular fusion was thought to be the most frequent type of tarsal coalition. This opinion derived from the fact that it is the one type of tarsal abnormality that is easily seen on conventional roentgenograms and is likely to be detected at routine examination of the foot.[29,32] The newer modalities of investigation (CT

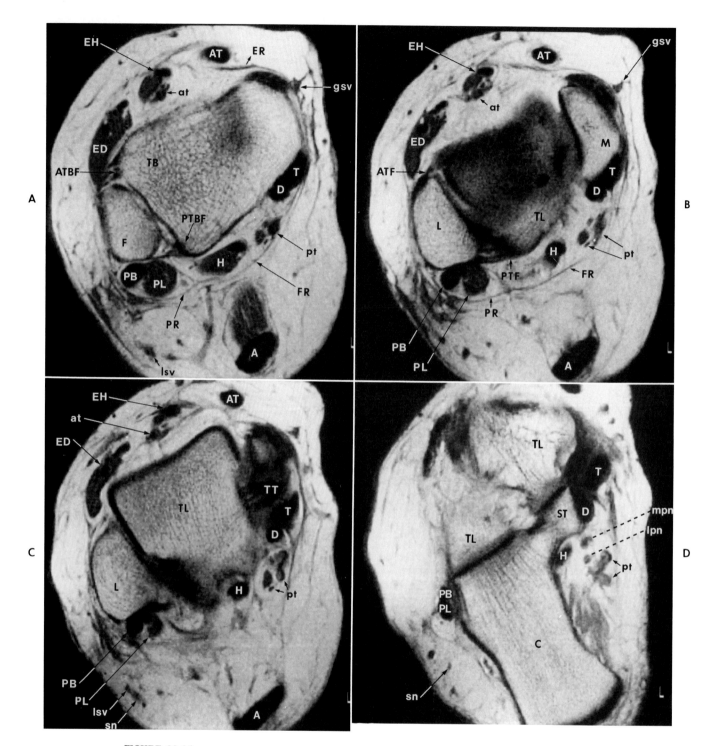

FIGURE 22-25
Axial MRI of the right ankle. Images are through, **A,** the syndesmosis, **B,** the tibiotalar joint, **C,** the dome of the talus, and, **D,** the calcaneus. Bone structures are the calcaneus *(C),* lateral malleolus *(L),* medial malleolus *(M),* tibia *(TB),* fibula *(F),* talus *(TL),* sustentaculum tali *(ST).* Ligaments are the anterior and posterior tibiofibular *(ATBF* and *PTBF),* anterior and posterior talofibular *(ATF* and *PTF),* tibiotalar *(TT),* also known as the deep layer of the deltoid ligament. Tendons are the posterior tibialis *(T),* flexor digitorum longus *(D),* flexor hallucis longus *(H),* peroneus brevis *(PB),* peroneus longus *(PL),* Achilles *(A),* anterior tibialis *(AT),* extensor hallucis longus *(EH),* and extensor digitorum longus *(ED).* Blood vessels and nerves are the anterior tibial artery *(at),* posterior tibial artery, vein, and nerve *(pt),* sural nerve *(s),* greater saphenous *(gsv)* and lesser saphenous *(lsv)* veins, and the medial *(mpn)* and lateral *(lpn)* plantar nerves. Also shown are the extensor retinaculum *(ER),* flexor retinaculum *(FR),* and peroneal retinaculum *(PR).*

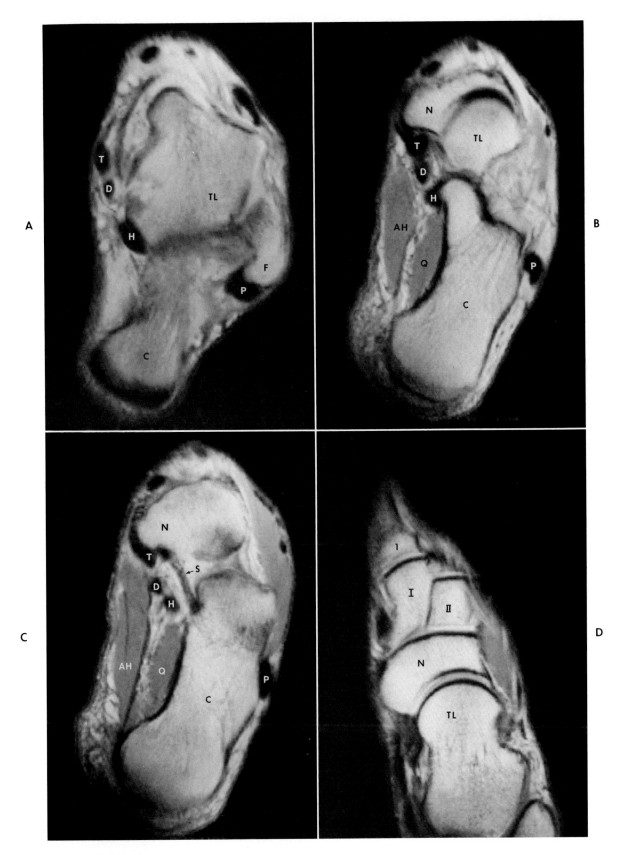

FIGURE 22-26
Axial MRI of the left foot. Sections are through, **A,** the talus, **B,** the calcaneus, **C,** the navicular, and, **D,** the cuneiforms. Bone structures are the calcaneus *(C)*, fibula *(F)*, talus *(TL)*, navicular *(N)*, medial cuneiform *(I)*, intermediate cuneiform *(II)*, first metatarsal *(1)*, and spring ligament *(S)*. Tendons are the tibialis posterior *(T)*, flexor digitorum longus *(D)*, flexor hallucis longus *(H)*, and peroneus brevis and longus *(P)*. Short muscles of the foot are the abductor hallucis *(AH)* and quadratus plantae *(Q)*.

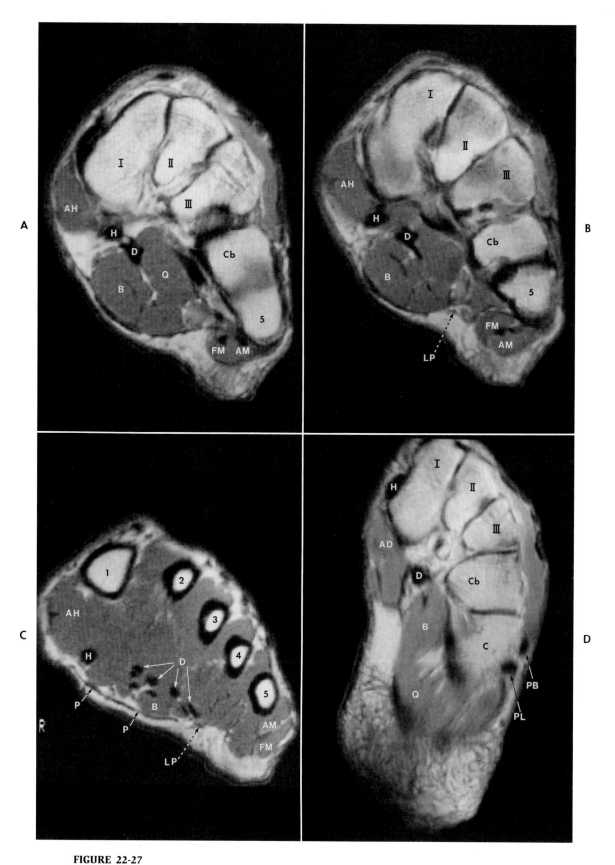

FIGURE 22-27

MRI of the left foot. **A** to **C,** Coronal and, **D,** axial images. Bone structures are the medial *(I),* intermediate *(II),* and lateral *(III)* cuneiforms, cuboid *(Cb),* metatarsals (1 to 5), and calcaneus *(C).* Tendons are flexor digitorum longus *(D),* flexor hallucis longus *(H),* peroneus brevis *(PB),* and peroneus longus *(PL).* Short muscles of the foot are the abductor hallucis *(AH),* flexor digitorum brevis *(B),* quadratus plantae *(Q),* abductor digiti minimi *(AM),* and flexor digiti minimi *(FM).* Also shown are the plantar fascia *(P)* and lateral plantar artery, vein, and nerve *(LP).*

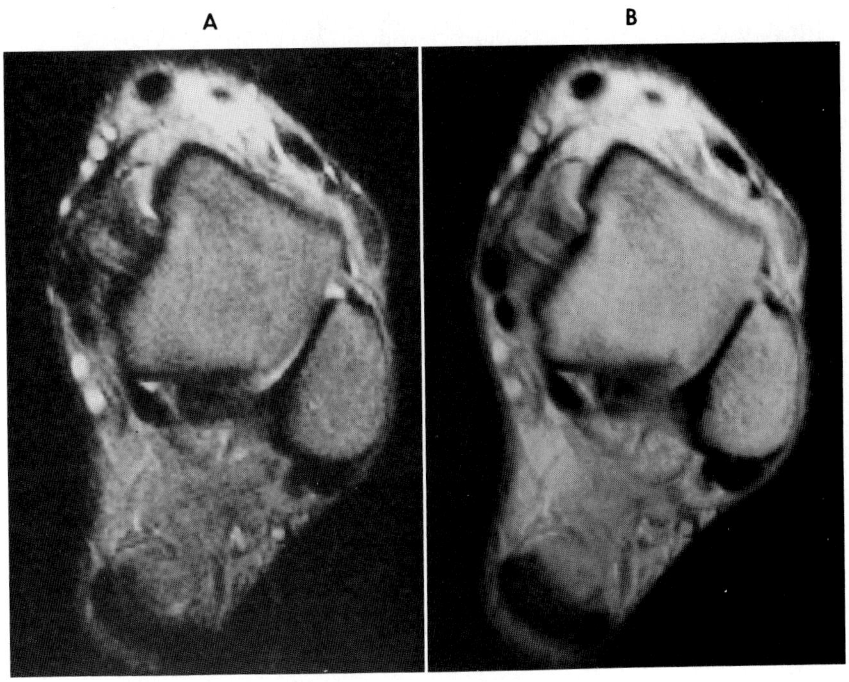

A   B

FIGURE 22-28
Axial image of the normal ankle. T2-weighted and proton density images of the same axial section. **A,** T2-weighted image (TR 2000 msec/TE 80 msec). Fluid in the joint and slow moving blood in superficial veins have high signal intensity. **B,** A proton density image (TR 2000 msec/TE 30 msec) shows better definition of the tendons.

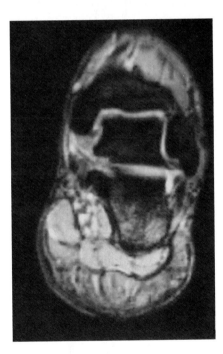

FIGURE 22-29
Gradient-recalled type of image (T2*) of the ankle (TR 600 msec/TE 20 msec, flip angle 20 degrees). The articular fluid has high signal, contrasting with the signal void of the articular cortex.

and MRI) have detected a large number of patients with tarsal coalition as having talocalcaneal fusion.[37-39] These modalities are also able to detect fibrocartilaginous or fibroosseous coalition, which were rarely diagnosed in the past and which may cause significant symptoms.

There are three varieties of talocalcaneal coalition: osseous, fibrocartilaginous, and fibroosseous.[40]

The *osseous* type is easiest to detect. On CT images it appears as a continuous band of bone with well-defined cortex uniting the medial margins of the talus and calcaneus. The medullary canal is seen in the center of the coalition segment, continuous with the medullary space of the talus and the calcaneus (Figs. 22-33 and 22-34).

Nonosseous coalitions of the subtalar joint are more difficult to detect. The *fibrocartilaginous* type is usually seen in children and is manifested as a segment of cartilage interposed between the osseous margins of the talus and calcaneus (Fig. 22-35). At the end of skeletal maturation this cartilaginous bar becomes osseous (Fig. 22-36). However, when first seen in children in its cartilaginous form, only subtle changes in the contour of the bone can be perceived as a sign of abnormality. Of all the tarsal coalitions, this specific variety of fibrocartilaginous union is the most difficult to detect, mainly because the cartilaginous element is not clearly visible on CT. Manifestations include hypoplasia or poor definition of the posterior margin of the sustentaculum tali and subtle irregularities in the articular surface of the middle facet of the subtalar joint. The *fibroosseous* type of coalition has a characteristic CT appearance. The segments of the articular margin that are united are usually hypertrophic and quite prominent on the medial side of the ankle. The margins of the bones united by fibroosseous coalition are irregular in contour. Very often these coalitions are discovered when bony sclerosis and marginal osteophytes are already present (Fig. 22-37).

The MRI appearance of talocalcaneal coalition is dependent upon the type of tissue that unites the two tarsal bones. In the osseous type a continuous bony bar

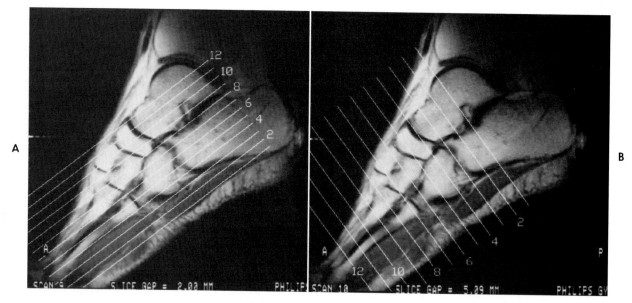

FIGURE 22-30
Technique of MRI of the foot. **A.** Slice orientation parallel to the plantar surface of the foot producing axial views. **B.** Slice orientation perpendicular to the plantar surface, producing coronal views.

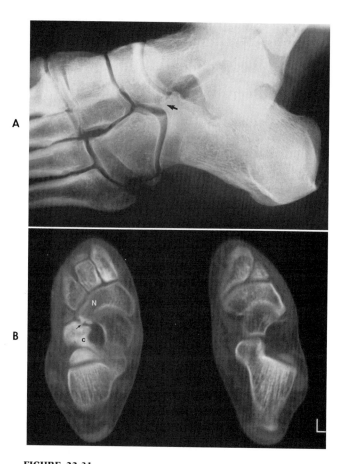

FIGURE 22-31
Calcaneonavicular osseous coalition. **A,** An oblique roentgenogram of the ankle demonstrates the coalition *(arrow).* **B,** An axial CT image of both feet demonstrates an osseous bar uniting the lateral margin of the navicular *(N)* with the distal part of the calcaneus *(C),* on the right side *(arrow).*

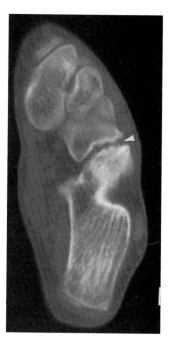

FIGURE 22-32
Fibroosseous calcaneocuboidal coalition. An axial CT image demonstrates the irregular margin of the calcaneus at the junction with the cuboid *(arrowhead).*

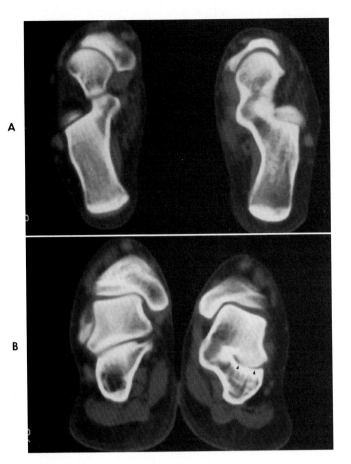

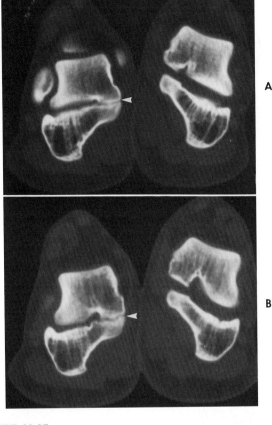

FIGURE 22-33
Osseous talocalcaneal coalition. **A,** An axial CT image of both ankles demonstrates an osseous bar uniting the medial side of the calcaneus with the talus, on the left. The medullary cavity of the coalition segment continues directly with that of the talus and calcaneus. A well-defined cortical margin is seen medially and laterally at this osseous segment. **B,** Coronal CT images of both ankles demonstrate the discrepancy between the normal right side and the osseous coalition on the left uniting the sustentaculum tali with the middle facet of the talus. The posterior facet of the calcaneus has an abnormal concave surface *(arrowheads)*.

FIGURE 22-35
Fibroosseous talocalcaneal coalition. **A,** Coronal CT image through the middle facet of the subtalar joint. The right ankle shows an abnormally narrow joint space between the sustentaculum tali and the medial facet of the talus, with an abnormal shape of these two segments of bone *(arrowhead).* **B,** A coronal image anterior to A demonstrates the characteristic zigzagging line of a fibroosseous coalition between the talus and calcaneus on the right side *(arrowhead).*

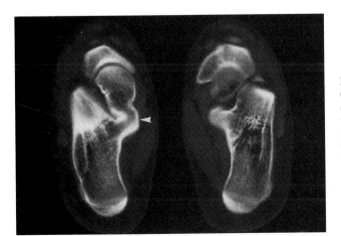

FIGURE 22-34
Osseous talocalcaneal coalition. An axial image of both ankles demonstrates an osseous bar uniting the medial side of the calcaneus with the talus on the right *(arrowhead).* The medullary cavity of the osseous segment of coalition continues in the medullary cavity of the talus and calcaneus. Cortical bone is seen extending from the talus through the bar and posteriorly in the calcaneus.

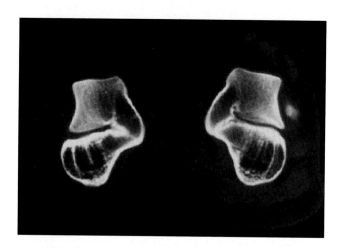

FIGURE 22-36
Bilateral talocalcaneal coalition. CT of the ankles in a 9-year-old girl with bilateral ankle pain. A coronal image of the subtalar joint shows the coalition: on the right osseous union, on the left a still visible line of separation (representing almost complete ossification of what might have been a fibrocartilaginous coalition).

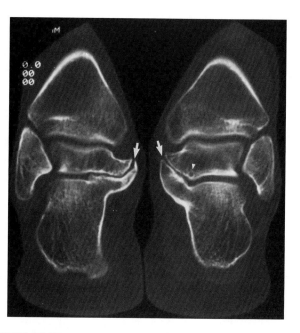

FIGURE 22-37
Bilateral fibroosseous talocalcaneal coalition. A coronal CT image shows the abnormal shape of the subtalar joint, beaklike projections protruding from the medial margin of the talus and calcaneus. Cystic erosion *(arrowhead)* and osteophytes *(arrow)* indicate that abnormal motion between these segments of bone has produced degenerative joint disease.

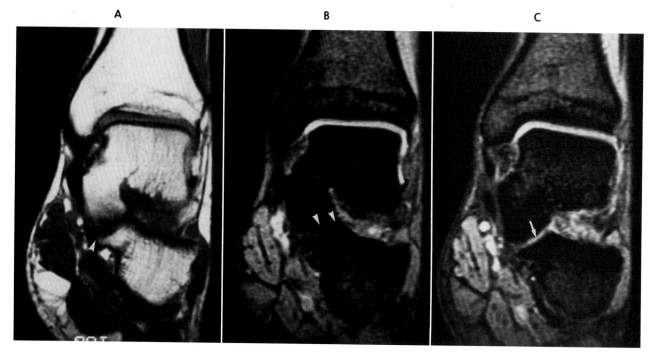

FIGURE 22-38
MRI of the talocalcaneal coalition. **A,** Coronal T1-weighted image. The sustentaculum tali is hypoplastic and has a slanted surface *(arrowheads)*. **B,** T2-weighted image, same location. Fibrocartilaginous coalition is seen as a low-signal band that obliterates the space between the sustenaculum tali and talus *(arrowheads)*. **C,** T2-weighted image anterior to **B.** The talus and sustentaculum are separated by a high-signal band *(arrow)* similar to the articular fluid in the mortise. This separation indicates that only the posterior part of the middle facet has the coalition. (A to C courtesy Dr. Ed Lubat.)

with bright signal in the medullary cavity is seen on the medial side of the talus and calcaneus. The fibrocartilaginous type must be detected by evaluating the shape of the middle facet of the subtalar joint. The fibrocartilaginous part that unites these two bone surfaces appears as an intermediate or low signal on T1-weighted and T2-weighted images and may be confused with the normal articular cortex. However, the sustentaculum is usually altered in shape, appearing hypoplastic, and its posterior border is ill-defined because it slopes gently into an oblique margin that is united by the cartilaginous bar

with the bone above (Figs. 22-38 and 22-39). The fibroosseous type of subtalar coalition is characterized by an irregular zigzagging margin of the bone surface and a band of low signal uniting the opposing articular margins. The low signal corresponds to the fibrous tissue (Fig. 22-40). The restriction of movement in the subtalar joint caused by the tarsal coalition produces an abnormal friction between articular surfaces and results in osteoarthritis. This is seen as erosions with a cystic appearance and large osteophytes formed mostly near the margin of the fibroosseous bar. The subchondral bony sclerosis,

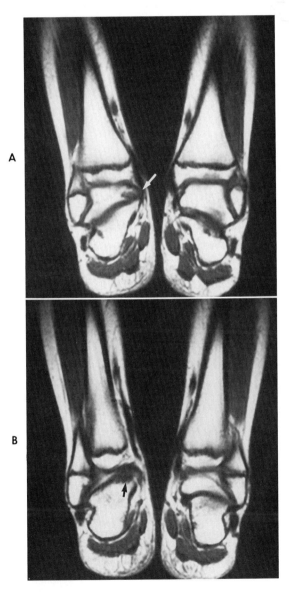

FIGURE 22-39
MRI of the fibrocartilaginous talocalcaneal coalition in an 11-year-old girl with right ankle pain. **A,** Coronal T1-weighted image of both ankles. There is abnormal tilt of the right subtalar joint surface with fibrocartilaginous union of the medial margin of the talus and calcaneus *(arrow)*. **B,** Image 8 mm posterior to **A.** The fibrocartilaginous union is attached to the posteromedial margin of the articular surface of the calcaneus *(arrow)*.

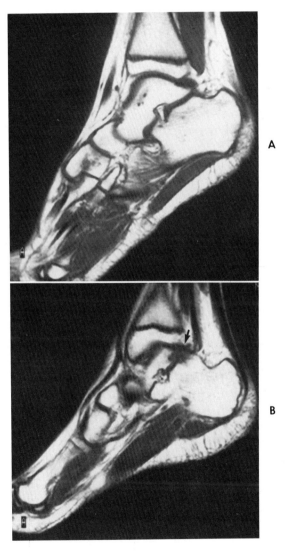

FIGURE 22-40
Fibrocartilaginous tarsal coalition, sagittal T1-weighted image of the patient in Fig. 22-39. **A,** Normal left ankle. **B,** Section through the medial side of the right ankle. A vertical slant of the posterior subtalar joint and a low-signal zone represent the coalition between talus and calcaneus *(arrow)*.

characteristic of the advanced stage of oseoarthritis, is seen on MR images as a low-signal zone. All these cortical abnormalities are better visualized on CT images than on MRI (Fig. 22-41).

One of the most important contributions that MRI has made in the evaluation of tarsal coalition is detection of abnormal position of the tendons on the medial side of the ankle. Specifically, in cases in which fusion of the calcaneus and talus has occurred posterior to the sustentaculum tali the flexor hallucis longus and occasionally flexor digitorum longus tendons are deviated posteriorly, coursing behind the synostosis. When the fibrous coalition reaches the stage of degenerative disease, with hypertrophic spur formation at its margin, it can entrap the posterior tibialis tendon between the margin of the tibia and the anterior border of the coalition (Fig. 22-42).

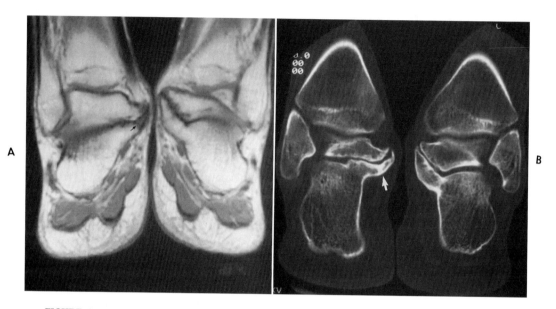

FIGURE 22-41
Fibroosseous talocalcaneal coalition. **A,** Coronal T1-weighted image. Bilateral prominences of the medial margin of the talus and calcaneus forming an upwardly oriented irregular joint surface. The bone marrow has focal zones of decreased signal intensity *(arrow)*. **B,** CT image at a level comparable to A. The osteophytic spurs *(arrow)*, cystic erosion, and reactive sclerosis at the site of the coalition are better defined in CT images than on MRI.

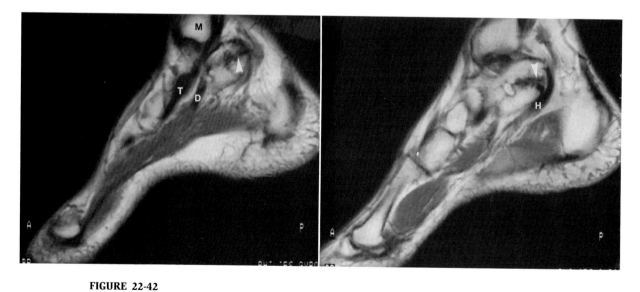

FIGURE 22-42
Tendon abnormalities associated with tarsal coalition, same patient as in Fig. 22-41. Adjacent sagittal T1-weighted images show the medial prominence of a fibroosseous coalition between the posterior margin of the talus and the calcaneus *(arrowhead)*. The posterior tibialis tendon *(T)* and flexor digitorum longus tendon *(D)* are trapped in the narrow space between the medial malleolus *(M)* and the coalition. The tendon of the flexor hallucis *(H)* is deviated as it curves behind the coalition.

MR images of this entrapment may explain the symptoms of chronic pain on the medial side of the ankle. In addition, they may explain why subtalar coalitions are perceived clinically as personeal spastic flatfoot. Specifically, the continuous pull and deviation of the medially located tendons have the action of turning the foot internally. As a result there is a continous contraction of the muscles of the peroneal side, in an attempt to compensate for this foot deviation. The continuous tension of the peroneal muscles leads to symptoms such as spastic contractures and pain.[41]

The treatment of tarsal coalitions depends upon their location and type. The calcaneonavicular bar is usually excised surgically, and complete recovery can be obtained.[42]

A talocalcaneal coalition can be resected if it is discovered early, in adolescence or young adulthood. [43] When planning treatment, the surgeon is greatly helped by imaging modalities that show the location, size, and type of coalition.[44] Precise osteotomy of the osseous coalition or excision of the synchondrosis must accomplish complete and permanent separation of the fused bones yet, at the same time, spare normal parts of the subtalar joint. Layers of soft tissue, especially fat, are interposed between the surfaces of the resected segments to prevent regrowth of the coalition[44]; but the rate of recurrence is so high that some authors[41] have advocated fusion of the entire subtalar joint as treatment for the painful spastic contractures of the peroneal tendons. Once the joint is fused in a normal position, the compensatory contraction of the peroneal muscles is stopped and the initial symptoms disappear. However, the mobility of the subtalar joint is an important factor in function of the ankle and foot; therefore fusion of this joint should be avoided if possible. It is hoped that early detection and full visualization of these coalitions by CT or MRI will promote surgical corrections of the congenital abnormality without impairment of the weight-bearing function. Talocalcaneal coalition discovered late, when complications such as osteoarthritis are already present, is treated by surgical fusion of the entire subtalar joint.

TRAUMATIC LESIONS
Ankle sprains

Injuries of the ankle are commonly encounterd in all emergency services involved in the care of acute trauma patients. In most cases the injury is limited to the ligaments (ankle sprain) and is caused by inversion with internal rotation of the foot. Seldom is the medial side of the ankle injured when trauma produces forceful eversion of the foot.

Ankle sprains are graded according to the degree of injury[45]: grade 1, stretching of the ligaments without disruption of their fibers or instability; patients with this type of injury have pain and swelling but can still ambulate; grade 2, an incomplete tear of a ligament; there is significant pain with swelling, making the physical examination difficult; grade 3, a complete ligament tear;

this causes significant ankle instability; grade 4, small avulsion fractures of a superficial layer of cortical bone representing the insertion site of a ligament.

It is difficult to determine clinically the grade of sprain, especially in the acute phase, when soft tissue swelling and echymosis may involve a large area, concealing the zone of ligament interruption.

Routine roentgenograms are usually not helpful in determining the degree of injury, except for grade 4, in which a small "flake of bone" can be seen on projections tangent to the surface of the injured area. In such cases on AP views a small fragment is seen in the soft tissue of the lateral ankle. This represents avulsion of the calcaneofibular ligament insertion site. Grade 4 injuries of the deltoid ligament are occasionally seen on coronal CT images as small cortical avulsions from the medial surface of the talus[46] (Fig. 22-43).

When roentgenographic signs of joint effusion (anterior teardrop sign) are seen in patients with acute trauma, the implication is that the capsule of the talocrural joint is intact and hence a grade 3 injury can be ruled out.[47] There is intimate association between the ankle joint capsule and the surrounding ligaments, which makes it unlikely that in the acute phase of an injury any ligament will be completely torn while the integrity of the capsule and its synovial lining is preserved. This is the rationale for performing arthrography in the acute stage of an ankle sprain — contrast material introduced into the synovial space leaks out through the rent in the capsule, at the site of the ligament tear.[48] The extravasation is sometimes subtle and better seen on CT performed immediately after

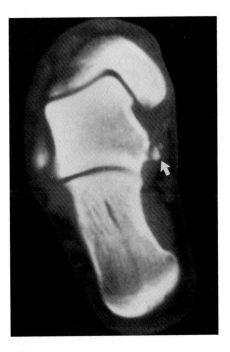

FIGURE 22-43
Deltoid ligament injury. A coronal CT image of the right ankle shows avulsion fracture fragments (*arrow*) at the inferior insertion of the tibiotalar ligament (deep layer of the deltoid ligament).

arthrography (Fig. 22-44). However, as early as 48 hours after injury a tear of the ligament may not be seen on arthrography because the synovium heals and seals off the initial traumatic rent, even though the adjacent ligament fibers remain torn and separated.[49] In such cases stress views of the ankle disclose the instability resulting from tears of the ligaments. The stress views are usually obtained in an anteroposterior position with medial and lateral tilt of the talus (valgus and varus stress). The angle formed by the lines drawn along the tibial plafond and talar dome is measured and compared with that on the normal side. The comparison is necessary because every individual has a certain inherent flexibility of the capsule and ligaments, permitting normal opening of the stressed joint space of between 5 and 23 degrees. Thus the test is considered positive when there is a difference of more than 10 degrees between the angles of the normal and the injured side. The stress should be performed with the foot in neutral and plantarflexed position. This is necessary to differentiate isolated tears of the anterior talofibular ligament (seen in stress applied only during plantarflexion) from combined tears of the anterior talofibular and calcaneofibular ligaments (seen in neutral position stress views).[47] However, all the stress tests have value only when positive. Normal stress views have been reported in 38% of patients proven to have ligament tears.[50]

The proximity of the peroneal tendons and calcaneofibular ligament predisposes to communications between a tear of the calcaneofibular ligament and peroneal tendon sheath on one side and the ankle joint on the other. Contrast injected into the peroneal tendon sheath (ankle tenogram) leaks through the tear and travels deep, entering into the tibiotalar joint space and assuming the distribution characteristic for ankle arthrograms. By using stress combined with tenography, it is possible to improve the diagnostic accuracy of calcaneofibular ligament tears up to 96%.[51]

Because the treatment of ankle sprains is controversial, precise diagnosis is especially important. Most authors writing on this subject prefer conservative treatment—consisting of a short interval of immobilization with a soft cast in grade 1 and grade 2 sprains and a walking cast for 3 to 6 weeks in grade 3 sprains. Complete ligament tears resulting in chronic instability require surgical treatment; if left uncorrected, they may lead to degenerative arthritis of the ankle joint.

Even though there are occasional reports of MRI detection of ligamentous abnormalities, MR has yet to be proven useful in the exact diagnosis of ligament tears. In MR images of healthy volunteers[26] the only ligament consistently seen was the anterior talofibular. Other important ligaments were not visualized in all cases. The multidirectional orientation of ligament fibers, especially the radiating pattern of multiple thin insertion bands (separated by layers of fat), makes it difficult to assess their integrity in any single plane of imaging. Possibly, in the near future, when the resolution of MR images is improved, thin slices will eliminate the effect of partial volume averaging between fat and thin obliquely oriented fibers. Until then, CT and MR can be used mostly only to rule out osseous injuries and tendon ruptures. In the absence of osseous or tendinous abnormalities the soft tissue swelling, edema, or hemorrhage seen in specific locations corresponding to the known arrangements of ligaments can be inferred indirectly as a sign of injuries to ligamentous structures supporting the ankle joint.[52] It is not yet possible, at least not in a constant and reliable way, to determine by CT and MRI whether these structures are separated, torn, or merely stretched.

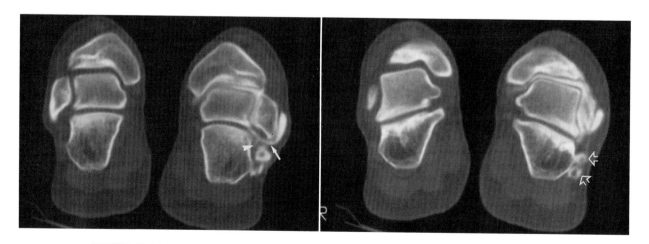

FIGURE 22-44
CT-arthrogram, coronal CT views of the mortise. Contrast introduced into the tibiotalar joint space leaks out laterally through a tear of the talofibular *(arrowhead)* and calcaneofibular ligaments *(arrow)*. The sleeves of the peroneal tendons contain contrast *(open arrows)*, another indication of tear of the calcaneofibular ligament.

Tendon injuries

ACHILLES TENDON TEAR

The Achilles tendon (calcaneus tendon), the largest tendon of the human body, is commonly torn in forceful dorsiflexion of the foot occurring in athletic activities requiring jumping with extended knees or rising up on the toes. Nonathletic injuries seen in middle-aged or older patients result most often from abrupt dorsiflexion of the foot when falling or landing on the forefoot. Certain conditions predispose to tendon fragility: rheumatoid arthritis, systemic lupus erthythematous, hyperparathyroidism, chronic renal failure, gout, and diabetes. Patients receiving chronic treatment with systemic steroids or local injections of steroids may have increased frequency of Achilles tendon tears.[53]

The most common location of such tears is the segment where the tendo Achillis is thinnest and least vascularized, approximately 3 to 5 cm superior to its calcaneal insertion. Occasionally tears will be seen at the musculotendinous junction.

Large complete tears do not need radiological investigations. Clinically they are characteristic: abrupt interruption of the tendon fibers can be observed on inspection and palpation of the ankle; plantarflexion of the ankle is impossible or greatly impaired. The history is also rather characteristic — a snap was felt in the ankle at the moment of injury, and intense pain followed. Several days after injury an echymosis may be observed on the skin in the calf or the heel area.

Roentgenograms of the ankle obtained in such patients may show in the lateral projection a gap or depression in the soft tissue band representing the tendon; often incomplete tears will be obscured by hemorrhage obliterating the pre-Achilles fat layer. Calcifications are occasionally seen at the site of scarring from an old tear and degenerative disease of the tendon.

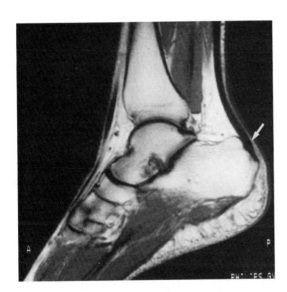

FIGURE 22-45
Normal Achilles tendon, MR appearance in sagittal section. A T1-weighted image shows the tendon as a band of signal void with smooth margins that inserts on the posterior surface of the calcaneus *(arrow)*.

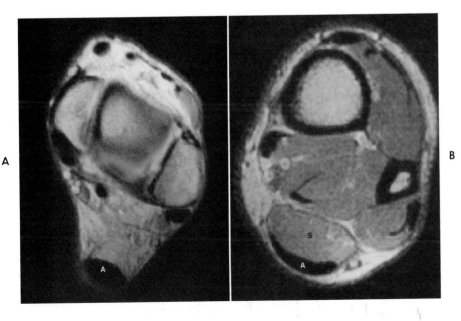

FIGURE 22-46
Normal Achilles tendon, MR appearance in axial section. **A,** Through the mortise. The tendon is seen as an oval signal void. **B,** At the musculotendinous junction. The soleus *(S)* inserts on the anterior surface of the tendon *(A)*.

Ultrasonography has been used to detect abnormalities of these tendons.[54] However, this method is observer dependent and not all institutions have enough personnel to perform and interpret such studies.

Most authors commenting on the radiology of Achilles tendon injuries have concluded that MRI is the best modality for studying this structure.[55-57]

On MR images the tendon appears as a band of signal void longitudinally traversing the posterior aspect of the calf and ankle. When normal, it has sharply defined margins and is homogeneously signalless (Fig. 22-45). On axial images of the calf the tendon is seen as a crescentic structure concave anteriorly where it receives the insertion of muscle fibers of the soleus (Fig. 22-46). Posteriorly the medial and lateral heads of the gastrocnemius interdigitate with the tendon fibers. As it travels inferiorly, this structure becomes oval in cross section and further down, at the ankle, assumes a flat bandlike configuration. Anterior to it is the fat layer, and posterior the crural fascia.

On T2-weighted images a tear of the Achilles tendon appears as a zone of abnormally high signal, representing fluid accumulated at the site of injury. Sagittal images demonstrate the longitudinal discontinuity and retraction of the torn fibers of the tendon (Fig. 22-47). Axial images give a better representation of hemorrhage in and around the tendon, often tracking up to the soleus and gastrocnemius. MR images, especially T2 weighted, show the accumulation of blood or edema in the peritendinous soft tissues; occasionally this extends up into the calf (Fig. 22-48). High pressure resulting from hemorrhage/edema beneath the fascia can produce a posterior compartment syndrome, leading to compression of the vascular and neural structures (Fig. 22-49).

The differential diagnosis of partial-thickness tears of the Achilles tendon includes tendinitis. Based on MRI findings, it is impossible to differentiate tendinitis from a minor intratendinous tear. Both are manifested in T2-weighted sequences as a zone of intermediate or high signal, contained within the tendon. In T1-weighted

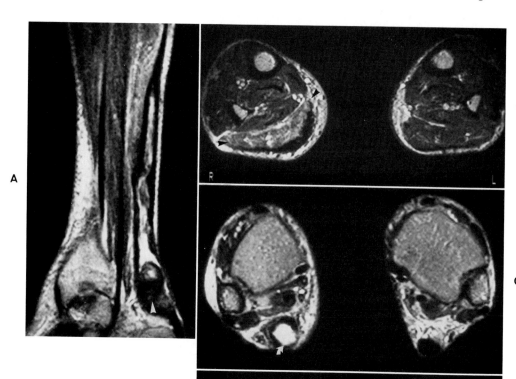

FIGURE 22-47
Partial tear of the Achilles tendon. **A,** Sagittal T2-weighted image. Longitudinal split of the tendon, containing a central collection of high-signal representing fluid. In the inferior end, a round zone of low signal represents retracted torn fibers and a fibrotic reaction *(white arrowhead).* **B** to **D,** Axial T2-weighted images. At the level of the musculotendinous junction **(B)** the tendon has an irregular anterior margin and there is increased signal in the soleus. This suggests edema *(black arrowheads).* At a more inferior level **(C)** fluid can be seen within the thin shell representing the torn Achilles tendon *(curved arrow).* At the ankle mortise **(D)** the retracted fibers of the tendon form a globe of low signal *(white arrowheads).* The anteroposterior dimension of the right tendon is markedly increased compared to the normal left side.

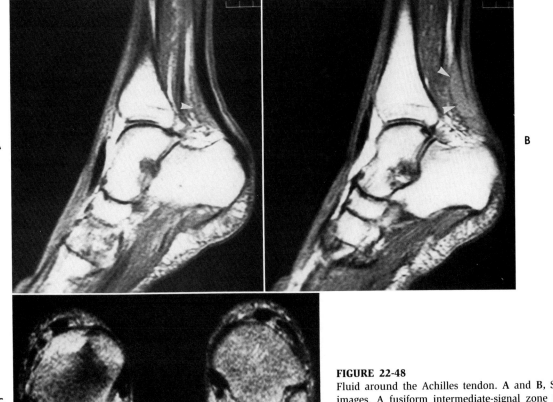

FIGURE 22-48
Fluid around the Achilles tendon. **A** and **B**, Sagittal T1-weighted images. A fusiform intermediate-signal zone represents the fluid *(arrowheads)*. **C**, Axial T2-weighted images of both ankles showing the circumferential collection of fluid on the left side.

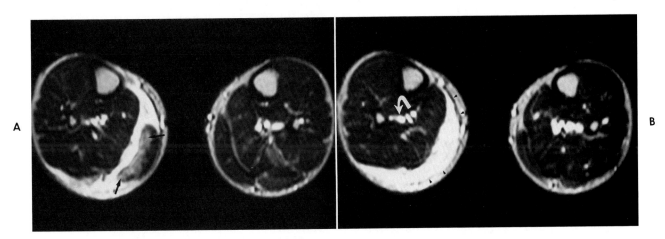

FIGURE 22-49
Tear of the Achilles tendon causing a posterior compartment syndrome. **A**, An axial T2-weighted image shows the tear of the musculotendinous junction in the right gastrocnemius, seen as an intermediate-signal zone in the posterior surface of the muscle *(arrows)*. **B**, Hemorrhage/edema beneath the crural fascia *(arrowheads)* has compressed the deep veins of the right calf *(curved arrow)*, which appear of smaller diameter compared to the normal left side. This is a sign of posterior compartment syndrome.

sequences the inflammatory edema surrounding the segment of tendonitis manifests as a low-signal zone in the fat layer anterior to the Achilles tendon. Subacute stage of a hematoma produced at the time of an anterior partial thickness tear may have a similar appearence. It remains to the clinical history for differentiation between these two conditions—specifically whether the pain started abruptly following an injury and whether a snap was felt, in which case a tear is more likely.

Treatment decisions depend upon the degree of tear, the activities that the patient expects to perform, and the existence of predisposing conditions (e.g., steroid treatment or underlying collagen disease). Minor tears of the Achilles tendon are treated with immobilization for several days followed by progressive return to normal activity using elevated heel pads placed in the shoe, with the aim of reducing tension in the tendon. Follow-up MRI examinations can be aimed at determining progression toward healing; resorption of fluid at the site of the tear is an indication that return to progressive activity can be safely attempted.

Incomplete tears of the Achilles tendon in young athletic individuals have been observed to progress to tendinous rupture (Fig. 22-50). Therefore in such patients surgical repair in the early stage of an injury prevents further progression to total interruption of the tendon fibers, a lesion much more difficult to repair. Surgical treatment of complete tears consists of suturing the ends of the torn tendon and/or placement of tendon grafts spanning the gap of the tear. A tendon that has been severed and repaired lacks normal flexibility and elasticity; the tear may recur at or adjacent to the site of surgery (Fig. 22-51).

In patients with compression of structures in the posterior compartment of the calf resulting from hemorrhage/edema that originated in a tear of the musculotendinous junction of the Achilles tendon, it may be necessary to relieve the pressure by draining the he-

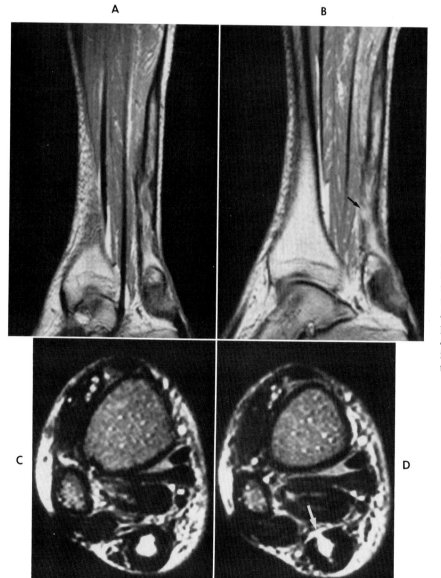

FIGURE 22-50
Progression of an Achilles tendon tear. **A,** Sagittal proton density image demonstrating the long intratendinous tear. **B,** Follow-up at 6 weeks. The anterior margin of the tendon appears interrupted *(arrow),* an indication of progression toward partial-thickness tear. **C** and **D,** Axial images show the change from an intratendinous to a partial-thickness tear of the anterior surface *(arrow).*

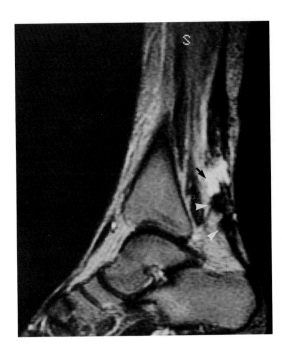

FIGURE 22-51
Recurrent tear of the Achilles tendon. A sagittal T2-weighted shows fluid collection at the site of a tear in the Achilles tendon *(arrow)*. More inferiorly there is distortion in the contour of the tendon at the site of previous surgical repair of a tear *(arrowheads)*.

matoma through percutaneous aspiration or surgical decompression.

POSTERIOR TIBIALIS TENDON TEAR

Tears of the posterior tibialis tendon are more frequently seen in women over the age of 50 and represent a cause of progressive flatfoot deformity in adults.[58,59]

In many patients the pathological process has an insidious onset and results from chronic degenerative disease of the tendon fibers rather then acute trauma. Rheumatoid arthritis or other collagen disease disorders predispose patients to such tears.[60] It is important to recognize tears of the posterior tibialis tendon; untreated, they produce progressive loss of the plantar arch and subsequent pain and limitation of activity, due especially to inability to rise onto the ball of the foot. A complete tear of this tendon leaves unopposed the pull of evertors of the ankle (peroneus brevis and longus). Thus it initiates a chain reaction leading to planovalgus deformity; the arch of the foot is also affected, because the posterior tibialis tendon is part of the medial strut of fibrous structures that keep the normal elevation of the arch by supporting the weight on the medial side.

The weak part of posterior tibialis tendon is the segment just posterior and inferior to the medial malleolus, where the structure changes direction from vertical to almost horizontal and is tightly contained within a limited space between the bone and the flexor retinaculum. No other supporting soft tissue structure is interposed medial to this tendon, a fact that diminishes its

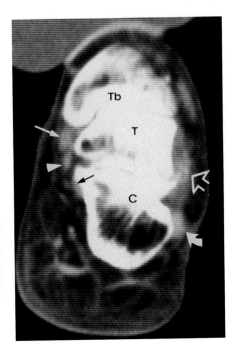

FIGURE 22-52
CT of ankle tendons. Coronal image of the left ankle. The tibia *(Tb)*, talus *(T)*, and calcaneus *(C)* can be identified. The posterior tibialis *(white arrow)* and flexor hallucis longus *(arrowhead)* tendons are located on the medial side, inferior to the medial malleolus. The flexor hallucis longus tendon *(black arrow)* is beneath the sustentaculum tali. The tendons of the peroneus brevis *(open arrow)* and peroneus longus *(curved arrow)* are seen in oblique section.

support and predisposes to dislocations in the subcutaneous fat layer on the medial side of the tibia.

In the chronic stage of a posterior tibialis tendon tear a small area of periosteal reaction is observed on the cortex of the medial malleolus. Osteophytes can be seen on the anterior lip of the tibial groove, in which the posterior tibialis tendon is located.[61] These are subtle roentgenographic changes; in general, conventional films have only limited value in detecting pathology of the posterior tibialis tendon.

CT images show the normal tendon to be the thickest of the dense soft tissue structures in the medial side of the ankle. It has an oval cross section and hugs the posterior margin of the medial malleolus (Fig. 22-52). When normal, its homogeneous density and sharp smooth margins are notable. Abnormalities can be manifested as changes in diameter and nonhomogeneity of its density.[62]

Three grades of posterior tibialis tendon rupture have been described [63]:

In grade 1 the tendon appears hypertrophic due to edema, hemorrhage, and cystic degeneration, causing accumulation of fluid inside the tendon itself.

In grade 2 there is marked attenuation of the tendon, which is partially torn. Retraction of its interrupted fibers leaves a segment that is abnormally thin. This becomes a weak spot that can transform itself with a minimum of stress into a complete tear.

In grade 3 there is a gap in the tendon, usually filled

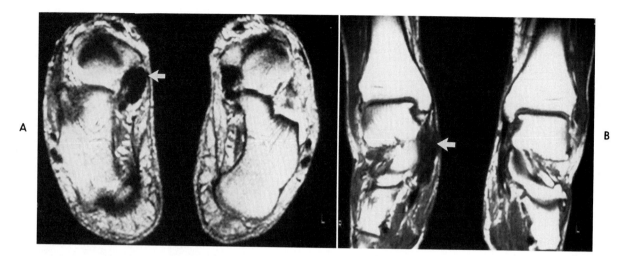

FIGURE 22-53
Grade I tear of the posterior tibialis tendon. **A,** A T2-weighted axial image through both ankles shows enlargement in the diameter of the tendon on the right side *(arrow)*. **B,** Coronal image. Enlargement of the posterior tibialis tendon and nonhomogeneous signal intensity, consistent with a grade I tear *(arrow)*.

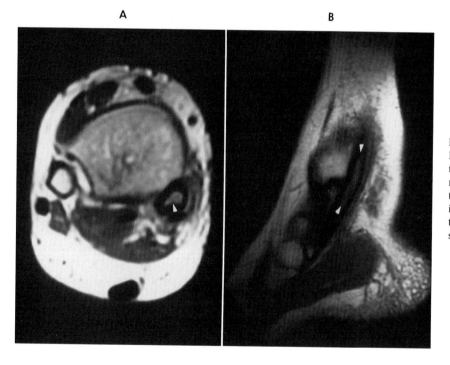

FIGURE 22-54
Intratendinous tear of the posterior tibialis tendon. **A,** An axial MR image (TR 1670 msec/TE 30 msec) shows increased diameter of the tendon with a zone of high signal in its center *(arrowhead)*. **B,** A sagittal image through the medial side of the right ankle shows the longitudinal tear *(arrowheads)*.

with fluid or fat, that represents a complete interruption of the tendon fibers. The proximal and distal ends of the torn tendon assume a bulbous rounded configuration due to retraction of the elastic fibers and the formation of granulation tissue at the margin of the tear.

At present, abnormalities of the posterior tibialis tendon in general are diagnosed radiologically by MRI, which offers better visualization of the length of segmental involvement and is more sensitive in depicting intratendinous tears and fluid collection.[63,64] The early stage of rupture shows a nonhomogeneous signal and

wider diameter of the involved tendon (Fig. 22-53). Vertical partial tears are manifested as lines of intermediate signal in T1-weighted images (Fig. 22-54). The fluid accumulated in these slits is best observed in T2-weighted images, owing to its high signal (which contrasts with the signal void of the normal part of the tendon) (Fig. 22-54). The synovial sleeve investing the tendon can be distended by fluid, also best seen on axial T2-weighted images (Fig. 22-55).

On MR images overestimation of the size of the cross section of the posterior tibialis tendon may be caused by summation of the signal void of the tendon with that of

A

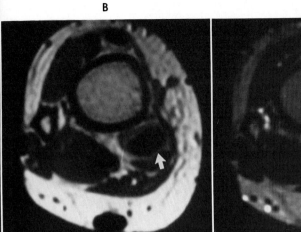

FIGURE 22-55
Fluid in the posterior tibialis tendon sleeve. **A,** A sagittal T2*-weighted image shows fluid in the sleeve and increased diameter of the tendon *(arrowheads).* **B** and **C,** Axial proton density and T2-weighted images above the ankle mortise show fluid in the tendon sleeve and increased diameter of the tendon *(arrow).*

B   C

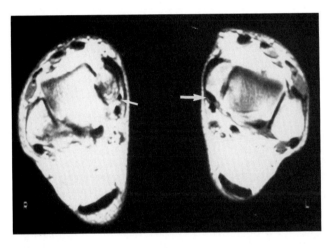

FIGURE 22-56
Grade 2 tear of the posterior tibialis tendon, MR appearance. Axial proton density images (TR 2200 msec/TE 30 msec) demonstrate an abnormally thin tendon on the right side *(small arrow)* compared to that on the opposite normal side *(large arrow).*

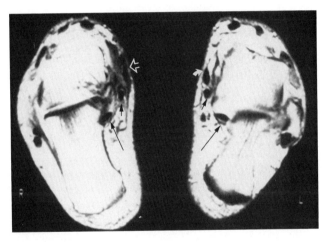

FIGURE 22-57
Grade 3 tear of the posterior tibialis tendon. An axial MR image of both ankles shows an ill-defined zone of low and intermediate signal in the subcutaneous fat layer on the medial side of the right talus. Tendons of the flexor hallucis longus *(long arrows)* and flexor digitorum longus *(short arrows)* are identified on each side and appear within normal limits. On the left the posterior tibialis tendon is well seen *(curved arrow).* In the corresponding location on the right no tendon structure is identified in the zone of low or intermediate signal, which represents edema and hemorrhage at the site of the complete tear *(open arrow).*

the tibial cortex immediately adjacent to it. Comparison with the asymptomatic side may help in detecting decreased diameter of the partially torn tendon, the hallmark of a grade 2 tear (Fig. 22-56).

In an acute grade 3 rupture, fluid and residual granulation tissue are represented on MR images by a high-signal zone replacing the gap in the tendon. In the chronic stage of a complete tear, fluid or fat replaces the torn tendon, appearing as a high-signal zone that completely replaces the signal void of the ligament (Fig. 22-57).

MR images have been found to provide 73% accuracy in detecting and classifying the types of posterior tibialis tendon tears in 22 patients who underwent surgical treatment.[63]

PERONEAL TENDON INJURIES

In the ankle the tendons of the peroneus brevis and longus are located in a groove on the posterior surface of the lateral malleolus, covered posterolaterally by the bands of fibrous tissue that forms the inferior and superior parts of the peroneal retinaculum (Fig. 22-6).

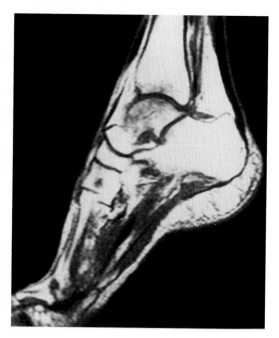

FIGURE 22-58

MRI of a stress fracture of the talus. This 60-year-old woman had had a prolonged immobilization in bed due to stroke. Two weeks after the resumption of weight-bearing activity, she began having ankle pain. A sagittal T1-weighted MR image demonstrates abnormally low signal in the bone marrow of the dome of the talus consistent with a stress fracture. It was assumed that the stress fracture had been a result of diminished mechanical resistance in the bone structures due to osteoporosis of disuse.

Variants of anatomy such as a shallow peroneal groove or a convex posterior surface of the fibula are factors predisposing to dislocations of these tendons, occasionally seen in skiing and ice skating injuries.[65] CT and MRI can detect these dislocations and reveal whether the contour of the fibular surface needs reconstruction, an important factor when corrective surgery is planned.[66-68]

Bone injuries
STRESS FRACTURES

Most fractures of the ankle and foot are easily diagnosed on routine roentgenograms. However, there are some that are difficult to detect mostly because they are obscured by the overlapping surfaces of the osseous structures of the tarsals and the distal tibia and fibula. The displacement of fragments and the resulting distortion of complex articular surfaces are sometimes difficult to visualize. Stress fractures are another category of abnormalities difficult to detect on conventional roentgenograms.

Roentgenographically occult fractures of the tarsal bones can be seen on radioisotope bone scans as focal or linear zones of increased uptake. However, these scans lack the spatial resolution necessary for an adequate morphological analysis of the abnormality. They can be used mainly just to rule out bone pathology or to locate the abnormality in a specific area. Tc99m bone scans give an indication for the next imaging modality, whether it be aimed at the specific segment of the osseous structures (when scan is positive) or be concentrated on soft tissues

A 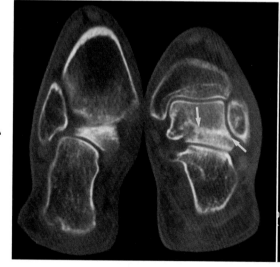 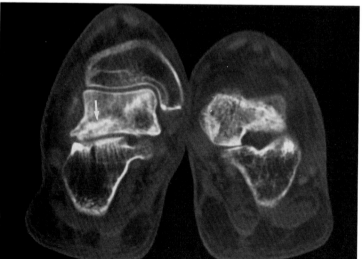 B

FIGURE 22-59

Bilateral stress fractures of the talus, CT images of the ankles of a 35-year-old woman who had had a pelvic fracture for which she was immobilized in bed several months. The rehabilitation period that followed included progressive weight-bearing and walking exercises. These produced increasing pain in both ankles. The CT examination was performed to determine the cause of the pain. **A,** A coronal image through both ankles demonstrates a horizontal line of density in the left talus representing the healing stage of a stress fracture *(arrows).* **B,** Another coronal image distal to A shows a similar band of density in the right talus, signifying a stress fracture *(arrow).* There is profound osteoporosis, especially evident in the calcaneus.

in the symptomatic site (when the scan shows no focal bone uptake).

Stress fractures of the ankle and foot can be produced by an unusually high degree of repetitive stress in the normal skeleton, occasionally seen when a person undertakes vigurous physical activities. Another, more unexpected, type of stress fracture is encountered in the patient who has been immobilized for a long time by a major brain injury or pelvic fracture. The lower extremities undergo profound disuse demineralization; the bone loss is more pronounced in spongy bone, which makes up a significant part of the talus and calcaneus, the two bones in direct vertical line of weight bearing. These brittle osteoporotic bones may not be able to sustain weight bearing in the early period of rehabilitation and resumption of walking. Stress fracture can appear when there is a too rapid advancement of weight-bearing exercises. Pain is the commonest manifestation of such stress fractures. The most advanced imaging modality for visualizing these stress fractures limited to spongy bone trabeculae is MRI. On T1-weighted images hemorrhage/edema of the fracture appears as bands or diffuse zones of increased signal, clearly seen against the background of bright signal of the fatty marrow (Fig. 22-58). On T2-weighted images or STIR pulse sequences the zone of hemorrhage/edema at the fracture site has increased signal intensity.[69]

CT can detect stress fractures only in the stage when increased density is present in the bones. This represents the phase of calcified callus formation, at the end of the normal repair process. These fractures appear as bands of density especially evident in osteoporotic bones (Fig. 22-59).

DISTAL TIBIAL AND FIBULAR FRACTURES

Fractures of the distal tibia and fibula often intersect the articular cortex. Those that extend to the weight-bearing surface of the tibial plafond or syndesmosis need careful treatment, aimed at reduction to anatomical position and alignment. Thus all fracture fragments and their relation to the articular space must be visualized, initially to plan the treatment and subsequently to verify whether the ideal reduction has been accomplished. The most thorough and rapid way to accomplish this task is by CT, which can be easily performed in acutely injured patients and in those who have a plaster cast or other means of immobilization already applied.

For evaluation of the distal tibia and fibula and their syndesmosis, axial CT images are the most informative. The alignment of articular surfaces and the proper "locking" of syndesmosis can be easily seen (Fig. 22-60). Fractures that intersect the articular surface of the tibial plafond or the dome of the talus are better seen on coronal CT images of the ankle mortise. The degree of distortion of the articular cortex that forms the weight-bearing surface can be directly perceived (Fig. 22-61).

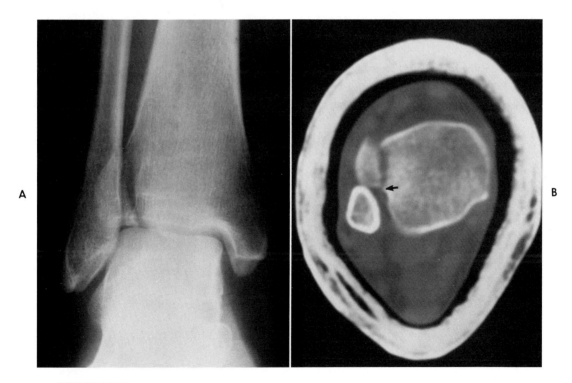

FIGURE 22-60
Intraarticular fracture of the distal tibia. **A,** An AP view of the right ankle demonstrates a vertically oriented fracture through the lateral margin of the distal tibia. **B,** After reduction of the fracture and casting, CT was performed to verify the alignment of fragments. An axial image through the distal tibia shows the fracture line and some external rotation of the fracture fragment. The fracture line intersects the surface of the syndesmosis *(arrow)*.

In complex comminuted fractures it is necessary to obtain axial as well as coronal CT images for better understanding of the spatial relationships of the fracture fragments. The alternative mode of scanning is to obtain thin axial slices, which can be reconstructed in sagittal, coronal, or oblique planes or can be used to produce three-dimensional representations of the ankle viewed from different angles.

The cartilaginous layer separating the epiphysis from the metaphysis in the immature skeleton represents a weak zone that is often fractured in injuries of the ankle. Fractures that involve the growth plate have been classified by Salter and Harris[70] into five types. In the ankle, injuries are commonly the result of torsion forces that produce Salter-Harris types II to IV fracture. These are fractures that traverse the growth cartilage and separate fragments of metaphysis (Type II), epiphysis (Type III), or both (Type IV). The younger the child, the more hazardous are the consequences that can derive from focal disturbances of the growth cartilage. Limited zones of the growth plate may become necrotic as a result of hemorrhage produced by the fracture and may stop generating new bone while the rest of the metaphysis and epiphysis continue to develop. Tilt or concavity of the growth plate can result from these focal abnormalities.

In the healing stage of Salter-Harris Type III and Type IV fractures bars representing mature callus can bridge the metaphysis to the epiphysis of the distal tibia, acting as a tether. The growth process in the uninjured part of the epiphyseal seam can generate new bone; the tibia grows in an asymmetrical fashion; and as a result, the ankle mortise becomes tilted. These abnormalities in the orientation of the growth plate and alignment of the ankle mortise are well seen on coronal images of both CT and MRI (Fig. 22-62).

In adolescents with ankle injuries a variant of Salter-Harris fractures is encountered, the triplane fracture of the distal tibia.[71] The spatial orientation of this fracture surface is complex: a horizontal fracture goes through the open cartilaginous growth plate, a sagittal fracture divides the epiphysis, and a coronally oriented fracture separates a fragment from the posterior margin of the metaphysis. Triplane fractures most commonly separate the lateral part of the distal tibia from the shaft fragment (two-part fracture); occasionally there is comminution of the epiphyseal fragment (three-part fracture).

Triplane fractures are usually seen in patients 12 to 15 years old, an age that corresponds to the beginning of ossification of the growth cartilage in the distal tibia. The first part to ossify is a limited zone, eccentrically located above the medial malleolus. From here the ossification spreads to the medial side and only later to the lateral part of the growth plate. This sequence of maturity explains why a 13-year-old child with an ankle fracture can have the medial fragment of the epiphysis left in a normal attachment to the metaphysis while the fracture line traverses only the lateral part of the nonossified cartilaginous growth plate and detaches the lateral side of the epiphysis (usually with a posterior tag of metaphysis attached to it). Each of the planes of fracture can be seen in a specific radiographic projection — sagittal fractures of the epiphysis in AP views, coronal fractures of the metaphysis in lateral views. The axial component of the fracture surface can be perceived on lateral projections as

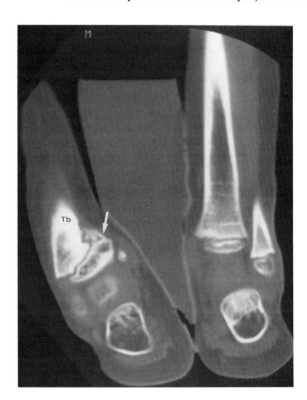

FIGURE 22-62
Salter-Harris Type II fracture. Coronal CT image of a 4-year-old child with progressive right ankle deformity following a fracture sustained at age 3. The tibial epiphysis is tilted and shifted medially. The posterior part of the fracture is still visible as a gap between the small fragment of the metaphysis *(arrow)* and the rest of the tibia *(Tb)*.

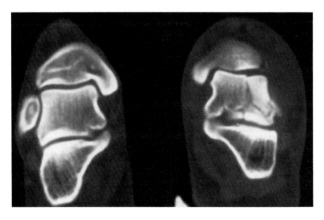

FIGURE 22-61
Fracture in the ankle mortise. A coronal CT shows depression and rotation of the fracture fragments forming the weight-bearing surface of the left talar dome.

abnormal widening of the anterior part of the growth plate. However, the complexity of this injury may create difficulty in comprehending the shape and position of the fragments. CT has been found most practical for visualizing all the fragments and their position.[71,72]

Sequential 3 to 5 mm sections through the distal tibia and fibula portray the exact size and position of these fragments (Fig. 22-63). Reformatted images in the coronal and sagittal planes may help define specific components of the fracture, especially important in planning its reduction, which is aimed at return to anatomical position and alignment. Any gap of 2 mm or more between the fragments forming the articular surface of the tibial plafond will cause joint incongruency, which results in traumatic osteoarthritis. This can be prevented by operative reduction and internal fixation of the displaced fracture fragments.

Pylon fractures of the ankle represent a clinical and radiological entity distinct from other types of ankle injuries.[73] They are produced by axial compression forces from a fall or a vehicular collision (as when there is impact between the foot of the driver and the brake pedal). At the moment of injury the talus is driven proximally and splits the horizontal surface of the distal tibia (plafond) into several fragments. This action has been likened to a pestle (the talus) hitting and breaking the mortar (tibial plafond).[74]

There are four radiological features of the pylon fracture: intraarticular fracture of the tibial plafond, extensive comminution with a centrifugal pattern of fragment displacement, frequent association with talus fracture, and preservation of the normal relation of the talus to the fibular malleolus (Fig. 22-64). This last distinguishes the pylon fracture from a trimalleolar

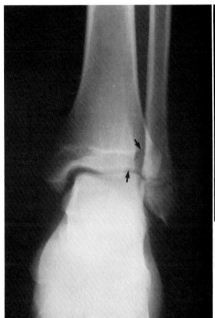

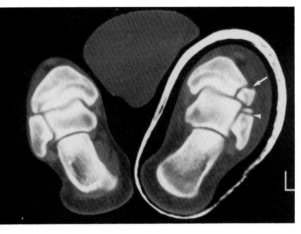

FIGURE 22-63
Triplane fracture of the distal tibia. **A,** An AP roentgenogram of the left ankle demonstrates a fracture line intersecting the lateral part of the growth plate of the distal tibia *(arrow);* it separates a lateral fragment from the epiphysis. **B,** A coronal CT image demonstrates the sagittal intraarticular fracture of the laterodistal tibia. The horizontal extension of this fracture widens the lateral part of the growth plate *(arrow)*. In addition, an unsuspected fracture is seen in the fibular margin at the surface of the syndesmosis *(arrowheads)*.

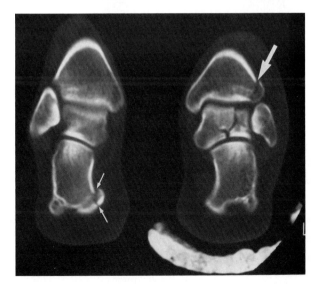

FIGURE 22-64
Pylon fracture of the left ankle, coronal CT of a patient who fell from a second floor window and landed on his heels. The left tibia has a sagittal fracture *(long arrow)*. The talus is comminuted in several fragments. The tibiofibular syndesmosis is normally aligned. The right calcaneus has a fracture of the medial side *(short arrows)*.

fracture, which usually is complicated by dislocation of the syndesmosis.

The prognosis for a pylon fracture is poor, mostly due to the marked comminution of the articular surface of the plafond. Surgical treatment is aimed at restoring the tibiofibular length and reconstructing the horizontal surface of the tibia. All the tibial fragments are anchored to the so-called surgical tibiofibular platform — represented by the fibula, bounded by the tibiofibular ligaments and the syndesmosis to the laterodistal tibial surface. Therefore, when surgical reduction and fixation is planned, it is important to know the exact size and position of the fracture fragments. This is best accomplished by CT.[73] When the tibial segment of the tibiofibular platform is small, reduction of the fracture and fixation of all the other fragments to the platform cannot be accomplished. In such cases fusion of the joint is a more practical alternative. Knowing the exact size of this fragment, from the axial images of CT, can help in deciding whether or not reduction and internal fixation of the fragments is feasible. When the tibial fragment of the platform is too small, internal fixation has a low chance of success and arthrodesis should be performed.

The trimalleolar fracture results from a twisting of the ankle in external rotation, with the foot supinated.[75] Fractures of the medial and lateral malleoli are easily seen on conventional roentgenograms and can be treated promptly with internal fixation.[76,77] However, the size of the posterior malleolar fragment is not estimated correctly on plain roentgenograms. CT has the advantage of producing axial images and thus can disclose the true size of the fragment detached from the posterior surface of

the tibia (Fig. 22-65). When this fragment represents 25% or more of the distal tibial cross section, the joint becomes inherently unstable.[73] It needs correction of the instability by means of anatomical reduction of the posterior malleolar fragment and internal fixation. This represents an additional step in the treatment of a trimalleolar fracture. It is therefore important to do CT examination in all cases to determine the exact size of the posterior fragment so an informed decision can be made as to the necessity of posterior malleolar internal fixation.

CALCANEAL FRACTURES

Comminuted fractures of the calcaneus are produced by impact of the heel with the ground (as when a person falls from a significant height). These fractures are often comminuted and the bone fragments may be compressed in a craniocaudal direction as well as displaced medially or laterally.[78] The restoration of alignment and position of the fragments forming the subtalar joint is the most important part of treatment.[79] CT can provide information regarding the number, size, and location of each fracture fragment[20,78,80,81] (Figs. 22-66 and 22-67). Lateral displacement of the calcaneal fragments may entrap the peroneal tendons.[82] Rotation of fragments or separation of the sustentaculum tali, detected by CT, indicates the need for surgical reduction (Fig. 22-68).

Calcaneal fractures that are too comminuted to be kept in normal position and alignment by orthopedic screws and plates have poor functional prognosis. The end result of incongruency of the subtalar joint is traumatic osteoarthritis (Fig. 22-69).

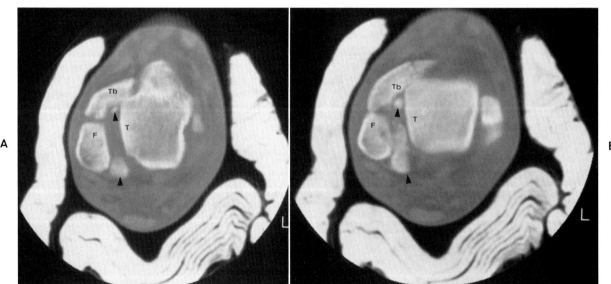

FIGURE 22-65
Trimalleolar fracture-dislocation of the right ankle. **A,** An axial image through the talus demonstrates the abnormally large space on the lateral side of the ankle mortise, where fracture fragments (*arrowheads*) displaced from the distal tibia (*Tb*) are interposed between the talus (*T*) and the lateral malleolus (*F*). **B,** Another axial image through the dome of the talus demonstrates marked comminution of the distal tibia (*arrowheads*) and an irreducible dislocation of the ankle mortise, secondary to interposition of fracture fragments between the fibula and the talus.

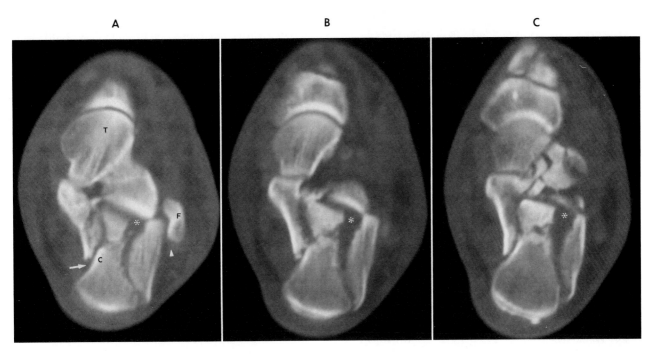

FIGURE 22-66

CT of a comminuted fracture of the os calcis. **A,** A CT axial image demonstrates the fracture with fragmentation of the subtalar joint articular surface and separation of the sustentaculum tali *(arrow)*. Lateral displacement of fragments causes entrapment of the peroneal tendons *(arrowhead)* posterior to the fibula *(F)*. **B** and **C,** CT axial images distal to **A** show marked comminution of the calcaneus and lateroanterior displacement of small fracture fragments. There is a gap in the articular surface of the subtalar joint *(asterisk)*.

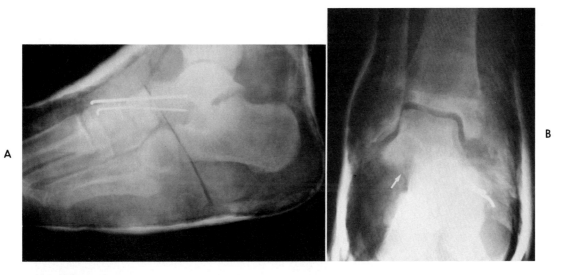

FIGURE 22-67

Fracture dislocation of the calcaneus. **A,** A lateral view of the right foot obtained through a plaster cast demonstrates slight enlargement of the joint space in the subtalar articulation. Orthopedic pins anchored in the head of the talus transfix the tarsal bones in a sagittal direction. **B,** Frontal view of the ankle obtained though the plaster cast. There is a medial shift of the tarsal bones in relation to the inferior surface of the talus *(arrow)*.

Continued.

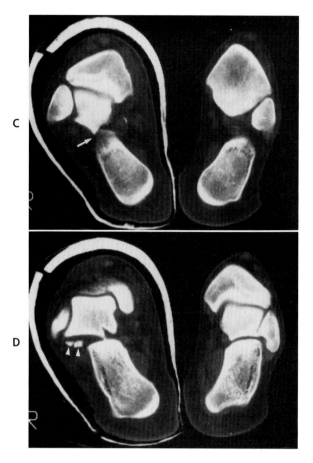

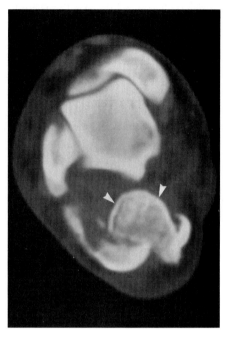

Occasionally in the healing phase of a displaced fracture CT will detect geode-like spaces between the fragments. These represent previous zones of hematoma at the fracture site; some of the blood is resorbed and replaced by fibrous callus or fat (Fig. 22-70).

TARSONAVICULAR FRACTURES

Nondisplaced navicular fractures may be difficult to see on plain films. CT images perpendicular and parallel to

FIGURE 22-67, cont'd
C, CT image representing a coronal view of the hindfoot in the plaster cast. Medial dislocation of the calcaneus relative to the articular surface of the talus *(arrow).* **D,** The CT image obtained further distally demonstrates again the dislocation of the subtalar joint and two distinct fracture fragments *(arrowheads)* interposed between the articular surface of the talus and the calcaneus. The presence of these trapped fragments in the joint prevented reduction of the dislocation.

FIGURE 22-68
Comminuted fracture of the calcaneus with rotation of the fracture fragments. A CT image of the hind foot shows a comminuted fracture of the calcaneus. A large fragment is rotated 180 degrees. The original plantar surface of the calcaneus is now directed toward the inferior articular surface of the talus *(arrowheads).*

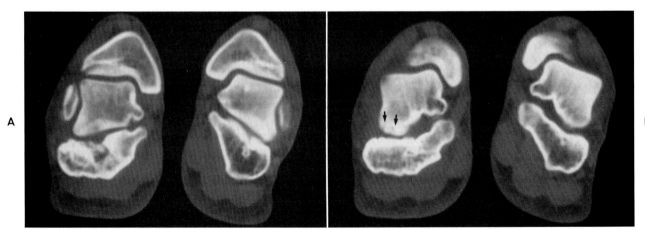

FIGURE 22-69
Osteoarthritis secondary to intraarticular fracture of the calcaneus, CT appearance. **A,** Deformity of the right os calcis secondary to the fracture. **B,** Osteoarthritis of the subtalar joint on the right side is manifested as erosions of the articular surface of the talus and subchondral bony sclerosis *(arrows).*

the plantar surface can easily detect these acute injuries (Fig. 22-71). It is important to establish their presence and to determine whether they progress to normal healing. Nonunion and aseptic necrosis are common complications and can be prevented by early surgical reduction, pinning, and immoblization (Fig. 22-72).

LISFRANK FRACTURE-DISLOCATIONS

The Lisfrank injury represents a fracture-dislocation of the second through fifth tarsometatarsal joints.[83] When the displacement is minor and mostly in the dorsal direction, it can be difficult to see on routine roentgenograms. Small fragments may be hidden by the zigzagging surfaces of the tarsometatarsal joints and go unrecognized.[84] CT is best at detecting these small fracture fragments and can establish their exact position[85] (Fig. 22-73), which facilitates their reduction to normal position in the articular surface.

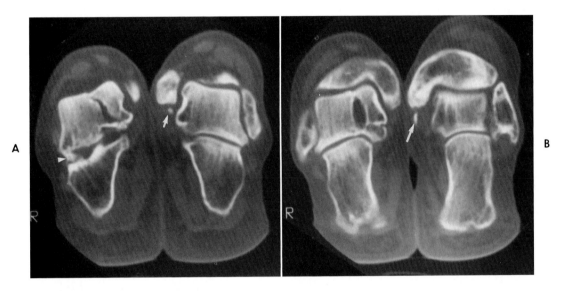

FIGURE 22-70
Sequelae of ankle fractures. A 38-year-old woman who had sustained bilateral fractures of the ankle 1 year earlier was having persistent pain with weight-bearing on the right side. **A,** A coronal CT image of both ankles shows deformity of the right talus secondary to an angulated intraarticular fracture. A segment of bone is interposed between the inferior surface of the talus and the calcaneus *(arrowhead)*. On the left side, calcification in the soft tissues indicates the site of injury in the deltoid ligament *(arrow)*. **B,** In the right talus a fat-containing cavity with sclerotic borders represents the space between the displaced fracture fragments. In the healing process fat has accumulated between the fragments. On the left side, calcification is again noted in the deltoid ligament *(arrow)* with deformity of the fibula secondary to the old injury.

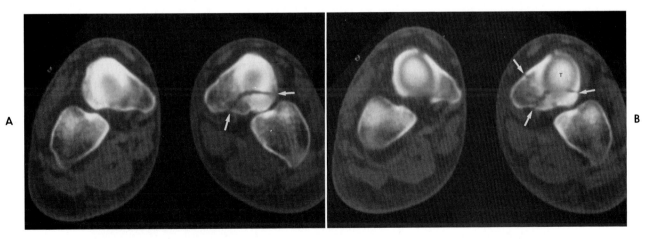

FIGURE 22-71
Fracture of the navicular. **A,** Axial CT image through the navicular. A fracture line *(arrows)* oriented in the horizontal plane traverses the navicular. **B,** CT image obtained 3 mm proximal to A. There is comminution of the medial side of the navicular *(arrows)*. The round structure in the center is a partial volume representation of the head of the talus.

MRI has played but a limited role in the evaluation of acute traumatic fractures of the ankle and foot, mainly because CT is more practical and rapid. However, it is expected that an increasing number of patients with acute injuries of the ankle and foot will undergo MR examination in the future. MRI has no deleterious biological effects, it offers the advantages of total freedom in selection of imaging plane, and it can provide simultaneous information about ligaments, tendons, and other soft tissues structures.[86,87] It is specifically indicated for comminuted impacted fractures of the calcaneus in patients with a fractured thoracolumbar junction. Spinal abnormalities, especially cord compression, are best seen and studied by MR images. It might be added at this point that while the patient is in the MR suite it is expeditious and practical to obtain an MR study of the ankles in two orthogonal planes, rather than transport the patient to the CT scanner[usually in a different location] for extremity imaging.)

On MR images a calcaneal fracture appears as an interruption in the contour of cortical bone signal void and hemorrhage/edema at the fracture site, manifested respectively as decreased and increased signal zones in T1- and T2-weighted sequences. Any disturbance in the longitudinal continuity of the subtalar joint surface is easily observed on sagittal images (Fig. 22-74).

• • •

OSTEOCHONDRITIS DISSECANS

Osteochondral fracture, transchondral fracture, and osteochondritis dissecans are terms used to describe radiologically similar talar lesions.[88-91] In patients with a distinct traumatic event this abnormality appears clinically as a fracture; in those with an insidious onset of symptoms, the osteonecrosis leading to detachment of bone is emphasized by calling the lesion osteochondritis *dissecans*.

There is a consensus in the orthopedic literature regarding the traumatic cause of osteochondritis dissecans. Inversion sprain of the ankle can produce a transchondral fracture of the talar dome laterally (when the foot is in dorsiflexion) or medially (when plantarflexion is present). The shearing/torsional force produces an interruption of the bone trabeculae, separating a superficial segment of bone from the rest of the talus. The elastic resilient articular cartilage may or may not be fractured at the margin of the fragment. The avulsed fragment, having lost its blood supply, is prone to aseptic necrosis. When this happens, a gradual increase in density, with reduction in volume secondary to compression, and fragmentation are seen. Motion between the

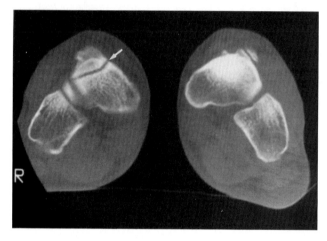

FIGURE 22-72
Nonunited fracture of the tarsal navicular, CT appearance. Coronal CT images through the tarsal bones show a horizontally oriented fracture through the right navicular *(arrow)*. Sclerosis at the fracture surface signifies nonunion.

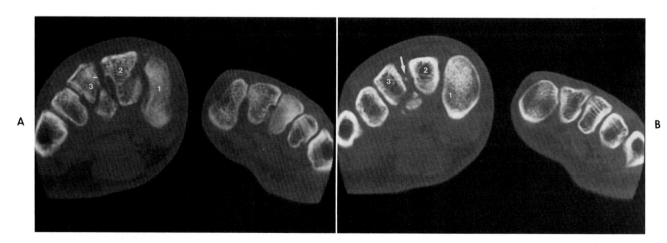

FIGURE 22-73
Lisfrank fracture-dislocation of the right foot. **A,** Axial CT image of the midfoot. Fractures on the plantar side at the base of metatarsal second and third. The joints between the first, second, and third metatarsals *(1 to 3)* are abnormally large. **B,** An axial CT image 5 mm proximal to **A** shows the abnormal space between the second and third metatarsals. In the joint space a fragment of bone is seen *(arrow)*. There is a fracture on the plantar surface of the third metatarsal.

fragment and its bed is the main reason for delayed healing or nonhealing of such lesions. The articular cartilage covering the necrotic fragment becomes soft, spongy, and frayed. Fracture of the cartilage surface, usually found at the margin of the fragment, permits access of synovial fluid in the fracture gap, with further impairment of callus formation. Ultimately, separation of the fragment from its bed is seen; the fragment "floats" in a layer of fluid and can be extruded as a free intrasynovial loose body that may further injure other cartilaginous surfaces and the synovium.

An advantageous sequence of events developing with osteochondral fractures would be as follows: lack of motion between the fragment and its bed promotes growth of capillaries from the bed into the separated fragment, which becomes slowly revascularized and thus maintains its intact articular cartilage. Healing can be very slow and may be interrupted at any stage when

motion between the fragment and the host bone is produced. The larger the fragment of osteochondral fracture, the more likely it is to receive a significant share of the weight-bearing forces. These intermittently applied can produce movement between the fragment and its bed, which leads to nonhealing.

Osteochondritis dissecans has been classified by Berndt and Hardy[88] into four types according to the degree of separation of the fragment: in type I, only depression of the articular surface is seen; in types II and III, the fragment is partially or totally detached but remains in its normal position; in type IV, the fragment is displaced from its surface of origin and moves freely in the joint.

All the imaging modalities have aimed not only at detecting osteochondritis dissecans but also at establishing the stage of this disease. The radiological detection of osteochondritis dissecans is usually simple.

Roentgenograms centered on the ankle mortise in

FIGURE 22-74
MRI of a calcaneal fracture. **A,** Lateral roentgenogram of the left foot. Fracture lines intersect the cortex of the calcaneus and talus. **B,** Axial T1-weighted image. Comminuted fracture with fragmentation of the sustentaculum tali *(large arrow).* The peroneal tendons *(small arrows)* are entrapped between the fracture fragments and surrounded by hemorrhage. **C** and **D,** Proton density and T2-weighted sagittal images show the fracture in the talus *(arrowhead)* and calcaneus *(large arrow)* with surrounding hemorrhage in the bone marrow. Joint effusion is seen as high signal on the T2-weighted and intermediate signal on the proton density–weighted images.

Continued.

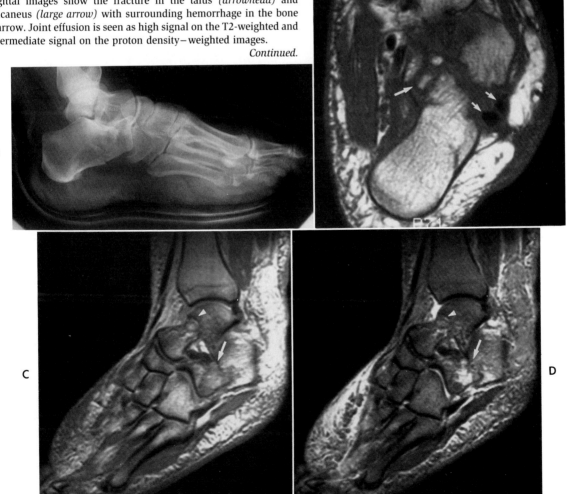

frontal, oblique, and lateral views portray a limited zone of increased density on the medial or lateral margin of the talus, separated by a lucent zone from the underlying bone (which appears sclerotic).

Coronal CT images of the ankle mortise can reveal whether or not the articular cortex is depressed; axial images are better at estimating the surface dimensions of a fragment of osteochondritis dissecans (Fig. 22-75).

Unfortunately, neither roentgenography nor tomography or CT can directly visualize the cartilage layer covering the dome of the talus. Therefore only indirect evidence of its interruption may be obtained when the necrotic fragment is grossly changed in shape, contour, or position. In such instances, however, the disease is advanced and preservation of the normal contour of the talus is beyond reach.

CT-arthrograms of the ankle have been used for determining the integrity of the articular cartilage layer. A double-contrast technique is preferred, mostly because it permits better visualization of small fragments against the background of air in a fully distended joint.

MRI has the advantage of providing, by a noninvasive method of study, information about the articular cartilage, necrotic segment, and underlying bone.[92] On T1-weighted images the necrotic segment of bone appears dark (Fig. 22-76). The normal articular cartilage is of intermediate signal intensity and appears as a smooth homogeneously gray layer covering the articular cortex of the dome.

Early-stage abnormalities of the articular cartilage nclude areas of nodularity, with thickening and nonhomogeneity of signal. Further progression of damage

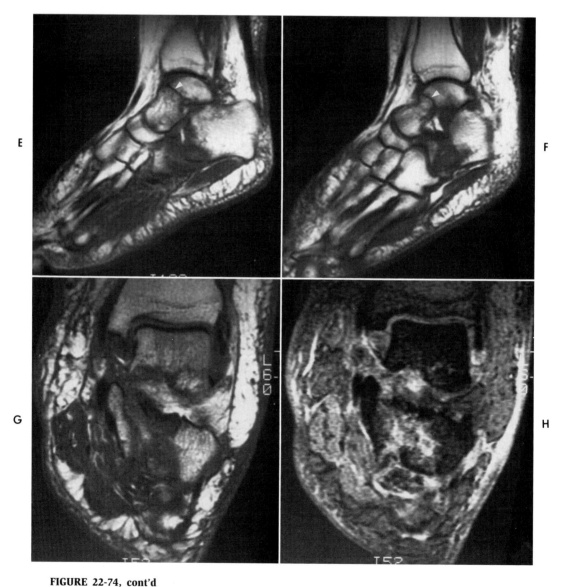

FIGURE 22-74, cont'd
E and **F,** Adjacent sagittal T1-weighted images show better definition of the talar fracture *(arrowhead).*
G and **H,** Coronal proton density and T2-weighted images at the same location. Marked comminution and spliting of the calcaneal fragments. (**A** to **H** courtesy Dr. Ed Lubat.)

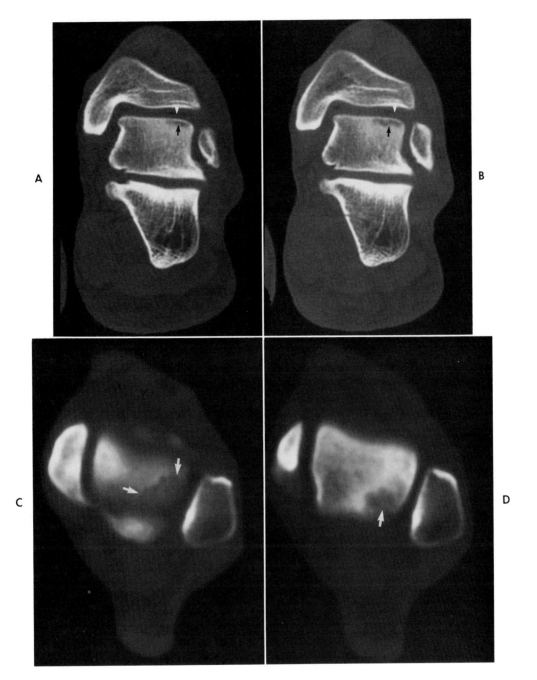

FIGURE 22-75
Osteochondritis dissecans of the talus. **A** and **B**, Coronal CT images through the ankle mortise. Defect in the subchondral bone on the lateral side of the talar dome *(arrow)*. The articular cortex appears intact. A small amount of air is seen in the joint space, produced by distraction of the joint and resulting in negative intraarticular pressure. The air outlines a normal layer of articular cartilage *(arrowhead)*. **C** and **D**, Axial CT images of the dome and articular cortex of the talus show the area of osteochondritis dissecans *(arrows)*.

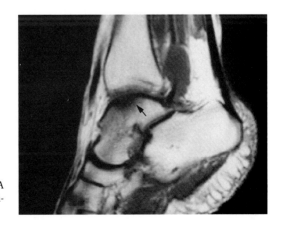

FIGURE 22-76
MRI of osteochondritis dissecans. Sagittal T1-weighted image. A low-signal zone in the dome of the talus represents the osteochondritis *(arrow)*.

produces thinning and fissures in the cartilage.

Reparative fibrocartilage filling in the fracture space also appears as a gray line of intermediate signal intensity. In such cases the necrotic bone fragment appears encircled by hyaline cartilage.[92]

Discontinuity of the articular cartilage covering an osseous lesion is a strong indication that the necrotic segment has become a loose fragment.[93] In such cases T2-weighted images may demonstrate articular fluid totally surrounding the loose fragment, including its deep surface, and appearing as a line of bright signal separating the bone fragment from its bed (Fig. 22-77). Partial separation of the osteochondral fragment may be seen (Fig. 22-78).

The underlying trabecular bone of the talus invariably has decreased signal intensity on T1- and T2-weighted MR images. At surgery it is found to correspond to reactive bony sclerosis seen in the normal viable bone that surrounds the focus of osteochondritis dissecans.

Occasionally, large cystic erosions filled with synovial fluid will be seen in the bed of osteochondritis; they appear on T2-weighted images as zones of homogeneously bright signal and on T1-weighted assume an intermediate intensity of signal.

Treatment of osteochondritis dissecans depends upon the presence or absence of mobility between the fragment and underlying bone as well as on the status of the covering cartilage.

In type I lesions immobilization may restore vascularity to the fragment, which is kept in position by the intact layer of overlapping articular cartilage.

In type II and type III lesions drilling from the normal talus across the line of separation and into the osteochondritis fragment has been observed to promote advancement of normal vascularity into the necrotic segment, thus promoting healing. Immobilization of the limb and non–weight bearing maintain the fragment in a constant relation to its bed, thus permitting vascularized granulation tissue to grow across the fracture line. The covering layer of cartilage may return to normal.

In type IV lesions removal of the necrotic loose body and curettage of the talar defect are necessary to prevent development of degenerative arthritis.[89,94]

AVASCULAR NECROSIS

In the ankle and foot avascular necrosis (AVN) of bone most commonly affects the talus, navicular, and metatarsals. In most cases it is due to trauma, either of the chronic repetitive type or following fractures and dislocations.[95,96]

In patients with lupus erythematous, sickle cell ane-

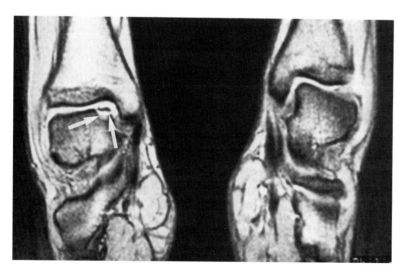
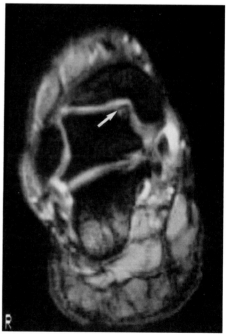

FIGURE 22-77
Osteochondritis dissecans (detached fragment). Coronal T2∗ image of both ankles. The medial side of the right talus has a detached osteochondral fragment surrounded by fluid *(arrows)*.

FIGURE 22-78
Osteochondritis dissecans, T2∗ image. Partial detachment of the necrotic fragment in the medial side of the talus *(arrow)*. Fluid in the posterior tibialis and flexor digitorum longus tendon sleeves.

mia, Gaucher's disease, or other disorders predisposing to bone marrow ischemia, avascular necrosis of the talus and navicular has been observed. Bilateral manifestations are often found.

Spontaneous osteonecrosis of the tarsal navicular is occasionally seen in obese adults with pes planus deformities. It is assumed that the medial shift of weight-bearing forces compromises the blood supply of the navicular by increasing the tension in the ligaments, capsule, and plantar aponeurosis.[96]

In the talus AVN can be encountered in the neck or head but most often is found in the dome, where it resembles advanced stages of osteochondritis dissecans.

The roentgenographic diagnosis of AVN is notoriously late. It has been established that the best method of detecting early stages of bone marrow ischemia is MRI. This is well documented in AVN of the femoral head. Similar data are being accumulated regarding AVN in other skeletal sites, including the talus.[95]

The MRI appearance of AVN is related to the stage of the disease. In the early phase the necrotic marrow has isointense signal; only the transition between normal and ischemic tissue appears as a zone of decreased signal on T1-weighted images. In later stages the necrotic marrow is hypointense. Eventually collapse of the dead bone leads to fractures of the cortical bone and covering cartilage. In some cases a "double line" sign can be seen — a separation of normal from ischemic bone by a band of low signal, and next to it and toward the ischemic bone a band of high signal. It is postulated that the low-signal band

represents the reactive bony sclerosis of healthy bone and the bright line represents edema and granulation tissue at the very margin of the necrotic bone. This orderly layering, described in Legg-Perthes disease, is rarely observed in AVN of the ankle and foot. In many cases the fractures or "bone bruises" seen with dislocations of the talus may produce signal abnormalities that predate and continue through to avascular necrosis (Fig. 22-79).

FOREIGN BODY DETECTION BY CT

Penetrating wounds of the foot are commonly encountered on emergency services. Most often thorns or wood splinters have pierced the skin and are embedded in the soft tissues of the plantar surface in patients who have been walking barefooted. Complete removal of superficial and visible foreign bodies can usually be accomplished without significant difficulty.

A different situation exists when the foreign body is not detectable by inspection, because either it is deeply seated or its point of entry has healed. Roentgenography has been used to detect radiopaque foreign bodies such as fragments of metal or glass or splinters of wood covered by lead-containing paint. Foreign bodies made of wood are not visible on roentgenograms.

When the diagnosis of retained foreign body has been made, finding its location is the most important step in preparing for its surgical removal. In the foot the multitudes of tendons and the complexity of osseous structures with interlocking surfaces make location by roentgenography difficult, even when the foreign bodies are radiopaque; obviously this is impossible when they are radiotransparent. Repeated surgical procedures often fail to retrieve such foreign bodies, which appear "lost in the haystack" of the complex anatomy of the foot.

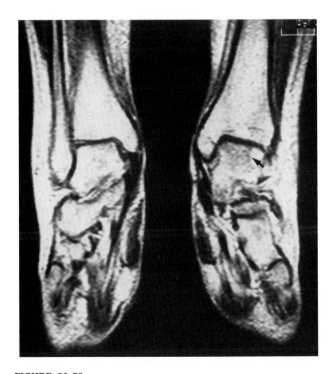

FIGURE 22-79
Avascular necrosis. Coronal T1-weighted image of both ankles in a patient with lupus erythematosus. Zones of decreased signal in the bone marrow of the talus represent the AVN *(arrow)*.

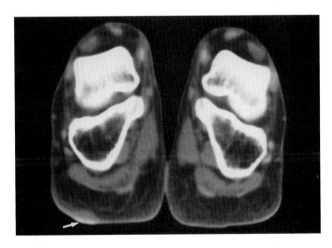

FIGURE 22-80
Foreign body granuloma. A 27-year-old woman with a 6-month history of persistent pain and swelling at the site of a puncture wound acquired when she stepped on a thorn. The CT image of both ankles shows a localized soft tissue swelling and thickening of the skin on the right plantar surface *(arrow)*. At surgery in the same location a 2 mm piece of wood was found, surrounded by a foreign body granuloma.

Computed tomography has been used for detection and precise location of foreign bodies in the extremities.[97-99] Compared with roentgenography, it has the double advantage of being able to detect nonmetallic foreign bodies and to locate them precisely in relation to bone as well as soft tissue structures. This facilitates their surgical removal with minimal trauma to normal structures (Figs. 22-80 to 22-82).

Occasionally the technique of scanning must be changed to accommodate marker placement at the point of best surgical entry for removal of a foreign body. Specifically, when the foreign body may still be in one of the plantar compartments, it is beneficial to scan the foot placed in a lateral recumbent position. This leaves the skin on the plantar surface exposed and free for marking. Once the foreign body has been detected, the most approachable point is identified on the skin with a radiopaque marker; a repeat CT image at this level confirms the correct spatial relation between the foreign body and the marker placed at the site of planned skin incision (Fig. 22-83).

On MR images foreign bodies of wood or glass appear as signal void zones with sharply circumscribed margins.[100] To avoid scanning patients with ferromagnetic foreign bodies, clinical history and plain roentgenographs must be used. Retained metal fragments may move in the tissue and produce further damage when the patients enter the magnetic field of the scanner.

OSTEOID OSTEOMA

Osteoid osteoma is a benign disease of unknown etiology characterized by a nidus containing highly vascular osteoid tissue. The typical clinical presentation is pain, worse at night, and usually relieved by salicylates.

When an osteoid osteoma is present in the metaphysis or diaphysis of a long bone, sclerosis and thickening of the cortex appear around the nidus.[101] These features make the diagnosis relatively easy on roentgenograms. However, when localized in cancellous bone, especially in a subperiosteal location, the nidus is difficult to detect roentgenographically; the characteristic sclerosis may be absent, and the nidus may contain calcification, making it isodense to the surrounding bone.[102]

The MRI features of osteoid osteoma in a short tubular bone are relatively nonspecific. On T1-weighted images a large zone of decreased signal intensity is seen in the marrow near the nidus. On T2-weighted images the same zone has increased signal intensity. These changes have been explained to be the result of hyperemia in the normal bone surrounding the nidus. When the reactive bony sclerosis is the dominant element around the nidus, then on both T1- and T2-weighted images the signal will be decreased in the marrow. The nidus itself is of intermediate or low signal intensity on T1- and T2-weighted images. The explanations for this signal change can be attributed to the presence of calcifications, a flow phenomenon in the richly vascularized nidus, or a combination of these.[103]

Occasionally the nidus will be too small and the signal contrast with the surrounding bone not great enough to make it visible. Even in such cases there is a benefit derived from MR imaging: the abnormal marrow signal establishes the existence and site of an abnormality. This narrows the search to a specific location. In a young patient presenting with pain worse at night and relieved by salicylates the clinical diagnosis is strongly in favor of osteoid osteoma. Finding the exact location of the nidus can be accomplished by subsequently obtaining a CT scan targeted specifically to the segmental abnormality seen on MR images. In the cancellous bone of the tarsals a zone of focal decreased density is easily seen on CT axial images.[104,105] Size estimation and precise location of the

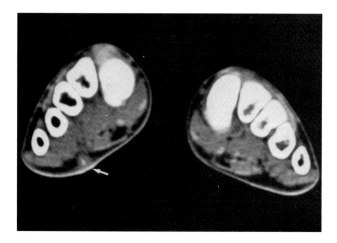

FIGURE 22-81
CT detection of a small foreign body. Coronal image of both feet. The radiopaque foreign body *(arrow)* is surrounded by soft tissue swelling in the right plantar surface. At surgery a piece of wood covered with paint was removed.

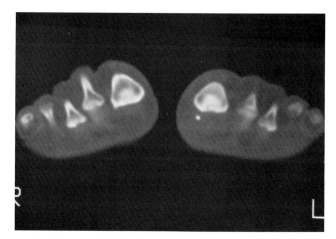

FIGURE 22-82
Locating a foreign body. CT image of both feet. A metallic density is located in the soft tissues on the plantar surface of the left proximal first phalanx.

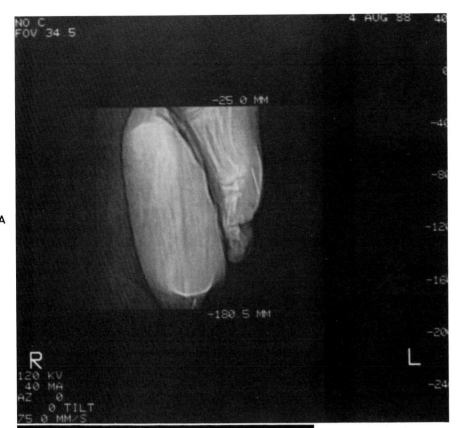

A

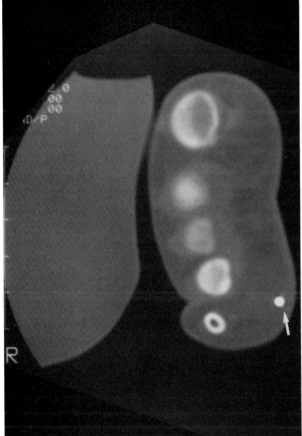

B

FIGURE 22-83
Metallic foreign body in the foot. **A,** Scout view of the foot in lateral decubitus immobilized with a water bag on the dorsal surface. The plantar surface was left free for placement of markers to indicate the best site of surgical approach for removal of the foreign body. A linear metallic density representing a needle embedded in the soft tissues on the plantar surface of the foot is visible. **B,** Axial image showing the most superficial location at the inferior end of the embedded foreign body *(arrow).*

nidus in relation to the bone surface make CT images an invaluable help in surgical planning. Thus targeting of surgery toward the nidus is possible with minimal distortion of unaffected tissues. Thorough curetting of the nidus is usually curative.

DIABETIC FOOT PATHOLOGY

Diabetes mellitus is estimated to affect 5% of persons in the United States, commonly producing complications that involve the feet and ankles—neuropathic joint disease, dystrophic ulcers, and infection of soft tissues and bones. Some of these complications coexist, merge with others, and lead to progressive disorganization of the ankle and foot, ultimately necessitating amputation.[106,107]

The overlap of roentgenographic manifestations has made the differential diagnosis between neuropathic joint disease and osteomyelitis rather difficult.[108-109] Newer imaging modalities are being used to resolve this dilemma. Scintigraphic evaluation of a pathological process in the feet of diabetic patients is a sensitive method of detecting abnormalities, but it lacks specificity and precision of anatomical location.[110-112]

Neuropathic bone and joint disease

The neuropathic joint and bone disease of diabetics is directly related to their peripheral neuropathy. Diminished pain sensation and impaired proprioception decrease the patient's awareness of minor or even major injuries to ligaments, articular capsule, and bone surfaces normally exposed to stress. Decreased pain sensation allows continuous use of the extremity when ligaments have been stretched or the articular capsule is loose and the joint unstable. The continuous use of unstable joints produces fragmentation of the articular surfaces. Fragments of bone floating free in the synovial space act as loose bodies, become trapped between opposing articular cartilage layers, and thus further damage the joint surfaces. The hemorrhage present at the surface of the fragmented bone seeps in the joint space and produces a chronic inflammatory reaction in the synovium. Synovial

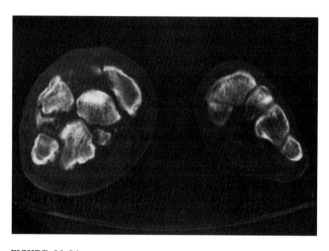

FIGURE 22-84
Neuropathic bone and joint disease, CT appearance. An axial image of both feet shows marked fragmentation and dislocation of the tarsal bones on the right side. The fragments retain some of their articular cortex, which is sharply defined. Soft tissue swelling is seen circumferentially around the tarsal bones.

fluid and blood accumulating in the joint space produce further stretching of the capsule and ligaments, enhancing instability of the joint; subluxations and frank dislocations appear. These, in turn, lead to further fragmentation of the osseous structures. The vicious circle of pathological effects of normal weight bearing proceeds ultimately to disorganization of the joints of the ankle and foot, transforming them into "a bag of bones." Bone resorption at the fracture contributes also to loss of the normal contour of articular surfaces. In the chronic phase of neuropathic joint disease attempts at healing produce sclerosis of bone and periosteal reaction. At this stage it is most difficult to differentiate the process from chronic osteomyelitis.

Computed tomography. CT images of neuropathic joint disease of the ankle and foot show diffuse soft tissue swelling, osteochondral fractures, and fragments of bone free in the joint space or embedded in the synovial lining.

The most frequently involved areas are the tarsometatarsal joints and the talonavicular, calcaneocuboidal, and cuboidocuneiform joints. A characteristic feature of this destructive form of neuroarthropathy is the relative preservation of cortex in the bone fragments splintered off the joint surface (Fig. 22-84). CT is particularly well suited to showing this feature of neuropathic joint disease because it displays thin slices of the complex structures, otherwise overlapped in the diseased joint transformed into a "bag of bones." Individual bone fragments can be analyzed and each of their surfaces evaluated in consecutive axial images (Fig. 22-85).

Another bone abnormality seen in the feet of diabetic patients is resorption of the distal diaphyses and epiphyses of the metatarsals. Slow but progressive bone loss produces deformities that have a "sharpened pencil" appearance.[113] On CT axial images of the forefoot this

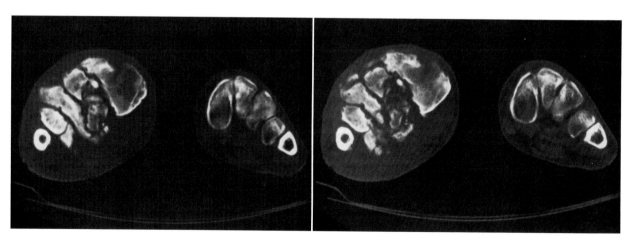

FIGURE 22-85
CT differentiation between infection and neuropathic joint disease. Axial images of both feet show fragmentation of the cuneiforms and navicular on the right side. Despite the fact that there is marked disorganization of bone structures, the splintered segments retain their intact cortex even at the margin of the fractures. This is in favor of mechanical trauma due to lack of proprioception, which has led to fragmentation of the joint surfaces but has not destroyed the untraumatized segments of cortex. An infectious process would produce indiscriminate generalized erosion and osteolysis of bone fragments.

appears as a decrease in metatarsal diameter, with obliteration of the medullary cavity by densely sclerotic and thickened cortical bone. Usually no soft tissue abnormalities are seen around these resorption sites in the metatarsals — an important feature distinguishing this process from chronic osteomyelitis.

Magnetic resonance. MR images of neuropathic joint disease of the foot and ankle show the same characteristic pattern of bone fragmentation and joint disorganization. Unlike other imaging modalities, MRI can directly detect hemorrhage/edema in the marrow, usually present at the margin of the fragmented bone and appearing as a zone of decreased signal on T1-weighted images and increased signal on T2-weighted images.

The joint effusion and inflammatory reaction in the synovium commonly present with neuropathic joint disease of the ankle appear on MR images very similar to the findings observed with infectious arthritis complicated by osteomyelitis. Both have increased signal on T2-weighted images. The preserved cortical bone of fragments with sharp intact margins is better demonstrated on CT images. In this particular situation CT apparently has the advantage over MRI by providing more precise information regarding cortical bone.

Infection

Diabetics, in general, have a propensity for infectious complications; it is not uncommon to see a severely disorganized neuropathic joint transformed into a site of osteomyelitis. The inflammatory and hemorrhagic fluid in the joint and the loose fragments of bone provide a good culture medium in which germs can multiply.[114] The microorganisms can gain access by direct spread from an ulceration in the adjacent soft tissue or through a hematogenous route. Once infected, the fluid quickly spreads the germs to the entire exposed fracture site, producing an osteomyelitis.

The hallmark of pyogenic osteomyelitis is rapid progression of osteolysis, involving indiscriminately cortical and spongy bone. Paraosseous soft tissue abscesses are common. Occasionally air is seen in the soft tissues or bone, signifying infection with gas-producing microorganisms. Usually the infection of soft tissues is propagated along the fascial compartments of the foot.[115] Occasionally the breakdown of tissue layers produced by the proteolytic enzymes of the pathogenic organisms will spread the infection through fascial septa to adjacent compartments. This specific information of the extent of soft tissue involvement of foot infections in diabetics is important for planning the level of amputation. Of all imaging modalities, MRI is best able to detect such abnormalities.[116,117]

Magnetic resonance. MRI of foot infections should consist of coronal T2-weighted and axial T1-weighted sequences.[118]

T2-weighted images of both feet obtained in a coronal plane are the best way to study soft tissue involvement: ulcerations of the skin are seen, and abscesses are portrayed as high–signal intensity collections.[119] The cellulitis commonly involving diabetic feet appears as a diffuse zone of increased signal; in the subcutaneous fat layer it assumes a criss-crossing pattern of lines with increased signal on T2-weighted images and decreased on T1-weighted[120-122] (Fig. 22-86).

Osteomyelitis of the metatarsal or tarsal bones is manifested on MR images as zones of abnormal signal in

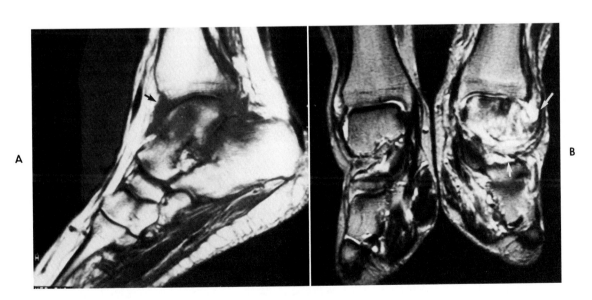

FIGURE 22-86
Osteomyelitis and septic arthritis. **A,** Sagittal T1-weighted images of the ankle show abnormally low signal in the marrow of the talus and calcaneus. Fluid in the tibiotalar joint is seen protruding anteriorly as an intermediate-signal zone *(arrow).* **B,** A coronal T2-weighted of both ankles shows the high-signal zone in the marrow of the talus at the site of osteomyelitis. There is fluid in the lateral mortise and in the subtalar joint *(arrows).* Diffuse soft tissue swelling and increased signal in the periarticular soft tissues of the left ankle are evident.

the bone marrow: increased signal on T2-weighted and decreased on T1-weighted images (Fig. 22-86). Interruption of the band of signal void representing the cortical bone is frequently seen adjacent to the focus of marrow infection (Fig. 22-87).

Computed tomography. CT images of infections in the feet display a multitude of abnormal findings, best seen when the images are obtained perpendicular to the plantar surface (coronal plane). Comparison with the opposite site helps to detect subtle abnormalities.[123]

The skin is usually thickened in the zone of active inflammatory process. A crisscrossing pattern of intermediate-density lines is seen in the subcutaneous fat layer. These findings signify the cellulitis that frequently presents around a focus of infection (Fig. 22-88).

Ulcerations of the skin and underlying soft tissue layers are easily seen on CT images; the exact relationship between the bottom of the ulcer and the deep bone structures can be readily established (Fig. 22-89).

Soft tissue abscesses are best seen on CT images obtained after the intravenous injection of contrast. The hyperemic layer of tissue that forms the wall of an abscess becomes denser on postenhanced images, contrasting with the low-density fluid center (Fig. 22-90). The osteolytic lesions of osteomyelitis are seen on CT images as zones of cortical bone destruction and low-density foci

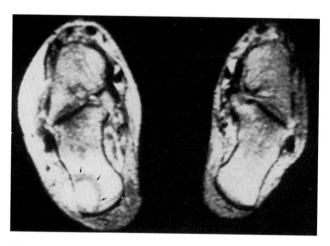

FIGURE 22-87
MRI of osteomyelitis. Proton density axial image of the calcaneus. A rim of abnormally low signal surrounds a focus of osteomyelitis *(arrows)*. The lateral cortex is destroyed; diffuse soft tissue swelling is present.

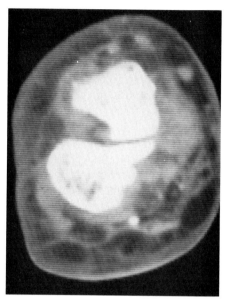

FIGURE 22-88
Cellulitis of the right foot, coronal CT image. The reticular pattern of dense lines in the soft tissue layers represents lymphangitis. The skin is abnormally thick, an indication of edema.

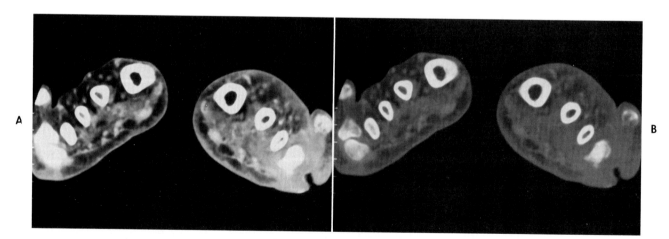

FIGURE 22-89
Osteomyelitis of the metatarsals in a diabetic. This 64-year-old man had had the distal part of his left fifth metatarsal amputated for osteomyelitis. Persistent ulceration in the soft tissues and pain in the lateral side of the left foot were the reasons for this CT examination. **A,** An axial CT image through the feet shows an ulceration in the lateral part of the soft tissues on the left side. Diffuse soft tissue swelling is seen around the fourth metatarsal, which appears abnormally dense. **B,** Same image viewed with bone windows showing the destruction of the posterior lateral margin of the left fourth metatarsal, in the vicinity of the soft tissue ulcer, an indication of osteomyelitis. The medullary cavity is obliterated by sclerotic dense bone, a sign of chronic infection.

in the spongy bone of the epiphyses and metaphyses. A calcified periosteal reaction appears on axial images as fuzziness of the cortical margins produced by the added layer of fluffy calcification on the external surface of the original cortex.

Spread of infection. The longitudinal spread of soft tissue infections in the forefoot is well documented on both CT and MR images.

The abnormalities in specific fascial compartments can be traced proximally on sagittal images or sequential axial sections. Infections propagated from the first or fifth toe are initially localized respectively to the medial or lateral compartment. When the infection originates at metatarsophalangeal joints II to IV, the middle compartment is affected.[123] Spread of such infections proximally can extend to the hindfoot and further into the calf, where it gains access along the course of the flexor tendons. The MR images will show continuous zones of increased signal intensity on the T2-weighted images. On T1-weighted images the fat layers separated by the normal fibrous septations lose their sharp borders and high signal. Similarly, in axial CT the soft tissue swelling of specific compartments can be traced proximally on sequential images (Fig. 22-91).

The strict division into three compartments applies only to the forefoot. In the ankle and just distal to it, these compartments are not well defined and the oblique course of some of the tendons creates routes of access for spread of infection in a multitude of directions.

Differential diagnosis. The differential diagnosis of infections and neuropathic disease of the feet in diabetic patients is occasionally difficult. Several features — periosseous edema, inflammatory reaction in the synovium, joint effusions — are common manifestions in both, even though to different degrees.[124] The infectious processes tend to have more focal soft tissue inflammation and periosseous abscesses. However, bone destruction assumes the characteristic pattern for each: in an infection

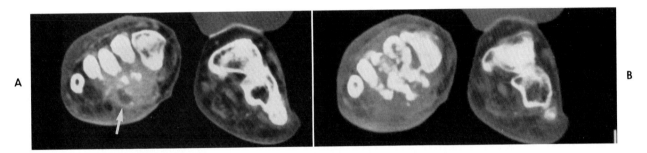

FIGURE 22-90
Soft tissue abscess and osteomyelitis of the metatarsals in a diabetic. Coronal CT images obtained after intravenous injection of contrast. **A,** Abscess in the soft tissues on the plantar side of the right foot *(arrow).* **B,** Osteomyelitis of the second, third, and fourth metatarsals is seen as marked fragmentation and destruction of bone. There is diffuse soft tissue swelling around the area of bone destruction. The skin is abnormally thick compared to the opposite side.

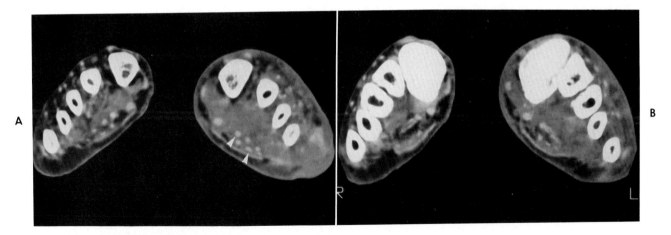

FIGURE 22-91
Spread of infection in the plantar compartments. **A,** An axial CT image through the metatarsal diaphysis shows tracking of the soft tissue infection in the middle compartment of the left foot, manifested as soft tissue swelling with displacement of the flexor tendons in a plantar direction *(arrowheads).* The fifth metatarsal is absent from this slice; it was amputated near its base. **B,** Another axial image, obtained at the base of the metatarsals, shows tracking of the soft tissue swelling further proximal in the middle compartment of the plantar spaces.

the entire joint is involved as a unit, most of the exposed surfaces of bone become eroded, and the amount of articular fluid is quite large; in neuropathic joint disease fragmentation of bone occurs, and there is dislocation with unexpectedly advanced disorganization of the joint for the amount of symptoms experienced by the patient. Even though some diabetics have pain as the presenting symptom of neuropathic bone and joint disease, the objective findings are always much more severe than the symptoms would predict. Preservation of intact cortex in the splintered fragments of bone is a strong sign against infection.

Occasionally the differentiation between osteomyelitis and neuropathic disease cannot be made with certainty by any of the imaging modalities; in such cases only aspiration of fluid and culture firmly establishes the diagnosis.

ARTHRITIS

The diagnosis of *rheumatoid arthritis* (RA) is usually made by correlation between the clinical and laboratory data and confirmed roentgenographically when characteristic erosions of articular cortex are seen. Rarely is there any need for CT and MRI in establishing the diagnosis.

MRI can depict the early manifestations of RA, especially erosions of the articular cartilage and abnormalities limited to the soft tissue structures (synovitis, pannus, joint effusions).[125] Even bone erosions may be seen better on CT and MR compared to plain films, mostly because the tomographic nature of these modalities permits visualization of thin sections of complex overlapping joint surfaces.[125,126] By detecting these minor erosions, MR can be used as a quantitative evaluation of response to different therapy regimens.[125] The noninvasive nature of MRI permits repeated follow-up examinations during the course of this prolonged chronic disease. Thus an objective image-based assessment of response to therapy can be made — especially important for patients treated with relatively toxic substances such as gold salts or antimalarial drugs. Those who do not respond positively can be detected in time, before leukopenia, thrombocytopenia, or retinopathy has developed.

The MR features of RA are nonspecific; it is mostly their location that contributes to the characterization of this arthritis. In the ankles and feet the intertarsal and metatarsophalangeal joints are most often affected.

The joints involved usually contain abnormally large amount of fluid, manifested as collections of bright signal on T2-weighted images (Fig. 22-92). The pannus may

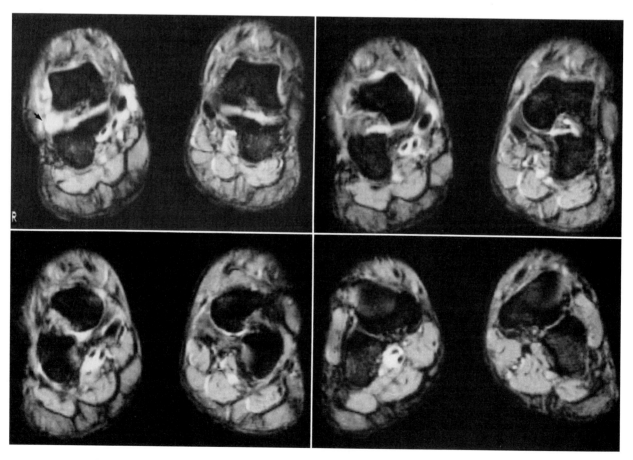

FIGURE 22-92
MRI of early-stage rheumatoid arthritis. Coronal T2* images of the right ankle and foot show fluid in the subtalar joint *(arrow)*, around the neck of the talus, and in the sleeves of the medial tendons.

appear of higher signal intensity when compared to synovial fluid. Occasionally hemosiderin deposited even in small amounts in the pannus of RA can give a relatively low signal intensity in both T1- and T2-weighted pulse sequences.[125] In this respect there is a similar appearance to the MRI of synovium in hemophilic arthritis.[127] The erosions of the articular cartilage and cortical bone appear as defects filled with either fluid or low-signal fibrin deposits.

The problem of differential diagnosis arises when other pathological processes (e.g., infection, neuropathic joint disease, pathological fractures) complicate the course of rheumatoid arthritis. In these instances MRI offers the benefit of visualization of fluid collections in the joint and tendon sleeve and direct visualization of pannus. CT images obtained in such cases demonstrate with better precision the location of fracture fragments and the amount of cortical bone destruction (Fig. 22-93).

Gout is one arthritic process that often involves the joints of the foot and ankle. The MRI manifestations of gouty arthritis parallel to a certain extent these seen on roentgenograms. Specifically erosions of bone are present at the sites where tophi develop, at the base of the great toe, or in the intertarsal joints. The tophus appears with an intermediate signal intensity in T1 and T2-weighted sequences (Fig. 22-94). There is usually a sharp zone of transition between the tophus and the adjacent normal bone marrow, when the scan is obtained in a quiscent stage of gouty arthritis. The overhanging edge of bone at the margin of the gouty tophus is seen in MRI similar to the appearence observed in roentgenographs. Whenever acute manifestations of disease are present, the inflammatory reaction around the tophus would give an increased signal intensity due to the high content of water in the flammatory infiltrate.

Infectious arthritis has nonspecific MR findings. Usu-

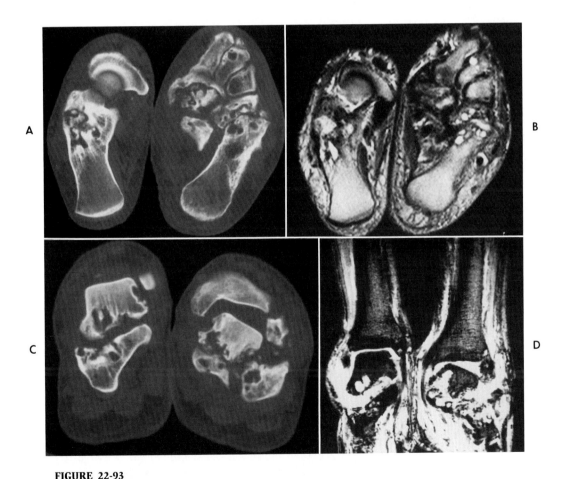

FIGURE 22-93
Rheumatoid arthritis complicated by infection and fracture. **A,** Axial CT images of both feet. **B,** A T2-weighted axial, same level as **A. C,** Coronal CT image of the subtalar joint. **D,** T2*-weighted coronal, same level as **C** (TR 630 msec/TE 20 msec, flip angle 20 degrees). There is bilateral erosive arthritis. The left calcaneus has been fractured and the talus is subluxated and rotated. The CT images better demonstrate the extensive amount of erosion of the articular cortex in the left subtalar joint, a sign of septic arthritis. The exact position and contour of each fractured fragment are better seen on the CT images. The MR images better outline the soft tissue edema and fluid in the joint space.

ally joint effusion is present, and there is a zone of abnormally low signal on T1-weighted images and increased signal on T2-weighted images in the marrow adjacent to the area of infection, a manifestation of hyperemia in the bone adjacent to the infectious process of the joint. When the disease is advanced and erosion of the articular cortex has taken place, the abnormality is

already in the stage of osteomyelitis complicating the infectious arthritis. (See Chapter 9.)

The erosions of articular cortex are better demonstrated by CT than by MRI. In the tarsal areas specifically, it is advantageous to obtain CT of the ankle and foot whenever early-stage cortical bone erosion needs to be detected in the subtalar articulation.[128] In the chronic stage of

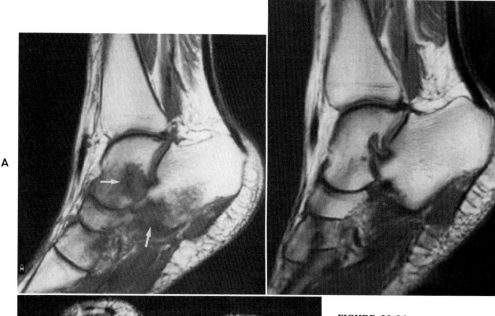

FIGURE 22-94
Tophaceous gout. **A,** Sagittal T1-weighted image of the right foot. Tophi are seen as well-circumscribed zones of intermediate signal intensity in the talus and calcaneus *(arrows)*. There is a zone of hyperemia in the marrow of the calcaneus posterior to them. Overhanging edges seen on MR images are similar to the characteristic roentenographic findings of gouty arthritis. **B,** A comparison MR image of the left foot shows the normal contour of the subtalar joint. **C,** An axial T2-weighted image shows the tophus, with intermediate signal intensity *(arrow)*. The hyperemic zone in the calcaneus has increased signal intensity *(arrowheads)*. There is diffuse soft tissue swelling, with edema and accumulation of fluid, in the tendon sleeves, consistent with the nonspecific inflammatory reaction of an acute attack of gout.

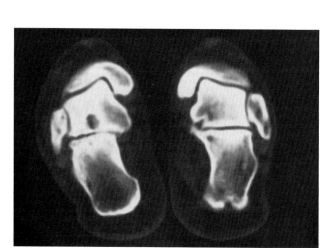

FIGURE 22-95
Chronic stage of pyogenic arthritis of the right subtalar articulation. A CT image of the ankles shows the joint space in the right subtalar articulation to be narrow. There is sclerosis of the subarticular bone with a large cystic erosion in the right talus, at the site of a chronic staphylococcal infection.

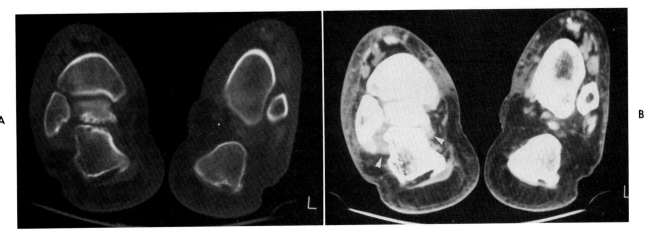

FIGURE 22-96
Infectious arthritis with *Candida albicans.* This 61-year-old woman with a long history of disseminated lupus erythematous treated with high doses of corticosteroids had had progressive pain in the right ankle for 3 months. A, A coronal CT image through the subtalar joint and ankle mortise shows erosive changes in the subchondral bone and the subtalar articular cortex. B, The same slice viewed with soft tissue windows shows fluid and synovial swelling at the margin of the subtalar joint protruding medially as well as laterally into the space between the calcaneus and fibula *(arrowheads)*. *Candida albicans* was isolated in fluid cultures.

pyogenic infections CT can detect the sclerotic reaction around a cortical erosion and the narrow and irregular articular space of the subtalar joint (Fig. 22-95).

Tuberculous arthritis is rarely seen in the ankle and foot. Delay in diagnosis is directly related to the difficulty of detection early stages of the disease using only roentgenograms. CT is the best modality for evaluating minimal erosions of the articular cortex. In most cases a large amount of fluid is present in the synovial spaces adjacent to the infectious process. Tuberculous arthritis produces marked periarticular osteoporosis, seen on CT images as decreased density of the adjacent bone structures.

Other rare chronic infections with organisms such as *Candida albicans* can produce nonspecific findings of bone erosion and fluid in the subtalar joint (Fig. 22-96). In these cases the role of CT and MRI is to detect the bone abnormalities and help determine the precise location of the fluid collections, which must be tapped for bacteriological diagnosis.

REFERENCES

1. Heger L, Wulff K: Computed tomography of the calcaneus: normal anatomy. AJR 1985;145:123-129.
2. Seltzer S, Weismann B, Braunstein EM, et al: Computed tomography of the hindfoot. J Comput Assist Tomogr 1986;8:488-497.
3. Solomon MA, Gilula LA: CT scanning of the foot and ankle: normal anatomy. AJR 1986;146:1192-1203.
4. Solomon MA, Gilula LA: CT scanning of the foot and ankle: clinical applications and review of the literature. AJR 1986;146:1204-1214.
5. Keyser CK, Gilula LA, Handy DC, et al: Soft tissue abnormalities of the ankle and foot: CT diagnosis. AJR 1988;150:845-850.
6. Middleton WD, Lawson TL: Anatomy and MRI of the joints: a multiplanar atlas. New York, Raven, 1988.
7. Beltran J. Noto AM, Mosure JC, et al: Ankle: surface coil MR imaging at 1.5T. Radiology 1986;161:203-209.
8. Hajek PC, Baker LL, Björkengren A, et al: High-resolution magnetic resonance imaging of the ankle: normal anatomy. Skeletal Radiol 1986;15:536-540.
9. Sartoris DJ, Resnick D: Pictorial review: cross-sectional imaging of the foot and ankle. Foot Ankle 1987;8:59-80.
10. Kneeland BJ, Macrandar S, Middleton WD, et al: MR imaging of the normal ankle: correlation with anatomic sections. AJR 1988;151:117-123.
11. Sartoris DJ, Resnick D: Cross-sectional imaging of the foot: test of anatomical knowledge. J Foot Surg 1988;27:374-383.
12. Crim JR, Cracchiolo A, Bassett LW, et al: Magnetic resonance imaging of the hindfoot. Foot Ankle 1989;10:1-7.
13. Noto AM, Cheung Y, Rosenberg ZS, et al: MR imaging of the ankle: normal variants. Radiology 1989;170;121-124.
14. Erickson SJ, Quinn SF, Kneeland JB, et al: MR imaging of the tarsal tunnel and related spaces: normal and abnormal findings with anatomic correlation. AJR 1990;155:323-328.
15. Clemente CD: Anatomy. A regional atlas of the human body, ed. Baltimore, Urban & Schwarzenberg, 1981, pp 424-449.
16. Pernkopf E: Atlas of topographical and applied human anatomy. Philadelphia, Saunders. 1964. Vol 2, pp 387-402.
17. Netter FH: Atlast of human anatomy. New York, Ciba-Geigy, 1989, pp 492-505.
18. Donaldon JS, Poznanski AK, Nieves A: CT of children's feet: an immoblization technique. AJR 1987;148:169-170.
19. Smith RW, Staple TW: Computerized tomography (CT) scanning technique for the hindfoot. Clin Orthop Rel Res 1983;177:34-38.
20. Guyer BH, Levinsohn EM, Frederickson BE, et al: Computed tomography of calcaneal fractures: anatomy, pathology, dosimetry, and clinical relevance. AJR 1985;145:911-919.
21. Mann FA, Gilula LA: Direct sagittal CT of the foot. (Letter.) AJR 1989;153:886.
22. Woolson ST, Dev P, Fellingham L, Vassiliadis A: Three-dimensional imaging of the ankle joint from computerized tomography. Foot Ankle 1985;6:2-6.
23. Magid D, Fishman EK: Imaging of musculoskeletal trauma in three-dimensions. An integrated two-dimensional/three-dimensional approach with computed tomography. Radiol Clin North Am 1989;27:945-956.

24. Ney DR, Fishman EK, Magid D, Kuhlman JE: Interactive real-time multiplanar CT imaging. Radiology 1989;170:275-276.

25. Magid D, Michelson JD, Ney D, Fishman EK: Adult ankle fractures: comparison of plain films and interactive two and three-dimensional CT scans. AJR 1990;154:1017-1023.

26. Beltran J, Munchow AM, Khabiri H, et al: Ligaments of the lateral aspect of the ankle and sinus tarsi: an MR imaging study. Radiology 1990;177:455-458.

27. Chieng PU, Davison PA Djukic S, et al: Optimisation of three-dimensional MR imaging reconstruction of the tendons and cortical bone in the ankle. Radiology 1989;173(P):356.

28. Rusineck H, Mourino MR, Firooznia H, et al: Volumetric rendering of MR images. Radiology 1989;171:269-272.

29. Cowell HR, Elener V: Rigid painful flatfoot secondary to tarsal coalition. Clin Orthop Rel Res 1983;177:54-60.

30. Wray JB, Herndon CN: Hereditary transmission of congenital coalition of calcaneus to the navicular. J Bone Joint Surg [Am] 1963;45:365-378.

31. Leonard MA: The inheritance of tarsal coalition and its relationship to spastic flatfoot. J Bone Joint Surg [Br] 1974; 56:520-526.

32. Stormont DM, Peterson HA: The relative incidence of tarsal coalition. Clin Orthop Rel Res 1983;181:28-36.

33. Wheeler R, Guevera A, Bleck EE: Tarsal coalitions: review of the literature and case report of bilateral dual calcaneonavicular and talocalcaneal coalitions. Clin Orthop Rel Res 1981; 156:175-177.

34. Elkus RA: Tarsal coalition in the young athelete. Am J Sports Med 1986;14(6):477-480.

35. Firooznia H, Golimbu C, Rafii M: Computerized tomography in detection of joint disorders. Orthop Rev 1983;12:69-82.

36. Herzenberg JE, Goldner JL, Martinez S, Silverman PM: Computerized tomography of talocancaneal tarsal coalition: a clinical and anatomic study. Foot Ankle 1986;6:273-289.

37. Sarno RC, Carter BL, Bankoff MS, Semine MC: Computed tomography of tarsal coalition. J Comput Assist Tomogr 1984;8:1155-1160.

38. Pineda C, Resnick D, Greenway G: Diagnosis of tarsal coalition with computed tomography. Clin Orthop Rel Res 1986; 208:282-288.

39. Bower BL, Keyser C, Gilula LA: Rigid subtalar joint — a radiographic spectrum. Skeletal Radiol 1989;17:583-538.

40. Lee MS, Harcke HT, Kumar SJ, Bassett GS: Subtalar joint coalition in children: new observations. Radiology 1989; 172:635-639.

41. Mosier KM, Asher M: Tarsal coalitions and peroneal spastic flatfoot. J Bone Joint Surg [Am] 1984;66:976-984.

42. Inglis G, Buxton RA, Macnicol MF: Symptomatic calcaneonavicular bars. The results 20 years after surgical excision. J Bone Joint Surg [Br] 1986;68:128-131.

43. Olney BW, Asher MA: Excision of symptomatic coalition of the middle facet of the talocalcaneal joint. J Bone Joint Surg [Am] 1987;69:539-544.

44. Scranton PE Jr: Treatment of symptomatic talocalcaneal coalition. J Bone Joint Surg [Am] 1987;69:533-539.

45. Kelikian H, Kelikian AS: Disorders of the ankle. Philadelphia, Saunders, 1985.

46. Meyer JM, Hoffmeyer P, Savoy X: High resolution computed tomography in chronically painful ankle sprain. Foot Ankle 1988;8:291-296.

47. Berquist TH, Johnson KA: Trauma. In Berquist TH (ed): Radiology of the foot and ankle. New York, Raven, 1989, pp 99-104.

48. Kaye JJ: The ankle. In Freiberger RH, Kay JJ (eds): Arthrography. New York, Appleton, 1979, pp 237-256.

49. Ala-Ketola L, Puramen J, Koivisto E, Puupera M: Arthrography in the diagnosis of ligament injuries and classification of ankle injuries. Radiology 1977;125:63-69.

50. Sausner DD, Nelson RC, Levine M, Wa CW: Acute injuries of the lateral ligaments of the ankle: comparison of stress radiography and arthrography. Radiology 1983;148:653-657.

51. Bleichrodt RP, Kingma LM, Binnendijk B, Klein JP: Injuries of the lateral ankle ligaments: classification with tenography and arthrography. Radiology 1989;173:347-349.

52. Kerr R, Forrester DM, Kingston S: Magnetic resonance imaging of the foot and ankle trauma. Orthop Clin North Am 1990; 21:591-601.

53. Kleinman M, Grass AE: Achilles tendon rupture following steroid injection. J Bone Joint Surg [Am] 1983;65:1345-1347.

54. Kaplan PA, Anderson JC, Norris MA, Metamoros A: Ultrasonography of post-traumatic soft tissue lesions. Radiol Clin North Am. 1989;27:973-982.

55. Beltran J, Noto AM, Herman LJ, et al: Tendon: high-field strength surface coil MR imaging. Radiology 1987;162:735-740.

56. Quinn SF, Murray WT, Clark RA, et al: Achilles tendon: MR imaging at 1.5T. Radiology 1987;174:767-770.

57. Keene JS, Lash EG, Fisher DR, DeSmet AA: Magnetic resonance imaging of Achilles tendon rupture. Am J Sports Med 1989;17:333-337.

58. Johnson KA: Tibialis posterior tendon rupture. Clin Orthop Rel Res 1983;177:140-147.

59. Funk DA, Cass RJ, Johnson KA: Acquired adult flat foot secondary to posterior tibial tendon pathology. J Bone Joint Surg [Am] 1986;68:95-102.

60. Downey DJ, Simkin DA, Mack LA, et al: Tibialis posterior tendon rupture. Arthritis Rheum 1988;31:441-446.

61. Norris SH, Mankin HJ: Chronic tenosynovitis of the posterior tibial tendon with new bone formation. J Bone Joint Surg [Br] 1978;60:523-526.

62. Rosenberg ZS, Jahss MH, Noto AM, et al: Rupture of the posterior tibialis tendon: CT and surgical findings. Radiology 1988;167:489-493.

63. Rosenberg ZA, Cheung Y, Jahss MH, et al: Rupture of posterior tibial tendon: CT and MR imaging with surgical correlation. Radiology 1988;169:229-235.

64. Alexander IJ, Johnson KA, Berquist TH: Magnetic resonance imaging in diagnosis of disruption of the posterior tibial tendon. Foot Ankle 1987;8:144-147.

65. Marti R: Dislocation of the peroneal tendons. Am J Sports Med 1977;5:19-22.

66. Szczukowski M Jr, St Pierre RK, Fleming LL, Somogyi J: Computerized tomography in the evaluation of peroneal tendon dislocation. Am J Sports Med. 1983;11:444-447.

67. Rosenberg ZS, Feldman F, Singson RD: Peroneal tendon injuries: CT analysis. Radiology 1986;161:743-748.

68. Zeiss J, Sademi SR, Ebraheim NA: MR imaging of the peroneal tunnel. J Comput Assist Tomogr 1989;13:840-844.

69. Unger EC, Summers TB: Bone marrow. Top Magn Reson Imag 1989;1:31-52.

70. Salter RB, Harris WR: Injuries involving the epiphyseal plate. J Bone Joint Surg [Am] 1963;45:587-622.

71. Cone RO III, Nguyen V, Flournoy M, Guerra J Jr: Triplane fracture of the distal tibial epiphysis: radiographic and CT studies. Radiology 1984;153:763-767.

72. Feldman F, Singson RD, Rosenberg ZS, et al: Distal tibial triplane fractures: diagnosis with CT. Radiology 1987;164:429-435.

73. Mainwaring BL, Daffner RH, Riemer BL: Plyon fractures of the ankle: a distinct clinical and radiologic entity. Radiology 1988;168:215.

74. Kellam JF, Waddel JP: Fractures of the distal tibial metaphysis with intra-articular extension: the distal tibial explosion fracture. J Trauma 1979;19:593-601.

75. Mitchell MJ, Ho C, Resnick D, Sartoris DJ: Diagnostic imaging of the lower extremity trauma. Radiol Clin North Am 1989;27:909-928.

76. Rogers LF: The ankle. In Rogers LF (ed): Radiology of skeletal trauma. New York, Churchill Livingstone, 1982, p 791.

77. Wilson FC: Fractures and dislocations of the ankle. In Rockwood CA Jr., Green DF (eds): Fractures in adults. Philadelphia, Lippincott, 1984, p 1667.

78. Crosby LA, Fitzgibbons T: Computerized tomography scanning of acute intra-articular fractures of the calcaneus. A new classification system. J Bone Joint Surg [Am] 1990;72:852-860.

79. Burdeaux BD: Reduction of calcaneal fractures by McReynolds medial approach technique and its experimental basis. Clin Orthop Rel Res 1983;177:87-103.

80. Heger L, Wulff K, Seddigi MSA: Computed tomography of calcaneal fractures. AJR 1985;145:131-137.

81. Rosenberg ZS, Feldman F, Singson RD: Intra-articular calcaneal fractures: computed tomographic analysis. Skeletal Radiol 1987;16:105-113.

82. Rosenberg ZS, Feldman F, Singson RD, Price GJ: Peroneal tendon injury associated with calcaneal fractures: CT findings. AJR 1987;149:125-129.

83. Hardcastle PH, Reschauer R, Kutscha-Lissberg E, Schoffman W: Injuries to the tarsometatarsal joint. Incidence, classification and treatment. J Bone Joint Surg [Br] 1982;64:349-356.

84. Faciszewski T, Burks RT, Manaster BJ: Subtle injuries of the Lisfrank joint. J Bone Joint Surg[Am] 1990;72:1519-1522.

85. Goiney RC, Connell DG, Nichols DM: CT evaluation of tarsometatarsal fracture-dislocation injuries. AJR 1985;144: 985-990.

86. Berger PE, Oftein RA, Jackson DW, et al: MRI demonstration of radiographically occult fractures: what have we been missing? Radiographics 1989;9:407-436.

87. Yao L, Lee JK: Occult intraosseous fracture: detection with MR imaging. Radiology 1988;167:749-751.

88. Berndt AL, Harty M: Transchondral fractures (osteochondritis dissecans) of the talus. J Bone Joint Surg [Am] 1959;41:988-1020.

89. Pettine KA, Morrey BF: Osteochondral fractures of the talus. J Bone Joint Surg [Br] 1987;69:89-92.

90. Canale T, Belding RH: Osteochondral lesions of the talus. J Bone Joint Surg [Am] 1980;62:97-102.

91. Anderson IF, Crichton KF, Crattan-Smith T, et al: Osteochondral fractures of the dome of the talus. J Bone Joint Surg [Am] 1989;71:1143-1152.

92. Yulish BS, Mulopulos GP, Goodfellow DB, et al: MR imaging of osteochondral lesions of the talus. JCAT 1987;11:296-301.

93. Mesgarzadeh M, Sapega AA, Bonakdarpour S, et al: Osteochondritis dissecans: anaylsis of mechanical stability with radiography, scintigraphy, and MR imaging. Radiology 1987;165: 775-780.

94. Bauer M, Jonsson K, Linden B: Osteochondritis dissecans of the ankle. A 20 year follow-up study. J Bone Joint Surg [Br] 1987;69:93-96.

95. Sierra A, Potchen EJ, Moore J, Smith HG: High field magnetic resonance imaging of aseptic necrosis of the talus. J Bone Joint Surg [Am] 1986;68:927-928.

96. Haller J, Sartoris DJ, Resnick D, et al: Spontaneous osteonecrosis of the tarsal navicular in adults: imaging findings. AJR 1988;151:355-358.

97. Firooznia H, Björkengren A, Hofstetter SR, et al: Computed tomography in localization of foreign bodies lodged in the extremities. Comput Radiol 1984;8:237-239.

98. Niska R, Pomeranz S, Porat S: The advantage of computed tomography in locating a foreign body in the foot. J Trauma 1986;26:93-95.

99. Kuhns LR, Borlaza GS, Siegel RS, et al: An in vitro comparison of computed tomography, xeroradiography and radiography in the detection of soft tissue foreign bodies. Radiology 1979;132:218-219.

100. Bodne D, Quinn SF, Cochran CF: Imaging foreign glass and wooden bodies of the extremities with CT and MR. J Comput Assist Tomogr 1988;12:608-611.

101. Swee RG, McLeod RA, Beabout JW: Osteoid osteoma. Detection, diagnosis and localization. Radiology 1979;130:117-123.

102. Kenzora JE, Abrams RC: Problems encountered in the diagnosis and treatment of osteoid osteoma of the talus. Foot Ankle 1981;2:172-178.

103. Yeager BA, Schiebler ML, Wertheim SP, et al: MR imaging of osteoid osteoma of the talus. J Comput Assist Tomogr 1987;11:916.

104. Pitman MI, Norman A: Value of CT scanning in differential pain diagnosis in runners. Am J Sports Med 1986;14:324-326.

105. Goranson K, Johnson RP: Osteoid osteoma of os calcis. Diagnosis made by computerized tomography. Orthop Rev 1986;15:98-102.

106. Jacobs RL, Karmody A: The diabetic foot. In Jahns MS (ed): Disorders of the foot. Philadelphia, Saunders, 1982, pp 1377-1398.

107. Zlatkin MB, Pathria M, Sartoris DJ, Resnick D: The diabetic foot. Radiol Clin North Am 1987;25(6):1095-1105.

108. Mendelson EB, Fisher MR, Deschler TW, et al: Osteomyelitis in the diabetic foot: a difficult diagnostic challenge. Radiographics 1983;3:248-261.

109. Thomasson JL, Saundaram M: The diabetic foot: radiographic appearances. Orthopedics 1985;8:668-677.

110. Park HM, Wheat AR, Burt RW, et al: Scintigraphic evaluation of diabetic osteomyelitis: concise communication. J Nucl Med 1982;23:569-573.

111. Maurer AH, Millmond SH, Knight LC, et al: Infection in diabetic osteoarthropathy: use of indium-labelled leukocytes for diagnosis. Radiology 1986;161:221-225.

112. Alazraki N, Dries D, Datz F, et al: Value of a 24-hour image (four-phase bone scan) in assessing osteomyelitis in patients. J Nucl Med 1985;26:711-717.

113. Kraft E, Spyropoulos E, Finby N: Neurogenic disorders of the foot in diabetes mellitus. AJR 1975;124:17-24.

114. Wheat LJ, Allen SD, Henry M: Diabetic foot infections: bacteriologic analysis. Arch Intern Med 1986;146:1935-1940.

115. Resnick D, Niwayama G: Diagnosis of bone and joint disorders. Philadelphia, WB Saunders, 1981, pp 1076-1078.

116. Beltran J, Noto AM, McGhee RB, et al: Infections of the musculoskeletal system: high-field strength MR imaging. Radiology 1987;164:449-454.

117. Quinn SF, Murray W, Clark RA, Cochran C: MR imaging of chronic osteomyelitis. J Comput Assist Tomogr 1988;12:113-117.

118. Beltran J: MRI: Musculoskeletal system. Philadelphia, Lippincott, 1990, pp 8.2-8.35.

119. Stoller DW: The ankle and foot. In Stoller DW (ed): Magnetic resonance imaging in orthopedics and rheumatology. Philadelphia, Lippincott, 1989, pp 62-96.

120. Santoro JP, Cachia VV, Sartoris DJ, Resnick D: Nonspecific inflammation in the foot demonstrated by magnetic resonance imaging. J Foot Surg 1988;27:478-483.

121. Unger E, Moldofsky P, Gatenby R, et al: Diagnosis of osteomyelitis by MR imaging. AJR 1988;150:605-610.

122. Tang JSH, Gold RH, Bassett LW, et al: Musculoskeletal infection of the extremities: evaluation with MR imaging. Radiology 1988;166:205-209.

123. Sartoris DJ, Devine S, Resnick D, et al: Plantar compartmental infection in the diabetic foot. Invest Radiol 1985;20:772-784.

124. Yuh WT, Corson JD, Baramiewski HM, et al: Osteomyelitis of the foot in diabetic patients: evaluation with plain films, 99mTc-MDP bone scintigraphy, and MR imaging. AJR 1989;152:795-800.

125. Beltran J, Caudill JL, Herman LA, et al: Rheumatoid arthritis: MR imaging manifestations. Radiology 1987;165:153-157.

126. Seltzer SE, Weisman BN, Braunstein EM, et al: Computed tomography of the hindfoot with rheumatoid arthritis. Arthritis Rheum 1985;28:1234-1242.

127. Yulish BS, Lieberman JM, Standjord SE, et al: Hemophilic arthropathy: assessment with MR imaging. Radiology 1987;164:759-762.

128. Kerr R: Computed tomography. In Forrester DM, Kricum ME, Kerr R (eds): Imaging of the foot and ankle. Rockville Md, Aspen, 1988, pp 247-281.

PART IV MRI SAFETY

23 MR Operational Safety Considerations

JEFFREY C. WEINREB

Because it uses no ionizing radiation or iodinated intravenous contrast medium, MR may be safer than CT. Hundreds of thousands of patient examinations with MR confirm its well-deserved reputation for safety.

Nevertheless, there are numerous potential and real health hazards associated with the unique environment it creates. In 1981 Budinger[1] outlined three potential sources of harmful health effects from MR: (1) static magnetic fields, (2) time-varying magnetic fields, and (3) radiofrequency (RF) heating. Subsequent clinical experience has shown that the greatest potential health hazard is from the interaction between the main magnetic field and ferromagnetic metals. To ensure the safety of clinical MR, the Food and Drug Administration (FDA)[2] established guidelines for acceptable exposure levels and mandated that certain safety considerations be specified in the labeling of MR systems by the manufacturers. This chapter will review the present knowledge with regard to potential hazards associated with MR and discuss practical safety considerations.

ABSOLUTE CONTRAINDICATIONS TO MRI

Examination by MR is contraindicated in patients with cardiac pacemakers, epicardial pacemaker wires, automatic cardioverter-defibrillators, neurostimulators, cochlear implants, bone-growth stimulators, internal infusion pumps, and any other electrically, magnetically, or mechanically activated or controlled implanted biomedical system, unless specific information has previously established its safety.[3] MRI is also contraindicated in some patients with intracranial aneurysm clips or metallic foreign bodies in the eye. A discussion of the rationale for these contraindications is discussed below.

BIOEFFECTS OF MRI
Static magnetic fields

Static magnetic fields have been shown to affect certain chemical reactions in vitro, and effects on physiological function and primate behavior in fields of several tesla seem to be reproducible. However, for the most part, no long-lasting hazardous bioeffects have been observed from short- or long-term exposure to static magnetic fields below 2 tesla.[4-12]

The movement of blood-borne electrolytes in the presence of a strong magnetic field can generate an electrical current. It was feared that if these currents were of sufficient magnitude, cardiac arrythmias could result, particularly in patients with underlying heart disease. In fact, it has been shown that high static magnetic fields create changes in T-wave amplitude. These changes increase linearly with the magnitude of the magnetic field. The effect is probably due to flow potentials generated within the aorta. Fortunately, they have no physiological significance and disappear as soon as magnetic field exposure is terminated.[13] Research and clinical experience have shown that there is no increase in ventricular vulnerability threshold in the presence of static magnetic fields and that even patients with recent cardiac infarcts and known arrhythmias can be safely studied by means of MRI.

Time-varying magnetic fields

Inside the bore of the main magnet is a second set of much smaller resistive electromagnets (gradient coils) that generate the momentary magnetic gradient fields used for spatial localization. Because the body may act as a stationary conducting medium, these time-varying magnetic fields, by means of Faraday's law of electromagnetic induction, can induce electrical currents in a patient. Theoretically, induction of currents in sensitive tissues (e.g., nerves, muscles, heart, and blood vessels) could interfere with normal function and present a significant danger. Similarly, electrical currents could be induced in implanted metallic hardware such as surgical clips and prostheses, and significant heating could result.[4,5,14,15] Fortunately, the exposure level for gradient fields recommended by the FDA for conventional MR seems to provide a wide margin of safety, and patients with "irritable" hearts, surgical clips, and large metallic prostheses have been studied with no heating sensation being reported.[6] However, patients with implanted metallic hardware require additional vigilance. For instance, it is conceivable that a potentially deleterious current could be induced in implanted pacemaker wires, and significant heating could occur in some of the older hip prostheses. Increased application of "fast-scanning" techniques such as echoplanar, which utilize greater time-varying magnetic fields than does conventional MR, and the use of higher–field strength magnets require further investigation with regard to health hazards.

Radiofrequency electromagnetic fields

Unlike traditional x-ray based medical imaging (e.g., CT), the relatively low radiofrequency (RF) used for MR is nonionizing. Thus the health considerations associated with RF exposure during MR are different from those with roentgen rays. The primary biological effect or the low RF of MR is tissue heating that results from deposition of RF energy. Excessive increases in local or body temperatures could overwhelm heat-dissipating mechanisms and be dangerous for the patient. This "thermal" effect is proportional to the square of the frequency. Since high-field strength (i.e., 1.5 T) systems use higher-frequency RF than do lower-strength units, this is a bigger concern at high field. However, the rate of RF energy deposition also depends upon a number of other factors, including the type of RF pulse, the pulse width, the pulse repetition time (TR), the duration of exposure, the type of RF coil, the patient's mass, the tissues imaged, and the ambient conditions.

Most studies[5,6,16-20] have shown that any temperature elevations that occur during MR are small and probably are physiologically inconsequential. In addition, the FDA has established guidelines for RF deposition, and commercial clinical imagers have safeguards to prevent the inadvertent use of excessively high RF power. However,

certain tissues, such as the testis and eye, and certain patients, such as neonates and those with peripheral vascular disease or diabetes, could theoretically be more susceptible to the adverse effects of temperature increases. These are areas that require further investigation.

RF radiation is also associated with "athermal" effects: biological changes that occur without an increase in temperature. These are not well understood, and their relevance to MRI is, at present, questionable.

MOVEMENT OF FERROMAGNETIC METALS

Unquestionably, the greatest potential hazard from MRI arises from magnetically induced motion of ferromagnetic metallic implants and particles within a patient or from ferromagnetic objects, such as pens, hairpins, or wrenches, which may be drawn into the magnet with great force and at high velocity. Ferromagnetic materials are those that have the inherent ability to concentrate magnetic lines and interact with magnetic fields. In other words, they are easily magnetized. These materials — iron, cobalt, nickel, and their various alloys — have the potential to move when placed within the magnetic field of the MR magnet. The motion may be either translational, so that metal outside of the magnet is drawn toward the magnet, or rotational, in which case metal within the magnet turns to align with the magnetic force lines. Both types of motion can present a serious risk to the patient.

The force of attraction between a ferromagnetic material and a magnet depends upon the local static magnetic field gradient (i.e., the change in static magnetic field with distance from the magnet). Because the magnetic field is intense but homogeneous within the center of the bore, neither magnetic gradient nor attractive force is exerted on metals placed in the center of the magnet. Outside the magnet the attractive force decreases at a rate proportional to r^3 (where r is the distance from the bore of the magnet). This means that the forces exerted on ferromagnetic objects are nonlinear with increasing distance from the magnet, and at the entrance to the MR imaging suite even highly ferromagnetic objects will not exhibit any appreciable attraction to the magnet. At a distance of 10 to 12 feet, where the magnetic field gradient is still fairly weak, the attractive force from a 1.5 T magnet may be sufficient to overcome the rolling friction of wheelchairs and patient carts. As an object is moved closer to the bore of the magnet, it may be suddenly and forcefully pulled in. For example, at a distance of 3 to 4 feet, the force of attraction is so great that a floor buffer or oxygen tank could be pulled into the magnet. The possibility of injury from flying projectiles is probably the most serious hazard of MR imaging systems, and there are many anecdotal reports of near disasters, such as a worker struck in the head by a flying wrench and an IV pole that flew into an empty magnet. A serious accident that did not involve a patient has been reported during the assembly of an MR site.[21,22] The MR staff must be on constant alert to the danger of flying missiles, and patients and staff must be carefully screened to prevent the entry of ferromagnetic objects into the magnet room (Fig. 23-1).

Once objects are within an MR imaging bore, no magnetic gradient exists and no force of attraction is experienced. However, a torque force, which is proportional to the magnetic field strength, will be present and will tend to turn the object and align it with the magnetic field lines. For example, a ferromagnetic neurological aneurysm clip may become magnetized in the MR magnet and align itself with the magnetic lines in a manner somewhat akin to that of a compass needle. The resultant force may be sufficient to cause dislodgment and subsequent subarachnoid hemorrhage or injury to sensitive adjacent tissues. Thus it is imperative to exclude patients with highly ferromagnetic intracranial aneurysm clips from MR.

Several investigators[23-25] have examined the ferromagnetic properties of aneurysm and hemostatic clips constructed of various metal alloys. They found that some of the commonly used vascular clips were only weakly ferromagnetic or nonferromagnetic and would not present any risk to a patient undergoing MRI.[26,27] Clips that do not exhibit ferromagnetism include those constructed of silver, aluminum, titanium, tantalum, or stainless steel alloys containing 10% to 14% nickel. However, the level of risk is proportional not only to the composition of the clip but also to the orientation of the clip relative to the field, the size and shape of the clip, the delicacy of the vascular wall, the degree of fixation, and the sensitivity of the tissues against which the clip may be forced. These factors should be considered carefully before a patient with a metallic medical implant undergoes MR imaging. For instance, a highly ferromagnetic surgical clip in the abdomen will not preclude an MR study because it is probably fixed firmly by fibrosis. Even if it moved slightly, it would not likely damage any vital structures. Thus surgical and vascular clips that are not in the brain are generally not contraindications for MRI (Fig. 23-2). Other types of metallic nonelectromagnetic implants, such as dental appliances, shunt tube connectors,

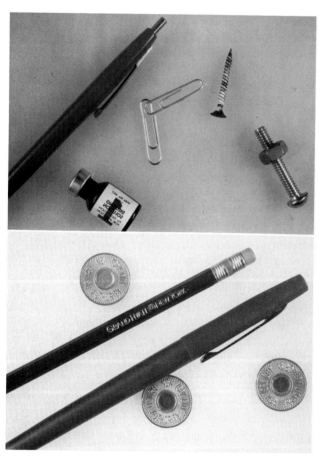

FIGURE 23-1
Common objects made of ferromagnetic materials may become hazardous high-velocity missiles in the strong magnetic field used for MRI. Despite careful screening of patients and vigilance of MRI staff, these ferromagnetic objects were pulled into a 1.5 T MRI unit. They include New York City subway tokens, a pencil, pens, paper clips, nuts and screws, and a medication bottle. Fortunately, there were no injuries.

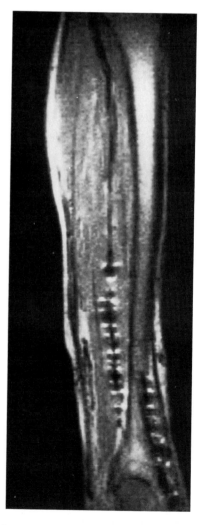

FIGURE 23-2
Artifacts due to surgical clips from extensive vascular surgery in the lower extremity. Surgical and vascular clips that are not in the brain are generally not contraindications for MRI.

and intravascular coils, filters, and stents, are also of little concern for similar reasons[28,29] (Fig. 23-3).

Many patients have bits of metal embedded in their body as a result of trauma (Fig. 23-4). In general, these do not pose significant risks to the patient, although there have been a few complaints of localized discomfort by patients with shrapnel embedded in their soft tissues. More worrisome is a situation such as the reported case of a former sheet metal worker with a clinically occult intraocular metal fragment who experienced a vitrous hemorrhage, with resulting blindness, at the conclusion of an MRI examination. According to the FDA, this case represents the first reported instance of a serious complication related to induced ferromagnetism.[30] As a result, candidates for MRI are currently screened for a history of occupational or traumatic exposure to airborne metal

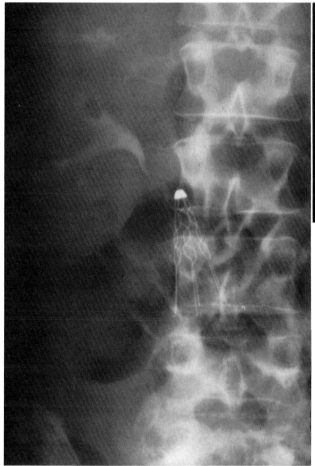

A

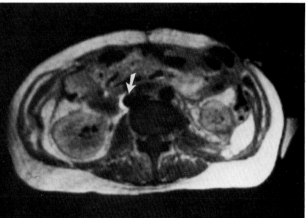

B

FIGURE 23-3
A patient with a Kimray-Greenfield vena cava filter may be safely examined with MRI. **A,** The roentgenogram from an intravenous urogram shows the metallic filter. **B,** MRI. Note the insignificant artifact produced by the titanium alloy filter in the inferior vena cava *(arrow).*

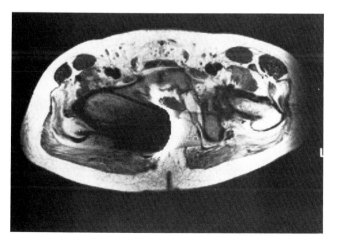

FIGURE 23-4
This patient had polymyositis (note atrophy of the posterior pelvic girdle muscles) and underwent MRI for left hip pain. A large metallic artifact can be seen emanating from the right side. The patient denied knowledge of any metal in the hip. A subsequent roentgenogram demonstrated the presence of shrapnel. Many patients have metal embedded in their body as a result of trauma.

particles. A history positive for such exposure should not automatically exclude a patient from undergoing an MRI examination; and if the patient has no ocular symptoms and AP and lateral roentgenograms of the orbits demonstrate no ocular metallic foreign body, MRI can be safely performed. This recommendation is based on the fact that any metallic foreign body massive enough to be moved through the ocular tissues by the magnetic force of a clinical MR system will be easily detected with conventional roentgenography.[31]

A number of different types of widely used metallic stapedectomy prostheses have been found to be unaffected by magnetic fields of 0.6 to 1.5 T. Thus, in most instances there is no danger that these prostheses will become displaced.[32,34] It is still possible, nevertheless, that other untested stapes prostheses made of different alloys could be moved, and in the absence of this information, affected patients should be excluded.

Cochlear implants consist of an external microphone and signal processor coupled across the skin to an internal nerve stimulator via a magnetic pickup coil. In the presence of electromagnetic fields, these patients may experience false auditory and temperature sensations.[33-35] Cochlear implants have also exhibited tremendous torque and deflection in magnetic fields as low as 0.6 T. Thus MRI is contraindicated in patients with cochlear implants.

Certain cosmetics, such as some brands of eye shadow, eyeliner, and mascara, contain metallic pigments that can act as conductors and result in significant heating as a result of RF energy deposition. These cosmetics should be removed prior to MRI. A more troublesome situation arises in patients with permanent eyeliners in which the eyelids are "tattooed" with metallic-based pigments that can cause swelling and puffiness of the soft tissues around the eye as a result of MR imaging.[36] Although this is not a contraindication to MRI, patients should be alerted to the fact that they may feel some discomfort after the examination.

ELECTROMAGNETIC DEVICES
Cardiac pacemakers

Many investigators have warned of the potential hazards to patients with implanted cardiac pacemakers. Normally a pacemaker functions in the demand mode, generating pacemaker impulses only when the patient's intrinsic heart rate drops below a predetermined rate. Pacemakers have a reed switch that can be activated by an external magnet for the purpose of periodic checks. Activation of the reed switch changes the operation of the pacer to the fixed-rate (asynchronous) mode, in which it operates independently of and competitively with the patient's intrinsic rhythm. Although exposure of a pacemaker to the magnetic field of an MR scanner can activate the reed switch and change the mode of pacing, this does not present a long-term or life-threatening risk to the patient. However, there are some genuine MR-related threats to patients with cardiac pacemakers. These electromagnetic devices can be temporarily or permanently reprogrammed or damaged by the RF pulses or the rapidly shifting magnetic fields used to generate the MR image. Furthermore, it is possible that the time-varying gradient magnetic fields used in the MR process will induce electrical currents in pacemaker leads that could mimic normal cardiac activity and inhibit pacemaker output. Another potential biohazard arises from the fact that some cardiac pacemakers contain numerous ferromagnetic components. Exposure to the intense magnetic fields used in MRI could result in permanent magnetization and malfunction and possibly to movement of the pacemaker inside the chest cavity. It is no surprise that, at present, MRI is contraindicated in all patients with cardiac pacemakers.[37,38]

The potential risks associated with the presence of epicardial pacemaker leads after removal of the pacemaker itself have received less attention. Theoretically, the rapid varying magnetic fields used in the MRI process could induce a closed-loop current, resulting in serious arrythmic disturbances. Thus, at present, it is prudent to exclude from MRI examination any patient with epicardial pacemaker lead wires.

Other devices

Similar concerns limit the use of MRI in all patients with almost any type of electromagnetic device, including TENS (transcutaneous electroneurostimulators), bone-growth stimulators, and drug infusion pumps.

ADDITIONAL CONSIDERATIONS
Prosthetic heart valves

Although there are measurable deflection forces for all prosthetic valves exposed to magnetic field strengths of 1.5 T, these are relatively minor compared to the forces exerted on the valves by the beating heart. With possible exception of the Pre-6000 Starr-Edwards valve,* implanted in the 1960s, patients with any type of prosthetic heart valve may be safely studied in MR systems up to 1.5 T.[25,29,39]

Orthopedic devices

The potential problems associated with MR in patients who have a metallic orthopedic device or implant are related to artifacts, dislodgment, heating, and induction of an electrical current.

Many modern metallic bioimplants can cause substantial image artifacts. Even nonferromagnetic devices may cause artifacts due to the induction of eddy currents by conductive materials. Usually areas of the body that are remote from the metallic device can be studied without significant image degradation.

---

*Baxter Healthcare Corp, Edwards Division, Santa Ana, Calif, 92711.

Most modern orthopedic implants are not ferromagnetic and will not become dislodged in the MR scanner.[40] Even in patients with older, bulky, ferromagnetic orthopedic implants, their fixation within the bone ensures little risk of movement (Figs. 23-5 to 23-7).

Another concern with metallic orthopedic implants is the possibility of heating. However, studies[41,42] have shown that, in general, temperature changes produced by MR imaging of metallic implants are negligible. In one study[44] an RF pulse sequence produced by a 1.5 T scanner was observed to increase the temperature of a large metallic orthopedic prosthesis by 25° C. Although

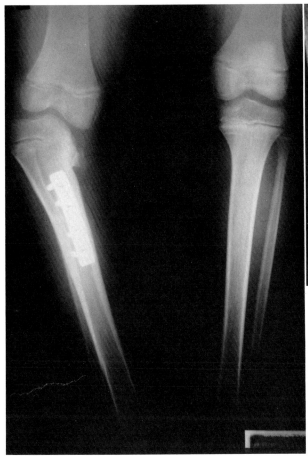

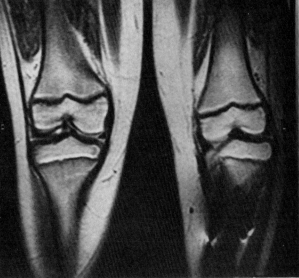

FIGURE 23-5
A 6-year-old girl who underwent osteotomy for Blount's disease. **A,** Radiography showing a stainless steel plate in the left tibia. (NOTE: The right and left sides were inadvertently switched during photography.) **B,** Coronal MRI showing an artifact from the metal plate. Most modern metallic orthopedic implants can be safely scanned with MRI.

FIGURE 23-6
A renal transplant patient with a metallic total hip prosthesis on the right and a metallic nail in the left femoral head. (NOTE: The right and left sides were inadvertently switched during photography.) **A,** CT. **B,** Coronal MRI.

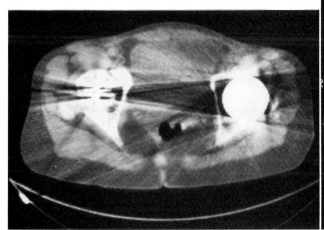

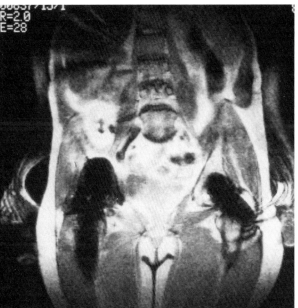

the patient with such an implant could experience a local heating sensation, this should not be a health hazard. In fact, numerous patients with metallic orthopedic implants are routinely scanned on systems operating at all clinical field strengths without incident [43-45] (Figs. 23-5 to 23-7).

Induction of currents in orthopedic implants is unlikely because of their shape and composition. However, there is still some concern about scanning patients with a halo vest or other other similar device used for stabilization of the cervical spine after trauma. Although many patients with such devices have undergone MRI without incident, it is possible that, because of their shape, mass, and composition, these devices could present a significant risk. Even though some commercially available halo devices are composed of nonferromagnetic materials, there is still the chance of inducing an electrical current in the ring portion of a halo composed of conductive materials due to Faraday's law of electromagnetic conduction (i.e., a current can be induced in a closed-loop conductor as it moves through a magnetic field). The patient could potentially be involved in part of this current loop and be subjected to an electrical or burn injury. Fortunately, there are commercially available halo vests that are both nonconductive and nonferromagnetic, and these will not cause any imaging artifacts or safety-related problems.

Acoustic noise

Some patients complain about the noise while undergoing MRI. This noise is caused by the force that is induced by the rapidly changing current pulsing through the gradient coils in the static magnetic field. The force is

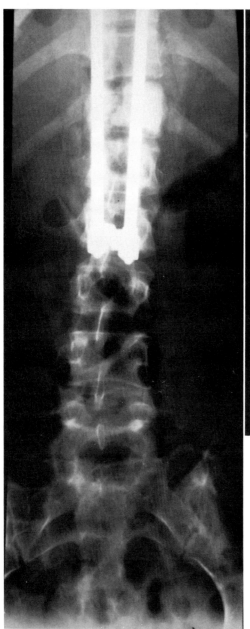

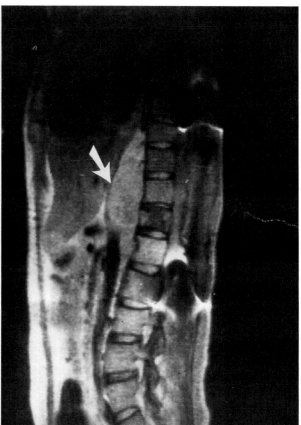

FIGURE 23-7
A patient with a Harrington rod in the lower thoracic spine following surgery for Ewing's sarcoma. **A,** Roentgenogram. **B,** Sagittal MRI. Note the artifacts from ferromagnetic fixation screws but not from the rod. There is abnormal low signal in the T12 vertebral body and the soft tissue mass *(arrow)* anterior to the spine.

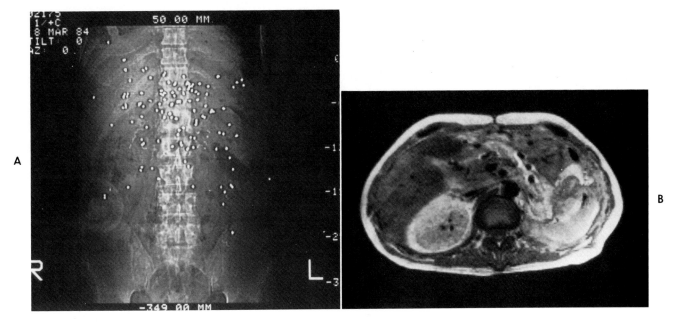

FIGURE 23-8
This patient with lead buckshot was safely studied with MR. Steel shot and other fired projectiles may be ferromagnetic and hazardous, depending upon their location in the body. A, Roentgenogram showing lead buckshot. B, MRI. Note the small artifacts from the buckshot.

transmitted to the MR unit as a vibration, which manifests as acoustic noise. Although loud sounds are usually tolerated without deleterious effect by most persons, they can cause temporary hearing deficits.[46] Protective ear plugs obviate this problem.

Pregnancy

Although no consistent teratogenic effects have been reported, possible mechanisms for embryological damage have been proposed.[47] However, there is no evidence that MRI interferes with human fetal development. Nevertheless, its use during pregnancy should be limited to instances of clear medical need and when it offers a definite advantage over other tests.[48]

Projectiles

One study[49] evaluated the potential ferromagnetic hazards of 21 fired missiles such as bullets and BBs; some of the bullets, BBs, and steel shot were deflected at the portal of a 1.5 T magnet. Thus, when located near a vital structure and not firmly embedded in bone, ferromagnetic fired projectiles represent a potential hazard.[49] Lead shot and pellets were not deflected, and these may be safely scanned with MRI (Fig. 23-8).

Sickle cell disease

Patients with sickle cell disease have a variety of musculoskeletal complications that may be assessed by means of MRI. A number of in vitro studies[50,51] raised the possibility of a health risk from MR imaging as a result of altered microcirculatory flow, but these concerns have been negated by a study[52] that showed no adverse effects on sickle cell blood flow during MR imaging in vivo. Numerous patients with sickle cell disease have undergone examination by MRI without incident.[53]

CONCLUSION

The results of hundreds of thousands of MRI examinations verify the widely held view that it is safe. However, constant vigilance is mandatory. Before entering the MR suite, the patient is asked to complete an MR safety information questionnaire (p. 886), which is evaluated by the MR staff. If the response to any of the questions has been affirmative, a knowledgeable physician or nurse is consulted to determine whether the patient is a candidate for MR. When there is doubt as to the safety of scanning a particular patient, it is best to err on the side of caution. When appropriate measures are taken, the safety record of MRI will be maintained.

REFERENCES

1. Budinger TF: Nuclear magnetic resonance (NMR) in vivo studies: known thresholds for health effects. J Comput Assist Tomogr 1981;5:800-811.
2. United States Food and Drug Administration: Guidelines for evaluating electromagnetic exposure risk for trials of clinical NMR systems. Rockville Md, Food and Drug Administration, Bureau of Radiologic Health, 1982.
3. Shellock FG, Crues JV: Safety considerations in magnetic resonance imaging. MRI Decisions 1989;Jan/Feb:25-30.
4. Budinger TF: Thresholds for physiological effects due to RF and magnetic fields used in NMR imaging. IEEE Trans Nucl Sci 1979;26:2821-2825.
5. Saunders RD, Smith H: Safety aspects of NMR clinical imaging. Br Med Bull 1984;40:148-152.
6. Shellock FG: Biological effects of MRI: a clean record so far. Diagn Imaging Clin Med 1987;Feb:96-101.
7. Prasad N, Lotsavá E, Thornby JI, et al: Effects of MR imaging on murine natural killer cell cytoxocity. AJR 1987;148:415-417.
8. Thomas SA, Morris PG: The effects on NMR exposure on living organisms: a microbial assay. Br J Radiol 1981;54:615-621.
9. Wolff S, James TL, Young GB, et al: Magnetic resonance imaging: absence of in vitro cytogenetic damage. Radiology 1985;155:163-165.
10. Schwartz JL, Crooks LE: NMR imaging produces no observable mutations or cytoxicity in mammalian cells. AJR 1982;139:583-585.
11. Withers HR, Mason KA, Davis CA: MR effect on murine spermatogenesis. Radiology 1985;156:741-742.
12. Jehenson P, Duboc D, Levergne T, et al: Change in human cardiac rhythm induced by a 2-T static magnetic field. Radiology 1988;166:227-230.
13. Doherty JU, Whitman GJR, Robinson MD, et al: Changes in cardiac excitability and vulnerability in NMR fields. Invest Radiol 1985;20:129-135.
14. Marino AA, Becker RO: Biological effects of extremely low frequency electric magnetic field: a review. Physiol Chem Phys 1977;9:131-147.
15. Davis PL, Crooks L, Arakawa M, et al: Potential hazards in NMR imaging: heating effects of changing magnetic fields and RF fields on small metallic implants. AJR 1981;137:857-860.
16. Shellock FG, Crues JV: Temperature, heart rate, and blood pressure changes associated with clinical MR imaging at 1.5 T. Radiology 1987;163:259-262.
17. Shellock FG, Crues JV: Temperature changes caused by MR imaging of the brain with a head coil. AJNR 1988;9:287-291.
18. Shuman WP, Haynor DR, Guy AW, et al: Superficial and deep tissue temperature increases in anesthetized dogs during exposure to high specific absorption rates in a 1.5 T MR imager. Radiology 1988;167:551-554.
19. Shellock FG, Crues JV: Corneal temperature changes induced by high-field-strength MR imaging with a head coil. Radiology 1988;167:809-811.
20. Slesin L: Power lines and cancer: the evidence grows. Technol Rev 1987;Oct:53-59.
21. Gangarosa RE, Minnis JE, Nobbe J, et al: Operational safety issues in MRI. Magn Reson Imaging 1987;5:287-292.
22. Pavlicek W: Safeguards help minimize potential MRI hazards. Diagn Imaging 1985;Nov:166-169.
23. New PF, Rosen BR, Brady TJ, et al: Potential hazards and artifacts of ferromagnetic and nonferromagnetic surgical and dental material and devices in nuclear magnetic resonance imaging. Radiology 1983;147:139-148.
24. Dujovny M, Kossovsky N, Kossowsky R, et al: Aneurysm clip motion during magnetic resonance imaging: in vivo experimental study with metallurgical factor analysis. Neurosurgery 1985;17:543-548.
25. Shellock FG, Crues JV: High-field-strength MR imaging and metallic biomedical implants: an ex vivo evaluation of deflection forces. AJR 1988;151:389-392.
26. Becker RL, Norfray JF, Teitelbaum GP, et al: MR imaging in patients with intracranial aneurysm clips. AJNR 1988;9:885-889.
27. Brown MA, Carden JA, Coleman E, et al: Magnetic field effects on surgical ligation clips. Magn Reson Imaging 1987;5:443-453.
28. Liebman CE, Messersmith RN, Levin DN, Lu CT: MR imaging of inferior vena cava filters: safety and artifacts. AJR 1988;150:1174-1176.
29. Shellock FG: MR imaging of metallic implants and materials: a compilation of the literature. AJR 1988;151:811-814.
30. Kelly WM, Paglen PG, Pearson JA, et al: Case report: ferromagnetism of intraocular foreign body causes unilateral blindness after MR study. AJNR 1986;7:243-245.
31. Williams S, Char DH, Dillo WP, et al: Ferrous intraocular foreign bodies and magnetic resonance imaging. Am J Ophthalmol 1988;105:398-401.
32. Applebaum EL, Valvossori GE: Effects of magnetic resonance imaging fields on stapedectomy prostheses. Arch Otolaryngol 1985;111:820-821.
33. Mattucci KF, Setzen M, Hyman R, Chaturvedi G: The effects of nuclear magnetic resonance imaging on metallic middle ear prostheses. Otolaryngol Head Neck Surg 1986;94:441-443.
34. Leon JA, Gabriele OF: Middle ear prosthesis: significance in magnetic resonance imaging. Magn Reson Imaging 1987;5:405-406.
35. Hepfner ST, Skelly MF: Radio-frequency interference in cochlear implants. (Letter.) N Engl J Med 1985;313:387.
36. Jackson JG, Acker JD, Sacco D: Permanent eyeliner and MR imaging. (Letter to the editor.) AJR 1987;149:1080.
37. Pavlicek W, Geisinger M, Castle L, et al: The effects of nuclear magnetic resonance on patients with cardiac pacemakers. Radiology 1983;147:149-153.
38. Erlebacher JA, Cahill PT, Pannizzo F, Knowles RJR: Effects of magnetic resonance imaging on DDD pacemakers. Am J Cardiol 1986;57:437-440.
39. Soulen RL, Budinger TF, Higgins CB: Magnetic resonance imaging of prosthetic heart valves. Radiology 1985;154:705-707.
40. Mesgarzadeh M, Revesz G, Bonakdapour A, Betz RR: The effect on medical metal implants by magnetic fields of magnetic resonance imaging. Skeletal Radiol 1985;14:205-206.
41. Davis P1, Crooks L, Arakawa M, et al: Potential hazards in NMR imaging: heating effects of changing magnetic fields and RF fields on small metallic implants. AJR 1981;137:857-860.
42. Shellock FG, Crues JV: High field MR imaging of metallic biomedical implants: an in vitro evaluation of deflection forces and temperature changes induced in large prostheses. Radiology 1987;165:150 (abstract).
43. Mechlin M, Thickman D, Kressel HY, et al: Magnetic resonance imaging of postoperative patients with metallic implants. AJR 1984;143:1281-1284.
44. Laakman RW, Kaufman B, Han JS, et al: MR imaging in patients with metallic implants. Radiology 1985;157:711-714.
45. Lemmens JAM, van Horn JR, den Boer J, et al: MR imaging of 22 Charnley-Muller total hip prostheses. ROFO 1986;145:311-315.
46. Brummett RE, Talbot JM, Charuhas P: Potential hearing loss resulting from MR imaging. Radiology 1988;169:539-540.

47. Delgado JMR, Leal J, Montegudo JL, Garcia MG: Embryological changes induced by weak, extremely low frequency electromagnetic fields. J Anat 1981;134:857-860.

48. Consensus Conference: Magnetic resonance imaging. JAMA 1988;259:2132-2138.

49. Teitelbaum GP, Yee CA, Van Horn DD, et al: Metallic ballistic fragments: MR imaging safety and artifacts. Radiology 1990;175:855-859.

50. Brody AS, Sorette MP, Gooding CA, et al: Induced alignment of flowing erythrocytes in a magnetic field: a preliminary report. Invest Radiol 1985;20:550-566.

51. Takashima S, Asakura T: Desickling of sickled erythrocytes by pulsed radio-frequency field. Science 1983;220:411-413.

52. Brody AS, Embury SH, Mentzer WC, et al: Preservation of sickle cell blood-flow patterns during MR imaging: an in vivo study. AJR 1988;151:139-141.

53. Rao VM, Fishman M, Mitchell DG, et al: Painful sickle cell crisis: bone marrow patterns observed with: MR imaging. Radiology 1986;161:211-215.

A Metallic Implants and Materials Tested for Deflection Forces: A Compilation of the Literature

Metallic Implant or Material	Deflection	Highest Field Strength (T)[a]
Aneurysm and Hemostatic Clips		
Drake (DR14, DR24) (Edward Weck, Triangle Park NJ)	Yes	1.44
Drake (DR16) (Edward Weck)	Yes	0.147
Drake (301 SS) (Edward Weck)	Yes	1.5
Downs multipositional (17-7PH)	Yes	1.44
Gastrointestinal anastomosis clip, Auto Suture SGIA (SS) (United States Surgical, Norwalk Conn)	No	1.5
Heifetz (17-7PH) (Edward Weck)	Yes	1.89
Heifetz (Elgiloy) (Edward Weck)	No	1.89
Hemoclip #10 (316L SS) (Edward Weck)	No	1.5
Hemoclip (tantalum) (Edward Weck)	No	1.5
Housepian	Yes	0.147
Kapp (405 SS) (V. Mueller)	Yes	1.89
Kapp curved (404 SS) (V. Mueller)	Yes	1.44
Kapp straight (404 SS) (V. Mueller)	Yes	1.44
Ligaclip #6 (316L SS) (Ethicon, Somerville NJ)	No	1.5
Ligaclip (tantalum) (Ethicon)	No	1.5
Mayfield (301 SS) (Codman & Shurtleff, Randolph Mass)	Yes	1.5
Mayfield (304 SS) (Codman & Shurtleff)	Yes	1.89
McFadden (301 SS) (Codman & Shurtleff)	Yes	1.5
Olivecrona	No	1.44
Pivot (17-7PH) (V. Mueller)	Yes	1.89
Scoville (EN58J) (Downs Surgical, Decatur Ga)	Yes	1.89
Stevens (50-4190, silver alloy)	No	0.15
Sugita (Elgiloy) (Downs Surgical)	No	1.89
Sundt-Kees (301 SS) (Downs Surgical)	Yes	1.5
Sundt-Kees Multi-Angle (17-7PH) (Downs Surgical)	Yes	1.89
Surgiclip, Auto Suture M-9.5 (SS) (United States Surgical)	No	1.5
Vari-Angle (17-7PH) (Codman & Shurtleff)	Yes	1.89
Vari-Angle McFadden (MP35N) (Codman & Shurtleff)	No	1.89
Vari-Angle Micro (17-7PM SS) (Codman & Shurtleff)	Yes	0.15
Vari-Angle Spring (17-7PM SS) (Codman & Shurtleff)	Yes	0.15
Yasargil (316 SS) (Aesculap)	No	1.89
Yasargil (Phynox) (Aesculap)	No	1.89
Dental Materials		
Brace Band (SS) (American Dental, Missoula Mont)	No	1.5
Brace Wire (chrome alloy) (Ormco, San Marcos Calif)	Yes[b]	1.5
Dental amalgam	No	1.44
Silver point (Union Broach, New York NY)	No	1.5
Permanent crown (amalgam) (Ormco)	No	1.5

From Shellock FG: AJR 1988; 151:812–813. © The American Roentgen Ray Society.

Note.— Names and locations of manufacturers are given if known. The location is given only once (the first time the manufacturer is mentioned); thereafter, only the name is given. SS = stainless steel; IVC = inferior vena cava.

[a]Numbers in this column refer to the highest static magnetic field strength (expressed in tesla [T]) at which the deflection force of an implant or material was evaluated. (See references for additional information.)

[b]Considered safe for MR imaging, even though it was deflected by the static magnetic fields. Certain prosthetic heart valves, for example, were deflected by the static magnetic fields, but the deflection forces were considered to be less than the force exerted on the valves by the beating heart.

Metallic Implant or Material	Deflection	Highest Field Strength (T)[a]
Intravascular Coils, Filters, and Stents		
Amplatz IVC filter (Cook, Bloomington Ind)	No	4.7
Cragg nitinol spiral filter	No	4.7
Gianturco embolization coil (Cook)	Yes	1.5
Gianturco bird nest IVC filter (Cook)	Yes	1.5
Gianturco zig-zag stent (Cook)	Yes	1.5
Greenfield vena caval filter (SS) (Medi-tech, Watertown Mass)	Yes[b]	1.5
Greenfield vena caval filter (titanium alloy) (Ormco, Glendora Calif)	No	1.5
Gunther IVC filter (William Cook Europe, Bjaeverskov Denmark)	Yes	1.5
Maas helical IVC filter (Medinvent, Lausanne Switzerland)	No	4.7
Maas helical endovascular stent (Medinvent)	No	4.7
Mobin-Uddin IVC/umbrella filter (American Edwards, Santa Ana Calif)	No	4.7
New retrievable IVC filter (Thomas Jefferson University, Philadelphia Pa)	Yes	1.5
Palmaz endovascular stent (Ethicon)	Yes	1.5
Prosthetic Ear Implants		
Cody tack	No	0.6
Cochlear implant (3M/House)	Yes	0.6
Cochlear implant (3M/Vienna)	Yes	0.6
House-type incus prosthesis	No	0.6
McGee stainless-steel piston	No	0.6
Reuter drain tube	No	0.6
Richards House-type wire loop (Richard's Company, Memphis Tenn)	No	1.5
Richards-McGee piston (Richard's)	No	1.5
Richards Plasti-pore with Armstrong-style platinum ribbon (Richard's)	No	1.5
Richards-Schuknecht Teflon wire (Richard's)	No	1.5
Richards Trapeze platinum ribbon (Richard's)	No	1.5
Schuknecht Gelfoam and wire prosthesis, Armstrong-style (Richard's)	No	1.5
Shea stainless-steel and Teflon wire prosthesis	No	1.5
Xomed stapes prosthesis, Robinson-style (Richard's)	No	1.5
Prosthetic Heart Valves		
Beall (Coratomic, Indiana Pa)	Yes[b]	2.35
Bjork-Shiley (convexo/concave) (Shiley, Irvine Calif)	No	1.5
Bjork-Shiley (universal/spherical) (Shiley)	Yes[b]	1.5
Bjork-Shiley, model MBC (Shiley)	Yes[b]	2.35
Bjork-Shiley, model 25 MBRC 11030 (Shiley)	Yes[b]	2.35
Carpentier-Edwards, model 2650 (American Edwards)	Yes[b]	2.35
Carpentier-Edwards (porcine) (American Edwards)	Yes[b]	2.35
Hall-Kaster, model A7700 (Medtronic, Minneapolis Minn)	Yes[b]	1.5
Hancock I (porcine) (Johnson & Johnson, Anaheim Calif)	Yes[b]	1.5
Hancock II (porcine) (Johnson & Johnson)	Yes[b]	1.5
Hancock extracorporeal, model 242R (Johnson & Johnson)	Yes[b]	2.35
Hancock extracorporeal, model M 4365-33 (Johnson & Johnson)	Yes[b]	2.35
Hancock Vascor, model 505 (Johnson & Johnson)	No	2.35
Ionescu-Shiley (Universal ISM)	Yes[b]	2.35
Lillehi-Kaster, model 300S (Medical, Inver Grove Heights Minn)	Yes[b]	2.35
Lillehi-Kaster, model 5009 (Medical)	Yes[b]	2.35
Medtronic-Hall (Medtronic)	Yes[b]	2.35
Medtronic Hall, model A7700-D-16 (Medtronic)	Yes[6]	2.35
Omnicarbon, model 3523T029 (Medical)	Yes[b]	2.35
Omniscience, model 6522 (Medical)	Yes[b]	2.35
Smeloff-Cutter (Cutter Laboratories, Berkeley Calif)	Yes[b]	2.35
Starr-Edwards, model 1260 (American Edwards)	Yes[b]	2.35
Starr-Edwards, model 2320 (American Edwards)	Yes[b]	2.35
Starr-Edwards, model 2400 (American Edwards)	No	1.5
Starr-Edwards, model Pre 6000 (American Edwards)	Yes	1.5
Starr-Edwards, model 6520 (American Edwards)	Yes[b]	2.35
St. Jude (St. Jude Medical, St Paul Minn)	No	1.5
St. Jude, model A 101 (St Jude Medical)	Yes[b]	2.35
St. Jude, model M 101 (St Jude Medical	Yes[b]	2.35

Metallic Implant or Material	Deflection	Highest Field Strength (T)[a]
Orthopedic Materials and Devices		
AML femoral component, bipolar hip prosthesis (Zimmer, Warsaw Ind)	No	1.5
Harris hip prosthesis (Zimmer)	No	1.5
Jewett nail (Zimmer)	No	1.5
Kirschner intermedullary rod (Kirschner Medical, Timonium Md)	No	1.5
Stainless-steel plate (Zimmer)	No	1.5
Stainlesss-steel screw (Zimmer)	No	1.5
Stainless-steel mesh (Zimmer)	No	1.5
Stainless-steel wire (Zimmer)	No	1.5
Penile implants		
Penile implant, AMS Malleable 600 (American Medical Systems, Minnetonka Minn)	No	1.5
Penile implant, AMS 700 CX Inflatable (American Medical Systems)	No	1.5
Penile implant, Flexi-Flate (Surgitek, Medical Engineering, Racine Wisc)	No	1.5
Penile implant, Flexi-Rod (standard) (Surgitek, Medical Engineering)	No	1.5
Penile implant, Flexi-Rod II (firm) (Surgitek, Medical Engineering)	No	1.5
Penile implant, Jonas (Dacomed, Minneapolis Minn)	No	1.5
Penile implant, Mentor Flexible (Mentor, Minneapolis Minn)	No	1.5
Penile implant, Mentor Inflatable (Mentor)	No	1.5
Penile implant, OmniPhase (Dacomed)	Yes	1.5
Miscellaneous Metallic Implants and Materials		
Artificial urinary sphincter, AMS 800 (American Medical Systems)	No	1.5
BB's (Daisy)	Yes	1.5
BB's (Crosman)	Yes	1.5
Cerebral ventricular shunt tube connector, Accu-Flow, straight (Codman & Shurtleff)	No	1.5
Cerebral ventricular shunt tube connector, Accu-Flow, right angle (Codman & Shurtleff)	No	1.5
Cerebral ventricular shunt tube connector, Accu-Flow, T-connector (Codman & Shurtleff)	No	1.5
Cerebral ventricular shunt tube connector (type unknown)	Yes	0.147
Contraceptive diaphragm, All Flex (Ortho Pharmaceutical, Raritan NJ)	Yes[b]	1.5
Contraceptive diaphragm, flat spring (Ortho Pharmaceutical)	Yes[b]	1.5
Contraceptive diaphragm, Koroflex (Young Drug Products, Piscataway NJ)	Yes[b]	1.5
Forceps (titanium)	No	1.44
Hakim valve and pump	No	1.44
Intraocular lens implant (Binkhorst, iridocapsular lens, platinum-iridium loop)	No	1.0
Intraocular lens implant (Binkhorst, iridocapsular lens, titanium loop)	No	1.0
Intraocular lens implant (Worst, platinum clip lens)	No	1.0
Intrauterine contraceptive device (IUD, Copper T) (Searle Pharmaceuticals, Chicago Ill)	No	1.5
Tantalum powder	No	1.44

B   Patient Information Safety Form

NYU MEDICAL CENTER
MAGNETIC RESONANCE IMAGING

IMPORTANT!!!

**THIS FORM MUST BE FILLED OUT BEFORE
UNDERGOING MRI STUDY**

Name: _____

Sex: _____ Age: _____ yr Weight: _____ lb Height: _____ ft _____ in

IF YOU HAVE ANY OF THE FOLLOWING, CHECK THE
APPROPRIATE BOX AND
DO NOT ENTER THE MRI ROOM

Cardiac pacemaker .... ☐
Cardiac defibrillator .... ☐
Previous cardiac pacemaker removed .... ☐
Aneurysm clip(s) in brain.. ☐
Implanted drug infusion device .... ☐
Bone growth stimulator... ☐
Neurostimulator (TENS unit) .... ☐
Any type of biostimulator .... ☐
Hearing aid .... ☐
Metal in eye .... ☐
Cochlear implant .... ☐
Any electrical device implanted in your body................ ☐

*If you have any questions, please consult with the nurse, doctor, technolgists, or
front desk before entering the MRI area*

(Continued on other side)

Please indicate if you have any of the following, as they may affect your scan:

Please mark the location of any metal inside your body on this drawing:

☐ Any type of surgical clip(s) or staple(s)
☐ Heart valve prosthesis
☐ Greenfield vena cava filter
☐ Gianturkle coil (spring embolus coil)
☐ Middle ear implant (stapes prosthesis)
☐ Penile prosthesis
☐ Orbital eye prosthesis
☐ Shrapnel or bullet
☐ Wire sutures
☐ Tatooed eyeliner
☐ Any dental item held in place by a magnet
☐ Any other implanted item _____

_____
_____

☐ Diaphragm or IUD
☐ Renal shunt
☐ Intraventricular shunt
☐ Wire mesh
☐ Artificial limb or joint
☐ Any orthopedic item (i.e., pins, rods screws, nails, clips, plates, wire, etc.)
☐ Dentures or dental braces
☐ Any type of removable dental item.

RIGHT   **LEFT**

Details _____

_____

Have you ever had a surgical procedure or operation of any kind?
☐ Yes   ☐ NO
IF yes, which type? _____

Are you pregnant?   ☐ Yes   ☐ No

I attest that the above information is correct to the best of my knowledge

_____
(Patient's signature)

Technologist _____

Index